Nephrology

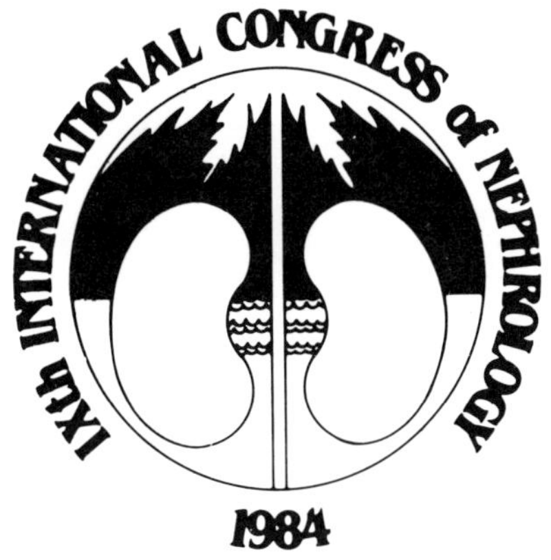

Nephrology VOLUME II

PROCEEDINGS OF THE
IXth INTERNATIONAL CONGRESS OF NEPHROLOGY

Editor
Roscoe R. Robinson

Associate Editors
Vincent W. Dennis · Thomas F. Ferris
Richard J. Glassock · Juha P. Kokko
C. Craig Tisher

With 220 Figures

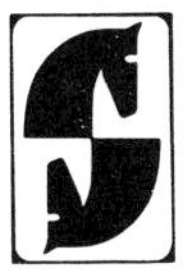

Springer-Verlag
New York Berlin Heidelberg Tokyo

Roscoe R. Robinson
Vanderbilt University Medical Center
Nashville, Tennessee, USA

Vincent W. Dennis, Duke University Medical Center, Durham, North Carolina, USA

Thomas F. Ferris, University of Minnesota Medical Center, Minneapolis, Minnesota, USA

Richard J. Glassock, Harbor-UCLA Medical Center, Torrance, California, USA

Juha P. Kokko, Southwestern Medical School, University of Texas Health Science Center, Dallas, Texas, USA

C. Craig Tisher, J. Hillis Miller Health Center, University of Florida, Gainesville, Florida, USA

Library of Congress Cataloging in Publication Data
International Congress of Nephrology (9th : 1984 : Los Angeles, Calif.)
   Nephrology : proceedings of the IXth International Congress of Nephrology.
   Includes bibliographies and index.
   Based on the proceedings of the IXth International Congress of Nephrology held in
Los Angeles, Calif., June 11–16, 1984.
   1. Kidneys—Diseases—Congresses.   2. Nephrology—Congresses.   I. Robinson,
Roscoe R.   II. Title.
[DNLM: 1. Nephrology—congresses.   W3 IN446 9th 1984n / WJ 300 I59 1984n]
RC902.A2I56   1984   616.6′1   84–22136

Typeset by Kingsport Press, Kingsport, Tennessee.
Printed and bound by Halliday Lithograph, West Hanover, Massachusetts.
Printed in the United States of America.

9 8 7 6 5 4 3 2 1

ISBN 0-387-96072-4 Springer-Verlag New York Berlin Heidelberg Tokyo
ISBN 3-540-96072-4 Springer-Verlag Berlin Heidelberg New York Tokyo

Foreword

For many reasons, as President of the International Society of Nephrology, I am happy and honored to write a brief introduction to *Nephrology,* the Proceedings of the IXth International Congress of Nephrology. One of these reasons is specially treasured: I edited the two books published after our first Congress (Geneva-Evian 1960).

The 1984 vintage will certainly be as good as the preceding ones. And, for any nephrologist, whatever his or her field of interest, many observations will be found in the Proceedings that will enhance their personal work. It is characteristic for our Congresses to be the converging point upon which many different orientations join together and form the nephrology that is researched and practiced throughout the world.

What could replace a State-of-the-Art lecture delivered by a selected nephrologist whose work is of the highest quality? At times, even more revealing are those presentations made by non-nephrologists, the basic scientists who bring us fresh data and new concepts far removed from the reader's daily world. But attending such a lecture is never enough. Their texts should be read and reread. Symposia and workshops, as sources of precise and up-dated knowledge espoused by experts, are often heart-breaking as they shake established dogma. Therefore, they should be neither neglected nor forgotten but scrutinized carefully. The evidence which could eventually lead to new concepts or hypotheses has to be weighed accurately and then either rejected, discarded temporarily, or accepted, even if the latter implies dramatic change. These Proceedings provide the necessary means by which such decisions can be made wisely. *La règle du jeu, ce n'est pas la mode, mais l'imagination controlée par la raison:* The rule of the game is not the mode but imagination controlled by reason.

Dig into that heap of genuine facts that awaits you and you might find a nugget that could intellectually enlighten and boost your research program.

What a hope for a miraculous draught of fishes! I wish you good fortune and remember to prepare your best results for presentation at the Xth Congress of Nephrology to be held in London in 1987.

Gabriel Richet
President
International Society of Nephrology
(1981–1984)

Preface

Nephrology represents a unique venture. It is based on the Proceedings of the IXth International Congress of Nephrology held in Los Angeles, California, June 11–16, 1984. However, it differs from the proceedings of almost all previous congresses, international or national.

When policy was established for the Congress two years ago, a commitment was made to achieve a level of scientific excellence that had never before been achieved in an International Congress. The Program Committee worked diligently for 18 months in this pursuit. Simultaneously, steps were taken to assure the transmission of the information to a worldwide audience in written form using the most authoritative and comprehensive presentations.

To accomplish the latter, it was essential that Dr. Roscoe R. Robinson serve as the Editor-in-Chief; for he is the member of our society who has a proven track record of dealing with large numbers of papers, of transforming them (when necessary) into a form consistent with his own high values, of creating the required degree of flow and transition, and finally, of never sacrificing quality for other considerations. The book would be not only contemporary but meritorious, and the substantive points made by the essayists would not be modified.

Dr. Robinson accepted the challenge and immediately appointed a distinguished board of associate editors: Vincent W. Dennis, Thomas F. Ferris, Richard J. Glassock, Juha P. Kokko, and C. Craig Tisher.

Working as a team, Dr. Robinson and his associate editors subjected submitted manuscripts not only to editorial scrutiny but to peer review by independent referees. Many were returned to the authors for substantive revisions; almost all of the manuscripts were subjected to editorial modification. The resultant synthesis has, I believe, set yet another record for editorial accomplishment by Dr. Robinson, father and editor of *Kidney International* for its first 13 years.

Renal disease is a new and rapidly growing area of medical science and practice. It has, in fact, undergone the transition from a "footnote in some textbooks of urology" to one of the most rapidly advancing and extensive areas of biomedical science and practice; and all of this has happened within 25 years. This is due, in no small way, to Dr. Robinson's impact on the field in his capacity as Editor of *Kidney International*. He is now about to step aside from that position. It thus seems fitting that he should end that portion of an exciting and innovative career with an award-winning presentation of the state-of-the-nephrologic-art in *Nephrology*. Thank you, Ike.

Neal S. Bricker
President
IXth International Congress of Nephrology
Los Angeles, 1984

Officers and Committees
IXth International Congress of Nephrology
Los Angeles, California, U.S.A.
June 11–16, 1984

OFFICERS

President	Neal S. Bricker
Vice-President	Shaul G. Massry
Secretary General	Richard J. Glassock
Treasurer	Michael A. Kirschenbaum

ORGANIZING COMMITTEE

Donald A. Adams   Harvey C. Gonick   Nachman Brautbar
Charles R. Kleeman   Jack W. Coburn   Joel D. Kopple
Leon G. Fine   Kiyoshi Kurokawa   Dominick E. Gentile
Donald J. Marsh   Morton H. Maxwell

SCIENTIFIC PROGRAM COMMITTEE

Neal S. Bricker, *Chairman*
Richard J. Glassock   Charles R. Kleeman   Rex L. Jamison
Donald J. Marsh   Michael A. Kirschenbaum   Shaul G. Massry

EDITORIAL COMMITTEE

Roscoe R. Robinson, *Chairman*
Vincent W. Dennis   Richard J. Glassock   Thomas F. Ferris
Juha P. Kokko   C. Craig Tisher

LIAISON COMMITTEE, INTERNATIONAL SOCIETY OF NEPHROLOGY

Gabriel Richet, *Chairman*
Vittorio Bonomini   Colin Johnston   Jugoro Takeuchi

ADVISORY COMMITTEE, INTERNATIONAL SOCIETY OF NEPHROLOGY

George E. Schreiner, *Chairman*
Michael J. Dunn   Gary E. Striker   Guy Lemieux
Robert L. Vernier   Robert T. McCluskey   Guillermo Whittembury
Victor E. Pollak   Curtis B. Wilson, Jr.

SOCIAL COMMITTEE

Donald A. Adams   Dominick E. Gentile

COUNSEL

Harvey Shapiro

ADMINISTRATIVE DIRECTOR

Mary Frances Armbruster

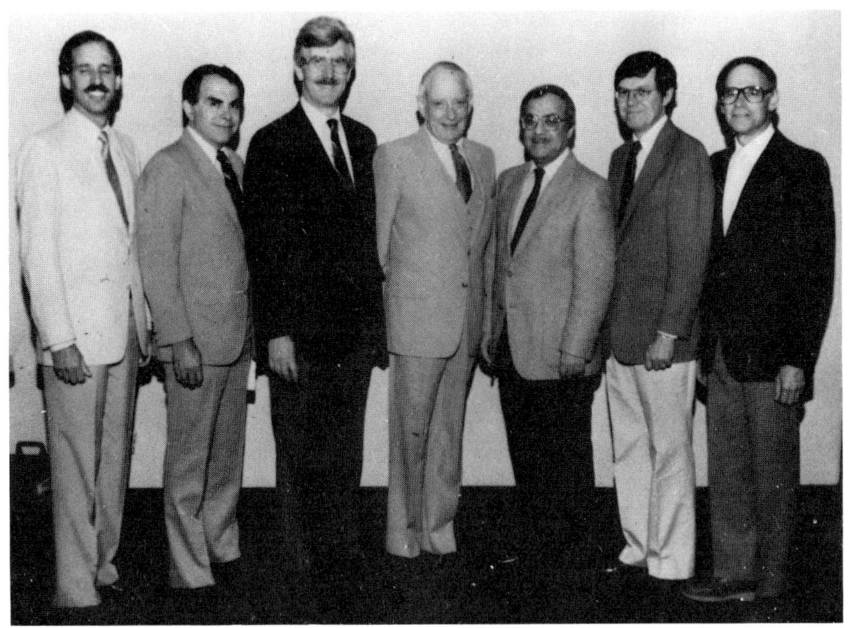

Scientific Program Committee (left to right): Michael A. Kirschenbaum, Donald J. Marsh, Richard J. Glassock, Neal S. Bricker (Chairperson), Shaul G. Massry, Rex L. Jamison, and Charles R. Kleeman.

Officers and Councillors
of the International Society of Nephrology
1981–1984

OFFICERS

President	Gabriel Richet, Paris
Immediate Past President	George E. Schreiner, Washington, D.C.
President-Elect	Donald W. Seldin, Dallas
Vice-President	Robert H. Heptinstall, Baltimore
Secretary General	John H. Moorhead, London
Treasurer	Robert W. Schrier, Denver
Editor, *Kidney International*	Roscoe R. Robinson, Nashville

COUNCILLORS

Stefan Angielski, Gdansk	Carl W. Gottschalk, Chapel Hill
Knut Aukland, Bergen	Renée Habib, Paris
A. William Asscher, Cardiff	Jean Hamburger, Paris
Jonas Bergstrom, Stockholm	Klaus Hierholzer, Berlin
Vittorio Bonomini, Bologna	Colin Johnston, Melbourne
J. Stewart Cameron, London	Guy Lemieux, Montreal
David P. Earle, Winnetka	Robert T. McCluskey, Boston
Laurence E. Earley, Philadelphia	E. J. Dorhout Mees, Utrecht
Carmelo Giordano, Naples	Floyd C. Rector, Jr., San Francisco
Richard J. Glassock, Torrance	Jugoro Takeuchi, Tokyo
Martin Goldberg, Cincinnati	Guillermo Whittembury, Caracas

Contents I

Volume I

Normal Structure and Function

Transport Processes and Epithelia

Determinants of Growth, Form, and Function in Epithelia
  Chairpersons: Joseph S. Handler and Marcelino M. Cereijido; *Discussants:*
  Maurice Burg, Mary Taub, Michael F. Horster, and John D. Valentich   3
Basolateral Membrane Properties of Sodium-absorbing Epithelia
  Stanley G. Schultz 7
Sodium-Glucose Cotransport Mechanisms
  R. James Turner 21
Cell Volume Regulation in Epithelia
  Chairpersons: Jared J. Grantham and Kenneth R. Spring; *Discussants:*
  Michael A. Linshaw, Guillermo Whittembury, Paola Carpi-Medina,
  Ernesto Gonzalez, Henry Linares, William B. Guggino, Kevin L. Kirk,
  James A. Schafer, Donald R. DiBona, and Peter M. Andrews . . . 34
Role of Cytosolic Calcium in Vasopressin-sensitive Epithelia
  Ann Taylor, Mirilee Pearl, Barbara Barber, and Beth Crutch. . . . 39
Role of Cytosolic Calcium in Renal Tubular Transport
  Erich E. Windhager and Gustavo Frindt. 51
Sodium Phosphate Cotransport: Studies with Vesicles and LLC-PK$_1$ Cells
  Heini Murer, Martin Amstutz, Jürg Biber, Piotr Gmaj, and
  Kerstin Malmström. 57

Two tables of contents have been provided. Contents I organizes the papers in a manner that provides the best sequential flow of content, irrespective of the order in which they were presented at the Congress or the type of presentation: State-of-the-Art lecture, Symposium manuscript, or Workshop summary. Contents II (see p. xxvii) is organized by the type of presentation.

Regulation of the Na$^+$/H$^+$ Antiporter in Cells of the Proximal Tubule
David G. Warnock and Harlan E. Ives   70

Renal Nerves

Functions of the Renal Nerves
Chairpersons: Gerald F. DiBona and Romulo E. Colindres; *Discussants:*
Luciano Barajas, Roger J. Summers, Nicholas G. Moss, Ulla C. Kopp,
and Richard E. Katholi   79

Renal Circulation

Organization of the Medullary Circulation: Functional Implications
Lise Bankir, Nadine Bouby, and Marie-Marcelle Trinh-Trang-Tan . .   84
Pathophysiology of the Medullary Circulation
June Mason   107
Intrarenal Control of Medullary Blood Flow and the Urinary Concentrating
Mechanism
Leon C. Moore   120

Glomerular Filtration

Intrarenal Control of Glomerular Filtration: Cellular Mechanisms of
Tubuloglomerular Feedback
P. Darwin Bell and L. Gabriel Navar.   130
Regulatory Role of the Tubuloglomerular Feedback Mechanism
Josephine P. Briggs and Jürgen Schnermann   143
Influence of Renal Nerves on the Glomerular Microcirculation
Valentina Kon and Iekuni Ichikawa   154

Structure and Transport Along the Nephron

Hydrogen Ion Transport Along the Nephron
Floyd C. Rector, Jr.   161
Proximal Tubule Transport
Chairperson: Harry R. Jacobson; *Co-Chairperson:* Jean Cardinal;
Discussants: Christine A. Berry, Bruno Corman, Dalon W. Barfuss,
Jacques Lapointe, Elsa Bello-Reuss, Sei Sasaki, Keith A. Hruska, and
Julian Seiffer   178
Transport Properties of the Pars Recta
James A. Schafer and Jack Work   186
Function of the Thin Limb of Henle's Loop
Masashi Imai, Matuhiko Hayashi, Masasuke Araki, and Kaoru Tabei.   196
Regulation of Sodium Chloride Transport by the Loop of Henle
John B. Stokes III   208
Sodium Chloride Reabsorption in the Thick Ascending Limb of the Loop
of Henle
Rainer Greger, Monika Wittner, Eberhard Schlatter, Brigitte Gebler,
Claudia Weidtke, and Antonio Di Stefano   224
Structural Heterogeneity of the Distal Nephron
Chairpersons: C. Craig Tisher and Brigitte Kaissling; *Discussants:*
Kirsten M. Madsen, Lise Bankir, Bruce Stanton, Dennis Brown, and
Michel Bergeron   243

Control of Acid and Electrolyte Excretion

Acidification Mechanisms
Chairpersons: Thomas D. DuBose, Jr. and Michel Paillard; *Discussants:*
Eberhard Frömter, Robert J. Alpern, David W. Good, and
Dennis K. Stone 251
Atrial Natriuretic Factor
Chairpersons: Adolfo J. de Bold and Harald Sonnenberg; *Discussants:*
Uwe Ackermann, Edward H. Blaine, Josephine P. Briggs,
Barbara R. Cole, Ralph Keeler, Sidney Solomon, Frank Spinelli,
Nick C. Trippodo, and Thomas Maack 257
Regulation of Potassium Excretion
Chairpersons: Gerhard Giebisch and Lawrence Rabinowitz; *Discussants:*
Fred S. Wright, Karol Bomsztyk, Stephen C. Hebert, Bruce Stanton,
John B. Stokes III, Bruce Koeppen, and Roger G. O'Neil 260

Renal Metabolism, Prostaglandins, and Renin

Contemporary Issues in Renal Metabolism
Chairpersons: Richard L. Tannen and Brian A. Ross; *Discussants:*
Anton C. Schoolwerth and Norman J. Siegel 269
Biochemistry of Renal Prostaglandins
Aubrey R. Morrison 277
From Molecular Biology to Antihypertensive Drugs: Current Research on
Renin Inhibitors
Edgar Haber 284
Inactive Renin
Jean E. Sealey. 302
The Renin Gene: Structure and Processing of Renin
Florent Soubrier, Joël Menard, and Pierre Corvol 318
Intracellular Actions of Renin
Tadashi Inagami, James C. McKenzie, Kailash Pandey,
Mitsuaki Nakamaru, Daniel L. Clemens, Tomio Okamura,
Mitsuhide Naruse, and Kiyoko Naruse 327

The Endocrine System and the Kidney

Similarity of the Effects of Antidiuretic Hormone, Parathyroid Hormone,
Calcitonin, and Glucagon on Rat Kidney
Christian de Rouffignac, Jean-Marc Elalouf, Nicole Roinel, Claire Bailly,
and Claude Amiel 340
Brush Border and Basal-Lateral Membranes in the Action of Thyroid
Hormone on the Proximal Tubule
Giovambattista Capasso and Rolf Kinne. 358
Binding of Aldosterone and Corticosterone Along the Nephron and Effects
on Na-K-ATPase
Adrian I. Katz, Marcia A. Chekal, and Salim K. Mujais 364
Localization of Aldosterone Receptors Along the Nephron
Nicolette Farman and Jean-Pierre Bonvalet. 372
Mechanism of Action of Aldosterone: Effects on Sodium, Potassium, and
Hydrogen Transport
Juha P. Kokko 380

Mechanism of Action of Aldosterone: Role of Na-K-ATPase
    Bernard C. Rossier, Käthi Geering, and Jean-Pierre Kraehenbuhl . . 388
Renal Actions by Which Vasopressin May Aid the Concentration of Urine
    Heinz Valtin 397
Cellular Modes of Action of Vasopressin
    Rui C. de Sousa 407
Specificity of Agonistic and Antagonistic Analogues of Vasopressin
    Wilbur H. Sawyer and Maurice Manning 417
Cardiovascular Effects of Vasopressin
    Colin I. Johnston, Masao Hiwatari, and Josephine M. Abrahams . . 426

Alterations of Extracellular Fluid Volume

Edema

Newer Concepts of Starling Equilibrium at the Capillary Level in the
Production of Edema
    Knut Aukland 435
Pathogenesis of Edema in Cirrhosis
    Murray Epstein 449
Renal Handling of Sodium in Hepatic Diseases Other than Cirrhosis
    J. Rapaport and Cidio Chaimovitz. 461
Primary Renal Sodium Retention in the Nephrotic Syndrome
    David B. Bernard 469

Causes and Mechanisms of Renal Injury

Immunologic Mechanisms in Renal Disease
    Alfred F. Michael 485
Cellular and Humoral Mediators of Renal Injury
    Chairpersons: D. Keith Peters and Curtis B. Wilson; *Discussants:*
    David J. Salant, Roland C. Blantz, Robert C. Atkins,
    Kym M. Bannister, Andrew J. Rees, George F. Schreiner,
    R. Bernd Sterzl, Michael J. Dunn, Raymond Ardaillou, and
    Roger C. Wiggins 504
Mechanisms of Immune Complex Formation and Deposition in Glomeruli
    William G. Couser, Stephen Adler, Patricia J. Baker, Richard J. Johnson,
    and Diana A. Perkinson 508
Characteristics of Circulating Immune Complexes That Deposit in Renal
Glomeruli
    Mart Mannik and V. Joyce Gauthier 527
Etiologic Factors in Immunologically Mediated Glomerulonephritis
    Philip J. Hoedemaeker, Gert J. Fleuren, and Jan J. Weening 540
Role of Antigen and Antibody Charge in Immune Complex Disease
    Wayne A. Border 550
Pathogenic Antigen of Heymann Nephritis (gp330): Identification, Isolation,
and Localization
    Dontscho Kerjaschki and Marilyn Gist Farquhar. 560
Monoclonal Antibodies as Probes of Normal and Abnormal Renal Structure
    Chairpersons: Gary E. Striker and Robert C. Atkins; *Discussants:*
    Wayne Hancock, John Hunt, Steven R. Holdsworth, Akira Y. T. Wu,
    Alfred F. Michael, Pierre Verroust, Dontscho Kerjaschki,
    Charles D. Pusey, Donna L. Mendrick, and Pierre Ronco. 575

Role of Proteoglycans in Glomerular Function and Pathology
   Marilyn Gist Farquhar, Margaret C. Lemkin, and Jennifer L. Stow . 580
Glomerular Arachidonic Acid Metabolism in Nephrotoxic Serum Nephritis
   Michael J. Dunn, Elias A. Lianos, and John E. Stork 601
Effects of Dexamethasone on Cultured Mesangial Cell Function During
Phagocytosis
   Laurent Baud, Joelle Perez, Diego Pujol, and Raymond Ardaillou . . 609

Diseases of the Kidneys

Primary Glomerular Diseases

Poststreptococcal Glomerulonephritis
   Bernardo Rodríguez-Iturbe 623
Minimal Change Disease, Mesangial Proliferative Glomerulonephritis and
Focal Sclerosis: Individual Entities or a Spectrum of Disease?
   Chairpersons: Renée Habib and Jacob Churg; *Discussants:* Jay Bernstein,
   J. Stewart Cameron, Arthur H. Cohen, Marie-France Gagnadoux, and
   Edmund J. Lewis 634
Pathogenetic Mechanisms of IgA Nephropathy from Studies of Experimental
Models
   Andrew J. Woodroffe and Jane D. Lomax-Smith 645
Immunologic Aspects of IgA Nephropathy in Humans
   Jesus Egido, Jaime Sancho, R. Blasco, L. Lozano, and Luis Hernando 652
Clinicopathologic Correlations in IgA Nephropathy
   Raja Sinniah and Gordon Ku 665
Natural History and Treatment of Idiopathic IgA Nephropathy
   Giuseppe D'Amico 686

Acute Renal Failure

Principles of Acute Renal Failure
   Michael Steinhausen and Niranjan Parekh 702
Pathology of Acute Renal Failure
   Ruth E. Bulger and Dennis C. Dobyan 711
Experimental Acute Renal Failure: Pathophysiology and Methods of
Protection
   Terrance A. Fried and Jay H. Stein 731
Control of Renal Regeneration After Acute Tubular Necrosis
   F. Gary Toback 748
Contribution of Proteases to Hypercatabolism in Acute Renal Failure
   August Heidland and Walter H. Hörl 763
Cellular Mechanisms of Protection in Nephrotoxic and Ischemic Acute
Renal Failure
   H. David Humes, Deborah A. Hunt, Mary J. Clark, Michael P. White,
   and Joel M. Weinberg 776
Clonidine, Propranolol, and the Prevention of Acute Renal Failure
   Kim Solez, Lorraine C. Racusen, and Andrew Whelton 784
The Role of Calcium Channel Blockers
   Thomas J. Burke, Patricia E. Arnold, and Robert W. Schrier. . . . 791
Adenine Nucleotides in the Prevention of Ischemic Acute Renal Failure
   Norman J. Siegel, Karen M. Gaudio, and Michael Kashgarian . . . 800

Nephrotoxicity

Mechanisms of Drug Nephrotoxicity
    William M. Bennett. 807
Nephrotoxicity of Nonsteroidal Anti-Inflammatory Drugs
    William L. Henrich 819
Renal Damage Induced by Radiologic Contrast Media
    Carl M. Kjellstrand, Robert O. Berkseth, and Paul A. Abraham . . 835
Antibiotic-Induced Nephrotoxicity
    Carlos A. Vaamonde 844
Nephrotoxicity Caused by Cancer Chemotherapy
    Richard E. Rieselbach 869

Volume II

The Kidney in Systemic Disease

Renal Involvement in Multiple Myeloma
    Manuel Martínez-Maldonado and Luis Báez-Díaz 885
Pathology of Light Chain Nephropathies
    Arthur H. Cohen 895
Glomerular Lesions in Lymphomas and Leukemias
    Liliane Morel-Maroger Striker, Françoise Mignon, David Dabbs, and
    Gary E. Striker 905
Sickle Cell Nephropathy
    Vardaman M. Buckalew, Jr. 916

Tubular Defects

Isolated Tubular Defects
    Chairpersons: Russell W. Chesney and Bernard S. Kaplan; *Discussants:*
    James C. M. Chan, Guido O. Perez, Juan Rodríguez-Soriano, and
    Robert L. Chevalier. 926

Obstructive Uropathy and Urinary Reflux

Pathophysiology of Obstructive Uropathy
    Chairpersons: Wadi N. Suki and Douglas R. Wilson; *Discussants:*
    A. Erik G. Persson, George A. Tanner, William E. Yarger, Saulo Klahr,
    Michael H. Humphreys, Adrian Spitzer, Ulla C. Kopp, and
    Elsa Bello-Reuss 932
Vesicoureteral Reflux and Renal Damage
    C. John Hodson 936
Renal Scars and Vesicoureteric Reflux: Pathology and Pathogenesis of
Segmental Atrophy
    Jay Bernstein and Billy S. Arant, Jr. 948
Natural History and Treatment of Reflux Nephropathy
    Priscilla S. Kincaid-Smith. 959

Urolithiasis

Pathogenesis of Calcium Renal Stones
    Fredric L. Coe and Joan H. Parks. 980

Physicochemical Factors in Calcium Oxalate Urolithiasis
 Lynwood H. Smith   990
Use of Thiazide Diuretics in Calcium Oxalate Nephrolithiasis
 Roger A. L. Sutton   999
Agents Other Than Thiazide Diuretics in the Treatment of Calcium Oxalate
Nephrolithiasis
 Ulla Backman.   1011
Urinary Inhibitors of Calcium Oxalate Crystallization
 Chairpersons: Charles Y. C. Pak and John L. Meyer; *Discussants:*
 Peter G. Werners, William B. Gill, Lawrence Resnick,
 William C. Thomas, and Michael J. Nicar   1025

Kidney Diseases in the Tropics

Nephrotic Syndrome in Tropical Africa: Glomerulonephritis in Zimbabwe
 Janet L. Seggie   1030
Renal Involvement in Leptospirosis
 Visith Sitprija.   1041

Diabetes Mellitus and the Kidney

Clinical and Renal Functional Studies of Diabetic Nephropathy in Humans
 Carl Erik Mogensen   1053
Altered Glomerular Metabolism in Diabetes Mellitus
 Pedro Cortes, Francis Dumler, and Nathan W. Levin   1074
Pathophysiology of Proteinuria in Diabetic Nephropathy
 Ovadia Shemesh, Henry W. Jones III, and Bryan D. Myers   1081
Early Markers of Diabetic Nephropathy: A Road to Prevention
 GianCarlo Viberti and Martin J. Wiseman   1094
Can the Insulin-Dependent Diabetic Patient Be Managed Without Kidney
Biopsy?
 S. Michael Mauer, Michael W. Steffes, Eileen N. Ellis, and
 David M. Brown.   1103
Pathogenesis as a Determinant of Therapy in Diabetic Nephropathy
 Eli A. Friedman   1109

Hypertension

Hypertension: Current Concepts of Mechanism and Management
 Austin E. Doyle.   1115
Effect of Dietary Fish Oils on Eicosanoid Formation in Platelets,
Neutrophils, and the Cardiovascular-Renal System
 Peter C. Weber, Sven Fischer, Reinhard Lorenz, Thomas Strasser,
 Clemens von Schacky, and Wolfgang Siess   1136
Calcium, Phosphate, and Parathyroid Hormone in Blood Pressure
Regulation
 Chairpersons: David A. McCarron and Kai Lau; *Discussants:*
 Roger L. Niser, Lawrence Resnick, Vito Campese, Johannes Mann,
 and David Bushinsky   1141
Role of Sodium and Other Dietary Factors in Hypertension
 Herbert G. Langford   1148

Hypertension in the Elderly
    Robert C. Tarazi. 1154
Mechanisms of Action and Use of Newer Antihypertensive Agents
    Chairpersons: David B. Case and Norman M. Kaplan; *Discussants:*
    Trefor O. Morgan, Richard de Zeeuw, Michael Weber, Keishi Abe,
    and Peter Weidmann 1163
An Analysis for and Against Treatment of Mild Hypertension
    Nemat O. Borhani 1168

Phosphate Depletion

Clinical Spectrum of Phosphate Depletion and Its Effects on Urinary
Acidification
    Sandra Sabatini 1183
Effect of Phosphate Depletion on Renal Tubular Transport
    Zalman S. Agus and Renée E. Garrick 1198
Phosphate Depletion and Renal Cell Metabolism
    Kiyoshi Kurokawa 1209
Mechanisms of Myocardial Injury in Phosphate Depletion
    Nachman Brautbar 1217

Pathogenesis and Consequences of Chronic Renal Failure

Mechanisms of Progression of Renal Disease
    Barry M. Brenner and Timothy W. Meyer 1233
Pathogenesis of Uremia
    Eberhard Ritz. 1247

Endocrine and Metabolic Abnormalities

Regulation of Parathyroid Gland Activity
    Joel F. Habener 1264
The Status of Parathyroid Hormone Measurements in Humans
    Jan A. Fischer, Ulrich Binswanger, Walter Born,
    Maximilian A. Dambacher, and Fritz A. Tschopp 1277
Parathyroid Hormone: Alterations in Chronic Renal Failure
    Eduardo Slatopolsky, Kevin J. Martin, Jeremiah J. Morrissey, and
    Keith A. Hruska. 1292
Vitamin D and Kidney Disease
    Jacob Lemann, Jr., Richard W. Gray, and Adel B. Korkor 1305
Endocrine and Metabolic Abnormalities in Acute Renal Failure
    Garabed Eknoyan 1322
Insulin, Glucose, Amino Acid, and Lipid Metabolism in Chronic Renal
Insufficiency
    Ralph A. DeFronzo, Anders Alvestrand, and Douglas J. Smith . . . 1334
Endocrine and Metabolic Abnormalities in the Nephrotic Syndrome:
Calcium and Carbohydrate Metabolism
    Giuseppe Maschio, Nicola Tessitore, Carmelo Loschiavo,
    Angela D'Angelo, Ermanno Bonucci, Bjarne Lund, and Birger Lund . 1349

Osteodystrophy

Renal Osteodystrophy: General Concepts and Current Issues
  Albert Fournier, Philippe Morinière, J. L. Sebert, B. Boudailliez,
  I. Grégoire, M. Garabédian, J. Guéris, and P. Meunier. 1357
Prevalence of Various Types of Bone Disease in Dialysis Patients
  Francisco Llach, Arnold J. Felsenfeld, Michael D. Coleman, and
  James A. Pederson 1374
Role of Aluminum Accumulation in Renal Osteodystrophy
  Jack W. Coburn, Henry G. Nebeker, Gavril Hercz, Dawn S. Milliner,
  Susan M. Ott, Dennis L. Andress, Donald J. Sherrard, and
  Allen C. Alfrey 1383
Treatment of Renal Osteodystrophy in Chronic Renal Failure
  Joseph M. Letteri 1396

Hematopoietic System

Prostanoid-Related Platelet Abnormalities in Renal Disease
  Ariela Benigni, Manuela Livio, and Giuseppe Remuzzi. 1406

Gastrointestinal

Intestinal Transport of Minerals in Renal Failure
  Chairpersons: David B. N. Lee and Carlo Gennari; *Discussants:*
  Zachariah Varghese, Herta C. Spencer, and Allen C. Alfrey 1412

Evaluation and Management of Kidney Diseases and Renal Failure

Microscopic and Biochemical Analysis of the Urine in the Evaluation of
Kidney Disease
  Chairpersons: Robert G. Narins and Kenneth F. Fairley; *Discussant:*
  Richard A. Zager 1425
Newer Imaging Techniques in Nephrology
  Chairpersons: Hedvig Hricak and Zoran L. Barbaric; *Discussants:*
  Richard M. Friedenberg, Hooshang Kangarloo, Bruce Hillman, and
  Bruce L. McClennan 1430
Are Randomized Trials in Kidney Disease Worthwhile?
  Chairpersons: Edmund J. Lewis and Cecil H. Coggins; *Discussants:*
  Clark D. West, Adrian Spitzer, Stephen W. Zimmerman, John Lachin,
  William Winslade, and Daniel C. Cattran 1437

Infections

Current Concepts in the Management of Urinary Tract Infections
  Chairpersons: A. William Asscher and Jan Winberg; *Discussants:*
  M. P. Glauser, Renée Kuytens, Roland Möllby, James A. Roberts,
  and Kate Verrier-Jones 1441

Treatment of Glomerular Diseases

Treatment of Glomerulonephritis Based on Knowledge of Its Pathogenesis
  J. Stewart Cameron. 1445

Use of Pulse Methylprednisolone in Primary and Multisystem Glomerular Diseases
    W. Kline Bolton 1464
Plasma Exchange for Glomerular Disease
    Charles D. Pusey and C. Martin Lockwood 1474
Treatment of Glomerular Disease with Anticoagulant, Antiplatelet, and Nonsteroidal Anti-inflammatory Agents
    James V. Donadio, Jr. 1486

Nutrition in Renal Failure

Causes of Catabolism and Wasting in Acute or Chronic Renal Failure
    Joel D. Kopple 1498
Influence of Nutritional Therapy on Progression of Renal Insufficiency
    William E. Mitch 1516

Dialysis

Advantages and Disadvantages of Current Dialysis Techniques
    Horst Klinkmann and Peter Ivanovich 1528
Vascular Access for Hemodialysis
    Chairpersons: Fred L. Shapiro and Robert Uldall; Discussants:
    Robert J. Anderson, Allan J. Collins, Howard Silberman,
    Raymond Vanholder, and Alex Heaton 1553
Anatomic and Physiologic Aspects of Peritoneal Dialysis
    Karl D. Nolph 1561
Efficacy and Adequacy of Continuous Ambulatory Peritoneal Dialysis
    George Wu, Donald Kim, and Dimitrios G. Oreopoulos 1581
Continuous Ambulatory Peritoneal Dialysis in Diabetic Patients
    Marcel C. Legrain, Jacques B. Rottembourg, Belkacem Issad,
    Pierre-Yves Cossette, and Amar Boudjemaa 1599
Long-Term Metabolic Consequences of Continuous Ambulatory Peritoneal Dialysis
    Bengt Lindholm, Anders Alvestrand, Hans Erik Norbeck, Anders
    Tranaeus, and Jonas Bergström 1611

Transplantation

Renal Transplantation: Current Status
    Peter J. Morris 1627
Endocrine and Metabolic Dysfunctions Following Kidney Transplantation
    Jacob Green and Ori S. Better 1644
Cyclosporine in Renal Transplantation
    Rolf Loertscher, Mario Abbud-Filho, and Terry B. Strom 1662
The Transfusion Effect in Renal Allograft Recipients
    Sondra Perdue and Paul I. Terasaki 1674
Antilymphocyte Globulin and Monoclonal Antibodies: Present Status as Therapy
    A. Benedict Cosimi 1681
Total Lymphoid Irradiation in Renal Transplantation: Reduction and Elimination of Maintenance Immunosuppressive Drugs
    Samuel Strober, Richard T. Hoppe, Barry Levin, and Derek Sampson. 1695
Adjuvant Methods of Immunomodulation for Transplantation
    Tadeusz Orłowski 1708

Immunological Monitoring and Renal Transplantation
    Chairpersons: Ronald D. Guttmann and Vittorio Bonomini; *Discussants:*
    Takahiro Oka, William E. Braun, Marvin R. Garovoy, Terry B. Strom,
    Fernando Valderrobano, Mark Waer, Louis Lanier, Wayne Hancock,
    and Mohammad Allajani 1715

Index 1725

Contents II

State-of-the-Art Lectures

Hydrogen Ion Transport Along the Nephron
 Floyd C. Rector, Jr. 161
Similarity of the Effects of Antidiuretic Hormone, Parathyroid Hormone,
Calcitonin, and Glucagon on Rat Kidney
 Christian de Rouffignac, Jean-Marc Elalouf, Nicole Roinel, Claire Bailly,
 and Claude Amiel 340
Immunologic Mechanisms in Renal Disease
 Alfred F. Michael 485
Mechanisms of Progression of Renal Disease
 Barry M. Brenner and Timothy W. Meyer 1233
Pathogenesis of Uremia
 Eberhard Ritz. 1247
Hypertension: Current Concepts of Mechanism and Management
 Austin E. Doyle 1115
Advantages and Disadvantages of Current Dialysis Techniques
 Horst Klinkmann and Peter Ivanovich 1528
Renal Transplantation: Current Status
 Peter J. Morris 1627

Symposia

Second Messengers and Epithelial Transport

Role of Cytosolic Calcium in Vasopressin-sensitive Epithelia
 Ann Taylor, Mirilee Pearl, Barbara Barber, and Beth Crutch. . . . 39
Role of Cytosolic Calcium in Renal Tubular Transport
 Erich E. Windhager and Gustavo Frindt. 51
Basolateral Membrane Properties of Sodium-absorbing Epithelia
 Stanley G. Schultz 7

Brush Border Transport Mechanisms

Sodium Phosphate Cotransport: Studies with Vesicles and LLC-PK$_1$ Cells
Heini Murer, Martin Amstutz, Jürg Biber, Piotr Gmaj, and
Kerstin Malmström.   57
Brush Border and Basal-Lateral Membranes in the Action of Thyroid
Hormone on the Proximal Tubule
Giovambattista Capasso and Rolf Kinne.   358
Sodium-Glucose Cotransport Mechanisms
R. James Turner.   21
Regulation of the Na$^+$/H$^+$ Antiporter in Cells of the Proximal Tubule
David G. Warnock and Harlan E. Ives   70

Regulation of Medullary Circulation

Organization of the Medullary Circulation: Functional Implications
Lise Bankir, Nadine Bouby, and Marie-Marcelle Trinh-Trang-Tan . .   84
Intrarenal Control of Medullary Blood Flow and the Urinary Concentrating
Mechanism
Leon C. Moore   120
Pathophysiology of the Medullary Circulation
June Mason   107

Intrarenal Control of Glomerular Filtration Rate

Influence of Renal Nerves on the Glomerular Microcirculation
Valentina Kon and Iekuni Ichikawa   154
Intrarenal Control of Glomerular Filtration: Cellular Mechanisms of
Tubuloglomerular Feedback
P. Darwin Bell and L. Gabriel Navar.   130
Regulatory Role of the Tubuloglomerular Feedback Mechanism
Josephine P. Briggs and Jürgen Schnermann   143

Transport Mechanisms in the Loop of Henle

Transport Properties of the Pars Recta
James A. Schafer and Jack Work   186
Function of the Thin Limb of Henle's Loop
Masashi Imai, Matuhiko Hayashi, Masasuke Araki, and Kaoru Tabei.   196
Sodium Chloride Reabsorption in the Thick Ascending Limb of the Loop
of Henle
Rainer Greger, Monika Wittner, Eberhard Schlatter, Brigitte Gebler,
Claudia Weidtke, and Antonio Di Stefano   224
Regulation of Sodium Chloride Transport by the Loop of Henle
John B. Stokes III   208

Aldosterone and the Kidney

Binding of Aldosterone and Corticosterone Along the Nephron and Effects
on Na-K-ATPase
Adrian I. Katz, Marcia A. Chekal, and Salim K. Mujais   364
Localization of Aldosterone Receptors Along the Nephron
Nicolette Farman and Jean-Pierre Bonvalet.   372

Mechanism of Action of Aldosterone: Effects on Sodium, Potassium, and
Hydrogen Transport
   Juha P. Kokko   380
Mechanism of Action of Aldosterone: Role of Na-K-ATPase
   Bernard C. Rossier, Käthi Geering, and Jean-Pierre Kraehenbuhl . .   388

Vasopressins: Diverse Action

Renal Actions by Which Vasopressin May Aid the Concentration of Urine
   Heinz Valtin   397
Cellular Modes of Action of Vasopressin
   Rui C. de Sousa   407
Specificity of Agonistic and Antagonistic Analogues of Vasopressin
   Wilbur H. Sawyer and Maurice Manning   417
Cardiovascular Effects of Vasopressin
   Colin I. Johnston, Masao Hiwatari, and Josephine M. Abrahams . .   426

Renin: Recent Advances

From Molecular Biology to Antihypertensive Drugs: Current Research on
Renin Inhibitors
   Edgar Haber   284
Inactive Renin
   Jean E. Sealey.   302
The Renin Gene: Structure and Processing of Renin
   Florent Soubrier, Joël Menard, and Pierre Corvol   318
Intracellular Actions of Renin
   Tadashi Inagami, James C. McKenzie, Kailash Pandey,
   Mitsuaki Nakamaru, Daniel L. Clemens, Tomio Okamura,
   Mitsuhide Naruse, and Kiyoko Naruse   327

Prostaglandins and the Kidney

Glomerular Arachidonic Acid Metabolism in Nephrotoxic Serum Nephritis
   Michael J. Dunn, Elias A. Lianos, and John E. Stork   601
Biochemistry of Renal Prostaglandins
   Aubrey R. Morrison   277
Effect of Dietary Fish Oils on Eicosanoid Formation in Platelets,
Neutrophils, and the Cardiovascular-Renal System
   Peter C. Weber, Sven Fischer, Reinhard Lorenz, Thomas Strasser,
   Clemens von Schacky, and Wolfgang Siess 1136
Prostanoid-Related Platelet Abnormalities in Renal Disease
   Ariela Benigni, Manuela Livio, and Giuseppe Remuzzi 1406

*Recent Advances in the Structure, Biochemistry and Function
of the Glomerulus*

Role of Proteoglycans in Glomerular Function and Pathology
   Marilyn Gist Farquhar, Margaret C. Lemkin, and Jennifer L. Stow .   580
Effects of Dexamethasone on Cultured Mesangial Cell Function During
Phagocytosis
   Laurent Baud, Joelle Perez, Diego Pujol, and Raymond Ardaillou . .   609
Pathogenic Antigen of Heymann Nephritis (gp330): Identification, Isolation,
and Localization
   Dontscho Kerjaschki and Marilyn Gist Farquhar.   560

Mechanisms of Immune Complex Formation and Deposition in Glomeruli

Mechanisms of Immune Complex Formation and Deposition in Glomeruli
William G. Couser, Stephen Adler, Patricia J. Baker, Richard J. Johnson, and Diana A. Perkinson 508
Etiologic Factors in Immunologically Mediated Glomerulonephritis
Philip J. Hoedemaeker, Gert J. Fleuren, and Jan J. Weening 540
Role of Antigen and Antibody Charge in Immune Complex Disease
Wayne A. Border 550
Characteristics of Circulating Immune Complexes That Deposit in Renal Glomeruli
Mart Mannik and V. Joyce Gauthier 527

Pathogenesis of Edema in Cirrhosis and Nephrotic Syndrome

Pathogenesis of Edema in Cirrhosis
Murray Epstein 449
Renal Handling of Sodium in Hepatic Diseases Other than Cirrhosis
J. Rapaport and Cidio Chaimovitz. 461
Newer Concepts of Starling Equilibrium at the Capillary Level in the Production of Edema
Knut Aukland 435
Primary Renal Sodium Retention in the Nephrotic Syndrome
David B. Bernard 469

IgA Nephropathy

Clinicopathologic Correlations in IgA Nephropathy
Raja Sinniah and Gordon Ku 665
Natural History and Treatment of Idiopathic IgA Nephropathy
Guiseppe D'Amico 686
Immunologic Aspects of IgA Nephropathy in Humans
Jesus Egido, Jaime Sancho, R. Blasco, L. Lozano, and Luis Hernando   652
Pathogenetic Mechanisms of IgA Nephropathy from Studies of Experimental Models
Andrew J. Woodroffe and Jane D. Lomax-Smith 645

Acute Renal Failure: Structure-Function Relationships

Principles of Acute Renal Failure
Michael Steinhausen and Niranjan Parekh 702
Pathology of Acute Renal Failure
Ruth E. Bulger and Dennis C. Dobyan 711
Experimental Acute Renal Failure: Pathophysiology and Methods of Protection
Terrance A. Fried and Jay H. Stein 731
Control of Renal Regeneration After Acute Tubular Necrosis
F. Gary Toback 748

New Frontiers in the Prevention of Acute Renal Failure

Cellular Mechanisms of Protection in Nephrotoxic and Ischemic Acute Renal Failure
H. David Humes, Deborah A. Hunt, Mary J. Clark, Michael P. White, and Joel M. Weinberg 776

Clonidine, Propranolol, and the Prevention of Acute Renal Failure
  Kim Solez, Lorraine C. Racusen, and Andrew Whelton 784
The Role of Calcium Channel Blockers
  Thomas J. Burke, Patricia E. Arnold, and Robert W. Schrier. . . . 791
Adenine Nucleotides in the Prevention of Ischemic Acute Renal Failure
  Norman J. Siegel, Karen M. Gaudio, and Michael Kashgarian . . . 800

Reflux Nephropathy: Current Status

Vesicoureteral Reflux and Renal Damage
  C. John Hodson 936
Renal Scars and Vesicoureteric Reflux: Pathology and Pathogenesis of
Segmental Atrophy
  Jay Bernstein and Billy S. Arant, Jr. 948
Natural History and Treatment of Reflux Nephropathy
  Priscilla S. Kincaid-Smith. 959

Pathogenesis and Treatment of Calcium Nephrolithiasis

Pathogenesis of Calcium Renal Stones
  Fredric L. Coe and Joan H. Parks. 980
Use of Thiazide Diuretics in Calcium Oxalate Nephrolithiasis
  Roger A. L. Sutton 999
Agents Other Than Thiazide Diuretics in the Treatment of Calcium Oxalate
Nephrolithiasis
  Ulla Backman. 1011
Physicochemical Factors in Calcium Oxalate Urolithiasis
  Lynwood H. Smith 990

Tropical Nephrology

Nephrotic Syndrome in Tropical Africa: Glomerulonephritis in Zimbabwe
  Janet L. Seggie 1030
Renal Involvement in Leptospirosis
  Visith Sitprija. 1041
Poststreptococcal Glomerulonephritis
  Bernardo Rodríguez-Iturbe 623
Sickle Cell Nephropathy
  Vardaman M. Buckalew, Jr. 916

The Kidney and Malignant Disease

Nephrotoxicity Caused by Cancer Chemotherapy
  Richard E. Rieselbach 869
Glomerular Lesions in Lymphomas and Leukemias
  Liliane Morel-Maroger Striker, Françoise Mignon, David Dabbs, and
  Gary E. Striker 905
Renal Involvement in Multiple Myeloma
  Manuel Martínez-Maldonado and Luis Báez-Díaz 885
Pathology of Light Chain Nephropathies
  Arthur H. Cohen 895

Nephrotoxicity and Drugs

Mechanisms of Drug Nephrotoxicity
William M. Bennett.   807
Nephrotoxicity of Nonsteroidal Anti-Inflammatory Drugs
William L. Henrich.   819
Renal Damage Induced by Radiologic Contrast Media
Carl M. Kjellstrand, Robert O. Berkseth, and Paul A. Abraham . .   835
Antibiotic-Induced Nephrotoxicity
Carlos A. Vaamonde   844

Diabetic Nephropathy: Concepts of Pathogenesis and Treatment

Pathogenesis as a Determinant of Therapy in Diabetic Nephropathy
Eli A. Friedman   1109
Clinical and Renal Functional Studies of Diabetic Nephropathy in Humans
Carl Erik Mogensen   1053
Can the Insulin-Dependent Diabetic Patient Be Managed Without Kidney
Biopsy?
S. Michael Mauer, Michael W. Steffes, Eileen N. Ellis, and
David M. Brown.   1103
Pathophysiology of Proteinuria in Diabetic Nephropathy
Ovadia Shemesh, Henry W. Jones III, and Bryan D. Myers   1081
Altered Glomerular Metabolism in Diabetes Mellitus
Pedro Cortes, Francis Dumler, and Nathan W. Levin   1074
Early Markers of Diabetic Nephropathy: A Road to Prevention
GianCarlo Viberti and Martin J. Wiseman   1094

Controversies in the Therapy of Hypertension

Hypertension in the Elderly
Robert C. Tarazi.   1154
An Analysis for and Against Treatment of Mild Hypertension
Nemat O. Borhani   1168
Role of Sodium and Other Dietary Factors in Hypertension
Herbert G. Langford   1148

Endocrine and Metabolic Abnormalities in Renal Diseases

Endocrine and Metabolic Abnormalities in Acute Renal Failure
Garabed Eknoyan   1322
Insulin, Glucose, Amino Acid, and Lipid Metabolism in Chronic Renal
Insufficiency
Ralph A. DeFronzo, Anders Alvestrand, and Douglas J. Smith . . .   1334
Endocrine and Metabolic Abnormalities in the Nephrotic Syndrome:
Calcium and Carbohydrate Metabolism
Giuseppe Maschio, Nicola Tessitore, Carmelo Loschiavo,
Angela D'Angelo, Ermanno Bonucci, Bjarne Lund, and Birger Lund .   1349
Endocrine and Metabolic Dysfunctions Following Kidney Transplantation
Jacob Green and Ori S. Better   1644

Parathyroid Hormone and Vitamin D in Uremia

Vitamin D and Kidney Disease
Jacob Lemann, Jr., Richard W. Gray, and Adel B. Korkor   1305

Regulation of Parathyroid Gland Activity
Joel F. Habener 1264
The Status of Parathyroid Hormone Measurements in Humans
Jan A. Fischer, Ulrich Binswanger, Walter Born,
Maximilian A. Dambacher, and Fritz A. Tschopp 1277
Parathyroid Hormone: Alterations in Chronic Renal Failure
Eduardo Slatopolsky, Kevin J. Martin, Jeremiah J. Morrissey, and
Keith A. Hruska. 1292

Renal Osteodystrophy: Recent Advances

Renal Osteodystrophy: General Concepts and Current Issues
Albert Fournier, Philippe Morinière, J. L. Sebert, B. Boudailliez,
I. Grégoire, M. Garabédian, J. Guéris, and P. Meunier. 1357
Role of Aluminum Accumulation in Renal Osteodystrophy
Jack W. Coburn, Henry G. Nebeker, Gavril Hercz, Dawn S. Milliner,
Susan M. Ott, Dennis L. Andress, Donald J. Sherrard, and
Allen C. Alfrey 1383
Prevalence of Various Types of Bone Disease in Dialysis Patients
Francisco Llach, Arnold J. Felsenfeld, Michael D. Coleman, and
James A. Pederson 1374
Treatment of Renal Osteodystrophy in Chronic Renal Failure
Joseph M. Letteri 1396

Renal and Vascular Consequences of Phosphate Depletion

Clinical Spectrum of Phosphate Depletion and Its Effects on Urinary
Acidification
Sandra Sabatini 1183
Effect of Phosphate Depletion on Renal Tubular Transport
Zalman S. Agus and Renée E. Garrick 1198
Phosphate Depletion and Renal Cell Metabolism
Kiyoshi Kurokawa 1209
Mechanisms of Myocardial Injury in Phosphate Depletion
Nachman Brautbar 1217

Nutritional Aspects of Renal Disease

Causes of Catabolism and Wasting in Acute or Chronic Renal Failure
Joel D. Kopple 1498
Influence of Nutritional Therapy on Progression of Renal Insufficiency
William E. Mitch 1516
Contribution of Proteases to Hypercatabolism in Acute Renal Failure
August Heidland and Walter H. Hörl 763

The Treatment of Glomerulonephritis

Treatment of Glomerulonephritis Based on Knowledge of Its Pathogenesis
J. Stewart Cameron. 1445
Use of Pulse Methylprednisolone in Primary and Multisystem Glomerular
Diseases
W. Kline Bolton 1464
Plasma Exchange for Glomerular Disease
Charles D. Pusey and C. Martin Lockwood 1474

Treatment of Glomerular Disease with Anticoagulant, Antiplatelet, and
Nonsteroidal Anti-inflammatory Agents
   James V. Donadio, Jr. 1486

Continuous Ambulatory Peritoneal Dialysis

Anatomic and Physiologic Aspects of Peritoneal Dialysis
   Karl D. Nolph 1561
Continuous Ambulatory Peritoneal Dialysis in Diabetic Patients
   Marcel C. Legrain, Jacques B. Rottembourg, Belkacem Issad,
   Pierre-Yves Cossette, and Amar Boudjemaa 1599
Efficacy and Adequacy of Continuous Ambulatory Peritoneal Dialysis
   George Wu, Donald Kim, and Dimitrios G. Oreopoulos 1581
Long-Term Metabolic Consequences of Continuous Ambulatory Peritoneal
Dialysis
   Bengt Lindholm, Anders Alvestrand, Hans Erik Norbeck,
   Anders Tranaeus, and Jonas Bergström 1611

Immunomodulation for Transplantation: New Approaches

Cyclosporine in Renal Transplantation
   Rolf Loertscher, Mario Abbud-Filho, and Terry B. Strom 1662
The Transfusion Effect in Renal Allograft Recipients
   Sondra Perdue and Paul I. Terasaki 1674
Antilymphocyte Globulin and Monoclonal Antibodies: Present Status as
Therapy
   A. Benedict Cosimi 1681
Total Lymphoid Irradiation in Renal Transplantation: Reduction and
Elimination of Maintenance Immunosuppressive Drugs
   Samuel Strober, Richard T. Hoppe, Barry Levin, and Derek Sampson   1695
Adjuvant Methods of Immunomodulation for Transplantation
   Tadeusz Orłowski 1708

Workshops

Determinants of Growth, Form, and Function in Epithelia
   Chairpersons: Joseph S. Handler and Marcelino M. Cereijido; *Discussants:*
   Maurice Burg, Mary Taub, Michael F. Horster, and John D. Valentich   3
Cell Volume Regulation in Epithelia
   Chairpersons: Jared J. Grantham and Kenneth R. Spring; *Discussants:*
   Michael A. Linshaw, Guillermo Whittembury, Paola Carpi-Medina,
   Ernesto Gonzalez, Henry Linares, William B. Guggino, Kevin L. Kirk,
   James A. Schafer, Donald R. DiBona, and Peter M. Andrews . . .   34
Functions of the Renal Nerves
   Chairpersons: Gerald F. DiBona and Romulo E. Colindres; *Discussants:*
   Luciano Barajas, Roger J. Summers, Nicholas G. Moss, Ulla C. Kopp,
   and Richard E. Katholi   79
Proximal Tubule Transport
   Chairperson: Harry R. Jacobson; *Co-Chairperson:* Jean Cardinal;
   Discussants: Christine A. Berry, Bruno Corman, Dalon W. Barfuss,
   Jacques Lapointe, Elsa Bello-Reuss, Sei Sasaki, Keith A. Hruska, and
   Julian Seifter   178

Structural Heterogeneity of the Distal Nephron
  Chairpersons: C. Craig Tisher and Brigitte Kaissling; *Discussants:*
  Kirsten M. Madsen, Lise Bankir, Bruce Stanton, Dennis Brown, and
  Michel Bergeron 243
Regulation of Potassium Excretion
  Chairpersons: Gerhard Giebisch and Lawrence Rabinowitz; *Discussants:*
  Fred S. Wright, Karol Bomsztyk, Stephen C. Hebert, Bruce Stanton,
  John B. Stokes III, Bruce Koeppen, and Roger G. O'Neil 260
Contemporary Issues in Renal Metabolism
  Chairpersons: Richard L. Tannen and Brian A. Ross; *Discussants:*
  Anton C. Schoolwerth and Norman J. Siegel 269
Acidification Mechanisms
  Chairpersons: Thomas D. DuBose, Jr. and Michel Paillard; *Discussants:*
  Eberhard Frömter, Robert J. Alpern, David W. Good, and
  Dennis K. Stone 251
Atrial Natriuretic Factor
  Chairpersons: Adolfo J. de Bold and Harald Sonnenberg; *Discussants:*
  Uwe Ackermann, Edward H. Blaine, Josephine P. Briggs,
  Barbara R. Cole, Ralph Keeler, Sidney Solomon, Frank Spinelli,
  Nick C. Trippodo, and Thomas Maack 257
Cellular and Humoral Mediators of Renal Injury
  Chairpersons: D. Keith Peters and Curtis B. Wilson; *Discussants:*
  David J. Salant, Roland C. Blantz, Robert C. Atkins,
  Kym M. Bannister, Andrew J. Rees, George F. Schreiner,
  R. Bernd Sterzl, Michael J. Dunn, Raymond Ardaillou, and
  Roger C. Wiggins 504
Monoclonal Antibodies as Probes of Normal and Abnormal Renal Structure
  Chairpersons: Gary E. Striker and Robert C. Atkins; *Discussants:*
  Wayne Hancock, John Hunt, Steven R. Holdsworth, Akira Y. T. Wu,
  Alfred F. Michael, Pierre Verroust, Dontscho Kerjaschki,
  Charles D. Pusey, Donna L. Mendrick, and Pierre Ronco 575
Minimal Change Disease, Mesangial Proliferative Glomerulonephritis and
Focal Sclerosis: Individual Entities or a Spectrum of Disease?
  Chairpersons: Renée Habib and Jacob Churg; *Discussants:* Jay Bernstein,
  J. Stewart Cameron, Arthur H. Cohen, Marie-France Gagnadoux, and
  Edmund J. Lewis 634
Current Concepts in the Management of Urinary Tract Infections
  Chairpersons: A. William Asscher and Jan Winberg; *Discussants:*
  M. P. Glauser, Renée Kuytens, Roland Möllby, James A. Roberts, and
  Kate Verrier-Jones 1441
Pathophysiology of Obstructive Uropathy
  Chairpersons: Wadi N. Suki and Douglas R. Wilson; *Discussants:*
  A. Erik G. Persson, George A. Tanner, William E. Yarger, Saulo Klahr,
  Michael H. Humphreys, Adrian Spitzer, Ulla C. Kopp, and
  Elsa Bello-Reuss 932
Isolated Tubular Defects
  Chairpersons: Russell W. Chesney and Bernard S. Kaplan; *Discussants:*
  James C. M. Chan, Guido O. Perez, Juan Rodríguez-Soriano, and
  Robert L. Chevalier 926
Urinary Inhibitors of Calcium Oxalate Crystallization
  Chairpersons: Charles Y. C. Pak and John L. Meyer; *Discussants:*
  Peter G. Werners, William B. Gill, Lawrence Resnick,
  William C. Thomas, and Michael J. Nicar 1025

Calcium, Phosphate, and Parathyroid Hormone in Blood Pressure
Regulation
Chairpersons: David A. McCarron and Kai Lau; *Discussants:*
Roger L. Niser, Lawrence Resnick, Vito Campese, Johannes Mann,
and David Bushinsky 1141
Mechanisms of Action and Use of Newer Antihypertensive Agents
Chairpersons: David B. Case and Norman M. Kaplan; *Discussants:*
Trefor O. Morgan, Richard de Zeeuw, Michael Weber, Keishi Abe,
and Peter Weidmann 1163
Intestinal Transport of Minerals in Renal Failure
Chairpersons: David B. N. Lee and Carlo Gennari; *Discussants:*
Zachariah Varghese, Herta C. Spencer, and Allen C. Alfrey 1412
Microscopic and Biochemical Analysis of the Urine in the Evaluation of
Kidney Disease
Chairpersons: Robert G. Narins and Kenneth F. Fairley; *Discussant:*
Richard A. Zager 1425
Newer Imaging Techniques in Nephrology
Chairpersons: Hedvig Hricak and Zoran L. Barbaric; *Discussants:*
Richard M. Friedenberg, Hooshang Kangarloo, Bruce Hillman, and
Bruce L. McClennan 1430
Are Randomized Trials in Kidney Disease Worthwhile?
Chairpersons: Edmund J. Lewis and Cecil H. Coggins; *Discussants:*
Clark D. West, Adrian Spitzer, Stephen W. Zimmerman, John Lachin,
William Winslade, Daniel C. Cattran 1437
Vascular Access for Hemodialysis
Chairpersons: Fred L. Shapiro and Robert Uldall; *Discussants:*
Robert J. Anderson, Allan J. Collins, Howard Silberman,
Raymond Vanholder, and Alex Heaton 1553
Immunological Monitoring and Renal Transplantation
Chairpersons: Ronald D. Guttmann and Vittorio Bonomini; *Discussants:*
Takahiro Oka, William E. Braun, Marvin R. Garovoy, Terry B. Strom,
Fernando Valderrobano, Mark Waer, Louis Lanier, Wayne Hancock,
and Mohammad Allajani 1715

Contributors

ABBUD-FILHO, MARIO. Department of Medicine, Beth Israel Hospital, Boston, Massachusetts, USA

ABE, KEISHI. Department of Internal Medicine, Tohoku University School of Medicine, Sendai, Japan

ABRAHAM, PAUL A. Regional Kidney Disease Program, Department of Medicine, Hennepin County Medical Center, Minneapolis, Minnesota, USA

ABRAHAMS, JOSEPHINE M. Department of Medicine, Monash University, Prince Henry's Hospital, Melbourne, Victoria, Australia

ACKERMANN, UWE. Department of Physiology, University of Toronto, Toronto, Ontario, Canada

ADLER, STEPHEN. Division of Nephrology, Department of Medicine, University of Washington, Seattle, Washington, USA

AGUS, ZALMAN S. Renal Section, Department of Medicine, University of Pennsylvania School of Medicine, Philadelphia, Pennsylvania, USA

ALFREY, ALLEN C. Medical and Research Services, Veterans Administration Medical Center, Denver, Colorado, USA

ALLAJANI, MOHAMMAD. Division of Renal Transplantation, Department of Surgery, Georgetown University Hospital, Washington, D.C., USA

ALPERN, ROBERT J. Department of Medicine, School of Medicine, University of California, San Francisco, California, USA

ALVESTRAND, ANDERS. Department of Renal Medicine, Karolinska Institute, Huddinge University Hospital, Stockholm, Sweden

AMIEL, CLAUDE. INSERM U 251, Département de Physiologie, Faculté de Médecine Xavier Bichat, Paris, France

AMSTUTZ, MARTIN. Department of Physiology, University of Zurich-Irchel, Zurich, Switzerland

ANDERSON, ROBERT J. Department of Medicine, University of Colorado Medical Center, Denver, Colorado, USA

ANDRESS, DENNIS L. Department of Medicine, University of Oklahoma Health Sciences Center, Oklahoma City, Oklahoma, USA

ANDREWS, PETER M. Department of Anatomy, School of Medicine, Georgetown University, Washington, D.C., USA

ARAKI, MASASUKE. Department of Anatomy, Jichi Medical School, Tochigi, Japan

ARANT, BILLY S., JR. Department of Pediatrics, Southwestern Medical School, University of Texas Health Science Center, Dallas, Texas, USA

ARDAILLOU, RAYMOND. Service d'Explorations Fonctionelles, Hôpital Tenon, Paris, France

ARNOLD, PATRICIA E. Department of Medicine, University of Colorado Medical School, Denver, Colorado, USA

ASSCHER, A. WILLIAM. Department of Renal Medicine, Welsh National School of Medicine, Royal Infirmary, Cardiff, Wales, UK

ATKINS, ROBERT C. Department of Nephrology, Prince Henry's Hospital, Monash University, Melbourne, Australia

AUKLAND, KNUT. Department of Physiology, University of Bergen, Bergen, Norway

BACKMAN, ULLA. Department of Internal Medicine, University Hospital, Uppsala, Sweden

BÁEZ-DÍAZ, LUIS. Departments of Medicine and Physiology, University of Puerto Rico School of Medicine, San Juan, Puerto Rico

BAILLY, CLAIRE. INSERM U 251, Département de Physiologie, Faculté de Médecine Xavier Bichat, Paris, France

BAKER, PATRICIA J. Division of Nephrology, Department of Medicine, University of Washington, Seattle, Washington, USA

BANKIR, LISE. INSERM U 90, Hôpital Necker, Paris, France

BANNISTER, KYM M. Department of Immunology, Research Institute of Scripps Clinic, La Jolla, California, USA

BARAJAS, LUCIANO. Department of Pathology, Los Angeles County Harbor-UCLA Medical Center, Torrance, California, USA

BARBARIC, ZORAN L. Department of Radiology, University of California at Los Angeles, Los Angeles, California, USA

BARBER, BARBARA. University Laboratory of Physiology, University of Oxford, Oxford, England, UK

BARFUSS, DALON W. Division of Nephrology, Department of Medicine, University of Alabama Medical Center, Birmingham, Alabama, USA

BAUD, LAURENT. Service de Néphrologie, Hôpital Tenon, Paris, France

BELL, P. DARWIN. Department of Physiology and Biophysics, University of Alabama Medical Center, Birmingham, Alabama, USA

BELLO-REUSS, ELSA. Department of Physiology, Washington University School of Medicine, St. Louis, Missouri, USA

BENIGNI, ARIELA. "Mario Negri" Institute for Pharmacological Research, Bergamo, Italy

BENNETT, WILLIAM M. Division of Nephrology, Department of Medicine, Oregon Health Sciences University, Portland, Oregon, USA

BERGERON, MICHEL. Department of Physiology, University of Montreal, Montreal, Quebec, Canada

BERGSTRÖM, JONAS. Department of Renal Medicine, Karolinska Institute, Huddinge University Hospital, Stockholm, Sweden

BERKSETH, ROBERT O. Regional Kidney Disease Program, Department of Medicine, Hennepin County Medical Center, Minneapolis, Minnesota, USA

BERNARD, DAVID B. Evans Memorial Department of Clinical Research, University Hospital and Renal Section, Department of Medicine, Boston University Medical Center, Boston, Massachusetts, USA

BERNSTEIN, JAY. Department of Anatomic Pathology, William Beaumont Hospital, Royal Oak, Michigan, USA

BERRY, CHRISTINE A. Division of Nephrology, Department of Medicine, University of California, San Francisco, California, USA

BETTER, ORI S. Department of Medicine, Rambam Hospital and Technion School of Medicine, Haifa, Israel

BIBER, JÜRG. Department of Physiology, University of Zurich-Irchel, Zurich, Switzerland

BINSWANGER, ULRICH. Section of Nephrology, Department of Internal Medicine, University of Zurich, Zurich, Switzerland

BLAINE, EDWARD H. Department of Renal Pharmacology, Merck Research Laboratories, West Point, Pennsylvania, USA

BLANTZ, ROLAND C. Division of Nephrology, Department of Medicine, Veterans Administration Medical Center, San Diego, California, USA

BLASCO, R. Servicio de Nefrología, Fundación Jiménez Díaz, Madrid, Spain

BOLTON, W. KLINE. Department of Internal Medicine, University of Virginia School of Medicine, Charlottesville, Virginia, USA

BOMSZTYK, KAROL. Department of Medicine, University of Washington School of Medicine, Seattle, Washington, USA

BONOMINI, VITTORIO. Department of Nephrology and Dialysis, St. Orsola University Hospital, Bologna, Italy

BONUCCI, ERMANNO. Dipartimento di Biopatologia Umana, Università di Roma, Rome, Italy

BONVALET, JEAN-PIERRE. INSERM U 246, Department of Biology, CEN/Saclay, Gif-sur-Yvette, France

BORDER, WAYNE A. Division of Nephrology, University of Utah Medical Center, Salt Lake City, Utah, USA

BORHANI, NEMAT O. Department of Community Health, School of Medicine, University of California, Davis, California, USA

BORN, WALTER. Research Laboratory for Calcium Metabolism, Balgrist Department of Orthopedic Surgery, University of Zurich, Zurich, Switzerland

BOUBY, NADINE. INSERM U 90, Hôpital Necker, Paris, France

BOUDAILLIEZ, B. Service de Néphrologie, Hôpital Nord, Amiens, France

BOUDJEMAA, AMAR. Department of Nephrology, Hôpital de la Pitie, Paris, France

BRAUN, WILLIAM E. Histocompatibility and Immunogenetics Laboratory, Cleveland Clinic Foundation, Cleveland, Ohio, USA

BRAUTBAR, NACHMAN. Division of Nephrology, Department of Medicine, University of Southern California, Los Angeles, California, USA

BRENNER, BARRY M. Renal Division, Department of Medicine, Brigham and Women's Hospital, Boston, Massachusetts, USA

BRIGGS, JOSEPHINE P. Physiology Institute, University of Munich, Munich, Federal Republic of Germany

BROWN, DAVID M. Division of Pediatric Nephrology, University of Minnesota Medical School, Minneapolis, Minnesota, USA

BROWN, DENNIS. Department of Morphology, Institute of Histology and Embryology, University of Geneva, Geneva, Switzerland

BUCKALEW, VARDAMAN M., JR. Departments of Medicine and Physiology and Pharmacology, Bowman Gray School of Medicine, Wake Forest University, Winston-Salem, North Carolina, USA

BULGER, RUTH E. Department of Pathology, University of Texas Medical School, Houston, Texas, USA

BURG, MAURICE. Laboratory of Kidney and Electrolyte Metabolism, National Heart, Lung, and Blood Institute, National Institutes of Health, Bethesda, Maryland, USA

BURKE, THOMAS J. Department of Medicine, University of Colorado Medical School, Denver, Colorado, USA

BUSHINSKY, DAVID. Division of Nephrology, Department of Medicine, University of Chicago Pritzker School of Medicine, Chicago, Illinois, USA

CAMERON, J. STEWART. Clinical Science Laboratories, Guy's Hospital Medical School, London, England, UK

CAMPESE, VITO. Division of Nephrology, University of Southern California, Los Angeles, California, USA

CAPASSO, GIOVAMBATTISTA. Department of Physiology, Albert Einstein College of Medicine, Bronx, New York, USA

CARDINAL, JEAN. Department of Physiology, University of Montreal, Montreal, Quebec, Canada

CARPI-MEDINA, PAOLA. Instituto Venezolano de Investigaciones Cientificas, Caracas, Venezuela

CASE, DAVID B. Cardiovascular Center, Department of Medicine, Cornell University Medical College, New York, New York, USA

CATTRAN, DANIEL C. University of Toronto, Toronto General Hospital, Toronto, Ontario, Canada

CEREIJIDO, MARCELINO M. Centro de Investigación y Estudios Avanzados, México City, Mexico

CHAIMOVITZ, CIDIO. Department of Nephrology, Soroka Medical Center and the Faculty of Health Sciences, Ben-Gurion University of the Negev, Beersheva, Israel

CHAN, JAMES C. M. Department of Pediatrics, Medical College of Virginia, Richmond, Virginia, USA

CHEKAL, MARCIA A. Department of Medicine, University of Chicago Pritzker School of Medicine, Chicago, Illinois, USA

CHESNEY, RUSSELL W. Department of Pediatrics, University of Wisconsin Hospitals, Madison, Wisconsin, USA

CHEVALIER, ROBERT L. Department of Pediatrics, University of Virginia Medical Center, Charlottesville, Virginia, USA

CHURG, JACOB. Department of Pathology, Mount Sinai Medical Center, New York, New York, USA

CLARK, MARY J. Department of Medicine, Veterans Administration Medical Center, Ann Arbor, Michigan, USA

CLEMENS, DANIEL L. Department of Biochemistry, Vanderbilt University School of Medicine, Nashville, Tennessee, USA

COBURN, JACK W. Research and Medical Services, Veterans Administration Medical Center, Wadsworth Division, Los Angeles, California, USA

COE, FREDRIC L. Renal Section, Department of Medicine, University of Chicago Pritzker School of Medicine, Chicago, Illinois, USA

COGGINS, CECIL H. Department of Medicine, Massachusetts General Hospital, Boston, Massachusetts, USA

COHEN, ARTHUR H. Department of Pathology, Harbor-UCLA Medical Center, Los Angeles, California, USA

COLE, BARBARA R. Department of Pediatrics, Washington University School of Medicine, St. Louis, Missouri, USA

COLEMAN, MICHAEL D. Holt-Krock Clinic, Fort Smith, Arkansas, USA

COLINDRES, ROMULO E. Department of Medicine, School of Medicine, University of North Carolina, Chapel Hill, North Carolina, USA

COLLINS, ALLAN J. Regional Kidney Disease Program, Hennepin County Medical Center, Minneapolis, Minnesota, USA

CORMAN, BRUNO. Department of Biology, INSERM U 246, CEN/Saclay, Gif-sur-Yvette, France

CORTES, PEDRO. Nephrology and Hypertension Division, Department of Medicine, Henry Ford Hospital, Detroit, Michigan, USA

CORVOL, PIERRE. INSERM U 36, Hôpital Broussais, Paris, France

COSIMI, A. BENEDICT. Department of Surgery, Massachusetts General Hospital, Boston, Massachusetts, USA

COSSETTE, PIERRE-YVES. Department of Nephrology, Hôpital de la Pitie, Paris, France

COUSER, WILLIAM G. Division of Nephrology, Department of Medicine, University of Washington, Seattle, Washington, USA

CRUTCH, BETH. University Laboratory of Physiology, University of Oxford, Oxford, England, UK

DABBS, DAVID. Department of Pathology, University of Washington, Seattle, Washington, USA

DAMBACHER, MAXIMILIAN A. Research Laboratory for Calcium Metabolism, Balgrist Department of Orthopedic Surgery, University of Zurich, Zurich, Switzerland

D'AMICO, GIUSEPPE. Division of Nephrology, San Carlo Borromeo Hospital, Milan, Italy

D'ANGELO, ANGELA. Department of Internal Medicine, University of Padova, Padova, Italy

DE BOLD, ADOLFO J. Department of Pathology, Queen's University, Kingston, Ontario, Canada

DeFRONZO, RALPH A. Department of Medicine, Yale University School of Medicine, New Haven, Connecticut, USA

DE ROUFFIGNAC, CHRISTIAN. Department of Biology, CEN/Saclay, Gif-sur-Yvette, France

DE SOUSA, RUI C. Departments of Physiology and Medicine, School of Medicine, University of Geneva, Geneva, Switzerland

DE ZEEUW, RICHARD. Section of Nephrology, Department of Internal Medicine, University of Groningen, Groningen, The Netherlands

DIBONA, DONALD R. Department of Physiology and Biophysics, University of Alabama Medical Center, Birmingham, Alabama, USA

DIBONA, GERALD F. Department of Internal Medicine, University of Iowa College of Medicine, Iowa City, Iowa, USA

DI STEFANO, ANTONIO. Max Planck Institute for Biophysics, Frankfurt, Federal Republic of Germany

DOBYAN, DENNIS C. Department of Pathology, University of Texas Medical School, Houston, Texas, USA

DONADIO, JAMES V., JR. Division of Nephrology, Department of Internal Medicine, Mayo Clinic and Mayo Foundation, Rochester, Minnesota, USA

DOYLE, AUSTIN E. Department of Medicine, University of Melbourne, Austin Hospital, Heidelberg, Victoria, Australia

DuBOSE, THOMAS D., JR. Division of Nephrology, Department of Medicine, University of Texas Medical Branch, Galveston, Texas, USA

DUMLER, FRANCIS. Nephrology and Hypertension Division, Department of Medicine, Henry Ford Hospital, Detroit, Michigan, USA

DUNN, MICHAEL J. Division of Nephrology, Department of Medicine, Case Western Reserve University School of Medicine, Cleveland, Ohio, USA

EGIDO, JESUS. Servicio de Nefrología, Fundación Jiménez Díaz, Madrid, Spain

EKNOYAN, GARABED. Renal Section, Department of Medicine, Baylor College of Medicine, Houston, Texas, USA

ELALOUF, JEAN-MARC. L.P.P.C., Department of Biology, CEN/Saclay, Gif-sur-Yvette, France

ELLIS, EILEEN N. Division of Pediatric Nephrology, University of Minnesota Medical School, Minneapolis, Minnesota, USA

EPSTEIN, MURRAY. Nephrology Section, Veterans Administration Medical Center, Miami, Florida, USA

FAIRLEY, KENNETH F. The Royal Melbourne Hospital, Parkville, Melbourne, Australia

FARMAN, NICOLETTE. INSERM U 246, Department of Biology, CEN/Saclay, Gif-sur-Yvette, France

FARQUHAR, MARILYN GIST. Department of Cell Biology, Yale University School of Medicine, New Haven, Connecticut, USA

FELSENFELD, ARNOLD J. Nephrology Section, College of Medicine, University of Oklahoma Health Sciences Center, Oklahoma City, Oklahoma, USA

FISCHER, JAN A. Research Laboratory for Calcium Metabolism, Balgrist Department of Orthopedic Surgery, University of Zurich, Zurich, Switzerland

FISCHER, SVEN. Department of Internal Medicine, University of Munich, Munich, Federal Republic of Germany

FLEUREN, GERT J. Department of Pathology, State University of Leiden, Leiden, The Netherlands

FOURNIER, ALBERT. Service de Néphrologie, Hôpital Nord, Amiens, France

FRIED, TERRANCE A. Division of Renal Diseases, Department of Medicine, University of Texas Health Science Center, San Antonio, Texas, USA

FRIEDENBERG, RICHARD M. Department of Radiology, University of California, Irvine, California, USA

FRIEDMAN, ELI A. Department of Medicine, State University of New York-Downstate Medical Center, Brooklyn, New York, USA

FRINDT, GUSTAVO. Department of Physiology, Cornell University Medical College, New York, New York, USA

FRÖMTER, EBERHARD. Max Planck Institute for Biophysics, Frankfurt, Federal Republic of Germany

GAGNADOUX, MARIE-FRANCE. Hôpital Necker Enfants-Malades, Paris, France

GARABÉDIAN, M. Hôpital Necker Enfants-Malades, Paris, France

GAROVOY, MARVIN R. Immunogenetics and Transplantation Laboratory, University of California School of Medicine, San Francisco, California, USA

GARRICK, RENÉE E. Renal Section, Department of Medicine, University of Pennsylvania School of Medicine, Philadelphia, Pennsylvania, USA

GAUDIO, KAREN M. Division of Nephrology, Department of Medicine, Yale University School of Medicine, New Haven, Connecticut, USA

GAUTHIER, V. JOYCE. Division of Rheumatology, Department of Medicine, University of Washington, Seattle, Washington, USA

GEBLER, BRIGITTE. Max Planck Institute for Biophysics, Frankfurt, Federal Republic of Germany

GEERING, KÄTHI. Pharmacology Institute, University of Lausanne, Lausanne, Switzerland

GENNARI, CARLO. Istituto di Semiotica Medica, Università di Siena, Siena, Italy

GIEBISCH, GERHARD. Department of Physiology, Yale University School of Medicine, New Haven, Connecticut, USA

GILL, WILLIAM B. Department of Urology, University of Chicago Pritzker School of Medicine, Chicago, Illinois, USA

GLAUSER, M. P. Division of Infectious Diseases, Department of Internal Medicine, CHU Vaudois, Lausanne, Switzerland

GMAJ, PIOTR. Department of Physiology, University of Zurich-Irchel, Zurich, Switzerland

GONZALEZ, ERNESTO. Instituto Venezolano de Investigaciones Cientificas, Caracas, Venezuela

GOOD, DAVID W. Laboratory of Kidney and Electrolyte Metabolism, National Heart,

Lung, and Blood Institute, National Institutes of Health, Bethesda, Maryland, USA

GRANTHAM, JARED J. Department of Medicine, University of Kansas Medical Center, Kansas City, Kansas, USA

GRAY, RICHARD W. Clinical Research Center, Froedtert Memorial Lutheran Hospital, Milwaukee, Wisconsin, USA

GREEN, JACOB. Department of Nephrology, Rambam Hospital and Technion School of Medicine, Haifa, Israel

GREGER, RAINER. Max Planck Institute for Biophysics, Frankfurt, Federal Republic of Germany

GRÉGOIRE, I. Service de Néphrologie, Hôpital Nord, Amiens, France

GUÉRIS, J. Laboratory of Radio-immunology, Hôpital Lariboisiere, Paris, France

GUGGINO, WILLIAM B. Department of Physiology, Johns Hopkins University, Baltimore, Maryland, USA

GUTTMANN, RONALD D. Royal Victoria Hospital, Montreal, Quebec, Canada

HABENER, JOEL F. Laboratory of Molecular Endocrinology, Massachusetts General Hospital and Howard Hughes Medical Research Institute, Harvard Medical School, Boston, Massachusetts, USA

HABER, EDGAR. Cardiac Unit, Massachusetts General Hospital and Department of Medicine, Harvard Medical School, Boston, Massachusetts, USA

HABIB, RENÉE. Hôpital Necker Enfants-Malades, Paris, France

HANCOCK, WAYNE. Department of Nephrology, Prince Henry's Hospital, Monash University, Melbourne, Victoria, Australia

HANDLER, JOSEPH S. Laboratory of Kidney and Electrolyte Metabolism, National Heart, Lung, and Blood Institute, National Institutes of Health, Bethesda, Maryland, USA

HAYASHI, MATUHIKO. Department of Pharmacology, Jichi Medical School, Tochigi, Japan

HEATON, ALEX. Department of Nephrology, Royal Victoria Hospital, Newcastle-upon-Tyne, England, UK

HEBERT, STEPHEN C. Department of Medicine, University of Texas Medical School, Houston, Texas, USA

HEIDLAND, AUGUST. Division of Nephrology, Department of Medicine, University of Würzburg, Würzburg, Federal Republic of Germany

HENRICH, WILLIAM L. Department of Internal Medicine, Southwestern Medical School, University of Texas Health Science Center, Dallas, Texas, USA

HERCZ, GAVRIL. Research and Medical Services, Veterans Administration Medical Center, Wadsworth Division, Los Angeles, California, USA

HERNANDO, LUIS. Servicio de Nefrología, Fundación Jiménez Díaz, Madrid, Spain

HILLMAN, BRUCE. Department of Radiology, University of Arizona, Tucson, Arizona, USA

HIWATARI, MASAO. Department of Medicine, Monash University, Prince Henry's Hospital, Melbourne, Victoria, Australia

HODSON, C. JOHN. Department of Diagnostic Radiology, Yale University School of Medicine, New Haven, Connecticut, USA

HOEDEMAEKER, PHILIP J. Department of Pathology, State University of Leiden, Leiden, The Netherlands

HOLDSWORTH, STEVEN R. Department of Medicine, Monash University, Prince Henry's Hospital, Melbourne, Victoria, Australia

HOPPE, RICHARD T. Department of Radiology, Stanford University Medical Center, Stanford, California, USA

HÖRL, WALTER H. Division of Nephrology, Department of Medicine, University of Freiburg, Freiburg, Federal Republic of Germany

HORSTER, MICHAEL F. Physiology Institute, University of Munich, Munich, Federal Republic of Germany

HRICAK, HEDVIG. Department of Radiology, University of California, San Francisco, California, USA

HRUSKA, KEITH A. Renal Division, Department of Internal Medicine, Washington University School of Medicine, St. Louis, Missouri, USA

HUMES, H. DAVID. Department of Medicine, Veterans Administration Medical Center, Ann Arbor, Michigan, USA

HUMPHREYS, MICHAEL H. Division of Nephrology, University of California School of Medicine, San Francisco General Hospital, San Francisco, California, USA

HUNT, DEBORAH A. Veterans Administration Medical Center, Ann Arbor, Michigan, USA

HUNT, JOHN. Department of Pathology. University of Otheo, Christchurch Clinical School of Medicine, Christchurch, New Zealand

ICHIKAWA, IEKUNI. Laboratory of Renal Physiology, The Children's Hospital, Boston, Massachusetts, USA

IMAI, MASASHI. Department of Pharmacology, National Cardiovascular Center, Research Institute, Osaka, Japan

INAGAMI, TADASHI. Department of Biochemistry, Vanderbilt University School of Medicine, Nashville, Tennessee, USA

ISSAD, BELKACEM. Department of Nephrology, Hôpital de la Pitie, Paris, France

IVANOVICH, PETER. Department of Medicine, Northwestern University School of Medicine, Chicago, Illinois, USA

IVES, HARLAN E. Nephrology Section, Department of Medicine, Veterans Administration Medical Center and Cardiovascular Research Institute and Department of Medicine, University of California, San Francisco, California, USA

JACOBSON, HARRY R. Department of Internal Medicine, Southwestern Medical School, University of Texas Health Science Center, Dallas, Texas, USA

JOHNSON, RICHARD J. Division of Nephrology, Department of Medicine, University of Washington, Seattle, Washington, USA

JOHNSTON, COLIN I. Department of Medicine, Monash University, Prince Henry's Hospital, Melbourne, Victoria, Australia

JONES, HENRY W., III. Department of Internal Medicine, Kaiser-Permanente Medical Center, Santa Clara, California, USA

KAISSLING, BRIGITTE. Anatomy Institute, University of Basel, Basel, Switzerland

KANGARLOO, HOOSHANG. Department of Radiology, University of California, Los Angeles, California, USA

KAPLAN, BERNARD S. Department of Pediatrics, McGill University, Montreal Children's Hospital, Montreal, Quebec, Canada

KAPLAN, NORMAN M. Department of Internal Medicine, Southwestern Medical School, University of Texas Health Science Center, Dallas, Texas, USA

KASHGARIAN, MICHAEL. Department of Pathology, Yale University School of Medicine, New Haven, Connecticut, USA

KATHOLI, RICHARD E. Department of Medicine, University of Alabama Medical Center, Birmingham, Alabama, USA

KATZ, ADRIAN I. Department of Medicine, University of Chicago Pritzker School of Medicine, Chicago, Illinois, USA

KEELER, RALPH. Department of Physiology, University of British Columbia, Vancouver, British Columbia, Canada

KERJASCHKI, DONTSCHO. Department of Pathological Anatomy, University of Vienna, Vienna, Austria

KIM, DONALD. Department of Medicine, Toronto Western Hospital and University of Toronto, Toronto, Ontario, Canada

KINCAID-SMITH, PRISCILLA S. Division of Nephrology, The Royal Melbourne Hospital, Parkville, Victoria, Australia

KINNE, ROLF. Max-Planck-Institut fur Systemphysiologie, Dortmund, Federal Republic of Germany

KIRK, KEVIN L. Department of Physiology and Biophysics, University of Alabama Medical Center, Birmingham, Alabama, USA

KJELLSTRAND, CARL M. Regional Kidney Disease Program, Department of Medicine, Hennepin County Medical Center, Minneapolis, Minnesota, USA

KLAHR, SAULO. Renal Division, Department of Medicine, Washington University School of Medicine, St. Louis, Missouri, USA

KLINKMANN, HORST. Department of Internal Medicine, Wilhelm-Pieck-University, Rostock, German Democratic Republic

KOEPPEN, BRUCE. Department of Medicine, University of Connecticut School of Medicine, Farmington, Connecticut, USA

KOKKO, JUHA P. Department of Internal Medicine, Southwestern Medical School, University of Texas Health Science Center, Dallas, Texas, USA

KON, VALENTINA. Laboratory of Renal Physiology, The Children's Hospital, Boston, Massachusetts, USA

KOPP, ULLA C. Department of Internal Medicine, University of Iowa School of Medicine, Iowa City, Iowa, USA

KOPPLE, JOEL D. Division of Nephrology and Hypertension, Harbor-UCLA Medical Center, Los Angeles, California, USA

KORKOR, ADEL B. Department of Medicine, Medical College of Wisconsin, Milwaukee, Wisconsin, USA

KRAEHENBUHL, JEAN-PIERRE. Biochemistry Institute, University of Lausanne, Lausanne, and Swiss Institute of Experimental Cancer Research, Epalinges, Switzerland

KU, GORDON. Department of Clinical Medicine, National University of Singapore, Singapore General Hospital, Singapore

KUROKAWA, KIYOSHI. Fourth Department of Medicine, Faculty of Medicine, University of Tokyo, Tokyo, Japan, and Department of Medicine, University of California, Los Angeles, California, USA

KUYTENS, RENÉE. Wilhelmina Kinderziekenhuis, Utrecht, The Netherlands

LACHIN, JOHN. Bio-statistics Center, Bethesda, Maryland, USA

LANGFORD, HERBERT G. Department of Medicine, University of Mississippi Medical Center, Jackson, Mississippi, USA

LANIER, LOUIS. Monoclonal Antibody Center, Becton Dickinson Company, Mountain View, California, USA

LAPOINTE, JACQUES. Department of Biochemistry, Laval University, Quebec City, Quebec, Canada

LAU, KAI. Renal Division, Michael Reese Hospital and University of Chicago, Chicago, Illinois, USA

LEE, DAVID B. N. Division of Nephrology, Sepulveda Veterans Administration Medical Center, Sepulveda, California, USA

LEGRAIN, MARCEL C. Department of Nephrology, Hôpital de la Pitie, Paris, France

LEMANN, JACOB, JR. Department of Medicine, Medical College of Wisconsin, Milwaukee, Wisconsin, USA

LEMKIN, MARGARET C. Department of Cell Biology, Yale University School of Medicine, New Haven, Connecticut, USA

LETTERI, JOSEPH M. Division of Nephrology, Department of Medicine, Nassau City Medical Center, East Meadow, New York, USA

LEVIN, BARRY. Renal Transplantation Service, Pacific Medical Center, San Francisco, California, USA

LEVIN, NATHAN W. Nephrology and Hypertension Division, Department of Medicine, Henry Ford Hospital, Detroit, Michigan, USA

LEWIS, EDMUND J. Department of Medicine, Rush-Presbyterian-St. Luke's Medical Center, Chicago, Illinois, USA

LIANOS, ELIAS A. Division of Nephrology, Department of Medicine, Medical College of Wisconsin, Milwaukee, Wisconsin, USA

LINARES, HENRY. Instituto Venezolano de Investigaciones Cientificas, Caracas, Venezuela

LINDHOLM, BENGT. Department of Renal Medicine, Karolinska Institute, Huddinge University Hospital, Stockholm, Sweden

LINSHAW, MICHAEL A. Department of Pediatrics, University of Kansas School of Medicine, Kansas City, Kansas, USA

LIVIO, MANUELA. "Mario Negri" Institute for Pharmacological Research, Bergamo, Italy

LLACH, FRANCISCO. Nephrology Section, Department of Medicine, College of Medicine, University of Oklahoma Health Science Center, Oklahoma City, Oklahoma, USA

LOCKWOOD, C. MARTIN. MRC Clinical Immunology Research Group, Department of Medicine, Royal Postgraduate Medical School, Hammersmith Hospital, London, England, UK

LOERTSCHER, ROLF. Department of Medicine, Beth Israel Hospital, Boston, Massachusetts, USA

LOMAX-SMITH, JANE D. Renal Unit, Royal Adelaide Hospital, Adelaide, South Australia, Australia

LORENZ, REINHARD. Department of Internal Medicine, University of Munich, Munich, Federal Republic of Germany

LOSCHIAVO, CARMELO. Division of Nephrology, University of Verona, Verona, Italy

LOZANO, L. Servicio de Nefrología, Fundación Jiménez Díaz, Madrid, Spain

LUND, BIRGER. Department of Orthopaedic Surgery, Rigshospital, Copenhagen, Denmark

LUND, BJARNE. Department of Orthopaedic Surgery, Rigshospital, Copenhagen, Denmark

MAACK, THOMAS. Department of Physiology, Cornell University Medical College, New York, New York, USA

MADSEN, KIRSTEN M. Division of Nephrology, Department of Medicine, J. Hillis Miller Health Center, University of Florida, Gainesville, Florida, USA

MALMSTRÖM, KERSTIN. Department of Physiology, University of Zurich-Irchel, Zurich, Switzerland

MANN, JOHANNES. Division of Nephrology, University of Heidelberg, Heidelberg, Federal Republic of Germany

MANNIK, MART. Division of Rheumatology, Department of Medicine, University of Washington, Seattle, Washington, USA

MANNING, MAURICE. Department of Biochemistry, Medical College of Ohio, Toledo, Ohio, USA

MARTIN, KEVIN J. Renal Division, Department of Internal Medicine, Washington University School of Medicine, St. Louis, Missouri, USA

MARTÍNEZ-MALDONADO, MANUEL. Medical Service, Veterans Administration Medical Center, San Juan, Puerto Rico

MASCHIO, GIUSEPPE. Istituto di Nefrologia Medica, Università di Verona, Verona, Italy

MASON, JUNE. Physiology Institute, University of Munich, Munich, Federal Republic of Germany

MAUER, S. MICHAEL. Department of Pediatrics, University of Minnesota Medical School, Minneapolis, Minnesota, USA

MCCARRON, DAVID A. Division of Nephrology and Hypertension, Department of Medicine, Oregon Health Sciences University School of Medicine, Portland, Oregon, USA

MCCLENNAN, BRUCE L. Department of Radiology, Washington University School of Medicine, St. Louis, Missouri, USA

MCKENZIE, JAMES C. Department of Biochemistry, Vanderbilt University School of Medicine, Nashville, Tennessee, USA

MENARD, JOËL. INSERM U 36, Hôpital Broussais, Paris, France

MENDRICK, DONNA L. Department of Pathology, Brigham and Women's Hospital, Boston, Massachusetts, USA

MEUNIER, P. INSERM U 234, University Alexis Carrel, Lyon, France

MEYER, JOHN L. Division of Research Grants, National Institutes of Health, Bethesda, Maryland, USA

MEYER, TIMOTHY W. Renal Division, Department of Medicine, Brigham and Women's Hospital, Boston, Massachusetts, USA

MICHAEL, ALFRED F. Departments of Pediatrics, Laboratory Medicine, and Pathology, University of Minnesota Medical School, Minneapolis, Minnesota, USA

MIGNON, FRANÇOISE. Service de Néphrologie, Hôpital Tenon, Paris, France

MILLINER, DAWN S. Division of Nephrology, Mayo Clinic, Rochester, Minnesota, USA

MITCH, WILLIAM E. Department of Medicine, The Brigham and Women's Hospital, Boston, Massachusetts, USA

MOGENSEN, CARL ERIK. Second University Clinic of Internal Medicine, Århus Kommunehospital, Århus, Denmark

MÖLLBY, ROLAND. National Bacteriological Laboratories, Stockholm, Sweden

MOORE, LEON C. Department of Physiology and Biophysics, Health Science Center, State University of New York, Stony Brook, New York, USA

MORGAN, TREFOR O. Department of Physiology, University of Melbourne, Parkville, Victoria, Australia

MORINIÈRE, PHILIPPE. Department of Nephrology, Hôpital Nord, Amiens, France

MORRIS, PETER J. Nuffield Department of Surgery, John Radcliffe Hospital, University of Oxford, Oxford, England, UK

MORRISON, AUBREY R. Department of Medicine and Pharmacology, Washington University School of Medicine, St. Louis, Missouri, USA

MORRISSEY, JEREMIAH J. Renal Division, Department of Internal Medicine, Washington University School of Medicine, St. Louis, Missouri, USA

MOSS, NICHOLAS G. Department of Physiology, School of Medicine, University of North Carolina, Chapel Hill, North Carolina, USA

MUJAIS, SALIM K. Department of Medicine, University of Chicago Pritzker School of Medicine, Chicago, Illinois, USA

MURER, HEINI. Department of Physiology, University of Zurich-Irchel, Zurich, Switzerland

MYERS, BRYAN D. Division of Nephrology, Department of Medicine, Stanford University School of Medicine, Stanford, California, USA

NAKAMARU, MITSUAKI. Department of Biochemistry, Vanderbilt University School of Medicine, Nashville, Tennessee, USA

NARINS, ROBERT G. Department of Medicine, Temple University Health Science Center, Philadelphia, Pennsylvania, USA

NARUSE, KIYOKO. Department of Biochemistry, Vanderbilt University School of Medicine, Nashville, Tennessee, USA

NARUSE, MITSUHIDE. Department of Biochemistry, Vanderbilt University School of Medicine, Nashville, Tennessee, USA

NAVAR, L. GABRIEL. Department of Physiology and Biophysics, University of Alabama Medical Center, Birmingham, Alabama, USA

NEBEKER, HENRY G. Research and Medical Services, Veterans Administration Medical Center, Wadsworth Division, Los Angeles, California, USA

NICAR, MICHAEL J. Department of Mineral Metabolism, University of Texas Health Science Center, Dallas, Texas, USA

NISER, ROGER L. Division of Nephrology, Department of Medicine, Veterans Administration Hospital, Miami, Florida, USA

NOLPH, KARL D. Division of Nephrology, Department of Medicine, University of Missouri Health Sciences Center, Columbia, Missouri, USA

NORBECK, HANS ERIK. Department of Renal Medicine, Karolinska Institute, Huddinge University Hospital, Stockholm, Sweden

OKA, TAKAHIRO. Department of Surgery, Kyoto Prefectural University of Medicine, Kamikyo-ku, Kyoto, Japan

OKAMURA, TOMIO. Department of Biochemistry, Vanderbilt University School of Medicine, Nashville, Tennessee, USA

O'NEIL, ROGER G. Department of Physiology, University of Texas Medical School, Houston, Texas, USA

OREOPOULOS, DIMITRIOS G. Department of Medicine, Toronto Western Hospital, University of Toronto, Toronto, Ontario, Canada

ORŁOWSKI, TADEUSZ. Transplantation Institute, Warsaw, Poland

OTT, SUSAN M. Department of Medicine, Harborview Medical Center, University of Washington, Seattle, Washington, USA

PAILLARD, MICHEL. Hôpital Louis Mourier, Colombes, France

PAK, CHARLES Y. C. Department of Internal Medicine, Southwestern Medical School, University of Texas Health Science Center, Dallas, Texas, USA

PANDEY, KAILASH. Department of Biochemistry, Vanderbilt University School of Medicine, Nashville, Tennessee, USA

PAREKH, NIRANJAN. Department of Physiology and Biophysics, University of Louisville Health Sciences Center, Louisville, Kentucky, USA

PARKS, JOAN H. Renal Section, Department of Medicine, University of Chicago Pritzker School of Medicine, Chicago, Illinois, USA

PEARL, MIRILEE. University Laboratory of Physiology, University of Oxford, Oxford, England, UK

PEDERSON, JAMES A. Nephrology Section, Department of Medicine, College of Medicine, University of Oklahoma Health Science Center, Oklahoma City, Oklahoma, USA

PERDUE, SONDRA. Tissue Typing Laboratory, UCLA School of Medicine, Los Angeles, California, USA

PEREZ, GUIDO O. Department of Medicine, University of Miami, Miami, Florida, USA

PEREZ, JOELLE. INSERM U 64, Hôpital Tenon, Paris, France

PERKINSON, DIANA A. Division of Nephrology, Department of Medicine, University of Washington, Seattle, Washington, USA

PERSSON, A. ERIK G. Departments of Physiology and Biophysics, University of Uppsala, Uppsala, Sweden

PETERS, D. KEITH. Department of Medicine, Royal Postgraduate Medical School, University of London, Hammersmith Hospital, London, England, UK

PUJOL, DIEGO. INSERM U 246, CEN/Saclay, Gif-sur-Yvette, France

PUSEY, CHARLES D. MRC Clinical Immunology Research Group, Department of

Medicine, Royal Postgraduate Medical School, University of London, Hammersmith Hospital, London, England, UK

RABINOWITZ, LAWRENCE. Department of Human Physiology, University of California, Davis, California, USA

RACUSEN, LORRAINE C. Department of Pathology, Johns Hopkins University School of Medicine, Baltimore, Maryland, USA

RAPAPORT, J. Department of Nephrology, Soroka Medical Center and the Faculty of the Health Sciences, Ben-Gurion University of the Negev, Beersheva, Israel

RECTOR, FLOYD C., JR. Cardiovascular Research Institute and Departments of Medicine and Physiology, University of California, San Francisco, California, USA

REES, ANDREW J. Department of Medicine, Royal Postgraduate Medical School, University of London, Hammersmith Hospital, London, England, UK

REMUZZI, GIUSEPPE. "Mario Negri" Institute for Pharmacological Research, Bergamo, Italy

RESNICK, LAWRENCE. Hypertension Center, New York Hospital-Cornell University Medical Center, New York, New York, USA

RIESELBACH, RICHARD E. Department of Medicine, Medical College of Wisconsin, Milwaukee, Wisconsin, USA

RITZ, EBERHARD. Section of Nephrology, University Medical Clinic, Heidelberg, Federal Republic of Germany

ROBERTS, JAMES A. Delta Regional Primate Center, Covington, Louisiana, USA

RODRÍGUEZ-ITURBE, BERNARDO. Renal Service and Laboratory, Hospital Universitario de Maracaibo, Maracaibo, Zulia, Venezuela

RODRÍGUEZ-SORIANO, JUAN. Department of Pediatrics, Hospital Infantile de la Seguridad Social, University School of Medicine, Cruces Bibao, Spain

ROINEL, NICOLE. L.P.P.C., Department of Biology, CEN/Saclay, Gif-sur-Yvette, France

RONCO, PIERRE. Service de Néphrologie, Hôpital Tenon, Paris, France

ROSS, BRIAN A. University of Oxford, Oxford, England, UK

ROSSIER, BERNARD C. Pharmacology Institute, University of Lausanne, Lausanne, Switzerland

ROTTEMBOURG, JACQUES B. Department of Nephrology, Hôpital de la Pitie, Paris, France

SABATINI, SANDRA. Section of Nephrology, Department of Medicine, University of Illinois College of Medicine, Chicago, Illinois, USA

SALANT, DAVID J. Department of Medicine, Boston University Medical Center, Boston, Massachusetts, USA

SAMPSON, DEREK. Renal Transplantation Service, Pacific Medical Center, San Francisco, California, USA (deceased)

SANCHO, JAIME. Servicio de Nefrología, Fundación Jiménez Díaz, Madrid, Spain

SASAKI, SEI. Department of Medicine, School of Medicine, University of California, San Francisco, California, USA

SAWYER, WILBUR H. Department of Pharmacology, College of Physicians and Surgeons of Columbia University, New York, New York, USA

SCHAFER, JAMES A. Department of Physiology and Biophysics, University of Alabama Medical Center, Birmingham, Alabama, USA

SCHLATTER, EBERHARD. Max Planck Institute for Biophysics, Frankfurt, Federal Republic of Germany

SCHNERMANN, JÜRGEN. Physiology Institute, University of Munich, Munich, Federal Republic of Germany

SCHOOLWERTH, ANTON C. Renal and Electrolyte Division, Department of Medicine, Pennsylvania State University, College of Medicine, Hershey, Pennsylvania, USA

SCHREINER, GEORGE F. Department of Pathology, Harvard Medical School, Boston, Massachusetts, USA

SCHRIER, ROBERT W. Department of Medicine, University of Colorado Medical Center, Denver, Colorado, USA

SCHULTZ, STANLEY G. Department of Physiology and Cell Biology, University of Texas Medical School, Houston, Texas, USA

SEALEY, JEAN E. Cardiovascular Center, New York Hospital-Cornell Medical Center, New York, New York, USA

SEBERT, J. L. Service de Néphrologie, Hôpital Nord, Amiens, France

SEGGIE, JANET L. Division of Nephrology, Department of Medicine, University of the Witwatersrand, Johannesburg, South Africa

SEIFFER, JULIAN. Laboratory of Kidney and Electrolyte Physiology, Brigham and Women's Hospital, Boston, Massachusetts, USA

SHAPIRO, FRED L. Regional Kidney Disease Program, Hennepin County Medical Center, Minneapolis, Minnesota, USA

SHEMESH, OVADIA. Division of Nephrology, Department of Medicine, Stanford University School of Medicine, Stanford, California, USA

SHERRARD, DONALD J. Department of Medicine, University of Washington School of Medicine, Seattle, Washington, USA

SIEGEL, NORMAN J. Department of Pediatrics, Yale University School of Medicine, New Haven, Connecticut, USA

SIESS, WOLFGANG. Department of Internal Medicine, University of Munich, Munich, Federal Republic of Germany

SILBERMAN, HOWARD. Department of Surgery, UCLA School of Medicine, Los Angeles, California, USA

SINNIAH, RAJA. Department of Pathology, National University of Singapore, Singapore

SITPRIJA, VISITH. Department of Medicine, Faculty of Medicine, Chulalongkorn University, Bangkok, Thailand

SLATOPOLSKY, EDUARDO. Renal Division, Department of Internal Medicine, Washington University School of Medicine, St. Louis, Missouri, USA

SMITH, DOUGLAS J. Section of Nephrology, Department of Medicine, Yale University School of Medicine, New Haven, Connecticut, USA

SMITH, LYNWOOD H. Nephrology Research Unit, Mayo Clinic and Mayo Foundation, Rochester, Minnesota, USA

SOLEZ, KIM. Department of Pathology, Johns Hopkins University School of Medicine, Baltimore, Maryland, USA

SOLOMON, SIDNEY. Department of Physiology, University of New Mexico School of Medicine, Albuquerque, New Mexico, USA

SONNENBERG, HARALD. Department of Physiology, Toronto General Hospital, Toronto, Ontario, Canada

SOUBRIER, FLORENT. INSERM U 36, Hôpital Broussais, Paris, France

SPENCER, HERTA C. Hines Veterans Administration Hospital, Hines, Illinois, USA

SPINELLI, FRANK. Ciba-Geigy Ltd., Basel, Switzerland

SPITZER, ADRIAN. Division of Pediatric Nephrology, Department of Pediatrics, Albert Einstein College of Medicine, Bronx, New York, USA

SPRING, KENNETH R. Laboratory of Kidney and Electrolyte Metabolism, National Heart, Lung, and Blood Institute, National Institutes of Health, Bethesda, Maryland, USA

STANTON, BRUCE. Department of Physiology, Yale University School of Medicine, New Haven, Connecticut, USA

STEFFES, MICHAEL W. Department of Chemistry, University of Minnesota Medical School, Minneapolis, Minnesota, USA

STEIN, JAY H. Division of Renal Diseases, Department of Medicine, University of Texas Health Science Center, San Antonio, Texas, USA

STEINHAUSEN, MICHAEL. Institute for Physiology, University of Heidelberg, Heidelberg, Federal Republic of Germany

STERZL, R. BERND. Department of Medicine, Veterans Administration Medical Center, Yale University School of Medicine, West Haven, Connecticut, USA

STOKES, JOHN B., III. Department of Internal Medicine, University of Iowa, Iowa City, Iowa, USA

STONE, DENNIS K. Department of Internal Medicine, Southwestern Medical School, University of Texas Health Science Center, Dallas, Texas, USA

STORK, JOHN E. Department of Medicine, Case Western Reserve University School of Medicine, Cleveland, Ohio, USA

STOW, JENNIFER L. Department of Cell Biology, Yale University School of Medicine, New Haven, Connecticut, USA

STRASSER, THOMAS. Department of Internal Medicine, University of Munich, Munich, Federal Republic of Germany

STRIKER, GARY E. Department of Pathology, University of Washington, Seattle, Washington, USA

STRIKER, LILIANE MOREL-MAROGER. Department of Pathology, University of Washington, Seattle, Washington, USA

STROBER, SAMUEL. Division of Immunology, Department of Medicine, Stanford University Medical Center, Stanford, California, USA

STROM, TERRY B. Department of Medicine, Beth Israel Hospital, Boston, Massachusetts, USA

SUKI, WADI N. Renal Section, Departments of Medicine and Physiology, Baylor College of Medicine, Houston, Texas, USA

SUMMERS, ROGER J. Department of Medicine, University of Melbourne, Austin Hospital, Heidelberg, Victoria, Australia

SUTTON, ROGER A. L. Department of Medicine, University of British Columbia, Vancouver, British Columbia, Canada

TABEI, KAORU. Department of Cardiology, Jichi Medical School, Tochigi, Japan

TANNEN, RICHARD L. Division of Nephrology, Department of Internal Medicine, University of Michigan Medical Center, Ann Arbor, Michigan, USA

TANNER, GEORGE A. Department of Physiology, Indiana University School of Medicine, Indianapolis, Indiana, USA

TARAZI, ROBERT C. Department of Clinical Science, Cleveland Clinic, Cleveland, Ohio, USA

TAUB, MARY. Department of Biochemistry, School of Medicine, State University of New York at Buffalo, Buffalo, New York, USA

TAYLOR, ANN. University Laboratory of Physiology, University of Oxford, Oxford, England, UK

TERASAKI, PAUL I. Tissue Typing Laboratory, UCLA School of Medicine, Los Angeles, California, USA

TESSITORE, NICOLA. Division of Nephrology, University of Verona, Verona, Italy

THOMAS, WILLIAM C. Division of Urology, Department of Surgery, J. Hillis Miller Health Center, University of Florida, Gainesville, Florida, USA

TISHER, C. CRAIG. Division of Nephrology, Department of Medicine, J. Hillis Miller Health Center, University of Florida, Gainesville, Florida, USA

TOBACK, F. GARY. Section of Nephrology, Department of Medicine, University of Chicago Pritzker School of Medicine, Chicago, Illinois, USA

TRANAEUS, ANDERS. Department of Renal Medicine, Karolinska Institute, Huddinge University Hospital, Stockholm, Sweden

TRINH-TRANG-TAN, MARIE-MARCELLE. INSERM U 90, Hôpital Necker, Paris, France
TRIPPODO, NICK C. Ochsner Medical Foundation, New Orleans, Louisiana, USA
TSCHOPP, FRITZ A. Research Laboratory for Calcium Metabolism, Balgrist Department of Orthopedic Surgery, University of Zurich, Zurich, Switzerland
TURNER, R. JAMES. Membrane Biology Group, Department of Medicine, University of Toronto, Toronto, Ontario, Canada
ULDALL, ROBERT. Renal Unit, Toronto Western Hospital, Toronto, Ontario, Canada
VAAMONDE, CARLOS A. Medical and Research Services, Veterans Administration Medical Center, Miami, Florida, USA
VALDERROBANO, FERNANDO. Nephrology Service, Hospital Provincial of Madrid, Madrid, Spain
VALENTICH, JOHN D. Department of Physiology and Cell Biology, University of Texas Medical School, Houston, Texas, USA
VALTIN, HEINZ. Department of Physiology, Dartmouth Medical School, Hanover, New Hampshire, USA
VANHOLDER, RAYMOND. Department of Nephrology, University Hospital, Ghent, Belgium
VARGHESE, ZACHARIAH. Royal Free Hospital, London, England, UK
VERRIER-JONES, KATE. Department of Renal Medicine, Welsh National School of Medicine, Royal Infirmary, Cardiff, Wales, UK
VERROUST, PIERRE. Service de Néphrologie, Hôpital Tenon, Paris, France
VIBERTI, GIANCARLO. Unit for Metabolic Medicine, Guy's Hospital Medical School, London, England, UK
VON SCHACKY, CLEMENS. Department of Internal Medicine, University of Munich, Munich, Federal Republic of Germany
WAER, MARK. Division of Immunology, Stanford University Medical Center, Stanford, California, USA
WARNOCK, DAVID G. Nephrology Section, Department of Medicine, Veterans Administration Medical Center and Cardiovascular Research Institute and Department of Medicine, School of Medicine, University of California, San Francisco, California, USA
WEBER, MICHAEL. Department of Medicine, Veterans Administration Medical Center, Long Beach, California, USA
WEBER, PETER C. Department of Internal Medicine, University of Munich, Munich, Federal Republic of Germany
WEENING, JAN J. Department of Pathology, State University of Leiden, Leiden, The Netherlands
WEIDMANN, PETER. Department of Medicine, University of Berne, Berne, Switzerland
WEIDTKE, CLAUDIA. Max Planck Institute for Biophysics, Frankfurt, Federal Republic of Germany
WEINBERG, JOEL M. Department of Medicine, Veterans Administration Medical Center, Ann Arbor, Michigan, USA
WERNERS, PETER G. Clinical Chemistry Laboratory, Mayo Clinic, Rochester, Minnesota, USA
WEST, CLARK D. Division of Nephrology, Children's Hospital Research Foundation, University of Cincinnati, Cincinnati, Ohio, USA
WHELTON, ANDREW. Department of Medicine, Johns Hopkins University School of Medicine, Baltimore, Maryland, USA
WHITE, MICHAEL P. Veterans Administration Medical Center, Ann Arbor, Michigan, USA
WHITTEMBURY, GUILLERMO. Instituto Venezolano de Investigaciones Cientificas, Caracas, Venezuela

WIGGINS, ROGER C. Department of Internal Medicine, University of Michigan School of Medicine, Ann Arbor, Michigan, USA

WILSON, CURTIS B. Department of Immunology, Research Institute of the Scripps Clinic, La Jolla, California, USA

WILSON, DOUGLAS R. Division of Nephrology, Toronto General Hospital, Toronto, Ontario, Canada

WINBERG, JAN. Department of Pediatrics, Karolinska Institute, Huddinge University Hospital, Stockholm, Sweden

WINDHAGER, ERICH E. Department of Physiology and Biophysics, Cornell University Medical College, New York, New York, USA

WINSLADE, WILLIAM. Program in Medicine, Law and Human Values, Neuropsychiatric Institute, School of Medicine, University of California, Los Angeles, California, USA

WISEMAN, MARTIN J. Unit for Metabolic Medicine, Guy's Hospital Medical School, London, England, UK

WITTNER, MONIKA. Max Planck Institute for Biophysics, Frankfurt, Federal Republic of Germany

WOODROFFE, ANDREW J. Renal Unit, Royal Adelaide Hospital, Adelaide, South Australia, Australia

WORK, JACK. Division of Nephrology, Department of Medicine, University of Alabama Medical Center, Birmingham, Alabama, USA

WRIGHT, FRED S. Department of Physiology, Yale University School of Medicine, New Haven, Connecticut, USA

WU, AKIRA Y. T. Department of Nephrology, National University of Singapore, Singapore General Hospital, Singapore

WU, GEORGE. Department of Medicine, Toronto Western Hospital and University of Toronto, Toronto, Ontario, Canada

YARGER, WILLIAM E. Department of Medicine, Duke University Medical Center and Veterans Administration Medical Center, Durham, North Carolina, USA

ZAGER, RICHARD A. Department of Medicine, Ohio State University Medical Center, Columbus, Ohio, USA

ZIMMERMAN, STEPHEN W. Division of Nephrology, University of Wisconsin Medical School, Madison, Wisconsin, USA

Acknowledgments

An International Congress of Nephrology is held triennially under the auspices of the International Society of Nephrology, and in accordance with its by-laws. The Officers and Organizing Committee of the IXth Congress acknowledge the support of the Officers and Councillors of the International Society of Nephrology and its Committees, as well as many other distinguished individuals who contributed so enormously of their time and energy to the organization of the Congress. Generous contributions were received from the following corporations: *Major Donors:* Boehringer-Ingelheim Ltd., Schering Laboratories, Travenol Laboratories, Inc.; *Additional Corporate Donors:* Abbott Laboratories, Beach Pharmaceuticals, Burroughs Wellcome Company, Pfizer Pharmaceuticals, E. R. Squibb and Sons, and USV Laboratories.

The Kidney in Systemic Disease

Renal Involvement in Multiple Myeloma

Manuel Martínez-Maldonado and Luis Báez-Díaz

Plasma cell dyscrasias are a group of disorders characterized by the clonal expansion of plasma cells or plasmocytoid lymphocytes. In over 95% of the patients with this disorder, an abnormal paraprotein can be detected in serum or urine samples. The clinical manifestations are related to the uncontrolled growth of plasma cells, which infiltrate tissues, and to the reduction of normal immunoglobulin production. The production of abnormal proteins can account for other unique manifestations of the disease, such as electrolyte disturbances, renal abnormalities, hyperviscosity, and glomerulopathy including amyloid deposition [1]. This last subject will be discussed elsewhere in this volume.

Electrolyte Disturbances

Electrolyte abnormalities can provide a clue to the diagnosis of paraproteinemias. Pseudohyponatremia may occur as a result of a decrease in total water per volume of plasma [2]. In these pseudohyponatremic patients, the measured plasma osmolality is normal but the calculated osmolality (serum or plasma sodium $\times$ 2) is abnormally low. Some paraproteinemias are associated with a low "anion gap"; this is because some myeloma proteins with high isoelectric points (7.5 to 9.0) will take up protons and become positively charged at a normal serum pH [3, 4]. The positive charges on these proteins must be neutralized by negatively charged particles such as chloride and bicarbonate, which leads to a low anion gap. This is most common in IgG paraproteinemias because IgA paraproteins are usually less cationic at a physiologic pH.

Occasionally, pseudohypercalcemia may be found in myelomatosis as a

---

This manuscript was presented as part of a Symposium on *The Kidney and Malignant Disease.*

Table 1. Renal abnormalities caused by paraproteins

Bence Jones proteinuria	Hyperviscosity syndrome
Myeloma kidney	Glomerulopathies
Renal tubular dysfunction	Systemic amyloidosis

result of the formation of complexes between the immunoglobulins and calcium [5]. True hypercalcemia is the most common electrolyte abnormality and occurs in 30 to 50% of all patients at the time of diagnosis.

Renal Abnormalities

Renal failure is second only to infection as a leading cause of morbidity and mortality in multiple myeloma [6, 7]. Frequently, the renal abnormalities are directly related to the abnormal paraprotein (Table 1), but disturbances in electrolyte and water metabolism contribute to the development of acute and chronic renal insufficiency (Table 2). Acute renal failure may be the presenting feature of the disease in about 8% of all patients and on occasions can precede the development of overt myeloma [8, 9].

Bence Jones Proteinuria

The immunoglobulin components found in normal urine are IgG, IgA, and polyclonal light chains (kappa and lambda). Light chains are synthesized by plasma cells and circulate in plasma as monomeric (mol wt, 22,000 daltons) or dimeric forms (mol wt, > 22,000 daltons) [10]. Most lambda light chains circulate as covalently linked dimers, whereas kappa chains exist primarily in monomeric form. The glomerular filtration rate (GFR) of light chains depends on the molecular weight of the circulating protein: monomeric forms are filtered freely; dimer forms are not—the GFR of dimers has been estimated to be about 8% that of inulin [11]. In normal individuals, the filtered load of lambda light chain is about 5 mg/kg/d, yet less than 1% appears in the urine. Most of the protein is reabsorbed and catabolized by proximal tubular cells.

Table 2. Other causes of renal abnormalities[a]

Hypercalcemic nephropathy (very common)	Uric acid nephropathy (very rare)
Dehydration or volume contraction (very common)	Obstructive uropathy (very rare)
Neoplastic infiltration of the kidney (rare)	Renal failure induced by contrast dyes (should not happen in any patient already known
Pyelonephritis (rare)	to have multiple myeloma)

[a] Very common would be over 30%; rare would be less than 1%; very rare would be less than 0.5%.

The mechanism of tubular reabsorption is similar to that of other proteins of equal molecular weight. The major site of protein reabsorption is the proximal tubule cell, but the distal tubule cells may also participate. The first step for the reabsorption of light chain is the adherence of the cationic zone to the negatively charged luminal membrane [12]. Infusion of positively charged amino acids leads to a competition with light chains for the binding sites to the tubule brushborder membrane, causing a decrease in the reabsorption and an increase in the urinary excretion of several proteins, including lambda and kappa light chains. After binding to the brushborder membrane, proteins are introduced to the interior of the cell by a process of pinocytosis [13]. The reabsorbed protein is degraded by hydrolytic lysosomal enzymes to amino acids and peptides. In patients with renal tubular diseases, large amounts of uncatabolized polyclonal light chains (lambda and kappa), microglobulins, and lysozymes can be found in the urine.

In patients with myelomatosis, large amounts of monoclonal light chains (kappa or lambda) will appear in the urine, sometimes in excess of 4 g/d. On the other hand, development of renal disease characterized by a decreased GFR will lead to decreased filtration and catabolism of Bence Jones proteins (BJPs). As a consequence, the plasma concentration of these proteins will rise. Any procedure or maneuver that improves GFR will increase catabolism and diminish urine excretion as long as tubular function is normal. Monoclonal light chains in the urine are designated BJPs because of their characteristic heat and solubility properties.

Bence Jones proteins normally are not detected during the routine screening of urine for protein (for example, the Albustix® test). Other reagents (sulfosalicylic acid, toluene, sulfuric acid) are more sensitive and specific, but urine electrophoretic studies are needed for the proper isotypic identification of the abnormal protein. The heat and solubility test lacks sensitivity and is dependent on a higher protein concentration ($>$ 200 mg/dl).

The causes of Bence Jones proteinuria are listed in Table 3. BJPs are almost invariably indicative of a malignant plasma cell disorder, but in rare instances, no evidence of myelomatosis is found on initial presentation (idiopathic). A follow-up of these patients (7 to 20 years) ultimately reveals the presence of plasma cell dyscrasia or amyloidosis [14]. The presence of large amounts ($>$ 4 g/d) of BJPs carries a poor prognosis. This is due to a higher incidence of acute and chronic renal failure, but it also relates to a higher myeloma cell tumor mass ($> 10^{12}$ cells/m^2) [15].

Table 3. Causes of Bence Jones proteinuria

Overt multiple myeloma	Heavy-chain disease (μ) (very rare)
Smoldering myeloma	Idiopathic (very rare)
Systemic light-chain disease	Chronic lymphoproliferative diseases (very rare)
Waldenstrom's macroglobulinemia	
Systemic amyloidosis	Benign monoclonal gammopathy (very rare)

[a] This represents a small contribution to the overall incidence of Bence Jones proteinuria, but two thirds of all patients with mu heavy-chain disease have Bence Jones proteins.

Myeloma Kidney

Myeloma kidney is a pathologic description of one of the various causes of renal failure in myeloma [16]. On light microscopy, the lesions consist of eosinophilic, homogeneous, frequently lamellated, proteinacious casts found mainly in the distal convolution, collecting tubules, and duct. There is usually a syncytial giant cell reaction with variable degrees of tubular atrophy and dilatation. On immunofluorescence examination, the presence of albumin, fibrinogen, IgG, as well as kappa and lambda chains are detected. Predominant kappa and lambda immunostaining correlates with the light-chain component of the M spike. Cytoplasmic hyaline droplets can be seen in tubular cells with positive fluorescence for kappa or lambda chains.

Factors that may contribute to myeloma cast nephropathy include the following: (1) direct toxicity of BJPs to tubular cells, (2) protein complex formation in the distal nephron, (3) tubule fluid pH, (4) reduction in renal plasma flow and GFR (reduced urine flow), and (5) systemic electrolyte abnormalities (hypercalcemia and dehydration).

Not all cases of myeloma kidney exhibit Bence Jones proteinuria, and not all patients will have significant cast formation to account for the degree of renal impairment, but tubule atrophy and epithelial thinning is a universal finding. These findings favor the hypothesis that a major component of the renal dysfunction is the toxic effects of light chains on cellular metabolism, rather than a mechanical obstruction secondary to intratubular cast formation. Nevertheless, as just mentioned, conditions that favor intratubular precipitation of BJPs (volume contraction, dehydration, acid urine) are known to induce or exacerbate renal failure. Clinical evidence, as well as laboratory evidence, indicates that volume expansion and urine alkalinization may prevent the development of myeloma kidney.

The nature of the nephrotoxicity of BJPs can be understood best if one considers a priori that both obstruction and direct nephrotoxicity are contributory factors. These facts can be deduced from the two most dramatic clinical presentations of these disturbances: the presence of myeloma kidney and tubular dysfunction such as proximal and distal tubular acidosis. Moreover, it has been shown that these proteins can directly affect the metabolic machinery of tubules in kidney slices in vitro and in isolated tubules [17–19]. In addition, recent studies have corroborated that cast formation will lead to reductions in GFR, at least in part, by reducing ultrafiltration pressure [20].

The influence of the isoelectric point (its cationic or anionic characteristics) of BJPs has been a major point of controversy. Clyne, Pesce, and Thomson [21], using a rat model and partially purified human Bence Jones protein, showed that the intraperitoneal administration of BJPs with high isoelectric points was more nephrotoxic. They were able to show in this rat model that the more cationic the protein (pI > 5.7), the greater the mean rise in serum urea nitrogen and creatinine as compared with the administration of BJPs having lower isoelectric points. They also showed that alkaluric rats (urine pH, > 8) injected with human lambda dimers showed less renal impairment as compared with aciduric rats (urine pH, < 5.5).

Weiss et al [20] failed, however, to confirm these findings using a different but comparable model. They did not find a correlation between the isoelectric point of human BJPs with nephrotoxicity induced by renal cast formation. Micropuncture and clearance techniques did show that the infusion of human BJPs into male Sprague-Dawley rats caused significant reductions in GFR and single-nephron GFR, which in part were the result of tubular obstruction by casts that contained these proteins.

Smolens, Venkatachalam, and Stein [22], using a rat myeloma tumor model developed by Bazin, Beckors, and Heremans [23], also could not find a correlation between the isoelectric point of rat myeloma BJPs and cast nephropathy. These studies assessed the development of renal failure in rats that had been implanted with immunoglobulin-secreting tumors and maintained on a diet designed to produce an acid urine and containing enough sodium to result in urine osmolalities of 2000 to 3000 mOsm/kg. Only a few of the rats infused with BJPs that had a pI of 7.6 and 6.7 developed renal failure, whereas all of those given BJPs with a pI of 5.2 developed distal nephron cast nephropathy and all those receiving BJP with a pI of 4.3 had either acute tubular necrosis (50%) or bland hyaline cast nephropathy (50%).

In this study as well as in that of Weiss et al [20], several points require further examination. Of interest is the finding that in neither of these models was giant cell formation nor round cell infiltration important. Thus, this finding, which is so common in humans, is: (1) unimportant in producing renal failure, (2) not seen in the short periods of observation (maximun 40 days) in these studies, or (3) is species-specific.

Moreover, the role played by Tamm-Horsfall protein (THP) in these models was not evaluated. Tamm-Horsfall is an anionic mucoprotein (pI, 3.5 to 4.8) produced by the cells of the thick ascending limb and has been found to be a component of tubular casts in human and mouse myeloma kidney. Its precipitation is more likely to occur when the salt content of the solution is raised because the proteins are "salted-out." Calcium in the medium also enhances the aggregation of macromolecules. For this reason, it is not difficult to recognize the need for maintaining calcium metabolism as close to normal as possible in clinical circumstances. It is also clear that the deposition of calcium, so frequently found in human kidney tissue, may be the result of calcium-protein complex formation [24, 25].

In a series of fundamental studies, Cotran, Hoyer, and their associates [24–26] have shown that ureteral obstruction leads to extravasation of THP into the interstitium without evidence (for the 3 weeks of observation in rats with unilateral ureteral obstruction) of humoral immune response, cellular immune response, or systemic humoral immunity. Thus, since BJP causes nephron obstruction, it is entirely possible that, in addition to intratubular interaction of the two proteins, they may lead to extravasation of THP into the interstitium and interaction with other proteins or ions such as calcium. If this occurs long enough, it is possible that immune or inflammatory responses might be observed eventually. Unfortunately, experiments have not been carried out for long enough to examine this point. Nor is it known if single-nephron obstruction, as compared with unilateral ureteral obstruction (UUO), can lead to THP extravasation. Since neither Weiss et al nor Smolens et al stained their sections for Tamm-Horsfall, it is not possible to evaluate the likelihood of this proposal or to assess whether the difference in the incidence of renal lesions was dependent on the intensity of Tamm-Horsfall secretion under the circumstances of their studies. Perhaps Tamm-Horsfall production was the factor determining beta-lactoglobulin toxicity in the Weiss study. Although neither study lends support to the pI as a predictive factor in nephrotoxicity, the role played by the interaction of Tamm-Horsfall and BJPs remains unexamined and unclarified.

Finally, it should be made clear that although increased intratubular pressure and the presence of casts were directly responsible for reductions in intratubular pressure and, thus, in net ultrafiltration pressure, the contribution of changes in ultrafiltration coefficient (K_f) or glomerular plasma flow in this process is unknown at present.

Renal Tubular Dysfunction

Abnormalities in proximal and distal tubule function including distal acidification and concentration defects have been described in patients with paraproteinemias [27, 28]. Adult Fanconi syndrome manifested by glucosuria, phosphaturia, aminoaciduria, uricosuria, bicarbonate wasting, and variable degrees of osteomalacia and pseudofractures can sometimes be present for years prior to the diagnosis of overt myeloma or amyloidosis. Most patients will have Bence Jones proteinuria (mostly kappa light chains). It has been suggested that this association (Bence Jones proteinuria and the Fanconi syndrome) represents a latent form of myeloma as a result of a very slow growth rate of the tumor, but that eventually most patients will develop an overt plasma cell dyscrasia [27].

Distal tubule dysfunction can occur in paraproteinemias, mostly in association with polyclonal gammopathies. A few patients have been described in whom proximal and distal tubule defects coexisted in association with Bence Jones proteinuria. This has been called *combined light chain nephropathy* by Smithline, Kassirer, and Cohen [29].

The mechanism of tubular dysfunction has not been elucidated. Most of the evidence favors a direct toxic effect of BJPs on tubular cells. In vitro studies by Preuss et al [17, 18] showed that BJPs can impair organic anion transport, gluconeogenesis, and other cellular functions in the tubular cells. Also, crystalline inclusions can be documented both clinically and experimentally in tubular cells exposed to BJPs. These probably represent a byproduct of their metabolism that may alter cellular metabolic functions. Moreover, McGeoch et al [19] have shown that human light chains can inhibit ouabain-sensitive Na-K-ATPase activity of renal plasma membranes isolated from rats. They also observed that gluconeogenesis from lactate was increased in isolated rat renal tubules. Because similar effects are obtained with ouabain, they concluded that light chains inhibit Na-K-ATPase in vivo. Of interest is the fact that this same group [30] perfused isolated rat kidneys with solutions to which light chains had been added in concentrations 4- to 10-fold greater than those seen in patients (10^{-4} moles/liter), but no changes in GFR or in sodium reabsorption were observed. Several explanations can be given for this outcome, including species specificity, duration of the experiment (2 hr) as compared to the disease in humans, or rapid loss (by catabolism) of light chain nephrotoxicity.

Hyperviscosity Syndrome

Symptoms and signs of hyperviscosity and hypervolemia will appear in most patients with macroglobulinemia sometime during the course of the disease. In contrast, less than 5% of myeloma patients will show symptoms attributable to hyperviscosity [31, 32]. This striking difference probably relates to the predominantly intravascular localization of the IgM globulin (> 80%); less than 50% of IgG is intravascular. Some physicochemical characteristics of the paraprotein in myeloma can predispose to the development of hyperviscosity. These include: (1) asymmetry of the molecule, (2) complex formation with other proteins, (3) polymerization, (4) cryoprecipitability, (5) euglobulin formation, and (6) cell-protein interaction.

The manifestations of this syndrome are attributed to the increased blood viscosity and hypervolemia and to the resulting stasis, sluggish blood flow, distention of capillary beds, and interference with coagulation. This clinical picture is at times confusing because of the multiple organ dysfunction (neurologic, ocular, cardiac, hematologic, and renal).

The renal manifestations include impaired urine concentration, azotemia, and (on occasions) hematuria. Rarely do acute renal failure or permanent renal dysfunction occur. Nevertheless, other causes of acute renal failure in myeloma can be potentiated by hyperviscosity. The diagnosis of hyperviscosity syndrome rests on the typical clinical findings and a measurement of "relative" serum viscosity. The appearance of symptoms usually correlates with a relative serum viscosity greater than 5 (relative to water; normal, 1.4 to 1.8), but each patient has his or her own threshold for overt symptoms.

Treatment

Long-term survival in multiple myeloma correlates well with three major prognostic factors: response to cytotoxic drugs, absence of renal failure, and absence of hypercalcemia [33]. Although renal failure carries a poor prognosis, a prolonged survival can at times be obtained with aggressive management [34]. The correction of hypovolemia and electrolyte imbalances should be undertaken immediately. The early institution of chemotherapy will help to lower the filtered load of proteins and the plasma viscosity. Plasmapheresis should be carried out if hyperviscosity is present; it can also be beneficial in some patients with acute renal failure despite normal relative serum viscosity [35]. Hemodialysis may be necessary to correct azotemia and water or electrolyte imbalances. Peritoneal dialysis can be beneficial, as it will help remove the abnormal paraprotein [36]. In the absence of anuria, urine alkalization and diuresis will benefit patients with cast nephropathy. Despite the above measures, a sizable number of patients will need long-term hemodialysis [37, 38]. If the systemic manifestation of the disease and the plasma cell tumor growth can be controlled, some patients may be candidates for renal transplantation. Isolated case reports have revealed post-transplant survival figures ranging from 15 to 105 months [39].

References

1. MARTINEZ-MALDONADO M, GARAYALDE G: Renal involvement in multiple myeloma, in *The Kidney in Systemic Diseases* (2nd ed.), edited by SUKI WN, EKNOYAN G, New York, John Wiley & Sons, 1981, p 197
2. FRICK PG, SCHMID JR, KISTLER HJ: Hyponatremia associated with hyperproteinemia in multiple myeloma. *Helv Med Acta* 33:317–329, 1967
3. SCHNUR MJ, APPEL GB, KARP G, OSSERMAN EP: The anion gap in asymptomatic plasma cell dyscrasias. *Ann Intern Med* 86:304–305, 1977
4. MURRAY T, LONG W, NARINS RG: Multiple myeloma and the anion gap. *N Engl J Med* 292(11):574–575, 1975
5. JAFFE JP, MOSHER DF: Calcium binding by myeloma protein. *Am J Med* 67:343–346, 1979
6. MARTÍNEZ-MALDONADO M, YIUM J, SUKI W, EKNOYAN GE: Renal complications in multiple myeloma: Pathophysiology and some aspects of clinical management. *J Chronic Dis* 24:221–237, 1971
7. DE FRONZO RA, HUMPHREY RL, WRIGHT JR, COOKE CR: Acute renal failure in multiple myeloma. *Medicine* 54:209–223, 1975
8. BORDER WA, COHEN AH: Renal biopsy diagnosis of clinically silent multiple myeloma. *Ann Intern Med* 93(part I):43–46, 1980
9. COHEN DJ, SHERMAN WH, OSSERMAN EF, APPEL GB: Acute renal failure in patients with multiple myeloma. *Am J Med* 78:247–256, 1984
10. SOLOMON A: Bence Jones proteins and light chains of immunoglobulins. *N Engl J Med* 294:17–23, 1976
11. MEYER F, PUTNAM FW: The fate of injected Bence Jones protein. *Nature* 200:223, 1963
12. MOGENSEN CE, SOLLING K: Studies on renal tubular protein reabsorption: partial and near complete inhibition by certain amino acids. *Scand J Lab Invest* 37:477–480, 1977
13. BONE F, POCKRANDT-HEMSTEDT H, BAUMANN K, KINNE R: Analysis of the pinocytic process in rat kidney: Isolation of pinocytic vesicles from rat kidney cortex. *J Cell Biol* 63:998, 1979
14. KYLE RA, GREIPP PR: Idiopathic Bence Jones proteinuria. *N Engl J Med* 306(10):564–567, 1982
15. DURIE B, SALMON SE: A clinical staging system for multiple myeloma. *Cancer* 36:841–854, 1975
16. BÁEZ-DIAZ L, MARTÍNEZ-MALDONADO M: The kidney in paraproteinemic disorder, in *Textbook of Nephrology,* New York, Elsevier North-Holland Inc., 1983, p 6.127
17. PREUSS HG, HAMMACK WJ, MURDAUGH HV: The effect of Bence Jones protein on the in vitro function of rabbit renal cortex. *Nephron* 5:210–216, 1967

18. PREUSS HG, WEISS FR, IAMMARINO RM, HAMMOCK WJ, MURDAUGH HV: Effects of rat kidney slice function in vitro of proteins from urine of patients with myelomatosis and nephrosis. *Clin Sci Mol Med* 46:283–294, 1974
19. MCGEOCH J, FALCONER SMITH J, LEDINGHAM J, ROSS B: Inhibition of active-transport sodium-potassium ATP-ase by myeloma protein. *Lancet* 2(8079):17–18, 1978
20. WEISS JH, WILLIAMS RH, GALLA JH, GOHSCHALL J, REED E, BHATHENA D, LUKE RG: Pathophysiology of acute Bence Jones protein nephrotoxicity in the rat. *Kidney Int* 20:198–210, 1981
21. CLYNE DH, PESCE AJ, THOMSON RE: Nephrotoxicity of Bence Jones protein in the rat: Importance of protein isoelectric point. *Kidney Int* 16:345–352, 1979
22. SMOLENS P, VENKATACHALAM M, STEIN JH: Myeloma kidney cast nephropathy in a rat model of multiple myeloma. *Kidney Int* 24:192–204, 1983
23. BAZIN HC, BECKORS A, HEREMANS JF: Transplantable immunoglobulin-secreting tumors in rats: General features of Lou/Vsl strain immunocytomas and their monoclonal proteins. *Int J Cancer* 10:568–580, 1972
24. HOYER JR, SERLER MW: Pathophysiology of Tamm-Horsfall protein. *Kidney Int* 16:279–289, 1979
25. COTRAN RS: Pathogenetic mechanisms in the progression of reflux nephropathy: The roles of glomerulo-sclerosis and extravasation of Tamm-Horsfall protein. *Proc Int Cong Nephrol, Athens, Greece,* Basel-Karger, 1981, p 374
26. DZIUKAS LJ, STERZEL RB, HODSON CJ, HOYER JR: Renal localization of Tamm-Horsfall protein in unilateral obstructive uropathy in rats. *Lab Invest* 47:185–193, 1982
27. MALDONADO JE, VELOSA JA, KYLE RA, WAGONER RD, HOLLEY KE, SALASSA RM: Fanconi syndrome in adults: A manifestation of a latent form of myeloma. *Am J Med* 58:354–364, 1975
28. LAZAR GS, FEINSTEIN DI: Distal renal tubular acidosis in multiple myeloma. *Arch Intern Med* 141:655–657, 1981
29. SMITHLINE N, KASSIRER JP, COHEN JJ: Light chain nephropathy: Renal tubular dysfunction associated with light chain proteinuria. *N Engl J Med* 294:71–74, 1976
30. FALCONER SMITH JF, VAN HEGAN RI, ESNOUF MP, ROSS BD: Characteristics of renal handling of human immunoglobulin light chain by the perfused rat kidney. *Clin Sci* 57:113–120, 1979
31. PRUZANSKI W, WATT JG: Serum viscosity and hyperviscosity syndrome in IgG multiple myeloma. *Ann Intern Med* 141:655–657, 1981
32. MESTECKY J, HAMMACK WJ, KOLHAVY R, WRIGHT GP, TOMANA M: Properties of IgA myeloma isolated from sera of patients with the hyperviscosity syndrome. *J Lab Clin Med* 89:919–926, 1977
33. KYLE AR: Long term survival in multiple myeloma. *N Engl J Med* 308:314–316, 1983
34. LAZARUS HM, ADELSTEIN DJ, HERZIG RH, SMITH MC: Long-term survival of patients with multiple myeloma. *Am J Kidney Dis* 2:521–525, 1983
35. MISIANI R, REMUZZI G, BERTANI T, LICINI R, LEVONI P, CRIPPA A, MECCA G: Plasmapheresis in the treatment of acute renal failure in multiple myeloma. *Am J Med* 66:684–688, 1979
36. YIUM J, MARTÍNEZ-MALDONADO M, EKNOYAN G, SUKI WN: Peritoneal dialysis in the treatment of renal failure in multiple myeloma. *South Med J* 64:1403–1405, 1971
37. LEECH SH, POLESKY HF, SHAPIRO FL: Chronic hemodialysis in myelomatosis. *Ann Intern Med* 77:239–242, 1972

38. BROWN WW, HUBERT LA, PIERING WF, PISCIOTTA AV, LIMANN J, GARANCIS JC: Reversal of chronic end-stage renal failure due to myeloma kidney. *Ann Intern Med* 90:793–794, 1979
39. HUMPHREY RL, WRIGHT JR, ZACHARY JB, STERIOFF S, DEFRONZO RA: Renal transplantation in multiple myeloma: A case report. *Ann Intern Med* 83:651–653, 1975

Pathology of Light Chain Nephropathies

Arthur H. Cohen

In 1848, Bence Jones [1] described an abnormal protein in the urine of a patient whose illness was later recognized as a malignancy of plasma cells. Since Bence Jones' original description, there has been considerable interest in renal abnormalities in multiple myeloma and other plasma cell dyscrasias, for his observation established at least a functional link between abnormal plasma cells and urinary alterations. Structural evidence of specific kidney damage in multiple myeloma was not reported until 1920, when Thannhauser and Krauss [2] described what we now know as myeloma kidney, a lesion of tubular precipitation of abnormal light chains, formation of characteristic casts, and a foreign body giant cell reaction to them [3]. For many years, this lesion or slight variants of it, including tubular luminal and cellular light-chain crystal localization, was thought to be the sole direct renal abnormality of light-chain deposits. Interest in other forms of renal damage in myeloma and plasma cells dyscrasias was rekindled in 1972–1974 with the report of Olsen [4] describing a different form of renal injury, nodular lesions of the glomerular mesangium, and the reports of Antonovych et al [5] and Randall et al [6] describing light-chain deposits in glomerular mesangium and basement membranes and tubular basement membranes. Since the mid-1970s, considerable work has been done to expand our knowledge of these two forms of renal disease in the plasma cell dyscrasias; this treatise will focus on advances, theories of pathogenesis, and controversies.

Myeloma Kidney

The lesion known as myeloma kidney (some have recently suggested the term Bence Jones cast nephropathy [7, 8]) is characterized by the presence of large, dense, homogeneous or lamellated casts with one or multiple fracture

This manuscript was presented as part of a Symposium on *The Kidney and Malignant Disease.*

lines that are usually surrounded intimately by multinucleated giant cells of the foreign body type. These casts occur in distal tubules, as well as occasionally in proximal tubules, the basement membranes of which may have large or small discontinuities [3] (Fig. 1). In a relatively small number of casts, clearly identifiable elongated rhomboid crystals may be present; occasionally, the crystals may be the dominant feature [8]. Whereas some studies have indicated that the peripheries of the casts are Congo red-positive and display an apple-green birefringence [9–11], some others have not [3, 12]. It is likely that amyloid is indeed formed by altered light chains in the casts, but that this phenomenon is by no means a universal occurrence. Degenerative changes of tubular epithelial cells are often observed; the cells may desquamate and be found in the lumina adjacent to the casts. In addition, various leukocytes, including monocytes, lymphocytes, and neutrophils, are also found in the tubules [3, 8]. The original descriptions of this lesion indicated that the multinucleated cells surrounding the casts were a foreign body type [2]; however, for many years following the postulate by Allen [13]—that they were a syncytium of tubule cells—most pathologists agreed with this, despite the previous observations and teachings. Four separate studies [3, 10, 14,

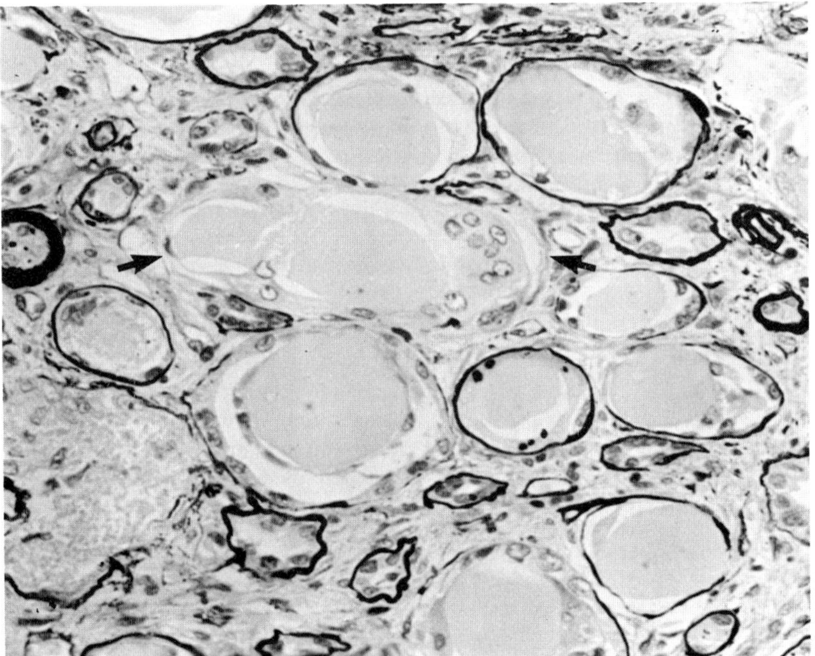

Fig. 1. Myeloma kidney (Bence Jones cast nephropathy). Most of the tubules contain dense casts. The tubule indicated by *arrows* has a cast that is "fractured" and surrounded by a multinucleated giant cell. The basement membrane has largely disappeared. Note the basement membrane defects in other tubules. (Periodic acid-silver methenamine stain; ×415)

15], based primarily on ultrastructure, have reaffirmed the initial descriptions. It appears that the giant cells form as a consequence of monocytes entering the tubules through the aforementioned basement membrane breaks and fusing. It is likely that free extravascular light chains can elicit cell-mediated immunity and, hence, a foreign body reaction. Whether the defects in the basement membrane result from the changes of tubular necrosis induced by the heavy light-chain load presented to the tubular cells or whether they evolve from increased intratubular pressure because of obstruction by casts is not known, although the latter has been suggested [16].

The casts were once thought to be composed of Bence Jones protein. But in 1968, when Levi, Williams, and Lindstrom [17] performed the first organized study by immunofluorescence, they demonstrated that the composition was mostly abnormal serum light chains with other serum proteins also included. Isobe et al obtained similar results [18], as did Cohen and Border in both a small series [3] and an unpublished larger series. Hill et al [16] and Levi et al [17] found that when no or occasional casts were present on light microscopy, there was no immunofluorescence staining of the tubular lumen contents.

The presence of Tamm-Horsfall protein (THP) in the casts has been demonstrated in human myeloma kidney by Cohen and Border [3] by both monospecific anti-THP antiserum and by ultrastructural examination [19]. It is well known that light chains can cause precipitation of THP [20]. THP was noted in casts in both distal and proximal tubules; inasmuch as THP is produced in the distal nephron, its presence in more proximal locations would indicate nephron obstruction by the casts and retrograde flow [20, 21]. Indeed, Cohen and Border [3] observed Tamm-Horsfall protein in glomerular urinary spaces, lending support to the hypothesis that renal insufficiency may be due, at least in part, to tubular obstruction by casts.

Experimental models of myeloma kidney [7, 22] have been produced mainly by injecting human Bence Jones proteins into animals, although recently Smolens, Venkatachalam, and Stein [23] described a unique rat model of multiple myeloma (vida infra). In general, these works have supported and supplemented many of the above observations on human myeloma kidney and, in addition, have addressed some other important problems. The initial success at the induction of this lesion in animals was attained by Koss et al [7], who injected varying dosages of purified lambda Bence Jones protein isolated from a patient with multiple myeloma. At the highest dose (200 mg), most mice developed cast nephropathy; initially (5 to 72 hr) the casts were composed only of the light chain, whereas after 3 days, increasing amounts of Tamm-Horsfall protein were identified in the casts. Initial (3 to 7 days) inflammation with neutrophils was followed by mononuclear cells and giant cells forming by about 1 to 2 weeks. It is of note that these lesions were not induced by lambda light chains isolated from two other patients with multiple myeloma. This study was notable for its reproduction of the human lesion, but it raised the question of why all abnormal light chains did not have this ability. This is pertinent to human disease, for it is well known that perhaps only 50% of myeloma patients develop renal insufficiency or cast formation [24]. Clyne et al [22] were unable to induce myeloma cast nephropathy using urinary kappa light chain isolated from a myeloma patient; they did, however, induce the formation of crystals containing kappa light chains in tubular cells and tubular dysfunction. On the basis of other experiments, Clyne et al [25] suggested that the nephrotoxicity of light chains depended largely on their isoelectric point, for those with high pIs were more likely to interact with and precipitate Tamm-Horsfall protein in the distal nephron. They, therefore, explained that the varying nephrotoxic potentials of light chains were related to their relative electrical charge, and that light chains with pI greater than 5.5 were more likely to induce cast formation and renal insufficiency. However, Smolens, Venkatachalam, and Stein [23], working with a unique model of rat myeloma, recently showed that animals excreting Bence Jones proteins of higher isoelectric points (pI, 6.7, 7.6) did not regularly develop myeloma casts, whereas those excreting light chains having a pI of 5.2 uniformly did; and those excreting light chains having a pI of 4.3 more commonly developed tubular necrosis and less severe myeloma cast nephropathy. Hill et al [16], in a study of human myeloma kidney, demonstrated a relation between cast formation and relative anionic charge of light chains at a physiologic pH. The lower the electrical charge, greater was the frequency of casts. It is obvious from these studies that not only charge but other properties of light chains, such as ability to aggregate, quantity, as well as host factors, including state of hydration, acid-base balance, tubular handling [26], and so forth, may play roles in determining the degree of renal damage.

In a few instances, the natural history of the lesion of myeloma cast nephropathy has been studied in humans, either by sequential renal biopsy examination or by biopsy–autopsy studies of the same patients. Although cast nephropathy is usually associated with severe renal insufficiency [27], the casts may disappear or be reduced in number consequent to chemotherapy and sometimes be associated with improved renal function [16]. There are several alterations that have been found with loss of casts. Hill et al [16] described three patients, one of whom developed massive renal amyloidosis whereas the other two had kidneys with kappa light-chain deposits, apparently in glomeruli and basement membranes. Ganeval et al indicated that with a disappearance of casts, tubular atrophy, and interstitial fibrosis supervened [28].

Light-Chain Nephropathy

The other major renal lesion in the plasma cell dyscrasias with abundant light-chain production concerns the deposition of light chains in various tissue components, most notably glomerular and tubular basement membranes. Unlike Bence Jones cast nephropathy, which, with rare exceptions, is associated with multiple myeloma, light-chain nephropathy (as this group of lesions will be called) occurs also in patients with a nonmyelomatous plasma cell dyscrasia. Furthermore, although this discussion is limited to the pathology of kidneys, it is important to realize that light chain tissue deposits may occur in other organs [6, 29].

A suggestion of abnormal tissue deposits in myeloma patients was first made by Kobernick and Whiteside [30] and Olsen [4], who described glomerular mesangial nodules in the absence of diabetes mellitus. It was not until the report of Antonovych et al [5], in which they showed that the glomerular nodules and renal basement membranes were the sites of a single class of light-chain deposits, that a glomerular lesion was demonstrated as being an integral part of disorders with abnormal light-chain production. Shortly thereafter, Randall et al [6] established the systemic nature of the tissue light-chain deposits. Subsequently, when appropriate studies were performed, virtually all initial reports indicated that the glomerular lesion was nodular in configuration and invariably associated with kappa light-chain deposition [31–35] (Fig. 2). However, glomerular hypercellularity [36–40], non-nodular mesangial enlargement without increase in cells [35], as well as virtually normal glomeruli [16] (Cohen AH, unpublished observations) were soon included in the spectrum of histologic abnormalities. Furthermore, it has been well established that this form of renal injury may also be induced by lambda light-chain deposits [29, 32, 41], although most patients have abnormal kappa chains. In addition, it has been established that these light-chain deposits may occur in the absence of classical multiple myeloma and that abnormally functioning plasma cells, with unbalanced immunoglobulin synthesis and excess free monoclonal light-chain production, may be the main bone marrow alteration [31, 42, 43].

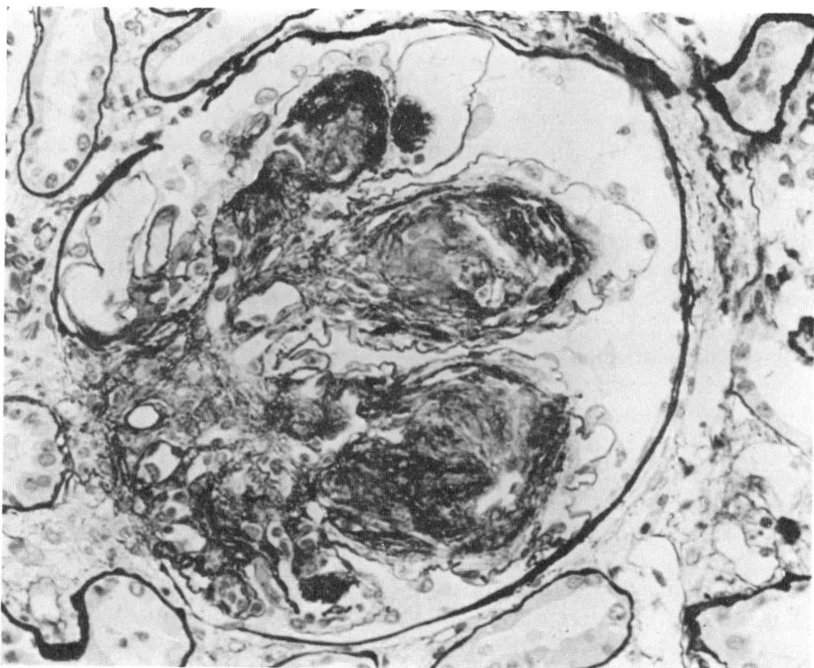

Fig. 2. Glomerulus in light chain nephropathy. There are prominent mesangial nodules, which are partially argyrophilic and capped by capillary microaneurysms. (Periodic acid-silver methenamine stain; ×360)

With this brief background, the renal pathologic features of light-chain nephropathy will be considered. Immunohistochemical studies have disclosed, in almost all cases, a localization of the abnormal monoclonal light chain to the basement membranes of tubules, the Bowman's capsules, and the glomerular capillaries in a linear pattern, and to the glomerular mesangial regions [8, 29, 31–33, 35]. Occasionally, the light chains have been described in the walls of arteries and arterioles [16]. There are, however, a number of instances in which the deposits are found only along tubule basement membranes, even when glomeruli are clearly abnormal [35]. In glomeruli with nodules by light microscopy, staining for light chains is often most heavy in the nodules, and less intense in the capillary walls. In non-nodular glomeruli, the mesangial staining is less bright. For reasons that are unclear, several investigators have documented monoclonal and normal immunoglobulin heavy chains and various complement components in the same sites as the abnormal light chains [16, 29, 34, 35]. Immunoelectron microscopy in one study has indicated the glomerular basement membrane deposits to be in the lamina rara interna, and the tubular basement membrane deposits to be "intramembranous" [32].

The light microscopic appearance of the glomeruli is usually that of a nodular "glomerulosclerosis," each glomerulus having one or more mesangial nodules with varying degrees of cellularity; in most, there are sparse numbers of cells within the mesangium. The staining characteristics of the nodules have been extensively described [29, 31, 33–35]. The most important features include their intensely positive reaction with eosin and periodic acid-Schiff (PAS), their partial argyrophilia with silver impregnation, and their completely negative reaction with any histochemical stains for amyloid. Although not widely recognized, there are aneurysmally dilated capillaries over many nodules [33, 34, 41]. The basement membranes may be normal or slightly thickened and are sometimes partially collapsed. A double contour, indicative of peripheral mesangial migration, is occasionally noted in scattered capillary walls [35, 41]. Non-nodular glomerular lobules may be normal or may have mesangial expansion with some degree of hypercellularity [28]. In a few patients, progression to nodules has been documented [28, 33]. It is of interest to note that in some of the patients reported to have various glomerular lesions with marked hypercellularity of the tufts or with crescents and no nodules, there was little or no glomerular light-chain localization, although the tubular basement membranes were regularly stained [29, 36, 37]. The appearance of affected tubule basement membranes can be quite striking. They are thickened, refractile [29, 35], and in our experience (Cohen AH, unpublished observations) have two layers best appreciated with PAS: an inner one, strongly positive, and an outer one, which is less densely stained and somewhat dull and homogeneous. It is uncommon to observe typical myeloma cast nephropathy in association with light-chain nephropathy, although a small number of patients have been described with the two light-chain lesions [16, 29, 44]. Repeat tissue examination on a small number of patients has disclosed varying results [16, 29]. Ganeval described serial data in four patients [29]. In one, glomerular hypercellularity diminished, although light-chain deposits persisted after chemotherapy. One patient with stable glomerular nodules had less intense tubular basement membrane light-chain staining. One patient's second biopsy displayed the new appearance of lambda light chains in glomerular and tubular deposits along with previously documented kappa deposits. And the fourth patient had a greater degree of interstitial fibrosis, but unchanged glomerular and tubular lesions and deposits. Hill et al described two patients whose initial lesion was myeloma kidney and whose subsequent tissue examination revealed no casts but tissue deposits of "presumed k-chain" [16]. Seymour et al [33] reported one patient with virtually no glomerular changes on initial biopsy who, 2 years later, had mesangial nodules. This form of renal disease has been infrequently transplanted. In a unique and well-described case, recurrence of glomerular nodules and mesangial and glomerular and tubular basement membrane kappa light-chain deposits were noted 20 months following allograft placement [44].

The ultrastructural features of light-chain nephropathy are also well characterized. There are finely granular continuous deposits of slight to deep electron density in the glomerular basement membranes, characteristically occupying the lamina rara interna or sometimes the lamina densa [31, 32, 34, 35, 41]; the deposits can, at times, be so prominent and conspicuous as to be confused with dense-deposit disease [37]. The mesangial nodules, likewise, contain granular deposits of varying electron density, often irregularly distributed. Some investigators [31] have observed that fibrils, 110 to 140 Å in diameter, are admixed in the deposits; it is likely that these fibrils are not part of the light chains, but are intrinsic to the glomerulus and are exaggerated in certain disease states [45]. The older nodules apparently contain increased mesangial matrix; a single report [46], which has not been confirmed by many subsequent studies, indicated long-spacing collagen as an integral component of the nodules. The tubular basement membrane deposits characteristically are on the outer (interstitial) aspects of these structures and appear as confluent finely or coarsely granular masses of differing electron densities. The deposits may be seen also in the interstitium and in vascular walls around smooth muscle cells [8, 34, 44].

The glomerular capillary wall changes can be quite striking in this disorder. As described by us [41] and mentioned in passing in few other reports [33, 34], capillary microaneurysms are a prominent and, perhaps, regular feature of the nodular form of injury. Although not commented upon, microaneurysms are illustrated in many reports of nodular light-chain glomerulopathy [6, 29, 31, 35, 44, 46]. Our study of this phenomenon has disclosed several changes that, in concert, appeared to explain the morphogenesis of the aneurysms. Neutrophils and monocytes accumulate in capillaries and infiltrate capillary walls in association with light chain deposits; possibly because of secretory products of these cells, the anchoring points between the peripheral portions of the mesangium and the basement membranes rupture. This injury, combined with endothelial cell degeneration, results in a ballooning of the capillary wall [41].

It is evident that there are many morphologic features of the glomerular abnormalities that may be virtually indistinguishable from the nodular glomerulosclerosis occurring in diabetes mellitus. These include acellular mesangial nodules and microaneurysms; as emphasized by several investigators [29,

35, 47], immunohistochemical studies using antisera monospecific for light-chain determinants are mandatory for separating these two glomerulopathies. It is more than likely that reports of Kimmelstiel-Wilson nodular glomerulosclerosis in the absence of diabetes mellitus represent light chain glomerulopathy.

Light chain nephropathy may occur in the absence of multiple myeloma; indeed, only about 50% of the reported cases have documented myeloma [29, 35, 41]. Furthermore, a serum or urine monoclonal intact immunoglobulin or light chain is also not demonstrated in every patient. Studies on bone marrow plasma cells from some patients without myeloma have disclosed a monoclonal population of cells; these produce abnormal immunoglobulins with normal heavy chains, but light chains that are abnormally large or small. Reasons for tissue deposition of the altered light chains are unknown, but it is speculated that polymerization and/or glycosylation of the light chains might play a role [29]. However, Gallo et al [31] described excess production of normal light chains in a patient with quantitatively normal plasma cells. Hill et al [16] noted that light chain nephropathy occurred in several patients whose abnormal serum light chains had a relatively high isoelectric point. At the present time, therefore, there are no precise explanations for why some patients with abnormal light-chain production develop cast nephropathy and why some develop light chain nephropathy (and why a few develop both, simultaneously or sequentially).

References

1. BENCE JONES H: On a new substance occurring in the urine of a patient with "mollities ossium." *Philos Trans R Soc Lond [Biol]* 138:55, 1848
2. THANNHAUSER SJ, KRAUSS E: Über ein degenerative Erkrankung der Harnkanalchen (Nephrose) bei Bence-Jones' scher Albuminurie mit Nierensch wund (kleine, glutte, Weisse Niere). *Dtsch Arch Klin Med* 133:183–192, 1920
3. COHEN AH, BORDER WA: Myeloma kidney: An immunomorphogenetic study of renal biopsies. *Lab Invest* 42:248–256, 1980
4. OLSEN S: Mesangial thickening and nodular glomerular sclerosis in diabetes mellitus and other diseases. *Acta Pathol Microbiol Scand [A]* 80 (Suppl 233):203–216, 1972
5. ANTONOVYCH T, LIN RC, PARRISH E, MOSTOFI K: Light chain deposits in multiple myeloma. *Abst 7th Annual Meeting, American Society of Nephrology,* 1973
6. RANDALL RE, WILLIAMSON WC JR, MULLINAX F, TUNG MY, STILL WJS: Manifestations of systemic light chain deposition. *Am J Med* 60:293–299, 1976
7. KOSS MN, PIRANI CL, OSSERMAN EF: Experimental Bence Jones cast nephropathy. *Lab Invest* 34:579–591, 1976
8. SILVA FG, PIRANI CL, MESA-TEJADA R, WILLIAMS G: The kidney in plasma cell dyscrasias: A review and a clinico-pathologic study of 50 Patients, in *Progress Surg Path,* edited by FENOGLIO CM, WOLFF M, New York, Masson, 1984, vol. 5, pp 131–176
9. LIMAS C, WRIGHT JR, MATSUZAKI M, CALKINS E: Amyloidosis and multiple myeloma: A re-evaluation using a control population. *Am J Med* 54:166–173, 1973
10. PAPADIMITRIOU JM, MATZ LR: The origin of multinucleate giant cells in my-

eloma kidney from mononuclear phagocytes: An ultrastructural study. *Pathology* 11:583–593, 1979

11. MELATO M, FALCONIERI G, PASCALI E, PEZZOLI A: Amyloid casts within renal tubules: A singular finding in myelomatosis. *Virchows Arch Path Anat* 387:133–145, 1980

12. ABRAHAMS C, PIRANI CL, POLLAK VE: Ultrastructure of the kidney in a patient with multiple myeloma. *J Pathol Bacteriol* 92:220–225, 1966

13. ALLEN AC: *The Kidney: Medical and Surgical Diseases.* New York, Grune and Stratton, 1951, p 280

14. JONES DB: Myeloma nephropathy, a light chain storage disease (*abstract*). *Am J Pathol* 78:49–50a, 1975

15. FACTOR SM, WINN RM, BIEMPICA L: The histiocytic origin of the multinucleated giant cells in myeloma kidney. *Hum Pathol* 9:114–120, 1978

16. HILL GS, MOREL-MAROGER L, MÉRY J-P, BROUET JC, MIGNON F: Renal lesions in multiple myeloma: Their relationship to associated protein abnormalities. *Am J Kidney Dis* 2:423–438, 1983

17. LEVI DF, WILLIAMS RC JR, LINDSTROM FD: Immunofluorescence studies of the myeloma kidney with special reference to light chain disease. *Am J Med* 44:922–933, 1968

18. ISOBE T, MATSUMOTO J, FUJITA T, MAEDA S, SUGIYAMA T: Localization of Bence Jones proteins in the kidney of myeloma patients. *Jpn J Med* 21:12–16, 1982

19. COHEN AH: Morphology of renal tubular hyaline casts. *Lab Invest* 44:280–287, 1981

20. HOYER JR, SEILER MW: Pathophysiology of Tamm-Horsfall protein. *Kidney Int* 16:279–289, 1979

21. McGIVEN AR, HUNT JS, DAY WA, BAILEY RR: Tamm-Horsfall in the glomerular capsular space. *J Clin Pathol* 31:620–625, 1978

22. CLYNE DH, BENDSTRUP L, FIRST MR, PESCE AJ, FINKEL PN, POLLAK VE, PIRANI CL: Renal effects of intraperitoneal kappa chain injection: induction of crystals in renal tubular cells. *Lab Invest* 31:131–142, 1974

23. SMOLENS P, VENKATACHALAM M, STEIN JH: Myeloma kidney cast nephropathy in a rat model of multiple myeloma. *Kidney Int* 24:192–204, 1983

24. DE FRONZO RA, COOKE CR, WRIGHT JR, HUMPHREY RL: Renal function in patients with multiple myeloma. *Medicine (Baltimore)* 57:151–166, 1978

25. CLYNE DH, PESCE AJ, THOMPSON RE: Nephrotoxicity of Bence Jones proteins in the rat: importance of protein isoelectric point. *Kidney Int* 16:345–352, 1979

26. FALCONER SMITH JF, ROSS BD, LEDINGHAM JGG: Nephrotoxicity of myeloma light chains (*abstract*). *Kidney Int* 18:535, 1980

27. BORDER WA, COHEN AH: Renal biopsy diagnosis of clinically silent multiple myeloma. *Ann Intern Med* 93:43–46, 1980

28. GANEVAL D, JUNGERS P, NOEL LH, DROZ D: La Néphropathie du Myélome Actualities Néphrologiques de l'Hôpital Necker. Paris, Flammarion, 1977, pp 309–347

29. GANEVAL D, MIGNON F, PREUD'HOMME JL, NOËL LH, MOREL-MAROGER L, DROZ D, BROUET JC, MÉRY JP, GRÜNFELD J-P: Visceral deposition of monoclonal light chains and immunoglobulins: A study of renal and immunopathologic abnormalities. *Adv Nephrol* 11:25–63, 1982

30. KOBERNICK SD, WHITESIDE JH: Renal glomeruli in multiple myeloma. *Lab Invest* 6:478–485, 1957

31. GALLO G, FEINER HD, KATZ LA, FELDMAN GM, CORREA EB, CHUBA JV, BUXBAUM JN: Nodular glomerulopathy associated with nonamyloidotic kappa

light chain deposits and excess immunoglobulin light chain synthesis. *Am J Pathol* 99:621–644, 1980

32. TUBBS RR, GEPHARDT GN, MCMAHON JT, HALL PM, VALENZUÈLA R, VIDT DG: Light chain nephropathy. *Am J Med* 71:263–269, 1981

33. SEYMOUR AE, THOMPSON AJ, SMITH PS, WOODROFFE AJ, CLARKSON AR: Kappa light chain glomerulosclerosis in multiple myeloma. *Am J Pathol* 101:557–580, 1980

34. GIPSTEIN RM, COHEN AH, ADAMS DA, ADAMS T, GRABIE MT: Kappa light chain nephropathy without evidence of myeloma cells. *Am J Nephrol* 2:276–281, 1982

35. MOREL-MAROGER L, VERROUST P, PREUD'HOMME J-L: Glomerular lesions in plasma cell dyscrasias, in *Pathology of Glomerular Disease*, edited by ROSEN S, New York, Churchill Livingstone, 1983, pp 207–224

36. SILVA FG, MEYRIER A, MOREL-MAROGER L, PIRANI CL: Proliferative glomerulopathy in multiple myeloma. *J Pathol* 130:229–236, 1979

37. KNOBLER H, KOPOLOVIC J, KLEINMAN Y, RUBINGER D, SILVER J, FRIEDLAENDER MM, POPOVTZER MM: Multiple myeloma presenting as dense deposit disease: Light chain nephropathy. *Nephron* 34:58–63, 1983

38. LAPENAS DJ, DREWRY SJ, LUKE RL III, LEEBER DA: Crescentic light-chain glomerulópathy: Report of a case. *Arch Pathol Lab Med* 107:319–323, 1983

39. RAO TKS, NICASTRI AD, CHEN CK, ROSENTHAL J, BROWN C, DELANO BG, FRIEDMAN EA: Membranoproliferative glomerulonephritis (MPGN), an unusual manifestation of multiple myeloma (*abstract*). *Kidney Int* 14:659, 1978

40. DHAR SK, SMITH EC, FRESCO R: Proliferative glomerulonephritis in monoclonal gammopathy. *Nephron* 19:288–294, 1977

41. SINNIAH R, COHEN AH: Glomerular capillary aneurysms in light chain nephropathy: An ultrastructural proposal of morphogenesis. *Am J Pathol* (in press, 1984)

42. SILVA F, MESA-TEJADA R, WILLIAMS GS, MOREL-MAROGER L, RAMANARAYANAN M, PIRANI CL: Light chain glomerulopathy (GN) as the first manifestation of plasma cell dyscrasia (*abstract*). *Lab Invest* 42:151A, 1980

43. PREUD'HOMME JL, MOREL-MAROGER L, BROUET JC, MIHAESCO E, CERF M, MIGNON F, MERY JP, GUGLIELMI P, SELIGMANN M: Synthesis of abnormal immunoglobulins in lymphoplasmacytic disorders with visceral light chain deposition. *Am J Med* 69:703–709, 1980

44. COLVIN R: Case records of the Massachusetts General Hospital (Case 1–1981). *N Engl J Med* 304:33–43, 1981

45. HSU H-C, CHURG J: Glomerular microfibrils in renal disease: a comparative electron microscopic study. *Kidney Int* 16:497–504, 1979

46. SCHUBERT GE, ADAM A: Glomerular nodules and long-spacing collagen in kidneys of patients with multiple myeloma. *J Clin Pathol* 27:800–805, 1974

47. HERF S, POHL SL, STURGILL B, BOLTON WK: An evaluation of diabetic and pseudodiabetic glomerulosclerosis. *Am J Med* 66:1040–1045, 1979

Glomerular Lesions in Lymphomas and Leukemias

Liliane Morel-Maroger Striker, Françoise Mignon, David Dabbs, and Gary E. Striker

In this chapter, we will consider the renal lesions that have been associated with hematologic malignancies. The hematologic conditions fall into the categories of lymphomas and leukemias. This is an extremely heterogeneous group of diseases, and the etiology of the renal lesions is poorly understood. Furthermore, the type of glomerular change is quite diverse within and between categories. Thus, we have chosen to present this review by discussing glomerular lesions as a function of the type of hematologic malignancy. The renal lesions associated with multiple myeloma will be considered in another section of this volume.

Herein, we present a brief summary of our personal experience based on 8000 renal biopsy examinations and a review of the Western literature. There have been several reviews of this subject [1–12]. This review is restricted to those patients with overt clinical or morphologic evidence of glomerular disease. The frequency of renal disease in hematologic malignancies may be underestimated. Renal lesions are often not the major presenting symptom. In addition, much of the data are in case reports or books, and the reported details of clinical or histologic findings are often incomplete.

The glomerular lesions associated with the following disorders will be described:

   I. Lymphomas
      A. Hodgkin's disease
      B. Other lymphomas
         1. Non-Hodgkin's lymphoma
         2. Angioimmunoblastic lymphadenopathy
         3. Burkitt's lymphoma
  II. Leukemias
      A. Chronic lymphocytic leukemia
      B. Myelogenous leukemia

This manuscript was presented as part of a Symposium on *The Kidney and Malignant Disease.*

III. Other hematologic malignancies
   A. Waldenstrom's macroglobulinemia
   B. Kaposi sarcoma

Lymphomas

Hodgkin's Disease

The first association between Hodgkin's disease and glomerular disease was recognized in 1930 in a patient with amyloidosis. Since then, a total of 40 cases have been recorded [9, 13–39]. The majority of these however, were recognized prior to 1962. The virtual disappearance of reported cases with this renal complication of Hodgkin's disease is unexplained, but may reflect the development of modern therapeutic measures. That this decrease is not an artifact is borne out by our personal experience. The last recognized patient with amyloidosis in our series occurred in 1967. It was a 9-year-old child who had been treated for Hodgkin's disease for 3 years and developed end-stage renal failure.

The heterogeneity in the composition of amyloid substance has only been recognized recently [38]. Therefore, its composition in Hodgkin's disease has been studied in few patients. In those examined, the deposits consisted of AA amyloid [38]. Since Hodgkin's disease is not usually accompanied by a monoclonal gammopathy, it seems reasonable that most of the other cases of amyloidosis would also have been of the AA type.

The most common pathologic lesion now associated with the nephrotic syndrome in patients with Hodgkin's disease is the minimal change lesion. To our knowledge, 40 patients with minimal change nephrotic syndrome have been reported, and we have seen one additional patient [1, 3, 5, 9, 10, 12, 32, 33, 40–59]. A general characteristic of these patients is that the nephrotic syndrome usually occurs early in the course of the disease and may even constitute a presenting symptom. Proteinuria parallels the evolution of the hematologic disorder; thus, the reappearance of proteinuria may herald the recurrence of Hodgkin's disease. Disappearance of proteinuria is often achieved by control of the disease, no matter whether the therapy is chemotherapeutic or irradiation, suggesting that the resolution is associated with loss of tumor rather than a direct effect of the therapy on the kidney.

Two patients with focal glomerulonephritis (focal GN) have been described [60, 61]. The first was a 26-year-old man with the nephrotic syndrome who also had lymphadenopathy and hepatomegaly. A diagnosis of Hodgkin's disease was made, and treatment resulted in a rapid remission of edema and proteinuria. In the second patient, a 27-year-old woman, the time sequence was unusual. This patient presented with a minimal change nephrotic syndrome that did not respond to corticosteroids. Seven months later, she developed progressive renal failure. A second renal biopsy examination disclosed focal GN, and within a few weeks Hodgkin's disease was discovered.

Membranous glomerulonephritis (membranous GN) has been reported in four patients [47, 62–64], and we have observed one additional patient in whom the nephrotic syndrome developed 4 months following successful chemotherapy and irradiation. The renal biopsy in the latter patient showed a stage II membranous nephrophathy. In addition to the subepithelial deposits, which contained IgG, C3, and Clq by immunofluorescence microscopy, there were also mesangial deposits of C3 and Clq. The presence of deposits in these two locations was confirmed by electron microscopy.

Membranoproliferative glomerulonephritis (MPGN) has been reported in two patients [6, 65], one of whom also had crescents [6].

Five patients with so-called proliferative GN have been reported [9–66]. The amount, distribution, and type of deposits varies widely.

Finally, six patients with crescentic GN with circulating antiglomerular basement membrane (GBM) antibody have been reported [67–69]. It should be pointed out that anti-GBM nephritis is an uncommon renal disease. Thus, even though the absolute number is not large, the relative number of patients with Hodgkin's disease and anti-GBM antibody-induced glomerulonephritis is several times higher than that found in patients without Hodgkin's disease. The factors responsible for this high incidence are unknown, but could be related to either the development of an autoantibody as a primary part of the malignant process or an abnormal immune response related to therapy.

Other Lymphomas

Non-Hodgkin's Lymphoma

There are fewer cases of glomerular lesions associated with non-Hodgkin lymphoma. To our knowledge, amyloid deposition has not been described in the glomeruli of these patients. As in Hodgkin's disease, the most frequent lesion is minimal change lesion. In contrast to the cases with Hodgkin's disease, there is little information about the relation between the onset of the disease and the recognition of the lymphoma. Where documented, the nephrotic syndrome lesion either precedes or occurs simultaneously with the lymphoma.

A total of 32 patients with glomerular disease have been reported in non-Hodgkin lymphoma, and we now report three others from our series. The minimal change lesion is relatively uncommon [3, 4, 5, 12, 72] and may precede the discovery of the malignancy [12]. Focal sclerosis, as in Hodgkin's disease, is exceptional, with only one case reported in the literature [73]. The proportion of patients with membranous GN is much higher than that reported in Hodgkin's disease: six patients have been reported previously [9, 12, 74, 75], and we have seen one additional patient.

Six patients with MPGN were reported in the literature, and we have seen one other [76, 77]. In addition, Helin et al [7] reported two patients with both mesangial and subendothelial deposits by electron microscopy. They probably fit within the category of MPGN although these patients did not have clear-cut lesions by light microscopy and had only minimal proteinuria. Three patients with crescentic GN have been reported [78, 79], and we have seen one additional patient. Immunofluorescence was not available in two patients, but in the two patients reported by Petzel et al [79] there were granular focal deposits of IgG, IgM, and β1c in a mesangial and capillary loop distribution in one patient. The second patient had only focal deposits of β1c in the mesangium.

Finally, in a report of 10 patients, Gupta found glomerular lesions in six [2]. We deduced from the light and immunofluorescence findings that two of them fit into the category of membranous GN and two were examples of MPGN. The remaining six were not sufficiently described to be placed into current diagnostic categories.

Angioimmunoblastic Lymphadenopathy

There have been two patients reported with angioimmunoblastic lymphadeno-pathy, and both presented with acute renal failure [81]. In one, this was associated with a necrotizing angiitis and proliferative GN without crescents. Prominent granular deposits of IgG and C3 in a diffuse pattern in both mesangial regions and peripheral loops were observed. In the other patient, no light microscopic lesions were seen, but diffuse granular deposits of IgM were noted in all glomeruli. The fluorescence and electron microscopic data in this communication suggested that the lesions best fit the category of MPGN, although this was not stated by the authors.

Burkitt's Lymphoma

There is one report of clinical renal disease in patients who present with Burkitt's lymphoma [66]. However, Oldstone et al [82] detected in two patients immunoglobulins and C3 on the glomerular basement membrane and in the mesangium, and a granular distribution consistent with a membranous lesion. Light and electron microscopic findings were not presented, and it was not stated whether the patients had clinical evidence of renal disease. The IgG eluted from renal biopsy samples of these two patients contained antibodies that bound to Epstein-Barr virus (EBV) antigens. In addition, these patients had circulating immune complexes containing EBV antigens. One reported patient developed the nephrotic syndrome 4 months after Burkitt's lymphoma was diagnosed and treated [66]. The histologic lesion by renal biopsy was type I membranoproliferative glomerulonephritis. There were deposits of IgG and C3 by immunofluorescence microscopy. The nephrotic syndrome regressed following cyclophosphamide therapy. The period of follow-up was only 6 months in this patient.

Leukemias

Chronic Lymphocytic Leukemia

An association between glomerular disease and chronic lymphocytic leukemia (CLL) used to be considered uncommon, but both the current literature and our personal experience no longer support this conclusion [5, 8, 10–12]. It appears that renal lesions may be associated as frequently with CLL as they are with other lymphoid malignancies. In addition, the type of associated renal lesions is equally diverse [8, 11–13, 37, 41, 83–89]. Amyloidosis was reported in two patients with untreated CLL [27, 83] and in one patient with hairy cell leukemia [84]. The composition of the amyloid was not studied. Unlike the patients with Hodgkin's disease, where it can be reasonably assumed that amyloidosis would be of the AA type, the same conclusions could not be reached in patients with CLL for the following reasons: (1) The mean age of patients with CLL is considerably higher than that in Hodgkin's disease. (2) More importantly, a relatively large number of patients with CLL develop a monoclonal gammopathy. Therefore, it seems likely that the amyloid deposits would be of the AL type. However, in the patient with hairy cell leukemia, the amyloid was of the AA type [84].

Feehally et al [8] reviewed 11 patients with CLL and the nephrotic syndrome, 6 of whom had proliferative and sclerosing (membranoproliferative) GN, 2 having amyloid, and 1 having membranous GN. It is noteworthy that only one patient with CLL had minimal change nephrotic syndrome, which is in sharp contrast to the patients with lymphomas and suggests that the etiology of the renal lesions differed. This is supported by the fact that in patients with proliferative lesions, both in our series and those in the literature, more than half had an associated cryoglobulinemia. In most cases, the cryoglobulin is a monoclonal immunoglobulin composed of either kappa or lambda light chains. Electron microscopic examination of the deposits in the kidneys in patients with CLL and cryoglobulinemia show a characteristic fibrillar substructure [8, 10, 11]. Gilboa et al [89] speculated that the fibrillar deposits were composed of IgG-anti IgG immune complexes. It is possible that the cryoglobulins commonly encountered in these patients are anti-idiotypic immunoglobulins induced by antigens deposited in the kidney. The nature of the initiating antigen is unknown, but one source may be viruses since kidneys from patients dying of leukemias or lymphomas [77] contain deposits of viral antigens. Thus, in the majority of patients with CLL, the nephrotic syndrome is associated with proliferative glomerular lesions that contain immune deposits.

Myelogenous Leukemias

In 1983, two patients with myelogenous leukemia, one acute and one chronic, and the nephrotic syndrome were recognized [90, 91]. Two patients with acute myelogenous leukemia had circulating and renal immune complexes containing antibodies directed against antigens on the leukemic cell membranes [92, 93]. One patient with chronic leukemia had a minimal change lesion, and the nephrotic syndrome responded to treatment with a diuretic and prednisone [90].

Other Hematologic Malignancies

Waldenstrom Macroglobulinemia

Overt renal symptoms do not usually accompany Waldenstrom macroglobulinemia. A characteristic of this disorder is a high serum concentration of
monoclonal IgM and serum hyperviscosity. Most patients excrete small
amounts of proteins bearing the antigenic determinants of μ chains, and
nearly one-half of the patients excrete urinary light chains. When the nephrotic
syndrome is present, it is most commonly associated with amyloidosis [37,
94, 95].

Although it is difficult to estimate the true incidence of amyloidosis in
Waldenstrom disease, in one series of 16 patients, 3 had amyloidosis [94].
The type of amyloid deposit is generally presumed to be of the AL type,
although one patient with the AA type has been reported [95].

The most specific histologic lesion by light microscopy is one that contains
amorphous intravascular aggregates (so-called thrombi) within the glomeruli
[37, 94]. The number is variable, but by immunofluorescence microscopy
they always contain IgM of the same light-chain type as that seen in the
serum monoclonal IgM. By electron microscopy, the aggregates are noted
to have a fibrillar substructure [37, 96].

Other glomerular lesions have been reported in Waldenstrom's disease,
including a nodular glomerulosclerosis similar to that noted in plasma cell
dyscrasia [37], membranous glomerulonephritis [97], minimal change [98],
and membranoproliferative nephritis [37, 99].

Kaposi's Sarcoma

Recently, a single case of Kaposi's sarcoma was reported in a 29-year-old
male who also had a serum cryoprecipitate containing IgM and heterogeneous
IgG and IgA proteins [100]. He excreted 5 g of protein/24 hr in the
urine. A test for hepatitis B surface antigen was positive, but no antibodies
were detected. A renal biopsy demonstrated a glomerular mesangial hypercellularity and a thickening of the capillary walls, with prominent deposits of
IgG, C3, and Clq in the peripheral vascular loops. In addition, there was
IgM in the mesangial regions, and HBsAg was positive in the mesangial
regions.

Summary

A variety of lesions may accompany lymphomas and leukemias. Amyloidosis,
the first lesion described in Hodgkin's disease, has nearly disappeared, to be
replaced by the minimal change nephrotic syndrome. In non-Hodgkin lymphomas, glomerular immune deposits are found more commonly. In lympho-

mas, the relation between glomerular lesions and malignancy is suggested by the fact that specific removal of tumor mass may result in disappearance of proteinuria. In leukemias, most of the glomerular lesions are of the proliferative type and are often associated with cryoglobulinemia.

References

1. PLAGER J, STUTZMAN L: Acute nephrotic syndrome as a manifestation of active Hodgkin's disease. *Am J Med* 50:56–66, 1971
2. GUPTA RK: Immunohistochemical studies of glomerular lesions in retroperitoneal lymphomas. *Am J Pathol* 71:427–433, 1973
3. GAGLIANO RF, COSTANZI JJ, BEATHARD GA, SARLES HE, BELL JD: The nephrotic syndrome associated with neoplasia: An unusual paraneoplastic syndrome. *Am J Med* 60:1026–1031, 1976
4. ROUTLEDGE RC, HANN IM, MORRIS JONES PH: Hodgkin's disease complicated by the neprotic syndrome. *Cancer* 38:1735–1740, 1976
5. EAGEN JW, LEWIS EJ: Glomerulopathies of neoplasia. *Kidney Int* 11:297–306, 1977
6. PASCAL RR: Renal manifestations of extrarenal neoplasms. *Hum Pathol* 11:7–17, 1980
7. HELIN H, PASTERNACK A, HAKALA T, PETTINEN K, WAGER O: Glomerular electron-deposits and circulating immune complexes in patients with malignant tumors. *Clin Nephrol* 14:23–30, 1980
8. FEEHALLY J, HUTCHINSON RM, MACKAY EH, WALLS J: Recurrent proteinuria in lymphocytic leukemia. *Clin Nephrol* 16:51–54, 1981
9. KRAMER P, SIZOO W, TWISS EE: Nephrotic syndrome in Hodgkin's disease. *Neth J Med* 24:114–119, 1981
10. GALLO GR, FEINER HD, BUXBAUM JN: The kidney in lymphoplasmacytic disorders. *Pathol Annu* 17:291–317, 1982
11. GOUET D, MARCHAUD R, TOUCHARD G, ABADIE JC, POURRAT O, SUDRE Y: Nephrotic syndrome associated with chronic lymphoid leukemia. *Nouv Pres Med* 16:3047–3049, 1982
12. MIGNON F, BEAUFILS H, MOREL-MAROGER L, CLAUVEL JP, VALLA D, AUBERT P: Glomerulopathies au cours des affections malignes, in *Seminaires d'Uronephrologie Pitie-Salpetriere,* Masson, Paris, 1982
13. WILKS S: Cases of lardaceous disease and some allied affections. *Guys Hosp Rep* 52:103–132, 1856
14. BANNICK EG, BARKER NW: Diffuse amyloidosis of unknown etiology. *Med Clinics N Am* 14:773–781, 1930
15. TOBIAS W, COLOMBI FA: Amiloidosis generalizada por linfogranulomatosis abdominal. *Rev Med Y Cien A Fines* 2:927–935, 1940
16. LEHMAN RG: Hodgkin's disease complicated by amyloidosis and a nephrotic syndrome: Case report. *Ohio State Med J* 39:232–233, 1940
17. CERVERA FG, PODESTA LD: La amiloidosis generalizada en la enfermedad de Hodgkin-Paltauf-Sternberg. *Prensa Med Argent* 33:2082–2085, 1946
18. JACKSON H: *Hodgkin's Disease and Allied Disorders.* New York, Oxford University Press, 1947
19. DAHLIN DC: Secondary amyloidosis. *Ann Intern Med* 31:105–119, 1949
20. SCOTT RB: The spleen and splenectomy. *Br Med J* 1:1063–1070, 1949
21. SHORT CL, MALLORY TB, CASTLEMAN B, PARRIS EE: Case records of the

Massachusetts General Hospital: Weekly clinicopathological exercises; case 35391. *N Engl J Med* 241:497–500, 1949

22. WALLACE SL, FELDMAN DJ, BERLIN I, HARRIS C, GLASS IA: Amyloidosis in Hodgkin's disease. *Am J Med* 8:552–557, 1950

23. GLEDHILL RC, SHILLITOE AJ: Purpura and amyloidosis in Hodgkin's disease. *Br Med J* 1:1336–1337, 1952

24. TEILUM G: Studies on the pathogenesis of amyloidosis: II. Effect of nitrogen mustard in inducing amyloidosis. *J Lab Clin Med* 43:367–374, 1954

25. SHERMAN MJ, MORALES JB, BAYRD ED, SCHIERMAN WD: Amyloid nephrosis secondary to Hodgkin's disease. *AMA Arch Intern Med* 95:618–621, 1955

26. SPAIN DM: Rapid and extensive development of amyloidosis in association with nitrogen mustard therapy. *Am J Clin Pathol* 26:52–55, 1956

27. LEONARD BJ: Chronic lymphatic leukemia and the nephrotic syndrome. *Lancet* 1:1356–1357, 1957

28. WINAWER SJ, FELDMAN SM: Amyloid nephrosis in Hodgkin's disease. *Arch Intern Med* 104:793–796, 1959

29. CARDELL BS: Role of cytotoxic agents in production of amyloidosis in Hodgkin's disease. *Br Med J* 1:1145, 1961

30. RICHMOND J, SHERMAN RS, DIAMOND HD, CRAVER LF: Renal lesions associated with malignant lymphoma. *Am J Med* 32:184–207, 1962

31. AZZOPARDI JG, LEHNER T: Systemic amyloidosis and malignant disease. *J Clin Pathol* 19:539–548, 1966

32. HAMBURGER J, RICHET G, CROSNIER J, FUNK-BRENTANO JL, ANTOINE B, DUCROT H, MERY JP, MONTERA H: *Nephrology*. Philadelphia, W.B. Saunders, 1968, vol. 1

33. KIELY JM, WAGONER RD, HOLLEY KE: Renal complications of lymphoma. *Ann Intern Med* 71:1159–1175, 1969

34. AACH R, KISSANE J: Clinicopathologic conference: Hodgkin's disease complicated by thrombocytopenia and nephrotic syndrome. *Am J Med* 51:109–120, 1971

35. FALKSON G, FALKSON HC: Amyloidosis in Hodgkin's disease. *S Afr J Med* 47:62–64, 1973

36. YUM MN, EDWARDS JL, KLEIT MS: Glomerular lesions in Hodgkin's disease. *Arch Pathol* 99:645–649, 1975

37. ZOLLINGER HU, MIHATSCH MJ: *Renal Pathology in Biopsy*. New York, Springer-Verlag, 1978, pp 216–217

38. GLENNER GG: Amyloid deposits and amyloidosis. *N Engl J Med* 302:1333–1343, 1980

39. CHAMPION M, RICHARD RL: Amyloidosis in Hodgkin's disease: A Scottish survey. *Scot Med J* 24:9–12, 1979

40. MILLER DG: The association of immune disease and malignant lymphoma. *Ann Intern Med* 66:507–521, 1967

41. BRODOVSKY HS, SAMUELS MI, MIGLIORE PJ, HOWE CD: Chronic lymphocytic leukemia, Hodgkin's disease, and the nephrotic syndrome. *Arch Intern Med* 121:71–75, 1968

42. HARDIN JG JR, COKER AS, BLANION JH: Medicine grand rounds from the University of Alabama Medical Center. *S Afr Med J* 62:1111–1118, 1969

43. GHOSH (BANERJI) L, MUEHRKE RC: The nephrotic syndrome: A prodrome to lymphoma. *Ann Intern Med* 72:379–382, 1970

44. PIESSENS WF, ZEICHER M: Hodgkin's disease causing a reversible nephrotic syndrome by compression of the inferior vena cava. *Cancer* 25:880–884, 1970

45. BICHEL J, BJORN JENSEN K: Nephrotic syndrome and Hodgkin's disease. *Lancet* 2:1425–1426, 1971

46. JACKSON RH, OO M: Nephrotic syndrome in Hodgkin's disease. *Lancet* 2:821–822, 1971
47. LOWRY WS, MUNZENRIDER JE, LYNCH GA: Nephrotic syndrome in Hodgkin's disease. *Lancet* 1:1127, 1971
48. HANSEN EH, SKOV PE, ASKJAER SA, ALBERTSEN K: Hodgkin's disease associated with the nephrotic syndrome without kidney lesion. *Acta Med Scand* 191:307–313, 1972
49. PERLIN E, POWERS JM, DICKSON LG, MOQUIN RB: The nephrotic syndrome in Hodgkin's disease. *Med Ann DC* 41:354–356, 1972
50. SHERMAN RL, SUSIN M, WEKSLER ME, BECKER EL: Lipoid nephrosis in Hodgkin's disease. *Am J Med* 52:699–706, 1972
51. CARPENTER CB, CASTLEMAN B, SCULLY RE, MCNEELY BU: Case records of the Massachusetts General Hospital. Weekly clinicopathological exercises. Case 49–1973. *N Engl J Med* 289:1241–1247, 1973
52. HAYSLETT JP, KASHGARIAN M, BENSCH KG, SPARGO BJ, FREEDMAN LR, EPSTEIN EH: Clinicopathological correlations in the nephrotic syndrome due to primary renal disease. *Medicine* 52:93–120, 1973
53. LARSON LS, FRITZ RD: Nephrotic syndrome in association with Hodgkin's disease. *Wis Med J* 75:14–17, 1976
54. MOORTHY AV, ZIMMERMAN SW, BURKHOLDER PM: Nephrotic syndrome in Hodgkin's disease: Evidence for pathogenesis alternative to immune complex disease. *Am J Med* 61:471–477, 1976
55. COUSER WG, BADGER A, COOPERBAND S, STILMANT M, JERMANOVITCH N, AURORA S, DONER D, SCHMITT G: Hodgkin's disease and nephrotic syndrome. *Lancet* 1:912, 1977
56. SHITARA T, SULLIVAN JP, BREWER ED, KOHL S, RICHIE E, BUTLER JJ: Hodgkin's disease complicated by nephrotic syndrome: New clinical observations on the response of both diseases to radiotherapy to the neck. *Am J Pediatr Hematol Oncol* 3:177–181, 1981
57. CALE WF, ULLRICH IH, JENKINS JJ: Nodular sclerosing Hodgkin's disease presenting as nephrotic syndrome. *South Med J* 75:604–606, 1982
58. CROWLEY JP, REE HJ, ESPARZA A: Monocyte-dependent serum suppression of lymphocyte blastogenesis in Hodgkin's disease: An association with nephrotic syndrome. *J Clin Immunol* 2:270–275, 1982
59. WALKER F, O'NEILL S, CARMODY M, O'DWYER WF: Nephrotic syndrome in Hodgkin's disease. *Int J Pediatr Nephrol* 4:39–41, 1983
60. CASE RECORDS OF THE MASSACHUSETTS GENERAL HOSPITAL: Weekly clinicopathological exercises; case 15–1983. *N Engl J Med* 308:888–896, 1983
61. WATSON A, STACHURA I, FRAGOLA J, BOURKE E: Focal segmental glomerulosclerosis in Hodgkin's disease. *Am J Nephrol* 3:228–232, 1983
62. FOTH R, BADFER K, KARK R: Development of nephrotic syndrome secondary to renal vein thrombosis with bronchogenic carcinoma and Hodgkin's disease. *Ill Med J* 125:505–509, 1964
63. FROOM DW, FRANKLIN WA, HANO JE, POTTER EV: Immune deposits in Hodgkin's disease with nephrotic syndrome. *Arch Pathol* 94:517–553, 1972
64. ROW PG, CAMERON JS, TURNER DS, EVANS DGH, WHITE RHR, OGG CS, CHANTLER C, BROWN CB: Membranous nephropathy: Long-term follow up and association with neoplasia. *Q J Med* 44:207–239, 1975
65. LOKICH JJ, GALVANEK EG, MOLONEY WC: Nephrosis of Hodgkin's disease. *Arch Intern Med* 132:597–600, 1973
66. HYMAN LR, BURKHOLDER PM, JOO PA, SEGAR WE: Malignant lymphoma and nephrotic syndrome. *J Pediatr* 82:207–217, 1973

67. MA KW, GOLBUS SM, KAUFMAN R, STALLY N, LONDER H, BROWN DC: Glomerulonephritis with Hodgkin's disease and herpes zoster. *Arch Pathol Lab Med* 102:527–529, 1978
68. KLEINKNECHT D, MOREL-MAROGER L, CALLARD P, ADHEMAR JP, MAHIEU P: Antiglomerular basement membrane nephritis after solvent exposure. *Arch Int Med* 140:230–232, 1980
69. WILSON CB: Anti-GBM glomerulonephritis, in *Pathology of Glomerular Disease*, edited by ROSEN S, New York, Churchill Livingstone, 1983, pp 171–194
70. ASAMER H, STUHLINGER W, DITTRICH P: Das paraneoplastiche nephrotische syndrom. *Dtsche Med Wochenschr* 99:573–575, 1974
71. KIY Y: Sindrome nefrotica associada a doenca de Hodgkin. *Rev Hosp Clin Fac Med Sao Paulo* 22:186–197, 1967
72. HERSKOWITZ LJ, GOTTLIEB RP, TRAVIS S: Nephrotic syndrome associated with non-Hodgkin's lymphoma: Complete remission with chemotherapy. *Clin Pediatr* 21:441–443, 1982
73. BELGHITI D, VERNANT JP, HIRBEC G, GUBLER MC, ANDRE C, SOBEL A: Nephrotic syndrome associated with T-cell lymphoma. *Cancer* 47:1878–1882, 1981
74. GLUCK MC, GALLO G, LOWENSTEIN J, BALDWIN DS: Membranous glomerulo-nephritis: Evaluation of clinical and pathologic features. *Ann Intern Med* 78:1–12, 1973
75. RABKIN R, THATCHER GN, DIAMOND LH, EALES L: The nephrotic syndrome, malignancy and immunosuppression. *S Afr Med J* 47:605–606, 1973
76. MUGGIA FM: Glomerulonephritis or nephrotic syndrome in malignant lymphoma, reticulum-cell type. *Lancet* 1:805, 1971
77. SUTHERLAND JC, MARTINEY MR: Immune complex disease in the kidneys of lymphoma-leukemia patients: The presence of an oncornavirus-related antigen. *J Natl Cancer Inst* 50:633–644, 1976
78. SAGEL J, MULLER J, LOGAN E: Lymphoma and nephrotic syndrome. *S Afr Med J* 45:79–80, 1971
79. PETZEL RA, BROWN DC, STALEY NA, MCMILLEN JJ, SIBLEY RK, KJELL-STRAND C: Crescentic glomerulonephritis and renal failure associated with malig-nant lymphoma. *Am J Clin Pathol* 71:728–732, 1979
80. SCHUPBACH J, SARNGADHARAN MG, BLAYNEY DW, KALYANARAMAN VS, BUNN PS, GALLO RC: Demonstration of viral antigen ^{24}P in circulating immune complexes of two patients with human T-cell leukaemia/lymphoma virus (HTLV) positive lymphoma. *Lancet* 1:302–305, 1984
81. WOOD WE, HARKINS M: Nephropathy in angioimmunoblastic lymphadenop-athy. *Am J Clin Pathol* 71:58–63, 1979
82. OLDSTONE MBA, THEOFILOPOULOS AN, GUNVEN P, KLEIN G: Immune com-plexes associated with neoplasia: Presence of Epstein-Barr virus antigen-antibody complexes in Burkitt's lymphoma. *Intervirology* 4:292–302, 1974
83. SCOTT RB: Leukemia. *Lancet* 1:1162–1167, 1957
84. LINDER J, SILBERMAN HR, CROKER BP: Amyloidosis complicating hairy cell leukemia. *Am J Clin Pathol* 78:864–867, 1982
85. CAMERON S, OGG CS: Nephrotic syndrome in chronic lymphocytic leukemia. *Br Med J* 4:164, 1979
86. MANDALENAKIS N, MENDOZA N, PIRANI CL, POLLAK VE: Lobular glomerulo-nephritis and membranoproliferative glomerulonephritis: A clinical and patho-logic study based on renal biopsies. *Medicine* 50:319–355, 1971
87. DATHAN JRE, HEYWORTH ME, MACIVER AG: Nephrotic syndrome in chronic lymphocytic leukemia. *Br Med J* 3:655–658, 1974

88. STRIPPOLI P, DE MARCO S, MARINOSCI A, SPEDICATO F, SCATIZZI A: Chronic lymphocytic leukemia and membranoproliferative glomerulonephritis. *Haemotologia* 67:805–807, 1982

89. GILBOA N, DURANTE D, GUGGENHEIM S, LACHER J, HOLMAN R, SCHORR W, GARFIELD D, MCINTOSH RM: Immune deposit nephritis and single-component cryoglobulinemia associated with chronic lymphocytic leukemia. *Nephron* 24:223–231, 1979

90. SUDHOLT BA, HEIRONIMUS JD: Chronic myelogenous leukemia with nephrotic syndrome. *Arch Intern Med* 143:168–169, 1983

91. DOSA S, PHILLIPS TM, ANTONOVYCH TT, SEGAL A, GUBA A, THOMPSON AM: Acute myelomonocytic leukemia associated with nephrotic syndrome: A case report with immunological studies. *Nephron* 43:125–129, 1983

92. JOTHY S, KNAACK J, ONERHEIM RM, BARRÉ PE: Renal involvement in malignant histiocytosis. An immunoperoxidase marker study. *Am J Clin Pathol* 76:183–189, 1981

93. MIYOSHI I, YOSHIMOTO S, OHTSUKI Y, FUJISHITA M, AKAGI T, YOSHIKI T, KOIKE T: Adult T-cell leukaemia antigen in renal glomerulus. *Lancet* 1:768–769, 1983

94. MOREL-MAROGER L, BASCH A, DANON F, VERROUST P, RICHET G: Pathology of the kidney in Waldenstrom's macroglobulinemia: A study of sixteen cases. *N Engl J Med* 283:123–129, 1970

95. MOYNER K, SLETTEN K, HUSBY G, NATVIG JB: An unusually large (83 amino acid residues) amyloid fibril protein AA from a patient with Waldenstrom's macroglobulinemia and amyloidosis. *Scand J Immunol* 11:549–554, 1980

96. SPARGO BH, SEYMOUR AE, ORDENEZ NG: *Paraproteinemia: Renal Pathology with Diagnostic and Therapeutic Implication,* New York, Wiley, 1980, p 374

97. LINDSTROM FD, HED J, ENESTROM JS: Renal pathology of Waldenstrom's macroglobulinemia with monoclonal antiglomerular antibodies and nephrotic syndrome. *Clin Exp Immunol* 41:196–204, 1980

98. FILLASTRE JP, BASCH A, VERGER D, MOREL-MAROGER L, DRUET P, RICHET G: Syndrome nephrotique revelateur d'une maladie de Waldenstrom. *J Urol Nephrol* 74:725–732, 1968

99. LIN JM, OROFINO J, SHERLOCK J, LETTER J, DUFFY JL: Waldenstrom's macroglobulinemia, mesangiocapillary glomerulonephritis, angiitis, and myositis. *Nephron* 10:262–270, 1973

100. SCULLY RE, MARK EJ, MCNEELY BU: Case records of the Massachusetts General Hospital: Case 11–1982. *N Engl J Med* 306:657–668, 1982

101. SHALHOUB RJ: Pathogenesis of lipoid nephrosis, a disorder of T-cell function. *Lancet* 2:556–559, 1974

102. LAGRUE G, XHENEUMONT S, BRANELLEC A, WEIL B: Lymphokines and nephrotic syndrome. *Lancet* 1:271, 1975

103. SUTHERLAND J, MARKHAM RV, RAMSEY HE, MARDINEY MR: Subclinical immune complex nephritis in patients with Hodgkin's disease. *Cancer Res* 34:1179–1181, 1974

104. SUTHERLAND J, MARKHAM RV, MARDINEY MR: Subclinical immune complexes in the glomeruli of the kidneys post mortem. *Am J Med* 57:536–541, 1976

105. PASCAL RR, KOSS MN, KASSEL RL: Glomerulonephritis associated with immune complex deposits and viral particles in spontaneous murine leukemia. *Lab Invest* 29:159–165, 1973

Sickle Cell Nephropathy

Vardaman M. Buckalew, Jr.

It has long been recognized that sickle cell anemia (SCA) is associated with a variety of disorders of renal morphology and function. Some abnormalities seem to be due to direct consequences of abnormal red blood cells, while others may represent random associations. Since there is no animal model for this relatively uncommon condition, understanding the pathophysiology of renal disease depends almost exclusively on studies in humans. In some cases, it may be possible to relate observations in patients to similar phenomena in experimental animals.

Several reviews of this topic have appeared [1–3], with the most recent one being in 1975 [3]. Since then, some new information has accumulated, both in patients with SCA and in the relevant experimental literature. As in our earlier review, we will summarize the various derangements of renal structure and function in SCA with an attempted synthesis of pathophysiologic mechanisms.

Renal Circulation

Renal Blood Flow and Glomerular Filtration Rate

Total renal blood flow (RBF) and glomerular filtration rate (GFR) are increased in young persons with homozygous SCA [4, 5]. Both RBF and GFR may be more than twice that of normal in some persons. The RBF usually is increased more than GFR, so that the filtration fraction is reduced. The extraction ratio for para-aminohippurate (E_{PAH}) is also reduced [4]. This was originally interpreted as being due to increased renal medullary blood flow [4]. However, decreased E_{PAH} is more likely due to the increase in cortical

---

This manuscript was presented as part of a Symposium on *Tropical Nephrology.*

blood flow, reducing transit time and tubular secretion of para-aminohippurate (PAH) [6]. Both RBF and GFR begin to decline about the second or third decade of life, and they may be reduced in older patients [7, 8].

The increase in GFR could be secondary to the high RBF. If so, it would suggest that GFR in these patients is dependent on the rate of renal plasma flow (RPF), as in the rat [9]. The mechanism of the increased RBF is not known. Acute reductions in hematocrit have been shown to increase RBF experimentally [10]. However, correction of anemia by blood transfusion had no effect of RBF in SCA patients [11, 12]. This suggests that anemia alone is not the cause. However, blood transfusions might increase blood volume and RBF [13], tending to cancel any effect of anemia correction to reduce RBF.

It has recently been shown that indomethacin reduces RBF and GFR in SCA [5]. Interestingly, RBF remained higher than in control groups, while GFR returned to normal. This study suggests that prostaglandins play some role in maintaining the elevated renal hemodynamics. However, urinary excretion of prostaglandin was not elevated [14]. Thus, it remains unclear whether there is increased synthesis of vasodilator prostaglandins in SCA, and as to what the stimulus might be.

Medullary Blood Flow

As noted above, the decreased E_{PAH} in young SCA patients led to the suggestion that renal medullary blood flow was increased. However, Van Eps et al [15] showed, via microangiographic techniques in autopsy material, that medullary perfusion was essentially absent in homozygous SCA patients. This observation is compatible with the suggestion of Perillie and Epstein that hypertonicity of the renal medulla increases sickling, which increases blood viscosity and reduces medullary blood flow [16].

Reduced medullary blood flow in the presence of increased total RBF might account for the dilated pelvic mucosal capillaries—the extravasation from which is thought to cause hematuria [17]. Efferent vessels from juxtamedullary glomeruli divide to form the vasa rectae, peritubular capillaries of juxtamedullary nephrons, and nutrient vessels of the renal pelvis [18, 19]. If resistance to flow in vasa rectae were increased, more blood would be shunted to juxtamedullary nephron and pelvic mucosal capillaries, thus causing the observed dilation and congestion of these vessels [2].

Tubular Function

Renal Concentrating Mechanism

Inability to concentrate urine maximally in response to fluid deprivation is a universal finding in a patient with SCA. The defect is not severe, and it usually is not clinically significant. In one series, maximum osmolality ranged from 369 to 767 mOsm/kg [20]. This defect improves strikingly when blood transfusions restore hematocrit to normal in young persons [20], while no improvement is seen in transfused older patients [12, 20].

It is not clear how transfusion might improve function of the renal counter-current mechanism. It probably increases renal medullary blood flow by reducing the percentage of sickled cells in the circulation, thereby reducing the viscosity of blood flowing through the renal medulla. Increased medullary blood flow might reduce the efficiency of the countercurrent mechanism [21]. However, it could be that a markedly reduced papillary blood flow might somehow prevent the vasa rectae from functioning as a countercurrent exchanger [22].

Increased medullary blood flow might increase oxygen delivery; however, this would be most important for the ascending limb, since metabolism of the inner medulla is largely anaerobic [23]. There are suggestions that thick ascending limb function may be normal in SCA patients, despite a decrease in maximum concentrating ability. Thus, in three studies, tubular reabsorption of free water ($T^c_{H_2O}$) was normal during solute diuresis induced by mannitol [22, 24, 25] and saline [25]. However, in a more recent study, Forrester and Alleyne found that $T^c_{H_2O}$ was reduced during solute diuresis induced by hypertonic sodium chloride [26]. The cause for the discrepancy is not certain.

These same authors found that the reduction of fractional excretion of sodium (FE_{Na}) after ethacrynic acid in SCA was comparable to normal groups. The reduction of FE_{Na} was due to the fact that GFR was higher in SCA patients. They suggested that reduced FE_{Na} in response to ethacrynic acid indicated an abnormal function of the thick ascending loop of Henle. However this argument is weak in view of the fact that absolute urinary sodium excretion was the same in SCA and normal groups. An increase in the filtered load of sodium would not necessarily cause absolute urinary sodium to be increased following administration of a loop diuretic. Thus, the weight of evidence continues to suggest that sodium reabsorption by the thick ascending loop of Henle is essentially normal in SCA patients.

DeJong et al have recently studied the effects of indomethacin on renal concentration and dilution in SCA patients [27]. They found that during water deprivation, prostaglandin inhibition had no effect on urine osmolality. This strongly suggests that prostaglandins play no role in the concentration defect. In water-loaded subjects, however, prostaglandin inhibition caused increased urine osmolality, decreased urine volume, but no change in GFR. Fractional sodium excretion was also reduced. Indomethacin had no effect on urine osmolality in normal control subjects. The mechanism of this indomethacin-induced impairment in water excretion is not known, and further studies including plasma vasopressin levels will be necessary. The fall in sodium excretion is similar to that reported in patients receiving nonsteroidal anti-inflammatory drugs (NSAIDs) therapeutically [28]—the mechanism of which is unknown.

Renal Acid Excretion

Several studies have demonstrated a defect in lowering urine pH in response to acid loading in many patients with SCA [29–31]. Since most of these patients do not have metabolic acidosis, they would be classified as having incomplete renal tubular acidosis [30], which is a variant of type I or "classic" renal tubular acidosis.

In addition, patients with SCA also have an inability to excrete potassium, which suggests a defect in distal tubular potassium secretion [32]. Rarely, the defect in potassium secretion leads to hyperkalemia and occurs in combination with metabolic acidosis—so-called type IV renal tubular acidosis [33, 34]. Type IV renal tubular acidosis is typically associated with urine pH below 5.5, indicating a normal ability to generate a distal hydrogen ion gradient. However, as noted above, patients with SCA usually have a type I defect in lowering urine pH. Therefore, the occasional SCA patient with type IV usually has type I renal tubular acidosis as well. Two patients with SCA have been reported with type IV renal tubular acidosis alone due to hypoaldosteronism [34]. The combination of types I and IV renal tubular acidosis is unusual, although not unique to SCA [33, 35]; and, it suggests a diffuse defect in collecting duct function.

Proximal Tubular Function

Uric acid production is increased in SCA patients due to chronic hemolysis. Most younger patients maintain normal serum urate levels, because tubular secretion of urate is increased [36]. However, hyperuricemia occurs with increasing frequency in older subjects, in association with return of RBF [36] to normal values. It appears that increased urate secretion is dependent on supernormal RBF.

Phosphate reabsorption was found to be increased in a series of SCA patients with mild elevations of serum phosphorus [37]. These same investigators reported increased tubular reabsorption of β-2 microglobulin, and they have suggested that SCA is associated with a diffuse abnormality in proximal tubular function [38]. The existence and possible significance of this postulated abnormality remains to be evaluated.

Glomerular Pathology

Increasingly, SCA patients are reported with glomerular insufficiency, nephrotic syndrome, and end-stage renal disease (ESRD) [39–43]. It now seems clear that renal insufficiency in SCA is not due to the fortuitous occurrence of glomerular disease, although this phenomenon undoubtedly does occur [39]. However, the relationship between abnormal red blood cells and glomerular pathology remains obscure.

Glomerular morphology in SCA patients who die without evidence of renal disease is well characterized. Glomeruli are enlarged (most prominently in the juxtamedullary area) and engorged with red blood cells, many of which appear sickled [17, 44, 45]. In addition, some appear to be mildly hypercellular on light microscopy [44]. Iron deposits may be seen in glomerular epithelial cells [2]. On electron microscopy, electron-dense deposits and a fibrillar-appearing material may be present in the mesangial matrix [44]. Varying degrees of mesangial proliferation [44] and reduplication of glomerular basement membrane (GBM) are also seen [39]. More extensive changes have been reported in patients with nephrotic syndrome. To a large extent, glomerular alterations in nephrotic syndrome represent more severe degrees of the abnormalities that are observed in patients without clinical evidence of renal disease. Mesangial cell proliferation, expansion of mesangial matrix, and reduplication of GBM are more prominent [39, 41]. Electron-dense deposits are more common, and they are seen in structures other than the mesangium [46]. Diffuse glomerular sclerosis may be seen [39].

Immunofluorescent studies of glomeruli give heterogeneous results. Elfenbein et al reported negative immunofluorescence in two cases with nephrotic syndrome [39]. However, Pardo et al described seven cases of glomerular disease, five of which had nephrotic syndrome and renal insufficiency with IgG and C3 in a granular pattern along the GBM and the mesangium [41]. IgM, Clq, C4, and C2 were also found. Renal tubular antigen was localized in the same pattern as immunoglobulins and C3 in two of the subjects [41].

The pathophysiology of glomerular lesions in SCA is unknown. McCoy suggested that mesangial cell proliferation and nephrotic syndrome might be due to iron deposits in the glomerulus. Elfenbein et al suggested that mesangial cell proliferation was caused by phagocytosis of red blood cell debris [39]. This suggestion is not unlike that of McCoy's, since red blood cell debris probably would contain iron. Pardo et al have made an entirely different suggestion. They proposed that patients with both SCA and nephrotic syndrome have a membranoproliferative glomerulonephritis due to immune complexes that contain renal tubular epithelial cells as antigen [41]. A third possible mechanism of glomerular sclerosis in SCA is chronic hyperperfusion of glomeruli with hyperfiltration of protein [47]. Increased GFR per nephron is surely present in young patients with SCA. If the hypotheses developed in rats have relevance to human disease, then SCA may offer a model for observing this phenomenon.

Possible causes of glomerular injury in SCA are summarized in Table 1. None of the mechanisms are mutually exclusive and all could be acting synergistically. It is possible that the decline in renal function with age is due to a combination of these mechanisms that operates over time to cause glomerular damage. However, the association between GFR and age in SCA is weak. Regardless of the pathophysiology, it seems clear that all patients with SCA have an underlying process tending to cause glomerular disease, which occasionally leads to heavy proteinuria and ESRD. Severe renal involvement seems to occur most frequently in patients with frequent, painful crises.

Table 1. Glomerular insults in SCA

Hyperfiltration
Phagocytosis by mesangial cells of
Iron
Red blood cell fragments
Immune complexes

Is There a Sickle Cell Nephropathy?

An entity called sickle cell nephropathy could be postulated if clinical syndromes could be attributed to abnormalities in structure and function due specifically to the presence of sickle hemoglobin in red blood cells.

Table 2 summarizes those abnormalities in renal function, which probably are due to sickle hemoglobin (as discussed earlier) and to the clinical syndromes that may be attributed to them. Marked medullary hypoperfusion due to sickled cells in the renal medulla may lead to a functional papillectomy, thus causing a renal concentrating defect and abnormal hydrogen ion and potassium secretion by the collecting duct. This abnormality may also occasionally lead to frank, acute papillary necrosis.

Cortical hyperperfusion may not be due specifically to sickle cells, but there is no comparable condition known in renal pathologic physiology. Regardless of the cause, overperfusion of blood vessels in juxtamedullary cortex, which supply nutrient vessels in the renal pelvic mucosa, probably accounts for intermittent hematuria. Glomerular hyperfiltration, which is probably secondary to cortical hyperperfusion, may contribute to development of the glomerular lesions that lead to a nephrotic syndrome and chronic renal failure. Other factors possibly involved are summarized in Table 1.

Clinical Management

Hematuria

Numerous therapies have been proposed for the treatment of hematuria. The most effective probably is aminocaproic acid [48], which can be used apparently without the problem of ureteral clotting and obstruction.

Nephrotic Syndrome

Most cases of nephrotic syndrome in SCA are associated with the lesions described above. Occasionally, "nil disease," or acute poststreptococcal glomerulonephritis, may occur coincidentally [39]. No cases of nephrotic syndrome due to sickle cell-related glomerular pathology have been reported to respond to steroid or other immunosuppressive therapy. Accordingly, steroids should not be used unless a renal biopsy specimen shows a nil lesion. This is not

Table 2. Sickle cell nephropathy

Functional disorder	Clinical syndrome
Medullary hypoperfusion	Polyuria Types I and IV renal tubular acidosis Papillary necrosis
Cortical hyperperfusion	Hematuria
Glomerular hyperfiltration	Nephrotic syndrome Renal failure

likely to occur in homozygous SCA, but it may occur in heterozygous SCA [39].

Renal Failure

Patients with ESRD can be maintained on dialysis and can be successfully transplanted, despite their tendency for intravascular clotting [40, 42, 43]. Thus, renal replacement therapy should be offered to them.

Papillary Necrosis

Acute papillary necrosis may occur with no provocation. Nonsteroidal anti-inflammatory drugs may cause acute papillary necrosis in some otherwise normal patients [49], and they probably should not be used in SCA.

Renal Tubular Acidosis

The rare patient who develops acidosis should be treated with adequate bicarbonate, since acidosis may precipitate sickle crises [50]. Alkali therapy may also control hyperkalemia, if that abnormality is present. Other standard methods of treating hyperkalemia, such as kayexalate, may also be necessary.

Summary

Several disorders of renal anatomy and function are found in patients with sickle cell anemia (SCA). Maximum urine osmolality is impaired, but urine dilution is intact and negative free water clearance during solute diuresis is normal. In young patients, overall renal blood flow (RBF) and glomerular filtration rate (GFR) are increased, whereas RBF and GFR are normal or reduced in older patients. The hyperdynamic renal circulation is dependent on the presence of prostaglandins, since prostaglandin inhibitors return RBF and GFR to normal. Papillary blood flow probably is reduced in all homozygous patients. Potassium excretion is impaired, and a defect in lowering urine pH is present in some patients. Increased tubular reabsorption of phosphate and increased secretion of uric acid have been reported.

The most common clinical disorder in SCA is hematuria, which probably is due to leakage of red blood cells from hyperemic, dilated renal pelvic blood vessels. Chronic renal failure, sometimes preceded by nephrotic syndrome, is observed—the prevalence of which is not known. Lesions associated with renal failure resemble glomerular sclerosis and membranoproliferative glomerulonephritis. Glomerular sclerosis may be secondary to chronic hyperfiltration. Patients with end-stage renal disease (ESRD) tolerate hemodialysis and transplantation with no increase in complications.

The constellation of renal abnormalities in SCA is unique; hence, the concept of "sickle cell nephropathy" seems to be justified.

References

1. SCHLITT LE, KEITEL HG: Renal manifestations of sickle cell disease: a review. *Am J Med Sci* 239:773–778, 1960

2. BUCKALEW VM JR, SOMEREN A: Renal manifestations of sickle cell disease. *Arch Intern Med* 133:660–669, 1974

3. ALLEYNE GAO, STATIUS VAN EPS LW, ADDAE SK, NICHOLSON GD, SCHOUTEN H: The kidney in sickle cell anemia. *Kidney Int* 7:371–379, 1975

4. HATCH FE, AZAR SH, AINSWORTH TE, NARDO JM, CULBERTSON JW: Renal circulatory studies in young adults with sickle cell anemia. *J Lab Clin Med* 76:632–640, 1970

5. DEJONG PE, DEJONG-VAN DEN BERG LTW, SEWRAJSINGH GS, SCHOUTEN H, DONKER AJM, STATIUS VAN EPS LW: The influence of indomethacin on renal hemodynamics in sickle cell anaemia. *Clin Sci* 59:245–250, 1980

6. VELASQUEZ MT, NOTARGIACOMO AV, COHN JN: Influence of cortical plasma transit time on p-aminohippurate extraction during induced renal vasodilation in anesthetized dogs. *Clin Sci* 43:401–411, 1972

7. ETTELDORF JN, SMITH JD, TUTTLE AH, DIGGS LW: Renal hemodynamic studies in adults with sickle cell anemia. *Am J Med* 18:243–248, 1955

8. MORGAN AG, SERJEANT GR: Renal function in patients over 40 with hemozygous sickle-cell disease. *Br Med J* 282:1181–1183, 1981

9. BRENNER BM, TROY JL, DAUGHARTY TM, DEEN WM, ROBERTSON CR: Dynamics of glomerular ultrafiltration in the rat: II. Plasma-flow dependence of GFR. *Am J Physiol* 223:1184–1190, 1972

10. SCHRIER RW, EARLEY LE: Effects of hematocrit on renal hemodynamics and sodium excretion in hydropenic and volume expanded dogs. *J Clin Invest* 49:1656–1667, 1970

11. KEITEL HG, THOMPSON D, ITANO HA: Hypostheruria in sickle cell anemia: a reversible renal defect. *J Clin Invest* 35:998–1007, 1956

12. STATIUS VAN EPS LW, SCHOUTEN H, LA PORTE-WIJSMAN LW, STRUYKER-BOUDIER AM: The influence of red blood cell transfusions on the hypostheruria and renal hemodynamics of sickle cell anemia. *Clin Chim Acta* 17:449–461, 1967

13. BAHLMAN J, MCDONALD SJ, DUNNINGHAM JG, DEWARDENER HE: The effect on urinary sodium excretion of blood volume expansion without changing the composition of blood in the dog. *Clin Sci* 32:403–413, 1967

14. DEJONG PE, SALEH AW, DEZEEUW D, DONKER AJM, VAN DER HEM GK, STATIUS VAN EPS LW: Prostaglandin-vasopressin interactions in sickle cell nephropathy (*abstract*). *Kidney Int* 23:277, 1983

15. STATIUS VAN EPS LW, PINEDO-VEELS C, DEVRIES CH, DEKONING J: Nature of the concentrating defect in sickle cell nephropathy: microradioangiographic studies. *Lancet* 1:450–452, 1970

16. PERILLIE PE, EPSTEIN FH: Sickling phenomenon produced by hypertonic solutions: a possible explanation for the hypothenuria of sicklemia. *J Clin Invest* 42:570–580, 1963

17. MOSTOFI KF, VORDER BRUEGGE CF, DIGGS LW: Lesions in kidneys removed for unilateral hematuria in sickle cell disease. *Arch Pathol* 63:336–351, 1957

18. MOFFAT DB, FOURRNAN J: The vascular pattern of rat kidney. *J Anat* 97:543–553, 1963

19. THORBURN GD, KOPALD HH, HERD JA, HOLLENBERG M, O'MORCHOE CCC, BARGER AC: Intrarenal distribution of nutrient blood flow determined with krypton[85] in the unanesthetized dog. *Circ Res* 13:290–307, 1963

20. KEITEL HG, THOMPSON D, ITANO HA: Hypostheruria in sickle cell anemia: a reversible renal defect. *J Clin Invest* 35:998–1007, 1956

21. BERLINER RW, BENNETT CM: Concentration of urine in the mammalian kidney. *Am J Med* 42:777–789, 1967

22. LEVITT MF, HAUSER AD, POLIMEROS D: The renal concentrating defect in sickle cell disease. *Am J Med* 29:611–622, 1960

23. SCAGLIONE PR, DELL RB, WINTERS RW: Lactate concentration in the medulla of rat kidney. *Am J Physiol* 209:1193–1198, 1965
24. WHITTEN CF, YOUNES AA: A comparative study of renal concentrating ability in children with sickle cell anemia and in normal children. *J Lab Clin Med* 55:400–415, 1960
25. HATCH FE, CULBERTSON JW, DIGGS LW: Nature of the renal concentrating defect in sickle cell disease. *J Clin Invest* 46:336–345, 1967
26. FORRESTER TE, ALLEYNE GAO: Excretion of salt and water by patients with sickle-cell anemia: effect of a diuretic and solute diuresis. *Clin Sci Mol Med* 53:523–527, 1977
27. DEJONG PE, DEJONG-VAN DEN BERG LTW, DE ZEEUW D, DANKER AJM, SCHOUTEN H, STATIUS VAN EPS LW: The influence of indomethacin on renal concentrating and diluting capacity in sickle cell nephropathy. *Clin Sci* 63:53–58, 1982
28. CLIVE DM, STAFF JS: Renal syndromes associated with nonsteroidal antiinflammatory drugs. *N Engl J Med* 310:563–572, 1984
29. HO PING KONG H, ALLEYNE GAO: Defect in urinary acidification in adults with sickle cell anemia. *Lancet* 2:954–955, 1968
30. GOOSENS JP, STATIUS VAN EPS LW, SCHOUTEN H: Incomplete renal tubular acidosis in sickle cell disease. *Clin Chim Acta* 41:149–156, 1972
31. OSTER JR, LESPIER LE, LEE SM, PELLEGRINI EL, VAAMONDE CA: Renal acidification in sickle cell disease. *J Lab Clin Med* 88:389–401, 1976
32. DEFRANZO RA, TAUFIELD PA, BLACK H, McPHEDRAN P, COOKE CR: Impaired renal tubular potassium secretion in sickle cell disease. *Ann Intern Med* 90:310–316, 1979
33. BATTLE DC, SEHY JT, ROSEMAN MK, ARRUDA JAL, KURTZMAN NA: Clinical and pathophysiologic spectrum of acquired distal RTA. *Kidney Int* 20:389–396, 1981
34. BATTLE DC, ITSARAYOUNGYUEN K, ARRUDA JAL, KURTZMAN NA: Hyperkalemic hyperchloremic metabolic acidosis in patients with sickle cell hemoglobin. *Am J Med* 72:188–192, 1982
35. BATTLE DC, ARRUDA JAL, KURTZMAN NA: Hyperkalemic distal renal tubular acidosis associated with obstructive uropathy. *N Engl J Med* 304:373–380, 1981
36. DIAMOND HS, MEISEL AD, HOLDEN D: The natural history of urate overproduction in sickle cell anemia. *Ann Intern Med* 90:752–757, 1979
37. DEJONG PE, DEJONG-VAN DEN BERG LTW, STATIUS VAN EPS LW: The tubular reabsorption of phosphate in sickle cell nephropathy. *Clin Sci Mol Med* 55:429–434, 1978
38. DEJONG PE, DEJONG-VAN DEN BERG LTW, SEWRAJSINGH GS, SCHOUTEN H, DONKER AJM, STATIUS VAN EPS LW: Beta-2-Microglobulin in sickle cell anemia. *Nephron* 29:138–141, 1981
39. ELFENBEIN IB, PATCHEFSKY A, SCHWARTZ W, WEINSTEIN AG: Pathology of the glomerulus in sickle cell anemia with and without nephrotic syndrome. *Am J Pathol* 77:357–374, 1974
40. FRIEDMAN EA, SREEPADA RAO TK, SPRUNG CL, SMITH A, MANIS T, BELLEVUE R, BUTT KMH, LEVERE RD, HOLDEN DM: Uremia in sickle-cell anemia treated by maintenance hemodialysis. *N Engl J Med* 291:431–435, 1974
41. PARDO V, STRAUSS J, KRAMER H, OZAWA T, McINTOSH RM: Nephropathy associated with sickle cell anemia: an autologous immune complex nephritis. *Am J Med* 59:650–659, 1975
42. CHATTERJEE SN: National study on natural history of renal allografts in sickle cell disease or trait. *Nephron* 25:199–201, 1980

43. GONZALES-CARRILLO M, RUDGE CJ, PARSONS V, BEWICK M, WHITE JM: Renal transplantation in sickle cell disease. *Clin Nephrol* 18:209–210, 1982
44. PITCOCK JA, MUIRHEAD EE, HATCH FE, JOHNSON JG, KELLY BJ: Early renal changes in sickle cell anemia. *Arch Pathol* 90:403–410, 1970
45. BERNSTEIN J, WHITTEN CF: A histologic appraisal of the kidney in sickle cell anemia. *Arch Pathol* 70:407–418, 1960
46. McCOY RC: Ultrastructural alterations in the kidney of patients with sickle cell disease and the nephrotic syndrome. *Lab Invest* 21:85–95, 1969
47. BRENNER BM, MEYER TW, HOSTETTER TH: Dietary protein intake and the progressive nature of kidney disease: the role of hemodynamically mediated glomerular injury in the pathogenesis of progressive glomerular sclerosis in aging, renal ablation, and intrinsic renal disease. *N Engl J Med* 307:652–659, 1982
48. BLACK WD, HATCH FE, ACCHIARDO S: Aminocaproic acid in prolonged hematuria of patients with sicklemia. *Arch Intern Med* 136:678–681, 1976
49. CARUANA RJ, SEMBLE EL: Renal papillary necrosis due to naproxen. *J Rheum* 11:90–91, 1984
50. BARRERAS L, DIGGS LW: Sodium citrate orally for painful sickle cell crisis. *JAMA* 215:762–768, 1971

Tubular Defects

Isolated Tubular Defects

Chairpersons: Russell W. Chesney and Bernard S. Kaplan
Discussants: James C. M. Chan, Guido O. Perez, Juan Rodríguez-Soriano, and Robert L. Chevalier

This Workshop focused on some of the more recently described syndromes that present as isolated defects in the renal tubular reabsorption of organic solutes, ions, and water. Emphasis was placed on methods of evaluation and diagnosis of these conditions, newer laboratory studies, pathophysiology, and management.

Renal Hypophosphatemic Rickets

Several recent studies suggest that there is a selective disorder of renal phosphate transport underlying X-linked hypophosphatemic rickets. It involves that component of phosphate transport that is responsive to parathyroid hormone (PTH), and it occurs as a transepithelial transport defect at the brushborder membrane of the kidney. In addition, however, there are associated defects in vitamin D metabolism.

Chesney and associates found that patients with hypophosphatemic rickets had a mean serum 1,25-dihydroxyvitamin D (1,25[OH]$_2$D) concentration of 16.9 pg/ml, which was significantly lower than the 47 pg/ml found in 27 healthy, age-matched controls. Their serum levels of PTH, calcium, and phosphate remained normal, however, suggesting a defect in the release of 1,25(OH)$_2$D. These observations were also seen in untreated adult patients with sex-linked dominant hypophosphatemic rickets. Acute phosphate deprivation augmented by phosphate binders in patients with familial hypophosphatemic rickets failed to evoke the expected rise in plasma concentration of 1,25(OH)$_2$D compared to normal controls. These recent data suggest that the renal 1-α-hydroxylase response to hypophosphatemia is defective.

Using the X-linked hypophosphatemic mouse model, many investigators

---

This is a summary of a Workshop by the same title.

found evidence that further supported a defective renal 1-α-hydroxylase activity as being central to this syndrome. Data derived in experimental animals may not apply fully to the human condition, however.

Based on currently available data, the following pathophysiologic sequence seems pertinent. The sex-linked dominant defect gives rise to a decreased renal tubular threshold for phosphorus as well as a defective renal 1-α-hydroxylase activity. PTH is among the humoral factors that modulate the decreased renal tubular threshold for phosphorus, resulting in hypophosphatemia. The defective renal 1-α-hydroxylase activity results in an inadequate production of serum $1,25(OH)_2D$ relative to the hypophosphatemia. It is possible that a partial end-organ resistance to $1,25(OH)_2D$, as well as PTH, may be present in this syndrome. However, the finding that renal tubular phosphate wasting occurs despite parathyroidectomy must also be considered.

A complete pathophysiologic sequence is difficult to construct at present. Any sequence, however, must explain rickets, bone deformities, short stature, dental pulp abnormalities, and osteomalacia.

Abnormalities of Renal Potassium Excretion

Hyperkalemia attributable to a decreased renal potassium excretion or to acidification abnormalities resistant to correction by exogenous mineralocorticoids has been described in patients exhibiting normal to moderately reduced glomerular filtration rate (GFR). This constellation of findings, referred to as "renal tubular hyperkalemia," has been reported as a transient abnormality in infants (pseudohypoaldosteronism), in patients with an unusual condition characterized by hyperkalemia, acidosis, hypertension, and normal GFR (chloride-shunt syndrome), and in patients with predominantly tubulointerstitial disease.

In the pseudohypoaldosteronism group, infants (type I) present with failure to thrive, renal sodium wasting, acidosis, and an elevated plasma renin activity and plasma aldosterone concentration. No structural abnormality of the kidney has been reported, and recent data suggest a genetic predisposition. The leading hypothesis is that the primary abnormality is a defect in renal sodium handling.

Patients with the "chloride-shunt" syndrome (type II) may show an abnormal increase in distal tubular chloride reabsorption such that the mineralocorticoid-induced, charge-dependent driving force for potassium and hydrogen ion secretion is attenuated by the voltage-shunting effect of excessive chloride reabsorption. It is believed that the increase in sodium chloride reabsorption also causes an expansion of the ECF volume, hypertension, and hypoaldosteronism. Of interest, a similar defect has been postulated as the pathogenic mechanism in patients receiving drugs that inhibit prostaglandin synthesis.

The third group of hyperkalemic patients (type III) includes those with tubulointerstitial renal disease and varying aldosterone levels. In patients with obstructive uropathy, it has been postulated that a failure of distal tubular sodium reabsorption reduces the transtubular potential difference, thus interfering with both potassium and hydrogen ion secretion. In contrast with patients who have hypoaldosteronism, these patients also may exhibit an inability to acidify the urine during acidosis, so that the condition also has been referred to as "hyperkalemic distal RTA." A similar defect may occur after the administration of diuretics that interfere with distal tubular sodium reabsorption, such as amiloride. Many patients in this group have been found to have reduced plasma renin and aldosterone levels. It is possible that both abnormalities arise independently as a consequence of structural renal damage; on the other hand, they may be causally related. For example, chronic hyperchloremia and acidosis might conceivably depress renin production, which in turn could lead to hypoaldosteronism.

Nephrogenic Diabetes Insipidus

Nephrogenic diabetes insipidus (NDI) includes a heterogeneic and heterogeneous group of conditions in which the kidneys are unable to concentrate urine despite having adequate levels of circulating antidiuretic hormone (ADH). ADH receptors are present in the basolateral portion of the collecting duct epithelium. Once ADH binds to the receptor, adenyl cyclase is stimulated, cyclic AMP is cleaved, and a protein kinase is stimulated. This results in a phosphorylation of plasma membranes, which enhances their permeability to water. Colchicine, intracellular calcium, and prostaglandins blunt the effect of ADH by inhibiting the aggregation of microtubules.

Hereditary NDI is usually an X-linked condition in which carrier females can have a mild concentrating defect. Polyuria beginning in infancy, polydipsia, dehydration, pyrexia, vomiting, and failure to thrive are the major clinical features. There appear to be at least two types of hereditary NDI based on urinary cyclic AMP responses to ADH administration. The more common form is "type I," with no increase in cyclic AMP. In "type II," urine cyclic AMP increases after ADH, and the inheritance may be autosomal-dominant. Administration of cyclic AMP or dibutyryl cyclic AMP does not reduce free-water clearance in hereditary NDI. Indomethacin inhibits prostaglandin synthesis and improves urine concentration. Indomethacin plus chlorothiazide further enhances urine concentration and reduces urine output. Acquired causes of NDI include: hypokalemia, hypercalcemia, amyloidosis, obstructive nephropathy, drugs (lithium, colchicine), chronic renal failure, and adrenal insufficiency.

Primary and Secondary Pseudohypoaldosteronism in Infancy

Pseudohypoaldosteronism is a rare disorder of electrolyte homeostasis. It is characterized by an apparent state of distal tubular insensitivity to the action of aldosterone, manifested by hyperkalemia, hyponatremia, metabolic acidosis, and a marked increase in plasma aldosterone concentrations.

Since first described in 1958, primary pseudohypoaldosteronism has been reported in some 50 patients. It is probably autosomal-dominant in nature. Infants present with failure to thrive, weight loss, vomiting, and dehydration. Variants of the syndrome with resistance to aldosterone in multiple organs (sweat and salivary glands and colon) have also been reported. Adrenal function and ordinary tests of renal function are normal. Primary pseudohypoaldosteronism is distinguished from primary hypoaldosteronism by a lack of patient improvement despite large doses of DOCA and by a normal ratio of tetrahydroaldosterone to 18-hydroxytetrahydro-compound A. Although the lesion persists, improvement may occur owing to maturation of proximal tubular function and development of salt appetite. A partial defect in the aldosterone receptor (either quantitative or qualitative), which can be offset by increasing the hormone levels, may be accounted for by a reduced Na-K-ATPase activity, which was found in microdissected tubules from one patient. A postulated defect in proximal tubular reabsorption of sodium is unlikely, since this would cause hypokalemia rather than hyperkalemia.

Secondary pseudohypoaldosteronism is rare in infancy. Tubular insensitivity to aldosterone probably accounts for the salt loss observed in many adult patients with chronic tubulointerstitial nephritis or after kidney transplantation. It may also occur in infancy, after renal vein thrombosis, or after medullary necrosis.

A syndrome of renal tubular resistance to aldosterone has been observed in infants with obstructive uropathy and urinary tract infection. They presented with fever, vomiting, polyuria, dehydration, and failure to thrive. They showed bacteriologic evidence of infection, radiologic evidence of hydronephrosis, as well as evidence of hyponatremia, hyperkalemia, and metabolic acidosis. Plasma aldosterone concentration was markedly elevated, and plasma renin activity was normal or high. Although the fractional excretion of potassium was not significantly different from control values, the fractional sodium excretion was significantly increased. Thus, the urinary potassium-to-sodium ratio was significantly lower in these patients. After medical or surgical therapy, all studies normalized. The possibility that a hyperkalemic salt-losing state may arise in infants with obstructive uropathy and urinary tract infection as a consequence of tubular unresponsiveness to aldosterone should be ruled out before making a diagnosis of primary pseudohypoaldosteronism.

Fanconi Syndrome with Hypercalciuria

Fanconi syndrome, a renal tubular disorder manifested by a decreased tubular reabsorption of phosphate, glucose, and amino acids, also has defects in the tubular reabsorption of protein, sodium, potassium, and uric acids. Occasionally, hypercalciuria (urinary calcium excretion greater than 4 mg/kg/d) also has been reported. Four boys have been described with rickets, short stature, phosphaturia, aminoaciduria, and hypercalciuria, but not glucosuria. More recently, Salti and Hemady reported a child with nephrolithiasis plus all the criteria of Fanconi syndrome. Unlike the two adults with Fanconi syndrome and nephrolithiasis who were found to have impaired renal acidification, all these children had normal urinary acid handling.

One explanation for the development of hypercalciuria in Fanconi syndrome is a reduced proximal tubular sodium reabsorption, as calcium and sodium excretion are correlated in hypercalciuric states. However, both sodium conservation and renal acidification were shown to be normal in a child with Fanconi syndrome and hypercalciuria. Furthermore, hypercalciuria in this patient was dependent on renal phosphate wasting, as urinary calcium excretion normalized following oral phosphate supplementation. The development of positive calcium balance also has been shown to result from phosphate supplementation in adults with Fanconi syndrome, and urinary calcium excretion decreases with phosphate replacement in certain types of idiopathic hypercalciuria. The mechanism for hypercalciuria in phosphate depletion states is not clear, but may result from decreased calcium reabsorption both in proximal and distal nephron segments or in deeper nephron populations. Although intestinal calcium absorption has been found to be increased in some patients with Fanconi syndrome, others have demonstrated persistent hypercalciuria during dietary calcium restriction. In addition, circulating $1,25(OH)_2D$ levels are reportedly low or normal in patients and in experimental models of Fanconi syndrome, despite the fact that hypophosphatemia is a potent stimulus for $1,25(OH)_2D$ synthesis. This implies a defect in the control of vitamin D metabolism. It is therefore likely that bone resorption contributes at least in part to urinary calcium losses and that it may be responsible for the progression of rickets or osteomalacia.

Although phosphate supplementation alone results in healing of rickets and correction of hypercalciuria in some patients with Fanconi syndrome, others may have hypercalciuria unrelated to phosphate balance or intestinal calcium absorption. Furthermore, the normal or low urinary calcium excretion of patients with hypophosphatemic rickets indicates that the hypercalciuria of Fanconi syndrome cannot be explained by a direct effect of hyperphosphaturia. It has been postulated that a humoral factor responsible for hypercalciuria is released in some patients with Fanconi syndrome, but not in those with hypophosphatemic rickets. It remains to be proven that phosphaturia in Fanconi syndrome can actually result in tissue phosphate depletion and hypercalciuria. Because Fanconi syndrome represents a heterogeneous group of renal tubular disorders, it is not surprising that hypercalciuria is an inconstant finding and that underlying mechanisms vary among patients. However, as vitamin D preparations are routinely administered to patients with Fanconi syndrome, urine calcium excretion should be monitored and reduced, with hydrochlorothiazide added if necessary.

Aminoaciduria

Aminoaciduria occurs when an excess amount of amino acid is excreted in the urine. This pathologic process can involve a single amino acid, a group of amino acids transported by a similar ("group-related") process, or virtually all amino acids ("generalized"). Aminoaciduria occurs by at least seven postulated (but unproven) mechanisms:

1. Whenever the filtered load of an amino acid exceeds the transport capacity of the renal tubule, an "overload" or a "prerenal" aminoaciduria can occur. Most inborn errors of amino acid metabolism exhibit this type of aminoaciduria, because the plasma concentration of individual amino acids that are poorly metabolized rises sharply.

2. When there is a defective proximal tubular system ("transport protein") for amino acid reabsorption, aminoaciduria occurs, leading to depletion of the amino acid involved.

3. When a single amino acid is reabsorbed poorly, reabsorption of other amino acids that are transported by the same system can be depressed, and this can lead to a more generalized aminoaciduria. Cystinuria is an example of this type of abnormality, because dibasic amino acids are excreted in excessive amounts even though the primary defect lies in cystine reabsorption.

4. When one amino acid accumulates because of impaired metabolism, it is filtered in excess amounts and can depress reabsorption of amino acids that are reabsorbed by the same transport system. An example of this occurred in a patient with hyper-β-alaninemia (presumably related to defective transamination of β-alanine) and led to the excretion of large amounts of taurine, β-aminoisobutyrate, and γ-alanine.

5. When the brushborder or basolateral membrane is "leaky," extensive back diffusion of reabsorbed amino acids can occur and overwhelm reabsorption. Such a mechanism has been postulated to account for the generalized aminoaciduria that occurs in some forms of the Fanconi syndrome.

6. When defective transport of amino acids across the basolateral membrane occurs, high intracellular amino acid concentrations could also lead to backflux of amino acids into the tubular lumen. This pathophysiologic sequence has been proposed to account for the defective lysine transport in lysinuric protein intolerance and for the aminoaciduria that occurs in "classical" cystinuria.

7. When a metabolic end-product accumulates in the tubule epithelium, it might lower reabsorption rates. Such a mechanism has been suggested as the cause of the generalized aminoaciduria of galactosemia and hereditary fructose intolerance, because galactose-1-phosphate or fructose-1-phosphate accumulates within the renal tubular cell in these disorders.

Exploration of amino acid transport has been hampered by the difficulty in obtaining sufficient renal tissue and membrane to explore these putative mechanisms. Recently, at least four techniques seem applicable: (1) measurement of amino acid accumulation by isolated brushborder membranes from animals; (2) measurement of efflux of amino acid from isolated tubules or slices; (3) uptake by long-term renal cortex cells grown in culture; and (4) examination of transport by human renal cortex grown in culture. Use of these techniques may improve our understanding of the mechanisms of aminoaciduria.

Obstructive Uropathy and Urinary Reflux

Pathophysiology of Obstructive Uropathy

Chairpersons: Wadi N. Suki and Douglas R. Wilson
Discussants: A. Erik G. Persson, George A. Tanner,
William E. Yarger, Saulo Klahr, Michael H. Humphreys,
Adrian Spitzer, Ulla C. Kopp, and Elsa Bello-Reuss

Obstruction of one or both kidneys results in a number of alterations in glomerular and tubular function, both during obstruction and following the release of obstruction. The early period following obstruction is accompanied by renal vasodilatation, which is followed subsequently by progressive renal vasoconstriction. These changes in renal hemodynamics are associated with changes in interstitial hydrostatic and oncotic pressures, which in turn appear to influence the setting of the tubuloglomerular feedback mechanism. The setting of tubuloglomerular feedback can be assessed by measuring proximal tubular stop-flow pressure while perfusing the loop of Henle and distal nephron at rates varying from subnormal to supranormal. In the normal kidney, when the perfusion rate exceeds the normal level, the stop-flow pressure falls sharply. Conditions such as extracellular fluid volume expansion, which increase interstitial hydrostatic pressure and/or decrease interstitial oncotic pressure, blunt the tubuloglomerular feedback by increasing the threshold perfusion rate at which stop-flow pressure would fall and by blunting the degree of reduction in stop-flow pressure. By contrast, conditions such as hypovolemia, which lower interstitial hydrostatic pressure and/or raise interstitial oncotic pressure, increase feedback sensitivity by lowering the threshold perfusion rate and by increasing the degree of decrement in stop-flow pressure. Ureteral occlusion for 1 to 2 hr reduces feedback sensitivity; in contrast, the feedback sensitivity is increased when ureteral occlusion is released after 2 hr of obstruction. These changes are explicable on the basis of the increased interstitial hydrostatic pressure and decreased interstitial oncotic pressure during the period of obstruction, whereas the opposite changes are seen following release of the obstruction. During 24 hr of unilateral ureteral occlusion, feedback sensitivity was increased, and in bilateral occlusion, it was reduced. These alterations are explained by the increased interstitial oncotic pressure and the increased interstitial hydrostatic pressure

---

This manuscript is a summary of the Workshop entitled *Current Concepts of the Pathophysiology of Obstructive Uropathy.*

in the two models, respectively. The feedback sensitivity is not changed after release of obstruction, whereas the distal delivery of fluid is increased, contributing to the occurrence of diuresis in the bilateral occlusion model, but not in the unilateral occlusion model.

Many of the changes observed following ureteral obstruction can be reproduced by the obstruction of single nephrons; a model that permits comparison of obstructed nephrons to their neighboring normal nephrons. After 1 day of nephronal obstruction, there is a small fall in glomerular capillary pressure and a larger fall in glomerular blood flow and single-nephron filtration rate, suggesting constriction of both afferent and efferent arterioles. This reduction in glomerular hemodynamics is ameliorated by captopril, the angiotensin converting enzyme inhibitor, and by saralasin, a competitive antagonist of angiotensin II (AII). Chronic saline administration and desoxycorticosterone also ameliorate the reduction in glomerular dynamics. These findings indicate that AII may play a role in the vasoconstriction that follows 24 hr of obstruction. After 1 week of nephron occlusion, there are even greater reductions in glomerular dynamics; blockade of the angiotensin system by captopril, or its antagonism with saralasin, produces small improvement. Thus, another vasoconstrictive mechanism must be operative in prolonged obstruction.

Increased production of PGE_2 is responsible for the initial vasodilatation. On the other hand, increased production of thromboxane has been proposed as an important factor in the subsequent vasoconstriction of the obstructed kidney. The role of thromboxane in this phenomenon has been investigated in the isolated perfused kidney. It was found that after 24 hr of unilateral ureteral obstruction, the baseline rate of thromboxane B_2 production by the kidney is increased and that this rate rises progressively with the duration of perfusion. In addition to this spontaneous increase in thromboxane production, the unilaterally obstructed kidney is hypersensitive to peptide hormones such as AII and bradykinin, which cause significantly greater increments in thromboxane B_2 production than in normal kidneys. Finally, both peptide hormones increase thromboxane B_2 production to a greater extent than they do prostaglandin E_2 production. Thus, in the 24-hr unilateral ureteral obstruction model, the spontaneous and hormone-induced production of vasoconstrictor prostanoids is preferentially increased. The possible role of thromboxane production in the reduced renal blood flow and glomerular filtration in the obstructed kidney in vivo was tested by infusing inhibitors of thromboxane synthetase, imidazole, and dazoxiben into the renal artery of the postobstructed kidney. Both agents had a dose-related beneficial effect on renal blood flow and glomerular filtration rate (GFR), indicating that thromboxane production in vivo must play a related role in the severe vasoconstriction that follows ureteral obstruction.

Other alterations in lipid metabolism have also been observed in the obstructed kidney. Following 24 hr of unilateral ureteral obstruction, the amount of triglycerides was found to be increased, both in the cortex and in the papilla. Phospholipids and free fatty acids were reduced in the cortex, but not in the papilla of the obstructed kidney. The reduction in phospholipids has been localized to the basolateral but not the brushborder membrane. The increase in triglyceride content of the kidney appears to be due to both an increase in the synthetic activity and a reduction in fatty acid oxidation. Thus, the incorporation of ^{14}C-oleic acid into triglycerides in the renal cortex is increased in the obstructed kidney. Similarly, the incorporation of ^{14}C-arachidonic acid into the triglyceride pool of the cortex and papilla of the obstructed kidney is increased. By contrast, the incorporation of ^{14}C-arachidonic acid into the phospholipid pool was markedly decreased in the cortex. The production of ^{14}C-CO$_2$ by the cortex of the obstructed kidney in the presence of ^{14}C-oleic acid is significantly decreased, indicating decreased oxidation. Thus, the triglyceride pool is increased by increased synthetic rate and reduced fatty acid oxidation. The phospholipid pool appears to be reduced by a reduction in the synthetic rate. These observations may account for the increased lipid storage observed histologically in the obstructed kidney.

These hemodynamic and biochemical changes in the obstructed kidney are associated with profound changes in tubular function. Some of these defects in tubular function include enhanced phosphate absorption with resistance to the phosphaturic effect of parathyroid hormone, sodium wasting, impaired urine concentration, impaired potassium excretion, and impaired distal renal acidification. The latter has been examined directly in the unilaterally obstructed kidney of the rabbit using the isolated renal tubule microperfused in vitro. Since the major site for distal acidification appears to be the medullary collecting tubule, this segment was chosen for study. At perfusion rates of 3 to 5 nl/min with symmetrical solutions containing 25 mM bicarbonate, tubules from unilateral obstructed kidneys exhibited a reduced bicarbonate absorption and a decreased lowering of bicarbonate concentration in the tubular fluid. However, when the tubules were perfused at 1 nl/min, their ability to lower bicarbonate concentration was not different from control. Thus, the obstruction appeared to cause a limitation in the capacity of the medullary collecting tubule to secrete hydrogen ion. Studies of the cortical collecting tubule using the same technique revealed a decrease in the voltage, the sodium transport, and the response to ADH after 4 hr of obstruction.

Not only does ureteral occlusion alter function in the obstructed kidney itself, but changes in function of the contralateral kidney are also observed. Following acute unilateral ureteral occlusion, an increase in cation excretion is observed in the contralateral intact kidney. This change in the function of the contralateral unobstructed kidney appears to be the result of a reno-renal reflex that is abolished by transection of the cord at T6. Denervation of the obstructed kidney abolishes the increased cation excretion from the contralateral kidney, indicating afferent renal nerves from the obstructed kidney must be involved in bringing about the cation diuresis. Conversely, denervating the contralateral unobstructed kidney prior to initiation of unilateral obstruction also abolishes the increased cation excretion observed after obstruction. This latter observation suggests that efferent renal nerves must be involved in causing the diuresis. Since changes in blood pressure, GFR, and renal blood flow were not observed, a direct tubular effect of the renal nerves must be invoked.

The effects of obstruction on the contralateral kidney appear to be age-related. Thus, compensatory hypertrophy and functional adaptation of the contralateral kidney are maximal when obstruction is produced in the newborn guinea pig, and they decline progressively when obstruction is produced, 1, 2, 3, or 4 weeks after birth. The effects of partial obstruction appear to be age-related also on the involved kidney itself. Thus, the reduction in GFR was most severe when obstruction was produced immediately after birth, and the effect became less severe with advancing age at the time of obstruction. Similarly, the effect on tubular function as manifested by the fractional excretion of sodium was greatest when the obstruction was produced at birth or at 1 week than when it was produced later. Perhaps because the majority of the juxtamedullary nephrons, which are most important for the process of concentration, are well developed at birth, the effect of partial obstruction to abolish the concentrating ability was not age-related.

It can be seen from the foregoing that complete or partial obstruction of the kidney results in profound alterations in the glomerular and tubular function of the obstructed kidney. Furthermore, the contralateral kidney also exhibits important changes in its function. The mechanisms for these alterations continue to provide an important focus for investigation.

Vesicoureteral Reflux and Renal Damage

C. John Hodson

Basic Pathophysiology

If a diluted, finely ground barium sulphate suspension is infused at slowly increasing pressure up a living pig's ureter, a point will be reached where equilibrium is established (about 60 to 70 cm H_2O). The pelvis and calices will be filled but not distended. If the pressure is further raised by small increments (5 cm) every 10 min, a second point will be reached (about 80 to 90 cm H_2O) where inflow recommences, but now in the form of pyelotubular reflux (IRR) into the renal parenchyma itself, and slowly extends along the nephrons until it fills the Bowman's capsules. The affected part of the kidney will be swollen and tense to palpation and will always be situated beyond a compound papilla, as these have been shown to possess ducts of Bellini with wide-open orifices (Fig. 1) [1–3]. If the pressure is now lowered, the infused barium sulfate will slowly drain out of the swollen areas, leaving no residue and no microscopically detectable residual damage. But if the pressure is slowly raised still further (100 to 120 cm H_2O), barium sulfate particles will remain in the kidney parenchyma and may be detected in scattered glomeruli, in a few tubules, in the interstitium beneath the capsule (sometimes within macrophages), and in adjacent lymph nodes 3 days after the pig has been sacrificed, although the vast bulk of the infused material will have drained away through the repaired ureter [4] (Hodson CJ, unpublished observations).

These observations indicate that refluxing fluid can enter the normal kidney through susceptible papillae, that it can do so and ebb away again without doing damage; but that if the pressure behind the reflux is maintained and

This manuscript was presented as part of a Symposium on *Reflux Nephropathy: Current Status.*

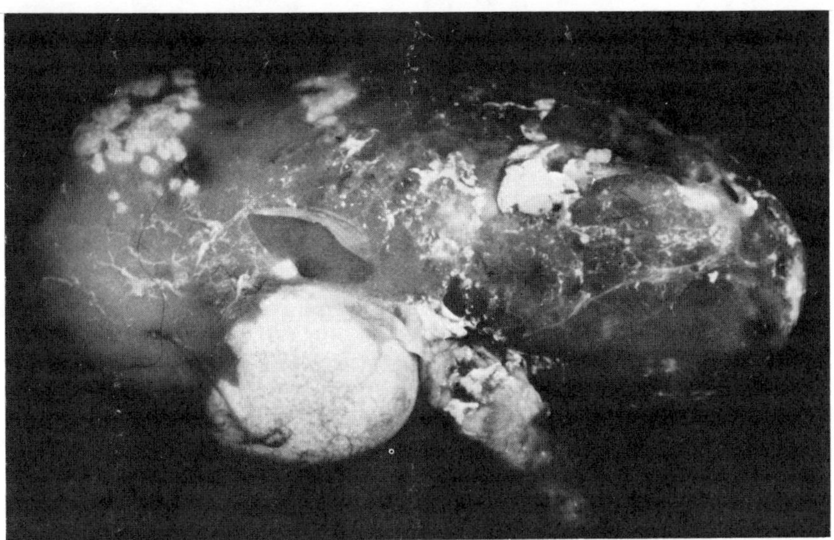

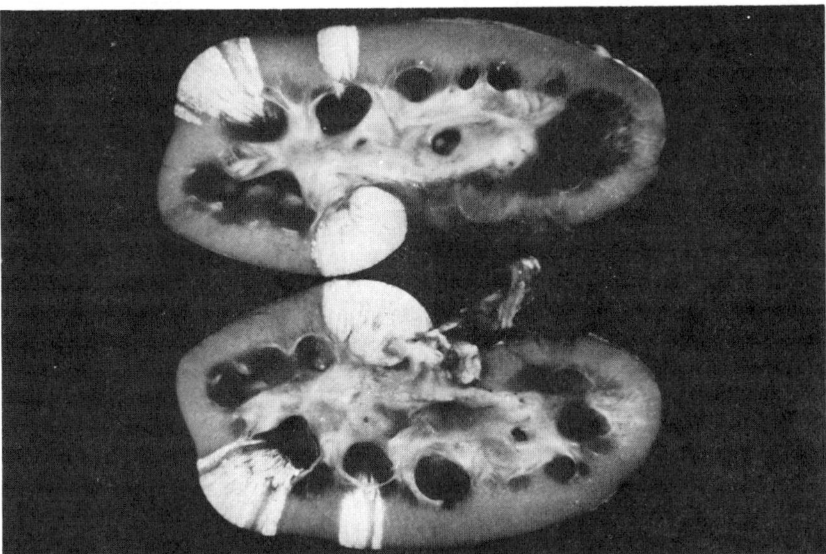

Fig. 1. Pig's kidney (outer and bivalved surfaces) 3 days after infusion of sterile barium sulphate suspension for 1 hr at a pressure of 80 cm. No postmortem shrinkage has occurred in intrarenal reflux zones. Histology showed widespread barium particles through interstitium [4]. Note capsular lymphatics filled with barium.

increased above a certain level, the tubules will rupture and urine will be extravasated into the interstitium and thence carried away by lymphatic drainage. That this can happen as the result of a single, sudden surge up a ureter is suggested by the radiographic evidence supplied by many retrograde pyelograms and by the observations of Brodeur using barium sulfate as a cystographic medium [4, 5].

The pressures involved in these methods were unknown, although they unlikely exceeded by much the pressures being documented today in children, as described later. These facts also serve as a framework for the interpretation of other experimental and clinical observations.

Further experiments in the living anesthetized animal (ketamine induction, IM followed by halothane and oxygen inhalation) confirmed that there is a lymphatic run-off through capsular, perivascular, and perureteral pathways [6] (Hodson CJ, unpublished observations). In these experiments, the contrast medium was barium sulfate, Evans blue, and India ink. Similarly, when Tamm-Horsfall protein was used as a marker, urine extravasation was demonstrated along the same pathways [6].

What appears necessary, therefore, to introduce infection into the kidney by the reflux of infected urine is a sustained plateau of bladder pressure or a series of pressure peaks lasting several minutes to overcome "kidney resistance," together with either the abolition of effective pelviureteral peristalsis or some change in the ureteral wall that interferes with the latter, such as some infections and the more severe grades of reflux so that bladder pressure is transmitted directly to the kidney and eventually results in tubular rupture. Evidence on both scores is slowly accruing in the clinical field [7, 8]. Once bacteria are introduced into the kidney by high-pressure reflux, they give rise to a focal inflammatory reaction, related to the extent of intrarenal reflux (IRR), and require very rapid treatment (within hours) for the treatment to be successful [9].

Finally, the status of a normal infant's urinary tract must be considered. At least three factors bear considering: (1) the normal, readily distendable nature of the ureters [10, 11], (2) the relatively large size of the "open" ducts of Bellini [3], and (3) Laplace's law as related to the bladder size together with the astonishingly high bladder pressures that can rapidly occur at this age [7]. All three would appear to render the young urinary tract particularly susceptible to reflux and may well account for the high incidence of renal damage when infection occurs at this age.

Clinical Age Groups

The Antenatal Period

Although a most recent conception, the possibilities for diagnosing and treating intrauterine obstructive processes should be mentioned. Ultrasound can detect an enlarged bladder, a thickened bladder wall, and an upper tract dilatation as early as week 16 of pregnancy; that is, only 3 to 4 weeks after urine is first formed. The bladder at this age (as in infants) is a superficial lower abdominal organ and accessible therefore by means of paracentesis through the mother's abdominal and uterine walls. By a relatively simple manipulation, a specially devised self-retaining catheter can be passed into the bladder and its outer end left draining into the amniotic space. The timing of this procedure may be important. In one case, an infant who was treated successfully at the uterine age of 24 weeks was born with dysplastic kidneys; in another case, an infant who was treated at the uterine age of 16 weeks, and the bladder likewise decompressed, was born at 30 weeks with what now, 12 months later, appear to be normal kidneys by ultrasound and physiological parameters [12, 13] (Glickman MG, personal communication). In susceptible families in which as many as 40% of the relatives may have reflux, a routine ultrasonography at 16 weeks could detect this anomaly and allow successful treatment. Indeed, all pregnancies might be so investigated. This is a new dimension opening up for high-risk pregnancies.

Birth to 2 Years

From birth to 2 years (or the "diaper age") is probably when most renal damage first occurs. Patients are normally detected because of their symptoms, fever mainly, but many have nonspecific symptoms; for example, convulsions or gastroenteritis. Urine cultures are mandatory in these patients, as in all ailing children. A long-term follow-up of infants with reflux showed that nearly half had renal damage by age 5 years, and most had ureteral reimplantation on this account [14]. This was in earlier years, however. In another series, in which symptomatic infection was treated early and effectively, the outlook appeared much better and surgery could often be avoided [15].

The problem here is to detect reflux *before* infection has occurred, and progress in this regard has been minimal. Two techniques seem promising. One is the parental monitoring of voiding patterns by a simple diaper technique, which proved extremely effective in one series and could probably detect reflux at an early stage [16]. The other is the detection of infection via a simple urine culture carried out by the parents in the home; a technique that provided remarkable results [17]. Both techniques should be more widely known.

At 2 to 5 Years

Most infants should be "bladder trained" by 2 years. It is possible this welcome milestone may be obtained in the future by the age of 6 months [18]. Any disturbance of voiding after 2 years, daytime or night-time enuresis or both, needs attention, because among these children are those with serious problems of bladder dysfunction. If these problems are neglected, these children may develop very high bladder pressures and, if refluxing and infected, consequent severe renal damage. This is thus the second age group to which more attention and analysis is being paid, with promising results [19, 20].

At 5 to 15 Years

The 5- to 15-year-old group includes those who have been missed previously and who now present with urinary infection, hypertension, and proteinuria and, occasionally, renal failure. The onset of uninformed sexual activity adds a further subgroup. However, the prognosis, because of early diagnosis, is already improving, and the principles of treatment are being better defined.

At 15 to 30 Years

Sex and pregnancy tend to dominate as predisposing factors in the 15- to 30-year-old age group, with neurogenic bladders secondary to trauma from road accidents adding a gradually increasing load. Sporadic fresh cases occasionally occur, sometimes secondary to other diseases such as diabetes or as a result of neurogenic bladder disease following trauma. The incidence of hypertension and renal failure increases. It is also in this age group, in particular, that severe bilateral disease with gross reflux is occasionally discovered in perfectly "fit" young men and women by routine medical examinations, which reveal mild hypertension or moderate (2 g/d) proteinuria. Left alone, their prognosis may be only 3 to 4 years [21].

Over 30 Years

The pattern of etiology is much the same, with hypertension and renal failure occurring more often, however. It is now being realized that the cause for this failure is a glomerulopathy, the onset of which is revealed by proteinuria recognizable by biopsy examination [22]. The nature of this complication has been much discussed, and the possibility of its being due simply to a scarcity of functioning glomeruli, as occurs in rats after five-sixths of the renal mass has been removed, has been shown to be moot [23, 24]. In many patients, the amount of surviving tissue greatly exceeds one-sixth of the total parenchymal mass. As well, in patients with unilateral kidney disease, the size and weight of the opposite kidney are often well above those of a single normal kidney; that is, above three-sixths of the original mass. Even so, the glomeruli in these apparently normal kidneys may show focal hyalinosis and sclerosis and have a bad prognosis [25–28]. Apart from the question what causes this severe complication, ignorance of its occurrence is possibly giving rise to false etiological statistics of the causes of renal failure, for glomerular disease is being mistaken for what is basically reflux nephropathy.

Other Clinical Groups

Mention has already been made of true neurogenic bladder disease. This occurs in infants with meningomyelocele or in older children with other congenital spinal abnormalities; for example, diastematomyelia. It may also result from any spinal injury affecting the cord, even in the absence of detectable bone injury or from central intervertebral disc protrusion. Peripheral neuritis of any etiology may cause neurogenic bladder disease, as may multiple sclerosis, syphilis, and other diseases of the central system. The previously poor outlook from this form of bladder dysfunction has been changed dramatically as the result of intermittent bladder catheterization and the use of antibiotics, ensuring normal upper urinary tracts. In contrast, when antibiotics are used alone and without due attention to bladder drainage, reflux, with both focal and generalized renal scarring, has occurred in the absence of infection (Rolleston GL, personal communication). In the older age groups, untreated prostatic enlargement can be associated with reflux, high bladder pressure, and consequent renal damage. In some families, the incidence of reflux may be as high as 40%, and among those individuals so discovered may be young people already in renal failure [29, 30]. Therefore, close relatives should always be investigated (preferably by ultrasound), and if any of these examinations are positive the whole family should be included in the search.

Advances in Diagnosis

For 25 years, the two clinical procedures on which the diagnosis of reflux nephropathy has been based are excretion urography (IVU) and voiding cystourethrography (VCU). By means of the former, it has been possible to determine kidney size, shape, and growth and the characteristic combination of large focal scars and papillary contraction with increasing elegance [31, 32]. It is from results of VCU that reflux has been graded and its significance thus based.

Both procedures have major drawbacks other than the involvement of X-radiation. The IVU requires an empty bowel, fluid restriction (not deprivation), a large bolus dose of contrast medium, and effective ureteric compression to give maximum information. It is rarely carried out properly as a routine and is particularly difficult to perform adequately in infants and young children. It has thus fallen into some degree of disrepute in this context. The VCU likewise suffers from difficulty of performance in the very young. Furthermore, its reliability has never been tested (ethically, it probably may not be), and most radiologists who have had extensive experience with it have the impression that different results (grades of reflux) may be obtained in the same child within days of one another. There are many ways of performing the examination, and multiple different objectives are often required of it, all of which simply cannot be achieved at the one examination, particularly in a squirming baby! It is an uncomfortable procedure at best and a traumatic and frightening one at worst. It is my opinion that no truly reliable physiologic data can be obtained from it; only a coarse quality of information. Furthermore, there are now six different ways of grading reflux, each with its firm band of disciples, and none of these ways is ever related to the patient's age, the presence or absence of infection, or the procedural method and contrast agent used. The incidence of reflux in *normal* children alone, as documented by the VCU, varies from 1 to 36% [33, 34], and yet it is on the result of one isolated VCU that the decision for or against surgery is often based. In one group of young children in which the VCU was repeated after a 6-month interval, 18% of those previously designated as grade III had ceased to reflux (Öbling H, personal communication). Further doubt is cast on the reliability of VCU by the results of combined simultaneous VCU and bladder pressure measurements. These have shown, among other things, that the point at which reflux occurs bears no relation to the pressure obtained in the bladder at the time and therefore to the propulsive force behind it [35].

Most VCUs represent one act of bladder filling and voiding carried out under completely unnatural circumstances. Also, unless fluoroscopy is maintained throughout the examination (an unwarranted X-ray exposure), the documented evidence will consist of only "spot" films representing a few points of time in an examination that may last 20 min; the limitations are obvious.

Cystography using radiopharmaceuticals consists of instilling a radioactive substance into the bladder, either by suprapubic injection (particularly suitable for infants) or by use of a small catheter that is then removed. The whole process of bladder filling and emptying can then be observed and recorded throughout on a computer-linked recording disc or tape without further disturbance to the child. Movement in small babies may be a problem, but can be overcome by "gating" the image. By this method, one can accurately measure the maximum bladder volume, the refluxing volume (that is, the volume at which reflux occurs, which is a reproducible constant, normally increasing with age, and the increase or otherwise of which has prognostic value [36]), and any residual urine. Furthermore, this method can be combined with the simultaneous recording of bladder pressure, if desired, and it is from these simultaneous image and pressure recordings that great advances in our knowledge of bladder behavior have been made [37, 38]. Reflux, and to a useful extent its degree, can also be documented by this method, but anatomic details are much less definite. However, there is little doubt that eventually this procedure will be preferred for most purposes, particularly for follow-up examinations for reflux.

Another isotope technique for identifying reflux, but not nearly so accurately measuring it, is called *indirect cystography*. In this technique, a radionuclide that is completely excreted by the kidneys in a short time is injected intravenously. Usually, 99^mTc = DPTA is the radionuclide used. Any sudden increase of activity in the upper tracts during or after voiding, or at any time during the actual excretion of the radionuclide, is due to reflux [36]. Perhaps as much as 25% of the lesser grades of reflux may be missed by this procedure. As well, a quantification of the data bearing on prognosis of the reflux [39, 40] cannot be obtained (and simultaneous bladder pressure measurements require catheterization anyhow). A further drawback is its use in patients with diminished renal function, in which the changes indicative of reflux may be lost against the high levels of "background" activity.

For parenchymal imaging, where an acute or chronic inflammatory lesion produces a negative area, at least two radiopharmaceuticals, technetium Tc 99m glucoheptonate and dimercaptosuccinic acid (DMSA), are in general use and can identify lesions not seen on good-quality IVUs [41, 42]. Gallium citrate (Ga 67) can also identify inflammatory conditions in the kidney, as elsewhere, as a positive accumulation after 24 hr. But these substances cannot give much detailed anatomic information and appear positive in renal infarcts [43].

Ultrasound is another relative newcomer to this field, but has enormous potential from fetal life onwards, as described earlier. It can accurately define renal size and shape, cortex, and medulla (when normal), the capacity of the pelvicalycine system and ureteral bladder, and sometimes urethral dilatation. Thickened bladder and pelvicalycine walls and both acute and chronic (scarred) parenchymal lesions above a certain size can also be detected. It is totally noninvasive and innocuous, and patient movement is no problem if "real-time" imaging is used [44].

Of the latter two imaging modalities, ultrasound is less expensive and simpler. Isotopes require special storage and disposal facilities, and image computerization is expensive in terms of personnel and hardware, but can be expected to be installed in all large- and medium-sized pediatric centers.

Computed tomography is another presently expensive diagnostic tool and can scarcely be anticipated to be available to even a minority of the very young patients under consideration. Nevertheless, it produces dramatic evidence in both acute and chronic states, particularly with regard to renal pathology [44]. Patient movement is a major problem in its use, and x-radiation is considerable.

Nuclear magnetic resonance (NMR) is still relatively untried. It may be of invaluable help in detecting diffuse lesions, particularly those found in glomerulopathy.

In summary, one might say that from the point of view of diagnosis, the present time is one of experimentation and shakedown, of comparison of old and new techniques. It may well be a decade before valid evaluation of the optimal use of these modalities in any given problem has been thrashed out. But it is likely that the nearer any method of imaging bladder function approaches a true physiologic representation, the greater will be its true clinical worth.

Early Diagnosis of Complications

Hypertension

As a rule, the likelihood of hypertension developing varies with the amount of scarring present, whether in one or both kidneys. It may become severe in degree as early as 4 years, but most often presents in the early teens. The conflicting reports regarding its relationship to increased renin production appear now to be settled, and serial plasma renin activity (PRA) assays have shown that at least in some children a persistent increase in PRA precedes clinical hypertension. But it is too early yet to know how often this happens. However, in view of the increased renal damage hypertension may cause in this disease, PRA estimation may enable early identification of patients at risk [45].

As well, renal vein sampling for renin levels, both from main and segmental veins, has been of value in determining the site of renin production and been used as valued evidence in the decision as to whether to carry out partial nephrectomy to obtain a permanent cure [46]. Again, only scanty information is yet available on this subject, particularly regarding at what stage surgery may be indicated and whether prophylactic total or partial nephrectomy for severe but strictly localized disease may prevent the onset of hypertension and, possibly, glomerulopathy [47].

The diagnosis of this glomerulopathy, with its usually sinister prognosis, depends on regular urinalysis (the degree of proteinuria commonly exceeding 1.5 g/d) and subsequent renal biopsy of an area of "normal" (that is, unscarred) parenchyma.

Perhaps the most recently known "complication" is that described by Kincaid-Smith, which occurs diffusely throughout "spared" tissue and in the apparently normal side in unilateral cases. It is associated both with hypertension and proteinuria and may therefore affect prognosis. Its diagnosis is by biopsy, and the main features are as follows: periglomerular fibrosis; chronic inflammatory cell infiltration, commonly cortical and focal in distribution; interstitial scarring around glomeruli; "typical" glomerular focal and segmental hyalinosis and sclerosis; dense, collagen scars; linear cortical scars; Tamm-Horsfall protein casts and interstitial deposits; and perivascular scarring [48]. Its significance is yet to be clarified, but in the experimental animal (pig), its cumulative effect is progressive focal ischemia, the scars following the course of the smaller (arcuate) arteries [49].

Summary

It is clear that reflux nephropathy is a disease that affects all age groups up to 50 years old, beyond which there are few survivors. Its symptoms are extremely varied at all ages; and it is a fact that in many instances, the diagnosis is only revealed by active clinical searching—by careful history taking and by routine blood pressure and urine examinations, the latter particularly for proteinuria or bacteriuria. The age when trouble begins is commonly below 3 years, and there is no doubt that the privacy of what might be termed the *diaper period* must be invaded and parents taught to be constantly on the alert for signs of bladder disturbance.

This is an extremely expensive and unpleasant disease, as the two main complications, hypertension and renal failure, occurring in young people lead not only to a greatly diminished life expectancy but also to a quality of life of a very low order.

References

1. HODSON CJ, MALING TMJ, MCMANAMON PJ, LEWIS MG: The pathogenesis of reflux nephropathy (chronic atrophic pyelonephritis). *Br J Radiol* 48(Suppl. 13), 1975
2. RANSLEY PG, RISDON RA: Renal papillary morphology and intrarenal reflux in the young pig. *Urol Res* 3:105–109, 1975
3. TAMMINEN TE, KAPIRO FA: The relation of the shape of the renal papillae and collecting duct openings to intrarenal reflux. *Br J Radiol* 49:345–350, 1977
4. BRODEUR AE, GOYER RA, MELICK W: A potential hazard of barium cystography. *Radiology* 85:1080–1085, 1965
5. HEPTINSTALL RH, HODSON CJ: Pathology of sterile reflux in the pig. *Contrib Nephrol* 39:344–345, 1984
6. BHAGAVAN BS, WEND RE, DUTTA D: Pathways of urinary backflow in obstructive uropathy demonstrated by pigmented gelatin injection and uromucoprotein markers. *Human Pathol* 10:669–683, 1979
7. VAN GOOL J, KRUITJEN RH, DONCKERWOLCKE RA, MESSER AP, VIVERBERG M: Bladder sphincter dysfunction, urinary infection and vesico-ureteral reflux with special references to bladder cognitive training. *Contrib Nephrol* 39:190–211, 1984
8. SVENSON SB, KÄLLENIUS G, KORHONEN TK, MÖLLBY R, ROBERTS JA, TULLUS K, WINBERG J: Initiation of clinical pyelonephritis: The role of P-fimbriae-mediated bacterial adhesion. *Contrib Nephrol* 39:252–273, 1984
9. RANSLEY PG, RISDON RA: Reflux nephropathy: The effects of antimicrobial therapy on the evolution of the early pyelonephritic scar. *Kidney Int* 20:733–742, 1981
10. CAMPBELL M: *Clinical Pediatric Urology.* Philadelphia, W.B. Saunders & Co., 1951, p 95
11. FRIEDLAND GW: *Reflux Nephropathy,* edited by HODSON CJ, KINCAID-SMITH P, New York, Masson USA, 1979, p 92
12. GOLBUS MS, HARRISON MR, FILLY RA, CALLEN PW, KATZ M: In utero treatment of urinary tract obstruction. *Am J Obstet Gynecol* (in press, 1984)
13. BERKOWITZ RL, GLICKMAN MG, WALKER-SMITH GJ, SIEGEL NJ, WEISS RM, MAHONEY MJ, HOBBINS JC: Fetal urinary tract obstruction: What is the role of surgical intervention in utero? *Am J Obstet Gynecol* 144:367–375, 1982
14. BAILEY RR: Long-term follow-up of infants with gross reflux. *Contrib Nephrol* 39:146–152, 1984
15. WINBERG J, ANDERSEN HJ, BERGSTROM T, JACOBSSON B, LARSON H, LINCOLN K: Epidemiology of symptomatic urinary tract infection in childhood. *Acta Pediatr Scand* 252(Suppl.):3–20, 1974
16. RANDOLPH MF, WOODS SE, HODSON CJ, KLAUBER GT: Home screening for the detection of urinary tract infection in children. *Am J Dis Child* 133:713–717, 1979
17. KLAUBER GT, MEARES EM: Evaluation of home monitoring for bacteriuria in children. *Contrib Nephrol* 39:378–382, 1984
18. DEVRIES MW, DEVRIES MP: Cultural relativity of toilet training readiness: A perspective from E. Africa. *Pediatrics* 60:170–177, 1977
19. KOFF SA, LAPIDES J, PIAZZA DH: Associations of urinary tract infection and reflux with uninhibited bladder contraction and voluntary sphincter obstruction. *J Urol* 122:373–376, 1979
20. GOLDRAICH NP, GOLDRAICH IH, ANSELMI OE, RAMOS OL: Reflux nephropa-

thy: The clinical picture in South Brazilian children. *Contrib Nephrol* 39:52–68, 1984

21. HODSON CJ: Scoring the damage, chap. 5 in *Reflux Nephropathy,* edited by HODSON CJ, KINCAID-SMITH P, New York, Masson USA, 1979

22. KINCAID-SMITH PS, BASTOS MG, BEAKER GJ: Reflux nephropathy in the adult. *Contrib Nephrol* 39:94–102, 1984

23. OLSON JL, HOSTETTER TH, RENNKE HG, BRENNER BM, VENKATACHALAM MA: Mechanisms of altered glomerular permselectivity and glomerulosclerosis following extreme ablation of renal mass. *Kidney Int* 16:857, 1979

24. ELEMA JD, ARENDS A: Focal and segmental glomerular hyalinosis in the rat. *Lab Invest* 33:554, 1975

25. BHATHENA DB, WEISS JH, HOLLAND NH, MCMORROW RG, CURTIS JJ, LUCAS BA, LUKE RG: Focal and glomerular sclerosis in reflux nephropathy. *Am J Med* 68:886–892, 1980

26. COTRAN RS: Glomerulosclerosis in reflux nephropathy. *Kidney Int* 21:528–534, 1982

27. KINCAID-SMITH P: Glomerular lesions in atrophic pyelonephritis and reflux nephropathy. *Kidney Int* 8(Suppl. 4):S81, 1975

28. BAILEY RR, SWAINSON CP, LYNN KL, BURRY AF: Glomerular lesions in the "normal" kidney in patients with unilateral reflux nephropathy. *Contrib Nephrol* 39:126–132, 1984

29. BAILEY RR, JANUS E, MCLOUGHLIN K, LYNN KL, ABBOTT GD: Familial and genetic data in reflux nephropathy. *Contrib Nephrol* 39:40–52, 1984

30. DEVARGAS A, EVANS K, RANSLEY P, ROSENBERG AR, ROTHWELL D, SHERWOOD T, WILLIAMS DI, BARRATT TM, CARTER CO: A family study of vesico-ureteric reflux. *J Med Genet* 15:85–90, 1978

31. EKLÖF D, RINGERTZ S: A method of kidney size measurement in children. *Acta Radiol (Diagn)* 17:617–625, 1976

32. CLAESSON I, JACOBSSON B, JODAL U, WINBERG J: Assessment of renal parenchymal thickness in normal children. *Acta Radiol (Diagn)* 22:305–314, 1981

33. BAILEY RR: Long-term follow-up of infants with gross vesico-ureteric reflux. *Contrib Nephrol* 39:146–152, 1984

34. KÖLLERMAN MW, LUDWIG H: Über den vesico-ureteralen Reflux bein normalen king im Sänglings und Kleinkind altur. *Z Kinderklinik* 100:185–191, 1967

35. MAIZELS M, WEISS S, CONWAY JJ, FIRLIT CF: The cystometric nuclear cystogram. *J Urol* 121:203–205, 1979

36. MELLER ST, WARD BCH, ECKSTEIN HB: Radionuclide cystography vs. micturating cysto-urethrography for diagnosing vesico-ureteric reflux in children. *Br J Radiol* 53:262–263, 1980

37. MERRICK MV, WILD SR, UTTLEY WS: Radionuclide cystography vs. micturating cysto-urethrography for diagnosing vesico-ureteric reflux in children. *Br J Radiol* 53:263–265, 1980

38. POLLETT JE, SHARP PE, SMITH FW: Radionuclide imaging for vesico-ureteric reflux using ^{99m}Tc DTPA. *Pediatr Radiol* 8:165–167, 1979

39. NASRALLAH PF, CONWAY JJ, KING LR, BELMAN AB, WEISS S: The quantitative nuclear cystogram: An aid in determining the spontaneous resolution of vesico-ureteral reflux. *Urology* 12:654–658, 1978

40. BINGHAM JB, MAISLEY MN: An evaluation of the use of 99 Tc dimercaptosuccinic acid (DMSA) as a static imaging agent. *Br J Radiol* 51:599–607, 1978

41. MCAFEE, JG: Radionuclide imaging in the assessment of primary chronic pyelonephritis. *Radiology* 138:203–206, 1979

42. LEONARD JC: Glucoheptonate imaging. *Clin Pediatr* 19:615–619, 1980

43. BRUGH R III: Gallium 67 scanning and conservative treatment in acute inflammatory lesions of the renal cortex. *J Urol* 121:232–235, 1979
44. HODDICK W, JEFFREY RB, GOLDBERG HI, FEDERLE MP, LAING FC: CT and sonography of severe renal and perirenal infection. *Am J Roentgenogr* 140:517–520, 1983
45. DILLON MJ, SMELLIE JM: Peripheral plasma renin activity, hypertension and renal scarring in children. *Contrib Nephrol* 39:68–81, 1984
46. DILLON MJ: Renal vein renin determination in evaluating hypertensive children, in *Paediatric Nephrology*, edited by GRUSKIN N, The Hague, Nijhoff, 1981, pp 127–133
47. DILLON MJ, GORDON I, SHAH V: 99Tc DMSA scanning and segmental renal vein renin estimations in children with renal scarring. *Contrib Nephrol* 39:20–28, 1984
48. KINCAID-SMITH PS: Diffuse parenchymal lesions in reflux nephropathy and the possibility of making a renal biopsy diagnosis in reflux nephropathy. *Contrib Nephrol* 39:111–116, 1984
49. KINCAID-SMITH PS, HODSON CJ: Lesions in the pig kidney with chronic reflux nephropathy, in *Reflux Nephropathy*, edited by HODSON CJ, KINCAID-SMITH P, New York, Masson USA, 1979, pp 197–213

Renal Scars and Vesicoureteric Reflux: Pathology and Pathogenesis of Segmental Atrophy

Jay Bernstein and Billy S. Arant, Jr.

Renal segmental atrophy is a form of severe renal scarring that results in parenchymal reduction and potentially in hypertension and chronic renal failure. The individual lesions appear typically as sharply demarcated shrunken lobes or clusters of lobes, with calyceal dilatation, medullary effacement, and nephronic depletion. Those features, which were localized to portions of undersized kidneys, had been attributed to segmental hypoplasia or maldevelopment and frequently were referred to as the Ask-Upmark kidney; however, it is now clear that the abnormality is acquired and that it carries a strong association with vesicoureteric reflux (VUR) [1]. Although it seems likely that there are other causes of segmental atrophy and that not all instances are accounted for by VUR, segmental atrophy stands in practice as a form of reflux nephropathy.

The pathogenesis of the segmental lesions is incompletely resolved. There is a general acceptance of the hypothesis that renal scarring follows intrarenal reflux [2, 3], perhaps [4–6] and perhaps not [7, 8] requiring concomitant infection. However, it is not clear how intrarenal reflux injures the kidney and how that injury progresses to gross scarring. Although radiographically obvious intrarenal reflux and gross scarring may be limited to susceptible segments—those with "refluxing" papillae [4, 5]—it seems possible that nonatrophic portions of scarred kidneys are also damaged by intrarenal reflux of milder degrees, with subclinical degrees of parenchymal atrophy. To explore that possibility, we have re-examined a series of scarred kidneys with an eye to changes that might be implicated in the pathogenesis of parenchymal scarring. We have also reviewed the clinical and radiographic data with emphasis on the evolution of renal scarring.

This manuscript was presented as part of a Symposium on *Reflux Nephropathy: Current Status.*

Methods

Cases were initially identified on the basis of either radiographic or morphologic evidence of renal segmental atrophy; and all cases were confirmed by histopathologic examination. All patients were demonstrated to have had VUR. Nephrectomies were performed because of severe hypertension, renal nonfunctioning, or persistent infection. One patient underwent a diagnostic open biopsy of a scar; 2 patients had segmental resections, 14 patients had unilateral nephrectomies, and 4 had bilateral nephrectomies. There were 25 renal specimens.

Vesicoureteric reflux was documented by low-pressure voiding cystourethrography, and it was graded as absent, mild, moderate, or severe (0 to 3+) according to the classification of Rolleston et al [9]. Hypertension was said to exist in children when diastolic blood pressure, which was measured with a cuff of an appropriate size on more than one occasion in an upper extremity, was > 2 SD above the mean pressure for the patient's age and sex [10]. Hypertension was said to be present in an adult when the diastolic pressure exceeded 95 mm Hg. Each patient was screened for evidence of urinary tract infection (UTI), and this diagnosis was made only after significant bacteriuria ($> 10^5$ organisms per milliliter of the same organism[s]) was found in two separately voided specimens or after bacterial growth occurred in one specimen obtained by suprapubic puncture. Glomerular filtration rate (GFR) was estimated from endogenous creatinine clearance (C_{CR}) [11] or from serum creatinine determinations [12]. Radiographic assessment of renal growth was done according to the method of Hodson et al [13]; values were compared to expected renal size for body height. Renal size in selected cases was also estimated from planimetric measurement of radiographic surface area. The weights of removed kidneys were compared to normal values for children and adults [14, 15]. Kidneys that fell below the mean for age by more than 2 SD by either standard were said to be small.

Tissue blocks were embedded in paraffin by routine methods, and histologic sections were stained with hematoxylin and eosin, periodic acid-Schiff (PAS), Gomori or Masson trichrome, and Verhoeff-van Gieson elastica stains. Sections were examined for vascular and inflammatory damage in nonatrophic portions of the kidneys.

Clinical Background

There were 21 patients, 12 of whom were female and 9 male. Nine of the patients, with a mean age of 15.7 (6 to 29) years, had normal blood pressure; 12 patients, with a mean age of 15.1 (7 to 48) years, had elevated blood pressure. Five patients (24%) sought medical attention after the discovery of hypertension, 7 (33%) initially had urinary tract infection, 4 (19%) had impaired renal function, 5 (24%) presented with flank pain, and 3 because of stones. None of the patients had more than mild proteinuria at any time in the course of disease. Associated genitourinary abnormalities included posterior urethral valves in 2 patients, bladder diverticula associated with ipsilateral VUR in 2, and double collecting systems in 3—of which 2 had double- and 1 had single-bladder insertions. Three patients had radiographic evidence of ureteropelvic junction obstruction, 1 had ureterovesical junction obstruction, and 1 patient was considered to have a mild form of prune-belly syndrome.

Radiographic studies showed the affected kidneys to be small. The lesion was bilateral in six patients—four of whom had bilateral nephrectomies in the course of this study, one of whom had a unilateral nephrectomy, and one of whom had the first kidney removed elsewhere at an earlier time for lithiasis. Two others had solitary kidneys because of contralateral agenesis. Five of the six patients with bilateral lesions and both of those with solitary kidneys had hypertension. By contrast, only 6 of 13 patients with radiographic or clinical evidence of unilateral involvement were hypertensive. Stated another way, the 12 hypertensive patients included 5 with bilateral involvement, 2 with involvement of a solitary kidney, and 5 with unilateral involvement. The nine normotensive patients included only one with bilateral involvement; the rest were unilateral. Impaired renal function (GFR $<$ 40 ml/min/1.73 m^2) was observed at the time of diagnosis in all six patients with bilateral involvement and in the two with solitary kidneys. Vesicoureteric reflux was more severe in hypertensive than in normotensive patients; of 12 hypertensive patients, 9 had severe VUR, whereas all normotensive patients had only moderate or mild reflux.

Of the 21 patients, 14 had bacteriologic evidence or a history that was suggestive of UTI at some time during their course. Seven patients, one-third of the total, did not have bacteriologic evidence or a history that was suggestive of UTI.

Evolution of Renal Scarring

The renal scars were seen radiographically as developing in 9 patients while under clinical observation [16]. Vesicoureteric reflux was detected at a mean age of 2.9 (0.1 to 10.0) years; and, in all patients, the renal size was initially normal with no radiographic evidence of scarring. The nine patients were followed for 5 to 14 years from the discovery of VUR, and renal scars were first observed at a mean age of 8.8 (3 to 19) years. Six patients developed unilateral scars and two had bilateral scars; one developed lesions in a single kidney. The interval between the discovery of VUR and the appearance of a renal scar in all nine patients was 6.1 (2.9 to 10.5) years. Renal function was normal in six patients having uncomplicated VUR and was 50 to 75% of normal in three having VUR combined with obstructive lesions. The worst degree of reflux ever observed in these patients was severe in five, moderate in two, and mild in two patients. All nine patients had a history of UTI at some time prior to correction of VUR.

All patients suffered failure of normal renal growth in affected kidneys. The mean radiographic length of affected kidneys at the same time that a scar was first observed was 92 ± 23% (mean ± SD) of the expected normal value for patient height [14]; at the time of surgical resection, the kidney length was 73 ± 14% of normal. Bilaterally scarred kidneys were nearly symmetric in that the mean ratio of left-to-right kidney lengths was 0.83 ± 0.07, whereas the ratio of affected-to-unaffected kidney length in unilateral disease was 0.64 ± 0.09. Planimetric measurements on excretory urograms of four cases showed that despite only modest decreases in lengths of affected kidneys, parenchymal surface areas were decreased by as much as 50% [16].

All nine patients developed renal scarring despite antireflux surgery; one other patient with scars at the onset also had progression of scarring after antireflux surgery (Table 1). Uncomplicated VUR was surgically corrected in six patients at the time of diagnosis; and, even though a seventh patient's VUR was reduced by the first attempted surgical correction, two additional procedures in 3 years were performed before the VUR was eliminated. Each of three patients with VUR and obstructive lesions had a diversionary procedure performed initially; two patients with posterior urethral valves subsequently had complete repair at 1 and 7 years of age, and the other with a solitary kidney had a diversion into an ileal pouch during the entire 14 years of observation. Three patients had recurrent UTI following repair of VUR, while the remaining seven had no demonstrable bacteriuria (four were cultured at 1- to 3-month intervals and three were occasionally cultured during the period of observation). Nephrectomies in the 10 patients were performed at a mean age of 11.8 (7 to 19) years.

Pathologic Observations

All of the intact kidneys were small by weight and all of the specimens contained segmental areas of severe atrophy. The abnormal segments were frequently, but not always, present as flat polar scars. Midrenal scars presented as transverse grooves.

All of the affected segments could be identified as lobes with a spectrum of histopathologic alteration. Some segments contained no glomeruli (or only

Table 1. Segmental renal atrophy: Progressive renal scarring in 10 patients following surgical correction of vesicoureteric reflux

Age at repair (mo)	Recurrent UTI	No clinical infection
< 24	2	1
25–72	1	3
73–120	0	2
> 120	0	1
	3	7

very few did), whereas others contained numerous hyalinized and obsolete glomeruli. Almost all of the persisting glomeruli within the atrophic segments were completely sclerotic, and a few were partially sclerotic, with lobules of patent capillaries. Some specimens contained only a few tubular remnants, whereas others contained numerous colloid-filled tubular microcysts. There were segments that contained both tubules and glomeruli, and segments that seemed to contain one or the other. The variability in histologic appearance existed both between adjacent scars and, to a lesser extent, within the confines of a single scar.

Vascular sclerosis also varied among specimens. The interlobular arteries were thickened principally by medial hypertrophy and occasionally also by intimal proliferation. Arterial mucoid intimal proliferation was present in one patient with moderate hypertension. However, very severe cortical atrophy, with extreme depletion of nephronic elements, was associated with small vessels. Venous dilatation was a common feature of the scarred cortical segments, which were present in all but two of the specimens. The dilated veins tended to be concentrated in the inner cortex, separating the residual tubules and arteries. The interlobar veins were also dilated, with medial muscular hypertrophy; and, the veins could be traced easily into the peripelvic fat with no evidence of obstruction, despite the occasional presence of nearby parapelvic fibrous scarring.

Tubular disruption with extravasation of PAS-positive material, presumably Tamm-Horsfall protein, was seen in only three specimens; only a single intravascular mass of PAS-positive material, presumably lying in an interlobar vein, was found in one other specimen.

Segments adjacent to the atrophic lobes were grossly sharply demarcated, although interstitial fibrosis focally extended into the margins of adjacent lobes. Histopathologic examination of the scars in the 25 specimens showed inflammatory cell infiltration to be negligible or lacking in 7, mild in 11, and moderate in 7 specimens; none of the scars contained heavy infiltrates. The sections were adequate for evaluating the medullary components of the scars in 24 of the specimens; in all specimens, there was severe atrophy, fibrosis, and depletion of tubules and blood vessels. Examination of the non-scarred tissue showed frequent injury with mild-to-moderate degrees of partial damage (Fig. 1). Adjacent medullary segments were available for examination in 18 specimens—the others being unsuitable for evaluation because of hydronephrosis. Although there was variation among the adjacent medullary pyramids in any specimen, the most severe degree of damage encountered in any specimen was moderate in eight and mild in nine; only one specimen showed no evidence of medullary damage in adjacent lobes available for examination. One specimen contained intramedullary calcification and lithiasis, and four specimens contained abnormal ducts that were suggestive of renal dysplasia. Cortical tissue immediately adjacent to the scars often consisted of partially damaged renal columns belonging to the affected lobes, and that tissue was not included in the following evaluation. The cortical portions of adjacent lobes also were focally damaged, commonly in a lobular distribution (Fig. 2). The affected lobules contained atrophic tubules, sclerotic glomeruli, and inflammatory cells—usually sharply demarcated from adjacent

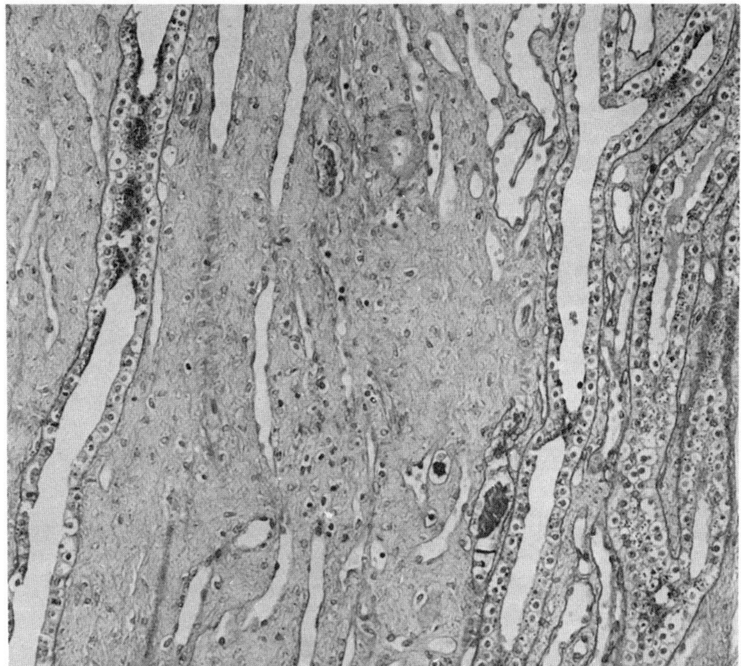

Fig. 1. The medulla contains areas of fibrosis with depletion of vasa recta and straight segments. The area of damage may be centered on a vascular bundle, with relative preservation of adjacent collecting ducts. (PAS stain; ×150)

normal parenchyma—and the lobular scars sometimes related to areas of medullary fibrosis. Seven specimens (five patients) contained relatively severe, apparently diffuse cortical damage with focal segmental glomerular sclerosis; all of those patients had renal insufficiency, but none had more than mild proteinuria or a history of more than mild proteinuria. One other specimen, a hydronephrotic kidney, had focal segmental glomerular sclerosis in association with relatively mild, diffuse cortical damage; that patient also had renal insufficiency without proteinuria. Focal cortical damage was moderate in two, mild in eight, and absent in five specimens; two specimens could not be evaluated because of insufficient material. Chronic inflammatory cell infiltration within the adjacent segments was severe in 1, moderate in 4, mild in 8, and negligible or lacking in 10 specimens; two specimens did not contain sufficient unscarred tissue for evaluation.

Discussion

The clinicopathologic aspects of this series reiterate the association between segmental scarring and VUR [1]. We were unable to confirm a history of

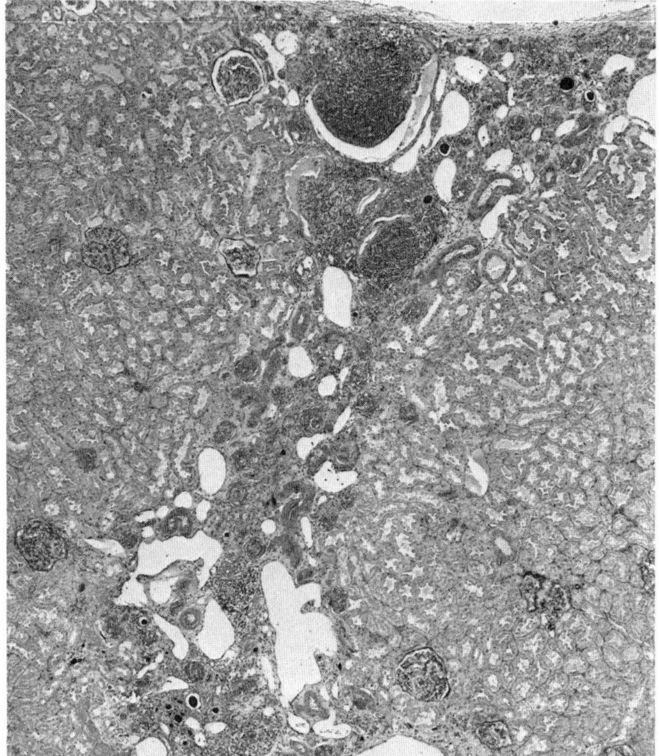

a

Fig. 2. A small area of scarring corresponds to a renal lobule. **a.** The cortex contains
a narrow area extending from capsule to medulla and containing hyalinized glomeruli,
a few tubular remnants, thick-walled arteries, and dilated veins. Inflammatory cell
infiltration is relatively sparse in the inner portion of the scar; the outer portion
contains lymphoid follicles. (PAS stain; ×40) **b.** The medulla contains a localized
area of scarring with tubular and vascular depletion corresponding to the atrophic
cortical lobe. Inflammatory cell infiltration is negligible. (Masson trichrome stain;
×50)

UTI in one-third of our patients, although we cannot exclude the possibility of silent infection. Nonetheless, the association between sterile reflux
and scarring is a recurrent observation in the literature [17] that is supported by experimental evidence [18]. We can say that despite uncertainty
about UTI at the onset of disease, renal scarring progressed in the absence
of infection. It probably also started in the absence of infection at least
in those patients whose kidneys showed evidence of renal dysplasia, indicating that reflux and the process of renal scarring began during fetal
life.

All of our patients suffered a failure of normal renal growth, in large
part because each kidney underwent a considerable loss of substance. There
also may have been retarded growth of seemingly unaffected segments—

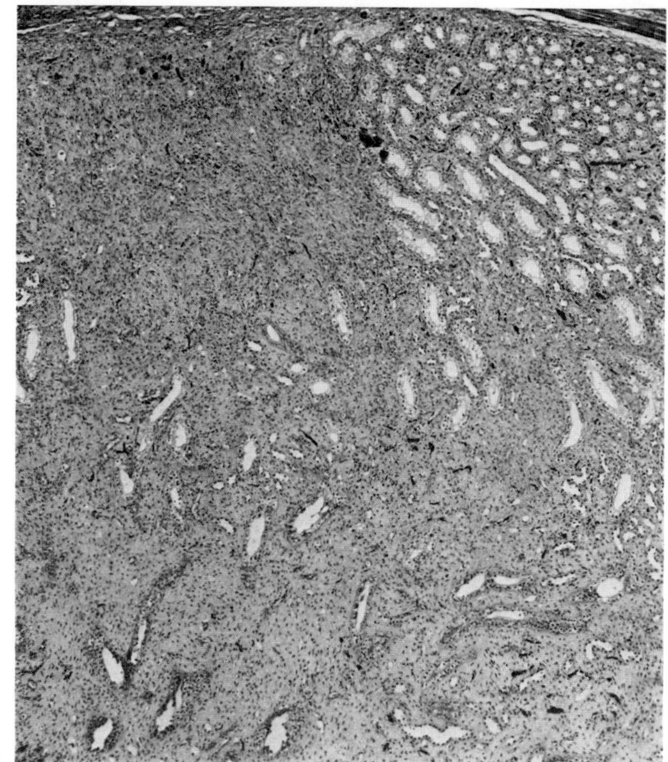

b

those with the focal or lobular lesions demonstrated in this study. Completely unaffected segments clearly underwent compensatory hypertrophy, with strikingly thickened cortices and often with realignment of their axes [1].

Nine patients (43%) had no renal scars when they came under clinical observation at a mean age of 2.9 years, and renal scars were first observed at a mean age of 8.8 years. We recognize the discrepancy between our observations and the belief that scarring is seldom seen developing in kidneys previously known to be normal [19]; but, our experience is not unique [20]. Renal scarring in patients with VUR is clearly not confined to the first few years of life [21], and progression of scarring continues into adulthood [22, 23].

It was discouraging to find that 10 of our patients had continued renal scarring despite surgical correction of their VUR and despite the absence of recurrent infection in seven of them. Other investigators have reported the progression of renal scarring after successful antireflux surgery [24], perhaps from damage incurred before surgery. If the abnormality, once initiated, does indeed progress inexorably over a period of several years—the "big bang" hypothesis [4]—it is necessary to identify the early changes that initiate and perpetuate the scar.

We were not surprised to find renal parenchymal damage outside of the scarred segments. It seems unlikely that intrarenal reflux either begins as or remains an all-or-none phenomenon [5, 25], devastating some segments and leaving others entirely unscathed. It also seems unlikely that the recruitment of new refluxing papillae under the pressure of continuing VUR, as proposed by Hodson [26], takes place all at once. Therefore, our finding of damage outside of the atrophic segments can be interpreted as evidence either of recruitment or of locally mild intrarenal reflux.

The areas of damage outside of the main renal scars are instructive in showing the patterns of injury. All of those medullary lesions, without suppuration or severe inflammation, included fibrosis with apparent loss of tubules and small blood vessels. The affected segments were hypovascular, like the scarred segments studied microangiographically by Ljungqvist and Lagergren [27]. We think it is likely that those abnormalities were initiated by extravasation of urine during intrarenal reflux. The initial injury may have been enhanced by bacterial infection; however, the inconsistent history of UTI in this study and in others [17] and the paucity of cellular infiltrates make continued bacterial infection an unlikely mechanism of progression. The paucity of inflammatory cell infiltration also militates against a continuing immune reaction; for example, to the hypothetic presence of extravasated Tamm-Horsfall protein [26]. Very few of our specimens contained extratubular inspissates of PAS-positive material.

If—as suspected clinically [17] and shown experimentally [18]—sterile intrarenal reflux results in scarring, how is the injury mediated? A strong clue lies in the demonstration of an acute and sharp loss of radiographic parenchymal opacification in refluxing segments [18, 26]. The immediate explanation lies either in rapid impairment of the renal circulation or in disruption of the tubular straight segments. Injury to the medullary microvasculature extends to the vascular bundles of the inner medulla, perhaps resulting in obstruction of inner cortical efferents with the occasional striking dilatation of small cortical vessels. Either direct injury to tubular straight segments or secondary ischemic injury following vascular damage can result in nephronic disruption. A complete account also includes damage to medullary interstitial cells, with functional consequences for the renal circulation. We prefer to claim primacy for a vascular pathway, because most loops of Henle in human kidneys turn in the outer medulla and seldom extend into the papilla [28]; therefore, injury to the long vasa recta is likely to be the initial event. The notion that segmental atrophy arises from localized circulatory disturbances is not exactly new; we can offer in support of that hypothesis the observation that affected medullary segments are devascularized with the loss of straight tubular segments and of ducts.

Summary

In a series of 21 patients who underwent nephrectomy for segmental renal atrophy in association with vesicoureteric reflux (VUR), we were able to examine 25 nephrectomy specimens. Based on the assumption that the segmental atrophy resulted from VUR and was a form of reflux nephropathy, we examined the nonatrophic portions of resected kidneys for damage that might be related to reflux. Focal medullary scarring, which was present in 17 of 18 specimens suitable for examination, consisted of interstitial fibrosis with loss of vessels and medullary tubules. Those lesions were seldom associated with significant inflammatory cell infiltrates, and they were interpreted as having resulted from localized intrarenal reflux. The cortical portions of those lobes also contained focal areas of scarring in a lobular distribution. The patterns of the small scars suggest a principal injury to the vasa recta with subsequent damage to, and disruption of, straight segments. We propose that microvascular injury following intrarenal reflux is responsible for the scarring in reflux nephropathy.

Acknowledgment. This work was supported by grant no. 81–32 from the William Beaumont Hospital Research Institute.

References

1. ARANT BS JR, SOTELO-AVILA C, BERNSTEIN J: Segmental "hypoplasia" of the kidney (Ask-Upmark). *J Pediatr* 95:931–939, 1979
2. ROLLESTON GL, MALING TMJ, HODSON CJ: Intrarenal reflux and the scarred kidney. *Arch Dis Child* 49:531–539, 1974
3. ROSE JS, GLASSBERG KI, WATERHOUSE K: Intrarenal reflux and its relationship to renal scarring. *J Urol* 113:400–403, 1975
4. RANSLEY PG: Vesicoureteric reflux: Continuing surgical dilemma. *Urology* 12:246–255, 1978
5. RANSLEY PG, RISDON RA: The renal papilla, intrarenal reflux, and chronic pyelonephritis, in *Reflux Nephropathy,* edited by HODSON J, KINCAID-SMITH P, New York, Masson Publishing, USA, 1979, chap 13, p 126
6. SMELLIE J, NORMAND C: Reflux nephropathy in childhood, in *Reflux Nephropathy,* edited by HODSON J, KINCAID-SMITH P, New York, Masson Publishing, USA, 1979, chap 2, p 14
7. BAILEY RR: The relationship of vesico-ureteric reflux to urinary tract infection and chronic pyelonephritis—reflux nephropathy. *Clin Nephrol* 1:132–141, 1973
8. BAILEY RR: End-stage reflux nephropathy. *Nephron* 27:302–306, 1981
9. ROLLESTON GL, SHANNON FT, UTLEY WLF: Relationship of infantile vesicoureteric reflux to renal damage. *Br Med J* 1:460–463, 1970
10. Report of the Task Force of Blood Pressure Control in Children (1977). *Pediatrics* 59(Suppl):802–803, 1977
11. ARANT BS JR, EDELMANN CM JR, SPITZER A: Congruence of inulin and creatinine clearances in children: Use of the Technicon AutoAnalyzer. *J Pediatr* 81:559–561, 1972
12. SCHWARTZ GJ, HAYCOCK GB, EDELMANN CM JR, SPITZER A: A simple estimate of glomerular filtration rate in children derived from body length and plasma creatinine. *Pediatrics* 58:259–263, 1976
13. HODSON CJ, DREWE JA, KARN MN, KING A: Renal size in normal children. A radiographic study during life. *Arch Dis Child* 37:616–622, 1962
14. OLIVER JT, RUBENSTEIN M, MEYER R, BERNSTEIN J: Congenital abnormalities

of the urinary system. III. Growth of the kidney in childhood—determination of normal weight. *J Pediatr* 61:256–261, 1962

15. LUDWIG J: *Current Methods of Autopsy Practice* (2 ed). Philadelphia, WB Saunders & Co, 1975, p 675

16. SHINDO S, BERNSTEIN J, ARANT BS JR: Evolution of renal segmental atrophy (Ask-Upmark kidney) in children with vesicoureteric reflux: Radiographic and morphologic studies. *J Pediatr* 102:847–854, 1983

17. BAILEY RR: Sterile reflux: Is it harmless? in *Reflux Nephropathy,* edited by HODSON J, KINCAID-SMITH P, New York, Masson Publishing, USA, 1979, chap 34, p 334

18. HODSON J, MALING TMJ, McMANAMON PJ, LEWIS MG: Reflux nephropathy. *Kidney Int* 8(Suppl):S50–S58, 1975

19. SMELLIE JM, NORMAND ICS: Bacteriuria, reflux, and renal scarring. *Arch Dis Child* 50:581–585, 1975

20. WINTER AL, HARDY BE, ALTON DJ, ARBUS GS, CHURCHILL BM: Acquired renal scars in children. *J Urol* 129:1190–1194, 1983

21. SMELLIE J, EDWARDS D, HUNTER N, NORMAND ICS, PRESCOD N: Vesicoureteric reflux and renal scarring. *Kidney Int* 8(Suppl):S65–S72, 1975

22. KINCAID-SMITH P, BECKER GJ: Reflux nephropathy in the adult, in *Reflux Nephropathy,* edited by HODSON J, KINCAID-SMITH P, New York, Masson Publishing, USA, 1979, chap 3, p 21

23. ARZE RS, RAMOS JM, OWEN JP, MORLEY AR, ELLIOTT RW, WILKINSON R, WARD MK, KERR DNS: The natural history of chronic pyelonephritis in the adult. *Quart J Med* 51:396–410, 1982

24. ELO J, TALLGREN LG, ALFTHAN O, SARNA S: Character of urinary tract infections and pyelonephritic renal scarring after antireflux surgery. *J Urol* 129:343–346, 1983

25. RANSLEY PG, RISDON RA: Reflux nephropathy: effects of antimicrobial therapy on the evolution of the early pyelonephritic scar. *Kidney Int* 20:733–742, 1981

26. HODSON CJ: Reflux nephropathy: A personal historical review. *AJR* 137:451–462, 1981

27. LJUNGQVIST A, LAGERGREN C: The Ask-Upmark kidney. A congenital renal anomaly studied by micro-angiography and histology. *Acta Pathol Microbiol Scand* 56:277–283, 1962

28. BEEUWKES R III: Vascular-tubular relationships in the human kidney, in *Renal Pathophysiology—Recent Advances,* edited by LEAF A, BOLIS L, GIEBISCH G, GORINI S, New York, Raven Press, 1980, p 155

Natural History and Treatment of Reflux Nephropathy

Priscilla S. Kincaid-Smith

Reflux nephropathy (or chronic atrophic pyelonephritis) emerged some 30 years ago as a clinical entity of particular importance in childhood. Its recognition was very largely due to the early work of one of the contributors to this Section, Dr. John Hodson [1], who has been delving into the problems of reflux nephropathy very effectively ever since then.

For a number of years, reflux nephropathy was thought to be a pediatric problem, primarily because coarse parenchymal scars rarely develop after childhood. Recently, it has become clear, however, that reflux nephropathy makes an important contribution to adult end-stage renal failure programs; and hence nephrologists have a major stake in defining those factors that cause the progressive renal damage and how they can be altered by treatment. I shall not address the question of prevention of reflux nephropathy in any detail, but clearly any methods aimed at prevention must be implemented in infancy because, by the time a first symptomatic infection occurs, 22% of kidneys in which vesicoureteric reflux is present already show parenchymal damage or reflux nephropathy [2]. Five aspects that are important in the natural history of this condition will be discussed: namely, progressive scar formation, hypertension, proteinuria, complications in pregnancy, and renal failure. Specific therapeutic approaches will then be discussed.

Progressive Scar Formation

Progressive, coarse renal scarring demonstrated radiologically has been the major focus of follow-up studies in childhood, perhaps because radiologists have played such an important part in recognizing reflux nephropathy and in documenting its progression.

This manuscript was presented as part of a Symposium on *Reflux Nephropathy: Current Status.*

That established scars are present at the time of presentation in 22% of infant kidneys [2] and in 33 to 36% of kidneys in children aged 0 to 12 with urinary tract infection [3] has significant implications for progressive scar formation. Kidneys that already show scars are much more likely to develop further scarring. Progressive scarring has been documented in children in over 60% of scarred kidneys with reflux by both Filly et al [4] and Lenaghan et al [5]. These studies are quoted rather than the prospective studies in which specific treatment methods were adopted, such as those of the U.C.H. group or the Göteborg group [3, 6] where the rate of progressive scarring was lower. The studies of Filly and Lenaghan et al [4, 5] are retrospective surveys and perhaps reflect what usually happens in reflux nephropathy.

Fewer progressive scars develop in kidneys that are normal at the first examination. Filly et al [4] found that new scars appeared in normal kidneys in only 5% of those managed conservatively, whereas Lenaghan et al [5] found progressive scars in 21%.

Most groups have also found a relation between the degree of progressive scarring and the grade of reflux [2, 3, 7–10]. Also, the very important findings of Winberg et al [6] must not be overlooked. In their "Göteborg study," in which the influence of vesicoureteric reflux on scar formation was not apparent, they stressed the importance of infection in scar formation and in growth arrest. They made careful measurements of the renal parenchyma 4.1 years after an episode of neonatal pyelonephritis. The renal parenchyma was significantly reduced irrespective of the presence or grade of reflux, comparing reflux grades 0 and I and reflux grades III and IV. In long-term follow-up studies in 20 girls who developed renal scars, there was again no correlation between the mean renal parenchymal area and the grade of reflux. Infection thus appears to have had more influence than reflux as a determinant of scar formation in the Göteborg study [6, 11].

Indeed, all the groups who have found a correlation between the degree of scar formation and the grade of reflux in children with reflux nephropathy also stress the importance of infection. Progressive disease in sterile reflux has been sparsely documented. Stephens [12] found no evidence of parenchymal damage in boys with prolonged sterile reflux over 5 to 15 years. Rolleston, Maling, and Hodson [13] documented scar formation in five patients with intrarenal reflux in whom no infection was documented over the period during which the scar appeared. In the vast majority of patients for whom fresh scars or progressive scars have been documented, infection has been invoked as an important contributing factor.

There is an important subgroup with vesicoureteric reflux and a sterile urine who have severe bilateral reflux and diffuse parenchymal atrophy. Heale [10] terms these the *thin-rim kidneys* and regards the lesions as being congenital rather than acquired. These patients may present with uremia and no history of infection [14].

Heale [10] documented deterioration in four boys with severe bilateral reflux and thin-rim kidneys in the absence of infection. Three of them had persisting severe reflux, but in the fourth, deterioration occurred in the absence of reflux, which had been corrected surgically.

Age is an important factor in the formation of new scars and in progressive scarring and impaired renal function [6, 15]. The kidney appears to be particularly susceptible in the neonatal period and in infancy. It has been commonly stated in the literature that fresh scar formation is rare over the age of 4. However, the study frequently quoted [13] actually stated that intrarenal reflux did not occur after the age of 4. In a recent study [9], more scars appeared in children over 5 than in those under 5. The same is true of the study by Smellie et al [3] in which 10 scars were documented in a follow-up of 75 children. Only 4 of the 10 scars could have developed before the age of 5. The study of Shah, Robins, and White [8] also documented new scars in two children over the age of 5.

The publications in which new scars in previously normal kidneys have been documented are summarized in Table 1. With the exception of the study by Rolleston et al [13], all were associated with infection, and only two studies [6, 9] reported acquired scars in the absence of vesicoureteric reflux. Perhaps with future studies, the reason for these differences will become apparent.

For many years, the pattern of coarse scars and their sharp demarcation from surrounding areas puzzled investigators in the field. The susceptibility of certain papillae, in particular the compound papillae, to intrarenal reflux was noted by Hodson soon after he commenced studies in the pig [19]. He pointed this out to Ransley, who subsequently, in a series of elegant studies carried out in conjunction with Risdon [20, 21], demonstrated the susceptibility of the gaping ducts of Bellini in compound papillae to intrarenal reflux.

Renal Function and Compensatory Renal Parenchymal Hypertrophy in Progressive Scar Formation

There is surprisingly little written about renal function in children with reflux nephropathy. One explanation for this is the rapid increase in glomerular

Table 1. Fresh scars developing in previously normal kidneys[a]

Reference	Normal kidneys with fresh scars	VUR	UTI	Age of scarring
	No. of children			
Penn and Breidahl [16]	9	9	9	2 to 8 yr
Smellie et al [3]	10	10	10	3 mo to 10 yr
Bergstrom et al 1972 [17]	3	—	3	0 to 6 mo
Rolleston et al [13]	3	3	+	10 days to 3 yr
Filly et al [4]	4	4	4	Under 10 yr
Lenaghan et al [5]	24	24	24	—
Shah et al [8]	5	5	5	2 to 9 yr
Heale and Ferguson [18]	44	44	44	4 to 10 yr
Winter et al [9]	41[b]	(50%)	41	1 to 16 yr
Winberg et al [6]	23	(30%)	23	0 to 16 yr

[a] Abbreviations are defined as follows: VUR, vesicoureteric reflux; UTI, urinary tract infection.

[b] Kidneys were normal or "minimally scarred" on initial study.

filtration rate (GFR) that accompanies unilateral loss of renal substance. This event is well documented in other situations [22, 23], which means that renal function tests fail to change as progressive scarring develops in one kidney or in areas of both kidneys while other areas hypertrophy.

Studies are now available on the function of individual kidneys in reflux nephropathy in children with clinical infections [24] and girls with asymptomatic bacteriuria [25]. Both studies were done at a single point in time. Aperia et al [24], on the basis of more serious impairment of function in older girls, concluded that "gradual deterioration in renal function" occurred if grade III vesicoureteric reflux persisted, but they did not consider the impact of renal scarring. Verrier-Jones et al [25] found that scarred kidneys were associated with a significant impairment of renal function, but that neither persisting vesicoureteric reflux nor covert bacteriuria appeared to be associated with progressive damage. In a study of symptomatic girls, Aperia et al [24] showed that by puberty, the GFR was reduced to 50% of normal in kidneys with persisting vesicoureteric reflux. In girls with asymptomatic bacteriuria, Verrier-Jones et al [25] showed that the GFR was reduced to 50% in individual scarred kidneys. Now that it is simple to estimate separate function of the two kidneys using labeling techniques and the gamma camera, prospective renal function studies will inevitably become available and may help to resolve some of the differences in these two studies. Impaired function is frequent if pyelonephritis develops under the age of 3 [15].

The morphologic equivalent of the increase in GFR that results from unilateral or segmental renal damage is hypertrophy of nephrons. Careful documentation of the renal parenchymal area has been carried out by Winberg et al [6] using the Eklöf and Ringertz method [26]. When one kidney is scarred, the other appears to compensate by increasing its size, so that by the age of 16 the total parenchyma of both is 99% of the predicted normal. The scarred kidney fails to grow and often decreases in size for some years, but it grows at puberty. In this study, persisting reflux did not influence compensatory growth, grade III reflux being compatible with considerable hypertrophy. Hypertrophy of noninvolved areas may maintain overall GFR at or near to normal levels in spite of extensive parenchymal loss.

In summary then, the factors that predispose to progressive scar formation are the following:

1. The age of the patient, the young being far more susceptible to the development of coarse segmental scars and functional impairment.
2. Infection, a major factor in most documented new scar or progressive scar formation.
3. The presence of existing scars.
4. The grade of reflux.

Hypertension

It has been known for many years that hypertension is present in 60 to 70% of the patients who have chronic atrophic pyelonephritis (reflux nephropathy) [27, 28]. A significant proportion of these cases have been associated with malignant hypertension. In children, reflux nephropathy is the most frequent underlying cause of severe hypertension [29, 30].

The cause of hypertension in chronic pyelonephritis is still a matter of debate, but because of the increased peripheral renin levels [31] and the increased renin levels in renal veins [32–36], the suggestion that renal ischemia may be a factor [27] has regained some popularity and has therapeutic implications. Only one study [37] failed to find a relation between renal vein renins and unilateral scarring from reflux nephropathy.

Several studies suggest that there is a relation between the degree of scarring and hypertension, although in a few cases hypertension has been present when only a small parenchymal scar can be demonstrated. A normal kidney at the time of correction of vesicoureteric reflux does not protect the patient from later development of hypertension [38].

In two long-term follow-up studies in children, hypertension was a prominent feature. Smellie and Normand [39] documented hypertension at the time of presentation in 13% of children. Half of these had malignant hypertension. During follow-up, 21% of the children had developed hypertension, two of them required treatment, one having a blood pressure of 180/120 at the age of 16.

Wallace et al [38] surveyed 141 patients in whom reflux had been repaired over 10 years before. Of them, 8% had a blood pressure consistently above 140/90 requiring treatment, and a further 5 had readings recorded over 140/90 but did not require treatment. Two of the hypertensive patients were in renal failure.

In Smellie and Normand's study [39], advanced scarring, what they termed the *end-stage type,* was present unilaterally (2 patients) or bilaterally (2 patients), and a further 2 had severe bilateral coarse scars. In the study of Wallace et al [38], 14 of 17 patients showed unilateral or bilateral scarring, but 3 had normal kidneys on preoperative radiographs.

In the adult, hypertension has been a prominent feature [40]. Of our patients, 21% of females and 23% of males presented with hypertension as their major clinical finding and were found to have reflux nephropathy during investigation for a cause of their hypertension. Among 217 patients, hypertension (a diastolic pressure greater than 90 mm Hg) was present in 42% at presentation (40% of females and 58% of males). Six (2.7%) had malignant hypertension. Hypertension developed during follow-up in a further 4%—a much lower figure than in Smellie and Normand's series [39].

There is a correlation between the presence of hypertension and both proteinuria ($P < 0.001$) and impaired renal function ($P < 0.0001$).

Malignant hypertension may greatly accelerate the rate of deterioration in renal function.

Reflux Nephropathy and Pregnancy

Adult women with reflux nephropathy often present as a result of urinary tract infection, hypertension, or proteinuria discovered during pregnancy.

Of our 184 female patients, 35 (19%) presented during pregnancy. Table 2 shows the complications that occurred during pregnancy in 72 patients. Although most women with reflux nephropathy do not develop serious complications during pregnancy, hypertension and urinary tract infection often require treatment.

Pregnancy may greatly accelerate the rate of progression to end-stage renal failure in patients with reflux nephropathy and impaired renal function. We have studied 5 such women during pregnancy in the past 10 years. Their progression to end-stage renal failure was much more rapid than that seen in other women with reflux nephropathy and impaired renal function. Malignant hypertension and pregnancy have a similar effect, both being associated with a very rapid decline to severe renal failure, which is not seen in other patients with reflux nephropathy in whom deterioration is gradual. We have documented this sudden deterioration related to pregnancy in patients who have previously remained relatively stable over periods of up to 10 years (Fig. 1).

Proteinuria

The potentially serious significance of proteinuria became apparent to us some 15 years ago. We had previously noted glomerular lesions in all nephrectomy specimens removed prior to transplantation. These had been attributed to the combined effects of severe hypertension and uremia: the so-called alterative glomerulitis. It was the documentation of proteinuria associated with glomerular lesions in the contralateral kidney in patients with apparent unilateral reflux scarring that first drew attention to a progressive glomerular lesion as a significant prognostic factor in reflux nephropathy [41, 42].

The occurrence of glomerular lesions in reflux nephropathy and their potential significance were reported at two international meetings in 1972 [41, 42]. Subsequently, biopsy and nephrectomy specimens from 103 patients with reflux nephropathy were reviewed. Glomerular lesions were found in 100%

Table 2. Complications during pregnancy in 72 women (152 pregnancies)

Complications	No.	Percentage of total pregnancies
Urinary infections	34	22.4
Pre-eclampsia	25	16.4
Hypertension	20	13.2
Miscarriage	12	7.9
Proteinuria	11	7.2
Impaired renal function	10	6.6
Stone	3	2.0
Fetal death in utero	2	1.3
No complications	47	31.0

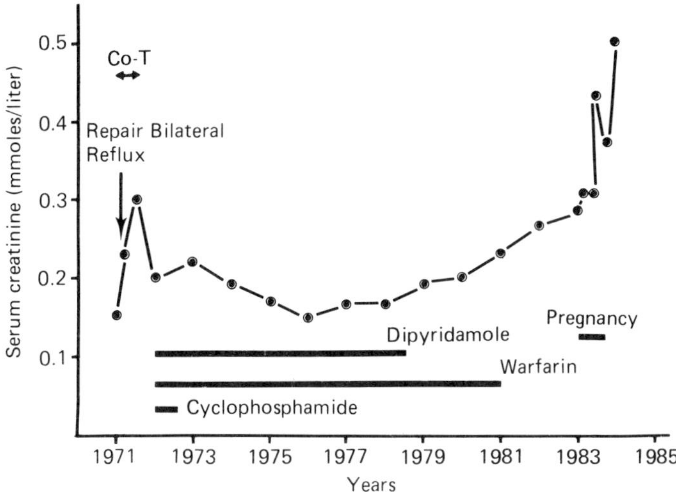

Fig. 1. Serum creatinine concentration in relation to other features over 12 years in a patient with bilateral vesicoureteric reflux and bilateral renal scars. At the time of correction of reflux in 1971, the function deteriorated sharply. Treatment of infection with cotrimoxazole could have been partly responsible. In 1972, a biopsy examination showed membranous glomerulonephritis, for which treatment with cyclophosphamide for 6 months and dipyridamole for 6 years and warfarin for 9 years was associated with relatively stable renal function. A gradual decline began after the dipyridamole was discontinued, but a greatly accelerated rate of decline accompanied pregnancy in 1984.

of the uremic patients and in over 80% of those with normal or only slightly abnormal serum creatinine concentrations and proteinuria [43]. Patients with proteinuria and glomerular lesions deteriorated to end-stage renal failure in spite of control of hypertension and infection and disappearance or surgical correction of vesicoureteric reflux. Progressive focal and segmental hyalinosis and sclerosis were demonstrated in most renal biopsy specimens from such patients, although a few showed membranous (Fig. 1) or diffuse proliferative glomerulonephritis. It became clear from these studies that proteinuria in patients with reflux nephropathy reflected a progressive glomerular lesion and was a poor prognostic sign [43–45].

Figure 2 illustrates our present findings in patients with reflux nephropathy and relates proteinuria to the outcome. It can be seen that proteinuria over 0.2 g in 24 hr is associated with a highly significant risk of developing renal functional impairment.

This association between a glomerular lesion and progressive disease in reflux nephropathy has now been confirmed by a number of other groups [46–49]. Cotran [49] believes that the glomerular lesion in reflux nephropathy is the counterpart of the progressive glomerular lesion documented in animal models in which five-sixths of the renal parenchyma is removed or infarcted [50, 51]. Progressive hyalinosis and sclerosis in glomeruli associated with hyperfiltration has recently received much attention [52].

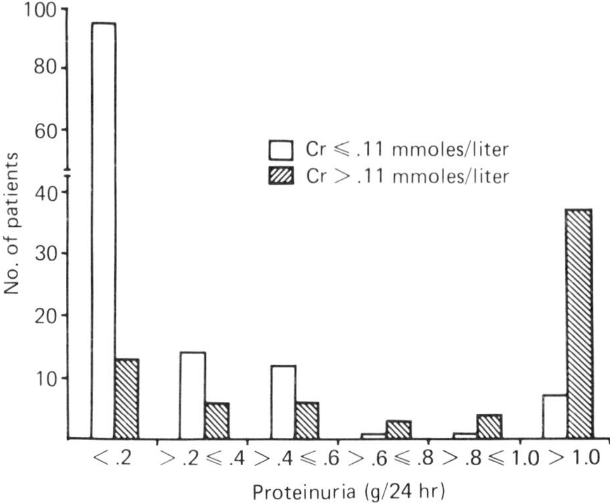

Fig. 2. Relation between protein excretion and renal functional impairment (plasma creatinine, > 0.11 mmoles/liter) at the end of follow-up in 211 patients followed prospectively for a mean of 62.8 months. Of this group, 108 (51.2%) had less than 0.2 g/d of urinary protein at presentation; these patients had a significantly ($P <$ 0.0001) greater chance of retaining normal renal function at the end of follow-up than did the patients with > 0.2 g/d of urinary protein at presentation.

Although, as Cotran points out [49], all the patients with reflux nephropathy and a glomerular lesion reported by other authors [46, 48] have had abnormal renal function, it was the occurrence of glomerular lesions in the contralateral kidney in patients with unilateral disease and normal renal function that first indicated to us that progression of this glomerular lesion was the most important factor in deterioration reflux nephropathy in adults [41, 42].

We have studied five such patients. Details are given in Table 3. In all, the contralateral kidney was normal in size or hypertrophied; in two patients, it measured over 16 cm in length. The course of one such patient is depicted in Figure 3.

If progressive obliteration of glomerular capillaries by hyalinosis and sclerosis is due to hyperfiltration of residual nephrons, its occurrence in patients with unilateral reflux nephropathy has important implications for patients who require nephrectomy or for living kidney transplant donors. It is also relevant that Kiprov, Colvin, and McCluskey [53] have found similar glomerular lesions in two of seven patients with unilateral renal agenesis, although they did not find glomerular disease in patients who died 8 to 46 years after unilateral nephrectomy in adulthood. Because the most serious forms of reflux scarring occur in early childhood, unilateral reflux nephropathy is potentially a very long-lasting form of "hyperfiltration" and should more closely resemble the renal agenesis group than an adult nephrectomy group. Proteinuria and progressive glomerular lesions were found in only 5 of our 102 patients with unilateral renal disease; a much lower proportion than

Table 3. Progressive renal deterioration in predominantly unilateral disease[a]

| Patient no. (sex/ age) | Radiology findings | | | | At presentation | | | At follow-up | | Comments |
| | Renal length (cm) | | Reflux grade | | P_{Cr} (mmoles/ liter) | Proteinuria (g/d) | Blood pressure | Period (mo) | Final P_{Cr} (mmoles/ liter) | |
	Right	Left	Right	Left						
1 (F,22)	5.0 Scarred	11.5 Normal	1	0	0.45	3.0	150/100	14	1.74	Deterioration precipitated by pregnancy and malignant hypertension
2 (F,27)	16.0 Normal	8.0 Scarred	0	0	0.07	<0.20	160/115	159	0.21	Developed proteinuria, mild controlled hypertension
3 (F,33)	12.7 ? Minor scarring	8.5 Scarred	0	3	0.09	1.20	220/130	122	1.20	Progressive deterioration despite reflux repair
4 (F,42)	11.0 Normal	17.0 ? Minor scarring	2	0	0.10	0.50	160/110	192	0.41	—
5(F,24)	6.0 Scarred	13.2 Minor scarring	1	0	0.12	0.45	130/80	180	1.92	Final deterioration accelerated by malignant hypertension

[a] P_{Cr} is the plasma creatinine concentration.

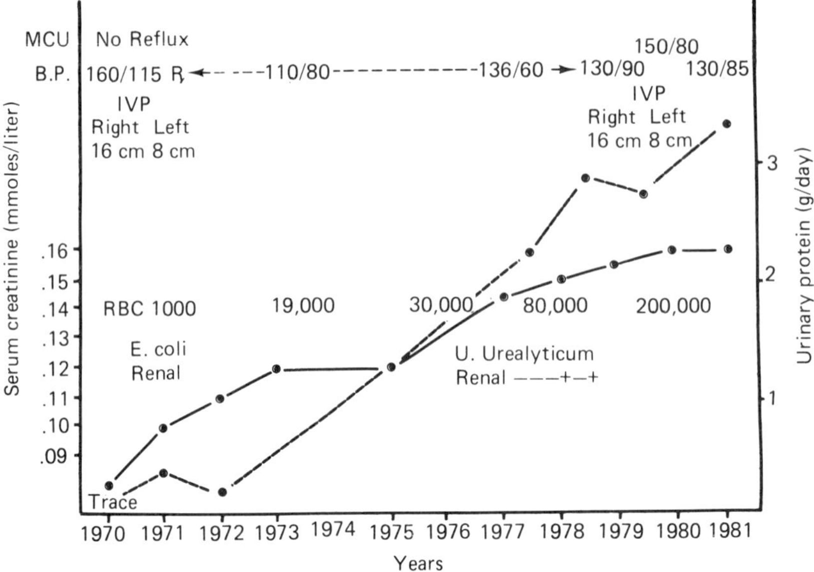

Fig 3. Course in a patient with scarring of reflux nephropathy in a small left kidney
and with a large (16 cm) right kidney. A trace of urinary protein (●- - - ●) in 1970
gradually increased over the following 11 years to 2.5 g/d, and over the same period
the serum creatinine (●———●) rose from 0.08 to 0.16 mmoles/liter. The urinary
erythrocyte count increased over the same period. Hypertension and infection were
controlled.

that reported by Kiprov et al in renal agenesis [53]. As might be expected,
proteinuria is more frequent in bilateral reflux nephropathy than it is in
unilateral reflux nephropathy: 17% of patients with unilateral scars and 41%
of patients with bilateral scars have greater than 0.6 g of proteinuria.

Renal Failure From Reflux Nephropathy

The most serious cases of reflux nephropathy are those that progress to end-
stage renal failure. Progression in adults is due to increasing destruction of
glomeruli by focal and segmental hyalinosis and sclerosis, although acute
deterioration caused by severe hypertension or pregnancy contributes in a
few patients.

Males have a significantly higher serum creatinine concentration at the
time of presentation than females do, and they have a higher percentage of
progression to end-stage renal failure.

One of the most tantalizing questions is the relation between the small
numbers presenting with end-stage renal disease and how this relates to the
prevalence of vesicoureteric reflux and parenchymal scarring in the community.

We can only calculate the prevalence among infants and children from population studies of bacteriuria, and so these exclude the nonbacteriuric cases, which may far exceed the numbers with bacteriuria. Bacteriuria is present in 1% of newborn infants; half of these have vesicoureteric reflux, a prevalence of 0.5% [54]. In infancy, both asymptomatic bacteriuria and symptomatic urinary tract infection are more frequent in males than in females, but we then lose sight of most males until a very small number (some 1 to 2 per million of the population per year) appear with renal failure.

The situation differs in females, in whom patients continue to develop urinary tract infection after the age of 1 year. Some 75% of children and adults in large clinical series with reflux nephropathy are female, and most of these are diagnosed as a result of symptoms of urinary tract infection. In apparently healthy schoolgirls, 1 to 2% have been found to have asymptomatic bacteriuria on screening studies. Between 19 and 34% of these have vesicoureteric reflux [55–59]. This means that vesicoureteric reflux is present in at least 0.4% of schoolgirls (it is probably more common than this, because it has only been identified in those with bacteriuria at one point in time). From 13 to 20% of the schoolgirls in the studies just mentioned had parenchymal scarring, so that the prevalence of reflux nephropathy in this age group is only a little lower than that of vesicoureteric reflux.

Bacteriuria screening studies in pregnant women [60, 61] have shown that 21% have vesicoureteric reflux and that 17 to 20% have parenchymal scars of reflux nephropathy, which means that 0.3 to 0.6% of women of childbearing age have reflux nephropathy. Studies in nonpregnant women with asymptomatic bacteriuria have demonstrated reflux nephropathy in 13% [62]. In the latter, radiographs were also done in controls, and 2% of these showed scars—another hint that reflux nephropathy is more frequent than is suggested from a study of bacteriuric subjects.

Reflux nephropathy can only be diagnosed with any confidence in patients with end-stage renal failure by an examination of nephrectomy specimens (or at autopsy). When nephrectomy was routinely performed prior to transplantation at the Royal Melbourne Hospital, we had the opportunity of examining 130 nephrectomy specimens from a consecutive series of patients presenting with end-stage renal failure. Of them, 18.5% showed classical lesions of chronic atrophic pyelonephritis or reflux nephropathy. Two-thirds of these were women. Thus, 3 women per million of the population per year present with end-stage reflux nephropathy. It is worth emphasizing that the parenchymal lesions are quite distinctive and cannot be confused with other lesions, such as analgesic nephropathy, when the whole kidney is available. Renal biopsy examinations, on the other hand, can be misleading.

Comparing the prevalence of reflux nephropathy in girls and young women with the numbers presenting in end-stage renal failure suggests that girls and young women with reflux nephropathy and bacteriuria have a 0.08% risk per year of developing end-stage renal failure—perhaps a lifetime risk as high as 5%. This calculation assumes that all those who develop end-stage renal failure would have been detected in screening studies; hence the risk may be much lower. Asscher et al, basing their calculation on observed progressive scarring, calculated that 1 in 1000 schoolgirls develop progressive renal damage [63]. Stamey [64], using again a different method of calculating those at risk of progression to end-stage renal failure, came up with a figure of 1 in 4000 girls under 12 having serious parenchymal scarring. Clinical studies in series of adults with reflux nephropathy are few, and the percentage of patients deteriorating to end-stage renal failure is influenced by those referred because of impaired renal function. If we exclude from our series the patients referred with uremic symptoms and those with a serum creatinine over 0.5 mmoles/liter at the time of presentation, 8% of our adult female patients and 11% of males have deteriorated to end-stage renal failure over a follow-up period of 2 to 20 years. All of these had proteinuria at the time of referral, indicating that they already had the glomerular lesion that accounts for progression in adults [43, 65].

There are a few large series in adults. The Newcastle study [40] does not mention end-stage renal failure, but from their Figure 6, eight patients must have been in end-stage renal failure or very close to it at the end of follow-up. This figure of 6% is a little lower than ours. The study from Portsmouth, which included children and adults, reported deterioration to end-stage renal failure in only 3 (5.4%) [66].

Clinical follow-up studies in children make little mention of renal function, let alone end-stage renal failure [4, 5, 10, 67]. As noted above, they concentrate on radiologic documentation of progression, from which one can infer relatively normal function; otherwise serial radiologic studies would not have been performed. Smellie and Normand [39] report 4 of 65 children developing renal failure during 5 to 30 years follow-up. This figure of 6% is not very different from that recorded above in adults, but no children had presented with normal renal function. Heale [10] mentions deteriorating renal function in four boys. None showed infection, three showed grade IV reflux, but in one this had been corrected surgically. This group with a very dilated system and thin rim of parenchyma may be a high-risk group in childhood because 18% in Heale's study had deteriorating renal function.

There is no doubt that reflux nephropathy makes a significant contribution to end-stage renal failure in childhood [68, 69]. In adults, the age of patients progressing to end-stage renal failure with reflux nephropathy is significantly lower than it is for adults with other causes of end-stage renal failure. Males presenting to our hospital developed end-stage renal failure at a mean age of 22 and females at a mean age of 33.

Specific Therapeutic Approaches in Reflux Nephropathy

Surgical Correction of Vesicoureteric Reflux

The greatest current controversy in the field of reflux nephropathy concerns the question of surgical repair of vesicoureteric reflux.

Vesicoureteric reflux disappears spontaneously in most children. This was first documented by Stephens and Lenaghan [70]. They reported that reflux ceased in 19 to 59 refluxing ureters and was greatly reduced in 17. They also reported a reduction in caliber of the ureter in 22 of 23 in which reflux persisted.

Since that time, many other groups have reported cessation of reflux. Normand and Smellie [71] reported the disappearance of vesicoureteric reflux in 79% of ureters and 71% of 75 children followed over 8 to 16 years. Reflux disappeared in 41% of ureters with grade IV vesicoureteric reflux.

Perhaps the strongest argument in favor of the conservative approach to the management of vesicoureteric reflux is this very high rate of spontaneous disappearance of reflux.

Those who argue in favor of surgical repair of vesicoureteric reflux do so on the basis of: (1) a reduction in the number of infective episodes and the need for long-term supervision of these; (2) the prevention of progressive scar formation or deterioration in renal function; (3) the restoration of normal renal growth.

Frequency of Infection After Surgical Correction of Vesicoureteric Reflux

At Stanford, Govan et al [72] divided girls with recurrent urinary tract infection into three groups: 61 with a vesicoureteric reflux that was corrected surgically, 42 with a vesicoureteric reflux that was not repaired, and 66 who had no vesicoureteric reflux. There was no difference in the rate of recurrence of infection in these three groups.

Huland, Scherf, and Köllerman [73] followed 21 females for up to 3 years after surgical correction of vesicoureteric reflux. Only 2 did not develop subsequent episodes of urinary tract infection, and the relapse rate was similar before and after surgery. There has been a suggestion that recurrent episodes after repair of vesicoureteric reflux are less likely to be renal [74]. While this may be important, clearly from the other two studies repair of reflux does not avoid the need to follow patients and to treat episodes of infection.

Prevention of Progressive Scar Formation or Functional Deterioration

Progressive scar formation and functional deterioration have both been documented after repair of vesicoureteric reflux and after spontaneous disappearance of vesicoureteric reflux.

In the literature, there are many examples showing that once renal function is impaired, surgical correction of vesicoureteric reflux is of no benefit in slowing the rate of decline in renal function. Although it is possible that the high rate of subsequent scarring observed in 66% of the children whose reflux was corrected surgically may have occurred in areas damaged prior to surgery [4], this is clearly a question that can only be answered by a controlled study. At least three controlled trials are being conducted at the present time.

The group with the highest risk of scar formation, infants under 1 year of age with gross vesicoureteric reflux, are being investigated at the Hospital for Sick Children in London. The current status of this trial is summarized in Table 4. A 5-year follow-up has shown no difference between the treated and control groups.

The results in a large study being conducted in Birmingham were published in 1983 [75]. In it, 149 children were allocated at random to surgery and nonsurgery groups. At entry, all patients had grade III reflux with or without renal scarring or grade II reflux with scarring. Of those followed for 2 years or longer, vesicoureteric reflux was abolished in 67 of 69 refluxing ureters in the surgery group.

All patients were receiving drug therapy to prevent infection. Breakthrough infection occurred in 12 of 49 in the surgery group and in 14 of 47 in the nonsurgery group. ^{51}Cr-EDTA clearances showed no significant difference at 2 years in any age group, and there was no difference in progressive scarring or new scar formation. New scars appeared in two kidneys in the surgery group and two in the nonsurgery group. One in each group was associated with breakthrough infection, and one was not.

At the present time, this is by far the best data available on which to base a decision about surgical treatment of vesicoureteric reflux. Present results suggest that, at least in the first 2 years, surgical correction has shown no advantages over conservative management.

Renal Growth

Hodson [76] first suggested that renal growth was impaired in children with urinary tract infection and vesicoureteric reflux. Many authors have subsequently documented this; however, the influence of infection has not usually been considered. Renal infection, without reflux, produces significant growth retardation [11]. In the case of neonatal pyelonephritis, this growth retardation is still demonstrable 4 years after the original infection, and Winberg [11] found that this was not influenced by the presence or degree of vesicoureteric reflux.

Two studies have demonstrated normal renal growth rates after surgical correction of vesicoureteric reflux [77, 78]. Smellie et al [79], however, have

Table 4. Controlled trial of surgical correction of vesicoureteric reflux[a]

Surgical correction	Conservative management
11[b]	12
At 5 years	
6	7
(No difference in GFR)	

[a] Data are from the report given by Ransley at the Workshop on Reflux Nephropathy, Santa Ynez, October, 1982.

[b] Three of these showed reflux after surgery.

documented normal growth rates in 100 of 111 kidneys drained by refluxing ureters in children on conservative management. Growth was impaired in only 10 of 111 kidneys, all of which were exposed to infection, and in a further kidney, which was probably infected. Impaired growth was independently associated with infection and renal scarring, but not independently associated with the severity of vesicoureteric reflux.

On balance, therefore, although the growth of kidneys is impaired when vesicoureteric reflux is associated with infection, impaired growth in association with sterile reflux is not well documented.

Only one controlled study is available to answer questions about renal growth rates after surgical correction of vesicoureteric reflux. This study from Birmingham [75] showed retarded renal growth at all ages, but no difference between surgery and nonsurgery groups after 2 years' observation.

Further data from this study and from the current international study [80] and study at the Hospital for Sick Children in London are awaited with interest, but on the basis of information presently available, there is no evidence that surgical repair of vesicoureteric reflux independently increases renal growth rate.

Treatment of Urinary Tract Infection

There is no real controversy as to whether urinary tract infection should be treated. The combination of urinary tract infection and vesicoureteric reflux is recognized as a threat to the preservation of normal function and structure of the kidney.

Almost all the evidence on progressive scar formation discussed above suggests that it occurs when both infection and reflux are present. Only a handful of cases have been reported in which new scars or progressive scarring has been documented in the absence of infection (Table 1).

The declining renal function in girls with urinary tract infection was clearly related to infection and not reflux by Berg and Johansson [15], although both factors were present in the study by Aperia et al [25].

Data from two groups [11, 71] shows that with prompt diagnosis and treatment of urinary tract infection and careful follow-up, the long-term course is benign, with few children developing scars or other serious manifestations of reflux nephropathy.

No controlled trial has compared the effects of intermittent treatment of infective episodes with the long-term prophylactic therapy as advocated by Normand and Smellie [71]. It is unlikely, however, that a controlled trial will be carried out. The rare development of new scars or progression of old scars in Smellie's series [3, 39, 71] stands in contrast with the frequency of scars in two other series [4, 5] in which no special attention was given to treatment of infection.

Even when infection did recur and when there was poor compliance with therapy, Verrier-Jones [25] was not able to document a difference in renal function in normal kidneys or scarred kidneys, nor in those with and without vesicoureteric reflux in relation to the number of infected urine samples over a 7-year period of follow-up. These findings contrast with some others (for example that of Aperia et al [24]), perhaps because Verrier-Jones et al [25] were following schoolgirls aged 4 to 11 at entry and 11 to 18 at the end of the study, whereas all the girls in the study of Aperia et al were under 12.

In spite of this benign course in girls with urinary tract infection and vesicoureteric reflux, most would probably recommend long-term prophylactic antibacterial treatment until puberty in children with reflux.

Treatment of Hypertension

Drug treatment of hypertension in reflux nephropathy is not a controversial issue. There is a general consensus that hypertension should be treated both to prevent the distant cardiovascular complications associated with it and to prevent the rapid deterioration in function that accompanies accelerated hypertension.

Rather more controversial is the role of surgery in removing scarred parenchyma in the hope of achieving a cure for hypertension. Recently, several groups [29–33, 81] have reported high renin levels in renal veins and segmental veins draining areas of scarring in reflux nephropathy. Surgical excision of scars has resulted in cure of hypertension.

Treatment of the Glomerular Lesion

Although it is now well accepted that progression of glomerular lesions of focal and segmental hyalinosis and sclerosis is the mechanism whereby deterioration of function occurs in reflux nephropathy, the reason why the glomerular lesion develops is still uncertain.

Certain antigens that gain access to the renal parenchyma in reflux nephropathy, such as Tamm-Horsfall protein [82] and bacterial antigens, may evoke an antibody response in patients with reflux nephropathy. Although interstitial deposits of Tamm-Horsfall protein are a regular finding in reflux nephropathy, there is no evidence to show that Tamm-Horsfall protein is an antigen involved in glomerular lesions in reflux nephropathy. Similarly, there is no evidence that bacterial antigen is present in glomeruli.

The most popular theory concerning the glomerular lesion is that it represents a "hyperfiltration" lesion owing to loss of renal parenchyma and hyperfiltration of residual nephrons. There is evidence in animals to show that certain therapeutic measures will halt or delay progression of the similar glomerular lesion of focal and segmental hyalinosis and sclerosis associated with hyperfiltration. The two animal models are the five-sixths nephrectomy model [50] and the model in which part of the renal cortex is oblated by embolization [51].

Protein loading aggravates the glomerular lesion in the five-sixths nephrectomy model, and protein restriction slows progression of the lesion.

In humans, no studies have been done in reflux nephropathy, but there is evidence that marked protein restriction will reduce the rate of progression in advanced renal failure.

In the model in which renal parenchyma is ablated by infarction, Purkeson, Hoffsten, and Klahr [51] have shown that both heparin and warfarin will delay progression of the glomerular lesion associated with hyperfiltration.

There would be merit in setting up trials to test both protein restriction and anticoagulants in progressive reflux nephropathy. In humans, measures such as repair of vesicoureteric reflux, treatment of infection, and treatment of hypertension do not halt progression. Once the glomerular lesion has appeared, progression to renal failure seems inevitable, although the decline in renal function is usually gradual over 8 to 10 years.

References

1. HODSON CJ, EDWARDS D: Chronic pyelonephritis and vesico-ureteric reflux. *Clin Radiol* 11:219–331, 1960
2. ROLLESTON GL, SHANNON GT, UTLEY WLF: Relationship of infantile vesico-ureteric reflux to renal damage. *Br Med J* 1:460–463, 1970
3. SMELLIE JM, EDWARDS D, HUNTER N, NORMAND ICS, PRESCOD N: Vesico-ureteric reflux and renal scarring. *Kidney Int* 8:S65–S72, 1975
4. FILLY R, FRIEDLAND GW, GOVEN DE, FAIR WR: Development and progression of clubbing and scarring in children with recurrent urinary tract infections. *Radiology* 114:145–153, 1974
5. LENAGHAN D, WHITAKER JG, JENSEN F, STEPHENS FD: The natural history of reflux and long-term effects of reflux on the kidney. *J Urol* 115:728–730, 1976
6. WINBERG J, BOLLGREN I, KÄLLENIUS G, MÖLBY R, SVENSON SB: Clinical pyelonephritis and focal renal scarring: A selected review of pathogenesis, prevention and prognosis. *Pediatr Clin North Am* 29:802–814, 1982
7. ROLLESTON GL, SHANNON FT, UTLEY WLF: Follow-up of vesicoureteric reflux in the newborn. *Kidney Int* 8:S59–S64, 1975
8. SHAH KJ, ROBINS DG, WHITE RHR: Renal scarring and vesicoureteric reflux. *Arch Dis Child* 53:210–217, 1978
9. WINTER AL, HARDY BE, ALTON DJ, ARBUS GS, CHURCHILL BM: Acquired renal scars in children. *J Urology* 129:1190–1194, 1983
10. HEALE WF: Age of presentation and pathogenesis of reflux nephropathy, in *Reflux Nephropathy*, edited by HODSON J, KINCAID-SMITH P, New York, Masson Publishing USA Inc, 1979, p 140
11. WINBERG J, CLAESSON I, JACOBSSON B, JODAL U, PETERSON H: Renal growth after acute pyelonephritis in childhood: An epidemiological approach, in *Reflux Nephropathy*, edited by HODSON J, KINCAID-SMITH P, New York, Masson Publishing USA Inc, 1979, p 309
12. STEPHENS FD: Preliminary follow-up study of 101 children with reflux treated conservatively, in *Renal Infection and Renal Scarring*, edited by KINCAID-SMITH P, FAIRLEY KF, Melbourne, Mercedes Publishing Services, 1970, p 283
13. ROLLESTON GL, MALING TMJ, HODSON CJ: Intrarenal reflux and the scarred kidney. *Arch Dis Child* 49:531–539, 1974
14. HUTCH JA, SMITH DR: Sterile reflux: Report of 24 cases. *Urol Int* 24:460–465, 1969
15. BERG UB, JOHANSSON SB: Age as a main determinant of renal functional damage in urinary tract infection. *Arch Dis Child* 58:963–969, 1983
16. PENN IA, BREIHDAL PD: Ureteric reflux and renal damage. *Aust NZ J Surg* 37:163–168, 1967

17. BERGSTRÖM T, LARSON H, LINCOLN K, WINBERG J: Studies of urinary tract infection in infancy and childhood: 1280 patients with neonatal infection. *J Pediatr* 80:866–959, 1972
18. HEALE WF, FERGUSON RS: The pathogenesis of renal scarring in children, in *Proc 3rd International Symposium on Chronic Pyelonephritis,* edited by BRUMFITT W, KASS ED, 1979
19. HODSON CJ: Reflux nephropathy: A personal historical review. *Am J Roentgenol* 137:451–462, 1981
20. RANSLEY PG, RISDON RA: Renal papillary morphology and intrarenal reflux in the young pig. *Urol Res* 3:105–109, 1975
21. RANSLEY PG, RISDON RA: Renal papillary morphology in infants and young children. *Urol Res* 3:111–113, 1975
22. LYTTON B, SCHWARTZ SJ, FREEDMAN LR, THOMPSON JW: The effects of ischemic injury on compensatory renal growth. *J Urol* 100:128–132, 1968
23. LYTTON B: Current problems in compensatory renal growth. *Bull NY Acad Med* 50:1147–1156, 1974
24. APERIA A, BROBERGER O, ERICSSON NO, WIKSTAD I: Effect of vesicoureteral reflux on renal function in children with recurrent urinary tract infections. *Kidney Int* 9:418–423, 1976
25. VERRIER-JONES K, ASSCHER AW, VERRIER-JONES ER, MATTHOLE K, LEACH K, THOMSON GM: Glomerular filtration rate in schoolgirls with covert bacteriuria. *Br Med J* 285:1307–1310, 1982
26. EKLÖF O, RINGERTZ H: Kidney size in children: Method of assessment. *Acta Radiol [Diagn] (Stockh)* 17:617–625, 1976
27. KINCAID-SMITH P: Vascular obstruction in chronic pyelonephritis kidneys and its relation to hypertension. *Lancet* 2:1263–1269, 1955
28. WEISS S, PARKER F JR: Pyelonephritis: Its relation to vascular lesions and to arterial hypertension. *Medicine (Baltimore)* 18:221–315, 1939
29. STILL JC, COTTOM D: Severe hypertension in childhood. *Arch Dis Child* 42:30–34, 1967
30. GILL DG, MENDES DE COSTA B, CAMERON JS, JOSEPH MC, OGG CS, CHANTLER C: Analysis of 100 children with severe and persistent hypertension. *Arch Dis Child* 51:951–959, 1976
31. SAVAGE JM, DILLON MJ, SHAH V, BARRATT TM, WILLIAMS DI: Renin and blood-pressure in children with renal scarring and vesicoureteric reflux. *Lancet* 2:441–444, 1978
32. POUTASSE EF, STECKER JF JR, LADAGA LE, SPERBER EE: Malignant hypertension in children secondary to chronic pyelonephritis: Laboratory and radiologic indications for partial or total nephrectomy. *J Urol* 119:264–267, 1978
33. STECKER JF, READ BP, POUTASSE EF: Paediatric hypertension as a delayed sequelae of reflux-induced chronic pyelonephritis. *J Urol* 118:644–646, 1977
34. LUSCHER TF, VETTER H, STUDER A, POULIADIO G, KUHLMANN U, GLÄNZER K, LARGIADER F, HAURI D, GRENINGER P, SIEGENTHALER W, VETTER W: Renal venous renin activity in various forms of curable renal hypertension. *Clin Nephrol* 15:314–320, 1981
35. SIAMOPOULOS K, SELLARS L, MISHRA SC, ESSENHIGH DM, ROBSON V, WILKINSON R: Experience in the management of hypertension with unilateral chronic pyelonephritis: Results of nephrectomy in selected patients. *Q J Med,* New Series 52:349–362, 1983
36. HOLLAND NH: Reflux nephropathy and hypertension, in *Reflux Nephropathy,* edited by HODSON J, KINCAID-SMITH P, New York, Masson Publishing USA Inc, 1979, p 257

37. Bailey RR, McCrae CH, Maling JMJ, Tisch G, Little PJ: Renal vein renin concentration in the hypertension of unilateral reflux nephropathy. *J Urol* 120:21–33, 1978
38. Wallace DMA, Rothwell DL, Williams DI: The long-term follow-up of surgically treated vesicoureteric reflux. *Br J Urol* 50:479–484, 1978
39. Smellie J, Normand C: Reflux nephropathy in childhood, in *Reflux Nephropathy*, edited by Hodson J, Kincaid-Smith P, New York, Masson Publishing USA Inc, 1979, p 14
40. Arze RS, Ramos JM, Owen JP, Morley AR, Elliott RW, Wilkinson R, Ward MK, Kerr DNS: The natural history of chronic pyelonephritis in the adult. *Q J Med*, New Series 51(204):396–410, 1982
41. Kincaid-Smith P, Mathew TH, Becker EL: *Glomerulonephritis*. New York, John Wiley & Sons, 1973, p 156
42. Kincaid-Smith P: The prevention of renal failure, in *Proc Vth International Congress of Nephrology, Mexico*, Basel, Karger, 1972, vol 3 (Clinical), pp 100–118
43. Kincaid-Smith P: Glomerular and vascular lesions in chronic atrophic pyelonephritis and reflux nephropathy, in *Actualites Nephrologiques de l'Hopital Necker*, edited by Hamburger J, Crosnier J, Funck-Bretano J, Paris, Flammarion, 1975, p 187
44. Kincaid-Smith P, Becker GJ: Reflux nephropathy in the adult, in *Reflux Nephropathy*, edited by Hodson J, Kincaid-Smith P, New York, Masson Publishing USA Inc, New York, 1979, p 21
45. Kincaid-Smith P, Becker GJ: Reflux nephropathy and chronic atrophic pyelonephritis: A review. *J Infect Dis* 138:774–780, 1978
46. Torres VE, Velosa JA, Holley KE, Kelalis PP, Stickler GB, Kurtz SB: The progression of vesicoureteral reflux nephropathy. *Ann Intern Med* 92:776–784, 1980
47. Bhathena DB, Weiss JH, Holland NH, McMorrow RG, Curtis JJ, Lucas BA, Luke RG: Focal and segmental glomerular sclerosis in reflux nephropathy. *Am J Med* 68:886–892, 1980
48. Senekjian HO, Stinebaugh BJ, Mattioli CA, Suki WN: Irreversible renal failure following vesicoureteral reflux. *JAMA* 241:160–162, 1979
49. Cotran RS: Glomerulosclerosis in reflux nephropathy. *Kidney Int* 21:528–534, 1982
50. Shimamura T, Morrison AB: A progressive glomerulosclerosis occurring in partial five-sixths nephrectomized rats. *Am J Pathol* 79:95–102, 1975
51. Purkerson ML, Hoffsten PE, Klahr S: Pathogenesis of the glomerulopathy associated with renal infarction in rats. *Kidney Int* 9:407–417, 1976
52. Olson JL, Hostetter TH, Rennke HG, Brenner BM, Venkatachalam MA: Altered charge and size selective properties of the glomerular wall: A response to reduced renal mass. *Kidney Int* 16:857, 1979
53. Kiprov DD, Colvin RB, McCluskey RT: Focal and segmental glomerulosclerosis and proteinuria associated with unilateral renal agenesis. *Lab Invest* 46:275–281, 1982
54. Abbott GD: Neonatal bacteriuria: A prospective study in 1460 infants. *Br Med J* 1:267–269, 1972
55. Kunin CM, Southall I, Paquin AJ: Epidemiology of urinary tract infections: A pilot study of 3057 school children. *N Engl J Med* 253:817–823, 1960
56. Newcastle Asymptomatic Bacteriuria Research Group: Asymptomatic bacteriuria in school-children in Newcastle-upon-Tyne. *Arch Dis Child* 50:90–102, 1975
57. Editorial: Covert bacteriuria: Peril or partnership. *Br Med J* 1:1649–1650, 1978

58. SAVAGE DCL, HOWIE G, ADLER K, WILSON MI: Controlled trial of therapy in covert bacteriuria of childhood. *Lancet* 1:358–361, 1975
59. LINDBERG U, CLAESSON I, HANSON LA, JODAL U: Asymptomatic bacteriuria in schoolgirls: VIII. Clinical course during a 3 year follow-up. *J Paediatr* 92:194–199, 1978
60. KINCAID-SMITH P, BULLEN M: Bacteriuria in pregnancy. *Lancet* 1:395–399, 1965
61. WILLIAMS GSL, DAVIES DKL, EVANS KT, WILLIAMS JE: Vesicoureteric reflux in patients with bacteriuria in pregnancy. *Lancet* 2:1202–1205, 1968
62. SUSSMAN M, ASSCHER AW, WATERS WE, EVANS JAS, CAMPBELL H, EVANS KT, WILLIAMS JE: Asymptomatic significant bacteriuria in the non-pregnant woman: I. Description of a population. *Br Med J* 1:799–803, 1969
63. ASSCHER AW, SUSSMAN M, WATERS WE, EVANS, JAS, CAMPBELL H, EVANS KT, WILLIAMS JE: Asymptomatic significant bacteriuria in the non-pregnant woman: II. Response to treatment and follow-up. *Br Med J* 1:804–806, 1969
64. STAMEY T: Urinary infections in infancy and childhood, in *Pathogenesis and Treatment of Urinary Tract Infections,* Baltimore, Williams and Wilkins, 1980, p 290
65. KINCAID-SMITH P: Glomerular lesions in atrophic pyelonephritis and reflux nephropathy. *Kidney Int* 8:S81–S83, 1975
66. MIHINDUKULASURIYA JCL, MASKELL R, POLAK A: A study of fifty-eight patients with renal scarring associated with urinary tract infection. *Q J Med,* New Series 49(194):165–178, 1980
67. EDWARDS D, NORMAND ICS, PRESCOD N, SMELLIE JM: Disappearance of vesicoureteric reflux during long-term prophylaxis of urinary tract infection in children. *Br Med J* 2:285–288, 1977
68. CAMERON JS: The treatment of chronic renal failure in children by regular dialysis and by transplantation. *Nephron* 11:221–251, 1973
69. DONCKERWOLCKE RA, BROYER M, BRUNNER FP, BRYNGER H, JACOBS C, KRAMER P, SELWOOD NH, WING AJ: Combined report on regular dialysis and transplantation of children in Europe, XI, 1981, Madrid. *Proc EDTA* 19:61, 1982
70. STEPHENS FD, LENAGHAN D: The anatomical basis and dynamics of vesicoureteral reflux. *J Urol* 87:669–680, 1962
71. NORMAND C, SMELLIE J: Vesicoureteric reflux: The case for conservative management, in *Reflux Nephropathy,* edited by HODSON J, KINCAID-SMITH P, New York, Masson Publishing USA Inc, 1979, p 281
72. GOVAN DE, FAIR WR, FRIEDLAND GW, FILLY RA: Management of children with urinary tract infections: The Stanford experience. *Urology* 6:273–286, 1975
73. HULAND H, SCHERF H, KÖLLERMAN MW: Zur infektanfalligkeit des Harntraktes nach erfolgreicher anti-refluxplastik (I). *Urologe A* 17:282–285, 1978
74. GOVAN DE, PALMER JM: Urinary tract infection in children—the influence of successful antireflux operations in morbidity from infection. *Pediatrics* 44:677–684, 1969
75. BIRMINGHAM REFLUX STUDY GROUP: Prospective trial of operative versus non-operative treatment of severe vesicoureteric reflux: Two years' observation in 96 children. *Br Med J* 287:171–174, 1983
76. HODSON CJ: The kidneys in urinary infection. *Proc Roy Soc Med* 59:416–417, 1966
77. WILLSCHER MK, BAUER SB, ZAMMUTO PJ, RETIK AB: Renal growth and urinary infection following antireflux surgery in infants and children. *J Urol* 115:722–725, 1976

78. McCrae CU, Shannon FT, Utley WLF: Effect on renal growth of reimplantation of refluxing ureters. *Lancet* 1:1310–1312, 1974
79. Smellie JM, Edwards D, Normand JCS, Prescod N: Effect of vesicoureteric reflux on renal growth in children with urinary tract infection. *Arch Dis Child* 56:593–598, 1981
80. International Reflux Study Committee: Medical versus surgical treatment of primary vesicoureteral reflux: A prospective international reflux study in children. *J Urol* 125:277–283, 1981
81. Dillon MJ: In *Proc Symposium on Reflux Nephropathy,* edited by Hodson J, (in press, 1984)
82. Fasth A, Jodal U: Analysis of autoantibodies to Tamm-Horsfall kidney glycoprotein to detect patients with urinary tract infection at risk to develop renal scarring. *Proc Allergy* 33:247–258, 1983

Urolithiasis

Pathogenesis of Calcium Renal Stones

Fredric L. Coe and Joan H. Parks

Excessive supersaturation, preformed nuclei, and crystallization inhibitors of less than normal efficacy are the main reasons for calcium renal stones. Most of these stones are predominantly calcium oxalate, but often they contain some apatite or brushite [1]. Supersaturation is increased because the daily urine excretion of calcium or oxalate is above normal, the urine volume is low, or, in the case of calcium phosphate, the urine pH is too high [2]. Uric acid, and perhaps urine proteins, may form an initial solid phase upon which calcium oxalate can grow. Acidic glycoproteins and perhaps carbohydrate polymers in urine reduce the growth rate of calcium oxalate [3]. Reduced amounts of inhibitors, or abnormal inhibitors, may predispose some patients to stone formation.

Supersaturation

Hypercalciuria

In general, a daily calcium excretion above 4 mg/kg of body wt or 140 mg/g creatinine is considered hypercalciuria [4]. In 50 to 75% of patients, it is due to an inherited disorder of metabolism called *idiopathic hypercalciuria,* in which serum calcium is normal and there is no evidence of renal or systemic disease except stones. About 5% of the patients have primary hyperparathyroidism [5]. Less than 1% have sarcoidosis, hyperthyroidism, immobilization, Paget disease, glucocorticoid excess, or renal tubular acidosis as a cause of hypercalciuria.

This manuscript was presented as part of a Symposium on *Pathogenesis and Treatment of Calcium Nephrolithiasis.*

Idiopathic Hypercalciuria

Urine calcium and intestinal calcium absorption are elevated equally; so the overall calcium balance is normal [6]. A low-calcium diet lowers calcium excretion, but less than normal, so urine calcium may exceed dietary intake (Fig. 1). Even when there is ongoing calcium depletion, serum parathyroid hormone (PTH) levels tend to be low, and serum calcium concentrations remain higher than they are in normal people eating the same diet. Serum 1,25-dihydroxy-vitamin D_3 (1,25-D_3) levels are normal despite low PTH levels and high serum calcium concentrations. The fasting urine calcium concentration tends to be higher than it is in normal persons [7]. Overall, these characteristics seem best explained by a disorder of 1,25-D_3 regulation, in which 1,25-D_3 production is inappropriately high. The elevated calcium absorption during a calcium-replete diet and the increased bone resorption when dietary calcium is low serve to down-regulate PTH. The final level of 1,25-D_3 results from the opposing effects of low PTH and the underlying tendency toward overproduction.

Treatment with thiazide lowers urine calcium excretion and urine supersaturation with respect to calcium oxalate. The drug increases renal tubule calcium resorption [8], but this alone could not lower calcium excretion chronically (see Sutton, this volume). Continued calcium absorption would raise the serum calcium and the filtered load of calcium until calcium excretion rose to match the net absorption. Calcium must enter bone or soft tissues at an increased rate, intestinal absorption must fall, or both. The drug may reduce absorption [9]. Bone calcium stores may increase [10]. This issue needs more study. New stone production falls, as we (Fig. 2) and others [11] have shown repeatedly.

Alternative treatment with a low-calcium diet or sodium cellulose phosphate has potential disadvantages (see Backman, this volume). Patients appear to lose calcium from skeletal stores when challenged with low-calcium diet (Fig. 1) for 9 days. The response to a prolonged challenge may be different, because the early losses may come from skeletal stores that are more readily mobilized than the bulk of bone mineral. Needed are measurements after months of a low-calcium diet regimen or cellulose phosphate. Orthophosphate could be the most rational of all treatments, for phosphate should suppress 1,25-D_3 production and lower urinary calcium excretion.

Hyperparathyroidism

Excessive secretion of PTH from a single adenoma (85%) or hyperplasia (15%) leads to high 1,25-D_3 and low serum phosphorus concentrations. The latter raises 1,25-D_3 further [12]. The result is hypercalciuria from calcium overabsorption. PTH stimulates osteoclastic bone resorption, and calcium removed from bone adds to the hypercalciuria. Hypercalcemia is a characteristic feature of primary hyperparathyroidism and distinguishes it from idiopathic hypercalciuria. Serum PTH is elevated, especially when compared

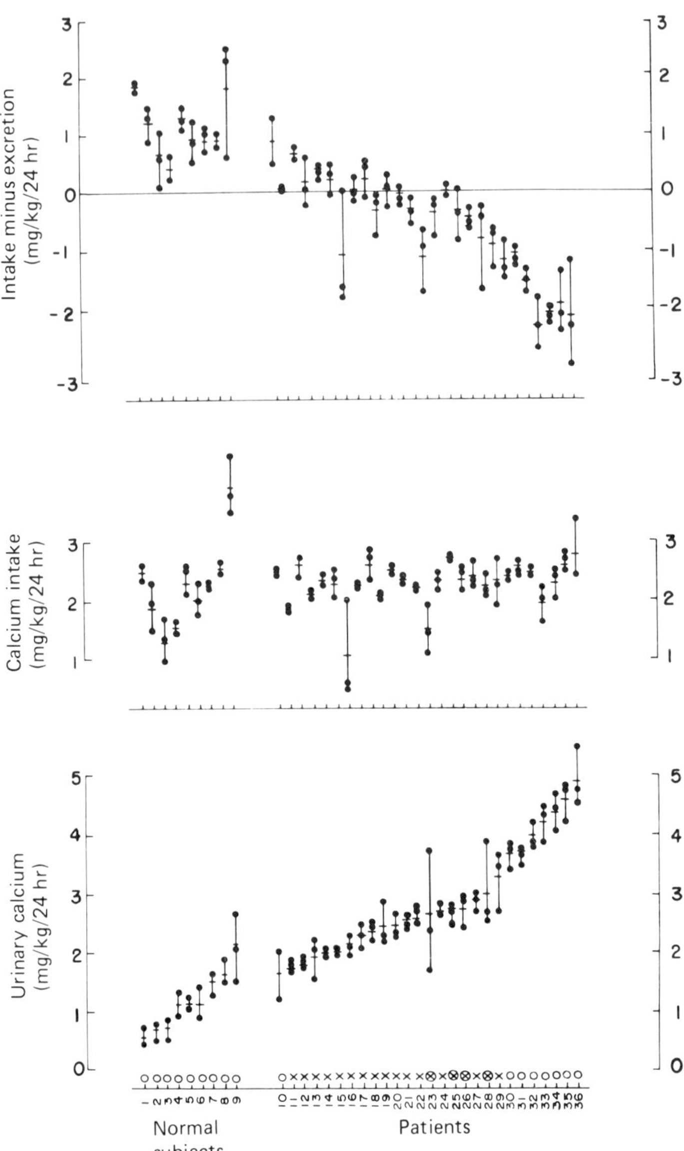

Fig. 1. Calcium intake and excretion values in patients and normal subjects ingesting a low-calcium diet. Mean calcium intakes of normal subjects (2.29 ± 0.15 SEM) and patients (2.31 ± 0.05) did not differ. During the low-calcium diet, mean excretion rates (1.18 ± 0.11 vs. 2.87 ± 0.11, $P < 0.001$) for normal subjects and patients, respectively, and values of intake minus excretion (1.14 ± 0.12 vs. −0.58 ± 0.11, $P < 0.001$) differed significantly from each other. Similarly, calcium excretion in normal subjects (1.78 ± 0.16) and patients (4.38 ± 0.15) during free-choice diet (not shown) differed from each other ($P < 0.001$) and from values during low-calcium diet ($P < 0.01$, both normal subjects and patients). Normal subjects and patients are shown in order of ascending mean calcium excretion. Patients 24 and 26 were mothers of patients 16 and 36, respectively. (Reproduced with permission from [7])

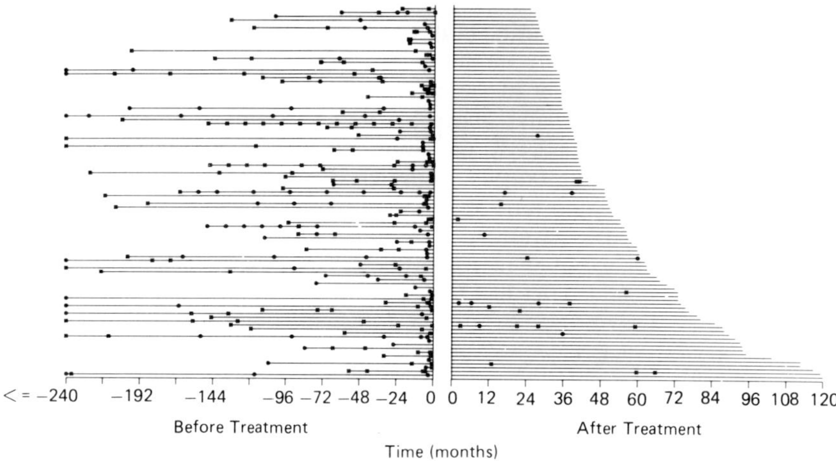

Fig. 2. Calcium stone formation before and during treatment of hypercalciuria with thiazide. Each patient is shown as a *horizontal line;* new stones, as *closed symbols;* multiple stones occurring in clusters, as *open symbols.* (Reproduced with permission from *Am J Med* 72:25–32, 1982)

to the low levels expected in hypercalcemic states. The reason hypercalcemia develops is that calcium reabsorption is stimulated in renal tubules [13]. Stone disease ceases in virtually everyone after parathyroidectomy [5].

Other Causes

Sarcoidosis, immobilization, Paget disease, hyperthyroidism, glucocorticoid excess, renal tubular acidosis, and vitamin D or calcium excess altogether account for less than 2% of the patients we have studied [14]. Sarcoidosis occasionally causes excessive 1,25-D$_3$ production, with consequent hypercalciuria and stones. Immobilization causes bone to demineralize. The calcium load causes hypercalciuria. Bone mineral loss is also the mechanism for hypercalciuria in Paget disease, hyperthyroidism, and glucocorticoid excess. Renal tubular acidosis causes systemic metabolic acidosis [15], which causes bone demineralization and also reduces renal tubule calcium reabsorption [16]. The resulting hypercalciuria is combined with an alkaline urine, so calcium phosphate stones form. Correction of the acidosis with alkali stops the stones [17] even though the urine becomes more alkaline.

Hyperoxaluria

Bowel Disease

Any cause of ileal malabsorption may increase absorption of oxalate by the colon and cause hyperoxaluria [18]. Oxalate is a metabolic end-product [19], and is excreted only in the urine [20]. Ileostomy prevents oxalate overabsorption, which can occur only in the colon. Normal colon mucosa is a size- and charge-selective barrier to the passive absorption of molecules [21]. The size barrier excludes molecules above 4 Å in radius, and additionally excludes anions. Oxalate is about 2.4 Å in radius, but carries two negative charges at a pH of 7.4, and normally is absorbed at a low rate. Malabsorption of fats allows medium-chain fatty acids, such as ricinoleate [22], and bile salts to enter the colon and increase permeability. The charge- and size-selective barrier remains intact, but all permeabilities are uniformly increased as though a nonselective second barrier had been disrupted. The resulting hyperoxaluria increases urine supersaturation and causes calcium oxalate stones. Treatment includes low-fat diet, calcium supplements that precipitate oxalate in the intestinal lumen, and cholestyramine that binds to oxalate and prevents its absorption [23].

Diet

Even if one excludes patients with bowel disease, patients with stones tend to have higher urine oxalate excretion rates than normal because of excessive dietary oxalate supply. The usual sources are pepper, nut products, chocolate, spinach, and rhubarb. Whereas enteric hyperoxaluria amounts to 70 to 150 mg per 24 hr in most cases, dietary excess leads to only 60 to 80 mg compared to the normal of 20 to 45 mg per 24 hr. Supersaturation is increased modestly. Treatment is with diet.

Inherited Oxalate Overproduction

Very rarely one encounters genetic hyperoxaluria. It occurs in at least two forms [24]. Stones may begin in childhood. Renal damage occurs and leads to renal failure in most cases. Pyridoxine, orthophosphate, and high-fluid intake together may reduce stone production, but the few cases available make a therapeutic trial impractical.

Low Urine Volume

We never have observed lower mean urine volumes in patients compared to normal people, so it is unclear that low volume is a sole reason for stones. More likely it contributes to stone formation by raising supersaturation at any level of calcium and oxalate excretion. The usual reason for low volume, below 1 liter daily of urine, is habitual dislike of water. Colectomy with ileostomy, a hot work environment, chronic diarrhea, and extreme exercise programs are reasons we have encountered. In general, we try to raise daily urine volume above 1.5 liter in all patients.

Heterogeneous Nuclei

Uric Acid

The formation of a new solid phase of calcium oxalate requires a higher supersaturation than is needed to cause growth of a surface that already exists [25]. For this reason, any material that forms a solid phase in the urinary tract could promote calcium oxalate stone if its surface fostered an overgrowth of calcium oxalate. Uric acid offers a surface that is well suited to such overgrowth. The spacing of charges on one face of the uric acid crystal conforms perfectly to that on one face of calcium oxalate, so calcium oxalate monohydrate tends to grow in an oriented way on a uric acid surface: a process called *epitaxial growth* [26]. Furthermore, microcrystals of calcium oxalate will tend to adhere to a uric acid surface so that all of the crystallites are oriented in the same way, forming a well-organized carpet upon which calcium and oxalate ions from the solution easily attach to produce orderly growth of the calcium oxalate phase.

Patients with calcium oxalate stones, especially men, tend to have higher urine uric acid excretion rates than normal, and lower urine pH [27]. Their urine is therefore abnormally supersaturated with respect to undissociated uric acid [27]. The cause is a high intake of meat, fish, and poultry, above 1 pound daily in many cases. Uric acid could promote stones by plugging occasional collecting ducts and offering to the urine a fixed surface of uric acid upon which calcium oxalate microcrystals can adhere, and calcium and oxalate ions can form a calcium oxalate overgrowth. The result would be an anchored papillary stone that needs contain little or no uric acid. Ideal treatment is reduced purine intake. Allopurinol reduces stone production (Fig. 3).

Protein Matrix

Often, protein will be found inside stones and has been considered a possible nucleus. The nature of the protein has never been determined. The role of protein as a promoter of stones remains to be determined.

Inhibitors of Crystal Growth

Glycoproteins

Urine retards the rate at which ions in solution enter the solid phase of calcium oxalate [28]. Most of the inhibition seems to arise from macromolecules (mol wts above 10,000 daltons). The main molecules isolated thus far are glycoproteins that are acidic, calcium binding, and have a high affinity for the calcium oxalate monohydrate crystal surface [3]. Normal urine has

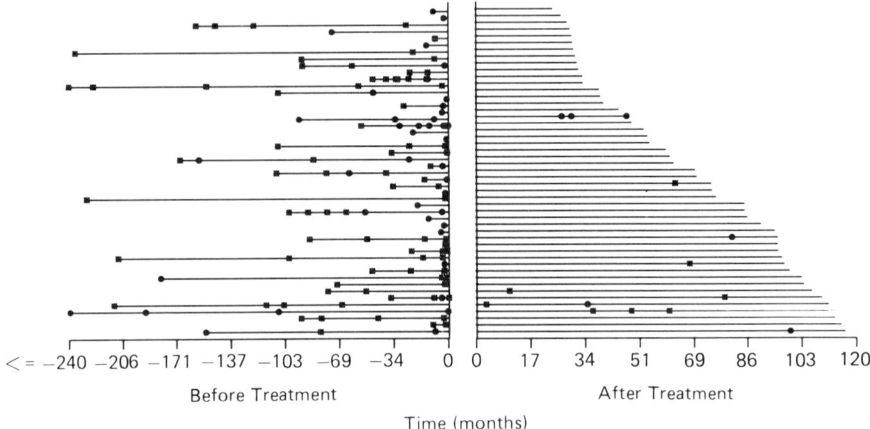

Fig. 3. Calcium stone formation before and during treatment of hyperuricosuria with allopurinol. Each patient is shown as a *horizontal line;* new stones, as *closed symbols;* multiple stones occurring in cluster, as *open symbols.* (Reproduced with permission from PARKS JH, COE FL, MILLMAN S: Stone disease in idiopathic hypocalciuria, in *Seminars in Nephrology,* 1981, vol. 4, p. 371)

four types of protein that are nearly identical in chemical composition, but differ in affinity for the crystal and in their elution from ion-exchange chromatography resins. Urine from stone-forming patients is less inhibitory of crystal growth than normal [29]. The glycoproteins form a very stable monolayer at an air-water surface, with a collapse pressure above 40 dynes/cm [30]. This suggests a strongly amphiphilic molecule that would tend to coat crystal surfaces and not easily re-enter the urine. The proteins have properties that make them easily confused with carbohydrate polymers. They contain few aromatic amino acid residues, and therefore show little light absorption at 280 nm. They react poorly with conventional protein stains and measurement systems [30].

Glycosaminoglycans

By the use of standard methods for their purification, glycosaminoglycans can be isolated from urine, and the fractions that contain them inhibit calcium oxalate crystal growth. This suggests a role for these compounds as inhibitors. However, the methods used will also concentrate the glycoproteins, which will not be easily detected as such because of their peculiar properties. The role of carbohydrate polymers in inhibition requires clarification through the use of methods that can separate them from the glycoproteins.

Pyrophosphate and Citrate

Urine contains pyrophosphate at about 10^{-6} M, which is sufficient to inhibit calcium oxalate crystal growth [31]. The importance of pyrophosphate is diminished by the fact that dialysis of urine has little effect upon inhibition, but the assays used usually require that urine be diluted. It may be that in whole urine pyrophosphate has an important role. Citrate is present in urine at about 10^{-3} M and at this concentration could reduce crystal growth. Like pyrophosphate, it may have more of a role in whole urine than in the dilute systems usually used for assay purposes.

Clinical Significance of Inhibitors

For most physicians, inhibitors are without meaning. They can be measured only in research settings and have an uncertain role in stone disease. There is no known way to increase their levels in urine safely on a long-term basis in patients. However, it is clear that urine from patients inhibits less well than normal, and it seems quite plausible that reduced inhibitors could predispose someone to form stones. For this reason, inhibitors have research interest. Synthetic analog could perhaps be fashioned if their structures were known. If people with low inhibitors could be easily detected, measures such as high fluid intake and reduced dietary purine could be used to prevent stone disease from beginning. In a deeper sense, the glycoproteins are mysterious because their exact biological meaning is unclear. They probably did not evolve to prevent stone formation, but they may be important in preventing local crystal formation at epithelial surfaces that contact fluids having high supersaturations with respect to calcium salts.

Overview

For the most part, stone disease seems to arise because of the interaction of culture with inheritance. Hypercalciuria appears inherited, in that urine calcium excretion varies over a wide range in human and even rat [32] populations so that some individuals have much higher levels than others. Likewise, urine inhibitors may vary in their effectiveness across a population. When calcium and oxalate are plentiful in the diet, people with high urine calcium concentrations, poorer inhibitors, or both will tend to form stones. In rich cultures that provide high meat intakes, uric acid excretion will also be high and promote crystal formation. Stones will be most prevalent when dietary calcium, oxalate, and purine all are high, as they are now in the Western hemisphere.

Acknowledgment. This work is supported by NIH Grant AM 39949.

References

1. HERRING LC: Observations on the analysis of 10,000 urinary calculi. *J Urol* 88:545–554, 1962

2. SUTOR DJ, WOOLEY SE, ILLINGWORTH JJ: Some aspects of the adult urinary stone problem in Great Britain and Northern Ireland. *Br J Urol* 46:275–279, 1974

3. NAKAGAWA Y, KAISER ET, COE FL: Isolation and characterization of calcium oxalate crystal growth inhibitors from human urine. *Biochem Biophys Res Commun* 84:1038–1044, 1978

4. ROBERTSON WB, MORGAN DB: The distribution of urinary calcium excretion in normal persons and stone formers. *Clin Chim Acta* 37:504–508, 1972

5. PARKS JH, COE FL, FAVUS MJ: Hyperparathyroidism in nephrolithiasis. *Arch Intern Med* 140:1479–1481, 1980

6. PAK CYC, EAST PA, SANZENBACKER LJ, DELEA CS, BARTTER FC: Gastrointestinal calcium absorption in nephrolithiasis. *J Clin Endocrinol Metab* 35:251–255, 1972

7. COE FL, FAVUS MJ, CROCKETT T, STRAUSS AL, PARKS JH, PORAT A, GANTT CL, SHERWOOD LM: Effects of low-calcium diet on urine calcium excretion, parathyroid function and serum $1,25(OH)_2D_3$ levels in patients with idiopathic hypercalciuria and in normal subjects. *Am J Med* 72:25–32, 1982

8. CONSTANZO LS, WEINER M: Relationship between clearances of Ca and Na: Effect of distal diuretics and PTH. *Am J Physiol* 230:67–73, 1976

9. FAVUS MJ, COE FL, KATHPALIA SC, PORAT A, SEN PK, SHERWOOD LM: Effects of chlorothiazide on 1,25 dihydroxy vitamin D3, parathyroid hormone, and intestinal calcium absorption in the rat. *Am J Physiol* 242:G575–G581, 1982

10. BUSHINSKY DA, FAVUS MJ, COE FL: Elevated $1,25(OH)_2D_3$, intestinal absorption, and renal mineral conservation in male rats. *Am J Physiol* 15:F140–F145, 1984

11. BACKMAN U, DANIELSON BG, JOHANSSON G, LJUNGHALL S, WIKSTROM B: Effects of therapy with bendroflumethiazide in patients with recurrent renal calcium stones. *Br J Urol* 41:175–177, 1979

12. POTTS JT JR, MURRAY TM, PEACOCK M, NIALL HO, TREAGER GW, KEUTMANN HT, POWELL D, DEFTOS LJ: Parathyroid hormone: Sequence, synthesis, immunoassay studies. *Am J Med* 50:639, 1971

13. LAFFERTY FW, PEARSON OH: Skeletal, intestinal and renal calcium dynamics in hyperparathyroidism. *J Clin Endocrinol Metab* 23:891, 1963

14. COE FL: *Nephrolithiasis: Pathogenesis and Treatment.* Chicago, Year Book Medical Publishers, 1978

15. BUCKALEW VM JR, PURVIS MD, SHULMAN MG, HERNDON N, RUCHMAN D: Hereditary renal tubular acidosis. *Medicine* 53:229–254, 1974

16. ALBRIGHT F, CONSOLAZIO WN, COOMBS FS, SULKOWITCH HW, TALBOTT JH: Metabolic studies and therapy in a case of nephrocalcinosis with ricketts and dwarfism. *Bull Johns Hopkins Hosp* 66:7–30, 1940

17. COE FL, PARKS JH: Stone disease in hereditary distal renal tubular acidosis. *Ann Intern Med* 93:60–61, 1980

18. DOBBINS JW, BINDER HJ: Importance of colon in enteric hyperoxaluria. *N Engl J Med* 296:298–300, 1977

19. HAGLER L, HERMAN JH: Oxalate metabolism. *Am J Clin Nutr* 26:758, 882, 1006, 1073, and 1242, 1973

20. HODGKINSON A, WILKINSON R: Plasma oxalate concentration and renal excretion of oxalate in man. *Clin Sci Mol Med* 46:61–65, 1974

21. FAVUS MJ, KATHPALIA SC, COE FL: Kinetic characteristics of calcium absorption and secretion by rat colon. *Am J Physiol* 240:G350–G354, 1981

22. KATHPALIA SC, FAVUS MJ, COE FL: Mechanism by which ricinoleate increases ascending colon oxalate absorption (*abstract*). *Clin Res* 30:452, 1982

23. SMITH LH: Enteric hyperoxaluria and other hyperoxaluric states, in *Contemporary*

Issues in Nephrology, edited by COE FL, BRENNER BM, STEIN JH, New York, Churchill Livingstone, 1980, vol 5 (Nephrolithiasis), p 136

24. WILLIAMS HE, SMITH LH JR: Primary hyperoxaluria, in The Metabolic Basis of Inherited Disease, edited by STANBURY JP, WYNGAARDEN JB, FREDRICKSON DS, New York, McGraw-Hill, 1972, p 196

25. COE FL, LAWTON RB, GOLDSTEIN RB, TEMBE V: Sodium urate accelerates precipitation of calcium oxalate in vitro. Proc Soc Exp Biol Med 149:926, 1975

26. DEGANELLO S, COE FL: Epitaxy between uric acid and whelwellite: Experimental verification. Neues Jahrbuch Minerologia H6:270–276, 1983

27. COE FL, STRAUSS AL, TEMPE V, DUN SL: Uric acid saturation in calcium nephrolithiasis. Kidney Int 17:662–668, 1980

28. ITO H, COE FL: Acidic peptide and polyribonucleotide crystal growth inhibitors in human urine. Am J Physiol 233:F455–F463, 1977

29. COE FL, MARGOLIS HC, DEUTSCH LH, STRAUSS AL: Urinary macromolecular crystal growth inhibitors in calcium nephrolithiasis. Mineral Electrolyte Metab 3:268–275, 1980

30. NAKAGAWA Y, ABRAM V, KEZDY FJ, KAISER EM, COE FL: Purification and characterization of the principal inhibitor of calcium oxalate monohydrate crystal growth in human urine. J Biol Chem 258:12594–12600, 1983

31. RUSSELL RGG, FLEISCH H: Inhibitors in urinary stone disease: Role of pyrophosphate in urinary calculi, in Urinary Calculi, edited by CIFUENTES-DELATTE L, RAPADO A, HODGKINSON A, Basel, Karger, 1973, p 307

32. FAVUS MJ, COE FL: Evidence for spontaneous hypercalciuria in the rat. Mineral Electrolyte Metab 2:150–154, 1979

Physicochemical Factors in Calcium Oxalate Urolithiasis

Lynwood H. Smith

The formation of calculi within the urinary tract is related to the balance between the ionic concentration in kidney and urine and the multiple physicochemical factors that may be present [1–6]. Elsewhere in this volume, Coe and Parks [7] outline the principal ions involved in this process and how disturbances in their metabolism and transport can lead to urinary calculi. Of special importance are those potential disturbances that produce an increased excretion rate and concentration of calcium and oxalate. This chapter reviews the various physicochemical factors that may influence the formation, retention, and growth of crystals within the urinary tract and ultimately produce urinary calculi.

Listed in Table 1 are the known and potential physicochemical factors that may be involved in the production and prevention of urinary calculi. The state of saturation, inhibitors of crystal formation, heterogeneous nucleation, and infection with bacteria that produce urease are factors that can be manipulated favorably with treatment currently available. In this review, I shall concentrate on these four factors, fully recognizing that many of the other known and potential physicochemical factors may be of equal or greater importance.

Table 1. Physicochemical factors in urolithiasis

Known factors	Possible factors
Supersaturation[a]	Site of crystal formation, retention, and growth
Inhibitors of crystal formation[a]	Crystal habit
Matrix	Crystal phase transformation and stabilization
Heterogeneous nucleation[a]	Promoters of crystal formation
Infection[a]	

[a] A factor that can be altered favorably with current treatment.

This manuscript was presented as part of a Symposium on *Pathogenesis and Treatment of Calcium Nephrolithiasis.*

Supersaturation

For calculi to form within the urinary tract, the urine must be supersaturated, at least intermittently, for the precipitating crystalline phase to occur. Outlined in Figure 1 are the potential states of saturation for any crystal system. If one begins with an undersaturated state of urine, there will be an energy for dissolution; crystals, if present, should dissolve. If one increases the ion product for a specific crystal system, one reaches the solubility product (K_{SP}). At that point, the solution is saturated for that crystal system. The ion product can be increased further, causing an energy for crystallization and a solution that is metastable for that crystal system. If crystals were present, they would grow and there would be a potential for heterogeneous nucleation. With a further increase of the ion product, the formation product (K_{FP}) would be reached. This is a less well-defined plateau above which the solution becomes unstable and has the potential for spontaneous nucleation. Patients who form urinary calculi have urine that has an ion product at/or near the formation product for the precipitating crystalline phase, at least on an intermittent basis. Most forms of treatment, at least in part, decrease the state of saturation for the precipitating crystalline phase. If these efforts can reduce the state of saturation below the solubility product, urinary calculi can dissolve within the urinary tract.

As with other biological fluids, urine is an extremely complex solution. The state of saturation for a specific crystal system is determined not only by the solute load, but also by ionic strength, complexation, and pH as they influence the specific crystal system. Ionic strength has an influence on the activity of a specific ion such as calcium or oxalate. This activity is the product of the ion concentration times the activity coefficient (f_2):

$$\text{Activity product} = (Ca \times f_2)(C_2O_4 \times f_2)$$

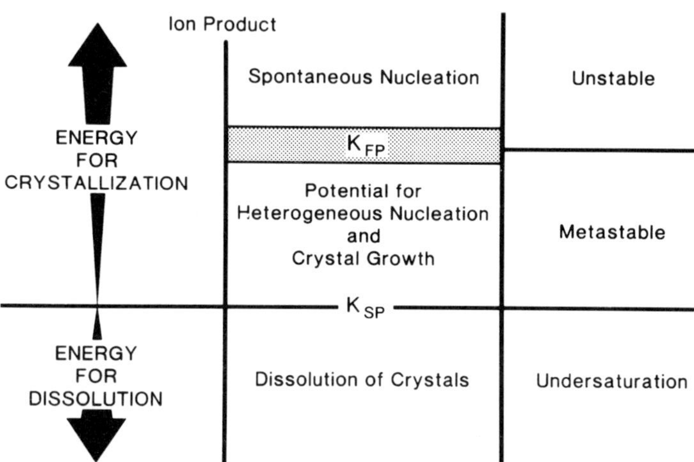

Fig. 1. States of saturation in biological fluids. The solubility product is denoted by K_{SP}; the formation product, by K_{FP}.

The activity coefficient is a function of ionic strength and decreases as ionic strength increases. Thus, the activity of a particular ion in a solution such as urine decreases as the ionic strength increases. The ionic strength of urine comes primarily from monovalent ions such as sodium, potassium, and chloride. Complexation occurs when ions form soluble complexes reducing the free ion activity; for instance, calcium combines with citrate and magnesium with oxalate as soluble complexes, which effectively removes a portion of these ions from solution and decreases their free ion activity:

$$Ca^{++} + Citrate^{3-} \rightleftharpoons CaCitrate^{-}$$
$$Mg^{++} + C_2O_4^{2-} \rightleftharpoons MgC_2O_4^{0}$$

In urine, approximately 50% of the total calcium and oxalate is complexed, and since the activity product is the product of the free ion activity in solution for a particular crystal, complexation directly affects supersaturation. The pH of urine, which varies over a wide range, can influence both complexation and free ion activity. An example of the effect of pH on complexation is shown with citrate. At a pH of 6.5 or greater, citrate is totally ionized and can complex three calcium ions [8]:

$$Ca^{++} + Cit^{-} \rightleftharpoons CaCit$$
$$2CaCit^{-} + Ca^{++} \rightleftharpoons Ca_3Cit_2$$

The effect of pH on free ion activity is illustrated below. As urine becomes more alkaline with a decrease in hydrogen ion content, there is a shift of the formula to the right, with an increase in free phosphate ion activity:

$$H_2PO_4 \rightleftharpoons HPO_4^{2-} + H^{+}$$
$$HPO_4^{2-} \rightleftharpoons PO_4^{3-} + H^{+}$$

To estimate supersaturation, one can measure the urine pH and the major ion species, which include sodium, potassium, chloride, calcium, magnesium, ammonium, phosphorus, sulfate, citrate, oxalate, and uric acid. The ionic strength, complexation, free ion activities, and ion activity products can be calculated with an iterative computer program [9, 10]. The relative supersaturation ratio is then estimated by dividing the calculated ion activity product by the thermodynamic solubility product.

$$Relative\ supersaturation\ ratio\ (SS) = \frac{ion\ activity\ product}{thermodynamic\ solubility\ product}$$

Similar results can be obtained by using the activity product ratio as described by Pak and Chu [11]. In dealing with the relative supersaturation of the major crystal systems present in urine, one confronts a special problem with hydroxyapatite, which is based on the fifth power of calcium activity and the cube of phosphate activity. These calculations result in a wide range of values for supersaturation that are difficult to visualize and compare. To avoid this problem, one can express the driving force for crystallization in terms of Gibbs-free energy of transfer from a supersaturated to a saturated solution, as expressed in the following equation:

$$\Delta G = \frac{-RT}{n} \ln SS$$

where R = 8.3114 joules per degree mole, T = temperature, n = number of ions in the molecule, and SS = supersaturation ratios. Using this expression of supersaturation, one can then compare the various crystal systems that may occur in urine [12].

Inhibitors of Crystal Formation

Specific inhibitors of crystal formation occur in normal urine for both the calcium oxalate and the calcium phosphate crystal systems (see Table 2) [13–15]. Characteristic of these compounds are their ability to have an effect on crystal formation at extremely low concentrations, eliminating the possibility that their major effect is due to complexation. Currently, it is felt that these compounds are adsorbed to active growth sites on the surface of crystals, effectively blocking crystal growth and, in some cases, aggregation; thus, a few molecules of inhibitor may tie up 1000 or more crystal molecules [5, 16]. A working hypothesis for the formation of urinary stones in patients with idiopathic calcium urolithiasis has been that there is a deficiency of inhibitor activity in the urine. Some workers have consistently demonstrated this deficiency for the calcium phosphate crystal system, owing perhaps in a large part to a decreased concentration in magnesium, citrate, and pyrophosphate [13, 17–20]. For the calcium oxalate crystal system, findings of an inhibitor deficiency in urine have been conflicting [20–24]. Recent studies in humans and animals suggest that the bladder may contribute a significant amount of inhibition for the calcium oxalate crystal growth [25, 26]. If subsequent studies document this phenomenon, then a deficiency of specific inhibitor activity for the calcium oxalate crystal system at the level of the kidney could go undetected because of the bladder contribution. At the same time, inhibitors that come from the kidney, such as citrate, pyrophosphate, and probably RNA fragments and acidic glycoproteins, may be more important in the inhibition involved in calcium oxalate crystal growth within the kidney.

Table 2. Urinary inhibitors of crystal formation

	Potency (moles/inhibitor unit)
Inhibitors of calcium oxalate	
Citrate	10^{-4}
Pyrophosphate	10^{-5}
Chondroitin sulfate	10^{-6}
RNA fragments	10^{-8}
Acidic glycoproteins	10^{-8}
Inhibitors of calcium phosphate	
Magnesium	10^{-4}
Citrate	10^{-5}
Pyrophosphate	10^{-6}

Heterogeneous Nucleation

That urinary calculi have a mixed crystalline composition has long been recognized [27, 28]. When one considers the constant variation in states of saturation between the various crystal systems present in urine throughout the day, it is easy to understand how stones could form with a mixed crystalline composition. Observations of this type led first Modlin [29] and then Lonsdale [30] to suggest that heterogeneous nucleation might be involved in the formation of urinary calculi. Coe and Raisen later applied this principle to hyperuricosuria and idiopathic calcium oxalate stone formation [31]. They suggested that the formation of uric acid crystals might cause the heterogeneous nucleation of calcium oxalate followed by calcium oxalate stone formation. To prevent this phenomenon, they gave patients with this apparent disorder allopurinol to reduce hyperuricosuria. It seemed to decrease the stone formation rate. Subsequent studies examining the potential for uric acid to nucleate calcium oxalate in in vitro systems questioned the role of uric acid in the nucleation of calcium oxalate [32]. As an alternative, monosodium urate was suggested as the needed component for heterogeneous nucleation, even though this is an extremely rare crystal in urinary calculi or freshly voided urine [33]. This alternative has been recently challenged [34].

Perhaps a more likely candidate for heterogeneous nucleation of calcium oxalate is calcium phosphate present as hydroxyapatite, carbonate apatite, and amorphous calcium phosphate. These phases of calcium phosphate are the most common types of crystals present in freshly voided urine and have the capacity to nucleate calcium oxalate at a level of supersaturation much lower than that required for homogeneous nucleation [12, 35]. Also supporting this hypothesis is the common finding of various phases of calcium phosphate in close association with matrix in otherwise pure calcium oxalate stones [36].

Infection

Another consideration is the effect of urinary infection with bacteria that produce urease [37]. Outlined below are the effects of urease on urine and the supersaturation of magnesium ammonium phosphate.

$$NH_2COHN_2 \text{ (urea)} + 2H_2O \xrightarrow{\text{urease}} 2NH_3 + H_2CO_3 \tag{1a}$$

$$2NH_3 + 2H_2O \longrightarrow 2NH_4^+ + 2OH^- \tag{1b}$$

$$H_2PO_4 \rightleftharpoons HPO_4^{2-} + H^+ \tag{2a}$$

$$HPO_4^{2-} \rightleftharpoons PO_4^{3-} + H^+ \tag{2b}$$

$$MgNH_4PO_4 \text{ (struvite)} \rightleftharpoons Mg^{2+} + NH_4^+ + PO_4^{3-} \tag{3a}$$

$$K_{SP} = (Mg^{2+})(NH_4^+)(PO_4^{3-}) \tag{3b}$$

Both the ammonium and phosphate ion activities are increased with the metabolism of urea and the alkalinization of urine. The changes increase the supersaturation of magnesium ammonium phosphate and produce the typical infection stone of struvite that may often occur as a secondary phenomenon with metabolic stones (for example, the calcium oxalate stone). To correct the abnormality in supersaturation, one must eradicate the bacteria that produces urease.

Other Physicochemical Factors

Matrix (the stone's skeleton) is always present in calculi formed within the urinary tract [36, 38, 39]. It is highly organized and in close association with crystals present in the stone. The chemical composition of matrix is amazingly similar in stones of varied crystal composition. In spite of its ubiquitous nature within urinary calculi, basic questions as to its source, exact chemical structure, and role in stone formation remain unanswered. To date, there is no specific treatment that can decrease or alter matrix.

A major void in our understanding of stone formation within the urinary tract relates to the site of initial crystal formation and the mechanism by which crystals are retained. Crystals that form are minute, much smaller than the container in which they form, and as one moves down the nephron into the collecting tubules, calyces, and renal pelvis, one is moving to containers of ever increasing size. In addition, the flow of urine potentially should push the crystals along. In spite of all of these factors that would favor passage of crystals that precipitate, stones do form, and the mechanism by which this occurs becomes a fundamental consideration in understanding urolithiasis. At least four theories have been advanced that could explain this mechanism. The first was suggested by Randall based on his observations of plaque-like deformities in the mucosal surfaces of the renal collecting system in patients with urinary calculi [40]. He suggested that these defects promoted crystal nucleation and growth, resulting in the formation of a stone. Carr observed initial stone formation at the fornices of the calyceal systems within the lymphatic channels and suggested that the channels had become blocked allowing stasis and stone formation [41]: the second theory. A third theory was proposed by Vermeulen and Lyon, who found rapid precipitation in the collecting ducts in the papillary tip with sledging, dilatation, and stone growth in several rat models when a high-solute load was given [42]. They found that if they induced this rapid precipitation for a short period of time when the activity product for the precipitating crystalline phase exceeded the K_{FP}, there followed a period when the urine was kept metastable for the same crystalline component. The stone formation was similar to that which occurred in animals that had high-solute loads. A fourth theory was proposed by Oliver et al [43] and later Malek and Boyce [44]. These investigators noted aggregates of crystals within the nephron in animals and patients with urolithiasis. These crystal deposits were in close association with amorphous material considered to be matrix, and the deposits were termed *intrane-*

phronic calculosis. Although each of these theories seem different in both mechanism and location, none are mutually exclusive, and examples of each would appear to occur in patients with urolithiasis.

Application to Treatment

As stated earlier, four of the known physicochemical factors can be altered in favorable ways to prevent calcium oxalate stone formation with current treatment. Treatment is often selected based on demonstrated abnormalities in these factors [45], and a favorable response to treatment in terms of prevention of further stone formation usually follows favorable changes in one or more of these factors [5, 46]. Application of these treatment principles is demonstrated in other chapters in this volume.

References

1. NORDIN BEC, ROBERTSON WG: Calcium phosphate and oxalate ion-products in normal and stone-forming urines. *Br Med J* 1:450–453, 1966
2. ROBERTSON WG, PEACOCK M, NORDIN BEC: Activity products in stone-forming and non-stone-forming urine. *Clin Sci* 34:579–594, 1968
3. PAK CYC: Physicochemical basis for formation of renal stones of calcium phosphate origin: Calculation of the degree of saturation of urine with respect to brushite. *J Clin Invest* 48:1914–1922, 1969
4. FINLAYSON B: Renal lithiasis in review. *Urol Clin North Am* 1:181–212, 1974
5. SMITH LH: Application of physical, chemical, and metabolic factors to the management of urolithiasis, in *Urolithiasis Research,* edited by FLEISCH H, ROBERTSON WG, SMITH LH, VAHLENSIECK W, New York, Plenum Press, 1976, pp 199–211
6. FINLAYSON B: Physicochemical aspects of urolithiasis. *Kidney Int* 13:344–360, 1978
7. COE FL, PARKS JH: Pathogenesis of calcium renal stones, this volume
8. MEYER JL: Formation constants for interaction of citrate with calcium and magnesium ions. *Anal Biochem* 62:295–300, 1974
9. MARSHALL RW, ROBERTSON WG: Nomograms for the estimation of the saturation of urine with calcium oxalate, calcium phosphate, magnesium ammonium phosphate, uric acid, sodium acid urate, ammonium acid urate and cystine. *Clin Chim Acta* 72:253–260, 1976
10. FINLAYSON B: Calcium stones: Some physical and clinical aspects, chapter 10 in *Calcium Metabolism in Renal Failure and Nephrolithiasis,* edited by DAVID DS, Toronto, John Wiley & Sons, Inc, 1977, pp 337–382
11. PAK CYC, CHU S: A simple technique for the determination of urinary state of saturation with respect to brushite. *Invest Urol* 11:211–215, 1973
12. SMITH LH, WERNESS PG: Hydroxyapatite: The forgotten crystal in calcium urolithiasis. *Trans Am Clin Climatol Assoc* (in press, 1984)
13. HOWARD JE: Studies on urinary stone formation: A saga of clinical investigation. *Johns Hopkins Med J* 139:239–252, 1976
14. FLEISCH H: Inhibitors and promoters of stone formation. *Kidney Int* 13:361–371, 1978

15. NAKAGAWA Y, ABRAM V, KEZDY FJ, KAISER ET, COE FL: Purification and characterization of the principal inhibitor of calcium oxalate monohydrate crystal growth in human urine. *J Biol Chem* 258:12594–12600, 1983

16. NANCOLLAS GH: The kinetics of crystal growth and renal stone-formation, in *Urolithiasis Research,* edited by FLEISCH H, ROBERTSON WG, SMITH LH, VAHLENSIECK W, New York, Plenum Press, 1976, pp 5–23

17. HOWARD JE, THOMAS WC JR: Some observations on rachitic rat cartilage of probable significance in the etiology of renal calculi. *Trans Am Clin Climatol Assoc* 70:94–103, 1958

18. BISAZ S, FELIX R, NEUMAN WF, FLEISCH H: Quantitative determination of inhibitors of calcium phosphate precipitation in whole urine. *Mineral Electrolyte Metab* 1:74–83, 1978

19. SMITH LH, MEYER JL, McCALL JT: Chemical nature of crystal inhibitors isolated from human urine, in *Urinary Calculi: Recent Advances in Aetiology, Stone Structure and Treatment,* edited by CIFUENTES DELATTE L, RAPADO A, HODGKINSON A, Basel, S Karger, 1973, pp 318–327

20. SMITH LH, WERNESS PG, WILSON DM: Metabolic and clinical disturbances in patients with calcium urolithiasis. *Scand J Urol Nephrol* 53(Suppl):213–220, 1980

21. ROBERTSON WG, PEACOCK M: Calcium oxalate crystalluria and inhibitors of crystallization in recurrent renal stone-formers. *Clin Sci* 43:499–506, 1972

22. ROBERTSON WG, PEACOCK M, MARSHALL RW, MARSHALL DH, NORDIN BEC: Saturation-inhibition index as a measure of the risk of calcium oxalate stone formation in the urinary tract. *N Engl J Med* 294:249–252, 1976

23. SALLIS JD, LUMLEY MF: On the possible role of glycosaminoglycans as natural inhibitors of calcium oxalate stones. *Invest Urol* 16:296–299, 1979

24. BOWYER RC, BROCKIS JG, McCULLOCH RK: Glycosaminoglycans as inhibitors of calcium oxalate crystal growth and aggregation. *Clin Chim Acta* 95:23–28, 1979

25. EDYVANE KA, RYALL RL, MARSHALL VR: Does the bladder mucosa contribute to urinary inhibitory activity? *Urol Res* 12:80, 1984

26. SMITH LH, MARTIN X, OPGENORTH T, WERNESS PG, ROMERO JC: Influence of the bladder on calcium oxalate crystal growth inhibition in dogs. *Kidney Int* 25:177, 1984

27. PRIEN EL, FRONDEL C: Studies in urolithiasis: I. The composition of urinary calculi. *J Urol* 57:949–994, 1947

28. HERRING LC: Observations on the analysis of ten thousand urinary calculi. *J Urol* 88:545–562, 1962

29. MODLIN M: The aetiology of renal stone: A new concept arising from studies on a stone-free population. *Ann R Coll Surg Engl* 40:155–178, 1967

30. LONSDALE K: The solid state: Epitaxy as a growth factor in urinary calculi and gallstones. *Nature* 217:56–58, 1968

31. COE FL, RAISEN L: Allopurinol treatment of uric acid disorders in calcium-stone formers. *Lancet* 1:129–131, 1973

32. MEYER JL, BERGERT JH, SMITH LH: The epitaxially induced crystal growth of calcium oxalate by crystalline uric acid. *Invest Urol* 14:115–119, 1976

33. COE FL, LAWTON RL, GOLDSTEIN RB, TEMBE V: Sodium urate accelerates precipitation of calcium oxalate in vitro. *Proc Soc Exp Biol Med* 149:926–929, 1975

34. MEYER JL: Nucleation kinetics in the calcium oxalate-sodium urate monohydrate system. *Invest Urol* 19:197–201, 1981

35. MEYER JL, BERGERT JH, SMITH LH: Epitaxial relationships in urolithiasis: The

calcium oxalate monohydrate-hydroxyapatite system. *Clin Sci Mol Med* 49:369–374, 1975

36. BOYCE WH: Organic matrix of human urinary concretions. *Am J Med* 45:673–683, 1968
37. GRIFFITH DP: Infection-induced renal calculi. *Kidney Int* 21:422–430, 1982
38. BOYCE WH, GARVEY FK: The amount and nature of the organic matrix in urinary calculi: A review. *J Urol* 76:213–227, 1956
39. FINLAYSON B, VERMEULEN CW, STEWART EJ: Stone matrix and mucoprotein from urine. *J Urol* 86:355–363, 1961
40. RANDALL A: An hypothesis for the origin of renal calculus. *N Engl J Med* 214:234–242, 1936
41. CARR RJ: New theory on formation of renal calculi. *Br J Urol* 26:105–117, 1954
42. VERMEULEN CW, LYON ES: Mechanisms of genesis and growth of calculi. *Am J Med* 45:684–692, 1968
43. OLIVER J, MACDOWELL M, WHANG R, WELT LG: The renal lesions of electrolyte imbalance: IV. The intranephronic calculosis of experimental magnesium depletion. *J Exp Med* 124:263–277, 1966
44. MALEK RS, BOYCE WH: Intranephronic calculosis: Its significance and relationship to matrix in nephrolithiasis. *J Urol* 109:551–555, 1973
45. PAK CYC, PETERS P, HURT G, KADESKY M, FINE M, et al: Is selective therapy of recurrent nephrolithiasis possible? *Am J Med* 71:615–621, 1981
46. SMITH LH: Enteric hyperoxaluria and other hyperoxaluric states, in *Contemporary Issues in Nephrology,* edited by COE FL, BRENNER BM, STEIN JH, vol 5, New York, Churchill Livingstone, 1980, pp 136–164

Use of Thiazide Diuretics in Calcium Oxalate Nephrolithiasis

Roger A. L. Sutton

Lamberg and Kuhlback [1] first reported a sustained reduction in urinary calcium excretion in patients treated with thiazide diuretics. They suggested that the most plausible explanation of this effect was a drug-induced enhancement of tubular calcium reabsorption associated with the familiar inhibition of sodium and chloride reabsorption. The mechanism of thiazide-induced hypocalciuria subsequently became the subject of intensive investigation. At the present time, it seems reasonable to conclude that the hypocalciuria results mainly from a direct stimulation by the thiazide diuretics of calcium reabsorption in the distal convoluted tubule [2].

Recent studies show that the addition of amiloride increases the hypocalciuric action of thiazides [3, 4] and that the actions of thiazide and amiloride on tubular calcium reabsorption probably occur at separate sites, in the early and late distal convoluted tubules, respectively [5]. It is possible that enhanced bulk reabsorption of fluid and ions in the proximal tubule, resulting from mild chronic volume depletion, may also contribute to thiazide-induced hypocalciuria [6]. Whether parathyroid hormone (PTH) is involved in the chronic hypocalciuric action of thiazides in man is uncertain [7].

The production of hypocalciuria by thiazides suggested their use for the prevention of recurrent calcium stones, which is the subject of this review. The use of thiazides for this purpose will be discussed with respect to efficacy, mode of action, indications, treatment regimens, side effects, and possible reasons for treatment failure.

Efficacy

Yendt and colleagues pioneered the use of thiazide diuretics in the management of idiopathic hypercalciuria and calcium nephrolithiasis (including cal-

This manuscript was presented as part of a Symposium on *Pathogenesis and Treatment of Calcium Nephrolithiasis.*

cium oxalate and calcium phosphate stones) and reported their experience in several publications [8–11]. By 1978 these investigators had treated 346 patients, usually with hydrochlorothiazide in dosages of 50 mg given twice daily. Stone progression occurred in only 11 fully treated compliant patients in whom other identifiable contributing causes of stone formation were absent. Treatment was also apparently effective in 28 patients who were not hypercalciuric. Similar favorable reports of uncontrolled studies of thiazide prophylaxis of calcium stones came from other investigators [12–15]. Coe [12] reported a highly significant reduction in the stone formation rate (compared with the pretreatment period) in 78 patients with "definite hypercalciuria" (>300 mg of calcium a day in men, >250 mg of calcium a day in women) and in 34 patients with "marginal hypercalciuria" (>150 mg of calcium per gram of creatinine in a 24-hr urine collection), most of whom received 4 mg daily of trichlormethiazide (equivalent to 33 mg/day of hydrochlorothiazide). Most of these patients had calcium oxalate stones. In the dosages used by Yendt et al, side effects necessitated discontinuation of the treatment in up to 10% of patients. Maschio et al [13] used a lower dose of hydrochlorothiazide in a combined preparation with amiloride (one-half tablet; 25 mg of hydrochlorothiazide plus 2.5 mg of amiloride given twice daily) with additional allopurinol (100 mg/day) in about 50% of their 519 patients. In this uncontrolled study, stone formation rate again fell to well below that observed in the pretreatment period. The treatment was noted to be effective even in 171 normocalciuric patients, in whom it was reported to have little effect on urinary calcium excretion. Backman et al [14] reported similar results, with a reduction from 1.0 to 0.16 stones per patient-year during treatment. Using metolazone in dosages of 2.5 to 10 mg/day to treat patients with calcium nephrolithiasis, Cunningham, Oliveros, and Nascimento [15] recently observed a decrease from 2.10 to 0.49 stones per patient-year. The decrease in urinary calcium excretion (averaging 51%) and the reduction of stone frequency occurred irrespective of the initial urinary calcium excretion.

Recently, some small double-blind controlled trials of thiazide therapy for calcium stones have been reported. Lockefeer, Juttmann, and Birkenhazer [16] compared the effects of treatment and no treatment in the same 14 hypercalciuric patients with recurrent stones: the duration of treatment (chlorthalidone, 100 mg, three times weekly) was an average of 34.5 months; the subsequent control period of no therapy was an average of 34 months. Stone growth or formation occurred in 7 patients during the control period, but in only 1 patient during the preceding treatment period. Brocks, Dahl, and Wolf [17] randomly allocated 62 calcium stone patients (with or without hypercalciuria) to either bendroflumethiazide (2.5 mg, three times daily) or placebo. De novo stone formation fell during a treatment period averaging 1.6 years, compared with a pretreatment period averaging 3 years, from 0.4 to 0.09 stones per patient-year with thiazide and from 0.7 to 0.1 with placebo, representing 5 new stones in each group. These investigators concluded that thiazide was no more effective than placebo. This study has been criticized with regard to the possible role of other factors (diet and fluid intake) and also the relatively low stone incidence [18]. Scholz, Schwille, and Sigel [19] compared hydrochlorothiazide (25 mg orally, twice daily) with placebo during 1 year in 51 patients in a double-blind study. Although urinary calcium excretion fell in the thiazide group (pretreatment mean 24-hr urinary calcium of 249 mg; after treatment, 153 mg) and not in the placebo group (272 and 235 mg, respectively), spontaneous passage of newly formed stones occurred in an equal number of patients (6) in each group. Wilson, Strauss and Manuel [20] in a preliminary report compared hydrochlorothiazide (100 mg/day) with "regular" treatment (extra fluids combined with a reduction in dietary calcium and oxalate) and with sodium phosphate or allopurinol or magnesium oxide treatment in patients with idiopathic calcium lithiasis. There were approximately 20 patients in each group, with average treatment periods of 2.8 years. Regular treatment reduced stone recurrences by 56% compared with the pretreatment period. Only thiazide was significantly more effective than regular treatment, reducing recurrences by 79%.

Most of these studies were not confined to patients with calcium oxalate stones, but included any recurrent idiopathic calcium stone formers. However, the great majority presumably had calcium oxalate stones.

In summary, although uncontrolled studies suggest that thiazides may reduce recurrences to 10% or less of the rate seen when there is no treatment, small controlled studies suggest that the contribution of thiazides over and above that of nonpharmaceutical treatments, including altered food and fluid intake, may be much smaller.

Mode of Action

The original rationale for attempting to prevent calcium stone formation with thiazide was the observed hypocalciuric action of these drugs. This action was first noted in patients without hypercalciuria [1]. With 50 mg of hydrochlorothiazide given twice daily, the reduction in urinary calcium averages 150 mg/day, but is sometimes much less [11].

This hypocalciuric action of thiazide diuretics is usually maximal within 6 days and is usually sustained for as long as the drug is taken [8, 11]. During long-term thiazide treatment, intestinal calcium absorption has been reported to remain unchanged (implying a shift toward overall positive calcium balance) or to decrease to offset reduced urinary calcium losses [11, 21–23]. The decrease in intestinal calcium absorption may take several months to occur and may be associated with a fall in serum $1,25(OH)_2D_3$ levels in some patients. Pak and his colleagues [22, 23] suggested that decreased intestinal calcium absorption occurs during thiazide therapy only in so-called "renal" hypercalciuria whereas in so-called "absorptive" hypercalciuria intestinal calcium hyperabsorption persists. Nevertheless, undesirable consequences of such a shift toward a positive overall calcium balance (such as metastatic calcification and osteosclerosis) are not seen with long-term thiazide therapy. Perhaps endogenous intestinal secretion of calcium increases so that significant overall positive calcium balance does not occur. In rat experiments [24], chlorothiazide did not prevent the increase in intestinal calcium absorption or in plasma $1,25(OH)_2D_3$ levels induced by a low-calcium diet. Chlorothiazide had no direct effect on intestinal calcium transport. Bone turnover has been reported to decrease with thiazide therapy in man [25]. A decrease in urinary hydroxyproline excretion has been observed in man [10] and in the rat [26].

Although the apparent beneficial effect of these drugs in preventing stones in both hypercalciuric and normocalciuric patients may be a result of the reduction in urinary calcium excretion, several other actions of the drugs may influence stone formation [11]. In short-term animal experiments, thiazides have little effect on magnesium excretion [27, 28]. A sustained increase in urinary magnesium excretion has been reported in some patients during thiazide therapy [8, 10, 29], and hypomagnesemia has been reported [11]. In contrast, other investigators have reported no change from the baseline magnesium excretion, whereas Scholz et al [19] observed a decrease in urinary magnesium excretion of comparable magnitude after a year of treatment wtih either hydrochlorothiazide or placebo. In view of these conflicting observations on urinary magnesium excretion, it seems unlikely that changes in magnesium output contribute significantly to stone prevention during thiazide therapy.

An increase in urinary zinc excretion has been observed with thiazides and may be sustained [30, 31]. Zinc may act as an inhibitor of calcification [32].

The long-term effect of thiazides on urinary oxalate excretion is controversial. A decrease in oxalate excretion has been reported [33, 34], which may take more than a year to become apparent [35] and could be a consequence of decreased intestinal calcium absorption [11]. Scholz et al [19] observed a similar decline in urinary oxalate excretion after one year in thiazide and placebo groups and suggested that this may have resulted from a reduced dietary oxalate intake in both groups.

Other potentially important effects of thiazide include an increase in urinary pyrophosphate [29], which is not sustained, and a reduction in urinary citrate [36], which could potentiate stone formation and may be secondary to potassium depletion [37, 38] or even possibly to magnesium depletion [39]. A reduction in urinary citrate was not observed with 25 mg of hydrochlorothiazide given twice daily for 1 year [19], but was recently reported after 1 month of hydrochlorothiazide at the same dosage (mean daily urinary citrate, 299 and 200 mg, respectively) and was not different (212 mg a day) with the addition of amiloride (2.5 mg twice daily) to the thiazide, despite an amelioration of the accompanying hypokalemia [4].

Thiazides do not alter the steady-state urinary uric acid excretion, though they do decrease the fractional urinary excretion of the filtered uric acid load, so that the plasma uric acid concentration rises, and gout may be precipitated.

A decrease in the urinary state of saturation with brushite [29] and calcium oxalate [40] has been observed in most thiazide-treated patients, mainly as a result of the hypocalciuric effect.

Indications for, and Choice of, Therapy

There is a lack of general agreement on the indications for use of prophylactic drug therapy in calcium stone formers. As discussed by Yendt and Cohanim [11], factors that influence this decision in a particular patient include the number and frequency of stone episodes, the presence of renal calcification, the history of stone surgery, the presence of hypertension (which may encourage the use of a thiazide diuretic), and the patient's own preference. If drug prophylaxis is chosen for the recurrent calcium stone former, Yendt and Cohanim recommend an initial therapy with hydrochlorothiazide (50 mg twice daily) and a switch to an alternative treatment if the thiazide is not tolerated. They recommend this approach irrespective of the presence or absence of hypercalciuria, irrespective of whether the hypercalciuria is the so-called "renal" or "absorptive" type, and irrespective of the presence or absence of hyperuricosuria, though it was in hyperuricosuric patients that many of their treatment failures occurred. Both Yendt and Cohanim [11] and Coe [12] have reported that thiazides are effective in stone prevention in the presence or absence of hypercalciuria. In 28 normocalciuric patients, of whom 17 had some degree of tubular ectasia or medullary sponge kidney, no new stones were observed during 103 patient-years of therapy with thiazides, and in several patients renal calcifications decreased without evidence of stone passage [11]. Pak [41] has suggested that treatment of idiopathic hypercalciuria should be influenced by the putative pathophysiologic defect, "renal" hypercalciuria being treated with thiazides and "absorptive" hypercalciuria with cellulose phosphate [42]. Although this is an apparently logical approach, there is currently considerable doubt as to whether there truly are different renal and absorptive types of hypercalciuria [43]. Furthermore, neither thiazide in presumed absorptive hypercalciuria (which might lead to calcium retention) nor cellulose phosphate in presumed renal hypercalciuria (which might promote negative calcium balance) has actually been observed to be associated with these putative undesirable side effects. Until recently, cellulose phosphate was not available for clinical use in the USA or Canada. It is somewhat less convenient to take than a thiazide diuretic and tends to increase the urinary oxalate excretion while reducing calcium excretion. Cellulose phosphate can also cause magnesium depletion [44] and has not been systematically investigated in normacalciuric calcium stone formers. Its ultimate place in the treatment of calcium stones is still unclear: it may prove to be a useful alternative in the hypercalciuric patient who is intolerant of thiazides, but should be accompanied by dietary oxalate restriction. Several other alternative forms of therapy are available, including increased water intake, which is probably advisable in all stone patients, and decreased calcium intake, which tends to be associated with an increase in alimentary oxalate absorption [42], so that dietary oxalate should also be restricted. In addition, treatment with orthophosphate (either as potassium acid phosphate or neutral phosphate) has been found effective in reducing calcium stone recurrence by some investigators [45, 46] but not by others [47, 48]. The form of phosphate may be important, since acid phosphate may increase urinary calcium excretion [49]. Recently renal prostaglandin E_2 has been shown to have calciuretic properties [50], and prostaglandin synthetase inhibitors have been suggested as a possible form of treatment for hypercalciuria and renal calculi [51].

Treatment Regimen

If thiazides are to be used, a decision has to be made regarding the drug dosage and the timing of its administration. Hydrochlorothiazide at 50 mg twice daily has been found to be effective by Yendt et al [11]; these authors suggest that in some patients a lower dosage may be less efficacious. In this dosage, early side effects related to volume depletion are frequent, and discontinuation of the drug may be needed in up to 10% of the patients. These investigators now suggest a starting dosage of 25 mg daily for one week, increasing by 25 mg per day each week until a dosage of 50 mg twice daily is achieved. If side effects occur, the dosage is reduced to 25 mg twice daily. Using this regimen, less than 7% of patients have needed to discontinue thiazide. Smaller dosages have been found to be effective by other authors, for example, 2 mg twice daily of trichlormethiazide (equivalent to 33 mg of hydrochlorothiazide daily) [12], or 25 mg of hydrochlorothiazide plus 2.5 mg of amiloride twice daily [13]. It is not possible from these studies to ascertain the minimum effective dosage of thiazide, but on the available evidence 25 mg twice daily of hydrochlorothiazide may be appropriate, and can be increased if ineffective. Yendt et al [11] and Pak [52] have suggested that a twice daily dosage of hydrochlorothiazide is necessary to achieve an optimal effect, but a formal comparison has not been conducted between the once and twice daily regimes. Trichlormethiazide [12] or chlorthalidone [16, 53] have a longer duration of action and may perhaps be given less frequently.

At these dosages of thiazide, potassium supplements generally are not given routinely. Patients should be seen after 4 to 8 weeks to determine serum calcium, sodium, potassium, and uric acid concentrations and 24-hour urinary calcium and sodium excretions. Thereafter, patients may be seen annually for repeat studies, including a plain abdominal film to assess renal calcification. If the serum potassium is below 3.0 mEq/liter, a potassium supplement is usually recommended; alternatively, the use of a thiazide-amiloride combination may be considered.

Recently, the effect of hydrochlorothiazide alone has been compared with the combined use of hydrochlorothiazide plus amiloride in the reduction of urinary calcium excretion in children receiving calcitriol [3] and in adults who have calcium stones [4]. The combination had a significantly greater hypocalciuric action, and the amiloride also prevented thiazide-induced hypokalemic alkalosis [3] but not the fall in urinary citrate excretion [4].

Hyponatremia is unlikely unless the patient is drinking very large amounts of water or has an additional disorder influencing urinary dilution; however, in the presence of untoward symptoms, it should be considered [54], as should magnesium depletion [11]. A high-salt intake can prevent the hypocalciuric action of thiazides [55]. Conversely, a low-salt intake can potentiate symptoms related to volume depletion. Accordingly, patients should be advised to maintain a fairly steady, moderate-salt intake [56], which can be monitored by determining the urinary sodium excretion.

Side Effects

The potential side effects of thiazides, including hypersensitivity, diabetes mellitus, hyperuricemia, potassium depletion, magnesium depletion, potentiation of cardiac arrhythmias, and possible promotion of atheroma are beyond the scope of this discussion. The possible long-term implications of some of these side effects are incompletely understood and may lead in the future to a reassessment of the role of these drugs in managing such a relatively benign disorder as recurrent calcium oxalate nephrolithiasis.

A side effect of particular interest in the calcium stone former is hypercalcemia. Its presence in a patient with renal calculi prior to the initiation of treatment raises the possibility of an underlying primary hyperparathyroidism or other rarer conditions, including sarcoidosis, which can be diagnosed by means of appropriate investigations. The appearance of hypercalcemia only after thiazide treatment is begun, however, is more difficult to interpret. It may represent the unmasking of previous "normocalcemic," "subtle," or intermittent hyperparathyroidism. Whether thiazides ever cause sustained hypercalcemia in patients with idiopathic hypercalciuria or with a normal antecedent calcium metabolism is uncertain. Yendt et al [11] reported a small initial rise in total plasma calcium concentrations during thiazide therapy, sometimes to a level above normal, but this appears to be related to hemoconcentration and is not accompanied by an elevation of the ionized or ultrafilterable plasma calcium concentration. A similar experience has been reported by others [57, 58]. Only in six of the patients of Yendt et al [11] did a rise above normal occur in ultrafilterable plasma calcium: three of these patients were proved to have primary hyperparathyroidism. Thiazides have been reported to induce hypercalcemia in other disorders such as juvenile osteoporosis [59].

Although thiazides are reported to cause parathyroid hyperplasia in the dog [60], evidence in man suggests, if anything, a parathyroid suppression during thiazide treatment of hypercalciuria [61]. The unmasking of autonomous hyperparathyroidism with thiazides in patients with apparent idiopathic hypercalciuria is unexpected, because an excess of parathyroid hormone should result in a reduction in the urinary calcium excretion in a normocalcemic patient. It is well recognized, however, that some patients with primary hyperparathyroidism have marked hypercalciuria despite minimal hypercalcemia [43], and several possible explanations have been suggested for this phenomenon [43]. Presumably, in those hypercalciuric patients whose hyperparathyroidism is unmasked by thiazides, the serum calcium concentration was borderline or only intermittently raised prior to the administration of thiazide, or perhaps its modest rise was insufficient to raise the total or ionized plasma calcium concentration above the conventionally accepted normal range. Thus, such unmasking may occur in patients with hyperparathyroidism because the suppression of parathyroid hormone secretion that normally occurs as a result of the tendency of thiazides to elevate the serum calcium concentration cannot occur because of a degree of parathyroid autonomy. The detection of patients with "subtle" primary hyperparathyroidism may be facilitated by measuring plasma ionized calcium concentrations [62] or by demonstrating parathyroid autonomy [63]. Evidence for the latter is hypercalcemia and a failure to suppress urinary cyclic AMP in response to an oral calcium load [63]. Improvements in parathyroid hormone assays [64] may also facilitate the separation of patients with primary hyperparathyroidism from those with idiopathic calcium stones.

Treatment Failures

Uncontrolled studies have suggested that most calcium stone formers are helped by thiazide prophylaxis [11, 12]. Some patients, however, do form new stones while on thiazide treatment. Yendt et al [11] observed that these patients frequently had tubular ectasia (medullary sponge kidney) and tended to have higher urinary calcium, phosphorus, and uric acid excretions than successfully treated patients. Hyperuricosuria (a 24-hour urinary uric acid >800 mg in males) was present in 9 out of 11 of these treatment failure patients, whereas it was present in only 13 of 31 successfully treated patients. Thus, for the successful thiazide prophylaxis of calcium stones, it may be important to control hyperuricosuria. Other conditions associated with treatment failure included urinary tract infection, failure to control hypercalciuria, and the use of a single daily dosage (rather than a twice daily dose) of hydrochlorothiazide.

Strauss et al [65] studied 57 patients in whom new stones formed during treatment, which was usually trichlormethiazide (2 mg twice daily) plus allopurinol (100 mg twice daily) for hyperuricosuria. These patients were compared with 189 others who were free of recurrence during at least 2 years of follow-up examinations. Relapses tended to occur early (more than 60% occurred within 3 years). Recurrence was associated with a short interval between the last stone and the commencement of treatment, and with a higher calcium excretion and a lesser increase in urine volume during therapy than that seen in the patients without recurrence. Other measured variables did not differ between groups. A urinary calcium excretion greater than 2.5 mg/kg of body wt per day during treatment was estimated to confer a probability of relapse of over 50% when the interval from the last pretreatment stone was less than one year.

References

1. LAMBERG BA, KUHLBACK B: Effect of chlorothiazide and hydrochlorothiazide on the excretion of calcium in urine. *Scand J Clin Lab Invest* 11:351–357, 1959

2. COSTANZO LS, WINDHAGER EF: Calcium and sodium transport by the distal convoluted tubule of the rat. *Am J Physiol* 235:F492–F506, 1978

3. ALON U, COSTANZO LS, CHAN JCM: Additive hypocalciuric effects of amiloride (AM) and hydrochlorothiazide (HCTZ) in children treated with calcitriol. *16th Ann Meeting Am Soc Nephrol Abstract,* 1983, p 1A

4. LEPPLA D, BROWNE R, HILL K, PAK CYC: Effect of amiloride with or without hydrochlorothiazide on urinary calcium and saturation of calcium salts. *J Clin Endocrinol Metab* 57:920–924, 1983

5. COSTANZO LS: Effects of diuretics on the distal convoluted tubular transport of calcium. *Proc 1st Int Conference on Diuretics, Miami Beach, Florida,* 1984 (in press, 1984)

6. SUKI WN, EKNOYAN G, SAMAAN N, DICHOSO C, JOHNSON PC, MARTINEZ-MALDONADO M: Idiopathic hypercalciuria: Its diagnosis, pathogenesis and treatment, in *Cornell Seminars in Nephrology,* edited by BECKER L, Wiley, New York, 1973

7. SUKI WN: Effects of diuretics on calcium metabolism. *Mineral Electrolyte Metab* 2:125–129, 1979

8. YENDT ER, GAGNE RJA, COHANIM M: The effects of thiazides in idiopathic hypercalciuria. *Trans Am Clin Climatol Assoc* 77:96–110, 1965

9. YENDT ER, GAGNE RJA, COHANIM, M: The effects of thiazides in idiopathic hypercalciuria. *Am J Med Sci* 251:449–460, 1966

10. YENDT ER, GUAY GF, GARCIA DA: The use of thiazides in the prevention of renal calculi. *Can Med Assoc J* 102:614–620, 1970

11. YENDT ER, COHANIM M: Prevention of calcium stones with thiazides. *Kidney Int* 13:397–409, 1978

12. COE FL: Treated and untreated recurrent calcium nephrolithiasis in patients with idiopathic hypercalciuria, hyperuricosuria, or no metabolic disorder. *Ann Intern Med* 87:404–410, 1977

13. MASCHIO G, TESSITORE N, D'DANGELO A, FABRIS A, PAGANO F, TASCA A, GRAZIANI G, AROLDI A, SURIAN M, COLUSSI G, MANDRESSI A, TRINCHIERI A, ROCCO F, PONTICELLI C, MINETTI L: Prevention of calcium nephrolithiasis with low-dose thiazide, amiloride and allopurinol. *Am J Med* 71:623–626, 1981

14. BACKMAN U, DANIELSON HG, LJUNGHALL S, WIKSTROM B: Effects of therapy with bendroflumethiazide in patients with recurrent renal calcium stones. *Br J Urol* 51:175–180, 1979

15. CUNNINGHAM E, OLIVEROS FH, NASCIMENTO L: Metolazone therapy of active calcium nephrolithiasis. *Clin Pharmacol Ther* 32:642–645, 1982

16. LOCKEFEER JHM, JUTTMANN JR, BIRKENHAGER JC: The effect of long-term chlorthalidone on stone formation and stone growth, intestinal absorption of calcium and secretion of parathyroid hormone in idiopathic hypercalciuria. *Neth J Med* 20:257–262, 1977

17. BROCKS P, DAHL C, WOLF H: Do thiazides prevent recurrent idiopathic renal calcium stones? *Lancet* 2:124–125, 1981

18. GRAZIANI G, AROLDI A, SURIAN M, COLUSSI G, PONTICELLI C: Do thiazides prevent recurrent idiopathic renal calcium stones. *Lancet* 2:578–579, 1981

19. SCHOLZ D, SCHWILLE PO, SIGEL A: Double-blind study with thiazide in recurrent calcium lithiasis. *J Urol* 128:903–907, 1982

20. WILSON DR, STRAUSS AL, MANUEL MA: Comparison of medical treatments for the prevention of recurrent calcium nephrolithiasis (*abstract*). *R Coll Physicians Surg Can Ann,* 1983, p 380

21. EHRIG U, HARRISON JE, WILSON DR: Effect of long-term thiazide therapy on

intestinal calcium absorption in patients with recurrent renal calculi. *Metabolism* 23:139–149, 1974

22. BARILLA DE, TOLENTINO R, KAPLAN RA, PAK CYC: Selective effects of thiazide on intestinal absorption of calcium in absorptive and renal hypercalciurias. *Metabolism* 27:125–131, 1978

23. ZERWEKH JE, PAK CYC: Selective effects of thiazide therapy on serum $1\alpha,25$-dihydroxyvitamin D and intestinal calcium absorption in renal and absorptive hypercalciurias. *Metabolism* 29:13–17, 1980

24. FAVUS J, COE FL, KATHPALIA SC, PORAT A, SEN PK, SHERWOOD LM: Effects of chlorothiazide on 1,25-dihydroxyvitamin D_3, parathyroid hormone, and intestinal calcium absorption in the rat. *Am J Physiol* 242:G575–G581, 1982

25. HARRISON JE, HITCHMAN JW, FINLAY JM, FRASER D, YENDT ER, BAYLEY TA, MCNEIL KG: Effect of treatment on calcium kinetics in metabolic bone disease. *Metabolism* 20:1107–1118, 1971

26. JORGENSEN FS, NEILSEN SP: Effects of long-term administration of bendroflumethiazide on bone metabolism in the rat. *Acta Pharmacol Toxicol* 31:521–528, 1972

27. EKNOYAN G, SUKI WN, MARTINEZ-MALDONADO M: Effect of diuretics on urinary excretion of phosphate, calcium, and magnesium in thyroparathyroidectomized dogs. *J Lab Clin Med* 76:257–266, 1970

28. WONG NLM, QUAMME GA, DIRKS JH: Effect of chlorothiazide on renal calcium and magnesium handling in the hamster. *Can J Physiol Pharmacol* 60:1160–1165, 1982

29. PAK CYC: Hydrochlorothiazide therapy in nephrolithiasis: Effect on urinary activity product and formation product of brushite. *Clin Pharmacol Ther* 14:209–217, 1973

30. PAK CYC, RUSKIN B, DILLER E: Enhancement of renal excretion of zinc by hydrochlorothiazide. *Clin Chim Acta* 39:511–517, 1972

31. COHANIM M, YENDT ER: The effects of thiazides on serum and urinary zinc. *Johns Hopkins Med J* 136:137–141, 1975

32. BIRD ED, THOMAS WC JR: Effect of various metals on mineralization in vitro. *Proc Soc Exp Biol Med* 112:640–643, 1963

33. GLAZENBURG J: The effect of hydrochlorothiazide on the renal excretion of oxalic acid and on the formation of oxalate stones in the urinary tract. *Arch Chir Neerl* 23:217–223, 1971

34. YENDT ER, COHANIM M: Ten years' experience with the use of thiazides in the prevention of kidney stones. *Trans Am Clin Climatol Assoc* 85:65–75, 1973

35. COHANIM M, YENDT ER: Reduction of urine oxalate excretion during chronic thiazide therapy (*abstract*). *Clin Res* 24:685A, 1976

36. GARCIA DA, YENDT ER: The effects of probenecid and thiazides and their combination on the urinary excretion of electrolytes and on acid-base equilibrium. *Can Med Assoc J* 130:473–483, 1970

37. EVANS BM, MACINTYRE I, MACPHERSON CR, MILNE MD: Alkalosis in sodium and potassium depletion: With especial reference to organic acid secretion. *Clin Sci* 16:53–65, 1957

38. SIMPSON DP: Citrate excretion: A window on renal metabolism. *Am J Physiol* 244:F223–F234, 1983

39. RUDMAN D, DEDONIS JL, FOUNTAIN MT, CHANDLER JB, GENON GG, FLEMING GA, KUTZNER MH: Hypocitraturia in patients with gastrointestinal malabsorption. *N Engl J Med* 303:657–661, 1980

40. WOELFEL A, KAPLAN RA, PAK CYC: Effect of hydrochlorothiazide therapy on the crystallization of calcium oxalate in urine. *Metabolism* 26:201–205, 1977

41. PAK CYC, ZERWEKH JE: Separate pathogenetic origins for absorptive and renal hypercalciurias: Different responses to treatment, in *Clinical Disorders of Bone and Mineral Metabolism,* edited by FRAME B, POTTS JH JR, Amsterdam, Excerpta Medica, 1983, pp 406–410

42. PAK CYC, DELEA CS, BARTTER FC: Successful treatment of recurrent nephrolithiasis (calcium stones) with cellulose phosphate. *N Engl J Med* 290:175–180, 1974

43. SUTTON RAL: Disorders of renal calcium excretion. *Kidney Int* 23:665–673, 1983

44. SUTTON RAL: Hypomagnesaemia and magnesium deficiency. *J R Coll Physicians Lond* 3:358–365, 1968

45. SMITH LH, THOMAS WC JR, ARNAUD CD: Orthophosphate therapy in calcium renal lithiasis, in *Urinary Calculi: Recent Advances in Etiology, Stone Structure, and Treatment,* edited by CIFUENTES DELATTE L, RAPADO L, HODGKINSON A, BASEL, KARGER, 1973, p 192

46. THOMAS WC JR: Use of phosphates in patients with calcareous renal calculi. *Kidney Int* 13:390–396, 1978

47. ETTINGER B, KOLB FO: Inorganic phosphate treatment of nephrolithiasis. *Am J Med* 55:32–37, 1973

48. ETTINGER B: Recurrent nephrolithiasis: Natural history and effect of phosphate therapy. *Am J Med* 61:200–206, 1976

49. LEMANN JJ JR: Idiopathic hypercalciuria, in *Nephrolithiasis: Contemporary Issues in Nephrology,* edited by COE FL, BRENNER BM, New York, Churchill Livingstone, 1980, vol. 5, p. 86

50. BUCK AC, LOTE CJ, SAMPSON WF: The influence of renal prostaglandins on urinary calcium excretion in idiopathic urolithiasis. *J Urol* 129:421–426, 1983

51. RAO PN, BLACKLOCK NG: An interim report of flurbiprofen for the control of idiopathic hypercalciuria. *J Int Med Res* 11(Suppl 2):24–27, 1983

52. PAK CYC: Hypercalciurias: Clinical response and side effects, chap. 3 in *Calcium Urolithiasis: Pathogenesis, Diagnosis, and Management,* edited by AVIOLI LV, New York, Plenum Medical Book Co, 1978, p 59

53. GURSEL E: Effects of diuretics on renal and intestinal handling of calcium. *NY State J Med* 399–405, 1970

54. ASHRAF N, LOCKSLEY R, ARIEFF AI: Thiazide-induced hyponatremia associated with death or neurologic damage in outpatients. *Am J Med* 70:1163–1168, 1981

55. BRICKMAN AS, MASSRY SG, COBURN JW: Changes in serum and urinary calcium during treatment with hydrochlorothiazide studies on mechanisms. *J Clin Invest* 51:945–954, 1972

56. COE FL: Idiopathic hypercalciuria, in *Nephrolithiasis: Pathogenesis and Treatment,* Chicago, Year Book Medical Publishers Inc, 1978, p 89

57. JORGENSEN FS, TRANSBOL I, BINDER C: The effect of bendroflumethiazide on total, ultrafiltrable and ionized calcium in serum in normocalcemic renal stoneformers and in hyperparathyroidism. *Acta Med Scand* 194:323–326, 1973

58. DUARTE CG, WINNACKER JL, BECKER KL, PACE A: Thiazide-induced hypercalcemia. *N Engl J Med* 284:828–830, 1971

59. PARFITT AM: Chlorothiazide-induced hypercalcemia in juvenile osteoporosis and hyperparathyroidism. *N Engl J Med* 281:55–59, 1969

60. PICKLEMAN JR, STRAUSS FH II, FORLAND M, PALOYAN E: Thiazide-induced parathyroid stimulation. *Metabolism* 18:867–873, 1969

61. COE FL, CANTERBURY JM, FIRPO JJ: Evidence for secondary hyperparathyroidism in idiopathic hypercalciuria. *J Clin Invest* 52:134–142, 1973

62. MULDOWNEY FP, FREANEY R, MCMULLIN JP: Serum ionized calcium and parathyroid hormone in renal stone disease. *Q J Med* 45:75–86, 1976
63. BROADUS AE, HORST RL, LITTLEDIKE ET, MAHAFFEY JE, RASMUSSEN H: Primary hyperparathyroidism with intermittent hypercalcemia: Serial observations and simple diagnosis by means of an oral calcium tolerance test. *Clin Endocrinol (Oxford)* 3:225–235, 1980
64. SEGRE GV: Amino-terminal radioimmunoassays for human parathyroid hormone, in *Clinical Disorders of Bone and Mineral Metabolism,* edited by FRAME B, POTTS JH JR, Amsterdam, Excerpta Medica, 1983, pp 14–17
65. STRAUSS AL, COE FL, DEUTSCH L, PARKS JH: Factors that predict relapse of calcium nephrolithiasis during treatment. *Am J Med* 72:17–24, 1982

Agents Other Than Thiazide Diuretics in the Treatment of Calcium Oxalate Nephrolithiasis

Ulla Backman

In many stone formers with metabolically active stone formation on conservative therapy, thiazide diuretics are often the first treatment of choice. Some patients, however, do not respond or cannot take thiazides. Also, depending on the underlying metabolic abnormality, some patients may even benefit more from some other drug. For these patients, there are several alternative drugs available, some of which have been used for many years (for example, orthophosphates) whereas others have not yet been fully evaluated.

One great drawback in assessing the preventive effectiveness of these drugs is that few controlled studies have been performed. Usually the results are compared with historical controls or with untreated groups of patients, or the patients are their own controls. Because the drugs act by different mechanisms, the indications for their use presume that some metabolic evaluation of the patients is being performed.

Orthophosphate

Inorganic phosphate has been used as a stone-preventing drug for many years. Albright noticed 40 years ago that orthophosphate reduced the calcium excretion in stone formers. More recently, it has been observed that orthophosphate changed not only the supersaturation of the urine but also had a beneficial effect on the inhibitors of stone formation.

Biochemical Effects of Orthophosphate

Orthophosphate reduces the urinary excretion of calcium by inhibiting the gastrointestinal absorption of calcium. This effect is most pronounced in pa-

This manuscript was presented as part of a Symposium on *Pathogenesis and Treatment of Calcium Nephrolithiasis.*

tients with hypercalciuria, whereas there is only a minimal reduction in normocalciuric patients. Theoretically, the reduced calcium absorption might lead to a negative calcium balance, but there is no evidence that the parathyroid glands are stimulated [1]. Oxalate excretion is unaffected by orthophosphate, but urinary phosphate excretion is increased. The stone inhibitory activity of urine is affected in several ways by orthophosphate. Citrate and pyrophosphate excretion increase, but magnesium excretion is reduced [2]. Thus, by affecting both the supersaturation and the stone inhibitory activity of urine, orthophosphate has a rather complex mode of action. Crystalluria decreases totally; the crystals become smaller, and crystal aggregation diminishes [2].

Orthophosphate is available in several forms: as acid, neutral, and alkaline salts. The neutral salts are the form used most often and are regarded as being the most effective. The acid salts have less of an effect on both calcium excretion and citrate excretion [3], and the alkaline salts increase to a greater extent both the pyrophosphate and the citrate excretion. However, the alkaline salts have not been used very much, probably owing to the large amount of sodium in the available mixtures. For an optimal effect, the drug must be given in sufficient dosages. A minimal dosage is usually considered to be 1.5 g/day, although success has been noted with only 1.0 g/day [1].

Clinical Effects

There is now strong evidence that orthophosphate has a stone preventive effect. Some studies maintained observation periods for up to 12 years [4]. Thomas concluded in his survey that about 90% of the patients treated with orthophosphate were free of recurrences [4], which is also our experience (Fig. 1). In one controlled study performed by Ettinger, there was no beneficial effect of orthophosphate [5], but an acid salt with a maximal daily dosage of 1.5 g was used. The reason for failure to demonstrate a beneficial effect could be attributed to the use of the acid salt.

Orthophosphate has been effective in both hypercalciuric and normocalciuric patients. Thiazides are considered the treatment of choice in the former group of patients as this therapy is less complex than orthophosphate [2]. Orthophosphate is also effective in patients with mild hyperoxaluria and in patients who have a reduced excretion of inhibitors. It has also been very effective in patients with primary hyperoxaluria for long-term control of stone formation [2].

Patients on therapy may pass old stones, which should not be a reason for discontinuing the drug or be interpreted as a sign of its ineffectiveness. A small group of patients have a very active stone formation against which neither orthophosphate nor thiazide alone is effective. By combining the two drugs it has been possible to prevent recurrences [7]. The action of these two drugs is additive in terms of the beneficial physico-chemical changes in the urine.

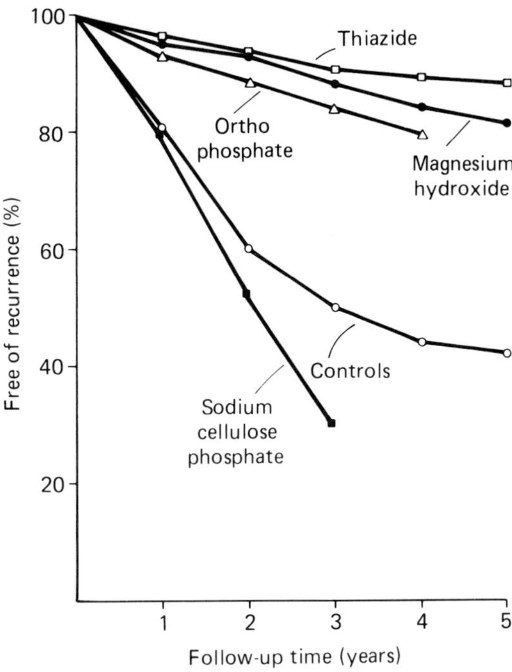

Fig. 1. Experience from Uppsala, Sweden, with different modes of prophylactic treatment for recurrent renal stone formation. Treatments were as follows: bendroflumethiazide, 2.5 mg twice a day ($N = 168$ patients); magnesium hydroxide, 250 mg twice a day ($N = 57$ patients); orthophosphate, 0.5 g three times a day ($N = 59$ patients); and cellulose phosphate, 5 g three times a day ($N = 35$ patients). The results were compared with a control group of 52 patients treated with diet and fluid alone.

Side Effects

Many patients suffer from the side effects of orthophosphate. Diarrhea is the most frequent side effect and is most pronounced during the first weeks of treatment. After this, it usually abates without further problems. When it persists, the dosage is halved until the diarrhea subsides; the dosage is then increased gradually to the full treatment level. Patients who have preexisting gastrointestinal problems, such as dyspepsia or duodenal ulcers, normally do not tolerate orthophosphate. In this regard, the acid salts of orthophosphate seem to give the most problems. Even if some patients can tolerate a lower dosage (and a daily dosage as low as 1 g of phosphorus may be effective), orthophosphate is probably not the first choice of treatment in these patients.

Hypertensive patients and those with a tendency for fluid overload should be treated with caution because the orthophosphates are sodium salts, especially the neutral and alkaline ones. If it is desirable to give orthophosphate to such patients, an acid potassium salt can be tried.

One of the main contraindications of orthophosphate is when the stone formation is due to infection or obstruction. In these disorders, an increased urinary excretion of phosphate may lead to a very rapid growth of the stone. This can happen with minimal symptoms, and thus very large staghorn calculi can be formed in a short time, leading to obstruction and stasis.

Orthophosphate should also be given with much caution in patients who have a reduced glomerular filtration rate (GFR). Treatment with orthophosphate to patients with renal insufficiency worsens the hyperphosphatemia with risk of metastatic calcifications, worsening of the renal function, secondary hyperparathyroidism, and uremic bone disease. Thus, orthophosphate is not recommended for patients whose GFR is below 30 ml/min.

Summary

It is well established that orthophosphate prevents the formation of stones by beneficially altering both the state of supersaturation and the stone inhibitory activity in the urine. The main indications for its use are patients with normocalciuria, hyperoxaluria, and those who have deficiencies of stone inhibitors.

Cellulose Phosphate

Hyperabsorption of calcium in the gut may be a common abnormality in hypercalciuric stone formers. The physiologically ideal drug for these patients should be cellulose phosphate, which binds and inhibits the gastrointestinal absorption of calcium. Cellulose phosphate is a nonabsorbable cation exchanger with a high affinity for calcium. Orally administered sodium cellulose phosphate acts by exchanging sodium for calcium, and the new calcium cellulose phosphate is excreted in the feces [8].

Biochemical Effects

The beneficial effects of cellulose phosphate in stone prevention are restricted to its ability to lower urinary calcium excretion. The reduced urinary calcium excretion appears soon after the start of the treatment, is in the range of 30% of the initial values, and is maintained after 3 to 4 years of follow-up [9]. However, its action is not confined to the inhibition of calcium alone, but to other divalent cations as well, above all magnesium and zinc, which are important inhibitors of stone formation. Magnesium is reduced to the same extent as calcium, which probably is a drawback of cellulose phosphate for it will influence the inhibitory system in a negative way [10]. It also affects oxalate. With a reduced amount of calcium available in the gut to bind oxalate, more oxalate is absorbed. Urinary excretion of oxalate will increase up to two or three times the pretreatment levels. The beneficial effect on calcium excretion will thus be counteracted by an increased excretion of oxalate, and the desirable reduction of supersaturation of calcium oxalate thus will not occur. Pak found that when precautions are also undertaken, such as dietary restriction of calcium and oxalate, the supersaturation for calcium oxalate and brushite decreased [9]. The excretion of phosphate is increased during treatment with cellulose phosphate. In Pak's study [9], this was observed only during the early treatment periods. Treatment with cellulose phosphate on a long-term basis might lead to a negative calcium balance and increase the risk of secondary hyperparathyroidism, especially if given to patients with renal hypercalciuria who have a compensatory hyperabsorption of calcium in the gut. Backman et al found that initially patients had an elevated excretion of cyclic AMP and increased levels of alkaline phosphatases; however, these never reached pathologic levels and were later normalized [10]. Pak also reported a normal level of parathyroid hormone (PTH) and a normal bone density, which did not change during a treatment period of 4 years [9]. Long-term follow-up studies should be conducted to fully evaluate the effect of cellulose phosphate on calcium metabolism and bone mineralization. Cellulose phosphate is given three times a day, with a maximal daily dosage of 15 g. Pak in later studies usually gave a lower dosage of 10 g a day. The drug should be given before or together with meals to attain the best effect on the calcium excretion.

Clinical Effects

In a small number of studies, the beneficial effect of the drug has been limited [9–11]. We used cellulose phosphate in a group of 35 patients who had a 47% recurrence rate after 2 to 3 years on the drug (Fig. 1). The recurrence rate was the same as that in a control group treated with the same dietary restrictions and fluid. The lack of a stone-preventive effect in spite of a reduction of the urinary excretion of calcium can probably be ascribed to the simultaneously reduced excretion of magnesium and the increased excretion of oxalate.

The beneficial effect of cellulose phosphate described by Pak is probably not due to the action of cellulose phosphate alone but to other measures undertaken in their study. Thus, the patients were instructed to maintain a low-oxalate diet and a restricted calcium intake. In addition, supplementation with magnesium gluconate (1 g, twice a day) was given separately from the intake of cellulose phosphate, before breakfast and at bedtime. With this regimen, a recurrence rate of only 22% was seen. As there were several instructions given to the patients, the nonspecific effects of diet may also have contributed to the clinical response. However, there was no control group, and the results were compared with the patients' pretreatment stone frequency. With the supplementation of magnesium, the urinary excretion of magnesium did not, however, change from pretreatment levels [9]. When all measures undertaken by Pak are followed, the metabolic changes that occur in the urine on treatment with cellulose phosphate seem to be favorable and prevent further stone formation. But on a long-term basis, such a program—with drugs to be taken five times a day in addition to adhering to a dietary regimen—is rather complex, and patient compliance may be inadequate, which also was the experience of Pak.

Side Effects

In our study, a great number of patients stopped taking cellulose phosphate not only because of its poor stone-preventive effect but also because of its side effects, the most common of which was diarrhea. This side effect may be dose-related because Pak did not see it with a lower dose of 10 g a day. In two of our patients, arthritis appeared, which subsided after the withdrawal of the drug. Another drawback of cellulose phosphate is that it is expensive, about $600 a year.

Summary

Cellulose phosphate has been used in a limited number of patients with a relatively short follow-up compared to that of thiazides and orthophosphate. Its stone-preventive effect is limited when given alone. Patients with proven absorptive hypercalciuria may benefit from this treatment when it is combined with a low-calcium and low-oxalate intake and when magnesium supplementation is given separately from the cellulose phosphate.

Magnesium

Magnesium as a stone-preventive agent has its origin in experimental studies. Several years ago, it was shown that there is a relation between magnesium deficiency and renal stone formation [12]. Rats which were kept on a magnesium-deficient diet very rapidly developed renal stones, mainly containing calcium phosphate. The earliest changes seen in the kidneys were calcifications in the proximal tubules. The same effect was achieved when the animals were given a diet without vitamin B_6, but when there was a high intake of magnesium at the same time, stone formation was prevented [13]. It was also shown that magnesium is able to increase the solubility of calcium oxalate in vitro, supporting its use for the prevention of renal stones [12]. Experimental studies have also shown a beneficial effect of treatment with magnesium on renal stone formation. The indications for its use in humans have generally not been based on any special metabolic abnormalities; instead, it has been given to recurrent stone formers without regard to pathogenesis.

Biochemical Effects

There are several mechanisms whereby magnesium exerts its beneficial effects on renal stone formation. Magnesium binds oxalate in the gut, thereby decreasing the gastrointestinal absorption of oxalate. It also binds to oxalate in the urine and is one of the inhibitors of both calcium oxalate and calcium phosphate crystallization. The solubility product for magnesium oxalate is greater than that for calcium oxalate.

Three forms of magnesium have been used in preventing stones: oxide, hydroxide, and gluconate. These forms may differ to some extent in their ability to increase the urinary excretion of magnesium. The absorption of magnesium occurs along the entire small intestine, although there may be differences in this respect between different compounds. We have given magnesium hydroxide in a daily dose of 500 mg divided in two doses.

Clinical Effects

Although there is strong experimental evidence that magnesium deficiency is related to renal stone formation, such a deficiency has not been confirmed clinically [14]. Nor did the stone formers in our study have a lower urinary magnesium excretion than healthy control persons [14]. But because many stone formers have a high excretion of calcium, an unfavorable relation between magnesium and calcium will be noted. With magnesium therapy, however, the ratio between magnesium and calcium will change in a favorable way.

There are relatively few clinical studies on magnesium as a stone preventive agent. Melnick reported in 1971 that 60% of 47 patients who were treated with magnesium oxide (600 mg) were free of recurrences during a 4-year follow-up study [15]. His conclusion was that magnesium could be used as a prophylactic agent for stone formation. In 1974, Prien and Gershoff reported a study in which they had treated stone formers with 300 mg of magnesium oxide and 10 mg of vitamin B_6 daily, to exclude a possible deficiency of vitamin B_6 [16]. After 5 years of treatment they stopped the study and concluded that their results were comparable to those of Melnick. However, the drop-out rate was 40%, making it difficult to evaluate the effectiveness of the drug.

Since 1976, we have treated 57 consecutive patients who have recurrent stones with magnesium hydroxide (250 mg twice a day). The recurrence rate fell to about 20%, which is relatively low (Fig. 1) [17]. During treatment we noticed an increased excretion of magnesium in the urine, differing in this respect from some of the studies using magnesium oxide [18]. The increase of the urinary magnesium was in the range of 1.6 to 2.0 mmoles/day. Initially, there was an increased serum magnesium, which normalized, however, during the first year and never reached pathologic levels. Another positive effect was an increased urinary excretion of citrate. The mechanism for this is unknown. The drop-out in our study has been low compared with the American studies.

Side Effects

Side effects have been few and never serious. Some patients have had loose stools and have discontinued the treatment for that reason. Hypermagnesemia has not been a problem. One contraindication to the use of magnesium for stone formers is probably urinary tract infections. In these instances, magnesium may lead to rapid growth of stones compared to that which occurs on treatment with phosphate for these patients.

Indications

In our experience, magnesium given as hydroxide has been an acceptable alternative to thiazides and orthophosphate. Besides, it probably should be used in those patients in whom there is a risk of developing magnesium deficiency, for instance, in patients with enteric hyperoxaluria. Also, patients who are on long-term treatment with thiazides may develop a negative magnesium balance and may benefit from supplementation with magnesium.

Summary

Magnesium has been used in a limited number of studies and seems to have a beneficial stone preventive effect. When it has been given as hydroxide, its effects have been comparable with those of thiazide and orthophosphate. However, further studies need to be performed to fully evaluate its effect and actions compared to other modes of treatment.

Allopurinol

Allopurinol has been used in two different conditions to prevent stone formation. The first use, not discussed here, is for patients who form pure uric acid stones, where the indications are quite clear. A more questionable indication is the use of allopurinol for patients who form calcium-containing stones. The reason for using allopurinol to treat patients who form calcium oxalate stones is that a disturbed metabolism of uric acid has been noticed in several stone formers.

Biochemical Background

Some experimental evidence supports the hypothesis that an increased urinary excretion of uric acid favors calcium stone formation. Uric acid and monosodium urate have a structure similar to calcium oxalate and would thus be able to induce heterogenous nucleation of calcium oxalate by a mechanism called epitaxy [19] (see also Coe and Parks, this volume). An increased excretion of uric acid and monosodium urate would favor the precipitation, growth, and aggregation of calcium oxalate crystals. Decreasing the urinary excretion of uric acid should stop this process and prevent further formation of calcium oxalate stones. However, monosodium urate crystals have not been identified in freshly voided urine, and monosodium urate is a very rare component of calcium-containing stones [20].

Another explanation is the influence of uric acid on the macromolecular crystal inhibition. It has been shown in vitro that sodium urate adsorbs the so-called glycosaminoglycans in the urine. The formation of a "colloidal urate" should lead to a decreased inhibitor activity [21]. This mechanism has not been confirmed in vivo. When the inhibition of this crystal system in the urine was studied in hyperuricosuric and normouricosuric patients, it was found to be higher in patients with hyperuricosuria.

Another mechanism of allopurinol is its effect on oxalate. Some authors have reported a reduction of the urinary excretion of oxalate [22]. Others, however, have not been able to confirm this change in the oxalate excretion.

Clinical Effects

Although it is difficult to explain the pathogenetic mechanism of the beneficial action of allopurinol on calcium stone formation, several studies have shown a reduced recurrence rate with this therapy. The indications to give allopurinol have usually been calcium oxalate stone formation in combination with hyperuricosuria. Studies with allopurinol have been reported by Coe [23]. He treated two groups of patients with recurring calcium oxalate stones. One group had hyperuricosuria and received allopurinol dosages of 300 mg daily. The other group had both hyperuricosuria and hypercalciuria and received a combination of allopurinol and thiazide. The results were compared with an untreated group. On treatment with a follow-up of about 4 years, there was a striking reduction of recurrences in both treated groups.

In another study by Smith a double-blind approach was used [24]. The indications, however, were based on a high serum uric acid above 65 mg/liter. In this way, some patients had a high urinary excretion of urate whereas others had a normal excretion. The results showed that only 60% of the treated patients were free of recurrences, which is comparable to the effect of treatment with diet and fluid alone. Other studies have also shown a beneficial effect of allopurinol to prevent calcium stone formation [25]. However, all these studies have been uncontrolled and the results are therefore difficult to interpret.

Our own studies with allopurinol are limited. We have treated a group of 65 consecutive stone formers with an observation period on therapy of up to 5 years. Our preliminary results show that patients who have hypercalciuria do not benefit from allopurinol alone. Recurring calcium stone formation is an approved indication for treatment with allopurinol in some countries such as Germany, England, and Australia, but not the United States.

Side Effects

The most common side effects of allopurinol are skin reactions and gastrointestinal tract disturbances. These can usually be avoided if the drug is given after meals. Leukopenia and hepatotoxicity are rare complications.

Summary

Patients who form calcium-containing renal stones and have hyperuricosuria may benefit from treatment with allopurinol. Patients who also have hypercalciuria need a combined therapy that includes some urinary calcium-reducing drug, such as thiazide or orthophosphate. The mechanism of allopurinol in preventing calcium stone formation is still obscure.

Alkali

Treatment with alkali is probably most used for patients who form pure uric acid stones or cystine stones where the aim is to increase their solubility by alkalinzing the urine. This mode of treatment has been very limited as a stone-preventing agent in calcium stone formers. Alkali has been given mainly to stone formers who have the complete form of renal tubular acidosis (RTA) [26]. As these patients have a manifest metabolic acidosis, alkali is given to correct the acidosis and reduce at the same time the stone formation.

Biochemical Effects

Alkali has a beneficial effect on the metabolic abnormalities that occur in the urine of patients with RTA. These patients have a low urinary excretion of citrate and a high excretion of calcium; both changes are closely related to the acidosis. Treatment with alkali will normalize these metabolic abnormalities in a favorable way in terms of stone formation. The most pronounced hypocitraturia is seen in renal tubular acidosis, but a low excretion has also been reported in idiopathic stone formers [27, 28]. The mechanism of hypocitraturia in idiopathic stone formers is unknown.

Clinical Effects

The stone preventive effect of alkali in patients with RTA is well known [26]. Few studies have been performed on treatment of the incomplete forms of RTA with alkali. We treated 19 patients with the incomplete form of RTA with sodium bicarbonate (3 to 4 g/day). On this therapy, the citrate excretion increased, and the calcium excretion decreased [27]. At the same time, there was a reduction of the stone frequency. Treatment with alkali in idiopathic stone formers has been tried in a small number of patients with a short follow-up [28]. The results were encouraging. All these patients had a low excretion of citrate, and some also had hypercalciuria. The short-term effect was a normalization of the metabolic abnormalities. The long-term follow-up was, however, only one year.

Side Effects

If the dosage of alkali is too high, there might be some gastrointestinal discomforts. Alkali should probably not be given to patients with stone formation combined with infection, in whom the urine is highly alkaline due to the urease-producing bacteria.

Summary

Alkali has a documented stone preventive effect when given to patients with the complete form of renal tubular acidosis. Preliminary experiences with alkali in patients with the incomplete form of renal tubular acidosis and idiopathic stone formers with hypocitraturia have been encouraging.

Investigational Treatments

Pyridoxine

Pyridoxine is commonly given to patients with primary hyperoxaluria because it reduces urinary oxalate. The dosages are usually large, 200 to 400 mg a day. Pyridoxine may also be effective in other forms of hyperoxaluria. In one study, in which hyperoxaluria was the only detectable metabolic disturbance, there was a reduction of the urinary excretion of oxalate to normal values and the reduction persisted after the therapy was discontinued [29]. This might be interpreted as a dietary deficiency of pyridoxine as a cause of the hyperoxaluria.

Diethyl-Amino-Ethanol (DEAE) Cellulose

In analogy with the use of a cation exchanger to treat absorptive hypercalciuria, the anion exchanger DEAE cellulose has been tried for decreasing the intestinal absorption of oxalate [30]. Like cellulose phosphate, its action is nonspecific and also binds other anions such as phosphate and sulfate. It was used in the study reported by Pinto and Bernshtam [30] for 22 patients with proven absorptive hyperoxaluria and no other metabolic abnormalities. The urinary excretion of oxalate decreased considerably to about one third of the pretreatment levels. There were no serious side effects. Stone formation was reduced or stopped during a follow-up period of 2 years. The indications for this type of treatment will probably be limited, and the program is as complex as it is with cellulose phosphate.

Summary

The medical treatment for renal stone formation should be directed, as far as possible, toward eliminating or reducing the underlying metabolic abnormalities. The different modes of medical treatment available today for patients

Table 1. Proposed medical treatments for calcium
urolithiasis

Metabolic disorder	Treatment
Primary hyperparathyroidism	Parathyroidectomy
Renal tubular acidosis	
Complete form	Alkali
	Orthophosphate
Incomplete form	Alkali
	Thiazide
	Orthophosphate
Idiopathic stones	Thiazide
	Orthophosphate
	Magnesium
	Cellulose phosphate?
	Allopurinol?
Hyperuricosuria	Allopurinol eventually
	combined with thiazide

with the heterogenous syndrome of calcium urolithiasis are summarized in
Table 1. As the tendency to form stones is often long-lasting it is important
that the medical program be effective and at the same time simple, safe,
well tolerated, and economical.

References

1. PEACOCK M, ROBERTSON WG, HEYBURN PJ, DAVIES AEJ, RUTHERFORD A:
   Phosphate treatment of idiopathic calcium stone disease, in *Urolithiasis: Clinical
   and Basic Research,* edited by SMITH LH, ROBERTSON WG, FINLAYSON TS,
   New York, Plenum Press, 1981, pp 259–265
2. SMITH LH, WERNESS PG, VAN DEN BERG CJ, WILSON DM: Orthophosphate
   treatment in calcium urolithiasis, in *Proceedings of the Symposium on Urolithiasis,*
   edited by DANIELSON BG, Stockholm, Almquist & Wiksell Periodical Company,
   1980, pp 253–263
3. LAU K, WOLF C, NUSSBAUM P, WEINER B, DE OREO P, SLATOPOLSKY E,
   AGUS Z, GOLDFARB S: Differing effects of acid versus neutral phosphate therapy
   of hypercalciuria. *Kidney Int* 16:736–742, 1979
4. THOMAS WC: Use of phosphates in patients with calcareous renal calculi. *Kidney
   Int* 13:390–396, 1978
5. ETTINGER B: Recurrent nephrolithiasis: Natural history and effect of phosphate
   therapy. *Am J Med* 61:200–206, 1976
6. DANIELSON BG, FAVUS MJ, LAPATSANIS P, SMITH LH: Alternative treatment
   in kidney stone disease, in *Proceedings of the Symposium on Urolithiasis,* edited
   by DANIELSON BG, Stockholm, Almquist & Wiksell Periodical Company, 1980,
   pp 273–284
7. KLEIN AS, GRIFFITH DP: Neutral potassium and thiazide: Combined treatment
   in recurrent stone formers, in *Urolithiasis: Clinical and Basic Research,* edited
   by SMITH LH, ROBERTSON WG, FINLAYSON TS, New York, Plenum Press,
   1981, pp 253–258

8. DENT CE, HARPER CM, PARFITT AM: The effect of cellulose phosphate on calcium metabolism in patients with hypercalciuria. *Clin Sci* 27:417–425, 1964
9. PAK CYC: Cautious use of sodium cellulose phosphate in the management of calcium nephrolithiasis. *Invest Urol* 19:187–190, 1981
10. BACKMAN U, DANIELSON BG, JOHANSSON G, LJUNGHALL S, WIKSTRÖM B: Treatment of recurrent calcium stone formation with cellulose phosphate. *J Urol* 123:9–13, 1980
11. BLACKLOCK NJ, McLEOD MA: The effect of cellulose phosphate on intestinal absorption and urinary excretion of calcium. *Br J Urol* 46:385–392, 1974
12. HAMMARSTEN G: On calcium oxalate and its solubility in the presence of inorganic salts with special reference to the occurrence of oxaluria. *CR Lab Carlsberg* 17:1–58, 1929
13. FARAGELLA FF, GERSHOFF SN: Interrelations among magnesium, vitamin B_6, sulphur and phosphorus in the formation of kidney stones in the rat. *J Nutr* 81:60–66, 1963
14. JOHANSSON G, BACKMAN U, DANIELSON BG, FELLSTRÖM B, LJUNGHALL S, WIKSTRÖM B: Magnesium metabolism in renal stone formers: Effects of therapy with magnesium hydroxide, in *Proceedings of the Symposium on Urolithiasis,* edited by DANIELSON BG, Stockholm, Almquist & Wiksell Periodical Company, 1980, pp 125–134
15. MELNICK I, LANDES RR, HOFFMAN AA, BURCH FF: Magnesium therapy for recurring calcium oxalate urinary calculi. *J Urol* 105:119–122, 1971
16. PRIEN EL, GERSHOFF SF: Magnesium oxide-pyridoxine therapy for recurrent calcium oxalate calculi. *J Urol* 112:509–512, 1974
17. JOHANSSON G, BACKMAN U, DANIELSON BG, FELLSTRÖM B, LJUNGHALL S, WIKSTRÖM B: Prophylactic treatment of renal stone disease with magnesium hydroxide during five years. *Fortschr Urol Nephrol* 20:313–317, 1982
18. GERSHOFF SN, PRIEN EL: Effect of daily MgO and vitamin B_6 administration to patients with recurring calcium oxalate kidney stones. *Am J Clin Nutr* 20:393–399, 1967
19. LONSDALE K: Epitaxy as a growth factor in urinary calculi and gallstones. *Nature* 217:56–58, 1968
20. WERNESS PG, BERGERT JH, SMITH LH: Crystalluria. *J Crystal Growth* 53:166–181, 1981
21. PAK CYC, HOLT K, ZERWEKH JE: Attenuation by monosodium urate of the inhibitory effect of glycosaminoglycans on calcium oxalate nucleation. *Invest Urol* 17:138–140, 1979
22. SCOTT R, PATERSON PJ, MATHIESON A, SMITH M: The effect of allopurinol on urinary oxalate excretion in stone formers. *Br J Urol* 50:455–458, 1978
23. COE FL: Hyperuricosuric calcium oxalate nephrolithiasis. *Kidney Int* 13:418–426, 1978
24. SMITH MJV: Placebo versus allopurinol for renal calculi. *J Urol* 117:690–692, 1977
25. SCHNEEBERGER N, BACH D, HESSE A, BECKS R, VAHLENSIECK W: Prophylaxe des Calcium-Oxalate-Stenleidens durch Beeinflussung der Harnsäurebildung mit Allopurinol, in: *Pathogenese und Klinik der Harnsteine VIII,* Darmstadt, Steinkopff, 1982, pp 414–418
26. MORRIS RC JR, SEBASTIAN A, McSHERRY E: Renal acidosis. *Kidney Int* 1:322–340, 1972
27. BACKMAN U, DANIELSON BG, JOHANSSON G, LJUNGHALL S, WIKSTRÖM B: The clinical importance of renal tubular acidosis in recurrent renal stone formers,

in *Urolithiasis: Clinical and Basic Research,* edited by SMITH LH, ROBERTSON WG, FINLAYSON BS, New York, Plenum Press, 1981, pp 67–70

28. BUTZ M: Oxalatesteinprophylaxe durch alkalitherapie. *Urologe* 21:142–146, 1982
29. HARRISON AR, KASIDAS GP, ROSE GA: Hyperoxaluria and recurrent stone formation apparently cured by short courses of pyridoxine. *Br Med J* 282:2097–2098, 1981
30. PINTO B, BERNSHTAM J: Diethylaminoethanol-cellulose in the treatment of absorptive hyperoxaluria. *J Urol* 119:630–632, 1978

Urinary Inhibitors of Calcium Oxalate Crystallization

Chairpersons: Charles Y. C. Pak and John L. Meyer
Discussants: Peter G. Werners, William B. Gill, Lawrence Resnick,
William C. Thomas, and Michael J. Nicar

It is well established that there are substances in the urine that delay or prevent the formation of the crystalline components of urinary stones. Some of these substances have been identified. Despite their effectiveness in vitro, their importance in preventing the initiation and growth of human urinary calculi has not been clearly established in vivo. It is the purpose of this workshop to summarize recent research in this field, to identify the research areas that require further investigation, and to attempt to put in perspective the role of these urinary stone inhibitors in the overall process of urolithiasis.

Topics to be considered will be glycosaminoglycans and RNA-like substances as inhibitors of calcium oxalate crystal growth, their potential origin in the bladder mucosa, the inhibitory properties of urothelial membrane surfaces, the functional role of urinary glycosaminoglycans, the metal citrate inhibitors of crystal growth, and the therapeutic role of the stimulated endogenous citrate excretion.

Urinary Calcium Oxalate Crystal Growth Inhibitors

Urine contains potent inhibitors of calcium oxalate crystal growth. In voided urine, about 80% of the inhibition is due to high-molecular-weight compounds, including glycosaminoglycans, RNA-like substances, and acidic glycoproteins. Pyrophosphate is estimated to contribute 20% of the inhibition.

It is estimated that, on the basis of weight, the glycosaminoglycans, mainly chondroitin sulfate, comprise most of the macromolecular inhibitory fraction. However, RNA-like materials and acidic glycoproteins are much more potent inhibitors than chondroitin sulfate and contribute significantly to the total amount of inhibition.

This is the summary of a Workshop of the same title.

Recent studies in dogs have shown that bladder washes also contain significant amounts of calcium oxalate inhibition. It should be noted that bladder urine may have factors inhibiting crystal growth from the kidney as well as the bladder. When urine was collected from both the bladder and the kidney, the bladder urine had twice as much inhibition as kidney urine did. This increase in inhibition was paralleled by an increase in Alcianblue-precipitable material (largely glycosaminoglycans), suggesting that glycosaminoglycans in voided urine may originate in the bladder rather than in the kidney. Therefore, the inhibitors that are renal in origin, such as pyrophosphate, may be more important than previously thought, and measurement of calcium oxalate crystal growth inhibition in voided urine may overestimate the inhibition present in the kidney.

However, another group has found similar inhibitor activity in voided urine and in ureteral urine in humans.

Inhibitory Properties of Urothelial Membrane Surfaces on Crystal Nucleation and Adhesion

The normal urothelial surfaces lining the urinary passages from the papillary duct, from the ostia to the distal urethra, are not only a barrier to water and urinary solutes, but they have uniquely inert surfaces to which stone crystals and solute ions do not bind or adhere. Following chemical injuries from high or low pH, detergents, enzymes, and bacterial toxins or physical injuries from crushing or osmotic alterations, calcium oxalate and struvite $(MgNH_4PO_4 \cdot 6H_2O)$ crystals adhere to injured urothelial surfaces but not to normal urothelium. Moreover, nucleation of calcium oxalate crystallization occurs at lower levels of metastable supersaturation in glass-lined or injured urothelial systems as contrasted with normal urothelial surfaces.

In the pathogenesis of urolithiasis, three events must occur in succession. First, there must be urinary supersaturation, an unstable excess of solute in solution over equilibrium solute levels. But unless the second event of crystal nucleation commences, the urine passes from the body as mere voided supersaturated urine. Crystal nucleation results in crystalluria, but unless the third event occurs—the retention of crystals—the crystals pass out in the urine from the body as mere crystalluria without resulting in urolithiasis. Retention of crystals could take place either by their lodgement at the papillary duct ostia, which is smaller in diameter than the crystals, or by their adhesion to the urothelial surfaces lining the urinary passages. The first of these possibilities would cause "free" particle growth; the next, "fixed" crystal particle growth.

Crystallization is a function of three major factors: (a) the nature of the solute, (b) the nature of solvent, and (c) the nature of the interfaces that contain the system. The liquid-to-solid interface is of fundamental importance, because it is here that nucleation preferentially occurs. Because interfaces are energetically favored sites, crystal adhesion to container surfaces is potentially a major problem both in industry (for example, "boiler scale") and in biologic disease states. Thus, it would appear that abnormal or injured urothelial surfaces could affect both nucleation and retention of crystals.

Techniques have been developed for studying crystallization in urothelial-lined "living test tubes." After bladders of anesthetized female rats are catheterized, crystallization can be induced by intravesical instillations of calcium and oxalate ions. The crystals can then be readily separated into free and adherent fractions. Chemical injuries to the urothelium can be produced by dilute acids, 5% Triton X100, a nonionic detergent, povidone iodine, Renografin, *Proteus* bacterial toxins, the proteolytic enzyme papain, the glycosidase neuraminidase, or hyperosmolar saline or urea, all of which result in marked crystal adhesion to the injured urothelium. Control bladders without urothelial injuries remain free of adherent crystals but form large numbers of small, free, filterable crystals of relatively uniform size.

Similar studies have been carried out with struvite ($MgNH_4PO_4 \cdot 6H_2O$) crystallization in urothelial containers in vivo. Again, crystals adhere only to injured urothelium but not to normal, uninjured urothelium.

Abnormal urothelial surfaces of bladder tumors have frequently been found to be the site of crystal adhesion in humans. Calcium oxalate has been found more frequently on human bladder tumor surfaces, but uric acid has also been seen.

The functional equivalency of upper and lower urinary tract urothelium with respect to crystal adhesions has been demonstrated in a catheterized rat ureter system in which the renal pelvis, calyces, and papillae are the urothelial-lined container surfaces. Again, crystals do not adhere unless there has been antecedent injury to the urothelial surfaces.

In studies on calcium oxalate nucleation, an elevation of the metastable limits and an absence of container-surface nucleation was found in urothelial-lined systems as contrasted to a lower metastable limit and a marked surface nucleation in glass containers. Also, a lowering of the metastable limit has been demonstrated in urothelium injured by povidone iodine.

A protective or restorative effect of heparin has been found. It prevents crystal adhesion of either calcium oxalate or struvite to many types of chemically injured urothelium. Several other sulfated glycosaminoglycans were not effective in restoring the antiadherence coat of the injured urothelial surfaces.

These studies demonstrate that normal urothelium has important inhibitory powers that prevent crystals from nucleating and adhering to its surfaces.

Glycosaminoglycans as Inhibitors of Calcium Oxalate Crystallization

Although glycosaminoglycans have always merited much biochemical attention as a characteristic component of vertebra connective tissues, they have recently begun to enjoy an accelerated amount of interest because of their numerous other biologic processes, both physiologic and pathologic. Glycosaminoglycans are located in structural tissue such as cartilage, nucleus pulposa, cornea, skin, blood vessel wall, as well as in "softer" tissues such as brain, kidney, and liver. They have been investigated extensively in the urine of normal people as well as in the urine of patients with mucopolysaccharidoses, such as Hurler's and San Filippo's syndromes. In normal urine, about 60% of the glycosaminoglycans is believed to be comprised of the chondroitin sulfates, with heparin sulfate and keratin sulfate accounting for about 15% each.

Within the genitourinary tract, the kidney is purported to have the major role in providing the urine with glycosaminoglycans. Since electrophoresis of serum shows a pattern of glycosaminoglycans similar to that of urine, it is presumed that most of the urinary glycosaminoglycans are filtered from the blood. The origin in serum is still unknown, but they may arise from the connective tissue ground substances with some contribution from vessel walls, leukocytes, and platelets.

Evidence exists that glycosaminoglycans are an important component of the organic matrix of urinary calculi. Recent evidence is most compelling for glycosaminoglycans acting as extremely potent inhibitors of crystal growth and aggregation and even, according to some investigations, spontaneous nucleation. There is, however, strong evidence that they act as promoters of nucleation. In fact, it is thought by some that it is the particular balance between nucleation, promotion, and aggregation/inhibition that will determine whether a person will form stones.

The mechanism of crystal inhibition is thought to involve binding of the inhibitor onto the crystal surface, disrupting the surface symmetry and inhibiting further growth as well as epitactic induction of growth. Aggregation inhibition probably involves binding of the inhibitor onto the crystal surface, inducing a change in zeta potential and thus causing a repulsion between crystals. Glycosaminoglycans are strongly bound to solid urate, a process that is enhanced by calcium and magnesium, so that an increase in urinary colloidal or crystalline uric acid or urate can lead to a decrease in the concentration of free glycosaminoglycans. This concept is supported in human studies by the finding that in hyperuricosuria the formation product for calcium oxalate is decreased.

Metal Citrate Inhibitors of Crystal Growth

Iron (III), aluminum (III), and chromium (III) interact uniquely with citrate to form potent inhibitors of hydroxyapatite crystal growth. This inhibition of phosphatic crystals is greatest when the concentration ratio of citrate to metal is high, for example, 20:1 or more. Interestingly, low concentration ratios of citrate to iron (III), but not aluminum or chromium, lead to the formation of a polymerized complex that inhibits the growth of calcium oxalate crystals at iron concentrations as low as 5 μM. Silicates prevent this interaction between citrate and iron. There is preliminary evidence indicating that much of the nonprotein-bound iron, aluminum, ad chromium in urine exist as complexes with citrate. The urinary excretion of nonprotein-bound aluminum and chromium is reduced in patients with medullary sponge kidneys or hyperparathyroidism and renal calculi but not in patients with idiopathic stones.

The identification of these unique metal citrate complexes in urine provides information on a new means whereby citrate may be effective in preventing crystal growth and possibly calculus formation. Ordinarily there is very little nonprotein-bound iron in urine. Therefore, if there is a protective effect against calcium oxalate stones by polyvalent metal citrate complexes in normal subjects, it would be expected to occur by the prevention of the formation of a phosphatic nidus for the principally calcium oxalate calculi.

Therapeutic Role of Potassium Citrate Therapy

The use of potassium citrate in the management of calcium nephrolithiasis is based on observations that (a) citrate is an important inhibitor of the crystallization of calcium oxalate and calcium phosphate, (b) urinary citrate is often reduced in calcium nephrolithiasis, and (c) oral potassium citrate is effective in restoring normal urinary citrate and retarding the crystallization of calcium salts.

When added in vitro, citrate reduces the saturation of calcium oxalate and calcium phosphate by complexing calcium and lowering calcium ion activity. Moreover, it directly inhibits spontaneous nucleation and crystal growth of calcium oxalate. The urinary excretion of this important inhibitor is reduced in many patients with nephrolithiasis, the reported incidence of hypocitraturia ranging from 19 to 63%. Hypocitraturia occurs not only in renal tubular acidosis and enteric hyperoxaluria, but also in patients with normal acidification and without intestinal disease. Thus, hypocitraturia may represent an important risk for calcium stone formation.

Oral potassium citrate therapy (60 mEq/day in divided doses) is usually effective in restoring normal urinary citrate in patients with hypocitraturic calcium nephrolithiasis. Moreover, it increases urinary pH (to between 6.3 and 6.8) and potassium. In some patients, urinary calcium significantly decreases during treatment. However, the excretion of phosphorus, magnesium, oxalate, and uric acid is not altered. Thus, the saturation of calcium oxalate decreases (because of reduced calcium activity), whereas that of brushite does not change (because the increased dissociation of phosphate is offset by citrate complexation of calcium). Moreover, the inhibitor activity against the crystallization of calcium salts is enhanced by stimulated citrate excretion.

Potassium citrate has been used during long-term treatment of hypocitraturic patients with calcium nephrolithiasis and in those with uric acid nephrolithiasis with complication of calcium nephrolithiasis. The treatment resulted in remission (no further stone formation) in approximately 74% of patients and reduced individual stone formation rate in 99% of patients. In patients who relapsed on thiazide therapy, the addition of potassium citrate prevented further stone formation.

Kidney Diseases in the Tropics

Nephrotic Syndrome in Tropical Africa: Glomerulonephritis in Zimbabwe

Janet L. Seggie

Zimbabwe shares with the rest of tropical Africa an extremely high incidence of glomerular disease (Fig. 1), along with a high endemicity for a variety of parasitic, bacterial, and viral infectious diseases. In view of the known

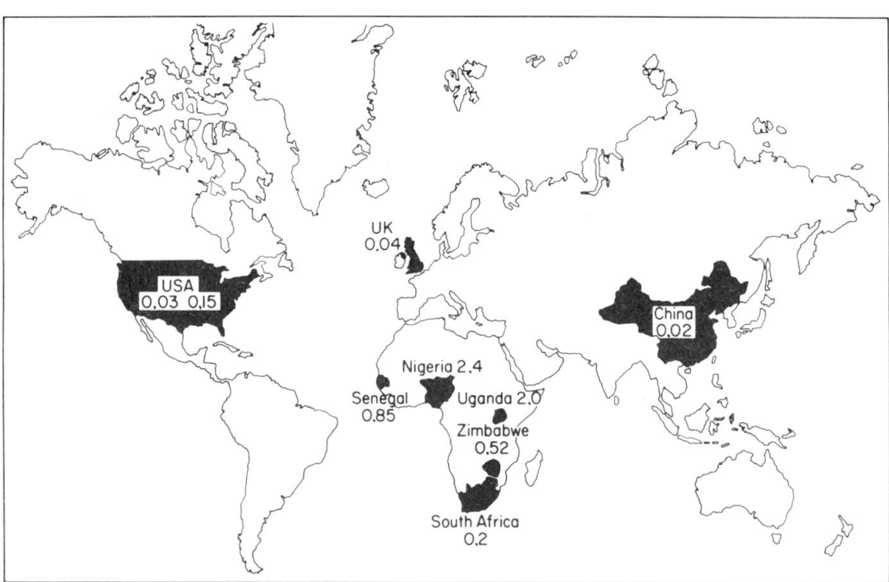

Fig. 1. Map of the world showing incidence rates of the nephrotic syndrome as a percentage of total medical admissions. Note the 20- to 80-fold greater incidence in tropical African countries when compared with the USA and Northern Europe.

This manuscript was presented as part of a Symposium on *Tropical Nephrology.*

glomerulonephritogenic potential of infections prevalent in the Zimbabwean environment, a study of the nephrotic syndrome was undertaken. It sought (1) to define the etiology of glomerular disease and, in particular, to elucidate the glomerulonephritogenic roles, if any, of schistosomiasis [1] and malaria [2] in the indigenous Zimbabwean population, (2) to analyze the histopathologic patterns of disease, and (3) during follow-up examination of patients for up to 3 years after presentation, to determine the natural history of different patterns of glomerulonephritis (GN) in this population.

Over an 18-month period (1979 to 1980), 98 patients with the nephrotic syndrome were admitted to hospitals of the University of Zimbabwe Medical School in the capital city of Harare and investigated. This report is based on the 87 patients who underwent renal biopsy examination. For ease and clarity in describing the results of the survey, patients are divided into children (aged 0 to 12 years) and adults (all patients over the age of 12 years).

The Nephrotic Syndrome in Children

In children, the nephrotic syndrome was associated with membranous GN in 7, proliferative GN in 7, focal glomerulosclerosis (FSGS) in 2, and congenital mesangial sclerosis in one (see Fig. 2).

In the majority of children (14 children), GN could be linked to infection:

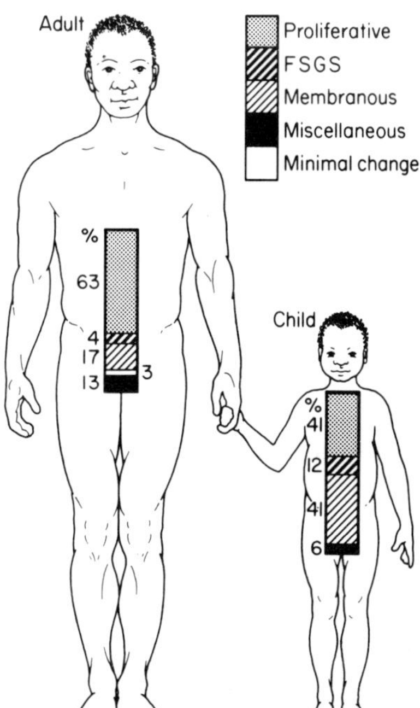

Fig. 2. Major histopathologic patterns of glomerulonephritis associated with the nephrotic syndrome in Zimbabwean children (aged 12 years and younger) and adults.

the hepatitis B virus in 8 and β-hemolytic streptococcus in a further six. In two children no etiologic factor could be defined: one had focal segmental proliferative disease with crescent formation and the other FSGS. The youngest child in the study (aged 2 years) had been ill for over a year, and biopsy examination showed neonatal or congenital mesangial sclerosis.

Minimal change nephropathy was entirely absent, but in spite of this the nephrotic syndrome in Zimbabwean children followed a generally benign course; most proceeded to full recovery. A few children with membranous GN were treated with corticosteroids, but this practice was abandoned when it became clear that it was not hastening resolution. Therapy thus continued to be maintaining a dietary intake high in protein, achieving a modest diuresis to relieve symptoms relating to peripheral edema, and being alert to and treating intercurrent infection and any concomitant parasitic infection discovered during investigation.

The striking absence of minimal change GN in Zimbabwean children deserves further discussion. Its rare occurrence in African children has been a constant characteristic of all surveys of childhood nephrosis undertaken in Africa to date [3–8] with the exception of that undertaken in Ghana [9]. Is there any explanation for this finding? The recent studies of Alfiler et al [10] and Ansquer et al [11] reveal that HLA DR7 is importantly associated with minimal change disease in European children, and a survey undertaken by Coovadia, Adhikari, and Morel-Maroger [5] in Natal, South Africa, provides circumstantial evidence in support of the "genetic factor" in determining the presence or absence of minimal change GN in African children. In Natal live three populations of children of European, Indian, and African descent. The patterns of disease giving rise to the nephrotic syndrome vary greatly between European and African children, but not as dramatically between European and Indian children. A survey of the genetic make-up of these populations (through study of their HLA antigen status) reveals that the genetic distance is greatest between the European and African populations and least between the European and Indian populations [12].

Membranous Glomerulonephritis and the Role of Hepatitis B Virus

Membranous GN in Zimbabwean children was exclusively associated with hepatitis B (HB) antigenemia [13], representing a 100% carrier rate for children with membranous nephropathy compared with a 5% carrier rate among healthy children who were used as controls. It proved impossible to demonstrate the presence of the surface antigen in biopsy material of these children (using a commercially prepared FITC antiserum), but the strong link between antigenemia and membranous GN constitutes circumstantial evidence for the role of the HB virus in the genesis of the NS in children.

The majority of them enjoyed complete remission of their nephropathy within one year of presentation. Steroid therapy, which was used for half our children, had no beneficial effect in terms of causing a reduction of proteinuria. (The steroids were used according to a modification of the protocol of the Collaborative Study of the Adult Idiopathic Nephrotic Syndrome [14].)

Based on this evidence, Zimbabwe therefore shares with South Africa [15] and Taiwan [16] this experience of a strong association between membranous glomerulopathy and hepatitis B viremia. Such is surely not surprising when one notes the extremely high carrier rates for the HB virus in the tropics [17]. Highest carrier rates for the HB surface antigen are noted in African children who are 2 to 9 years old [18], which ties in with the finding that most children developing HB-related nephrosis are 3 to 12 years old [13, 16].

It appears that HB-induced glomerulopathy is immune complex (IC) mediated [19], and the demonstration by immunofluorescence of glomerular deposits containing the surface [16, 20], core [21], or e antigen [22, 23] is regarded as corroborative evidence. That few patients exhibit circulating immune complexes (CICs), however, has led to the suggestion [16] that in situ glomerular IC formation takes place [24].

It is notable that membranous GN dominates patterns of nephrosis in African children in countries in which *Plasmodium malariae* has not been etiologically implicated [3–5], and it is likely that much of this may be due to this HB infection. Moreover, it seems certain that the nephrotic syndrome will be increasingly associated with this infection. The reasons for this are the rising carrier rates of the HB virus owing to its parenteral spread by blood-sucking insects and practices such as tattooing and scarification with unsterile instruments, and its nonparenteral spread associated with unhygienic living conditions. Immunization programs, on the face of it, seem to provide a ready answer. But alas, this cannot be so in Africa until much cheaper vaccines are synthesized.

In 6 children with proliferative patterns of GN, the presence of serologic markers of streptococcal infection suggested that their nephrosis was a manifestation of poststreptococcal GN (PSGN). These cases are discussed later in this report.

Role of Malaria

One of the purposes of this survey was to determine whether *P. malariae* was etiologically significant in the genesis of the nephrotic syndrome, which has been shown to be the case amongst Nigerian and Ugandan children [6, 7]. It must be noted, however, that epidemiologic surveys have shown that *P. malariae* causes only about 15% of clinical cases of malaria treated in Zimbabwe's hospitals and clinics [25].

Although 13 patients in the series had elevated titers of malarial antibody ranging from 1:20 to 1:2560, there was no statistical difference between patients and healthy controls ($P > 0.05$). In only one patient, a young male adult, was a parasitemia due to *P. malariae* demonstrated; since his nephrotic syndrome was associated with an underlying focal sclerosing glomerular lesion, it is probable that he represents a single case in the entire series of quartan malarial nephropathy (QMN). However, electron microscopic examination of his biopsy sample failed to reveal a splitting or flaking ("feuilletage") of the glomerular basement membrane, which has been shown by Hendrickse et al [26] to be typical of QMN. *P. malariae* clearly played no role in the etiology of childhood nephrosis in Zimbabwe underlining what other workers in tropical Africa have found [3, 4, 9]: *P. malariae* is not common as a cause of childhood nephrosis except in Nigeria and Uganda.

The Nephrotic Syndrome in Adults

In adults, patterns of GN associated with the nephrotic syndrome were not greatly different from those in children (Fig. 2). Minimal change GN found representation here, but in each of two patients was associated with malignant lymphoma. When compared with their counterparts in the First and Second Worlds, Zimbabwean adults exhibited a very much more proliferative GN.

Proliferative (Postinfectious) Glomerulonephritis

In our study population, 42 adults exhibited either diffuse endocapillary proliferative GN (22 patients) or mesangial proliferative GN (20 patients). In 21 patients, elevated antistreptolysin (ASO) and antideoxyribonuclease B (anti-DNAse B) titers and a frequent clinical association with scabies pyoderma [27] suggested a poststreptotoccal etiology for the glomerulopathy.

"Nephritic" features of microhematuria, renal insufficiency, and hypertension were common. Biopsy samples showing diffuse proliferative GN were characterized by neutrophil polymorph infiltration of glomeruli, presence of subepithelial electron-dense deposits, and heavy capillary loop fluorescence for IgG (frequently accompanied by IgM) and C3. In those showing mesangial proliferation, deposits of IgG, IgM, and C3 were demonstrated in the mesangial matrix. Thus, these patients superficially resembled typical cases of acute postinfectious GN, but the striking feature was that all were nephrotic with heavy proteinuria, ranging from 3 to 23 g per square meter of body surface per day, hypoalbuminemia, and hypercholesterolemia.

Recently, Sorger et al [28, 29] have drawn attention to subcategories of postinfectious GN, which they term the *garland, starry sky,* and *mesangial* patterns. Zimbabwean patients exhibited many of the clinical and histopathologic features said to be characteristic of the former two Sorger categories: patients were older having "already passed through childhood." They ranged in age from 6 to 69 (mean, 26 years) and males predominated (male:female ratio, 3:2); heavy proteinuria (resulting in the nephrotic syndrome) was common to both categories; and histopathologic patterns (outlined above) closely resembled those delineated by Sorger and colleagues. As these authors stressed, IgM deposits were frequently demonstrated, especially in patients having the garland pattern.

A distressing feature of Zimbabwean patients was the tendency for clinical manifestations such as renal insufficiency and heavy proteinuria to persist (this was the case in 11 of 22 patients with the garland pattern, 5 of whom progressed to end-stage renal failure and death, and in 3 out of 20 patients with the starry sky pattern). This mirrors the experience of Sorger et al [29] and coincidentally that of Wing, Hutt, and Kibukamusoke [30] in young adult Ugandans in whom postinfectious GN manifested also as the nephrotic syndrome.

Every survey of the nephrotic syndrome in adults contains a cohort of patients with idiopathic proliferative GN, but the African population appears to display the greatest proportion of such patients [8, 31]. The supposition would be that such patterns of disease in tropical Africa represent the encounter between susceptible hosts and infective agents within the environment, which, so far, remain unidentified.

It seems important to attempt to explain why postinfectious GN in Zimbabweans should have followed an essentially malignant course in so many individuals. First, it is acknowledged that such progression is more common in adults than in children [29, 32], and our patients were older children and young adults. Second, the histology provided some forewarning: although no patients exhibited crescentic GN, which might have been expected to follow a rapidly progressive course, 6 patients (5 of whom subsequently died) showed varying degrees of glomerulosclerosis at the initial biopsy examination. Rodriguez-Iturbe et al [32] and Gallo et al [33] have already alerted us to the potentially ominous significance of such a finding in follow-up biopsy examination of patients with PSGN.

In light of work by Brenner, which was reviewed recently [34], we may be able to relate the progression of renal failure in our patients to a hemodynamically mediated glomerular injury. Pursuing this line of thought, we would have to surmise that the initial attack of GN led to immunologically mediated glomerular injury and glomerular destruction, to a level that resulted in sustained hyperfiltration by remaining nephrons and progressive nonimmunologically mediated glomerular sclerosis.

A third possibility exists, that concomitant parasitism in African patients might have predisposed them to a more severe initial glomerular injury than usually occurs in the course of the average episode of postinfectious GN affecting a patient living, say, in industrialized Europe or America. In this context, it is noteworthy that 22 (52%) Zimbabwean patients had schistosomiasis and that circulating and complexed schistosomal antigen was demonstrated in the serum of the majority of these individuals. Such parasite-derived macromolecular material as this might saturate reticuloendothelial clearance mechanisms, setting the stage for severe glomerular injury during the course of nephritogenic infections.

Syphilitic Glomerulonephritis

In 4 adult patients, the nephrotic syndrome occurred as a manifestation of secondary syphilis. The renal lesion was typically marked by glomerular hypercellularity and variable thickening of the glomerular basement membrane [35], and all patients rapidly recovered with penicillin treatment [36].

Studies of incidence rates for venereal disease in tropical Africa [37] reveal that syphilis is at least 50 times more common than it is in the UK and 5 times more common than it is in the USA. Syphilis is therefore likely to always be represented in any survey of the nephrotic syndrome in tropical Africa.

Membranous Glomerulonephritis

In contrast to the situation in children, membranous GN in adults was unrelated to hepatitis B. In one patient, it was due to lupus nephritis. Among our study population, 6 adults had membranous GN. Five patients with stage-1 or -2 disease were treated with high-dose alternate-day corticosteroids [14]. Two of them had complete resolution of proteinuria, and two had partial resolution (reduction of proteinuria to < 1 g/day).

Role of Schistosomiasis

Schistosomiasis, often caused by mixed infestation with *Schistosoma mansoni* and *Schistosoma hemotobium,* is rife in Zimbabwe, spread of infection being encouraged by the development of large irrigation schemes in all parts of the country. It is not uncommon to find infection rates of 96% for *S. hemotobium* and 85% for *S. mansoni* in the same population of children between the ages of 5 and 12 [38]. Furthermore, schistosomiasis mansoni is the major cause of hepatosplenomegaly in the Zimbabwean population [39].

In view of what has been learned from the work of Andrade and Rocha in Brazil [1], namely, that individuals with hepatosplenic schistosomiasis with complicating heavy *S. mansoni* infection may develop a mesangial glomerulo-pathy and the nephrotic syndrome, it seemed important to investigate whether such nephropathy ever develops in Zimbabweans. It appears from clinical studies, corroborated by animal studies [40], that the evolution of portosystemic shunts accompanying schistosomal "cirrhosis" of the liver is crucial to the establishment of glomerular disease. It is supposed that circulating schistosomal antigenic and immune complex material is thus able to gain access to the renal circulation and glomeruli by bypassing the normal clearing mechanisms vested in the Kuppfer cell system of the liver.

The major antigen associated with schistosomal glomerulopathy appears to be a high-molecular-weight polysaccharide (referred to as circulating anodic-antigen by Deelder et al [41]). There is evidence that this antigen is derived from the digestive tube mucosa of the adult worm and is constantly regurgitated into the blood stream of the infected host [41, 42].

Among all Zimbabwean patients with nephrosis, 53 (61%) had evidence of schistosomiasis (based on a positive bilharzial fluorescent antibody test [43] or the presence of schistosome ova in urine, stool, or rectal snip biopsy specimens). The incidence of schistosomiasis among patients was not, however, significantly different from that in healthy controls ($P > 0.05$). More importantly, no case of hepatosplenic schistosomiasis and the nephrotic syndrome was diagnosed.

When subjected to fluorescence testing with a bank of FITC schistosomal antisera, biopsy material of schistosomiasis-positive patients yielded uniformly negative results. (The antisera was generously donated by A. M. Deelder, Laborotorium voor Parasitologie, Rijks Universiteit to Leiden, Netherlands; these included anticirculating anodic-antigen; antisecretory and excretory antigens; antiadult-worm antigens, and antitegument antigens.)

Thus, it was concluded, on the basis of this survey at least, that glomerular disease in Zimbabweans was not *primarily* related to schistosomal infection.

Whether schistosomal macromolecular material (free circulating and complexed adult worm antigen), which was demonstrated (using an ELISA sandwich technique) in 29 (55%) of the 53 patients with schistosomiasis, had any *secondary* role in determining the severity of glomerular disease in patients—for example, those with postinfectious GN (vide supra)—must remain a matter for speculation and future investigation.

Conclusion

In common with the rest of tropical Africa, the Zimbabwean experience showed an extremely high incidence of the nephrotic syndrome, at least ten times that of the USA and Northern Europe. Clear explanations for this remarkable difference between tropical and nontropical populations are not immediately obvious, but certain clues emerge from this study of Zimbabwean Africans.

The high prevalence of a variety of potentially glomerulonephritogenic infections within the African environment is clearly important. Thus, the disease in a third of Zimbabwean patients could be linked to hepatitis B, β hemolytic streptococcal, and syphilitic infection. A further 25% of them exhibited clinical and histopathologic features suggestive of postinfectious GN.

Immunity deficiency [44] in Africans—first by virtue of malnutrition [45–47] and second as a consequence of chronic, often multispecific, parasitic illness (for example, schistosomiasis and malaria in the same individual) [48]—is likely also to play a role. It is recognized that parasitic infection by virtue of its stimulation of polyclonal B cell proliferation [48] and thence of immunoglobulin [49] and autoantibody [50] synthesis may induce a state of relative exhaustion of the circulating macrophage and reticuloendothelial systems with respect to their macromolecular clearance function.

Thus, a picture may be conjured up of an African living in the tropics, immuno-compromised by virtue of malnutrition and parasitic disease, and falling prey to glomerulonephritogenic infections that characterize his natural environment. Poor antigen elimination because of an acquired reticuloendothelial "block" might result in severe and protracted glomerular injury [51], explaining the poor prognosis with which the nephrotic syndrome in Africans is so often associated.

References

1. ANDRADE ZA, ROCHA H: Schistosomal glomerulopathy. *Kidney Int* 16:23–39, 1979

2. KIBUKAMUSOKE JW: *Nephrotic Syndrome of Quartan Malaria*. London, Edward Arnold, 1973

3. MOREL-MAROGER L, VERROUST P, SLOPER JC, SAIMOT JC: Extramembranous proliferative glomerulonephritis in West African children, in *Proc 6th Int Congr Nephrol*, 1975, pp 457–461

4. MOREL-MAROGER L, SAIMOT AG, SLOPER JC, WOODROW DF, ADAM C, NIANG I, PAYET M: "Tropical nephropathy" and "tropical extramembranous glomerulonephritis" of unknown etiology in Senegal. *Br Med J* 1:541–546, 1975

5. COOVADIA HM, ADHIKARI M, MOREL-MAROGER L: Clinico-pathological features of the nephrotic syndrome in South African children. *Q J Med* 48:77–91, 1979

6. HENDRICKSE RG, GILLES HM: The nephrotic syndrome and other renal diseases in children in Western Nigeria. *East Afr Med J* 40:186–201, 1963

7. KIBUKAMUSOKE JW, HUTT MSR, WILKS NE: The nephrotic syndrome in Uganda and its association with quartan malaria. *Q J Med* 36:393–407, 1967

8. KUNG'U A, SITATI SM: Glomerulopathies in Kenya: A histopathological study. *East Afr Med J* 57:525–539, 1980

9. ADU D, ANIM-ADDO Y, FOLI AK, BLANKSON JM, ANNOBIL SH, REINDORF CA, CHRISTIAN EC: The nephrotic syndrome in Ghana: Clinical and pathological aspects. *Q J Med* 50:297–306, 1981

10. ALFILER CA, ROY LP, DORAN T, SHELDON A, BASHIR H: HLA DRW7 and steroid responsive nephrotic syndrome of children. *Clin Nephrol* 14:71–74, 1980

11. ANSQUER JC, LAURENT J, LAGRUE G, DE MOUZON CAMBON A, BRACQ C: HLA DRW7 in adult lipoid nephrosis patients: Significant difference according to age of onset. *Nephron* 34:270, 1983

12. HAMMOND MG, APRADOO B, BRAIN P: Subdivision of HL-A5 and comparative studies of the HLA polymorphism in South African Indians. *Tissue Antigens* 4:42–49, 1974

13. SEGGIE J, NATHOO K, DAVIES PG: Association of hepatitis B (HB$_s$) antigenaemia and membranous glomerulonephritis in Zimbabwean children. *Nephron*, in press

14. A controlled study of short-term prednisone treatment in adults with membranous nephropathy: Collaborative study of the adult idiopathic nephrotic syndrome. *N Engl J Med* 301:1301–1306, 1979

15. ADHIKARI M, COOVADIA HM, CHRYSTAL V: Extramembranous nephropathy in Black South African children. *Ann Trop Pediatr*, in press

16. HSU H-C, LIN G-H, CHANG M-H, CHEN C-H: Association of hepatitis B surface antigenaemia and membranous nephropathy in children in Taiwan. *Clin Nephrol* 20:121–129, 1983

17. SOBESLAVSKY O: HBV as a Global Problem in Viral Hepatitis, edited by VYAS GN, COHEN SH, SCHMID R, New York, Franklin Institute Press, 1978, pp 347–356

18. WANKYA BM, HANSEN DP, NGINDU AMN, FEINSTONE SF, PURCELL RH: Seroepidemiology of hepatitis A and B in Kenya: A rural population survey in Machakos District. *East Afr Med J* 56:134–138, 1979

19. KLEINKNECHT C, LEVY M, PEIX A, BROYER M, COURTECUISSE V: Membranous glomerulonephritis and hepatitis B surface antigen in children. *J Pediatr* 95:946–956, 1979

20. BRZOSKO WJ, KRAWCZYNSKI K, NAZAREWICZ T, MORZYCKA M, NOWOSLAWSKI A: Glomerulonephritis associated with hepatitis B surface antigen immune complexes in children. *Lancet* 2:478–482, 1974

21. SLUSARCZYK J, MICHALAK T, NAZAREWICZ DE MEZER T, KRAWCZYNSKI K, NOWOSLAWSKI A: Epimembranous glomerulonephritis associated with hepatitis B core antigen immune complexex. *Am J Pathol* 98:29–39, 1980

22. FURUSE A, HATTORI S, TERASHIMA T, KARASHIMA S, MATSUDA I: Circulating immune complexes in glomerulopathy associated with hepatitis B virus infection. *Nephron* 31:212–218, 1982
23. TAKEKOSHI Y, TANAKA M, MIYAKAWA Y, HOSHIZAWI H, TAKAHASH K, MAYUMI M: Free "small" and IgG-associated "large" hepatitis B 'e' antigen in the serum of and glomerular capillary walls of 2 patients with membranous glomerulonephritis. *N Engl J Med* 300:814–818, 1979
24. COUSER WG, SALANT D: In situ immune complex formation and glomerular injury. *Kidney Int* 17:1–13, 1980
25. SCHMITZ B, GELFAND M: A study of the clinical features of malaria in Rhodesia: Part 1. *Cent Afr J Med* 22:83–88, 1976
26. HENDRICKSE RG, ADENIYI A, EDINGTON GM, GLASGOW EF, WHITE RHR, HOUBA V: Quartan malarial nephrotic syndrome: Collaborative clinicopathological study in Nigerian children. *Lancet* 1:1143–1149, 1972
27. WHITTLE HC, ABDULLAHI MT, FAKUNLE F, PARRY EHO, RAJKOVIC AD: Scabies pyoderma and nephritis in Zaria, Nigeria. A clinical and epidemiological study. *Trans R Soc Trop Med Hyg* 67:349–363, 1973
28. SORGER K, GESSLER FK, HÜBNER FK, KÖHLER H, SCHULZ W, STÜHLINGER W, THOENES GH, THOENES W: Subtypes of acute postinfectious glomerulonephritis: Synopsis of clinical and pathological features. *Clin Nephrol* 17:114–128, 1978
29. SORGER K, BALUN J, HÜBNER FK, KÖHLER H, OBLING H, SCHULZ W, SEYBOLD D, THOENES GH, THOENES W: The garland type of acute postinfectious glomerulonephritis: Morphological characteristics and follow-up studies. *Clin Nephrol* 20:17–26, 1983
30. WING AJ, HUTT MSR, KIBUKAMUSOKE JW: Poststreptococcal glomerulonephritis and the nephrotic syndrome in Uganda. *Trans R Soc Trop Med Hyg* 65:543–548, 1972
31. SEEDAT YK: Clinicopathological features of nephrotic syndrome in the Africans and Indians of South Africa. *South Afr J Hosp Med* J:219–222, 1979
32. RODRIGUEZ-ITURBE B, GARCIA R, RUBIO L, CUENCA L, TRESER G, LANGA K: Epidemic glomerulonephritis in Maracaibo: Evidence for progression to chronicity. *Clin Nephrol* 5:197–206,1976
33. GALLO GR, FEINER HD, STEELE JM, SCHACHT RG, GLUCK MC, BALDWIN DS: Rule of intrarenal vascular sclerosis in progression of poststreptococcal glomerulonephritis. *Clin Nephrol* 13:49–57, 1980
34. BRENNER BM, MEYER TW, HOSTETTER TH: Dietary protein intake and progressive nature of kidney disease: The role of hemodynamically mediated glomerular injury in the pathogenesis of progressive glomerular sclerosis in aging, renal ablation, and intrinsic renal disease. *N Engl J Med* 307:652–659, 1982
35. BRAUNSTEIN GD, LEWIS EJ, GAVANEK EG, HAMILTON A, BELL WR: The nephrotic syndrome associated with secondary syphilis: An immune deposit disease. *Am J Med* 48:643–648, 1970
36. FALLS WF, FORD KL, ASHWORTH CT, CARTER NW: The nephrotic syndrome in secondary syphilis: Report of a case with renal biopsy findings. *Ann Intern Med* 63:1047–1058, 1965
37. ARYA OP, BENNET FJ: Role of medical auxiliaries in the control of sexually transmitted disease in a developing country. *Br J Vener Dis* 52:116–121, 1976
38. CLARKE V DE V: Patterns of transmission of bilharziasis in Rhodesia. *Cent Afr J Med* 23:2–6, 1977
39. WILES WA: The etiology of gross splenomegaly in Rhodesia and the significance of bilharzia. *Centr Afr J Med* 26:3–5, 1980
40. VAN MARCK EAE, JACOBS W, DEELDER AM, GIGASE PLJ: Experimental schisto-

somal glomerulopathy in mice and its relation to porto-systemic collateral circulation: A light and electron microscope study. *Ann Soc Belge Med Trop* 59:33–47, 1979

41. DEELDER AM, KLAPPE HTM, VAN DEN AARDWEG GJMJ, VAN MEERBEKE EHEM: *Schistosoma mansoni:* Demonstration of the circulating antigens in infected hamsters. *Exp Parasitol* 40:189–197, 1976

42. NASH TE, PRESCOTT B, NEVA FA: The characteristics of the circulating antigen in schistosomiasis. *J Immunol* 112:1500–1507, 1974

43. NASH TE: Localization of the circulating antigen within the gut of *Schistosoma mansoni. Am J Trop Med Hyg* 23:1085–1087, 1974

44. PETERS DK, LACHMANN PJ: Immunity deficiency in pathogenesis of glomerulonephritis. *Lancet* 1:58–61, 1974

45. SMYTHE PM, BRETON-STILES GG, GRACE HJ, MAYFYOANE A, SCHONLAND M, COOVADIA HM, LOEWING WEK, PARENT MA, VOS GH: Thymolymphatic deficiency and depression of cell mediated immunity in protein-calorie malnutrition. *Lancet* 2:939–943, 1971

46. CHANDRA RK: Immunocompetence in undernutrition. *Pediatrics* 81:1194–1200, 1972

47. PASSWELL JH, STEWARD MW, SOOTHILL JF: The effects of protein malnutrition on macrophage function and the amount and affinity of antibody response. *Clin Exp Immunol* 17:491–495, 1974

48. CLAYTON CE: Immunosuppression in trypanosomiasis and malaria, in *The Role of the Spleen in the Immunology of Parasitic Disease* (Tropical Research Series 1), Basel, Scwabe and Co AG, 1979, pp 97–115

49. TURNER MW, VOLLER A: Studies on immunoglobulins of Nigerians: 1. The immunoglobulin levels of a Nigerian population. *J Trop Med Hyg* 69:99–103, 1961

50. GREENWOOD BM: Autoimmune disease and parasitic infections in Nigerians. *Lancet* 2:380–382, 1968

51. STERZEL RB, KRAUSE PH, KREGELER M: Experimental changes in the mesangial capacity to handle glomerular immune deposits in rats. *Contr Nephrol* 2:66–75, 1976

Renal Involvement in Leptospirosis

Visith Sitprija

Leptospirosis is an infectious disease caused by leptospires. *Leptospira interrogans* is the only species, but it is divided into two complexes. The interrogans complex is pathogenic, whereas the biflexa complex is saprophytic. Although the disease of leptospirosis is predominantly tropical, it is in fact worldwide. It is common in Thailand because of the tropical climate, the heavy rainfall, and the geographical low land. Various serotypes have been recovered, but bataviae predominates, especially in Bangkok, the capital city. The organisms enter a host through an abrasion in the skin or mucosa. Penetration through the intact skin is unlikely, although it is possible that prolonged exposure to contaminated water may provide an opportunity for invasion. Rodents, especially rats, are the most important reservoir.

Leptospirosis is characterized by a sudden onset of fever, with chills, headache, conjunctivitis, muscular pains, and jaundice. In the less severe form, jaundice is absent, and the disease can be subclinical [1]. The kidney is usually involved. Leptospirosis is a common cause of acute renal failure in the tropics. In one report, leptospiral renal failure accounted for nearly 40% of tropical acute renal failure [2]. Weil's syndrome represents leptospirosis, with renal failure and jaundice indicating severe infection. Myocarditis, the hemolytic uremic syndrome, and acute respiratory failure may occur rarely.

This review of renal involvement in leptospirosis is based on a long-term experience with the disease in Thailand. It is intended to cover the clinical aspects and pathophysiology of the disease.

Clinical Renal Manifestations

Urinary Abnormalities

Renal symptoms may not be apparent, especially in the mild form of the disease. In most patients, urinalysis reveals cellular elements during the septi-

This manuscript was presented as part of a Symposium on *Tropical Nephrology*.

cemic phase. Abnormal urinary findings are noted in 70 to 80% of patients. Microscopic hematuria and leukocyturia are common. Granular casts are noted frequently; bile pigmented casts and hemoglobin casts may be found. Mild proteinuria is often present and myoglobinuria may be observed. Leptospires can be detected in the urinary sediment by dark field microscopy. Urinary abnormalities disappear with recovery, but leptospiruria may continue for as long as 4 weeks.

Renal Failure

Acute renal failure occurs in 44 to 67% of patients [3, 4]. Renal failure may appear as early as 3 to 4 days after the onset of the disease. Certain characteristics deserve mentioning. Renal failure is usually catabolic in nature, with a rapid rise of blood urea nitrogen giving a high blood urea nitrogen and serum creatinine ratio. Hyperkalemia, hyperuricemia, hyperphosphatemia, and hyperbilirubinemia may be present. It is of note that alterations of renal function may be profound and out of proportion to the renal histologic changes. Para-aminohippurate clearance may be decreased despite normal glomerular filtration, a finding suggestive of proximal tubular dysfunction [5].

Relevant to the renal manifestations is the presence of intravascular hemolysis and coagulation. Serum C3 is variable but often decreased during the acute phase of the disease. The plasma fibrinogen concentration and the erythrocyte sedimentation rate are increased. Thrombocytopenia is a well-known complication of leptospirosis, and renal failure was observed in 72% of thrombocytopenic patients in one series [6].

Anicteric Renal Failure

Renal failure in leptospirosis need not be associated with jaundice. Anicteric renal failure often represents a mild form of renal dysfunction. Nonoliguric acute renal failure is not uncommon, although oliguric renal failure may be present in certain patients.

Renal failure in this group may also be prerenal [7], and in this respect urinalysis and urinary indexes are helpful in establishing the diagnosis. Impaired renal function is mild and readily resolves following fluid therapy.

Anicteric renal failure constitutes the majority of acute renal failure cases in leptospirosis.

Icteric Renal Failure

Icteric renal failure is usually described as Weil's syndrome. Previously the syndrome was believed to be specific for icterohemorrhagiae infection. It is no longer type-specific and can be seen in any severe infection. Vascular collapse, hemorrhage, and alteration of consciousness may be observed. Jaundice is usually cholestatic in type, with high serum alkaline phosphatase out of proportion to the rise of transaminases. Jaundice can even be more severe in the patient with hemolysis owing to G-6-PD deficiency. Renal failure is often severe and more catabolic than it is in the anicteric group, and it is not surprising to find striking hyperuricemia and hyperphosphatemia in this group. Of interest is the high urine uric acid and urine creatinine ratio over unity in patients with severe jaundice [8]. Although occasional patients may be severely oliguric or anuric, most patients are nonoliguric. When associated with hyperbilirubinemia with a total bilirubin of over 25 mg/dl, renal failure can be severe and sometimes may be accompanied by severe oliguria or even anuria [9].

Hemolytic Uremic Syndrome

The syndrome is observed rarely. It is characterized by the presence of disseminated intravascular coagulation, thrombocytopenia, bizarre erythrocytes, reticulocytosis, hemolysis, and renal failure. The possible causes are multiple, including immune mechanisms, endotoxemia, prostacycline deficiency, vascular injury, and alteration of red cell membrane [10]. There is no evidence that an immune mechanism plays a role in the pathogenesis of renal lesions in human leptospirosis [11]. Theoretically, the occurrence of hemolytic uremic syndrome in leptospirosis is plausible because of vascular and membrane injuries caused by leptospires [12, 13]. Endothelial swelling and vacuolation followed by necrosis have been shown in leptospirosis. Platelet aggregation has been noted. In our experience, the syndrome is less severe, and spontaneous recovery follows only conventional treatment. Residual renal damage has been observed.

Treatment

Treatment of renal failure in leptospirosis does not differ from that for acute renal failure attributable to other causes. Of great importance is the specific treatment of infection. Antibiotics should be given during the febrile period or within 4 to 7 days after the onset of the disease when the patients are septicemic. Penicillin, streptomycin, and tetracycline are among the antibiotics known to kill leptospires. Penicillin is preferred since the others are nephrotoxic. Parenteral aqueous penicillin G at a dosage of 1,000,000 units at 6-hour intervals for a period of one week is recommended in adult patients. Erythromycin can be used in the patient who is allergic to penicillin.

Maintenance of the patient's state of hydration is important since renal failure may be prerenal. Good urine flow may follow fluid administration. In parenchymal renal failure, dialysis, when indicated, should be performed frequently because of hypercatabolism. A high dose of furosemide or bumetanide may be helpful in converting oliguric to nonoliguric renal failure, which is easier for the clinical management. The clinical course of renal failure, however, is unchanged [14]. A high urine flow is desirable, especially

in the presence of a high urine uric acid to creatinine ratio. In hyperbilirubinemia (total bilirubin, over 25 mg/dl), exchange blood transfusion has been
useful in decreasing the degree of jaundice and improving the renal function
[9, 15, 16].

On a theoretical basis, heparinization, plasmapheresis, fresh plasma transfusion, and prostaglandin I_2 (PGI_2) administration are of value in the management of the hemolytic uremic syndrome. However, in my experience, conservative treatment is sufficient when the syndrome is mild in degree.

With the use of dialysis and the present understanding of pathophysiology
of the disease, the prognosis of leptospirosis, in general, is good except when
complicated with myocarditis or acute respiratory distress syndrome. The
mortality is reduced to almost negligible.

Renal Pathologic Changes

All structures of the kidney are involved in leptospirosis. Tubulointerstitial
changes are important and account for renal failure. Glomerular and vascular
changes are usually mild and do not interfere with renal function. These
changes are reversible and do not run a chronic course.

Leptospires in the Lesions

Leptospires can be seen in the renal lesions by Levaditi's stain. Since renal
biopsy is usually performed late in the course of the disease because of bleeding
tendency, it is therefore difficult to demonstrate the organisms in the lesions.
In hamsters, the organisms are demonstrated in the glomeruli and interstitium
a few hours after inoculation. After 9 hours, they are found in increased
number in the interstitium and proximal tubules. The organisms are detectable
in the antigen form 5 days following inoculation. The antigen is initially
seen in the interstitium and is later found in increasing amount in proximal
and distal tubular cells over a period of 2 to 3 weeks [11].

Glomerular Changes

Glomerular lesions are usually mild. Mild mesangial hypertrophy or proliferation, or both, are observed. The changes are similar to those seen in the
other infectious diseases [17–19]. Early in the course of the disease, polymorphonuclear cells may be present in the glomeruli, but this is a transient
phenomenon [11].

By electron microscopy, focal fusion of foot process and focal thickening
of the basement membrane may be noted. Prominent Golgi complexes and
dilated endoplasmic reticulum are seen in the cytoplasm of visceral epithelial
cells. Pseudovilli, which represent the long slender projections of the visceral

epithelial cells into the urinary space, are noted [20]. Fibrin deposition in the paramesangial area is observed occasionally.

Deposition of C3 in the mesangial areas and in the capillary loop is noted by immunofluorescence. IgM deposition in the mesangial region is seen in occasional cases [11, 21], but in most cases immunoglobulins are not demonstrable.

Vascular Lesions

Hemorrhage is common in leptospirosis because of the bacterial toxin-induced increased fragility of the capillary walls. Yet, vascular changes in the kidney are usually not noticeable by light microscopy. Only C3 deposition without immunoglobulins is seen in the glomerular afferent arterioles. The significance of this finding is not clear. It might represent trapping of C3 at the site of injury in the blood vessels. This finding is also shared by other infectious diseases [17, 19].

Nonspecific swelling and vacuolation of the endothelial cells are seen by electron microscopy. The endoplasmic reticulum is dilated and the mitochondria are enlarged. Endothelial necrosis is demonstrable in the peritubular capillaries, allowing the escape of erythrocytes. Platelet aggregation is also noted. These changes are mostly in the corticomedullary area [12, 22]. Vascular lesions are believed to be due to cytotoxin.

Tubular Lesions

Tubular changes are minimal in the absence of renal failure. Cloudy swelling of the tubular cells may be seen. An experimental study in guinea pigs without renal insufficiency has shown edema of proximal tubular cells with dilatation of endoplasmic reticulum [22]. Mitochondria and the brush border are intact.

In renal failure, tubular degeneration and necrosis are seen in both proximal and distal convoluted tubules. Proximal tubules are affected first. Distal tubules are involved with progression of the disease. The basement membrane may be disrupted. These changes may be focal. Bile and heme casts are often demonstrable in the tubular lumen in jaundiced patients. Increased mitoses may be noted in the tubular epithelial cells. By histochemic technique, impairment of tubular enzyme activities such as alkaline phosphatase, glutamic, isocitric, lactic, malic, and glucose 6-phosphate dehydrogenases may precede the pathologic changes [23]. By electron microscopy, an increased number of cytosomes and an active system of apical vesicles and vacuoles are observed. Focal dilatation of intercellular space is noticeable.

Interstitial Changes

Interstitial changes form the basic renal lesion in leptospirosis [20]. They are observed even in the mild case of leptospirosis without renal failure.

Interstitial edema and cellular infiltration are noted. Cellular infiltration may be diffuse or may be focal around the glomeruli and venules. The infiltrates are mainly mononuclear cells, with few eosinophils. Polymorphonuclear cells are present during the early stage of the disease. There may be interstitial hemorrhage. Complements and immunoglobulins are not detectable in the interstitium [11]. In contrast, immune complex deposition has been demonstrated in canine leptospirosis [24]. Although interstitial changes may be considered as a secondary phenomenon to acute tubular necrosis, in my experience (mostly with bataviae serotype) interstitial changes are noted even before tubular necrosis. This is true both in man and hamsters. In this respect, leptospirosis is one of the bacterial models of interstitial nephritis.

Pathogenesis

Several clinical features of leptospirosis suggest toxemia as the cause of manifestation. As in many infectious diseases, renal failure can occur in severe infection. Renal damage is believed by many investigators to be attributed to renal ischemia, which results in focal distribution of renal lesions. Differing from the other diseases, this disease requires the presence of leptospires for the renal lesion to develop. Three mechanisms have been proposed to explain the pathogenesis of renal lesions [11].

Nonspecific Effects of Infection

Several nonspecific factors related to infection can compromise renal function, either by their direct effects or by hemodynamic alterations that lead to decreased renal blood flow.

Hypovolemia

Blood volume determination is infectious diseases has given varying results. Hypervolemia may be observed in less severe infection. This has been attributed to the effect of antidiuretic hormone and a shift of water from cells. However, in severe infection, especially in the patient who does not receive intravenous fluid, hypovolemia has been observed. Hypovolemia has been shown in both leptospirosis [11] and malaria [25]. Several factors including an increased fluid loss from fever, increased sweating, diarrhea, decreased fluid and salt intake, and increased vascular permeability can lead to hypovolemia. Increased vascular permeability is often seen in inflammation, and is brought about by a number of chemical mediators released during the process of inflammation. These mediators include kinins, prostaglandins, serotonin, and histamine [26]. Increased plasma kinin activity and histamine have been reported in infectious diseases [27–29]. Fibrinopeptides, fibrin degradation products, and catecholamines can also increase vascular permeability. In leptospirosis, cytotoxin, which is present in the circulation during the early stage of the disease, has an injurious effect on the vascular endothelium, thus increasing vascular permeability [30, 31].

Blood Hyperviscosity

Increased blood viscosity is commonly observed in infectious diseases. The rise in plasma fibrinogen is a normal response to acute infection and can account for the increase in blood viscosity [32]. Plasma viscosity is markedly increased in leptospirosis [11]. The erythrocyte sedimentation rate is also increased in the disease [33]. In addition to the rise in plasma fibrinogen, hypovolemia and hemoconcentration secondary to increased vascular permeability and fluid loss further contribute to blood hyperviscosity. Because of the inverse relationship between laminar blood flow and blood viscosity, blood hyperviscosity would decrease renal blood flow unless there is compensatory vasodilatation.

Catecholamine Effects

Catecholamine release is often noted in severe infectious diseases. In septicemia and malaria, this has been well documented [34] in response to hypovolemia and kinin stimulation [35]. Blood flow to the kidney is therefore compromised. The renin-angiotensin system can be activated. Catecholamines can also increase vascular permeability, allowing leakage from the intravascular compartment [36]. Although catecholamine metabolism has not yet been studied in leptospirosis, an increase in its release is a possibility.

Intravascular Coagulation

Intravascular coagulation can occur in leptospirosis because of hyperfibrinogenemia, hemoconcentration, and vascular injury. Increased serum fibrin degradation products [11] and decreased platelets [6] have been documented. However, in most cases, intravascular coagulation is of low grade and local [11]. Unless disseminated intravascular coagulation or hemolytic uremic syndrome occurs, which is uncommon, in ordinary cases of leptospirosis, renal blood flow is unlikely to be compromised by this low grade intravascular coagulation.

Intravascular Hemolysis

In leptospirosis, there is usually mild intravascular hemolysis because of bacterial hemolysin [37]. Hemolytic anemia may also result from membrane injury [13]. Severe intravascular hemolysis is seldom; yet, it may be observed in the patient with G-6-PD (glucose-6-phosphate dehydrogenase) deficiency or in disseminated intravascular coagulation. Intravascular hemolysis of mild degree in leptospirosis would not ordinarily alter renal blood flow unless there is severe intravascular hemolysis.

Jaundice

Jaundice may or not be present in leptospirosis. The presence of jaundice indicates severe infection. Mild jaundice does not affect renal function, but in severe jaundice renal function can be easily compromised. The association between severe jaundice and renal failure in surgery is well recognized [38]. The mechanism is not clearly understood. Unconjugated bilirubin [39], conjugated bilirubin [40], bile acids [41] and endotoxin [42] have been implicated. Natriuresis has been shown in the patient with hyperbilirubinemia [43]. The ability of the kidney to conserve sodium is diminished in the patient with severe jaundice resulting in hyponatremia. A high concentration of unconjugated bilirubin in the renal medulla [39] might interefere with sodium chloride reabsorption in the ascending limb of Henle's loop. Furthermore, jaundice has been shown to increase vascular response to catecholamine [44] and increase plasma renin activity [45], causing renal vasoconstriction.

In addition, jaundice has an effect on uric acid excretion. There is uricosuria [46], resulting in an increased urine uric acid to urine creatinine ratio over unity [8]. With oliguria and acid urine, this might further compromise renal function. Fortunately, in most jaundiced cases the patient is nonoliguric.

In support for the adverse effects of jaundice on renal function, exchange blood transfusion decreases jaundice and improves renal function [9, 15, 16].

All the above factors are nonspecific for leptospirosis and are shared by many infectious diseases. They can produce renal ischemia and renal failure. Thus, any severe infection is capable of causing acute renal failure through these multiple factors. Hyperpyrexia [47], myoglobin released from inflamed muscles [48], and decreased renal blood flow from carditis [1] could further enhance tubular injury in leptospirosis.

Immunologic Mechanisms

Nephropathy in canine leptospirosis has been shown to be immune mediated. The evidence for this is lacking in man. Immune complex deposition is not demonstrable in the kidney lesions. Only C3 is seen in the glomerular afferent aterioles and occasionally in the glomeruli. There may be faint deposition of IgM in the mesangial region which is rather nonspecific [11, 21]. Circulating immune complexes have been detected in a few instances, and must be interpreted with caution and again may be nonspecific. Experimental leptospirosis in hamsters also failed to show immunologic evidence [11].

Interstitial nephritis with mononuclear cell infiltration would favor cell-mediated immune response as a mechanism of the lesion. However, no deposition of immune complexes in the lesion is demonstrated both in man and hamsters [11]. On the contrary, immune complex deposition is evident in canine leptospirosis [24]. There are no data concerning the onset of renal interstitial changes in man. In hamsters these changes occur within 3 hours after an intraperitoneal inoculation of leptospires. The onset appears to be too short for the delayed type of hypersensitivity. The difference in findings in various models could reflect the difference in immune response and the clinical course of the disease in different hosts. In canine leptospirosis, the disease may run a chronic course leading to chronic renal failure [49]. Although autoimmune response to the epithelial antigens released by degenerated tubules could lead to chronic renal disease, antikidney antibodies cannot be detected in the chronic stage of renal lesions [50]. Chronic renal disease in man because of leptospirosis has not been observed, although residual renal damage may occasionally occur when the disease is severe. It is therefore unlikely that immunologic mechanisms are involved in the pathogenesis of renal lesions in man.

Direct Nephrotoxicity

Experiments in hamsters have shown that renal lesions are associated with the presence of leptospires. Glomerular changes occur a few hours after inoculation [11]. This is followed by interstitial changes, whch become more marked at the later stage. Tubular degeneration occurs at the 6th hour. Glomerular changes, interstitial lesion, and tubular necrosis occur with the presence of leptospires or leptospire antigen in the lesion. It is interpreted that leptospires enter the kidney by blood stream, causing initially a glomerular injury that is benign and transient. The organisms then circulate to the peritubular capillaries and penetrate into the interstitium and later to the tubules, causing interstitial nephritis and tubular necrosis. Proximal tubules are primarily involved, whereas distal tubules are affected later. The organisms are then eliminated in the urine with recovery of the lesions. Cellular reaction in the interstitium is a response to bacterial invasion. Cellular infiltrates are primarily polymorphonuclear cells but later are mononuclear cells. These mononuclear cells are essential for phagocytosis [51].

However, it is unclear whether the lesions are caused by leptospire invasion itself or whether they are due to factors related to bacterial virulence, such as toxins and enzymes, or to metabolites. Both are likely implicated. In animal experiments pathologic changes were caused only by viable leptospires [52]. Injection of killed organisms failed to cause the renal lesion. Attempts to demonstrate the presence of endotoxin have not met with success except in some serotype [53]. The role of endotoxin of intestinal bacteria had been considered, but was later excluded. Infection of germ-free guinea pigs with serotype icterohaemorrhagiae produced the lesions similar to those observed in control animals [54]. Vascular changes have been attributed to cytotoxic substance from leptospires or from leptospire and host interaction [30, 31]. Although vascular damage is not evident in light microscopy, C3 deposition in the glomeruli and afferent arterioles would suggest complement activation, perhaps through the alternative pathway with trapping of C3 by the injured blood vessels.

Clinical and experimental evidence therefore suggests that renal lesions and renal dysfunction in leptospirosis are caused by both nonspecific effects of infection and direct nephrotoxicity. Tubular necrosis with acute renal failure is both toxic and ischemic in origin. Interstitial nephritis is caused by bacterial invasion. The broad spectrum of renal lesions with some discrepancy among the pathology reports could reflect the predominance of factors involved, the difference in host response, and the time of study.

References

1. SITPRIJA V: Leptospirosis, in *Oxford Textbook of Medicine,* edited by WEATHER-ALL DJ, LEDINGHAM JGG, WARRELL DA, Oxford, Oxford University Press, 1983, vol 1, pp 5.297–5.300
2. SITPRIJA V, BENYAJATI C: Tropical diseases and acute renal failure. *Ann Acad Med (Suppl)* 4:112–114, 1975
3. SUNDHARAGIATI B: Leptospirosis in man and animal in Thailand. *Report to the National Research Council of Thailand,* 1967, p 6
4. CHAROONRUANGRIT S, BOONPUCKNAVIG S: Leptospirosis at Chulalongkorn Hospital: A report of 54 cases. *J Med Assoc Thai* 47:653–659, 1964
5. AREAN VM: Studies on the pathogenesis of leptospirosis: II. A clinicopathologic evaluation of hepatic and renal function in experimental leptospiral infections. *Lab Invest* 11:273–288, 1962
6. EDWARDS CN, NICHOLSON GD, EVERARD COR: Thrombocytopenia in leptospirosis. *Am J Trop Med Hyg* 31:827–829, 1982
7. SITPRIJA V: Renal involvement in human leptospirosis. *Br Med J* 2:656–658, 1968
8. TUNGSANGA K, BOONWICHIT D, LEKHAKULA A, SITPRIJA V: Urine uric acid and urine creatinine ratio in acute renal failure. *Arch Intern Med,* in press
9. SITPRIJA V, CHUSILP S: Renal failure and hyperbilirubinaemia in leptospirosis: Treatment with exchange transfusion. *Med J Aust* 1:171–172, 1973
10. MOREL-MAROGER L: Adult hemolytic-uremic syndrome. *Kidney Int* 18:125–134, 1980
11. SITPRIJA V, PIPATANAGUL V, MERTOWIDJOJO K, BOONPUCKNAVIG V, BOONPUCKNAVIG S: Pathogenesis of renal disease in leptospirosis: Clinical and experimental studies. *Kidney Int* 17:827–836, 1980
12. DE BRITO T, BÖHM GM, YASUDA PH: Vascular damage in acute experimental leptospirosis of the guinea-pig. *J Pathol* 128:177–182, 1979
13. TROWBRIDGE AA, GREEN JB, BONNETT JD, CHOHET SB, PONNAPPA BD, McCOMBS WB: Hemolytic anemia associated with leptospirosis: Morpholigic and lipid studies. *Am J Clin Pathol* 76:493–498, 1981
14. BORIRAKCHANYAVAT V, VONGSTHONGSRI M, SITPRIJA V: Furosemide and acute renal failure. *Postgrad Med J* 54:30–32, 1978
15. POCHANUGOOL C, SITPRIJA V: Hyperbilirubinemic renal failure in tropical disease: Treatment with exchange transfusion. *J Med Assoc Thai* 61 (Suppl):75–77, 1978
16. PECCHINI F, BORGHI M, BODINI U, COPERCINI B, GRUTTA D'AURIA C, ROMANINI GL, ROMANO C: Acute renal failure from leptospirosis: New trend of treatment. *Clin Nephrol* 18:164, 1982
17. SITPRIJA V, BOONPUCKNAVIG V: Malarial nephropathy in Thailand. *Proc 1st Asian-Pacific Congress of Nephrology, Tokyo, 1979,* pp 126–130

18. SITPRIJA V, PIPATANAGUL V, BOONPUCKNAVIG V, BOONPUCKNAVIG S: Glomerulitis in typhoid fever. *Ann Intern Med* 81:210–213, 1974

19. SITPRIJA V, KEOPLUNG M, BOONPUCKNAVIG V, BOONPUCKNAVIG S: Renal involvement in human trichinoisis. *Arch Intern Med* 140:544–545, 1980

20. SITPRIJA V, EVANS H: The kidney in human leptospirosis. *Am J Med* 49:780–788, 1970

21. LAI KN, AARONS I, WOODROFFE AJ, CLARKSON AR: Renal lesions in leptospirosis. *Aust NZ J Med* 12:276–279, 1982

22. DAVILA DE ARRIAGA AJ, ROCHA AS, YASUDA PH, DE BRITO T: Morphofunctional patterns of kidney injury in the experimental leptospirosis of the guineapig (L. icterohaemorrhagiae). *J Pathol* 138:145–161, 1982

23. AREAN VM, HENRY JB: Studies on the pathogenesis of leptospirosis: IV. The behaviors of transaminases and oxidative enzymes in experimental leptospirosis; a histochemical and biochemical assay. *Am J Trop Med Hyg* 13:430–442, 1964

24. MORRISON WJ, WRIGHT NG: Canine leptospirosis: An immunopathological study of interstitial nephritis due to leptospira canicola. *J Pathol* 120:83–89, 1976

25. SITPRIJA V, VONGSTHONGSRI M, POCHYACHINDA V, ARTHACHINTA S: Renal failure in malaria: A pathophysiologic study. *Nephron* 18:277–287, 1977

26. GRAEME RB, MAJNO G: Acute inflammation: A review. *Am J Pathol* 86:185–276, 1977

27. STUCHLY Z, FAL W: The level of kinins in the blood plasma in the course of experimental trichinosis in white rat. *Wiad Parazytol* 15:698–699, 1969

28. TELLA A, MAEGRAITH BG: Studies on bradykinin and bradykininogen in malaria. *Ann Trop Med Parasitol* 60:304–317, 1966

29. SRICHAIKUL T, ARCHARARIT N, SIRIASWAKUL T, VIRIYAPANICH T: Histamine changes in Plasmodium falciparum infection. *Trans R Soc Trop Med Hyg* 70:36–38, 1976

30. KNIGHT LL, MILLER NG, WHITE RJ: Cytotoxic factor in the blood and plasma of animals during leptospirosis. *Infect Immun* 8:401–405, 1973

31. MILLER NG, ALLEN JE, WILSON RB: The pathogenesis of hemorrhage in the lung of the hamster during acute leptospirosis. *Med Microbial Immunol* 160:269–278, 1974

32. CARR WP: Acute-phase proteins. *Clin Rheum Dis* 9:227–239, 1983

33. CHEAH JS, RANSOME GA: The erythrocyte sedimentation rate in leptospirosis. *Med J Aust* 1:1233–1234, 1971

34. SKIRROW MB, CHONGSUPHAJAISIDDHI T, MAEGRAITH BG: The circulation in malaria: II. Portal angiography in monkeys (Macaca Mulatta) infected with Plasmodium knowlesi and in shock following manipulation of the gut. *Ann Trop Med Parasitol* 58:502–510, 1964

35. FELDBERG W, LEWIS GP: Action of peptides on adrenal medulla: Release of adrenalin by bradykinin and angiotensin. *J Physiol (London)* 171:98–108, 1964

36. ROSELL S: Neural control of microvessels. *Ann Rev Physiol* 42:359–371, 1980

37. FEIGIN RD, ANDERSON DC: Human leptospirosis. *CRC Crit Rev Clin Lab Sci* 5:413–467, 1975

38. BETTER OS: Acute renal failure complicating obstructive jaundice, in *Acute Renal Failure,* edited by BRENNER BM, STEIN JH, New York, Churchill Livingstone, 1980, pp 108–122

39. ODELL GB, NATZSCHKA JC, STOREY GNB: Bilirubin nephropathy in the Gunn strain of rat. *Am J Physiol* 212:931–938, 1967

40. BAUM M, STERLING GA, DAWSON JL: Further study into obstructive jaundice and ischaemic renal damage. *Br Med J* 2:229–231, 1969

41. AOYAGI T, LOWENSTEIN LM: The effect of bile acids and renal ischemia on renal function. *J Lab Clin Med* 71:686–692, 1968
42. BAILEY ME: Endotoxin, bile salts and renal function in obstructive jaundice. *Br J Surg* 63:774–778, 1976
43. SITPRIJA V: Renal failure in obstructive jaundice: A pathophysiologic consideration. *J Med Assoc Thai* 62 (Suppl 3):46–49, 1978
44. BLOOM D, McCALDEN TA, ROSENDORFF C: Effect of jaundiced plasma on vascular sensitivity to noradrenalin. *Kidney Int* 8:149–157, 1975
45. MELMAN A, WEINBERGER MH: Alterations of renin-angiotensin system in bile duct ligated dogs on varied sodium diet. *Clin Res* 24:407, 1976
46. MICHELIS MF, WARMS PC, FUSCO RD, DAVIS BB: Hypouricemia and hyperuricosuria in Laennec cirrhosis. *Arch Intern Med* 134:681–683, 1974
47. ELKON D, FECHNER RE, HOMZIE M, BAKER DG, CONSTABLE WC: Response of mouse kidney to hyperthermia: Pathology and temperature-dependence of injury. *Arch Pathol Lab Med* 104:153–158, 1980
48. KAHN JB: A case of Weil's disease requiring steroid therapy for thrombocytopenia and bleeding. *Am J Trop Med Hyg* 31:1213–1215, 1982
49. TAYLOR PL, HANSON LE, SIMON J: Serologic, pathologic and immunologic features of experimentally induced leptospiral nephritis in dogs. *Am J Vet Res* 31:1033–1049, 1970
50. KROHN K, MERO M, OKSANEN A, SANDHOLM M: Immunological observations in canine interstitial nephritis. *Am J Pathol* 65:157–172, 1971
51. BANFI E, CINCO M, BELLINI M, SORANZO MR: The role of antibodies and serum complement in the interaction between macrophages and leptospires. *J Gen Microbiol* 128:813–816, 1982
52. AREAN VM, SARASIN G, GREEN JH: The pathogenesis of leptospirosis: Toxin production by Leptospira icterohaemorrhagiae. *Am J Vet Res* 24:836–843, 1964
53. FINCO DR, LOW DG: Endotoxin properties of Leptospira canicola. *Am J Vet Res* 128:1863–1872, 1967
54. HIGGINS R, DESCÔTEAUX JP, DEGRÉ R: Pathogenesis of experimental leptospira interrogans serotype icterohaemorrhagiae infection in the guinea pig: Possible role of endotoxin of intestinal bacteria in the development of lesions. *Can J Comp Med* 44:304–308, 1980

Diabetes Mellitus and the Kidney

Clinical and Renal Functional Studies of Diabetic Nephropathy in Humans

Carl Erik Mogensen

Renal disease that is primarily located in the glomerulus and is found after many years of metabolic aberrations in diabetes is now one of the main causes of end-stage renal failure in Europe and North America. Insulin-dependent as well as noninsulin-dependent patients are at risk of developing diabetic nephropathy; however, the course often is more dramatic in young patients, and progression of the disease probably is more rapid than in type II diabetic patients [1–3]. In principle, nephropathy in these two types of patients is not very different, but severity of diabetes, age, and hemodynamic alterations may considerably modify the course and make development different in the two types of diabetes mellitus. Also, in the elderly noninsulin-dependent patient, cardiovascular disease often determines the fate of the patient before the development of the uremic phase [4]. These have been serious problems for many years, because diabetic patients live longer due to insulin treatment; however, the realities of the situation have become more and more apparent in recent years. Diabetic patients are being increasingly accepted for end-stage renal failure treatment [5].

As many as 40 to 45% of insulin-dependent diabetic patients treated with insulin, diet, and general measures develop (after a variable span of years) the characteristic pattern of proteinuria, increasing blood pressure, and subsequent fall in kidney function ending with uremia—which for many years was believed to be the last event. [1, 3, 6]. The risk of developing nephropathy may be lower at present due to the fact that a more intensive treatment of diabetes mellitus has been the rule over the last 1 or 2 decades.

The number of diabetic patients that are accepted for dialysis and for transplantation has increased considerably during the late 1970s and early 1980s; however, it is still likely that in many countries, a sizable number of patients neither has been offered nor has been accepted for these programs due to capacity problems [7].

This manuscript was presented as part of a Symposium on *Diabetic Nephropathy: Concepts of Pathogenesis and Treatment.*

These are the late events in the drama that seem to begin with the diagnosis of diabetes mellitus. In fact, changes in the diabetic kidney occur very early in the course of disease; abnormalities are present even at the time of clinical diagnosis, where marked changes in the structure and function of the kidney have been documented [8, 9]. Diagnostic and prognostic methods, as well as therapy, have improved considerably during the last few years. It is now possible to predict overt nephropathy early in the course of disease in both the insulin-dependent [10–12] and noninsulin-dependent patient [4], giving rise to the concept of *incipient diabetic nephropathy* [13–16]. At the same time, early therapy is possible, especially with respect to early antihypertensive treatment; in the future, earlier therapy may also be possible with the increasingly widespread use of insulin pumps or other intensified insulin treatment modalities. However, the effectiveness of such therapeutic measures with respect to prevention of diabetic nephropathy remains to be documented.

Both types of diabetes mellitus will be discussed in this survey, with emphasis on the role of so-called persistent "microalbuminuria" in predicting renal disease as well as early mortality.

Methods

Kidney Function Tests

In research on diabetic renal disease, very exact methods for the evaluation of kidney function are required [8]. These include classic methods, such as measurement of glomerular filtration rate (GFR) and renal plasma flow (RPF) that were developed by Homer Smith, as well as newly developed methods of measuring excretion rates of plasma proteins. ^{51}Cr-EDTA-clearance as a single-shot method that does not depend on urine collections has been used in many studies; however, exact measurement of renal function can only be done by employing a constant infusion technique with urine collection by using inulin or ^{125}I-iothalamate as test substances. Renal plasma flow is measured by a constant infusion technique that uses ^{131}I-hippuran/or para-aminohippurate (PAH) as marker [8]. Measurement of the excretion rates of albumin and beta-2-microglobulin has been used extensively over the last decade since the development of radioimmunoassay and other sensitive methods [17, 18]. It has been shown that urinary albumin excretion (UAE) is a key parameter in the evaluation of early renal involvement in diabetes [14]. Precision collections of urine with patients at rest is essential. Serum creatinine and creatinine clearance (C_{cr}) values also can be used in the evaluation of kidney function in diabetic patients, but these methods do not provide any exact assessment of renal function [19–21].

Measurement of Progression

Using the methods indicated previously, it has been shown that progression of renal disease in diabetes mellitus is a rather well-defined process in the individual patient who has proteinuria or persistent microalbuminuria. The rate of reduction in GFR, which is expressed in ml/min/mo, is a very useful parameter. The reduction-rate approaches linearity in most patients. In this way, the natural history—and more importantly the effect of new treatment modalities—can be evaluated [21–23].

In the early phase of renal disease (incipient diabetic nephropathy), GFR is well preserved and even supranormal. The progression rate must be evaluated by measuring the increased rate of UAE expressed as μg/min/yr or percentage increase per year, or possibly as decline in GFR, from the supranormal level [14].

Provocation Tests

A provocation test utilizing increases in protein excretion might be useful in the early evaluation of predicting renal disease in diabetes; that is, before baseline values are abnormal [17, 18]. It is possible that the well-known stimulatory effect of physical exercise on proteinuria can be used, thus pinpointing patients prone to diabetic renal disease very early in its course, for example, diabetic children or teenagers [24]. However, this remains to be established. Other provocative tests may be developed in the future, with a perspective of early prognostic evaluation and early intervention. Of course, such minor abnormalities are likely to depend much more on both acute and long-term elevations of the blood glucose level and associated abnormalities.

Stages of Renal Involvement in Diabetes

Systematic studies over the last decade using the methods indicated above have allowed definition of a number of stages in the development of renal function changes in diabetes (Table 1). The following stages can be described in the development of insulin-dependent patients, but the classification may also (at least partly) be used in noninsulin-dependent patients.

1. *The early hyperfunction-hypertrophy stage with nephromegaly.* These abnormalities are found at the time of clinical diagnosis of diabetes. Hypertrophy and hyperfunction may only exist in insulin-dependent patients; however, microalbuminuria, which is also related to poor metabolic control, is found in both types of diabetes.
2. *The silent stage with development of renal lesions*—without clinical and laboratory signs of renal disease. Urinary albumin excretion is within normal limits.
3. *The incipient diabetic nephropathy.* This important stage is characterized by persisting elevation of UAE despite good metabolic control, but without clinical proteinuria. The increase rate in UAE is slow, from normal values up to the level of clinical proteinuria. It is the forerunner of the well-known overt nephropathy [12].

Table 1. Stages in diabetic renal disease in insulin-dependent (type I) and noninsulin-dependent (type II) diabetes

Stage	Urinary albumin excretion (UAE)		Glomerular filtration rate (GFR)		Blood pressure	
	Insulin-dependent	Noninsulin-dependent	Insulin-dependent	Noninsulin-dependent	Insulin-dependent	Noninsulin-dependent
1 Changes at clinical diagnosis	Increased and rapidly reversible	Increased (and possibly reversible)	Increased by 30 to 40% (as is kidney size)	C_{cr} normal	Normal	Without obesity: normal
2 Renal lesions without clinical or laboratory sign of disease	Usually in the normal range. Increased at poor control and at exercise	Normal or slightly increased	Increased by 20 to 30% during ordinary control (as is kidney size)	C_{cr} normal	Normal. May increase at moderate ketosis	Without obesity: normal
3 Incipient nephropathy (or persistent microalbuminuria)	Increased, but not clinical proteinuria. Announces stage 4	Increased, but not clinical proteinuria. Announces stage 4	Still increased, but GFR starts to fall (when UAE > 70 $\mu g/min$)	Probably declining	Slightly increased (140/90 *mm Hg*) more pronounced at exercise	Unknown
4 Overt nephropathy with proteinuria	Without antihypertensive treatment: increasing	Less dramatic course	Fall rate ~ 1 *ml/min/mo*, reduced by 60% during antihypertensive treatment	Declining. Patients often die from nonrenal diabetic complications	Increased (~ 160/100), but readily reduced by "triple therapy"	Increased, but readily reduced by "triple therapy"

Abbreviations: UAE = urinary albumin excretion; C_{cr} = creatinine clearance

4. *Overt diabetic nephropathy.* This is characterized by proteinuria, an increase in blood pressure, and a fall in kidney function.
5. *The end-stage renal failure stage.* This is characterized by severely reduced kidney function. Dialysis or transplantation must be considered.

The majority of diabetic patients only go through the first two stages, which means that they never develop clinically important renal disease. There can be no question that marked structural changes are present in the kidney. It is an open question whether such patients, by unidentified mechanisms, are "protected" against renal disease or whether renal disease would develop in all if they live long enough [1, 25].

The remaining patients develop into stages 3 and 4. So far, it is not known why some patients develop increased proteinuria after 10 to 15 years of diabetes, whereas other patients after 30 or more years of diabetes preserve normal albumin excretion [25, 26]. Of course, sustained poor metabolic control must be suspected, but other factors probably also play a role, for example, genetic patterns, the degree of early involvement in kidney function, the level of blood pressure, and heavy smoking.

In the following discussion, the individual stages of renal involvement will be discussed in detail, both in insulin-dependent patients and in noninsulin-dependent patients in whom the picture is less clear. Renal data for insulin-dependent patients are given in Table 2.

Stage 1: Renal Hyperfunction-Hypertrophy

This entity was described in newly diagnosed insulin-dependent diabetic patients who did not exhibit dehydration or acidosis at clinical presentation. The GFR is increased by about 30 to 40% with concomitant increase in renal size. The RPF may be increased, but this is not the case in all studies [8, 9]. Clinical proteinuria is only present in the case of severe ketoacidosis. However, by using sensitive methods, the UAE rate is clearly increased (Table 2), which is an increase that is further aggravated during light-to-moderate physical exercise [27]. The abnormalities are clearly of glomerular origin, since beta-2-microglobulin excretion is normal, both at rest and at exercise. These abnormalities are at least partially reversible with strict insulin treatment.

Noninsulin-dependent patients have not been studied intensively, but recent studies that used C_{cr} suggest that GFR is not increased in newly diagnosed patients, as shown in the Fredericia survey study [28]. Renal size has not been assessed in these patients. However, UAE is increased at clinical presentation; also, when compared to a background population of the same age, sex, and living conditions [28].

When diabetic control is imperfect for several years in both insulin-dependent and noninsulin-dependent patients, elements of stage 1 will be found in the kidney function-structure pattern. Complete normalization of the metabolic state (for instance, by insulin pump) may be able to normalize these abnormalities completely.

Table 2. Renal function and blood pressure (BP) in the stages of renal involvement in diabetes

	C ($N = 18$)	D_I ($N = 12$) Before treatment	During treatment	D_{II} ($N = 23$)	D^f_{III} ($N - 15$)	D_{IV} ($N = 10$)
Age (yr)	28.6 ± 4.8	28.3 ± 4.6		27.6 ± 4.7	27.4 ± 4.9	31.0 ± 4.9
Duration (yr)	—	At clinical diagnosis	10 d	15.7 ± 4.9	14.9 ± 5.6	20.0 ± 4.3
Albumin excretion (μg/min)	$4.3 \times/\div 1.3$	$10.5^{\Phi} \times/\div 2.2^b$	$4.4 \times/\div 1.5^a$	$4.8 \times/\div 1.4$	$30.4 \times/\div 1.4^{d,e}$	$2705.1 \times/\div 2.6$
Systolic blood pressure (mm Hg)	115 ± 10	123 ± 7	108 ± 3	122 ± 6^c	$130 \pm 12^{d,e}(a)$	167 ± 19
Diastolic blood pressure (mm Hg)	73 ± 8	76 ± 11	73 ± 7	80 ± 7^c	$86 \pm 7^{d,e}$	109 ± 15
GFR (ml/min)	123 ± 12	151 ± 18^b	126 ± 15^a	$132 \pm 9^c(a)$	$149 \pm 17^{d,e}$	89 ± 26
RPF (ml/min)	546 ± 55	555 ± 70	562 ± 55	533 ± 81 ($N = 21$)	546 ± 67	383 ± 92

Filtration fraction	0.227 ± 0.020	0.27 ± 0.03[b]	0.22 ± 0.04[a]	0.251 ± 0.031[c]	0.274 ± 0.028[d,e](a)	0.236 ± 0.056
Renal vascular resistance	0.162 ± 0.022	0.165 ± 0.022	0.151 ± 0.022	0.180 ± 0.025[c](a)	0.186 ± 0.024	0.357 ± 0.113
Plasma glucose at examination (mg/dl)	Normal	256 ± 14	151 ± 42[a]	180 ± 90	184 ± 120	174 ± 50

[a] Significant fall during treatment ($p < 0.01$).

[b] Elevated compared to C ($p < 0.01$).

[c] Elevated compared to C ($p < 0.01$); (a) $= p < 0.05$.

[d] Elevated compared to C ($p < 0.01$).

[e] Elevated compared to D_{II} ($p < 0.01$); (a) $= p < 0.05$.

[f] Only patients with UAE of 15 to 70 are included.

All BP and renal values for D_{IV} patients were abnormal when compared to C, D, D_{II}, and D_{III}.

C, Healthy controls; D_I, diabetics examined at diagnosis before and during treatment; D_{II}, diabetics with normal albumin excretion; D_{III}, diabetics with incipient nephropathy; D_{IV}, diabetics with overt nephropathy; UAE, urinary excretion rate.

The results are given in mean $\pm$ SD except for albumin excretion, which is given in geometric mean $\times/\div$ tolerance factor because of calculations after log transformation.

Φ, Range: 3.0 to 31.8 μg/min.

Stage 2: Glomerular Lesions Without Signs of Disease

This is "the silent stage," which may last many years in some cases, and even a lifetime in some diabetic patients with a diabetes duration of 30 to 40 years [26]. The GFR is still increased with concomitant nephromegaly, at least in insulin-dependent patients. Urinary albumin excretion is within the normal range, both in insulin-dependent and noninsulin-dependent patients [15]. Small abnormalities in UAE may be explained by imperfect metabolic control.

Neither UAE nor GFR and RPF is correlated with the actual plasma glucose concentration in cross-sectional studies; this suggests that the fluctuation in plasma glucose is not reflected by fluctuation in kidney function, or at least only to a limited extent. However, when glucose is given intravenously, but not orally, a slight increase in GFR is found. Likewise, administration of glucagon and growth hormone also produces a minor increase in GFR. Growth hormone is not able to increase renal function in acute experiments [29, 30].

The elevation in GFR of about 30 to 40%, therefore, is not explainable on the basis of abnormal glucose, abnormal glucagon, and growth hormone levels alone. The major cause of the elevated kidney function probably is the nephromegaly—including the increased glomerular size—found in these patients [8]. The cause of the diabetic nephromegaly is not known.

Patients with a long duration of diabetes (for example, more than 15 years) and with normal baseline UAE exhibit clear abnormalities in exercise-induced protein excretion. Abnormal exercise-induced albumin excretion may be the first sign announcing a subsequent development of renal disease, but further follow-up studies are needed [24].

Stage 3: Incipient Diabetic Nephropathy

This stage has been characterized in recent studies [13, 14]. Urinary albumin excretion is persistently elevated despite fair clinical control of diabetes. An albumin excretion rate of more than 15 μg/min in resting condition is clearly abnormal. Young, normal, and healthy subjects rarely excrete more than 10 μg/min. It has recently been shown that an increased rate of $>$ 15 μg/min has a strong predictive value with respect to development of overt nephropathy (Fig. 1). A recent study [12] has shown that 80% of patients with an excretion rate above 15 developed clinical nephropathy over the next 10 years. Patients in the early phase of incipient diabetic nephropathy, which is defined as UAE between 15 and 70 μg/min, also exhibit a clearly elevated GFR that often is more than 150 ml/min (Table 2 and Fig. 2). At the same time, blood pressure is slightly to moderately increased when compared to healthy young subjects and diabetic patients with strict normal baseline UAE (Table 2). Therefore, an extremely high GFR, as well as an elevated blood pressure, may be involved at an early stage in the process which leads to clinically important diabetic renal disease [12].

The rate of progression in incipient diabetic nephropathy is slow [14], as outlined in Figure 3. It is also characteristic that the progression rate, as

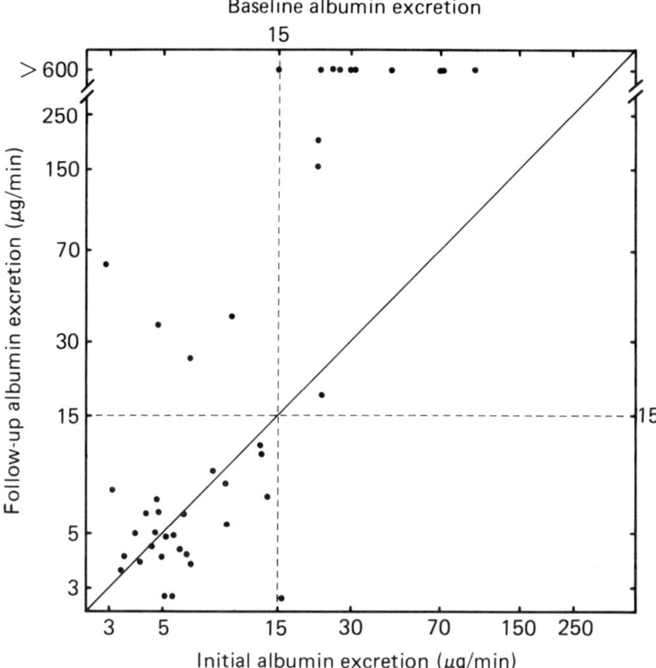

Fig. 1. Follow-up albumin excretion as a function of initial albumin excretion in 43 young male diabetics followed for 7–14 yr, mean 10.4 yr ± 3 (SD). Patients with initial albumin excretion above 15 μg/min exhibit a highly significant risk in developing overt diabetic nephropathy. Conversely, none of the patients below 15 μg/min developed overt diabetic nephropathy, but four patients increased to the microalbuminuria range. (10-yr follow-up studies.) (From *N Engl J Med,* 311:89–93, 1984)

measured by yearly percentage increase, is quite variable from patient to patient. The increase rate is associated with blood pressure levels, as well as with renal vascular resistance as shown in Figure 4.

Since both an elevated GFR and an elevated UAE may be related to poor metabolic control, long-term elevation of plasma glucose levels is likely to be involved in the pathogenesis of these abnormalities.

Defining the progression of disease is clearly important in describing the natural history of renal involvement in diabetes. However, measurements of the rate of progression also appear to be extremely important when evaluating therapeutic measures such as supercontrol of metabolism (for example, by insulin pumps or early antihypertensive treatment) in diabetic patients with marginal blood pressure elevation.

In type II diabetes, microalbuminuria also appears to be an important predictor, both with respect to development of renal disease and also with respect to early mortality [4]. The picture probably is less clear in noninsulin-dependent patients, because microalbuminuria may be due to a variety of abnormalities besides poor metabolic control of diabetes. Nondiabetic renal

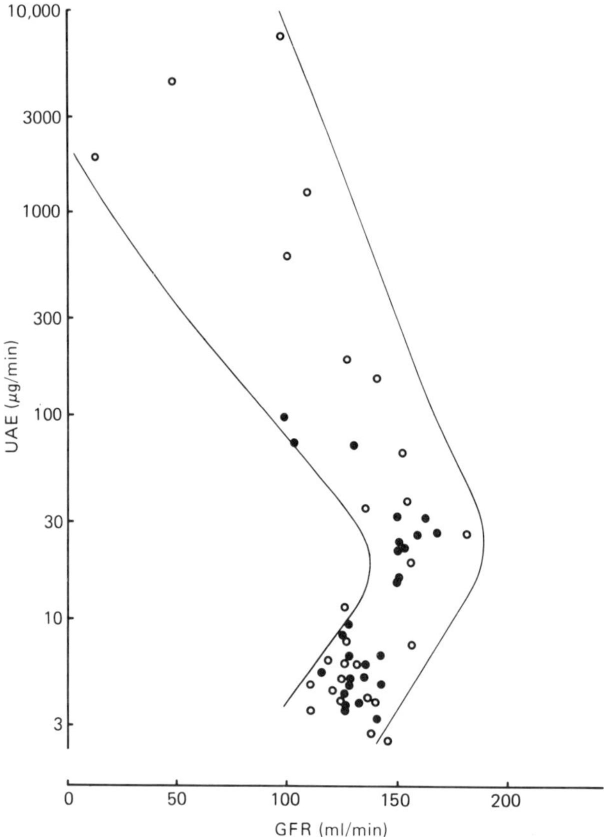

Fig. 2. Urinary albumin excretion plotted against GFR in 39 patients. ● indicate initial measurement of kidney function ($N = 27$); ○ indicate follow-up measurements ($N = 28$). (From *N Engl J Med,* 311:89–93, 1984)

disease and systemic diseases, including congestive heart failure and hypertension, may be involved in such patients. Urinary tract infection (UTI) also should be taken into consideration, although patients with signs of UTI only exhibit marginally elevated excretion rates compared to patients with no infection [28].

In noninsulin-dependent patients, a 10-year follow-up study showed that 22% of patients with microalbuminuria develop proteinuria compared to only 6% of patients with low albumin concentration (Table 3). In the noninsulin-dependent patients, increased urinary albumin concentration is also strongly associated with early mortality. When urinary albumin concentration is in the normal range (≤ 15 µg/ml), mortality is only 37% higher than in a comparable background population at 10-year follow-up. With an increase in urinary albumin concentration, the 10-year mortality increases dramatically; it is 76% when the urinary albumin concentration is 16 to 29 µg/ml and 148% when concentrations are between 30 to 140 µg/ml. A further

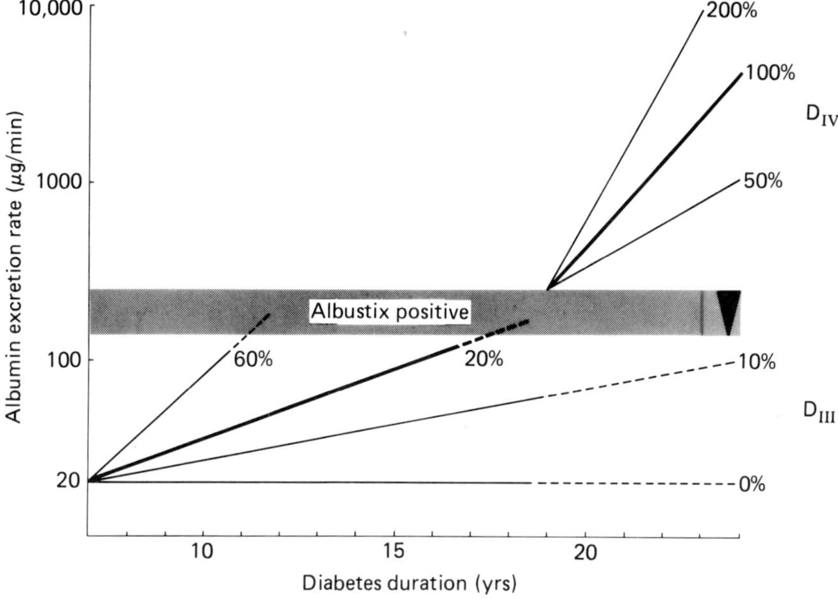

Fig. 3. Sketch of the development of renal changes in diabetes mellitus. In incipient diabetic nephropathy, the yearly percentage increase rate is a mean of 20% with a wide range. The increase rate is positively related to the blood pressure level. In overt nephropathy, it is necessary to correct excretion to the GFR. Also, in overt diabetic nephropathy, there is a wide range with respect to progression. An increase in proteinuria is associated with a decline in GFR. (D_{III}, different rates of progression in incipient diabetic nephropathy; D_{IV}, different rates of progress in overt diabetic nephropathy.)

increase in urinary albumin concentration is not associated with a further increase in mortality. In this study, identity with respect to age, diabetes duration, blood glucose level, weight, and mortality was ensured for all groups [4].

Thus, the development of the implementation of radioimmunoassays for albumin has formed the basis for the definition of a new entity; that is, the incipient diabetic nephropathy in diabetes. It can be concluded that the stan-

Table 3. The 10-year development of overt nephropathy and 10-year mortality in microalbuminuria patients

	Development of nephropathy (stage 4)		10-yr mortality	
	Insulin-dependent (%)	Noninsulin-dependent (%)	Insulin-dependent (%)	Noninsulin-dependent (%)
Microalbuminuria	~ 80	~ 22	~ 20	~ 75
Normal UAE[a]	0	~ 6	0	~ 40

[a] UAE, urinary albumin excretion.

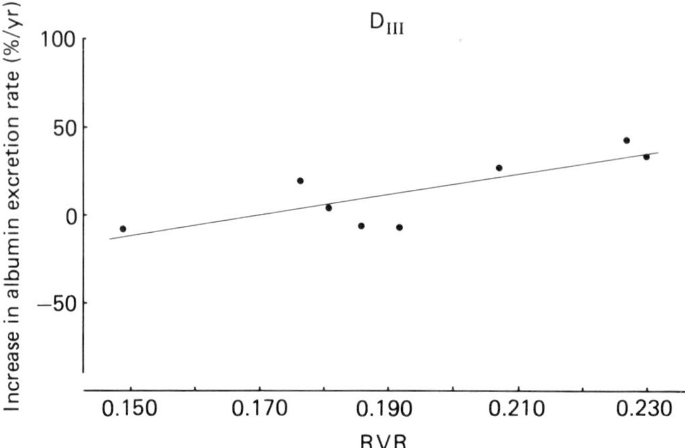

Fig. 4. Percentage of yearly increase in urinary albumin excretion plotted against renal vascular resistance (RVR). A significant association is found, suggesting that progression in nephropathy is related to normalities both in systemic pressures as well as blood flow to the kidney. ($r = 0.80$; $N = 8$; and $y = 580x - 99$.)

dard methods for detection of proteinuria are no longer sufficient in evaluating diabetic patients. A report from the clinical laboratory indicating that there is no protein in the urine is, of course, incorrect. It only reflects the fact that routinely used laboratory methods are unable to accurately measure not only normal, but also elevated, levels of urinary albumin.

Stage 4: Overt Diabetic Nephropathy

This is the classic entity characterized by permanent proteinuria, increased blood pressure, and fall in GFR. It has been shown that the rate of progression in overt diabetic nephropathy is a rather well-defined process; in many patients, in fact, it follows a linear course. Without treatment, the decline rate is about 1 ml/min/mo; however, with a large range, which means that some patients exhibit a slow progression compared to a very rapid progression in other patients. The patients with rapid progression generally exhibit high blood pressure, which is also found in some studies of unsatisfactory control of diabetes [31, 32].

Increasing protein excretion is also a prominent feature in these patients. On a log scale, the increase rate is fairly linear; however, excretion has to be related to the level of GFR, since there is a marked decline in GFR in this stage of the disease [21, 33]. An increase in blood pressure is a prominent feature in overt diabetic nephropathy. Control studies have documented that blood pressure continues to increase during this phase of the disease [34].

Importantly, blood pressure during exercise reaches very high levels in diabetic patients with nephropathy, including the incipient phase of nephropathy [13, 35].

Only a few studies are available on clinically overt nephropathy in type 2 patients, but it is likely that the pattern is not too different in these patients. Clinically, however, the impression is that progression is slower. Cardiovascular disease often is a prominent feature in these patients, and it represents the main cause of death [4].

Notes on Pathogenesis

General Concepts

There is now overwhelming evidence indicating that both the microvascular and macrovascular lesions in the kidney, and elsewhere, are secondary to the metabolic aberrations found in diabetes. The characteristic electron microscopic lesions in the kidney—namely, the increase in thickness of the basement membrane and mesangial expansion—are not found at diagnosis; they develop after a few years of diabetes [36]. Moreover, in the animal model, a number of changes in the kidney are reversed after normalization of glucose metabolism [37]. Lesions in the kidney are preventable with strict metabolic control in streptozotocin-diabetic rats [38]. How exactly these changes are generated in diabetes has not been established. Nonenzymatic glycosylation and enzyme-induced increases in basement membrane synthesis may play a role, as well as decreased degradation of basement membrane material [36]. Of interest are a number of possible modulating factors that may influence the metabolically induced, approximately "linear rate" in morphogenesis, such as charge depletion in the glomerular barrier, locally elevated pressures in the glomerulus, and (finally) increases in systemic blood pressure.

Linear Rate in Morphogenesis

A number of studies suggests that structural lesions, as indicated above, progress in an approximately linear fashion as a function of duration of diabetes—at least early in the course [36]. However, this progression rate may be extremely varied from patient to patient [39]. Unfortunately, only a few studies have employed an examination of serial renal biopsy specimens taken at intervals over the years. What happens with respect to morphology when clinically important renal disease develops has not been clarified thus far. Recent studies suggest that rather pronounced changes may be present without evidence of clinically important renal disease [25].

Decrease of Anionic Charge in the Glomerular Barrier

Deckert et al [40] have recently proposed that the onset of incipient diabetic nephropathy could be due to a decrease of anionic charge in the glomerular barrier that is mainly brought about by depletion of heparan sulphate concentration. The loss of negative charges should explain the increase in UAE. Also of note is that the neutral IgG molecules are excreted in early or incipient diabetic nephropathy [41]. At present, there is no firm evidence for this hypothesis in human diabetes, but it is potentially testable if exact quantitation of anionic charges on the glomerulus is possible in biopsy specimens.

Aggravation by Increased Intraglomerular Pressure

This hypothesis is mainly generated by the work of Brenner et al [42]. The model is derived from experimental observations in kidney tissue that remains after extensive removal of kidney substance. Since renal hyperfunction already exists in diabetes, the process leading to additional damage in remaining glomeruli may be more easily established in diabetes—after damage has already occurred in a number of glomeruli. It is also possible that the early hyperfunction, which is present at clinical diagnosis in diabetes, plays a role early in the course. However, it seems likely that metabolically induced damage must have occurred before hemodynamic changes can induce notable glomerulopathy. This concept is based on the fact that clinically important glomerulopathy does not seem to occur after unilateral nephrectomy in humans, in whom hyperfunction and hypertrophy also prevail as in diabetes. The recent observations of high GFR in incipient diabetic nephropathy favor the view that extreme glomerular hyperfunction may set the stage for late glomerular damage [12]. However, the hemodynamic or metabolic changes are interwoven in a complex way, also with changes in systemic blood pressure.

Aggravation by Increased Systemic Blood Pressure

A number of clinical studies show that a high blood pressure seems to accelerate glomerular damage [8, 22, 23, 31–33, 43] (Table 4). High blood pressure develops along with an increase in albumin excretion. Morphologically the changes in blood pressure are associated with considerable expansion of mesangial volume [39] and also with the extent of diffuse glomerular lesions in general [44]. A case history of a patient with unilateral stenosis of the renal artery may underline the role of abnormal hemodynamics [45]. Extensive changes were found in the kidney exposed to high pressures, whereas the poststenotic kidney exhibited only minor lesions. Studies of a similar nature have been carried out in experimental animals after induction of Goldblatt hypertension [46].

These observations are potentially of major clinical importance; and, indeed, studies already have documented the beneficial effect of antihypertensive treatment in diabetic nephropathy associated with hypertension.

It is clear that the above-mentioned mechanisms may operate simultaneously when extensive accumulation of basement membrane material is associated both with charge defects and with locally increased glomerular pressures, as well as with an increase in the systemic blood pressure.

Table 4. Blood pressure level and rate of decline in renal function in diabetic nephropathy

	Treatment	No. of subjects	Age (yr)	Duration of diabetes (yr)	Observation period (mo)	GFR before treatment (ml/min)	BP (mm Hg)		Decrease in GFR (ml/min/mo)	Albumin or protein excretion (yearly increase)
Mogensen (1982)	Before treatment				28		162/103	(123)	1.23	107%
		6	30	18		86				
	During treatment				73		144/95	(111)	0.49	5%
Parving et al (1983)	Before treatment				29		144/97	(113)	0.91	Further increase
		10	29	16		80				
	During treatment				39		128/84	(99)	0.39	Reversed
Viberti et al (1983)	Before insulin pump treatment				17			(107)	1.35	Increasing
		6	47	22		65				
	During insulin pump treatment				21			(102)	0.69	Increasing

Table 4. (*continued*)

	Treatment	No. of subjects	Age (yr)	Duration of diabetes (yr)	Observation period (mo)	GFR before treatment (ml/min)	BP (mm Hg)	Decrease in GFR (ml/min/mo)	Albumin or protein excretion (yearly increase)
	Controls without pumps (run in)				17		(107)	1.24	Increasing
		6	40	19		?			
	Controls without pumps (experimental)				18		(105)	0.91	Increasing
Cataland et al (1983)	During insulin pump treatment (progression in proteinuria)	6	31	18	12	82[a]	(110)	0[a]	90%[b]
	During insulin pump treatment (stability or decline in proteinuria)	6	30	21	12	92[a]	(98)	0[a]	−38%[b]

[a] Creatinine clearance.
[b] Different by definition.
BP values in parentheses are those for mean blood pressure (BP).

The Perspective of Insulin Pump Treatment

Treatment with a continuous subcutaneous insulin infusion system (CSII)—the insulin pump—brings about a near normalizaton of plasma glucose values in selected diabetic subjects [47]. When begun rather late—that is, in patients with rather advanced background eye lesions—the results of insulin pump treatment have been disappointing. It has not appeared to be possible to effectively influence progression in such patients as compared to control patients treated with conventional insulin treatment [47, 48]. Probably, intervention with insulin pumps must start much earlier in the course. At present, studies are being carried out in both stage 2 and stage 3 of diabetic renal disease. In stage 4, recent studies from Great Britain suggest that insulin pump treatment is unable to modify the course, although there was a tendency toward reduced progression during pump treatment [49].

Recent work has shown that long-term insulin pump treatment is able to normalize the elevated GFR, as well as to reduce a slightly increased UAE rate [50]. Since elevation in these parameters is associated with future progression in nephropathy, the results presently are to some extent encouraging. However, long-term follow-up studies have to be carried out.

Antihypertensive Treatment in Diabetic Nephropathy

Recent studies have shown that effective antihypertensive treatment is able to reduce the rate of decline in glomerular filtration in diabetic patients with overt nephropathy (Table 4). In two studies [22, 23], the rate of decline in GFR was reduced by about 60% during antihypertensive treatment. There also was a dramatic decline in the inceased rate of proteinuria or albumin excretion, which is a further indication of a beneficial effect on the kidney. The studies by Nyberg et al [32] and Cataland et al [31] also show that progression of renal disease is associated with an insufficiently treated blood pressure level. Cataland et al studied the effect of insulin pump treatment on kidney function in young patients with overt diabetic nephropathy. Blood pressure appeared to be an important factor with respect to progression of proteinuria. In this study, GFR (as measured by C_{cr}) remained stable for 1 year, but protein excretion increased only in the hypertensive pump-treated diabetic patient. In the study by Viberti et al [49], blood pressure was kept at approximately similar levels before and during pump therapy. However, blood pressure tended to be lower in the experimental situation; therefore, it is difficult to assess whether the lower mean values in progression rate, although statistically insignificant, may be related to more effective control of blood pressure. The fact that both blood pressure and metabolic control seem to be relevant for progression creates problems in our experimental designs.

Viewed together, evidence from the above-mentioned studies indicate that effective control of blood pressure is as essential for the postponement of end-stage renal failure in patients with diabetic nephropathy as it probably is in other renal disorders [43]. It is likely that blood pressure should be at a level comparable to that obtained by Parving et al; namely, about 140/85 to 90 mm Hg [23].

At present, studies are being carried out to clarify whether antihypertensive treatment, in the phase of incipient diabetic nephropathy, is able to postpone or even to prevent progression in disease before decline in GFR has even started. Preliminary studies suggest that effective antihypertensive treatment has a clear effect on protein excretion, but control studies over several years have to be carried out.

Acknowledgments. These studies were supported by The Danish Medical Research Foundation, the Research Fund of the University of Aarhus and Landsforeningen for Sukkersyge.

References

1. ANDERSEN AR, CHRISTIANSEN JS, ANDERSEN JK, KREINER S, DECKERT T: Diabetic nephropathy in type I (insulin-dependent) diabetes: An epidemiologic study. *Diabetologia* 25:496–501, 1983
2. FABRE J, BALANT LP, DAYER PG, FOX HM, VERNET AT: The kidney in maturity onset diabetes mellitus: A clinical study of 510 patients. *Kidney Int* 21:730–738, 1982
3. McCRARY FF, PITTS TO, PUSCHETT JB: Diabetic nephropathy. Natural course survivorship, and therapy. *Am J Nephrol* 1:206–209, 1981
4. MOGENSEN CE: Microalbuminuria predicts clinical proteinuria and early mortality in maturity-onset diabetes. *N Engl J Med* 310:356–360, 1984
5. FRIEDMAN EA: Diabetic nephropathy. Strategies in prevention and management. *Kidney Int* 21:780–791, 1982
6. WEINER RB: Observations of diabetic, hypertensive physician following renal transplantation. *Diabetic Nephrop* 1:20–21, 1982
7. JACOBS C, BRUNNER FP, BRYNGER H: The first five thousand diabetics treated by dialysis and transplantation in Europe. *Diabetic Nephrop* 2:12–16, 1983
8. MOGENSEN CE: Pathophysiology of diabetic complications. Abnormal physiological processes in kidney, in *Handbook of Diabetes: Biochemical Pathology* (vol 4), edited by BROWNLEE M, New York, Garland STPM Press, 1981, pp 23–85
9. CHRISTIANSEN JS, GAMMELGAARD J, TRONIER B, SVENDSEN PAA, PARVING HH: Kindey function and size in diabetics, before and during initial insulin treatment. *Kidney Int* 21:683–685, 1982
10. PARVING HH, OXENBØLL B, SVENDSEN PAA, CHRISTIANSEN JS, ANDERSEN AR: Early detection of patients at risk of developing diabetic nephropathy. A prospective study of urinary albumin excretion. *Acta Endocrinol* 100:550–555, 1982
11. VIBERTI GC, HILL RD, JARRETT RJ, ARGYROPOULOS A, MAHMUD Y, KEEN H: Microalbuminuria as a predictor of clinical nephropathy in insulin-dependent diabetes mellitus. *Lancet* 1:1430–1432, 1982
12. MOGENSEN CE, CHRISTENSEN CK: Predicting diabetic nephropathy in insulin dependent patients. *N Engl J Med,* in press
13. MOGENSEN CE, CHRISTENSEN CK, VITTINGHUS E: Changes in renal function and blood pressure control in diabetes mellitus. With special reference to exercise-

induced changes in albumin excretion and blood pressure, in *Second Diabetic Renal/Retinal Syndrome,* edited by FRIEDMAN EA, L'ESPERANCE FA, New York, Grune & Stratton, 1982, pp 41–58

14. MOGENSEN CE, CHRISTENSEN CK, VITTINGHUS E: The stages in diabetic renal disease. With emphasis on the stage of incipient nephropathy. *Diabetes* 32(Suppl 2):64–78, 1983

15. MOGENSEN CE, CHRISTENSEN CK, BECK-NIELSEN H, VITTINGHUS E: Early changes in kidney function, blood pressure and the stages in diabetic nephropathy, in *Prevention and Treatment of Diabetic Nephropathy,* edited by KEEN H, LEGRAIN M, Boston, MTP Press Limited, 1983, pp 57–83

16. MOGENSEN CE: The incipient diabetic nephropathy. Introduction. *Diabetic Nephrop* (in press, 1984)

17. MOGENSEN CE, CHRISTENSEN CK, CHRISTENSEN NJ, GUNDERSEN HJG, JACOBSEN FK, PEDERSEN EB, VITTINGHUS E: Renal protein handling in normal, hypertensive, and diabetic man. *Contr Nephrol* 24:139–142, 1981

18. MOGENSEN CE, SØLLING K, VITTINGHUS E: Studies on mechanisms of proteinuria using amino acid-induced inhibition of tubular reabsorption in normal and diabetic man. *Contr Nephrol* 26:50–55, 1981

19. PARVING HH, ANDERSEN AR, SMIDT UM: Monitoring kidney function in insulin-dependent diabetics with diabetic nephropathy. *Diabetic Nephrop* (in press, 1984)

20. MOGENSEN CE, CHRISTENSEN CK: Serum creatinine level in incipient diabetic nephropathy. *Diabetic Nephrop* (in press, 1984)

21. MOGENSEN CE: Preazotemic diabetic nephropathy. Inhibited by antihypertensive treatment, in *Diabetic Renal/Retinal Syndrome,* edited by FRIEDMAN EA, L'ESPERANCE FA, New York, Grune & Stratton, 1980, pp 183–196

22. MOGENSEN CE: Long-term antihypertensive treatment inhibiting progression of diabetic nephropathy. *Br Med J* 285:685–688, 1982

23. PARVING HH, ANDERSEN AR, SMIDT UM, SVENDSEN PAA: Early and aggressive antihypertensive treatment reduces the rate of decline in kidney function in diabetic nephropathy. *Lancet* I:1175–1177, 1983

24. DAHLQUIST G, APERIA A, PERSSON B: Renal function and albuminuria in diabetic children—relation to metabolic control and duration. *Diabetic Nephrop* (in press, 1984)

25. DECKERT T, PARVING HH, ANDERSEN AR, CHRISTIANSEN JS, OXENBØLL B, SVENDSEN PAA, TELMER S, CHRISTY M, LAURITZEN T, THOMSEN OF, KREINER S, ANDERSEN JR, BINDER C, NERUP J: Diabetic nephropathy. A clinical and morphometric study, in *Advances in Diabetes Epidemiology. INSERM Symposium Number 22,* edited by ESCHWEGE E, New York, Elsevier Biomedical Press BV, 1982, pp 235–243

26. MOGENSEN CE: A complete screening of urinary albumin concentration in an unselected diabetic out-patient clinic population (1082 patients). *Diabetic Nephrop* 2:11–18, 1983

27. VITTINGHUS E, MOGENSEN CE: Graded exercise and protein excretion in diabetic man and the effect of insulin treatment. *Kidney Int* 21:725–729, 1982

28. DAMSGAARD EM, MOGENSEN CE, NIELSEN JR: Excretion of albumin and beta-2-microglobulin before and after exercise in 60–74 yr old subjects with newly diagnosed fasting hyperglycemia, previously known diabetics, and non-diabetic control subjects. *Diabetic Nephrop* (in press, 1984)

29. CHRISTIANSEN JS: On the pathogenesis of the increased glomerular filtration rate in short-term insulin-dependent diabetes. *Dan Med Bull* (in press, 1984)

30. PARVING HH, VIBERTI GC, KEEN H, CHRISTIANSEN JS, LASSEN NA: The

haemodynamic origin of diabetic microangiopathy. *Metabolism* 32:943–949, 1983
31. CATALAND S, O'DORISIO TH: Diabetic nephropathy. Clinical course in patients treated with the subcutaneous insulin pump. *JAMA* 249:2059–2061, 1983
32. NYBERG G, BLOHME G, NORDEN G: Constant glomerular filtration rate in diabetic nephropathy — correlation to blood pressure and blood glucose control. *Diabetic Nephrop* (in press, 1984)
33. MOGENSEN CE: Progression of nephropathy in long-term diabetics with proteinuria and effect of initial anti-hypertensive treatment. *Scand J Clin Lab Invest* 36:383–388, 1976
34. PARVING HH, ANDERSEN AR, SMIDT UM, CHRISTIANSEN JS, OXENBØLL B, SVENDSEN PAA: Diabetic nephropathy and arterial hypertension. The effect of antihypertensive treatment. *Diabetes* 32(Suppl 2):83–87, 1983
35. KARLEFORS T: Circulatory studies during exercise with particular reference to diabetics. *Acta Med Scand* (Suppl) 1966, p 449
36. ØSTERBY R: Basement membrane morphology in diabetes mellitus, in *Diabetes Mellitus. Theory and Practice* (3 ed), edited by ELLENBERG M, RIFKIN H, New York, Medical Examination Publishing Co, 1983, pp 323–341
37. BROWN DM, ANDRES GA, HOSTETTER TH, MAUER SM, PRICE R, VENKATACH-ALAM MA: Kidney complications. *Diabetes* 31(Suppl 1):71–81, 1982
38. RASCH R: Prevention of diabetic glomerulopathy in streptozotocin diabetic rats by insulin treatment. Glomerular basement membrane thickness. *Diabetologia* 16:319–324, 1979
39. MAUER SM, STEFFES MW, ELLIS EN, SUTHERLAND DER, BROWN DM, GOETZ FC: Structural-functional relationships in diabetic nephropathy. *J Clin Invest* (in press)
40. DECKERT T, FELDT-RASMUSSEN B, MATHISEN ER, BAKER L: Pathogenesis of incipient nephropathy. *Diabetic Nephrop* (in press, 1984)
41. VIBERTI GC, MACKINTOSH D, BILOUS RW, PICKUP JC, KEEN H: Proteinuria in diabetes mellitus: Role of spontaneous and experimental variation of glycaemia. *Kidney Int* 31:714–720, 1982
42. BRENNER BM: Hemodynamically medicated glomerular injury and the progressive nature of kidney disease. *Kidney Int* 23:647–655, 1983
43. HASSLACHER CH, RAMBAUSEK M, RITZ E: Genesis and management of hypertension in diabetic nephropathy, in *Prevention and Treatment of Diabetic Nephropathy*, edited by KEEN H, LEGRAIN M, Boston, MTP Press Limited, 1983, pp 177–190
44. GELLMAN DD, PIRANI CL, SOOTHILL JF, MUEHRCKE RC, MADUROS W, KARK RM: Structure and function in diabetic nephropathy. The importance of diffuse glomerulosclerosis. *Diabetes* 8:251–256, 1959
45. BERKMAN J, RIFKIN H: Unilateral nodular diabetic glomerulosclerosis (Kimmelstiel-Wilson): Report of a case. *Metab Clin Exp* 22:715–718, 1974
46. MAUER SM, STEFFES MW, AZAR S, SANDBERG SK, BROWN DM: The effect of Goldblatt hypertension on the development of glomerular lesions of diabetes mellitus in the rat. *Diabetes* 27:738–744, 1978
47. TAMBORLANE WV, PUKLIN JE, PRESS MC, ETKIND EL, SHERWIN RS: Continuous subcutaneous insulin infusion, in *Prevention and Treatment of Diabetic Nephropathy*, edited by KEEN H, LEGRAIN M, Boston, MTP Press Limited, 1983, pp 129–138
48. LAURITZEN T, FORST-LARSEN K, LARSEN HW, DECKERT T, THE STENO STUDY GROUP: Effect of 1 year of near-normal blood glucose levels on retinopathy in insulin-dependent diabetics. *Lancet* I:200–203, 1983
49. VIBERTI GC, BILOUS RW, MACKINTOSH D, BENDING JJ, KEEN H: Long-term

correction of hyperglycaemia and progression of renal failure in insulin dependent diabetes. *Br Med J* 286:598–600, 1983
50. BECK-NIELSEN H, MOGENSEN CE, RICHELSEN B, CHARLES P: Normalization of glomerular filtration rate and urinary albumin excretion in insulin dependent diabetes induced by improved metabolic control for 1 year. *Diabetes* (in press, 1984)

Altered Glomerular Metabolism in Diabetes Mellitus

Pedro Cortes, Francis Dumler, and Nathan W. Levin

Thickening of the peripheral glomerular basement membrane (GBM) and prominence of the mesangium due to increased mesangial matrix are characteristic of early glomerular damage in long-standing diabetes [1]. These changes have been considered to be the morphologic result of the altered metabolism of basement membrane material leading to its progressive accumulation [2, 3]. Recent investigations have identified functional glomerular changes associated with insulin-deficient diabetes that, if perpetuated, may be factors initiating and maintaining the abnormal glomerular metabolism [4].

Detailed analysis of glomerular morphology in young diabetic patients has demonstrated significant thickening of the GBM in the first 2 years of the disease [5]. In experimentally induced insulin-deficient diabetes in rats, there is a rapid increase in glomerular content of basement membrane material during the first 4 days of the disease [6]. This change is associated with early enhancement of precursor incorporation into the GBM [2]. Therefore, glomerular metabolic alterations leading to increased synthesis and deposition of GBM material are changes occurring soon after the onset of diabetes.

Characteristically, early in the course of juvenile diabetes, renal size is increased and glomeruli are enlarged [7, 8]. Similarly, in the rat, induction of diabetes is rapidly followed by renal growth, increased renal cortical content of RNA, and glomerular hypertrophy [9–11]. The increase in RNA content is associated with enhanced synthesis of uracil ribonucleotides [12]. Although this metabolic alteration is associated with other types of renal growth, such as after unilateral nephrectomy [13], it also could be of pathogenetic significance in diabetes if it occurs in glomeruli. Since sugar derivatives of uridine triphosphate (UTP) are specific glycosyl donors in the formation of GBM components, increased bioavailability of UTP in diabetic glomeruli may facilitate enhanced synthesis of GBM material.

To assess UTP synthesis during glomerular hypertrophy in early diabetes,

---

This manuscript was presented as part of a Symposium on *Diabetic Nephropathy: Concepts of Pathogenesis and Treatment.*

we have studied the incorporation of orotate (an intermediate in the de novo pathway for pyrimidine synthesis) into UTP and have measured the cellular pool of UTP in diabetic glomeruli incubated in vitro.

Methods

Diabetes was induced in male Fischer rats by the intravenous injection of 50 mg/kg of streptozotocin. Animals injected with acidified 0.15 M sodium chloride (NaCl) served as controls. Glomeruli were isolated by graded sieving from 90 to 120 pooled renal cortices by using buffered 0.15 M NaCl: A purity of 98% or greater was obtained in all glomerular isolates. Pooled glomeruli were suspended in media containing 20 mM glucose, 10 μM sodium orotate, 11.6 μCi/ml of [³H]orotic acid, and 10% dialyzed fetal calf serum in Krebs-Ringer bicarbonate buffer, pH 7.40. The tissue in each glomerular suspension was divided equally into seven to nine samples, each containing $150 \pm 18 \times 10^3$ SD glomeruli in 2 ml of media and incubated at 37°C. Incubations were terminated by immersion of the vials in liquid nitrogen. All studies were carried out 48 hr after the induction of diabetes.

The frozen contents of the incubation vials were mixed with frozen 1 N perchloric acid after pulverization in a stainless steel mortar precooled in liquid nitrogen, and the mixture was allowed to melt. After addition of [¹⁴C]UTP as the internal standard, the samples were homogenized at 2°C in a final acid concentration of 0.24 N. The tissue fraction that was soluble in cold perchloric acid was neutralized and lyophilized for further nucleotide analysis. The acid-insoluble material was submitted to alkaline and acid hydrolysis to extract RNA and DNA, respectively [14]. RNA was quantified by its ribose content [15], and DNA was measured according to its ultraviolet absorption [16] by using calf thymus DNA as a reference. Uridine triphosphate was separated by anion exchange, high-pressure liquid chromatography (HPLC) by using 22 μl of the lyophilized acid-soluble fraction after its suspension in a volume of 160 μl [12]. Column effluents were collected in separate fractions for radioactive measurement. Uridine triphosphate was quantified according to its absorbancy at 254 nm; its peak area was compared to that generated by known amounts of purified standards. The UTP found in the whole sample containing tissue and incubation media was considered to have originated intracellularly, since this nucleotide is not transported into the media [17].

Results were expressed as per unit DNA, because this is the only renal component that remains constant during early diabetic renal growth [10]. Relationships between two variables were studied by polynomial regression analysis.

Results

The cellular content and specific radioactivity of UTP and RNA were measured in control and diabetic glomeruli at different intervals during a 4-hr incubation period.

In control glomeruli, RNA content decreased gradually during the first 90 min of the incubation period to about two-thirds of its initial value; it remained unchanged thereafter (Fig. 1). Despite this apparent inhibition of RNA formation, RNA-specific activity increased steadily. This increase was linear for the initial 2 hr of incubation, and then it slowed gradually (Fig. 1). The content of UTP, which is a precursor required for RNA synthesis, progressively increased and reached a maximum at about 3 hr (Fig. 1). The specific activity of UTP reached its highest value within the first 30 min of incubation (Fig. 1), and it did not change with longer periods of incubation; this value was about 1/20th of the specific activity of the orotate added to the incubation media as a pyrimidine precursor. Since UTP-specific activity

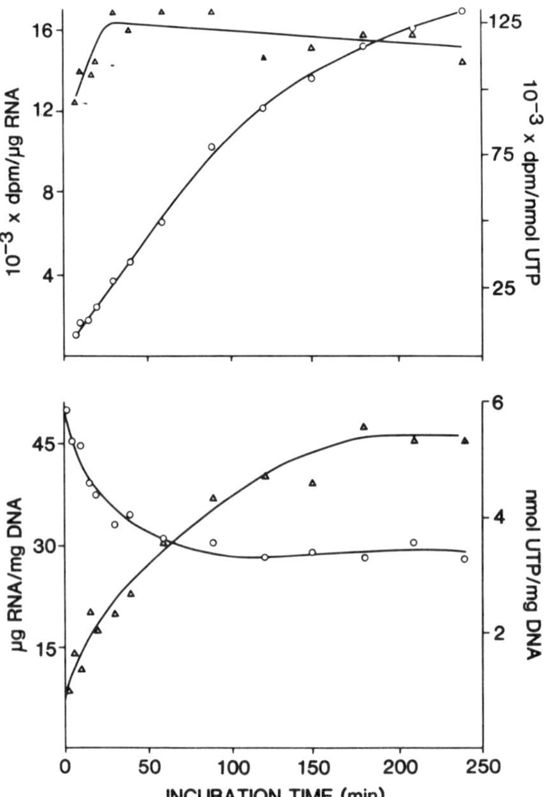

Fig. 1. Synthesis of UTP and RNA in control glomeruli after different periods of incubation in vitro. Renal cortices were pooled and their glomeruli were isolated and divided into seven samples. Incubations were carried out in media containing 10 μM orotate and [^{3}H]orotic acid. The value for one sample that was not incubated is plotted at 0 time. Results represent data obtained in two successive experiments. Changes in RNA- (○) and UTP- (△) specific radioactivity (*upper panel*) and cellular content (*lower panel*) are shown.

remained unchanged after the first 30 min and RNA-specific activity increased linearly, it is unlikely that breakdown products originating during the initial loss of RNA were used for nucleotide synthesis.

In separate experiments with glomeruli obtained from diabetic rats, changes were demonstrated in RNA content and in RNA-specific activity during the 4-hr incubation period, which resembled the pattern found in controls (Figs. 1, 2). However, UTP content did not reach a plateau, but it increased steadily during the entire incubation period. The UTP-specific activity increased to its maximum value more rapidly than in controls (Fig 2); however, as in controls, once the maximum activity was reached, it remained constant. In addition to qualitative dissimilarities between control and diabetic glomeruli, there were important quantitative differences both in the rates of increase in UTP content and in the incorporation of exogenous precursors into nucleo-

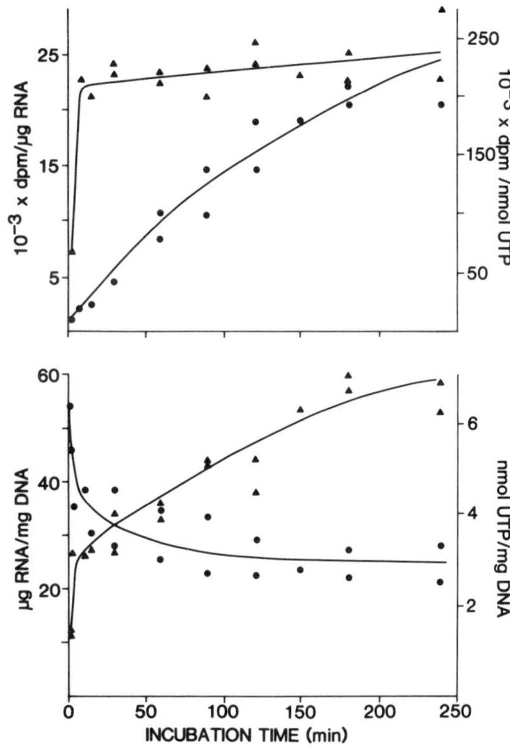

Fig. 2. Synthesis of UTP and RNA in diabetic glomeruli after different periods of incubation in vitro. Kidneys were obtained 48 hr after the i.v. injection of 50 mg/kg streptozotocin. Renal cortices were pooled and their glomeruli were isolated and divided into nine samples. Incubations in media containing [³H]orotic acid were carried out, as in Figure 1. Results represent data obtained in two successive experiments. Changes in RNA- (●) and UTP- (▲) specific radioactivity (*upper panel*) and cellular content (*lower panel*) are shown.

tides and RNA. For example, the steady state of UTP-specific activity was about 1/10th the specific activity of the orotate in the incubation media—approximately double the control value. Furthermore, UTP cellular content at 3 to 4 hr of incubation was about 20% greater than in controls (Figs. 1, 2).

Additional studies, in which control and diabetic glomeruli were compared in the same experiment after 3 hr of incubation, revealed the importance of the time period required for obtaining and purifying the glomerular preparations on their capacity to synthesize UTP with incubation. In experiments in which glomeruli were incubated within 40 min of the beginning isolation, greater amounts of UTP were produced in diabetic and control glomeruli. Nevertheless, greater UTP-specific radioactivity (72%), RNA-specific radioactivity (69%), and UTP cellular content (20%) were obtained in diabetic patients as compared to control patients.

Discussion

In previous work performed in our laboratory, in vivo incorporation of exogenous orotate into nucleotide extracts of glomeruli was shown to be increased 2 days after the induction of diabetes [9]. These observations are confirmed in the present studies using isolated glomeruli incubated in vitro. In addition, the excessively incorporated orotate is present in UTP and probably in other uracil ribonucleotides. Since the enhanced incorporation of precursor is associated with expansion of the cellular pool of UTP, it is likely that in early diabetes there is accelerated synthesis and turnover of uracil ribonucleotides. However, increased cellular transport of exogenous orotate cannot be excluded as a reason for augmented incorporation of radiolabel into UTP.

There is evidence relating the bioavailability of specific uridine diphosphate (UDP)-sugars and UDP-aminosugars to the rate of formation of glycoproteins [18–20]. Depletion of the cellular pool of these UTP derivatives results in decreased glycosylation of secreted and tissue glycoproteins [19, 20]. In cultured fibroblasts, insufficient glycosylation of newly formed glycoproteins and procollagen decreases the net secretion of these compounds by retardation of their intracellular processing and by enhancement of proteolytic degradation of these less stable underglycosylated proteins [21, 22]. Therefore, in conditions of increased synthesis of precursors of GBM material (as in diabetic glomeruli), greater bioavailability of UTP derivatives may be necessary to maintain-optimal glycosylation of newly formed proteins and their increased extracellular deposition.

The glomerular alteration in nucleotide metabolism in diabetes is limited to pyrimidine nucleotide, since the in vivo uptake of exogenous adenine into total glomerular nucleotides or RNA remains unaltered; this suggests normal purine nucleotide metabolism [9]. In addition, the enhanced incorporation of orotate into pyrimidine nucleotides is related to insulin deficiency or its consequences, since insulin infusion in vivo prevents the metabolic change [9].

In the diabetic kidney, the increased synthesis of uracil ribonucleotides is not limited to the glomeruli, since similar metabolic changes have been demonstrated in the whole renal cortex of the intact animal [9, 12]. Exaggerated incorporation of orotate into UTP and UDP sugars and expansion of the pools of UTP, UDP hexoses and UDP hexosamines have been shown in the renal cortex of 2-day diabetic animals [23]. In addition, the increased tissue content of UDP hexoses is rather specific for the kidney, since (except for the testis) it is not found in other diabetic tissues [24].

Since glomerular filtration rate is not increased in the diabetic rat for the first 3 days after the injection of streptozotocin [25], metabolic changes precede measurable functional alterations. Therefore, glomerular hyperfunction is not a likely cause for the metabolic alterations described in this study.

References

1. KIMMELSTIEL P, KIM OJ, BERES J: Studies on renal biopsy specimens with the aid of the electron microscope. I. Glomeruli in diabetes. *Am J Clin Pathol* 38:270–279, 1962.
2. BROWNLEE M, SPIRO RG: Glomerular basement membrane metabolism in the diabetic rat. In vivo studies. *Diabetes* 28:121–125, 1979
3. COHEN MP, VOGT C: Evidence for enhanced basement membrane synthesis and lysine hydroxylation in renal glomerulus in experimental diabetes. *Biochem Biophys Res Comm* 49:1542–1546, 1972
4. HOSTETTER TH, RENNKE HG, BRENNER BM: The case for intrarenal hypertension in the initiation and progression of diabetic and other glomerulopathies. *Am J Med* 72:357–380, 1982
5. ØSTERBY R: Early phases in the development of diabetic glomerulopathy. A quantitative electron microscopic study. *Acta Med Scand* 574(Suppl):1–82, 1975
6. ØSTERBY R, GUNDERSEN HJG: Fast accumulation of basement membrane material and the rate of morphological changes in acute experimental diabetic glomerular hypertrophy. *Diabetologia* 18:493–500, 1980
7. MOGENSEN CE, ANDERSEN MJF: Increased kidney size and glomerular filtration rate in early juvenile diabetes. *Diabetes* 22:706–712, 1973
8. ØSTERBY R, GUNDERSEN HJG: Glomerular size and structure in diabetes mellitus. I. Early abnormalities. *Diabetologia* 11:225–229, 1975
9. CORTES PF, DUMLER F, VENKATACHALAM KK, GOLDMAN J, SASTRY KSS, VENKATACHALAM H, BERNSTEIN J, LEVIN NW: Alterations in glomerular RNA in diabetic rats. Roles of glucagon and insulin. *Kidney Int* 20:491–499, 1981
10. SEYER-HANSEN K: Renal hypertrophy in streptozotocin-diabetic rats. *Clin Sci Mol Med* 51:551–555, 1976
11. SEYER-HANSEN K, HANSEN J, GUNDERSEN HJG: Renal hypertrophy in experimental diabetes. A morphometric study. *Diabetologia* 18:501–505, 1980
12. CORTES P, LEVIN NW, DUMLER F, RUBENSTEIN AH, VERGHESE CP, VENKATACHALAM KK: Uridine triphosphate and RNA synthesis during diabetes-induced renal growth. *Am J Physiol* 238:E349–E357, 1980
13. CORTES P, LEVIN NW, MARTIN PR: Ribonucleic acid synthesis in the renal cortex at the initiation of compensatory growth. *Biochem J* 158:457–470, 1976
14. MUNRO HN, FLECK A: The determination of nucleic acids. *Methods Biochem Anal* 12:113–176, 1966
15. MCKAY E: Pentose estimation by the orcinol method with particular reference to plasma pentose. *Clin Chem Acta* 10:320–329, 1964

16. TSANEV R, MARKOV G: Substances interfering with spectrophotometric estimation of nucleic acids and their elimination by the two-wavelength method. *Biochem Biophys Acta* 42:442–452, 1960
17. PLAGEMANN PGW, WOHLHUETER RM: Permeation of nucleotides, nucleic acid bases, and nucleotides in animal cells. *Curr Topics Membr Transp* 14:225–330, 1980
18. DATEMA R, SCHWARTZ RT, JANKOWSKI AW: Fluoroglucose-inhibition of protein glycosylation in vivo. Inhibition of mannose and glucose incorporation into lipid-linked oligosaccharides. *Eur J Biochem* 109:331–341, 1980
19. DECKER K, KEPPLER D: Galactosamine hepatitis: Key role of the nucleotide deficiency period in the pathogenesis of cell injury and cell death. *Rev Physiol Biochem Pharmacol* 71:77–106, 1974
20. BATES CJ, ADAMS WR, HANDSCHUMACHER RE: Control of the formation of uridine diphospho-N-acetyl-hexosamine and glycoprotein synthesis in rat liver. *J Biol Chem* 241:1705–1712, 1966
21. HOUSLEY TJ, ROWLAND FN, LEDGER PW, KAPLAN J, TANZER ML: Effects of tunicamycin on the biosynthesis of procollagen by human fibroblasts. *J Biol Chem* 255:121–128, 1980
22. OLDEN K, PRATT RM, YAMADA KM: Role of carbohydrates in protein secretion and turnover: Effects of tunicamycin on the major cell surface glycoprotein of chick embryo fibroblasts. *Cell* 13:461–473, 1978
23. CORTES P, DUMLER F, SASTRY KSS, VERGHESE CP, LEVIN NW: Effects of early diabetes on uridine diphosphosugar synthesis in the rat renal cortex. *Kidney Int* 21:676–682, 1982
24. SPIRO MJ: Effect of diabetes on the sugar nucleotides in several tissues of the rat. *Diabetologia* 26:70–75, 1984
25. CARNEY SL, WONG NLM, DIRKS JH: Acute effects of streptozotocin diabetes on rat renal function. *J Lab Clin Med* 93:950–961, 1979

Pathophysiology of Proteinuria in Diabetic Nephropathy

Ovadia Shemesh, Henry W. Jones, III, and Bryan D. Myers

Diabetic glomerulopathy is a complex disorder associated with a diffuse expansion of collagenous components of the glomerulus, and it is the predominant cause of end-stage renal disease (ESRD) in the United States [1]. The natural history of diabetic glomerulopathy has been best documented in patients with type I diabetes mellitus who have been subjected to prolonged serial observations. Although early abnormalities of glomerular function and structure appear to be invariable in all type I diabetic patients [2], only 30 to 50% will go on to develop a progressive, proteinuric form of diabetic glomerulopathy [3]. The evolution of the glomerulopathy in this subset of type I diabetic patients may be thought of as a continuum of glomerular injury. As illustrated in Fig. 1, the continuum may be divided into three stages.

Stage 1: Occult Diabetic Glomerulopathy

The first stage of occult glomerulopathy cannot be diagnosed by conventional laboratory techniques, and it lasts for approximately 10 years. The most striking laboratory finding is a 20 to 40% elevation of the glomerular filtration rate (GFR) above that found in age-matched normal control populations. The glomerular hyperfiltration is accompanied by a subtle increase in urinary albumin excretion that is not measurable by conventional techniques for detecting proteinuria [4]. Using a sensitive radioimmunoassay, it has been shown that healthy adolescents and young adults excrete albumin in their urine at rates of up to 15 μg/min. Among patients with type I diabetes of short duration, a substantial proportion excrete immunoassayable albumin at rates below those detectable by conventional techniques, or 100 μg/min, but in excess of 15 μg/min [5]. To distinguish this phenomenon from overt protein-

This manuscript was presented as part of a Symposium on *Diabetic Nephropathy: Concepts of Pathogenesis and Treatment.*

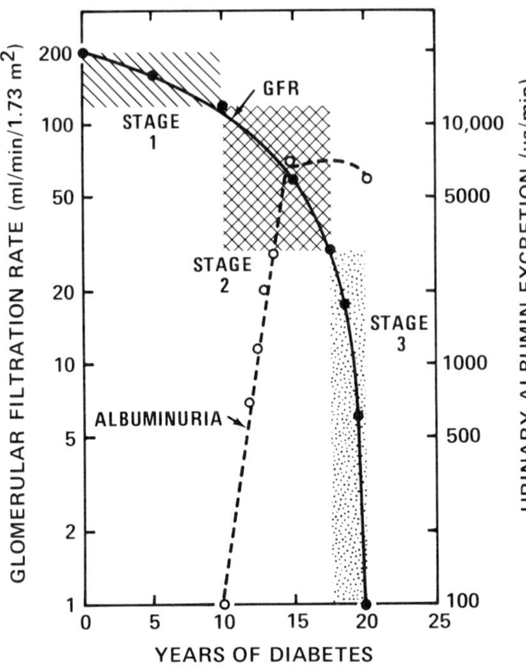

Fig. 1. The GFR (●——●) and albumin excretion rate (○- - -○) have been plotted against time to chart a hypothetic course that is typical of diabetic glomerulopathy. The course of the disease has been divided into three stages, which are described in the text.

uria, it has been termed microalbuminuria. It is inferred to represent an increase in the transglomerular filtration of albumin, rather than a decrease in tubular reabsorption of a normal filtered albumin load. That microalbuminuria may have a hemodynamic basis is suggested by its association with the most striking degrees of hyperfiltration observed among type I diabetic patients. Furthermore, it is exaggerated by exercise, which causes an increase in the intraluminal hydraulic pressure of the glomerular capillaries [6]. Conversely, it is blunted—although not abolished—by restoration of normoglycemia, which is a maneuver that lowers the perfusion rate and pressure of glomerular capillaries [5].

Stage 2: Intermediate Diabetic Glomerulopathy

This stage is heralded by the development of persistent, easily measurable proteinuria. Once proteinuria has become manifest, its magnitude tends to reflect the rate of deterioration of glomerular capillary wall (GCW) function that typifies the second stage of diabetic glomerulopathy. As indicated in Fig. 1, proteinuria tends to increase exponentially with time and to be related inversely to GFR [7]. After several years of proteinuria, urinary losses reach nephrotic proportions (> 3.5 g/24 hr) and the patient will frequently become edematous. The proteinuria is also paralleled by an increasing prevalence of hypertension. Thus, stage 2 is characterized by increasing proteinuria, declining GFR, and the development of hypertension and edema.

Stage 3: Advanced Diabetic Glomerulopathy

The third stage represents the terminal 2 or 3 years of what is (in the prototypic case) a 20- to 25-year process. Its onset is delineated by the development of azotemia. Retention in the serum of urea nitrogen, creatinine, and other nitrogenous compounds generally will become apparent once the GFR has declined to less than one-third of normal levels. As with the intermediate stage that preceded it, GFR in the third and terminal stage of diabetic glomerulopathy has been observed to decline at rates approaching 1 ml/min/mo [8, 9]. Thus, in the prototypic case illustrated in Fig. 1, GFR is predicted to decline from a normal value approximating 120 ml/min at the onset of stage 2 to zero at the end of stage 3 over a period of 10 years. Not only does GFR decline irrevocably, resulting in progressive azotemia, but edema and hypertension tend to worsen in the third and final stage of the disease. Similarly, proteinuria continues to be massive; finally, hypoproteinemia eventuates. Although reduced plasma protein concentration and the lowered GFR serve to diminish the filtered protein load, the urinary protein excretion rate is maintained at massive levels, reflecting increasing leakiness of the glomerular capillary wall to large plasma proteins.

The purpose of the present study was to characterize the derangement of glomerular capillary wall (GCW) function that underlies the progression of diabetic glomerulopathy in the prototypic case illustrated in Fig. 1.

Methods

Patient Population

Ideally, longitudinal evaluation would be required to elucidate the pathophysiology of the progressive injury to the GCW illustrated in Fig. 1. However, longitudinal study of the entire course of diabetic glomerulopathy is impractical for a variety of reasons. These include: (1) our inability to predict with any degree of certainty that a subset of patients among a diabetic population is destined to develop glomerulopathy, (2) the difficulty for both patient and investigator of sustaining an investigative effort over a 20- to 30-year period, and (3) the likelihood that those techniques used to evaluate glomerular capillary function at the outset of a longitudinal investigation will become obsolete long before the project can be completed. For these reasons, we have attempted to evaluate the pathophysiology of progressive diabetic glomerulopathy by studying a large, susceptible population of type I diabetic patients in cross-sectional fashion. With the aid of colleagues in our respective institutions, we recruited for study 62 patients with type I diabetes mellitus that was complicated by ophthalmoscopic evidence of proliferative diabetic retinopathy. The retinopathic form of diabetic microangiopathy has been strongly correlated with the presence of either overt clinical glomerulopathy or histopathologic evidence of intercapillary glomerulosclerosis [10]. Therefore, we reasoned that the presence of proliferative retinopathy was the single diabetic phenomenon most likely to identify the patient subset with an occult (stage 1) or overt (stages 2 and 3) form of diabetic glomerulopathy.

Study Protocol

Each patient was studied by a differential macromolecule clearance technique described in earlier publications [7, 11]. The study protocol was approved by the Committee for the Protection of Human Subjects in Research at Stanford University. Each patient gave informed consent before the study was done.

Clearances were performed during water or furosemide diuresis. A priming dose followed by a constant infusion of inulin and para-aminohippuric acid (PAH) was administered. Dextran-40 (130 mg/kg) was infused i.v. immediately after the inulin prime. After a 60-min equilibration period, three carefully timed urine collections were taken. The GFR was expressed as the mean inulin clearance of all three timed collections. It has been shown that renal PAH extraction is normal in stage 1 glomerulopathy [12], but it declines progressively with increasingly severe proteinuric glomerulopathy [13]. Based on these direct determinations, we assumed that the extraction ratio for PAH (E_{PAH}) was 0.9, 0.7, and 0.5 in patients with stages 1, 2, and 3 glomerulopathy, respectively. Renal plasma flow (RPF) was then estimated by dividing the measured mean PAH clearance by the assumed estimates of E_{PAH}.

Fractional clearances (θ) of macromolecule probes (relative to inulin clearance, C_{in}) were determined during the first timed collection. The macromolecules used were albumin, IgG, and dextran-40. Albumin and IgG have effective molecular radii (r) of 36 and 55 Å, respectively. Dextran-40 is polydispersed over an r-range of 20 to 60 Å. Albumin and IgG concentrations were determined by radial immunodiffusion. Dextran and inulin (the reference molecule) were assayed by an autoanalyzer anthrone technique. To permit θ for narrow dextran fractions to be determined (r interval $= 2$ Å), a protein-free filtrate of plasma and a urine sample were subjected to gel permeation chromatography before assay. The chromatographic technique and assay procedures employed in this study have been described previously [7, 11]. Deviation of the foregoing clearance values from normal was evaluated via comparison with corresponding values of an age-matched group of 20 healthy volunteer controls.

Theoretic Considerations

The extent to which the GCW limits the transmural passage of a given test macromolecule is expressed most conveniently as the Bowman's space to plasma concentration ratio for that macromolecule, which is a quantity known as a sieving coefficient [14]. The biologically inert and polydispersed dextran preparation used in the present study is filtered passively at the glomerulus and is neither reabsorbed nor secreted by the tubule [15]. Therefore, the sieving coefficient for a given dextran macromolecule of known size is equal to its fractional clearance, which is defined as the clearance of that dextran divided by the clearance of a freely permeable reference solute; in this case, inulin. Because dextran is uncharged, its θ is a function only of its molecular radius (r); and, the relationship between θ and r may be used to characterize the size-selective properties of the glomerular filter.

It has been shown that the endogenous proteins, albumin and immunoglobulin G (IgG), can also be used as macromolecule probes of the glomerular filter under conditions in which their filtered loads are massively enhanced. Under these conditions, the process by which filtered protein is removed from tubular fluid via endocytotic uptake into proximal tubular cells is overwhelmed [16]. Therefore, at high-filtered loads that are typical of states of heavy proteinuria, only a minor fraction of filtered protein is reabsorbed ($< 20\%$) and the fractional clearance of a given protein approaches its sieving coefficient [17, 18]. The test proteins used in the present study have been shown to differ not only in size, but also in their molecular charge [11]. Whereas albumin is strongly anionic in physiologic solution, the larger protein IgG has subclasses that are (for the most part) either neutral or cationic [11].

Theoretic calculations (based on fractional clearances of neutral dextrans) indicate that the normal GCW behaves, to good approximation, as an isoporous filter with a pore radius of 50 to 55 Å [14]. Therefore, it is theoretically possible that anionic albumin ($r = 36$ Å) could gain access to Bowman's space in proteinuric diabetic subjects because of a loss of electrostatic barrier function by a GCW depleted of its fixed, negatively charged components. By contrast, the large size of IgG ($r = 55$ Å) makes it likely that its leakage into Bowman's space—and, hence, into urine—is a function of the extent to which the size-selective properties of the GCW have become impaired. In the hope that its transglomerular passage would reflect impaired size selectivity in an unambiguous fashion, the fractional clearance of IgG, rather than albumin, was used to characterize injury to the filtration barrier in the diabetic population.

Results

Classification of Glomerular Capillary Wall Injury

Fractional IgG clearance is plotted as a function of GFR in Fig. 2. Three stages of progressively severe diabetic glomerulopathy that correspond to those postulated for the prototypic case of diabetic glomerulopathy in Fig. 1 can be identified from the relationship between the two. These are:

Stage 1, or occult glomerulopathy: no immunoglobulinuria ($N = 14$);
Stage 2, or intermediate glomerulopathy: fractional IgG clearance < 0.001
($N = 23$); and

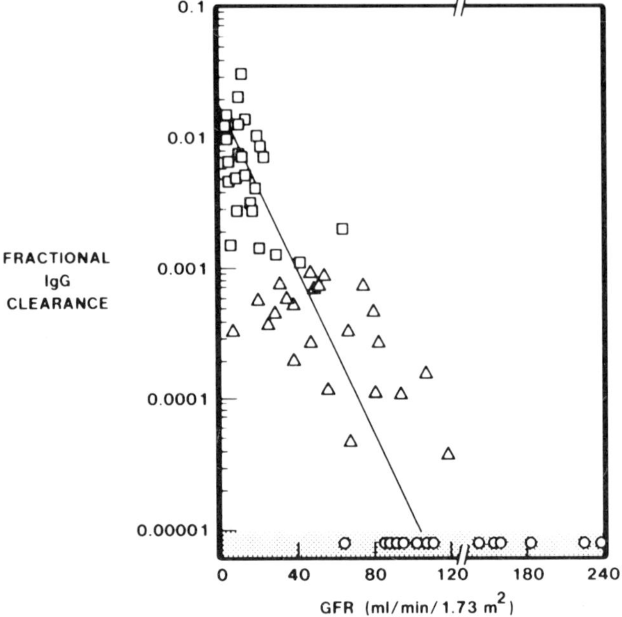

Fig. 2. Fractional IgG clearance plotted as a function of GFR. Stage 1 patients are indicated along the *abscissa* and do not have immunoglobulinuria. ○, stage 1 DG; △, stage 2 DG; □, stage 3 DG; $r = 0.78$.

Stage 3, or advanced glomerulopathy: fractional IgG clearance > 0.001 ($N = 25$).

As shown in Fig. 2, immunoglobulinuria was undetectable in the 14 patients classified as having occult stage 1 glomerulopathy. These patients had microalbuminuria that was not usually detectable by conventional tests for proteinuria, or 34 ± 19 μg/min (Table 1). Despite the presence of diabetic retinopathy, and in keeping with the findings of other investigators in patients with

Table 1. Clinical and laboratory features

	Stage 1 $(\theta_{IgG} = 0)$	Stage 2 $(\theta_{IgG} < 0.001)$	Stage 3 $(\theta_{IgG} > 0.001)$
Number of patients	14	23	25
Duration of diabetes (yr)	16 ± 2	20 ± 1	20 ± 2
GFR (ml/min/1.73 m²)	132 ± 15	$56 \pm 2*$	$16 \pm 3*^+$
RPF (ml/min/1.73 m²)	501 ± 56	$280 \pm 42*$	$80 \pm 6*^+$
Incidence of hypertension (%)	21	$72*$	$100*^+$
Plasma oncotic pressure (mm Hg)	24.9 ± 0.8	$22.8 \pm 0.7*$	$20.3 \pm 0.7*^+$
Urinary albumin excretion rate (μg/min)	34 ± 19	$3174 \pm 574*$	$5914 \pm 651*^+$

* and + = p-value significantly different from stages 1 and 2, respectively.

microalbuminuria [8], the GFR was in a normal range or was elevated to supernormal levels. On the average, the GFR in these 14 patients was elevated to a level above that observed in the nondiabetic control population: 132 ± 15 versus 103 ± 7 ml/min/1.73m^2, respectively.

Proteinuria was heavy and immunoglobulinuria was easily detectable in the remaining 48 subjects. A value for fractional IgG clearance below and above 0.001 has been selected arbitrarily to divide the patients into an intermediate second stage and an advanced third stage, respectively. As shown in Fig. 2, the presence of measurable immunoglobulinuria was associated (with three exceptions) with depression of the GFR to subnormal values below 80 ml/min/1.73m^2. More importantly, the magnitude of GCW hyperpermeability to IgG (judged by the fractional IgG clearance) was strongly coupled to the extent to which GFR was depressed (correlation coefficient $= -0.78$). On the average, GFR in those patients with moderate urinary IgG leakage (stage 2) was 56 ± 2 ml/min/1.73m^2, while that in patients with massive urinary IgG leakage (stage 3) averaged only 16 ± 3 ml/min/1.73m^2. Also in keeping with the hypothetic schema in Fig. 1, urinary albumin losses were at the lower end of the nephrotic range in stage 2 patients and were of massive proportions in stage 3 patients: 3174 ± 574 and 5914 ± 651 μg/min, respectively (Table 1). Not surprisingly, serum albumin concentration was related inversely to the urinary albumin excretion rate in the three stages. The profound hypoalbuminemia (2.9 ± 0.2 g/dl) that characterized the third stage of advanced glomerulopathy was associated invariably with the presence of edema.

Nature of the Glomerular Capillary Wall Injury

Glomerular Barrier Function

That increasing GCW permeability to IgG (and very likely also to albumin) is indeed associated with impaired glomerular barrier size selectivity is elucidated by examination of the mean fractional dextran clearance profiles in each designated stage of the glomerulopathy in Fig. 3. In stage 1 patients without immunoglobulinuria, transglomerular dextran transport was restricted relative to that of normal control subjects over the entire range of molecular sizes examined (24 to 58Å, left panel). Therefore, the size-selective barrier in these patients appears to have retained its integrity. The transglomerular passage of smaller dextrans ($r < 40$ Å) was also reduced below normal in proteinuric stages 2 and 3 patients. However, for dextrans larger than 54 Å in stage 2 (middle panel) and larger than 44 Å in stage 3 (right panel), fractional clearances were elevated above normal control values. Moreover, the extent to which the fractional clearances of larger dextrans exceeded normal values increased with increasing size of the dextran molecules. This selective enhancement of the transglomerular sieving of large, nearly impermeant dextrans indicates a loss of size selectivity by the glomerular filtration barrier, with greater impairment of this property of the filter in stage 3 patients with advanced glomerulopathy than in those with intermediate stage 2 glomer-

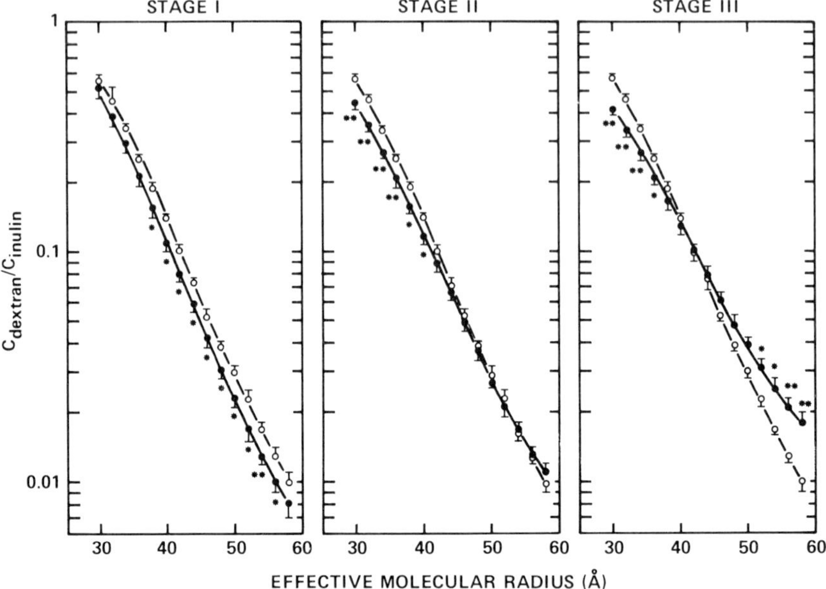

Fig. 3. The mean sieving curve for each stage of diabetic glomerulopathy (*closed circles*) is compared to that of healthy, age-matched volunteers (*open circles*). All results are expressed as the mean $\pm$ SEM. (*, $P < 0.05$; **, $P < 0.01$.)

ulopathy. From the large size of the dextran molecules undergoing enhanced transport and the similarity of their gel chromatographic radii to that of IgG, it is likely that a growing subset of large, protein-premeable pores or defects has developed in the GCW with progressively severe diabetic glomerulopathy [7, 11].

Glomerular Filtration Dynamics

That an increasing derangement of glomerular membrane-pore structure is linked to a loss of ultrafiltration capacity by the GCW in diabetic glomerulopathy is suggested by examination of the pattern of filtration dynamics in the three stages of glomerular injury (Table 1). The progressive reduction of GFR from stage 1 through stage 2 to stage 3 glomerulopathy was accompanied by a parallel, but proportionately smaller, fall in RPF. Thus, the filtration fraction was depressed from 0.26 in stage 1 to 0.14 and 0.10 in stages 2 and 3 patients, respectively, which suggests that factors besides reduced RPF must be implicated in the progressive hypofiltration that was observed. The increasingly heavy proteinuria in stage 2 and 3 patients was accompanied by a progressive decline in plasma oncotic pressure (π), which is taken to be the same as that in the afferent arteriole (π_a, Table 1). Given the falling filtration fraction, corresponding decrements in oncotic pressure at the efferent end of the glomerular capillary network are predicted to be even larger than at its afferent end [19]. On the other hand, arterial hypertension was found to be more prevalent in stage 2 patients than in stage 1 patients, and also to be invariable in stage 3 glomerulopathy (Table 1). Arterial hypertension is predicted to be accompanied by glomerular capillary hypertension and, hence, by an increase in the transmembrane hydraulic pressure differences (ΔP) [20, 21]. These findings, although indirect, strongly suggest that net transcapillary ultrafiltration pressure ($\triangle P - \pi$) increases as diabetic glomerulopathy advances. By exclusion, declining GFR is most likely to be explained by a progressive reduction in the intrinsic ultrafiltration capacity of the GCW in subjects with diabetic glomerulopathy [19].

Discussion

Because of the uncontrolled manner in which our type I diabetic population was selected for study, the observed abnormalities of glomerular filtration should not be regarded as necessarily representative of all patients with diabetic retinopathy. Nevertheless, it is apparent that retinopathy may be associated with a spectrum of functional changes in the GCW, ranging from virtual normality to extreme loss of ultrafiltration capacity and hyperporosity. The similar duration of diabetes in the three graded stages of progressive glomerular injury (Table 1) confirms that this factor also is a poor predictor of the presence and extent of diabetic glomerulopathy. It remains an enigma as to why after 2 decades of type I diabetes some patients develop extreme glomerular damage, while others retain the integrity of the glomerular filter despite microangiopathic changes in the retinal circulation.

Although the variability in the rate of progression of diabetic glomerulopathy among individual patients remains unexplained, our cross-sectional analysis of filtration properties of the GCW provides insights into the nature of progressively severe injury. The inverse relationship between GFR and the extent to which the glomerular filtration barrier has become leaky to proteins and to large, nearly impermeant dextrans suggests that loss of untrafiltration capacity is linked to impairment of barrier size selectivity.

The intrinsic ultrafiltration capacity of all glomerular capillaries in the two human kidneys is best expressed as an ultrafiltration coefficient (K_f), which is equated with the product of hydraulic permeability and the total capillary surface area available for filtration. The product of K_f and the net transcapillary ultrafiltration pressure in turn, determines the rate of transcapillary water flux, or GFR [19]. Because ultrafiltration pressure appears to increase with increasingly severe diabetic glomerulopathy, it appears that a progressive decrement in K_f must account uniquely for the graded hypofiltration that was observed (Fig. 2, Table 1). Although morphologic studies were not performed during the course of this study, other investigators have shown that diffuse intercapillary glomerulosclerosis is strongly correlated with progressive deterioration of the GFR in diabetic patients [22, 23]. The greatly expanded mesangial matrix associated with this pathologic lesion would—

by obliterating many capillary lumina—result in a reduction of capillary surface area for filtration, and hence in K_f.

Progressive widening of the glomerular basement membrane (GBM) constitutes a second common ultrastructural abnormality of the glomerulus in diabetic glomerulopathy. It has been proposed that a diffuse increase in the size of the functional pores in the hydrated interior of this widened basement membrane renders the GCW hyperpermeable to plasma proteins [24]. That this is unlikely to be the case is suggested by our finding that the transglomerular passage of neutral dextran macromolecules of broad size distribution (radii 28 − 44 Å) is actually depressed, even in stage 3 patients with massive proteinuria (Fig. 3). As stated previously, the normal GCW generally has been represented as a membrane perforated by cylindrical pores of identical size (isoporous) [14]. While this representation may also be consistent with the GCW of nonproteinuric patients with stage 1 injury (left panel, Fig. 3), no single population of pores of identical size can account for the simultaneous reduction in the transport of smaller dextrans and in enhanced transport of larger dextrans observed in proteinuric stage 2 or 3 glomerulopathy (middle and right panel, Fig. 3). Rather, it is necessary in these latter instances, to postulate a heteroporous membrane that contains a subset of pores that are sufficiently large to account for the selective enhancement in transport of large, nearly impermeant dextrans. Theoretic analysis of the dextran filtration data observed in stage 3 injury, which uses a model of solute transport through a heteroporous membrane, reveals that the fraction of the glomerular membrane occupied by enlarged pores is less than 2% of total pore area [7]. Presumably, the loss of barrier size selectivity in diabetic glomerulopathy is due to isolated defects in a GCW that are otherwise characterized by normal porosity. That even the development of these types of isolated defects in the glomerular filter is unassociated with the process by which the glomerular basement membrane becomes widened is suggested by a recent morphometric analysis showing a lack of correlation between basement membrane width and the magnitude of proteinuria [23]. Indeed, striking membrane widening has been observed in diabetic patients without proteinuria [22, 23].

The ultrastructural counterpart of functional GCW defects—through which a protein-rich fraction of glomerular filtrate might be shunted into Bowman's space in diabetic glomerulopathy—must remain conjectural. Nevertheless, it is interesting to note that an ubiquitous injury that might cause a focal disruption of the glomerular filtration barrier has been observed in several proteinuric glomerulopathies in experimental animals [25, 26]. This injury is characterized by a focal foot process degeneration, with detachment of epithelial cells from, and denudation of, the underlying GBM. Where electron-dense tracers have been injected, they have been observed to penetrate the GBM at these denuded sites exclusively, and also to enter Bowman's space via the abnormal space beneath the detached epithelial layer [25, 26]. Although a similar injury has been reported in proteinuric humans with either diabetic glomerulopathy or focal glomerular sclerosis, such reports are rare [27]. It may be that the development of functional defects or shunts that do not restrict the passage of proteins in the human GCW are not resolvable by conventional electron microscopy. It is also possible that the derangement of the GCW membrane-pore structure attending proteinuric diabetic glomerulopathy may be caused by biophysical influences, such as altered glomerular perfusion characteristics or charge depletion of the GCW, rather than by a consequence of structural disruption of the filtration barrier.

Summary

A cross-sectional analysis of glomerular capillary wall (GCW) function was undertaken in 62 type I diabetic patients with proliferative retinopathy. The magnitude of fractional clearance (θ) of the large protein IgG, which is a measure of impaired glomerular barrier function, correlated inversely with the glomerular filtration rate (GFR) (r value -0.78). This relationship was used to delineate three stages of progressively severe GCW injury: stage 1: $\theta_{IgG} = 0$, GFR 131 ± 14 ml/min ($N = 14$); stage 2: $\theta_{IgG} < 0.001$, GFR 56 ± 6 ml/min ($N = 23$); and stage 3: $\theta_{IgG} > 0.001$, GFR 16 ± 3 ml/min ($N = 25$). Mean θ for neutral dextrans of a small size (radii $20 - 40$ Å) was reduced, while the corresponding θ for larger dextrans ($40 - 60$ Å) was elevated in stages 2 and 3 versus stage 1 with the changes in stage 3 > stage 2. There also was an increasing prevalence of hypertension combined with a declining plasma oncotic pressure in stages 1 through 3, suggesting a progressive rise in ultrafiltration pressure with increasing injury and, by exclusion, a loss of ultrafiltration capacity by the GCW. We conclude that increasingly severe injury to the diabetic GCW can be ascribed to progressive loss of filtration surface area accompanied by a parallel loss of barrier size selectivity. The presence of retinopathy per se does not predict the presence or extent of this GCW injury.

Acknowledgments. This study was supported by a grant from the National Institutes of Health (AM29985) and, in part, by grants from the Kroc Foundation and the Kaiser Foundation Research Institute.

References

1. GOLDSTEIN DA, MASSRY SG: Diabetic nephropathy. *Nephron* 20:386–396, 1978
2. ØSTERBY R, GUNDERSON, HJB, HØLYCK A, KOUSTRUP JP, NYBERG G, WESTBERG G: Diabetic glomerulopathy: Structural characteristics of the early and advanced stages. *Diabetes* 32:79–82, 1983
3. KNOWLES HC JR: Magnitude of the renal failure problem in diabetic patients. *Kidney Int* 4(Suppl 1):52–57, 1974
4. PARVING HH: Increased microvascular permeability to plasma protein in short-term and long-term juvenile diabetics. *Diabetes* 25(Suppl 2):884–889, 1976
5. VIBERTI GC, PICKUP JC, JARRETT RJ, KEEN H: Effect of control of blood glucose on urinary excretion of albumin and B_2 microglobulin in insulin-dependent diabetes. *N Engl J Med* 300:638–641, 1979
6. MOGENSEN CE, VITTINGHUS E, SØLLING K: Abnormal albumin excretion after two provocative renal tests in diabetes: Physical exercise and lysine injection. *Kidney Int* 16:385–393, 1979

7. MYERS BD, WINETZ JA, CHIU F, MICHAELS AS: Mechanisms of proteinuria in diabetic nephropathy: A study of glomerular barrier function. *Kidney Int* 21:96–105, 1982

8. MOGENSEN CE: Progression of nephropathy in long-term diabetics with proteinuria and effect of initial anti-hypertensive treatment. *Scand J Clin Lab Invest* 36:383–388, 1976

9. PARVING HH, ANDERSEN AR, SMIDT UM, SANDAHL CHRISTIANSEN J, OXENBØLL B, SENDSEN PA: Diabetic nephropathy and arterial hypertension: The effect of antihypertensive treatment. *Diabetes* 32:83–97, 1983

10. THOMSEN AC: *The Kidney in Diabetes Mellitus. A Clinical and Histological Investigation Based on Renal Biopsy Material.* Copenhagen, Munksgaard Press, 1965, p. 214

11. MYERS BD, OKARMA TB, FRIEDMAN S, BRIDGES C, ROSS J, ASSEFF S, DEEN WM: Mechanisms of proteinuria in human glomerulonephritis. *J Clin Invest* 70:732–746, 1982

12. NYBERG G, GRANERUS G, AURELL M: Renal extraction ratios for ^{51}Cr-EDTA, PAH and glucose in early insulin-dependent diabetic patients. *Kidney Int* 21:706–708, 1982

13. BUCHT H, EK J, WERKO L: Renal function studies in diabetic nephropathy. *Scand J Clin Lab Invest* 8:309–318, 1956

14. DEEN WM, MYERS BD, BRENNER BM: The glomerular barrier to macromolecules: Theoretical and experimental considerations, in *Contemporary Issues in Nephrology: Nephrotic Syndrome,* edited by BRENNER BM, New York, Churchill Livingstone, 1982, pp 1–29

15. CHANG RLS, UEKI IF, TROY JL, DEEN WM, ROBERTSON CR, BRENNER BM: Permselectivity of the glomerular capillary wall to macromolecules. II. Experimental studies in rats using neutral dextran. *Biophys J* 15:887–895, 1975

16. OKEN DE, KIRSCHBAUM BB, LANDWEHR DM: Micropuncture studies of the mechanisms of normal and pathologic albuminuria, in *Contribution to Nephrology* (vol. 24), edited by BERLYNE GM, Basel, Karger, 1981, pp 1–8

17. EISENBACH GM, VAN LIEW JB, BOYLAN JW: Effect of angiotensin on the filtration of protein in the rat kidney. A micropuncture study. *Kidney Int* 8:80–87, 1975

18. GALASKE RG, BALDAMUS CA, STOLTE H: Plasma protein handling in the rat kidney: Micropuncture experiments in the acute heterologous phase of anti-GBM nephritis. *Pflügers Arch* 375:269–277, 1978

19. DEEN WM, ROBERTSON CR, BRENNER BM: A model of glomerular ultrafiltration in the rat. *Am J Physiol* 223:1178–1183, 1972

20. NAVAR LG, BELL PD, WHITE RW, WATTS RL, WILLIAMS RH: Evaluation of the single nephron filtration coefficient in the dog. *Kidney Int* 11:137–149, 1977

21. AZAR S, JOHNSON MA, HERTEL B, TOBIAN L: Single-nephron pressures, flows and resistances in hypertensive kidneys with nephrosclerosis. *Kidney Int* 12:28–40, 1977

22. GELLMAN DD, PIRANI CC, SOOTHILL JF, MUEHRCKE RC, KARK RM: Diabetic nephropathy. A clinical and pathologic study based on renal biopsies. *Medicine* 38:321–367, 1959

23. MAUER SM, STEFFES MW, ELLIS EN, SUTHERLAND DER, BROWN DM, GOETZ FC: Structural-functional relationships in diabetic nephropathy (*abstract*). *Kidney Int* 25:225, 1984

24. SPIRO RG: Search for a biochemical basis of diabetic microangiopathy. *Diabetologia* 12:1–14, 1976

25. OLSON JL, RENNKE HG, VENKATACHELAM MA: Alterations in the charge and

size-selectivity barrier of the glomerular filter in aminonucleoside nephrosis in rats. *Lab Invest* 44:271–279, 1981

26. OLSON JL, HOSTETTER TH, RENNKE HG, BRENNER BM, VENKATACHALAM MA: Altered glomerular permselectivity and progressive sclerosis following extreme ablation of renal mass. *Kidney Int* 22:112–126, 1982

27. COHEN AH, MAMPASO F, AMBONI L: Glomerular podocyte degeneration in human renal disease. An ultrastructural study. *Lab Invest* 37:40–42, 1977

Early Markers of Diabetic Nephropathy: A Road to Prevention

GianCarlo Viberti and Martin J. Wiseman

In 1840, Richard Bright first recognized the poor prognosis associated with the appearance of proteinuria in his diabetic patients [1]. Almost 150 years later, the development of proteinuria exceeding 0.5 g/24 hr in a diabetic patient without other obvious causes of renal disease still heralds a progressive, relentless, and inexorable decline in renal function to end-stage renal failure [2]. The social and economic impact of diabetic nephropathy is staggering. In the United States, one of every four patients entering renal support programs is diabetic [3, 4]. Approximately 43% of insulin-dependent patients will develop diabetic nephropathy, with the peak incidence being 16 to 17 years after the onset of diabetes mellitus. After 35 years of diabetes mellitus, only a small proportion (approximately 4%) develop nephropathy [5, 6]. The reason(s) for this selection is not entirely clear, but it suggests susceptibility in a group of patients. Environmental factors, however, play a necessary role [7], and poor glycemic control has been shown to be associated with a higher incidence of clinical proteinuria [8].

Elevation of arterial blood pressure has been found to be an early event in proteinuric diabetic patients, preceding the appearance of low glomerular filtration rates (GFR) [9]. By the time GFR is significantly reduced, almost all patients have significant arterial hypertension. Once persistent proteinuria is established, a fall in GFR that is linear with time sets in. The rate of decline varies in different subjects, ranging between 0.6 to 2.4 ml/min/mo, and it appears to be irreversible [10, 11]. The risk factors responsible for the different speeds of fall are little known; long-term correction of hyperglycemia has proved to be of little value in slowing the progression of renal impairment in these patients [11]. Although treatment of elevated arterial pressure has proved to be successful in reducing albuminuria, and in some cases retarding the loss of glomerular function, it has failed to arrest (let alone reverse) this process [12, 13]. Thus, by the time the diabetic state has resulted in

This manuscript was presented as part of a Symposium on *Diabetic Nephropathy: Concepts of Pathogenesis and Treatment.*

clinically detectable renal damage, present therapeutic maneuvers appear to be inadequate, and patients are consigned to the salvage processes of renal support programs. Although other therapeutic measures that are potentially capable of affecting the progressive deterioration of renal function should not be neglected (for example, low-protein diet), it is natural that endeavors at prevention (rather than treatment) of diabetic nephropathy should become prominent.

Identification of Early Markers

The clinical hallmark of diabetic nephropathy is proteinuria, predominantly albuminuria (roughly 50% of total protein excretion [14]); until recently, it was thought that the increase in albumin excretion above the detection threshold of current clinical methods (for example, the Albustix® test) was a sudden event that was preceded by years of normal protein excretion [15]. Moreover, high blood pressure was thought to be an accompaniment only of advanced nephropathy [16]. Recent work has challenged both of these notions.

Proteinuria

The development of a specific and sensitive radioimmunoassay [17] has allowed the detection of very small concentrations of albumin in the urine of normal and diabetic subjects who are without clinically evident renal disease. As albumin is the plasma protein contributing the largest amount to total urinary proteins, its measurement has become a standard for proteinuria in diabetes [14]. Several studies have shown that 30 to 45% of insulin-dependent diabetic persons excrete albumin in the urine in amounts in excess of the upper limit of the normal range (about 18 mg/24 hr, calculated as mean + 2 SD), while still remaining negative to conventional clinical tests for proteinuria (such as the Albustix test) [14, 18, 19]. These subclinical elevations of albumin excretion rates have been termed microalbuminuria [14]. When diabetic subjects with microalbuminuria were intensively treated by continuous subcutaneous insulin infusion (CSII), to achieve levels of near-normoglycemia, the albumin excretion rate was found to be significantly reduced and even normalized in several cases. Control microalbuminuric diabetic subjects treated with conventional insulin therapy failed to show any significant change in the albumin excretion rate over the same period (Fig. 1). The response of albumin excretion to improved diabetic control in these patients is in sharp contrast to the lack of effect of strict blood glucose control on the heavier albuminuria in diabetic subjects with nephropathy [11]. The importance of these findings lay fallow until it was shown that certain degrees of microalbuminuria could predict the later development of Albustix-positive proteinuria [20, 21]. In a cohort study of 63 insulin-dependent diabetic subjects

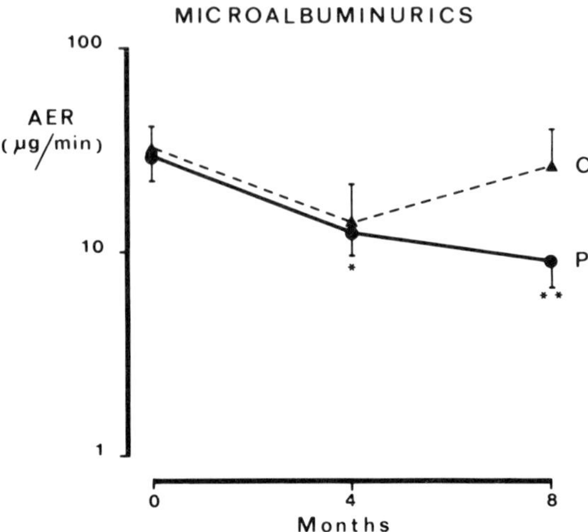

Fig. 1. Albumin excretion rates in a group of microalbuminuric IDDs made nearly normoglycemic by continuous subcutaneous insulin infusion (*P*) and a group of microalbuminuric IDDs on unchanged conventional treatment (*C*) over an 8-mo period. (* = $P < 0.05$, ** = $P < 0.02$ for change from baseline.)

(IDDs) screened in 1966–1967, seven of the eight IDDs with overnight albumin excretion in excess of 30 µg/min developed persistent Albustix-positive proteinuria by the time of follow-up 14 years later, while only two of the remaining 55 IDDs did so too (Fig. 2). This is approximately a 20-fold increase in risk.

The interpretation of this difference in risk is not yet entirely clear. The heavier degrees of microalbuminuria (that is, > 30 µg/min) may simply indicate the diabetic subjects who are further along the track and/or proceeding faster towards nephropathy. The mean duration of diabetes was indeed longer in this group, although the difference could have arisen by chance. An important alternative interpretation is that microalbuminuria of this degree is a glomerular marker of susceptibility to ultimate clinical nephropathy. Variations in levels of metabolic control appear to explain some, but not all, of the variations in the risk of nephropathy in diabetic patients. Those patients who survive more than 30 years of diabetes without developing Albustix-positive proteinuria appear to be almost free of subsequent risk [5, 6]. The transition from micro- to macroalbuminuria appears to occur through a progressive (perhaps self-accelerating) increase in albumin excretion, but the time course of the transition differs markedly between patients [20, 21]. The factors determining the transition are presently unknown. These findings support the view that microalbuminuria of a certain degree represents an early phase of the nephropathic process and is not a separate entity from clinical nephropathy. These degrees of microalbuminuria are responsive to glycemic correction and are reversible—a fact that lends support to the idea that strict blood glucose control in these patients may hinder or even prevent

Fig. 2. Overnight albumin excretion rates (AER) in 63 IDDs at screening and after up to 14 yr follow-up. Only 2 of 55 IDDs with AER at screening < 30 μg/min (*inner square*) developed Albustix-positive proteinuria by the time of follow-up, compared to seven out of eight IDDs with screening AER > 30 μg/min. *Outer square* delimits the level above which the Albustix test (*Alb*) is likely to be positive. (*D*, deaths plotted against screening AER.)

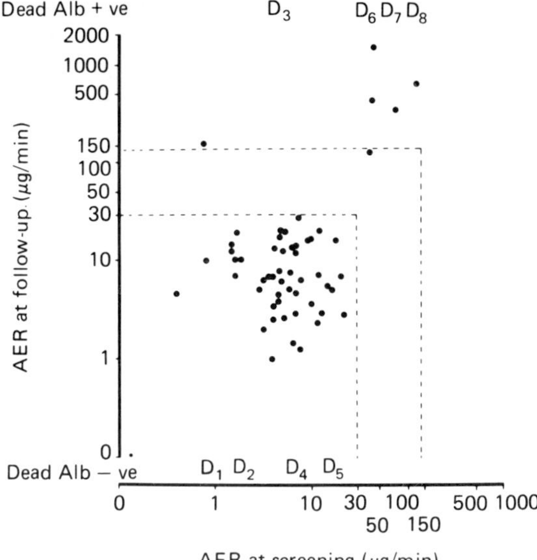

the development of established nephropathy. Only prospective trials of both diabetic control and renal complications will establish this point. However, the possibility of early identification [22] and treatment of these "diabetic susceptibles" should encourage the use of new resources towards this at-risk population.

Blood Pressure

The prevalence of both arterial hypertension and diabetes mellitus in Caucasian populations is high, and opinions differ on whether diabetic populations have similar or higher blood pressure than nondiabetic populations [23, 24].

The almost invariable concurrence of hypertension with advanced diabetic nephropathy led Parving, in a prospective study, to investigate patients with persistent proteinuria whose GFR was still in the normal range and whose blood pressure was still within conventionally accepted limits of normality (< 160/95 mm Hg) [9]. Over a 2-year period, there was a significant rise in blood pressure, in some cases to hypertensive levels far in excess of that expected. The GFR fell concomitantly, but the mean value at the end of the study was still 87 ml/min. These findings led us to consider the possibility that a relationship between arterial pressure and the albumin excretion rate might exist, even before the onset of clinical proteinuria. We have investigated this aspect cross-sectionally in a group of 28 microalbuminuric insulin-dependent diabetic subjects and in a group of 28 IDDs with a normal albumin excretion rate who were matched for age, sex, and duration of diabetes (25).

Microalbuminuric patients were divided into two subgroups according to the degree of albumin excretion. The low-risk microalbuminurics (LM) had an albumin excretion rate below 30 μg/min, while the high-risk microalbuminurics (HM) excreted more than 30 μg/min of albumin. Figure 3 diagrammatically shows the matching procedures. The microalbuminuric diabetic subjects had worse glycemic control than the matched control diabetic subjects, irrespective of the degree of microalbuminuria. This was demonstrated not only by the diurnal glucose profile, which was consistently higher in the microalbuminurics, but also by glycosylated hemoglobin concentrations (Table 1). Moreover, it was found that the "low-risk" group had mean blood pressures that were indistinguishable from their matched normoalbuminuric diabetic control group. However, the "high-risk" group had significantly higher blood pressures, both systolic and diastolic, than both their control and "low-risk" microalbuminuric subjects (Table 1). Most of these subjects had blood pressures within conventionally accepted normal limits; only one had both systolic and diastolic blood pressures exceeding these levels (172/100 mm Hg). It is impossible to establish from a cross-sectional study whether the higher blood pressures are the result of existing kidney disease (although subclinical) or whether it is those diabetic subjects with blood pressures in the upper reaches of the normal distribution who are more likely to develop microalbuminuria, thus initiating the vicious circle of hypertension and kidney disease characteristic of late nephropathy. These data pose the question of whether conventional levels of hypertension are set too high to detect potentially reversible kidney damage; also, whether lower treatment thresholds for blood pressure should be applied to diabetic populations, or even whether a rising blood pressure within the normal range should be recognized as an indication for intervention. While reduction in blood pressure has been shown

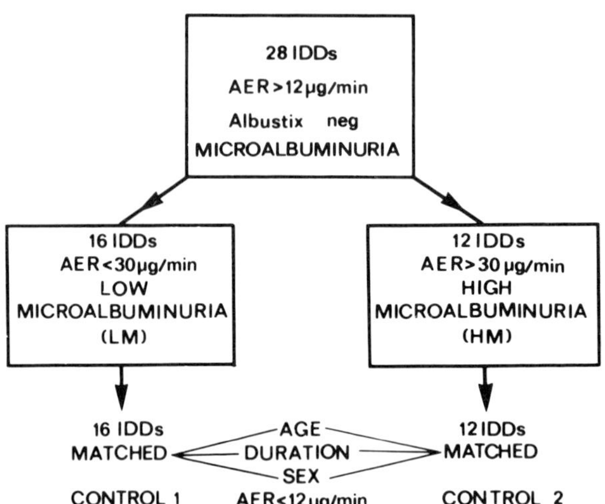

Fig. 3. Diagrammatic representation of the matching procedures and study design employed in the cross-sectional study of glycemia and arterial pressure in microalbuminuria.

Table 1. Mean (± SD) blood pressure and glycosylated hemoglobin concentrations in low-risk (LM), high-risk microalbuminuric IDDs (HM) and matched control groups (C)

	LM (N = 16)	C (N = 16)	HM (N = 12)	C (N = 12)
Glycosylated hemoglobin (%)	12.1[a] ± 2.1	10.5 ± 1.8	12.2[b] ± 1.4	9.8 ± 1.2
Mean blood pressure (mm Hg)	92.5 ± 8.2	90.0 ± 9.9	102.8[b] ± 11.7[c]	86.8 ± 6.9

[a] $P < 0.05$.

[b] $P < 0.001$ for difference from control group.

[c] $P < 0.02$ for difference from LM group. Mean blood pressure is calculated as diastolic pressure plus one-third of pulse pressure.

to normalize the microalbuminuria in essential hypertension [26] and to reduce the heavier proteinuria in established nephropathy [13], hypotensive treatment has not yet been applied to subjects who do not have conventionally accepted "hypertension." This point must remain speculative, until studies addressing this specific problem clarify the issue.

Are There Even Earlier Indicators of Renal Damage?

While both microalbuminuria and higher blood pressure are earlier signs of diabetic kidney involvement than were previously recognized, they may not be the earliest ones.

Since 1959, it has been known (27) that insulin-dependent diabetic patients may have a hugely elevated GFR, and this has been confirmed by several investigators (28, 29, 30). This is associated with an increase in renal plasma flow (RPF), although to a lesser extent (30). Even in 1959, it was postulated that this high GFR might, in some way be a precursor of the well-known late kidney disease; however, the theoretic basis and the experimental evidence for this possibility have only recently become available. Studies in experimentally diabetic animals have demonstrated that hyperfiltering nephrons in diabetic rats develop characteristic pathologic lesions more rapidly and more severely than nonhyperfiltering nephrons (31). Moreover, the hyperfiltration and hyperperfusion of the remnant kidney in the one and 5/6-nephrectomized rat leads to renal failure with histologic lesions that are not dissimilar from those of diabetes (32). An occasional "experiment of nature" in humans has shown that in a diabetic subject with coincident unilateral renal artery stenosis, classic diabetic lesions were confined to the nonstenosed kidney; the stenosed kidney showed only ischemic changes (33). Although prospective data in humans are presently not available, it is possible that the hyperperfused-hyperfiltering kidneys are those proceeding to severe structural damage and clinical nephropathy (34–36). Identification and prospective investigation of such patients with hyperfiltration may clarify the problem.

The cause of this hyperfiltration is not entirely clear. It occurs in 25 to 35% of nonproteinuric insulin-dependent diabetic subjects [37]; the reasons for the sparing of the remaining subjects are obscure.

It is uncertain whether the hemodynamic abnormalities can be ascribed simply to the metabolic and hormonal disturbances of diabetes or whether only susceptible subjects would respond to "diabetes" by raising their GFR. In other words, it remains speculative whether the diabetes only uncovers a latent renal hemodynamic instability or whether the diabetes itself causes the dysfunction. Regardless of the mechanism, it has been shown that the elevated GFR can be normalized by intensive insulin treatment and by near-normalization of glycemia [38].

Conclusions

Thus, early markers of the process leading to clinical nephropathy in diabetes have been identified, and they have been shown to be amenable to correction. It is a reasonable and attractive assumption to think that normalization of indices that are prognostic of renal failure may prevent its occurrence. The detection of these risk indicators is relatively simple, as is their treatment. This opens the road for controlled studies attempting prevention of clincial diabetic nephropathy.

Acknowledgments. We would like to thank Professor H. Keen for his help and encouragement. These studies were supported by the Wellcome Trust and the National Medical Research Fund.

References

1. BRIGHT R: Dr. Bright's cases of renal disease. *Guy's Hospital Reports* 5:157–161, 1840
2. JONES RH, HAYAKAWA H, MACKAY JD, PARSONS V, WATKINS PJ: Progression of diabetic nephropathy. *Lancet* 1:1105–1106, 1979
3. FRIEDMAN EA: Is diabetic microangiopathy preventable? A billion dollar question. *Diabetic Nephropathy* 1:1, 1982
4. FRIEDMAN EA, L'ESPERANCE FA JR: Pragmatic realities in the diabetic renal-retinal syndrome, in *Diabetic Renal-Retinal Syndrome,* edited by FRIEDMAN EA, L'ESPERANCE FA JR, New York, Grune & Stratton, 1982, pp 1–2
5. DECKERT T, POULSEN JE, LARSEN M: Prognosis of diabetics with diabetes onset before the age of thirty-one. *Diabetologia* 14:363–370, 1978
6. ANDERSEN AR, SANDAHL CHRISTIANSEN J, ANDERSEN JK, KREINER S, DECKERT T: Diabetic nephropathy in type 1 (insulin-dependent) diabetes: An epidemiological study. *Diabetologia* 25:496–501, 1983
7. MAUER SM, BARBOSA J, VERNIER R, ET AL: Development of diabetic vascular lesions in normal kidneys transplanted into patients with diabetes mellitus. *N Engl J Med* 295:916–920, 1976

8. PIRART J: Diabète et complications dégénératives. Presentation d'une étude prospective portant sur 4,400 cas observés entre 1947 et 1973 (three parts). *Diabète Metab* 3:97–107, 173–182, 245–256, 1977

9. PARVING H-H, SMIDT UM, FRIISBERG B, BONNEVIE-NIELSEN V, ANDERSEN AR: A prospective study of glomerular filtration rate and arterial blood pressure in insulin-dependent diabetics with diabetic nephropathy. *Diabetologia* 20:457–461, 1981

10. VIBERTI GC, BILOUS RW, MACKINTOSH D, KEEN H: Monitoring renal function in diabetic nephropathy. A prospective study. *Am J Med* 74:256–264, 1983

11. VIBERTI GC, BILOUS RW, MACKINTOSH D, BENDING JJ, KEEN H: Long term correction of hyperglycaemia and progression of renal failure in insulin dependent diabetes. *Br Med J* 286:598–602, 1983

12. MOGENSEN CE: Long-term antihypertensive treatment inhibiting progression of diabetic nephropathy. *Br Med J* 285:685–688, 1982

13. PARVING HH, ANDERSEN AR, SMIDT UM, SVENDSEN PA: Early aggressive antihypertensive treatment reduces rate of decline in kidney function in diabetic nephropathy. *Lancet* 1:1175–1179, 1983

14. VIBERTI GC, WISEMAN MJ: The natural history of proteinuria in insulin dependent diabetes mellitus. *Diabetic Nephropathy* 2:22–25, 1983

15. MOGENSEN CE: Renal function changes in diabetes. *Diabetes* 25:872–879, 1976

16. IRELAND JT, VIBERTI GC, WATKINS PJ: The kidney and the urinary tract, in *Complications of Diabetes*, edited by KEEN H, JARRETT J, London, Edward Arnold Publishers, 1982, pp 137–178

17. KEEN H, CHLOUVERAKIS C: An immunoassay method for urinary albumin at low concentrations. *Lancet* ii:913–916, 1963

18. MOGENSEN CE, STEFFES MW, DECKERT T, CHRISTIANSEN JS: Functional and morphological renal manifestations in diabetes mellitus. *Diabetologia* 21:89–93, 1981

19. VIBERTI GC, PICKUP JC, JARRETT RJ, Keen H: Effect of control of blood glucose on urinary excretion of albumin and β_2-microglobulin in insulin-dependent diabetes. *N Engl J Med* 300:638–641, 1979

20. VIBERTI GC, HILL RD, JARRETT RJ, Argyropoulos A, Mahmud U, Keen H: Microalbuminuria as a predictor of clinical nephropathy in insulin-dependent diabetes mellitus. *Lancet* 1:1430–1432, 1982

21. PARVING H-H, OXENBØLL B, SVENDSEN PAA, CHRISTIANSEN JS, ANDERSEN AR: Early detection of patients at risk of developing diabetic nephropathy. A longitudinal study of urinary albumin excretion. *Acta Endocrinol* 100:550–555, 1982

22. VIBERTI GC, VERGANI D: Detection of potentially reversible diabetic albuminuria. *Diabetes* 31:973–975, 1982

23. KEEN H, TRACK NS, SOWRY GSC: Arterial pressure in clinically apparent diabetics. *Diabète Metab* 1:159–178, 1975

24. JARRETT RJ, KEEN H, CHAKRABARTI R: Diabetes, hyperglycaemia and arterial disease, in *Complications of Diabetes*, edited by KEEN H, JARRETT J, London, Edward Arnold Publishers, 1982, pp 179–203

25. WISEMAN MJ, VIBERTI GC, JARRETT RJ, KEEN H: Glycaemia, arterial pressure and microalbuminuria in type I (insulin-dependent) diabetes. *Diabetologia,* in press

26. PEDERSEN EB, MOGENSEN CE: Effect of antihypertensive treatment on urinary albumin excretion, glomerular filtration rate and renal plasma flow in patients with essential hypertension. *Scand J Clin Lab Invest* 36:231–237, 1976

27. STALDER C, SCHMID R: Severe functional disorders of glomerular capillaries and renal haemodynamics in treated diabetes mellitus during childhood. *Ann Paediat* 193:129–138, 1959

28. DITZEL J, SCHWARTZ M: Abnormally increased glomerular filtration rate in short-term insulin treated diabetic subjects. *Diabetes* 16:264–267, 1967

29. MOGENSEN CE, ANDERSEN MJF: Increased kidney size and glomerular filtration rate in untreated juvenile diabetes: Normalization by insulin treatment. *Diabetologia* 11:221–224, 1975

30. SANDAHL CHRISTIANSEN J, GAMMELGAARD J, FRANDSEN M, PARVING H-H: Increased kidney size, glomerular filtration rate and renal plasma flow in short-term insulin dependent diabetics. *Diabetologia* 20:451–456, 1981

31. STEFFES MW, BROWN DM, MAUER SM: Diabetic glomerulopathy following unilateral nephrectomy in the rat. *Diabetes* 27:35–41, 1978

32. HOSTETTER TH, OLSON JL, RENNKE HG, VENKATACHALAM MA, BRENNER BM: Hyperfiltration in remnant nephrons: A potentially adverse response to ablation. *Am J Physiol* 241:F85–F93, 1981

33. BERKMAN J, RIFKIN H: Unilateral nodular diabetic glomerulosclerosis (Kimmelstiel-Wilson). *Metabolism* 22:715–722, 1973

34. KEEN H, WISEMAN MJ, VIBERTI GC: Diabetic microvascular disease and metabolic dysregulation, in *Biology and Pathology of the Vessel Wall,* edited by WOOLF N, Eastbourne and New York, Praeger, 1982, pp 189–196

35. PARVING H-H, VIBERTI GC, KEEN H, CHRISTIANSEN JS, LASSEN NA: Haemodynamic factors in the genesis of diabetic microangiopathy. *Metabolism* 32:943–949, 1983

36. HOSTETTER TH, RENNKE HG, BRENNER BM: The case for intrarenal hypertension in the initiation and progression of diabetic and other glomerulopathies. *Am J Med* 72:375–380, 1982

37. WISEMAN MJ, VIBERTI GC, KEEN H: Threshold effect of plasma glucose in the glomerular hyperfiltration of diabetes. *Nephron* (in press, 1984)

38. CHRISTIANSEN JS, GAMMELGAARD J, TRONIER B, SVENDSEN PA, PARVING HH: Kidney function and size in diabetics before and during initial insulin treatment. *Kidney Int* 21:683–688, 1982

Can the Insulin-Dependent Diabetic Patient Be Managed Without Kidney Biopsy?

S. Michael Mauer, Michael W. Steffes, Eileen N. Ellis, and David M. Brown

Diabetic nephropathy is the most important single disorder leading to renal failure in adults [1]. At the outset, we emphasize our view that the emergence of knowledge that could be of great help in understanding and treating this problem has been hampered by reluctance to perform renal biopsy procedures in patients with insulin-dependent diabetes mellitus (IDDM). The procedure has been seen by the diabetologist as risky, meddlesome, unwarranted, and not helpful. The nephrologist tends to view the renal biopsy procedure as diagnostic rather than prognostic; this opinion is supported by studies suggesting that there exists, at best, only a vague relationship between renal structure and function. Herein, we argue that there may be a role for renal biopsy procedure in the process of decision making regarding the care of the IDDM patient. Although written to be controversial, this position is based on arguments we believe to be valid.

Diabetic Nephropathy and Diabetes Mellitus

Diabetic nephropathy does not occur without diabetes; that is, without persistent or intermittent hyperglycemia [2]. Østerby showed that glomerular basement membrane (GBM) thickness and mesangial area are normal at the onset of IDDM [3]. These studies strongly argue that there is no linkage between the genetic tendency to develop diabetes and the tendency to develop microvascular diabetic lesions. We do not mean to dispute that individuals with diabetes vary greatly in the rate at which their lesions develop, and that this may be partly genetically determined. In fact, there is evidence to suggest that the rate at which lesions develop or the "sensitivity" may be dependent on end-organ susceptibility to diabetic injury (see below). Nor

This manuscript was presented as part of a Symposium on *Diabetic Nephropathy: Concepts of Pathogenesis and Treatment.*

do we suggest that patients with "mild" diabetes cannot develop severe nephropathy. However, it is our interpretation of the literature that there is no substantive evidence that diabetic nephropathy develops in the absence of the diabetic state [2]. Therefore, one would presume that adequate treatment of the diabetic state, at least before the lesions are far advanced, would arrest or reverse the progression of the nephropathogy.

Glycemic Control and Diabetic Renal Lesions

Abundant animal experiments support the presumption that glycemic control influences the rate at which renal lesions develop [2]. Information from humans that addresses this issue currently is totally inadequate. However, what minimal information is available is consistent with the view provided by animal studies. Thus, it has recently been demonstrated (in parallel with animal studies [4]) that kidneys with diabetic nephropathy lesions transplanted into nondiabetic recipients undergo resolution of the lesions [5]. Furthermore, preliminary observations in IDDM patients with successful pancreas transplantation indicate a reversibility of moderate mesangial expansion (personal observations of the authors).

It is not known whether there is a uniform level of glycemic control that will prevent nephropathy from developing in humans. It appears that some patients do not develop nephropathy despite decades of IDDM with levels of glycemia that are not different (at least superficially) from patients with advanced nephropathy. Furthermore, there may be discordance in as many as 45% of patients between the appearance of serious retinopathy and nephropathy, indicating that different organs may need different metabolic environments in the same patient to develop microvascular complications [6]. Logically, these observations suggest that glycemic control may have to be individualized to prevent diabetic complications and to avoid treatment that could add significant morbidity with uncertain benefit.

It is not known at what point the lesions of diabetic nephropathy are no longer reversible. Viberti et al showed that the hyperfiltration and microalbuminuria of patients without established clinical nephropathy can be normalized by precise glycemic regulation, with continuous subcutaneous insulin infusion and home glucose monitoring [7]—while patients with overt proteinuria continue on a downhill course despite the institution of identical therapy [8]. However, the anatomic substrate in these patients was not examined. Viberti et al [9] and Mogensen et al [10] both have suggested that patients with microalbuminuria in the range of 30 to 300 μg/min have a much increased risk of developing clinical nephropathy compared to patients with lesser quantities of urinary albumin. Since the higher levels of urinary albumin excretion (UAE) can be reduced towards normal by careful glucose regulation, they have suggested that this "incipient" nephropathy may be amenable to treatment. However, there are several suppositions in this hypothesis that require detailed confirmation before it can be accepted. First, urinary albumin excretion is directly related to Hgb A_1C levels [8]. The study of "incipient" nephropathy [9, 10] did not describe glycemic control. Thus, the patients with microalbuminuria may have been those with the worst control; that is, the control may have been so poor as to be unacceptable on any terms. Second, there is no evidence that glycemic control that is sufficient to reduce UAE is adequate to prevent progression of lesions. Finally, as described in detail below, we can find no relationship between microalbuminuria and the severity of underlying diabetic glomerulopathy. It should be self-evident that progression of clinical diabetic nephropathy does not occur without progression of pathologic lesions. Thus, if microalbuminuria predicts future lesions in patients with minimal changes on a kidney biopsy specimen, this would suggest that an additional factor(s) may be operative that is independent of current renal pathology. Nonetheless, these issues will not be resolved without carefully performed prospective studies of the natural history of diabetic nephropathy relating structure, function, and time.

Structural-functional Relationships in Diabetic Nephropathy

Our ongoing (as yet unpublished) studies indicate that clinical diabetic nephropathy—as manifested by Albustix®-positive proteinuria and fixed hypertension, with or without a decline in glomerular filtration rate (GFR)—is always associated with advanced glomerular structural changes. These clinical findings predict, with great certainty, the presence of marked mesangial expansion and associated diminution in capillary lumenal area and peripheral capillary filtration surface. Parenthetically, patients with 20 or more years of IDDM who have large kidneys and markedly increased GFR predictably have only minimal or modest lesions. This, along with the highly specific nature of the diabetic renal lesions [2], argues against the concept that "hyperfiltration" per se is a sufficient explanation for the cause of diabetic nephropathy. Thus, it is only within these two groups (those with established clinical nephropathy and those with marked hyperfiltration despite 2 decades of disease) that structure is predictable from function. In all other patients (the majority studied by us), we found that knowledge of kidney size, GFR, UAE, and duration of IDDM were not helpful in predicting the severity of the underlying lesions. Furthermore, we are unable, as yet, to find a significant correlation between muscle capillary basement membrane thickness and the serious pathologic changes of diabetic nephropathy. Thus, to our knowledge, there exists no indirect test that can replace the renal biopsy procedure in providing an assessment of renal status in the majority of patients who have had IDDM for several years.

Lessons from the Transplanted Kidney (the Kidney or the Body)

We have had the opportunity to study kidney biopsy specimens in 19 patients who had received renal allografts from nondiabetic donors 6 to 13 years ago (work in progress). Some patients developed little or no changes in the graft, some had mild-to-moderate lesions of diabetic nephropathy, and some had advanced changes that sometimes were associated with proteinuria, hypertension, and decreasing GFR. We found no predictive relationship between duration of IDDM prior to end-stage renal failure, donor source, HLA match, or a rough estimate of glycemic control and the severity of recurrent lesions in the allograft. Thus, allografts residing in the diabetic environment may not develop lesions of diabetic nephropathy despite the fact that in essentially the same milieu, the patient's original kidneys had been destroyed by the diabetic process—despite the renal allograft recipient having a single kidney, which is a situation known to be associated with the accelerated development of glomerular lesions in animals [11]. One hypothesis, which is consonant with these preliminary observations, is that diabetic nephropathy develops as a consequence of both the diabetic state and a separate end-organ "sensitivity" to this state. If correct, this could explain why some patients escape certain complications while others do not, and why there often is a marked discordance between different complications (for example, eye and kidney) in the same IDDM patient. This presents a confounding situaton. If glycemic control can influence these complications, there is no reason to suppose that the level of control sufficient to positively influence eye lesions will be sufficient for the kidney.

Strategies for the Future

There are several approaches that one could adopt towards the management of the patient with IDDM. Given the indirect nature of the evidence supporting improved glycemic control as a means of preventing complications, one might argue that the current treatment of IDDM patients should continue. The second approach might be that all patients should receive strict glycemic control despite the fact that the risk-benefit ratio for a given patient is unknown. Clearly, patients who are not at risk for complications with current "standard" control would be exposed to the added inconvenience, expense, and risks of precise glycemic management without potential benefit, while those patients highly susceptible to complications still might not be receiving adequate therapy. A further choice that is currently being exercised by the National Institutes of Health is a large, collaborative controlled trial examining the influence of control on complications. Although potentially of great value, this type of trial has limitations. By design, patient management cannot be individualized. The primary focus on the eye may not answer questions that are relevant to nerve and kidney complications. Furthermore, as argued previously, the incorporation of indirect measures of renal lesions as endpoints in such trials runs a high risk of proving to be inadequate.

Therefore, it is argued here that IDDM patients should be considered for a baseline kidney biopsy procedure after approximately 10 years of disease. If careful study reveals little or no abnormalities, and if eye and nerve evaluations are not worrisome, then continuation of "standard" care would seem to be appropriate and a repeat biopsy procedure could be contemplated approximately 5 years later. If more advanced abnormalities are present, consideration should be given to efforts to improve glycemic control. The effectiveness of these efforts might be best evaluated by a repeat renal biopsy procedure within 3 to 5 years. It appears reasonable to us that the intensity of glycemic management should be matched to the potential benefits in the individual patient, at least until broader principles emerge from experiences in controlled trials or other sources. It has been argued that difficulty in both achieving and maintaining patient compliance for strict control is such that this recommended scheme is impractical. However, this begs the question. The same fundamental issues exist in the long-term management of patients with hypertension, systemic lupus erythematosus, and other chronic diseases in which an effort is made to tailor the therapy to the seriousness of the disease process despite recognition that the patient's cooperation is largely not within the physician's power of control. Nonetheless, from the perspective of the complexity of management for the blind diabetic patient in end-stage renal failure, we suggest that the effort outlined in this chapter may be less burdensome than the current alternatives.

Summary

It is clear that kidney failure in diabetic nephropathy is consequent to the development of advanced renal lesions. These lesions, which in their aggregate are unique to diabetes, are almost certainly the result of the dysmetabolism of the diabetic state. There is evidence from animal studies that precise control of hyperglycemia can prevent, arrest, or reverse the renal histopathology of diabetes. However, only approximately 40% of patients with type I diabetes develop renal failure. When early clinical nephropathy (Albustix-positive proteinuria) is present, lesions are uniformly very far advanced. However, to date, we have found no indirect test of kidney function that allows accurate delineation as to which individual patient is progressing towards serious renal lesions. Furthermore, there is nearly a 50% discordance between the occurrence of serious complications within the classic end-organs of eye, kidney, and nerve. Thus, except for patients with overt clinical nephropathy, a renal biopsy procedure is the only accurate method of quantifying the severity of nephropathy. Rational treatment decisions in the individual patient may not be possible without this information.

Acknowledgments. This work was supported, in part, by National Institutes of Health Grant No. AM17697 and by Juvenile Diabetes Foundation Grant No. 82R237.

References

1. RAO TKS, FRIEDMAN EA: Diabetic nephropathy in Brooklyn, in *Diabetic Retinal Syndrome* (vol 2), edited by FRIEDMAN EA, L'ESPERANCE FA JR, New York, Grune & Stratton, 1982, pp. 3–8

2. MAUER SM, STEFFES MW, BROWN DM: The kidney in diabetes. *Am J Med* 70:603–612, 1981
3. ØSTERBY R: Early phases in the development of diabetic glomerulopathy. *Acta Med Scand* 574:1–82, 1975
4. LEE CS, MAUER SM, BROWN DM, SUTHERLAND DER, MICHAEL AF, NAJARIAN JS: Renal transplantation in diabetes mellitus in rats. *J Exp Med* 139:793–800, 1974
5. ALBOUNA G, KREME G, DADDAH S, AL-ADNANI M, KUMAR S, KUSMA HG: Reversal of diabetic nephropathy in human cadaveric kidneys after transplantation into non-diabetic recipients. *Lancet* 2:1274–1276, 1983
6. MARKS HH: Longevity and mortality of diabetics. *Am J Publ Health* 55:416–423, 1965
7. VIBERTI GC, PICKUP JC, JARRETT RJ, KEEN H: Effect of control of blood glucose on urinary excretion of albumin and B2-microglobulin in insulin-dependent diabetes. *N Engl J Med* 300:638–641, 1979
8. VIBERTI G, MACKINTOSH D, BILOUS RW, PICKUP JC, KEEN J: The proteinuria of diabetes mellitus. The role of spontaneous and experimental variation of glycaemia. *Kidney Int* 21:714–720, 1982
9. VIBERTI GC, HILL RD, JARRETT RJ, ARGYNOPOULOS A, MAHMUD U, KEEN H: Microalbuminuria as a predictor of clinical nephropathy in insulin-dependent diabetes mellitus. *Lancet* 1:1430–1432, 1982
10. MOGENSEN CE, CHRISTENSEN CK, UTTENGHUS E: The stages in diabetic renal disease: With emphasis on the stage of incipient diabetic nephropathy. *Diabetes* 32(Suppl 2):64–78, 1984
11. STEFFES MW, BROWN DM, MAUER SM: Diabetic glomerulopathy following unilateral nephrectomy in the rat. *Diabetes* 27:35–41, 1978

Pathogenesis as a Determinant of Therapy in Diabetic Nephropathy

Eli A. Friedman

Clinical management of the patient with diabetes mellitus and uremia has improved remarkably since 1980. Rehabilitated type I (insulin-dependent) diabetic patients constitute a growing minority of the 100,000 Americans who have benefited from large-scale governmental support for dialysis or kidney transplant regimens [1]. Although Najarian, Starzl, and others demonstrated during the 1970s that selected patients with type I diabetes could survive for ten or more years following kidney transplantation [2], nephrologists and surgeons remained generally wary about their treatment. To this day, a negative view of the potential for useful life extension in the uremic diabetic patient seems to prevail in Great Britain. In the United States and the remainder of Western Europe, however, formulation of a successful clinical strategy for these patients (Table 1) has gradually replaced an attitude of futility with optimism. During this decade, their survival, whether they are treated by dialysis or by kidney transplantation, has improved steadily. In mid-1984, at least a 50% 3-year survival can be anticipated for type I diabetic patients who are beginning maintenance hemodialysis or receiving a first kidney transplant [3].

Coinciding with the progress in devising a clinical regimen to extend life in the uremic patient with diabetes mellitus, there has been an unraveling of the pathogenesis of nephropathy in this disorder (Table 2). Throughout the first ten or more years following the onset of insulin dependence, type I diabetic patients have enlarged kidneys functioning at a supernormal glomerular filtration rate (GFR) [4]. According to some theorists (extrapolating from experiments in rats with reduced renal mass) [5], sustained glomerular hyperfiltration is injurious to the nephron. In this construction, hyperglycemia or excess protein ingestion causes glomerular hyperfiltration, which (by an undefined mechanism) leads to glomerular sclerosis and obliteration. Alverstrand and Bergström speculate that a supernormal GFR both in diabetes

---

This manuscript was presented as part of a Symposium on *Diabetic Nephropathy: Concepts of Pathogenesis and Treatment.*

Table 1. Clinical advances in diabetic nephropathy

1. Recognition of adverse effect of hypertension on renal function.
2. Self-monitoring of blood glucose to effect euglycemia.
3. Interventive ophthalmology (laser + vitrectomy + lensectomy) applied early in the course of nephropathy.
4. Potent diuresis (furosemide + metolazone) to manage resistant anasarca in nephrotic stage of nephropathy.
5. Metoclopramide premeal and at bedtime for gastroparesis.
6. Ultrafiltration hemodialysis to control hypertension.
7. Continuous ambulatory peritoneal dialysis (CAPD).
8. Cyclosporine + low-dose prednisone for kidney transplants.
9. Incorporation of podiatric defensive foot care.

and after protein ingestion is induced by glomerulopressin, a liver hormone with a mol wt of less than 500 daltons [6].

If glomerular hyperfiltration is the root cause of glomerulosclerosis in diabetes, then as observed by Alverstrand and Bergström, ". . . it would raise interesting therapeutic possibilities both in chronic renal failure and in diabetes" [6]. Experiments in the induced-diabetic rat, for example, show that establishing euglycemia by islet of Langerhans transplantation or insulin treatment will reduce the GFR and forestall glomerular damage [7]. Unfortunately, no long-term controlled studies of the effect of strict glucose control on glomerular function and structure have been performed in type I diabetic patients. Lacking controlled studies of strict versus "conventional" control of diabetes mellitus, treatment protocols for either preazotemic or uremic diabetics must be based on clinical judgment and intuition rather than syllogistic reasoning from facts. Partisans debating the value of rigorous glucose regulation must interpret skimpy evidence selectively without reaching a firm and defensible conclusion [8, 9].

Adding to the complexity of devising a strategy to prevent macro- and micro-vasculopathy is the observation by Mogensen that not all type I diabetic patients lose renal function at the same rate [10]. From Mogensen's studies, it may be inferred that factors in addition to hyperglycemia contribute to glomerular damage. Those type I diabetic children and young adults followed for seven or more years who will develop renal injury manifest microalbu-

Table 2. Enhanced understanding of pathophysiology of diabetic nephropathy

1. Recognition of early glomerular hyperfiltration.
2. Value of microalbuminuria in predicting later glomerulopathy.
3. Dual injury to glomerular basement membrane (charge + size).
4. Rat glomerulopathy associated with hyperglycemia (corrected by transplant into nondiabetic or by insulin or islets).
5. Appreciation that factors other than duration of diabetes are associated with progression.
6. Discovery that in the rat, and dog, modifications in dietary protein content may alter course of glomerulopathy.
7. Demonstration in type I diabetic patients that reduction of hypertensive pressures slows deterioration.

minuria before azotemia or other evidence of renal damage is apparent. Identification of type I patients who though having a normal or supernormal GFR are nevertheless at high risk of developing nephropathy may prove important to health planners. Proffering intensive glucose control measures such as implantable closed-loop insulin pumps to patients at high risk of microvasculopathy may minimize the overall cost of diabetes care. It has yet to be learned, however, how late after the onset of insulin dependence, glomerulopathy (and retinopathy) may be arrested by careful glucose regulation.

Castells et al underscored a dissociation between functional and morphologic changes in diabetic glomeruli by reporting that kidney biopsy specimens from short-duration type I diabetic adolescents (with normal and supernormal glomerular filtration) evince advanced glomerulosclerosis [11]. It follows that euglycemia regimens begun in patients expressing only "mild" clinical nephropathy may fail to normalize either renal structure or function because extensive irreversible glomerular damage was present at the initiation of tight control.

Lacking the ability to regenerate nephrons with sclerotic glomeruli, there are nevertheless compelling reasons to normalize blood glucose concentrations in diabetic patients who have become uremic. First, type I diabetic patients who use an insulin pump or split insulin doses along with self-monitoring of blood glucose consistently report an admittedly subjective benefit of overall mood and well-being. Furthermore, euglycemic diabetic patients are more likely than poorly regulated diabetic patients to manage intercurrent infections to which they are made susceptible by the immunosuppression of uremia. Second, inferences from studies in induced-diabetic rat kidney transplant recipients suggest that maintaining a euglycemic milieu will protect against the development of glomerulopathy in the allograft [7]. Diabetic glomerulosclerosis, which destroyed the patient's native kidneys, may be preventable in the renal allograft by a tight glucose control program.

Until the controversy over the value of strict glucose regulation in preventing or modifying glomerulopathy is resolved, it seems prudent to base clinical management of the type I diabetic patient on a combination of striving toward euglycemia and control of hypertension. Should it be subsequently learned that glucose regulation has little to do with the genesis of microvasculopathy, then patients subjected to rigorous self-monitoring will have expended time and money for glucose strips without the sought after benefit. They will also have suffered sore finger tips and more frequent hypoglycemic reactions. On the other hand, should the "hyperglycemia-induces-glomerulopathy" argument prove valid [12], patients progressing toward blindness and renal insufficiency under conventional glucose regulation will have been needless casualties in the struggle against a no longer inexorable illness.

Before this decade ends, it is probable that simplified inexpensive measures for diabetes regulation will be devised. By the turn of the century, extensive multicenter studies of strict versus conventional glucose regulation will have been completed. Key questions in diabetes understanding (Table 3) will prove answerable in the next few years. What is certain about the future of diabetes, diabetatologists, and nephrologists, is that incremental advances in patient care will continue. Diabetic nephropathy may well become the first high prevalent cause of renal insufficiency to yield to the new discipline of preventive nephrology.

Table 3. Vital questions in diabetic nephropathy

1. Does nodular or diffuse intercapillary glomerulosclerosis occur in the absence of hyperglycemia?
2. Is hyperglycemia alone sufficient to induce characteristic diabetic glomerulopathy (nodular and diffuse intercapillary glomerulosclerosis)?
3. Will normalization of blood glucose concentration level in diabetic patients prevent or at least retard microvasculopathy?
4. Given the absence of a clear answer to question 3, is it reasonable in 1984 to pursue a regimen of tight glucose control in (a) azotemic diabetics or (b) nonazotemic diabetics?
5. Should discovery mandate that microalbuminuria be construed as an indication for urgent normalization of blood glucose levels in type I diabetic patients?
6. Are inferences drawn from type I diabetes about pathogenesis and timing of therapy applicable to type II diabetes?
7. Does i.p. insulin administration retard rate of progression in terms of microvasculopathy?
8. Given groups of type I diabetic patients matched for severity of illness, can an advantage in terms of survival or morbidity be demonstrated for maintenance hemodialysis, continuous ambulatory peritoneal dialysis, or kidney transplantation?

References

1. FRIEDMAN EA: Planning therapy for diabetic nephropathy. *Diabetic Nephropathy* 3(1):1, 1984
2. SUTHERLAND DER, FRYD CE, GOETZ FC, FERGUSON RM, SIMMONS RL, NAJARIAN JS: Kidney transplantation in diabetics at the University of Minnesota: An analysis of results by era. *Transplant Proc* 15:1110–1113, 1983
3. KJELLSTRAND C, COMTY C, SHAPIRO F: A comparison of dialysis and transplantation in insulin-dependent diabetic patients, in *Diabetic Renal-Retinal Syndrome,* edited by FRIEDMAN EA, L'ESPERANCE FA JR, New York, Grune & Stratton, 1982, vol 2, pp 309–320
4. MOGENSEN CE: Renal functional changes in diabetes. *Diabetes* 25:872–879, 1976
5. BRENNER BM: Hemodynamically mediated glomerular injury and the progressive nature of kidney disease. *Kidney Int* 23:647–655, 1983
6. ALVERSTRAND A, BERGSTROM J: Hypothesis: Glomerular hyperfiltration after protein ingestion, during glucagon infusion, and in insulin-dependent diabetes is induced by a liver hormone. *Lancet* 1:195–197, 1984
7. MAUER SM, STEFFES MW, BROWN DM: The kidney in diabetes. *Am J Med* 20:603–612, 1981
8. CAHILL GF: Diabetic control and complications. *Diabetes Care* 6:310–311, 1983
9. VIBERTI GC, BILOUS RW, MACKINTOSH D, BENDING JJ, KEEN H: Long term correction of hyperglycemia and progression of renal failure in insulin dependent diabetes. *Br Med J* 286:598–602, 1983
10. MOGENSEN CE: Microalbuminuria predicts clinical proteinuria and early mortality in maturity onset diabetes. *N Engl J Med* 310:356–360, 1984
11. CASTELLS S, TEJANI A, NICASTRI A, CHEN CK, FUSI M-A, SEN D: Diabetic nephropathy: Early renal changes in adolescent insulin-dependent diabetics. *Diabetic Nephropathy* 3(1):15–18, 1984
12. FRIEDMAN EA: Diabetic nephropathy is a hyperglycemic glomerulopathy. *Arch Intern Med* 142:1269–1270, 1982

Hypertension

Hypertension: Current Concepts of Mechanisms and Management

Austin E. Doyle

During the last 25 years, there have been major developments in both the management and the concepts relating to the mechanism of hypertension. The term "essential hypertension" was based on what now appears to be a false concept [1]. An early pathologic finding was that arteries or arterioles within the kidney in patients with hypertension showed hyaline changes and narrowing; and, the term "essential hypertension" was used to imply that the rise in blood pressure was essential to maintain tissue and (particularly) renal perfusion. This concept led to the belief that any attempt to reduce blood pressure would be dangerous, because the high blood pressure was an essential response to the underlying disorder that, at that time, was widely supposed to be of renal origin.

Following the introduction of the ganglion blocking drugs in 1950, it became apparent that reducing blood pressure had an extremely favorable impact on the course of severe hypertension. The manifestations of retinopathy resolved, hypertensive heart failure improved, and cerebral hemorrhage became much less common [2]. Moreover, it generally became clear that in the great majority of patients, reduction of blood pressure to almost normal levels was not associated with clinical manifestations of reduced tissue perfusion, such as progressive renal failure or cerebral or cardiac infarction. These findings led to the concept, which was only slowly accepted, that the manifestations of hypertensive vascular disease were, in most cases, the result of the high arterial pressure itself—rather than the high blood pressure being a compensatory and essential response to arterial disease. In recent years, it has been demonstrated that even in mild hypertension, effective antihypertensive therapy can reduce the incidence of cardiovascular complications [3, 4], with the result that a progressively increasing proportion of the population is being considered as needing antihypertensive therapy.

The use of antihypertensive drug therapy thus far has been largely empiric, with the primary aim being to reduce blood pressure, rather than to provide

---

This manuscript was presented as a State-of-the-Art lecture of the same title.

specific therapy directed towards the mechanism of the disease. Rather than being used for specific indications, the use of various antihypertensive drugs (such as diuretics, the angiotensin-converting enzyme inhibitors, or the centrally acting drugs) has advanced knowledge of the mechanisms involved in the pathogenesis of hypertension. In particular, it has become clear that there are many mechanisms that may operate to produce hypertension, and that interference with any of these mechanisms may lead to compensating responses of the others. While it is convenient to discuss the various mechanisms separately, it is important to realize that essential hypertension almost certainly is multifactorial in origin, and it involves the interaction of the numerous control mechanisms concerned, such as the autonomic nervous system, the renin-angiotensin system, the peripheral resistance vessels, and circulating volume. Disturbances in these may be genetic or environmental in origin.

The Resistance Vessels

The smallest arteries or arterioles are vessels with an internal diameter of 20 to 90 μm. They have medial layers of smooth muscle cells arranged concentrically, so that constriction or relaxation of the smooth muscle layer gives rise to corresponding changes in internal diameter. Because resistance to flow is inversely proportional to the caliber, changes in the state of smooth muscle contraction alter resistance to the flow, which is a major determinant of the arterial pressure.

In all forms of hypertension, there is evidence for an increase in total peripheral resistance (TPR), presumably due to excessive shortening of vascular smooth muscle. While this may be due, in some instances, to an excess of vasoconstrictor influences (such as increased levels of either circulating angiotensin or the neurotransmitter norepinephrine), it may be (and probably often is) the result of factors that are present within the arterial wall itself and lead to an abnormally large response to vasoconstrictor influences. Such an increase in vascular reactivity has been found to be present both in human hypertension [5] and in experimental hypertension of various etiologies in animals [6, 7].

There is no doubt that a major factor leading to increased vascular reactivity is hypertrophy of vascular smooth muscle. Folkow [8] has pointed out that hypertrophy of vascular smooth muscle leads to increased wall thickness and to exaggerated luminal changes for given shifts in muscular activity. These changes may be reinforced if the medial hypertrophy induces narrowing of the lumen. Depending on its extent, this structural change in the resistance vessels would provide either a raised or a normal baseline, from which exaggerated luminal narrowing would provide an increased resistance at unchanged levels of vasoconstrictor input. While this concept of structural change provides a satisfactory mechanism for the maintenance and progression of the hypertensive process once initiated, it does not provide a convincing explanation for the initiation of the process—since it is likely that medial hypertrophy and the consequent structural vascular redesign occur mainly as a consequence of the raised blood pressure, rather than an initiating cause. Probably, some other mechanism must provide the stimulus for both the initial rise in blood pressure and the consequent vascular change.

The question as to whether abnormalities in vascular reactivity may also be due to functional—as well as to structural—changes in vascular smooth muscle, therefore, is of considerable importance, since such functional changes could provide an initiating mechanism by preceding rather than following hypertension. In humans, Doyle and Fraser [9] found increased reactivity of forearm blood vessels in the normotensive children of hypertensive parents, which suggests that hyper-reactivity might be an inherited characteristic that preceded the development of hypertension. Similarly, in spontaneously hypertensive rats (SHR), enhanced vascular reactivity can be demonstrated in the prehypertensive phase [10]. Moreover, in some vascular beds, increased reactivity can be demonstrated to some pressor agents, but not to others [10–12]. These observations all lead to the conclusion that a functional change in vascular smooth muscle (in some instances, genetic changes and in others, acquired ones) may cause vascular hyper-reactivity before the development of structural medial hypertrophy. These changes probably initiate hypertension, which in turn leads to the structural vascular change that will reinforce or replace the original disturbance. There are many factors that might be responsible for increased vascular smooth muscle responsiveness. These can be subdivided into disturbances of local hormones, autonomic neurotransmitter availability, and membrane disturbances of vascular smooth muscle itself.

There is considerable evidence for the presence and production of locally active vasoactive substances within arterial smooth muscle. Most, if not all, of the components of the renin-angiotensin system have been found in the arterial wall [13, 14]; there is evidence for conversion of angiotensin I to angiotensin II within vascular tissue [15]. Evidence that increased local levels of angiotensin II exist in hypertensive vascular tissue is not available; however, such a situation would clearly cause vasoconstriction, both directly and via the augmentation of release of norepinephrine from sympathetic nerve endings [16]. There also is considerable evidence that arterial endothelium also can form the potent vasodilator prostacyclin via the release and conversion of arachidonic acid from membrane phospholipids. Interestingly, angiotensin II stimulates prostacyclin release [17]. The presence of these two substances with their opposing actions within vascular tissue strongly suggests that their interaction may be a mechanism that regulates blood flow at a local level. The factors controlling this possible interaction are not yet understood; yet, it may plainly be that the normal equilibrium is shifted to produce excessive contraction in hypertensive arteries. Although such evidence currently available suggests that hypertensive vascular endothelium produces more, rather than less, prostacyclin from exogenous arachidonate [18], it remains possible that a defect in arachidonic acid release from precursor phospholipid exists in hypertension.

The resistance vessels are richly innervated by the sympathetic nervous system. In response to nerve stimulation, norepinephrine is released from nerve terminals by a process of exocytosis into the neural cleft. The released neurotransmitter initiates vascular smooth muscle contraction, and it is either inactivated by local monoamine oxidase or retaken up by the nerve ending. The magnitude of contraction partly depends on the concentration of neurotransmitter reaching the receptor. Augmentation of vascular responses would occur, if release of norepinephrine were augmented or if inactivation or reuptake were impaired. Release of norepinephrine is increased by angiotensin II, and it is also under inhibitory and facilitory influences of the alpha and beta prejunctional receptors, respectively. It has been proposed by Rand et al [19] that epinephrine originally released from the adrenal medulla may be taken up and subsequently released by sympathetic nerve terminals; with the consequence that the released epinephrine may stimulate beta prejunctional receptors, thus inducing a positive feedback release of augmented amounts of neurotransmitter. There is some evidence for an increase in exocytotic release of norepinephrine in both the hypertensive rabbit [20] and the young spontaneously hypertensive rat [21].

In human hypertension, there is evidence that plasma norepinephrine levels are elevated in some patients [22]. Furthermore, plasma norepinephrine levels are reduced by ganglion blocking drugs and by the centrally acting drug, clonidine [23]—observations suggesting that the plasma norepinephrine gives an indication of the amounts of neurotransmitter spilling over into the peripheral circulation following release at sympathetic nerve endings. It is not clear whether the finding of an elevated plasma norepinephrine level is due to increased release or to diminished neuronal reuptake; and, also whether either process represents a defect in local mechanisms or reflects an increased sympathetic tone. The former mechanism might certainly include increased vascular responsiveness.

Finally, there recently has been renewed interest in the possible influence that disturbances in ionic permeability of the membrane of the vascular smooth muscle cell may have inducing changes in vascular reactivity. Over 30 years ago, Tobian and Binnion reported an increased sodium content in vascular tissue in both experimental and human hypertension [24, 25]. Since those early observations, it has become widely accepted that an important determinant of vascular smooth muscle contractility relates to the transmembrane distribution of sodium, potassium and calcium [26]. In the SHR [27] and in desoxycorticosterone (DOC) hypertension [28], there is evidence for an increased inward leak of sodium into vascular smooth muscle cells. Such a leak could be of genetic origin in the SHR. Both DOC and aldosterone induce increases in intracellular sodium [29]. Moreover, most vasoconstrictor agents promote the inward movement of sodium. Friedman [26] has suggested that the increased intracellular sodium stimulates protein synthesis by the vascular smooth muscle, thus leading to medial hypertrophy and structural change. There is also increased synthesis of the Na-K-ATPase, which by increased activity restores intracellular sodium to normal or near-normal levels. The link between increased cellular sodium and increased vascular reactivity has been suggested to occur via a Na^+/Ca^{++} exchange mechanism [30], which would result in increased availability of activator calcium in the intracellular stores. Finally, another mechanism leading to increased intracellular sodium has been proposed by McGregor and de Wardener [31].

This proposal postulates the presence of a circulating natriuretic hormone that operates as an inhibitor of the Na-K-ATPase pump—the secretion of which is favored by sodium retention. This putative material is supposed to induce vascular smooth muscle contraction. In support of this hypothesis, substances with actions resembling cardiac glycosides (which inhibit pump activity) have been found in the plasma of some hypertensive patients.

There recently has been great interest in the natriuretic peptides now termed atriopeptins, which appear to be derived from granular cells contained within the walls of the atria. The precise nature of this material has not been finally established, although several peptides have been identified, each with natriuretic activity [32, 33]; and, at least one has been synthesized [34]. While it seems clear that these substances are natriuretic and while they are postulated to be elaborated as a result of the activity of the volume receptors present within the atria, their other physiologic actions are not yet clear. In particular, the possible effects as inhibitors of Na-K-ATPase and any corresponding effects on vascular smooth muscle responsiveness have not yet been reported. Early data suggest that they are potent vasodilators.

In addition to evidence concerning the increased rate of sodium efflux from vascular smooth muscle, there also is evidence that ^{42}K turnover in aortic smooth muscle cells in SHR is almost twice that of similar cells from WKY rats [35]. The resting potential of smooth muscle cells has been found to be about 6-mv lower in hypertensive cells than in those from WKY [36]. Sodium and potassium turnover rates are linked by the Na-K-ATPase pump, and also by the Na-K-cotransport mechanism [37].

Since the movement of calcium through potentially dependent channels is determined, to an important degree, by the resting potential, changes in monovalent cation fluxes may be a factor leading to increased availability of activator calcium in cell cytoplasm [38].

The question as to whether the $Na^+:C^{++}$ exchange mechanism is of relevance to vascular smooth muscle has been challenged. Postnov [39] has produced evidence that in SHR, calcium binding by membranes is reduced in erythrocytes, adipose tissue, and vascular smooth muscle cells; this has been suggested as being the primary cause of the increased permeability for sodium and potassium ions. More importantly, alterations in intracellular concentration of calcium may be due to adenosine triphosphate-dependent calcium accumulation in mitochondria and cytoplasmic retriculum. It has been claimed by Postnov that in both SHR and essential hypertension in humans, there are defects in membrane control over intracellular calcium concentration. This may act as a primary agent in the pathogenesis of hypertension, since these can be demonstrated in the prehypertensive state [40].

In humans, observations on vascular smooth muscle cell ionic transport are not available. However, studies in human red blood cells have confirmed that there are disturbances in sodium transport in hypertension [41]. Although there are considerable discrepancies between the reported changes in red blood cell transport systems, the balance of evidence suggests that there is an increased intracellular sodium content in red blood cells of hypertensive patients. It remains uncertain whether this is due to a passive leak, to a defect in the Na-K cotransport system [42], or to the presence of a circulating inhibitor of the Na-K-ATPase sodium pump [43, 44]. However, sufficient evidence has been found to suggest that a disturbance in transmembrane sodium transport (perhaps linked to calcium transport) may be pathogenetically important as either a genetic or acquired cause of the increased vascular reactivity found in human hypertension.

The Autonomic Nervous System

In established hypertension in humans, there is very clear evidence that the autonomic nervous system is actively involved in the regulation of the blood pressure to its high level—since hypertensive patients regulate blood pressure as competently as normotensive people in response to factors tending to reduce blood pressure, such as the erect posture or the administration of vasodilator drugs. The response to the upright posture involves reflex vasoconstriction of both resistance and capacitance vessels. Patients given ganglion blocking drugs or patients with autonomic degeneration lose the capacity to adjust blood pressure in response to posture, whereas hypertensive patients can do so without difficulty.

The capacity to regulate blood pressure in hypertension involves resetting the baroceptor reflexes. This resetting occurs within a few days of the onset of hypertension in experimental animals [45, 46], and it can be demonstrated to be present in hypertensive patients [47]. The resetting involves an increase in the threshold blood pressure at which afferent baroreceptor nerve impulses appear in recordings from the carotid sinus or aortic arch. The reflexes are also dependent on the integrity of the coordinating centers in the brainstem, which are responsible for providing a coordinated response of the cardiovascular system [48]. Regardless of whatever the mechanism for baroreceptor resetting may be, it is clear that it can be rapidly reversed following the removal of a single cause of hypertension. For example, following surgical relief of renal artery stenosis, blood pressure falls to normal levels and the regulation of blood pressure to normotensive levels again is achieved within a few hours or days.

Plainly, the autonomic nervous system is actively engaged in the regulation of blood pressure in most forms of hypertension. It is less clear whether hypertension can be initiated by autonomic hyper-reactivity. Baroreceptor denervation certainly causes increased variability of blood pressure without usually causing a sustained rise in blood pressure. While complete destruction of the nucleus of the solitary tract produces severe and fulminating hypertension [49], partial destruction produces increased variability without a sustained increase in blood pressure [50].

There have been recent major advances in understanding the anatomy and function of the medullary centers that regulate blood pressure, and also in the supramedullary centers that provide integrated cardiovascular responses. The nucleus of the solitary tract appears to be the site of the first synapses of the baroreflex nerves [51]. This nucleus gives projections to groups of noradrenergic and adrenergic cell bodies within the pons and medulla.

Recent evidence suggests that the adrenergic groups of cells at the pontine medullary junction may be a major efferent pathway for cardiovascular responses [52]. There also are numerous connections between the medullary and suprabulbar centers, notably the hypothalamus, basal ganglia, limbic system, and cerebral cortex [53]. It seems likely that inputs from the cerebral cortex or limbic system may influence baroreceptor reflexes, and it may also have the capacity to stimulate the cardiovascular system to initiate hypertension [48].

In experimental animals, psychosocial stress has been reported to induce hypertension in mice; operant conditioning to painful or unpleasant stimuli is followed by hypertension in the squirrel monkey. There seems to be strong evidence that in the SHR, there is evidence of increased autonomic activity early in the hypertensive process. Direct evidence of increased sympathetic nerve firing rates have been found in these animals [54]. The SHR kept in social isolation have lower blood pressures than those reared in a conventional manner [55]. There is some evidence to suggest that autonomic factors may also be responsible for human hypertension in some instances. Borderline hypertension in humans is characterized by an elevated cardiac output [56, 57] and by a hemodynamic pattern similar to that seen in the defense reaction, with increases in cardiac output and muscle blood flow accompanied by renal and splanchnic vasoconstriction [58]. There is some evidence from long-term follow-up studies that these early changes are followed by the later development of persistent hypertension with an increased peripheral resistance. Both these findings and the pharmacologic effectiveness of drugs that act via autonomic mechanisms certainly suggest that in many instances, the autonomic nervous system may initiate essential hypertension. The natural history of essential hypertension in humans reveals that in many instances, higher than average blood pressures have been recorded for many years. There is no doubt that in normal people, blood pressure is very variable, and that rises in blood pressure occur in response to pain, anxiety, and probably to other factors [59]. It is not certain whether rises in blood pressure induced by autonomic factors are larger in individuals who are genetically prone to hypertension. If they are, it is not difficult to envision a situation in which repeated rises in blood pressure might induce progressive changes in vascular reactivity, with progressively larger responses. Sooner or later, baroreceptor resetting would raise the level to which pressure was regulated. Whether this pattern, in fact, does occur as a cause of hypertension is not clear.

The Kidney and Hypertension

The kidney has been traditionally regarded as central to the problem of hypertension. From the clinical point of view, almost all types of chronic renal disease are associated with hypertension; and, from the experimental viewpoint, the classic experiments of Goldblatt [60] demonstrated conclusively that interference with renal blood supply is a predictable cause of experimental hypertension. Thus, there is no doubt about the capacity of the kidney to initiate hypertension. However, the mechanisms involved are certainly not finally resolved; in particular, it is not yet established whether or in what way the kidney is concerned with the pathogenesis of essential human hypertension.

The discovery of the renin-angiotensin system by Page [61] and by Braun-Menendez [62] in 1939 seemed to have solved the problem of the pathogenesis of renal hypertension; yet, it now seems clear that the original idea that circulating angiotensin II might cause hypertension by causing a vasoconstriction of peripheral blood vessels is unlikely to be true, except in malignant hypertension and in renovascular hypertension. In essential hypertension, plasma renin activity (PRA) has a wider range than in normotensive subjects, and the mean value in hypertensive subjects is somewhat lower [63]. While about 25% of hypertensive patients have renin values below the normal range, their arbitrary division into low-, normal-, and high-renin group has doubtful validity [64]. Plasma renin levels fall with age, both in normotensive and hypertensive subjects [65]. Although few studies of angiotensin II levels have been reported, most hypertensive subjects have values within the normal range [66]. Patients with renal artery stenosis often have elevated PRA, but many have levels within the normal range [67]. In the Goldblatt 2-kidney 1-clip model in the rat, PRA is not always elevated in hypertensive animals [68]. Plasma renin activity and angiotensin levels are commonly raised in malignant (accelerated) hypertension, but this often is associated with hyponatremia polyuria and weight loss; and, the activation of the renin-angiotensin system seems likely to be due, at least in part, to sodium loss in this syndrome [69]. From these findings, it would seem unlikely that the renin-angiotensin system is actively involved in the pathogenesis of essential hypertension. However, although the angiotensin receptor blocking drug, saralasin, rarely reduces blood pressure in patients unless they have marked elevation of PRA [70], angiotensin-converting enzyme inhibitors often do [71]. This finding suggests that the renin-angiotensin system may be playing a pathogenetic role in essential hypertension in a more subtle way than via the direct vasoconstricting effects of angiotensin II on the peripheral circulation.

The renin-angiotensin system has an important physiologic role in the regulation of sodium and water balance. Both sodium depletion and hemorrhage stimulate renin release, with the consequent production of angiotensin II. During hypovolemic stimuli, this system mediates a complex series of responses consisting of arteriolar and venous constriction, stimulation of aldosterone production, and stimulation of centers in the hypothalamic area that result in thirst and increased water intake.

In addition to these actions, there is a strong probability that the renin-angiotensin system has important actions within the kidney; thus, it may be operating as a local intrarenal hormone. This local action is almost certainly concerned with the regulation of renal vascular resistance, and there also is evidence for angiotensin having important effects on the regulation of sodium excretion [72]. With the possible exception of renin substrate, all the components of the renin-angiotensin system are present within the kidney. Preformed angiotensin can be extracted from the kidney in very large amounts [73].

Moreover, micropuncture studies of renin levels within the efferent arteriole suggest that factors causing renin release lead to the release of renin and perhaps angiotensin, into renal interstitial tissue, rather than into the efferent arteriole [74]. This suggests that the intrarenal effects of this system often are of greater importance than the remote circulatory effects.

In normal animals, angiotensin II causes both a fall in renal sodium excretion and a rise in renal vascular resistance [74]. Chronic low-dose angiotensin infusion in dogs causes a marked shift to the right in the renal sodium excretion/blood pressure relationship, which implies that higher levels of blood pressure are required to establish equilibrium between salt and water intake and output [75]. There also is evidence for an angiotensin-mediated renal vasoconstriction in the renal circulation of the kidney—the artery to which has been clipped. This vasoconstriction can be blocked by angiotensin-converting enzyme inhibitors, and these agents induce a natriuresis. This vasoconstriction distal to the clip appears to provide a mechanism for the preservation of glomerular filtration rate (GFR) in the presence of reduced renal arterial pressure; and, it additionally promotes sodium and water reabsorption from the ischemic kidney [76].

An early manifestation of essential hypertension is an increase in the filtration fraction, which is a reduced renal blood flow (RBF) with a normal GFR. The reduced RBF is most likely due to constriction of the efferent arteriole. This raises the possibility that a selective vasoconstriction of the renal efferent arterioles may be an initiating factor in essential hypertension [77]. This type of selective vasoconstriction might be due to changes in reactivity to constrictor stimuli. It is also possible that there may be a local disturbance of the renin-angiotensin system within the kidney, causing increased renal vascular resistance with a consequent shift in the relationship between renal sodium excretion and blood pressure. The recent finding of high concentrations of angiotensin II-specific receptors within the vasa recta [78] would be consistent with a possible role of angiotensin as a mediator of RBF. Finally, there also is evidence that both renal vascular resistance and renal sodium excretion can be influenced by the autonomic nervous system [79], so that these changes could be initiated primarily by the central nervous system. There is also evidence that structural change in the renal blood vessels, secondary to hypertension, may be an important sustaining mechanism. For example, in the two-kidney rat model, blood vessels within the clipped kidney (which are protected from the high pressure) remain structurally normal. Removal of both the clip and contralateral kidney restores blood pressure to normal levels. Removal of the clipped kidney, leaving the contralateral kidney as the sole remaining renal tissue, does not restore blood pressure to normal levels; this is due presumably to the presence of structural changes of the arteries of the clipped kidney that have been exposed to the raised pressure [80].

Therefore, it seems likely that an abnormal constriction of the renal vasculature could lead to essential hypertension. Indeed, as Guyton et al [81] have pointed out, a resetting of the relationship between blood pressure and sodium excretion probably is essential for the development of hypertension.

Further evidence that the kidney is essential for the development of hypertension has been provided by evidence from the transplantation of kidneys between normotensive and hypertensive rats. In the Dahl salt-sensitive strain of rats, initial experiments using parabiosis suggested that genetic factors were responsible for the effects of the kidney in producing hypertension. Rats of the resistant (R) and sensitive (S) strains were joined in parabiosis, after which one rat was nephrectomized. When the S partner was nephrectomized, blood pressure failed to rise when a high-sodium diet was fed, but it did so when the R partner was nephrectomized [82]. Furthermore, in the absence of nephrectomy, a high-sodium diet induced hypertension that occurred first in the R rat [83]. These studies indicate that an agent-inducing hypertension produced by a kidney from an S rat, or requiring a functioning S kidney, was transmitted across the parabiotic junction.

In transplantation experiments in rats on low-sodium diets, R rats had kidneys that retarded the development of hypertension, while kidneys transplanted from S to R rats induced hypertension. The results were much less clear-cut when the recipients received high-sodium diets—a discrepancy attributed to "subclinical rejection" as a result of the anoxia induced by the procedure [84].

More clear-cut, although less dramatic, changes along the same lines were reported by Bianchi et al using the Milan hypertensive strain of rats (MHS) and normotensive rats (NR) [85]. Kidney cross-transplantation between adult rats of both strains demonstrated that the recipients of MHS kidneys had significantly higher pressures than those receiving NR kidneys. A major problem in interpreting these studies arises from the fact that kidneys from the hypertensive animals might well exhibit acquired vascular changes as a result of the hypertension, rather than due to purely genetic factors. This possibility has been partly excluded by later studies in the MHS strain, in which cross-transplantation was performed at the early age of 1 month, when there was little or no difference in blood pressure levels between the two strains [86].

Even though these studies emphasize the primacy of the kidney in inducing hypertension, they leave the mechanism uncertain. Tobian [87] was able to demonstrate a marked shift in the pressure: natriuresis ratio in the two strains of Dahl rats, to the degree that S rats excreted much less sodium than R rats for any given level of inflow pressure.

It may well be that due to either local vascular abnormality within the kidney or other unknown factors, there is a defective capacity for excreting sodium in these hypertensive animals. Such a situation would be consistent with many clinical situations.

There is a great deal of evidence supporting the concept that factors leading to impaired sodium excretion regularly cause hypertension. Anephric patients or animals often show marked rises in blood pressure as sodium intake is increased; similar changes occur in patients with chronic renal failure [88]. Both excess secretion of aldosterone or the administration of deoxycorticosterone acetate (DOCA) regularly induce hypertension that seems to be dependent on sodium retention. It is not unreasonable to suggest that, in most instances, renal hypertension represents a situation where due to a loss of renal tissue, abnormal sodium-retaining influences, or vascular disturbances within the kidney, sodium excretion becomes difficult—except at high arterial perfusion pressure. In a few instances, which usually are related to sodium depletion, the extra renal effects of the renin-angiotensin system are involved.

Concepts of Management

During the past 30 years, ideas about the treatment of hypertension have evolved from a nihilistic approach through agreement about the need for treatment of life-threatening complications of severe hypertension; now, they have evolved to the current situation, in which the treatment of even mildly raised blood pressure is widely perceived to be an appropriate measure for preventing the early onset of cardiovascular disease. To a very important extent, this evolution of the concept of appropriate management has resulted from the availability of improved drugs. An important additional factor has been the demonstration of efficacy. In these days of the almost universal belief in the indispensibility of the controlled therapeutic trial, it is interesting to realize that the widespread acceptance of the desirability of reducing blood pressure preceded, by some years, the first controlled demonstration of its efficacy. Early studies by Smirk 1951 [89] and McMichael 1975 [90] concentrated largely on the effects within malignant (accelerated) hypertension. Smirk reported as early as 1951, on the basis of open studies, the resolution of retinopathy, relief of congestive heart failure, and reduced incidence of cerebral hemorrhage. The first partly successful attempt at a controlled therapeutic trial was reported by Hamilton in 1964 [91]; however, it was the classic Veteran's Administration Cooperative Studies [92, 93], published between 1967 to 1970, that finally established the efficacy of antihypertensive drug treatment. For mild hypertension, acceptable evidence was delayed until the Australian Therapeutic Trial [3] and the Hypertension Detection and Followup Program (HDFP) [4] reported their results in 1980.

Nevertheless, the early studies established some important and enduring concepts; notably, that reduction of blood pressure improved the clinical manifestations and appeared not to cause ischemic complications. Other notable concepts that have persisted were the synergistic effects of drugs of different types, such as the ganglion blocking drugs, with reserpine [94] and the diuretics [95]. From this observation arose the principle of combining different types of drugs to reduce adverse effects, which remains the basis of the so-called "stepped-care" approach. From what is known of the pathogenesis of hypertension, it is obvious that attempts to devise specific methods of management for hypertensive patients will prove to be difficult. In the great majority of patients, hypertension is multifactorial. Since the final common pathway appears to be constriction of the resistance vessels, the use of drugs that specifically relax vascular smooth muscle (such as hydralazine, minoxidil, or nifedipine) might seem logical as first therapeutic agents. Unfortunately, as is well known, the use of vasodilating drugs provokes reflex tachycardia and fluid retention, because the vasodilatation is opposed by an increased response of both the antonomic nervous system and the regulators of body fluid volume. The simultaneous use of beta-blocking drugs and diuretics are needed to block these responses to vasodilating drugs.

Since sodium retention is widely considered as playing an important role in the pathogenesis of hypertension, diuretic drugs might also appear to be a logical monotherapeutic agent. As with the vasodilating drugs, however, attempts to induce sodium depletion usually induce compensatory changes. The most common of these is stimulation of the renin-angiotensin system and the secretion of aldosterone, which limit the antihypertensive response and also lead to hypokalemia. These compensating responses can be blocked by the concurrent administration of angiotensin-converting enzyme inhibiting drugs, or less reliably, by beta-blocking drugs.

Sodium and water retention are two of the most common responses to the administration of antihypertensive drugs; they lead to the development of "false tolerance," [96] with a progressive diminution of the antihypertensive response. This reaction particularly occurs in response to the peripherally or centrally acting drugs that interfere with autonomic mechanisms. This compensatory response can be blocked by small doses of diuretic drugs.

These compensatory responses make it very difficult to establish pathogenetic features, which indicate specific forms of treatment. The measurement of PRA in relation to urinary sodium excretion—the so-called renin-profiling method—has been advocated as a means by which the most effective therapy can be selected for any particular individual [97]. While it is generally true that very high levels of PRA usually are associated with sodium-losing states, and markedly suppressed renin levels are associated with mineralocorticoid hypertension, these situations are rather uncommon; in the great majority of patients, plasma renin levels are not markedly different from those in normal patients. Treatment with diuretics commonly induces a rise in PRA, which (as mentioned above) then increases the sensitivity to specific inhibitors of the renin-angiotensin system. Perhaps the most controversial aspect of the renin-profiling method is the idea that high-renin patients respond specifically well to beta-adrenoceptor drugs. While in some cases—particularly in renal failure—such patients do respond well to the very small doses required to reduce PRA, much larger doses are required in most instances. Moreover, as discussed above, many patients with low-to-normal PRA respond adequately to both angiotensin-converting enzyme inhibitors and beta-blocking drugs.

Furthermore, the desirability of treating patients with a single drug (rather than several) has not been established. The practical advantages of administering a single tablet, rather than two or more types of tablets, to patients are not well documented. It has been claimed that simplification may improve patient compliance in following the drug regimen. While there is considerable evidence that failure by patients to take their medication is a major problem in managing hypertension [98], there is (unfortunately) little evidence that any of the available measures solves this problem, including reduction of tablet numbers. Nevertheless, combination tablets are widely prescribed, particularly beta-adrenoceptor blocking drugs and a diuretic. An alternative approach is the synthesis of drugs with combined actions such as labetalol, which combines alpha- and beta-blocking properties.

For the last 15 years, at least in Europe, the most widely used regimen has been the combined use of diuretic and beta-adrenoceptor blocking drugs, with the addition of vasodilating drugs such as hydralazine or (more recently) prazosin when necessary. However, the recent development of newer types of drugs seems to be changing this practice. In mild hypertension, the angiotensin-converting enzyme inhibitors combined with diuretics seem to be effective antihypertensive drugs in most patients [99]. While they probably are little, if any more, effective as are the beta blockers in mild hypertension, they induce a fall—rather than a rise—in peripheral vascular resistance, do not block exercise-induced tachycardia, and seem better tolerated by most patients than the beta blockers. However, the differences are not decisive.

It is particularly interesting that the angiotensin-converting enzyme inhibitors are often effective in the absence of any evidence of raised PRA in both humans and animals. In the SHR, which is not a high-renin hypertensive model, angiotensin-converting enzyme inhibition induces a slow fall of blood pressure over several hours—in distinction to the very rapid blockade of plasma-converting enzyme inhibition and in contrast to their very rapid effects in animals with high PRA and peripheral angiotensin levels [100]. Similarly, in humans, although angiotensin-converting enzyme inhibitors do not reduce blood pressure in primary aldosteronism, they do so in patients with essential hypertension [101]. It is very tempting to conclude that these drugs reduce blood pressure by inducing selective renal vasodilatation because of the intrarenal action of angiotensin in mediating this. If this indeed is their mode of action, they may be reversing a fundamental defect in pathogenesis. It also raises the possibility that the antihypertensive action of the beta-blocking drugs, which has never really been adequately explained, may similarly operate to reduce the intrarenal effects of angiotensin that is locally released as a result of activity of the sympathetic nervous system.

An alternative possibility is that angiotensin-converting enzyme inhibitors may be acting via mechanisms operating within the autonomic nervous system [102]. There is much evidence for the actions of angiotensin in the control of drinking behavior [103]; and, centrally administered captopril reduces blood pressure in the SHR [104]. It is possible, but as yet not proven, that the brain renin-angiotensin system may play an important pathogenetic role in hypertension.

Calcium channel-blocking drugs are composed of two main types. Verapamil and gallapomil are moderately powerful vasodilating drugs, but they have a major action at the sinoatrial node. Probably as a result of this action, reflex tachycardia and fluid retention are not major features of their action. In clinical trials, these drugs have proven to be about as effective as beta-blocking drugs [105, 106]; and, like angiotensin-converting enzyme inhibitors, they induce vasodilatation with little effect on exercise tolerance. Apart from inducing constipation, these drugs are well tolerated. The dihydropridine drugs, of which nifedipine is the prototype, are very powerful vasodilators with little, if any, effect on cardiac muscle in the doses that are used clinically.

Like other vasodilators, they induce tachycardia, sometimes raise plasma renin, and induce edema. They probably are best used in combination with beta-blocking drugs [107].

Since these drugs apparently act at vascular smooth muscle levels by inhibiting the entry of calcium into the smooth muscle cell, they also may be interfering with a specific pathogenetic mechanism. In particular, they may be reversing the increased vascular reactivity, which is doubtlessly a potent maintaining factor in hypertension; evidence of this is not yet available. However, in spontaneously hypertensive rats, these drugs do not reduce blood pressure in the early phases; but, they do so in the later stages [108], which suggests that they may, (in effect) be antagonizing the increased vascular responses due to structural smooth muscle hypertrophy.

Perhaps the most interesting antihypertensive drug yet produced is the centrally acting drug, clonidine. It appears to act via an alpha-adrenergic agonist effect on the medullary control centers [109], is much more effective in reducing blood pressure in hypertensive humans or animals than in normotensive ones, and induces large falls in blood pressure without an orthostatic effect and without major disturbances of cardiovascular-regulating responses. It often is effective without other drugs. The major problems relate to its often severe side effects of sedation and dryness of the mouth, which appear to be dose-related. Discontinuation of therapy, often even temporarily, may induce rebound hypertension of quite marked severity. Recent studies suggest that this latter effect may be due to its alpha-1 agonistic properties, whereas the antihypertensive action is predominantly an alpha-2 effect. Interesting new prototypes of clonidine-like drugs are now being synthesized that hold considerable promise for the future.

Finally, a matter of major importance in the treatment of hypertension is the relationship between hypertension and atheromatous vascular disease. There is no doubt that effective reduction of blood pressure reduces the incidence of cerebral hemorrhage, congestive heart failure, and malignant hypertension—all of which are directly caused by high blood pressure. By contrast, atherosclerotic complications, particularly myocardial infarction, are much less dramatically (if at all) reduced in frequency. This may be partly due to multiple factors being responsible for atheroma. On the other hand, the demonstration that secondary recurrence of myocardial infarction is substantially reduced by beta-adrenoceptor blocking drugs raises the possibility that these drugs have a cardioprotective effect, even in the absence of hypertension. There is presently no evidence that these drugs have a specific role in the primary prevention of myocardial infarction in hypertensive patients. However, if this should prove to be the case, this would provide a decisive reason for the continued use of these drugs.

A present source of some anxiety is the possibility that some metabolic effects of diuretics may have contributed to the failure of most studies to demonstrate a conclusive reduction in the incidence of complications of ischemic heart disease. Some degree of hypokalemia is a common consequence of the administration of most diuretics. This is certainly dose-related; however, even with the small doses used in Europe and Australia, hypokalemia is frequently observed. The major anxiety raised by this is the possibility of the development of arrhythmias and sudden death. There is no doubt that hypokalemia following myocardial infarction is associated with an increased incidence of tachyarrhythmias. Interestingly, not all hypokalemia is drug-related, but much of it is. The possibility that diuretic-induced hypolakemia may cause sudden death is a real one; however, hypertension and ischemic heart disease also cause sudden death, and any association with diuretic drugs may well be hidden by the underlying disease process.

Other metabolic effects are common, such as interference with glucose tolerance, elevation of serum uric acid, the occurrence of gout, and elevation of serum cholesterol. While the relationship between these effects and ischemic heart disease is not definitively established in hypertension, the possibility certainly is present.

Nevertheless, diuretic drugs remain extremely valuable agents in antihypertensive drug treatment. While they need to be used in the smallest effective doses with close monitoring of their metabolic side effects, the present evidence does not justify abandoning their wide use in the treatment of hypertension.

Summary and Conclusions

Essential hypertension is a complex disorder that involves disturbances in autonomic regulation, vascular smooth muscle, and regulatory mechanisms of body fluid volume.

The pathogenetic mix of these factors varies from patient to patient, and in individuals from time to time.

Interference with any single control mechanism usually leads to compensatory stimulation of other mechanisms.

It is probable that in the majority of instances, the primary abnormality is in the nervous system; however, there is also evidence that the process sometimes can be predominantly renal in origin. Management of hypertension is directed towards reduction of blood pressure, because high blood pressure seems to cause many of the vascular complications characteristic of the illness. In most instances, drugs that interfere with a single mechanism have proven to be less effective than combinations of drugs that block several mechanisms.

Knowledge of the pharmacology of antihypertensive drugs and observations of their effects in both human and experimental hypertension have contributed greatly to concepts of both pathogenesis and treatment.

References

1. GULL WR, SUTTON HC: On the pathology of the morbid state commonly called chronic Bright's disease with contracted kidney. *Med Chir Trans* 55:273–326, 1872
2. SMIRK FH: Results of methonium treatment of hypertensive patients. Based on 250 cases treated for periods up to 3½ years including 28 with malignant hypertension. *Br Med J* 1:717–723, 1954

3. REPORT OF THE MANAGEMENT COMMITTEE: The Australian therapeutic trial in mild hypertension. *Lancet* 1:1261–1267, 1980

4. HYPERTENSION DETECTION AND FOLLOW-UP PROGRAM COOPERATIVE STUDY GROUP: Five year findings of the hypertension detection and follow up program. Reduction in mortality of persons with high blood pressure, including mild hypertension. *JAMA* 242:2562–2571, 1979

5. DOYLE AE, FRASER JRE, MARSHALL RJ: Reactivity of forearm vessels to vasoconstrictor substances in hypertensive and normotensive subjects. *Clin Sci* 18:441–454, 1959

6. HINKE JAM: In vitro demonstration of vascular hyperresponsiveness in experimental hypertension. *Circ Res* 17:359–371, 1965

7. McQUEEN EG: Vascular reactivity in experimental renal and renoprival hypertension. *Clin Sci* 15:523–532, 1956

8. FOLKOW B: Cardiovascular structural adaptation: Its role in the initiation and maintenance of primary hypertension. The fourth Volhard lecture. *Clin Sci Mol Med* 55(Suppl):3s–22s, 1978

9. DOYLE AE, FRASER JRE: Essential hypertension and inheritance of vascular reactivity. *Lancet* 2:509–511, 1961

10. BERECEK KH, SWERTSCHLAG V, GROSS F: Alterations in renal vascular resistance and reactivity in spontaneous hypertension of rats. *Am J Physiol* 238:H287–H293, 1980

11. LAIS LT, BRODY MJ: Mechanism of vascular hyperresponsiveness in the spontaneously hypertensive rat. *Circ Res* 36(Suppl 1):1-216–1-222, 1975

12. McGREGOR DD, SMIRK FH: Vascular responses to 5-hydroxy-tryptamine in genetic and renal hypertensive rats. *Am J Physiol* 219:687–690, 1970

13. GOULD AB, SKEGGS LT, KAHN JR: The presence of renin activity in blood vessel walls. *J Exp Med* 119:389–399, 1964

14. GANTEN D, HAYDUCK K, BRECHT MH, BOUCHER R, GENEST J: Evidence of renin release or production in splanchnic territory. *Nature* 226:551–552, 1970

15. AIKEN JW, VANE JR: Inhibition of converting enzyme of the renin angiotensin system in kidneys and hindlegs of dogs. *Circ Res* 30:263–273, 1972

16. VANHOUTTE PM, WEBB RC, COLLIS MC: Pre and post junctional adrenergic mechanisms and hypertension. *Clin Sci* 59:211s–223s, 1980

17. DUSTING GJ, MULLENS EM, NOLAN RD: Prostacyclin (PGI_2) release accompanying angiotensin conversion in rat mesentery. *Eur J Pharmacol* 70:129–137, 1981

18. DUSTING GJ, DAVIES W, DRYSDALE T, DOYLE AE: Increased conversion of arachidonic acid to vasodilator prostanoids in spontaneously hypertensive rats. *Clin Exp Pharmacol Physiol* 8:435–440, 1981

19. MAJEWSKI H, TUNG LH, RAND MJ: Adrenaline induced hypertension in rats. *J Cardiovasc Pharmacol* 3:179–185, 1981

20. BEVAN RD, PURDY RE, SU C, BEVAN JA: Evidence for an increase in adrenergic nerve function in blood vessels from experimental hypertensive rabbits. *Circ Res* 37:503–508, 1975

21. WEBB RC, VANHOUTTE PM, BOHR DF: Adrenergic transmission in vascular smooth muscle from spontaneously hypertensive rats. *Hypertension* 3:93–103, 1981

22. deQUATTRO V, CHANG S: Raised plasma catecholamines in some patients with primary hypertension. *Lancet* 1:806–809, 1972

23. LOUIS WJ, DOYLE AE, ANAVEKAR SN: Plasma norepinephrine levels in essential hypertension. *N Engl J Med* 288:599–601, 1973

24. TOBIAN L, BINNION JT: Tissue cations and water in arterial hypertension. *Circulation* 5:754–758, 1952

25. TOBIAN L, BINNION JT: Arterial wall electrolytes in renal and DOC hypertension. *J Clin Invest* 33:1407–1414, 1954
26. FRIEDMAN SM: The transmembrane distribution of sodium, potassium and water in vascular smooth muscle and the hormonal regulation of vascular tone and reactivity, in *The Role of Salt in Cardiovascular Hypertension,* edited by FREGLY M, KARE M, New York, Academic Press, 1982
27. FRIEDMAN SM: Evidence for enhanced sodium transport in the tail artery of the spontaneously hypertensive rat. *Hypertension* 1:572–582, 1979
28. FRIEDMAN SM, NAKASHIMA N: Evidence for enhanced Na transport in hypertension induced by DOCA in the rat. *Can J Physiol Pharmacol* 56:1029–1035, 1978
29. FRIEDMAN SM: Evidence for an enhanced transmembrane Na^+ gradient induced by aldosterone in the incubated rat tail artery. *Hypertension* 4:230–237, 1982
30. BLAUSTEIN MP: Sodium ions, calcium ions, blood pressure regulation and hypertension: A reassessment and hypothesis. *Am J Physiol* 323:C165–C173, 1977
31. McGREGOR GA, DEWARDENER HE: Is a circulating sodium transport inhibitor involved in the pathogenesis of essential hypertension? *Clin Exp Hypertension* 3:815–830, 1981
32. THIBAULT G, GARCIA R, CAUTIN M, GENEST J: Atrial natriuretic factor: Characterization and partial purification. *Hypertension* 5(Suppl I):1-75–1-80, 1983
33. CURRIE MG, GELLER DM, COLE BR, SIEGEL NR, FOK KF, ADAMS SP, EUBANKS SR, GALLUP GR, NEEDLEMAN P: Purification and sequence analysis of bioactive atrial peptides (Atripeptins). *Science* 222:67–69, 1984
34. WINQVIST RJ: Characterization of synthetic atrial natriuretic factor: Vasodilator-profile and decreased vascular sensitivity in hypertensive rats. *Proc 10th Int Soc Hypertension,* in press
35. JONES AW: Altered ion transport in vascular smooth muscle from spontaneously hypertensive rats. Influences of aldosterone norepinephrine and angiotensin. *Circ Res* 33:563–572, 1973
36. HERMSMEYER K: Cellular basis for increased sensitivity of vascular smooth muscle in spontaneously hypertensive rats. *Circ Res* 38(Suppl II):II-53–II-57, 1976
37. WILEY JS, COOPER RA: A furosemide-sensitive cotransport of sodium plus potassium in the human red cell. *J Clin Invest* 53:745–755, 1974
38. BOHR DF, SEIDEL C, SOBIESKI J: Possible role of sodium-calcium pumps in tension development of vascular smooth muscle. *Microvasc Res* 1:335–343, 1969
39. POSTNOV YV, ORLOV SN, POKUDIN NI: Alteration of the intracellular calcium pool of adipose tissue in spontaneously hypertensive rats. No effect of peripheral immunosympathectomy. *Pflügers Arch* 390:256–259, 1981
40. POSTNOV YV, ORLOV SN: Alteration of cell membranes in primary hypertension, in *Hypertension, Pathophysiology and Treatment* (2 ed), edited by GENEST J, KUCHEL O, HAMET P, CAUTIN P, New York, McGraw-Hill, 1983, pp 95–108
41. LOSS H, WEHMEYER H, WESSELS F: Der wasser und Elektrolytgehalt von Erthrozyten bei arterieller Hypertonie. *Klin Wochenschr* 38:393–395, 1960
42. GARAY RP, DAGHER C, PERNOLLET M-G, DEVYNK MA, MEYER P: Inherited defect in a Na^+K^+ co-transport system in erythrocytes from essential hypertensive patients. *Nature* 284:281–283, 1980
43. POSTON L, JONES RB, RICHARDSON PJ, HILTON PJ: The effect of antihypertensive therapy on abnormal leucocyte sodium transport in essential hypertension. *Clin Exp Hypertension* 3:693–701, 1981
44. MORGAN T, MYERS J, FITZGIBBON W: Sodium intake, blood pressure and red cell sodium efflux. *Clin Exp Hypertension* 3:641–653, 1981

45. McCubbin JW, Green JH, Page IH: Baroreceptor function in chronic renal hypertension. *Circ Res* 4:205–210. 1956
46. Angel-James JE: Characteristics of single aortic and right subclavian baroreceptor fiber activity in rabbits with chronic renal hypertension. *Circ Res* 32:149–161, 1973
47. Mancia G, Ludbrook J, Ferrari A, Gregorini L, Zanchetti A: Baroreceptor reflexes in human hypertension. *Circ Res* 43:170–177, 1978
48. Korner PI: Integrative neural cardiovascular control. *Physiol Rev* 51:321–367, 1971
49. Doba N, Reis DJ: Acute fulminating neurogenic hypertension produced by brainstem lesions in the rat. *Circ Res* 32:584–593, 1973
50. Nathan MA, Reis DJ: Chronic labile hypertension produced by lesions of the nucleus tractus solitarrii in the cat. *Circ Res* 40:72–81, 1977
51. Muira M, Reis DJ: Termination and secondary projections of carotid sinus nerve in the cat brain stem. *Am J Physiol* 217:142–153, 1969
52. Reis DJ: Biochemical neuroanatomy of blood pressure control. *Hypertension,* in press
53. Gebber GL, Snyder DW: Hypothalamic control of baroreceptor reflexes. *Am J Physiol* 218:124–131, 1970
54. Judy WV, Farrell SK: Arterial baroreceptor reflex control of sympathetic nerve activity in the spontaneously hypertensive rat. *Hypertension* 1:605–614, 1979
55. Hallback M: Consequence of social isolation on blood pressure, cardiovascular reactivity and design in spontaneously hypertensive rats. *Acta Physiol Scand* 93:455–465, 1975
56. Julius S, Schark MA: Borderline hypertension—a critical review. *J Chronic Dis* 23:723–754, 1971
57. Lund-Johansen P: Haemodynamics in essential hypertension. *Clin Sci* 59(Suppl):343S–354S, 1980
58. Hilton SM: Hypothalamic control of the cardiovascular responses in fear and rage. *Lect Sci Basis Med* 8:217–238, 1976
59. Mancia G: Methods for assessing blood pressure values in humans. *Hypertension* 5(Suppl III):III-5–III-11, 1983
60. Goldblatt H, Lynch J, Hanzal RF, Summerville WW: Studies on experimental hypertension. 1. The production of persistent elevation of systolic blood pressure by means of renal ischemia. *J Exp Med* 59:347–379, 1934
61. Page IH, Helmer OM: A crystalline pressor substance, angiotonin, result from reaction of renin and renin activator. *J Exp Med* 71:29–42, 1940
62. Braun-Menendez E, Fasciolo JC: Accion vasoconstrictora e hipertensora de la sangre venosa del rinon en isquenianicompleta agnda. *Rev Soc Argent Biol* 15:161–172, 1939
63. Brown JJ, Davies DL, Level AF, Robertson JIS: Plasma renin concentration in human hypertension: Renin in relation to aetiology. *Br Med J* 2:1215–1219, 1965
64. Doyle AE, Jerums G: Sodium balance, plasma renin and aldosterone in hypertension. *Circ Res* 26, 27(Suppl II):267–275, 1971
65. Tuck M, Williams GH, Cain JP, Sullivan DM, Dluby RG: Relation of age, diastolic pressure and known duration of hypertension to the presence of low renin hypertension. *Am J Cardiol* 32:637–642, 1973
66. Catt KJ, Cran E, Zimmet PZ, Best JB, Cain MD, Coghlan JP: Angiotensin blood levels in human hypertension. *Lancet* 1:459–463, 1971

67. BROWN JJ, DAVIES DL, LEVER AF, ROBERTSON JIS: Variations in plasma renin concentration in several physiological and pathological states. *Can Med Assoc J* 90:201–206, 1964

68. MACDONALD GJ, BOYD GW, PEART WS: Effect of the angiotensin II blocker 1-sar-8-Ala-angiotensin II on renal artery clip hypertension in the rat. *Circ Res* 37:640–646, 1975

69. MOHRING J, MOHRING B, NAUMANN HJ, PHILLIPI A, HOMSY E, ORTH H, DAUDA G, KAZDA S, GROSS F: Salt and water balance and renin activity on renal hypertension of rats. *Am J Physiol* 228:1847–1855, 1975

70. CASE DB, WALLACE JM, KEVIN HJ, SEALEY JE, LARAGH JH: Usefulness and limitations of saralasin, a partial competitive agonist of angiotensin II, for evaluating the renin and sodium factors in hypertensive patients. *Am J Med* 60:825–836, 1976

71. GAVRAS H, WEBER B, GAVRAS I, BIOLLAS J, BRUNNER HR, DAVIES RO: Antihypertensive effects of the new oral angiotensin converting enzyme inhibitor, "MK421." *Lancet* 2:543–546, 1981

72. THURAU K: Intra renal action of angiotensin, in *Angiotensin,* edited by PAGE IH, BUMPUS FM, Berlin, Springer-Verlag, 1974, pp 475–489

73. MENDELSOHN FAO: A method for measurement of angiotensin II in tissues and its application to rat kidney. *Clin Sci Mol Med* 51:111–125, 1976

74. LOUIS WJ, DOYLE AE: The effects of varying doses of angiotensin on renal function and blood pressure in man and dogs. *Clin Sci* 29:489–504, 1965

75. DECLUE JW, COLEMAN TG, COWLEY AW, MCCAA RE, GUYTON AC: Influence of angiotensin II (AII) on the long term renal excretion of sodium (abstract). *Fed Proc* 35:397, 1976

76. ANDERSON WP, KORNER PI, JOHNSTON CI: Acute angiotensin II mediated restoration of distal renal artery pressure in renal artery stenosis and its relationship to the development of sustained one kidney hypertension in conscious dogs. *Hypertension* 1:292–298, 1979

77. HOLLENBERG NK, BORUCKI LJ, ADAMS DF: The renal vasculature in early essential hypertension. Evidence for a pathogenetic role. *Medicine* 57:167–178, 1978

78. MENDELSOHN FAO, AGINLERA G, SAAVEDRA JM, GUIRUM R, CATT KT: Characteristics and regulation of angiotensin II receptors in pituitary, circumventricular organs and kidney. *Clin Exp Hypertension* A57, 8:1081–1097, 1983

79. OSBORN JL, HOLDAAS H, THAMES MD, DIBONA GF: Renal adrenoceptor mediation of anti-natriuretic and renin secretion responses to low frequency renal neurostimulation in the dog. *Circ Res* 53:298–305, 1983

80. TAKATA Y, DOYLE AE: Effect of DOCA-salt on angiotensin dependency and surgical reversal of hypertension in two-kidney, one-clip renal hypertensive rats. *J Hypertension* 1:57–63, 1983

81. GUYTON AC, COLEMAN TG, COWLEY AW, MANNING RD, NORMAN RA, FERGUSON JD: A systems analysis approach to understanding long range arterial blood pressure control and hypertension. *Circ Res* 23:479–491, 1968

82. IWAI J, KNUDSEN KD, DAHL LK, HEINE M, LEITL G: Genetic influences on the development of hypertension in parabiotic rats: Evidence for a humoral factor. *J Exp Med* 129:507–522, 1969

83. KNUDSEN KD, IWAI J, HEINE M, LEITL G, DAHL LK: Genetic influences on the development of hypertension in parabiotic rats: Evidence that a humoral hypertensinogenic factor is produced in kidney tissue of hypertension-prone rats. *J Exp Med* 130:1353–1363, 1969

84. DAHL LK, HEINE M, THOMPSON K: Genetic influence of the kidneys on blood pressure: Evidence from chronic renal homografts in rats with opposite predispositions to hypertension. *Circ Res* 34:94–101, 1974

85. BIANCHI G, FOX U, DIFRANCESCO DF, GIAVONETTI AM, PAGETTI D: Blood pressure changes produced by kidney cross-transplantation between spontaneously hypertensive rats and normotensive rats. *Clin Sci Mol Med* 47:435–448, 1974

86. FOX U, BIANCHI G: Primary role of the kidney in causing the blood pressure difference between the Milan hypertensive strain (MHS) and normotensive rats. *Clin Exp Pharmacol Physiol* 3(Suppl 7):71–74, 1976

87. TOBIAN L JR: Viewpoint concerning the enigma of hypertension. *Am J Med* 52:595–609, 1972

88. MORGAN TO: in *Pharmacological and Therapeutic Aspects of Hypertension* (vol 1), edited by DOYLE AE, MENDELSOHN FAO, MORGAN TO, Boca Raton, Florida, CRC Press, 1980

89. SMIRK FH, ALSTAD KS: Treatment of arterial hypertension by penta- and hexamethonium salts based on 150 tests on hypertensives of varied aetiology and 53 patients treated for periods of two to fourteen months. *Br Med J* 1:1217–1228, 1951

90. MCMICHAEL J, MURPHY EA: Methonium treatment of severe and malignant hypertension. *J Chronic Dis* 1:527–535, 1955

91. HAMILTON M, THOMPSON EN, WISNIEWSKI TKM: The role of blood pressure control in preventing complications of hypertension. *Lancet* 1:235–238, 1964

92. VETERAN'S ADMINISTRATION COOPERATIVE STUDY GROUP ON ANTIHYPERTENSIVE AGENTS: Effects of treatment on morbidity in hypertension: I. Results in patients with diastolic blood pressures averaging 115 through 129 mmHg. *JAMA* 202:1028–1034, 1967

93. VETERAN'S ADMINISTRATION COOPERATIVE STUDY GROUP ON ANTIHYPERTENSIVE AGENTS: Effects of treatment on morbidity in hypertension: II. Results in patients with diastolic blood pressures averaging 90 through 114 mmHg. *JAMA* 213:1143–1152, 1970

94. DOYLE AE, MCQUEEN EG, SMIRK FH: Treatment of hypertension with reserpine, with reserpine in combination with pentapyrrollodinium, and with reserpine in combination with veratrum alkaloids. *Circulation* 11:170–181, 1955

95. FREIS ED: Acute antihypertensive effects of chlorothiazide. *Am J Cardiol* 8:880–883, 1961

96. GERBER JC, NIES AS: in *Hypertension, Pathophysiology and Treatment* (2 ed), edited by GENEST J, KUCHEL O, HAMET P, CAUTIN M, New York, McGraw-Hill 1983, pp 1093–1126

97. LARAGH JH: Personal views on the mechanisms of hypertension, in *Hypertension, Pathophysiology and Treatment* (2 ed), edited by GENEST J, KUCHEL O, HAMET P, CAUTIN M, New York, McGraw-Hill 1983, pp 615–631

98. SACKETT DL, HAYNES RB, GIBSON ES, HACKETT B, TAYLOR DW, ROBERTS RS, JOHNSON AL: Randomized clinical trial of strategies for improving medication compliance in primary hypertension. *Lancet* 1:1205–1207, 1975

99. BRUNNER HR, GAVRAS H, WAEBER B, TEXTOR SL, TURINI CA, WARTERS JP: Clinical use of an orally acting converting enzyme inhibitor, Captopril. *Hypertension* 2:558–566, 1980

100. TAKATA Y, DINICOLANTONIO R, MENDELSOHN FAO, HUTCHINSON JS, DOYLE AE: A comparison of the activity of the angiotensin converting enzyme inhibitors SQ14225, SA446 and MK421. *Clin Exp Pharmacol Physiol* 10:131–145, 1983

101. VETERAN'S ADMINISTRATION COOPERATIVE STUDY GROUP ON ANTIHYPERTENSIVE AGENTS: Low-dose captopril for the treatment of mild to moderate hypertension. *Hypertension* 5(Suppl III):III-139–III-144, 1983
102. SEVERS WB, DANIELS-SEVERS AE: Effects of angiotensin on the central nervous system. *Pharmacol Rev* 25:413–449, 1973
103. DINICOLANTONIO R, MENDELSOHN FAO, HUTCHINSON JS: Central angiotensin converting enzyme blockade and thirst. *Pharmacol Biochem Behav* 18:731–735, 1983
104. HUTCHINSON JS, MENDELSOHN FAO, DOYLE AE: Blood pressure responses of conscious normotensive and spontaneously hypertensive rats to intracerebroventricular and peripheral administration of captopril. *Hypertension* 2:546–559, 1980
105. LEONETTI G, PASOTTI C, PERRARI GP, ZANCHETTI A: Double blind comparison of the antihypertensive effects of verapamil and propranolol, in *Calcium Antagonism in Cardiovascular Therapy*, edited by ZANCHETTI A, KRIKLER DM, Amsterdam, Excerpta Medica, 1981, pp 260–263
106. DOYLE AE: Comparison of beta-adrenergic blockers and calcium antagonists in hypertension. *Hypertension* 5(Suppl II):II-103–II-108, 1983
107. LEDERBALLE PEDERSON O, CHRISTENSEN CK, MIKKELSEN E, RAMSCH KD: Relationship between the antihypertensive effect and steady state plasma concentration of nifedipine given alone or in combination with a beta-adrenoceptor blocking agent. *Eur J Clin Pharmacol* 18:287–293, 1980
108. TAKATA Y, HOWES LG, HUTCHINSON JS: Antihypertensive effect of diltiazem in young or adult rats of genetically hypertensive strains. *Clin Exp Hypertension Theory Prac* A5:455–468, 1983
109. KOBINGER W: Central alpha adrenergic systems as targets for antihypertensive drugs. *Rev Physiol Biochem Pharmacol* 81:40–100, 1978

Effect of Dietary Fish Oils on Eicosanoid Formation in Platelets, Neutrophils, and the Cardiovascular-Renal System

Peter C. Weber, Sven Fischer, Reinhard Lorenz, Thomas Strasser, Clemens von Schacky, and Wolfgang Siess

Many physiologic and pathophysiologic reactions (such as vascular resistance, thrombosis, wound healing, inflammation, and allergy) are modulated by oxygenated metabolites of arachidonic acid and related polyunsaturated fatty acids that are collectively termed eicosanoids. These compounds include prostaglandins, prostacyclin, thromboxane, leukotrienes, and hydroxylated derivatives of arachidonic acid. In the kidney, which is a rich source of eicosanoid-synthesizing and degrading enzymes [1, 2], these mediators modulate a variety of processes that include the release of renin [3], vascular and tubular responses to peptide hormones [4–6], glomerular filtration and renal electrolyte handling [7, 8]—as well as hemodynamic and inflammatory responses to immunologic [9] and mechanical [10] stimuli.

Dietary Fatty Acids and Eicosanoid Formation

Thromboxane, prostaglandins, prostacyclin, and leukotrienes are all synthesized from essential fatty acids that must be provided in the diet [11]; production of eicosanoids is controlled by cellular mechanisms for the uptake, release, and oxygenation of the eicosanoid precursor fatty acids. Interference with eicosanoid synthesis is the basis for many therapeutic agents, including antihypertensives and diuretics, anti-inflammatory drugs, and antithrombotic agents. However, a change of eicosanoid production and eicosanoid-dependent cellular functions also may be achieved by altering eicosanoid precursor availability. Under our Western dietary conditions, arachidonic acid (AA, C20:4w6) is by far the dominant precursor fatty acid of biologically highly active eicosanoids of the two series. The major source of AA in our food chain is linoleic acid (C18:2w6). At variance with fatty acids of the linoleic or w-6 family in terrestrial animals and in most plant seeds—which are the major sources

---

This manuscript was presented as part of a Symposium on *Prostaglandins and the Kidney.*

of our eicosanoid precursor fatty acids—the fatty acids of the linolenic or w-3 family predominate in green leaves and especially in marine lipids [12].

Effects of w-3 Polyunsaturated Eicosanoid Precursor Fatty Acids

Several independent lines of evidence suggest that changes in the natural history of hypertensive, atherothrombotic, and inflammatory disorders may be achieved by altering the eicosanoid precursor availability. Native Greenland Eskimos [13] and Japanese fishermen [14] have a high dietary intake of long-chain w-3 polyunsaturated fatty acids obtained from seafood and have a low incidence of myocardial infarction, even when compared with their westernized ethnic counterparts. Diets containing w-3 polyunsaturated fatty acids reduce the severity of experimental cerebral [15] and myocardial [16] infarction, and they protect NZB $\times$ NZW F_1 mice from developing autoimmune nephritis [17].

We have evaluated in humans the effects of diets enriched with w-3 polyunsaturated fatty acids on plasma and cellular fatty acid composition, platelet function and thromboxane formation, blood pressure control, kidney function, urinary prostanoid excretion, prostacyclin synthesis, and leukotriene formation—to determine if these factors could be favorably influenced by changes in dietary fatty acids.

Substitution of w-6 Polyunsaturated Fatty Acid by Dietary w-3 Polyunsaturated Fatty Acids

In 1980, we demonstrated that it is possible to induce, in Caucasians, less reactive platelets and reduced formation of proaggregatory and vasoconstrictive thromboxane A_2 (TXA_2) via substituting mackerel (which is a rich source of w-3 polyunsaturated fatty acids) as the sole source of their dietary fat [18]. In plasma and platelet membrane phospholipids, w-3 fatty acids increased at the expense of w-6 fatty acids, thus inducing an "Eskimo-like" pattern of fatty acids that is characterized by a low content of AA (C20:4w6) and a high content of eicosapentaenoic acid (EPA) (C20:5w3). The results suggested that both the decrease of AA in platelet membranes and the reduction in its release and metabolism to proaggregatory TXA_2 might be a mechanism by which the EPA-enriched diet reduced platelet aggregability.

Supplementation of Western Diet with w-3 Polyunsaturated Fatty Acids

In a subsequent study [19], the Western diet (which almost exclusively supplies w-6 polyunsaturated fatty acids) was supplemented with 40 ml/d of cod liver oil, providing about 4 to 5 g of EPA and about 5 to 6 g of docosahexaenoic acid (DHA, C22:6w3)—the other major w-3 polyunsaturated fatty acid in marine lipids. Both EPA and DHA were incorporated in platelet and erythrocyte membrane phospholipids at the expense of the w-6 polyunsaturated fatty acids, C18:2w6 and C20:4w6. Bleeding time increased ($P < 0.001$) platelet count ($P < 0.05$) and platelet aggregation on adenosine diphosphate and collagen ($P < 0.01$ to 0.05) decreased and associated TXB_2 formation ($P < 0.01$). Blood pressure ($P < 0.05$) and pressure response to both norepinephrine ($P < 0$ to 0.01) and angiotensin II (not significant) fell without major changes in plasma catecholamines and red blood cell cation fluxes, but with slight decreases in renin, urinary aldosterone, kallikrein, and prostaglandins E_2 and $F_{2\alpha}$. Biochemical and functional changes were reversed 4 weeks after cessation of the fish oil supplement. Both formation of prostaglandins derived from EPA and interference of EPA with formation and action of prostaglandins derived from AA were evident in vitro. The conclusion was that this moderate supplement of w-3 polyunsaturated fatty acids markedly changed membrane phospholipids and prostanoid formation; and, it was associated with a shift towards less reactive platelets and a blunted circulatory response to pressor hormones.

Formation of Eicosanoids of the Three Series After Diets Enriched with Eicosapentaenoic Acid

Previous in vitro experiments had shown that TXA_3 derived from C20:5w3 (EPA) is not proaggregatory and is not vasoconstrictive, as is the potent TXA_2 derived from C20:4w6 (AA). By contrast, prostaglandin I_3 (PGI_3) derived from EPA is as antiaggregatory as PGI_2 derived from AA [20]. Therefore, a shift of prostanoid formation from the dienoic to the trienoic series may have changed the TXA/PGI balance in our dietary studies, resulting in a less thrombogenic state and in reduced blood pressure. In addition, EPA-derived leukotriene B_5 (LTB_5) is one order of magnitude less chemotactic than LTB_4 derived from AA [21]; and, leukotriene C_5 (LTC_5) is less active than LTC_4 in constricting smooth muscle cells [22]. Therefore, a diet enriched with C20:5w3 may also modify the contribution of leukotrienes in the cellular responses to inflammatory and immune reactions.

Thus, although dietary manipulation of eicosanoid formation seemed to be an attractive approach, it had been uncertain whether trienoic eicosanoids are indeed formed from dietary EPA in vivo in humans.

Therefore, we studied this question in detail. We found that less active TXA_3 is formed ex vivo in human platelets after dietary enrichment with EPA [23]. In parallel, the formation of TXA_2 was diminished, as was the content of AA in membrane phospholipids and the aggregability of platelets.

We then demonstrated [24] that the major urinary metabolite of endogenous prostaglandin I_3 (PGI_3) is present in subjects that have ingested either cod liver oil ($\sim 4g$ EPA/d) or mackerel (~ 10 to 15 g EPA/d). It is important to note that in these dietary studies, formation of PGI_2 was not reduced, as evidenced by an unchanged or even increased excretion rate of its major urinary metabolite. This finding indicates that in the endothelial cell (or other cells responsible for the in vivo formation of PGI_3 and PGI_2), EPA obviously does not impair the release and cyclo-oxygenation of AA to PGI_2. This observation contrasts with the findings in platelets, where dietary EPA reduced the ex vivo formation of TXA_2 from endogenous AA.

Finally, we also demonstrated [25] that LTB_5 is easily formed by human neutrophils, in addition to LTB_4, after dietary supplementation of cod liver oil ($\sim$ 4g EPA/d) to an otherwise unchanged Western diet.

These results prove that it is possible, in humans, to change the spectrum of biologically highly active eicosanoids by nutritional means and to alter it into a favorable direction. This may be a mechanism by which diets enriched with w-3 polyunsaturated fatty acids can induce a lower blood pressure, less reactive platelets, and blunt inflammatory and immunologic reactions. We suggest that the supplementation of w-6 eicosanoid precursor fatty acids prevailing in our Western nutrition with w-3 eicosanoid precursor fatty acids may represent a fresh approach in evaluating processes related to eicosanoid formation and eicosanoid-modulated cellular functions, including hypertension, atherothrombosis, and inflammatory and immunologic reactions.

References

1. LARSSON C, ÄNGGÅRD E: Regional differences in the formation and metabolism of prostaglandins in the rabbit kidney. *Eur J Pharmacol* 25:326–332, 1973
2. FOLKERT VW, SCHLÖNDORFF D: Prostaglandin synthesis in isolated glomeruli. *Prostaglandin* 17:79–86, 1979
3. WEBER PC, LARSSON C, ÄNGGÅRD E, HAMBERG M, COREY EJ, NICOLAOU KC, SAMUELSSON B: Stimulation of renin release from rabbit renal cortex by arachidonic acid and prostaglandin endoperoxides. *Circ Res* 39:868–874, 1976
4. MCGIFF JC, MALIK KU, TERRAGNO NA: Prostaglandins as determinants of vascular reactivity. *Fed Proc* 35:2382–2387, 1976
5. KIRSCHENBAUM KM, LOWE AG, TRIZNA W, FINE LG: Regulation of vasopressin action by prostaglandins. *J Clin Invest* 70:1193–1204, 1982
6. SCHOR N, ICHIKAWA I, BRENNER BM: Mechanism of actions of various hormones and vasoactive substances on glomerular ultrafiltration in the rat. *Kidney Int* 20:442–451, 1981
7. SCHNERMANN J, BRIGGS JP, WEBER PC: Tubuloglomerular feedback, prostaglandins and angiotensin in the autoregulation of glomerular filtration rate. *Kidney Int* 25:53–64, 1984
8. WEBER PC, LARSSON C, SCHERER B: Prostaglandin E_2 9-keto-reductase as a mediator of salt intake-related prostaglandin-renin interaction. *Nature* 266:65–66, 1977
9. LIANOS EA, ANDRES GA, DUNN MJ: Glomerular prostaglandin and thromboxane synthesis in rat nephrotoxic serum nephritis. *J Clin Invest* 72:1439–1448, 1983
10. MORRISON AR, NISHIKAWA K, NEEDLEMAN P: Unmasking of thromboxane A_2 synthesis by ureter obstruction in the rabbit kidney. *Nature* 269:259–260, 1977
11. CRAWFORD MA: Background to essential fatty acids and their prostanoid derivatives. *Bri Med Bull* 39:210–213, 1983

12. TINOCO J: Dietary requirements and functions of α-linolenic acid in animals. *Prog Lipid Res* 21:1–45, 1982

13. DYERBERG J, BANG HO: Haemostatic function and platelet polyunsaturated fatty acids in Eskimos. *Lancet* II:433–435, 1979

14. HIRAI A, HAMAZAKI T, TERANO T, NISHIKAWA T, TAMURA Y, KUMAGAI A, SAJIKI J: Eicosapentaenoic acid and platelet function in Japanese. *Lancet* II:1132–1133, 1980

15. BLACK KL, CULP B, MADISON D, RANDALL OS, LANDS WEM: The protective effects of dietary fish oil on focal cerebral infarction. *Prostaglandins Leukotrienes Med* 5:257–268, 1979

16. CULP BR, LANDS WEM, LUCCHESI BR, PITT B, ROMSON J: The effect of dietary supplementation of fish oil on experimental myocardial infarction. *Prostaglandins* 20:1021–1031, 1980

17. PRICKETT JD, ROBINSON DR, STEINBERG AD: Dietary enrichment with the polyunsaturated fatty acid eicosapentaenoic acid prevents proteinuria and prolongs survival in NZB $\times$ NZW F_1 mice. *J Clin Invest* 68:556–559, 1981

18. SIESS W, ROTH P, SCHERER B, KURZMANN I, BÖHLIG B, WEBER PC: Platelet-membrane fatty acids, platelet aggregation, and thromboxane formation during a mackerel diet. *Lancet* 1:441–444, 1980

19. LORENZ R, SPENGLER U, FISCHER S, DUHM J, WEBER PC: Platelet function, thromboxane formation and blood pressure control during supplementation of the Western diet with cod liver oil. *Circulation* 67:504–511, 1983

20. NEEDLEMAN P, RAZ A, MINKES MS, FERRENDELLI JA, SPRECHER H: Triene prostaglandins: Prostacyclin and thromboxane biosynthesis and unique biological properties. *Proc Natl Acad Sci USA* 76:944–948, 1979

21. GOLDMAN DW, PICKETT WC, GOETZL EJ: Human neutrophil chemotactic and degranulating activities of leukotriene B_5 (LTB$_5$) derived from eicosapentaenoic acid. *Biochem Biophys Res Commun* 117:282–288, 1983

22. HAMMARSTRÖM S: Leukotriene C_5: A slow reacting substance derived from eicosapentaenoic acid. *J Biol Chem* 255:7093–7094, 1980

23. FISCHER S, WEBER PC: Thromboxane A_3 (TXA$_3$) is formed in human platelets after dietary eicosapentaenoic acid (C20:5w3). *Biochem Biophys Res Commun* 116:1091–1099, 1983

24. FISCHER S, WEBER PC: Prostaglandin I_3 is formed in vivo in man after dietary eicosapentaenoic acid. *Nature* 307:165–166, 1984

25. STRASSER T, FISCHER S, WEBER PC: Leukotriene B_5 (LTB$_5$) is formed in human peripheral polymorphonuclear neutrophils (PMN) after dietary eicosapentaenoic acid (EPA) (*abstract*). *Washington Spring Symposium,* 1984

Calcium, Phosphate, and Parathyroid Hormone in Blood Pressure Regulation

Chairpersons: David A. McCarron and Kai Lau
Discussants: Roger L. Niser, Lawrence Resnick, Vito Campese, Johannes Mann, and David Bushinsky

This workshop addressed current issues surrounding calcium, phosphate, and parathyroid hormone (PTH) metabolism in blood pressure regulation. The intent of the workshop was to draw upon the experience of investigators currently involved in research addressing the individual effects of these factors on blood pressure control and their relation to other nutrient and hormonal factors. The discussion of current data was highlighted by the complex interactions among: (1) the disturbances in calcium metabolism in hypertension; (2) the effect of modification of calcium balance on blood pressure; (3) the cardiovascular actions of PTH; and (4) the relation of these factors to, and the influence of, alterations in hormones and ions closely related to calcium and PTH. In the final segment, the implication of these observations to the therapy of high blood pressure was assessed.

The data presented and the discussion that is summarized represent the current state of this expanding area of clinical and basic investigation. Because of the multifaceted relations among calcium, phosphorus, magnesium, sodium, PTH, vitamin D, catecholamines, and prostaglandins, it is apparent that fruitful investigative work will follow in the future. The results of those investigative efforts will potentially provide additional therapeutic modalities for the management of hypertension in humans.

Calcium

Vascular Smooth Muscle Etiology

The ion calcium is critical for the normal regulation of the vascular smooth muscle cell. Calcium is an essential factor in the initiation of contraction,

---

This is the summary of a Workshop of the same title.

producing increased peripheral resistance and ultimately an increase in blood pressure. Calcium affects vasoconstriction via its transmembrane influx, inducing the release of sarcoplasmic reticulum calcium and activating myosin light-chain kinase, the enzyme that mediates crossbridge linking of the contractile proteins actin and myosin. Equally as important, though less well appreciated, is the fact that calcium also serves to regulate factors that mediate relaxation of vascular tissue. This includes a membrane-stabilization or inhibition of calcium fluxes by calcium itself. In addition, calcium, in association with calmodulin, induces a phosphorylation of myosin light-chain kinase, which reduces that enzyme's activity by 10- to 1000-fold. The enzyme's ability to catalyze the actin and myosin interaction in thereby inhibited. The permeability of the cell membrane to calcium appears to be a critical factor in the cation's initiation of contraction. Conversely, the cation's ability to stabilize and down-regulate its own fluxes is critical to this regulation of vasorelaxation.

Calcium is also a factor in stimulating the synthesis and release of circulating vasoconstrictors and vasodilators. The ion is a cofactor in the binding of circulating vasoactive substances to the sarcolemmal membrane. Additionally, calcium modifies intravascular volume and thereby blood pressure regulation via direct effects upon the heart and cardiac output and the kidney through regulation of glomerular filtration and sodium and water reabsorption.

Calcium Disturbances in Human and Experimental Hypertension

Disordered calcium metabolism has been characterized in a variety of ways in both human and experimental hypertension. These include reductions in extracellular ionized calcium, enhanced secretion of parathyroid hormone, increased urinary calcium excretion, altered intestinal calcium transport, and increased intracellular platelet calcium. In vascular tissue, primary disorders of calcium binding, transport, and sequestration have also been reported. More recent observations suggest that Ca-ATPase activity of red blood cells (RBCs) in humans with hypertension is suppressed. This suppression of pump activity is, in part, independent of observed variations in either Na-K-ATPase activity or Mg-ATPase activity. The low ionized calcium values encountered in human hypertension follow the renin and sodium status of the subjects. Low renin and high urinary sodium in human hypertension is associated with low ionized calcium values. To the degree that increased sodium intake suppresses serum calcium, the greater will be the antihypertensive effect of modifying calcium intake.

Blood Pressure Response to Calcium Modification

Acute Hypercalcemia

The infusion of calcium acutely causes blood pressure to rise in animals and humans. This increase in blood pressure is associated with the magnitude of the PTH suppression that is induced. Parathyroidectomized animals that are infused with calcium do not experience a rise in blood pressure. These collective observations suggest that the pressor response to acute hypercalcemia is, in part, dependent upon the suppression of the endogenous peptide vasodilator, PTH.

Chronic Hypercalcemia

The long-term administration of calcium to experimental animals lowers blood pressure. This reduction in blood pressure is observed in both parathyroid-intact and parathyroidectomized animals. In humans, the administration of calcium lowers both systolic and diastolic blood pressure. This has been confirmed in trials of oral calcium supplementation for periods lasting 8 to 26 weeks. The greatest impact appears to be on systolic blood pressure. Older age and female gender are associated with a greater response. Likewise, greater urinary sodium excretion and greater degrees of pretreatment suppression of ionized calcium are also associated with a greater reduction in blood pressure with oral calcium. These observations are in agreement with several reports characterizing low-calcium dietary intake as a predictor of blood pressure status in the United States. Greater calcium intake is associated with a lower mean arterial pressure and a reduction in an individual's risk of being hypertensive for her or his peer group.

The chronic administration of calcium to animals is associated with an increase in plasma volume concurrent with the reduction in blood pressure. Calcium's primary systemic hemodynamic effect appears to be direct vasodilation without a significant effect on cardiac output. Long-term net sodium balance, as measured by exchangeable sodium ions, is affected by the administration of calcium, as exchangeable sodium increases following chronic increased ingestion of calcium.

Interrelation of Ionized Calcium and PTH with Phosphorus, Magnesium, and Sodium

Phosphorus

Phosphorus disorders have been implicated in human hypertension. Serum phosphorus has been noted to be depressed in both humans and animals. Paradoxically, the induction of chronic phosphorus depletion is associated with a reduction in blood pressure. This appears to be primarily an alteration in energy metabolism directly adversely modifying cardiac output. Conversely, the parenteral administration of phosphorus to animals who are chronically receiving supplemental dietary calcium reverses the antihypertensive effect of calcium. This pressor effect of phosphorus has not been shown with dietary manipulations of phosphorus.

Magnesium

The relation of magnesium metabolism to blood pressure regulation has been suggested from earlier observations that noted higher serum magnesium values in subjects with high blood pressure. Intracellular magnesium values are low in hypertensive patients. This is the converse of the findings with calcium, when increases in intracellular platelet free calcium have been documented in the setting of low extracellular calcium concentrations.

The provision of magnesium to mature spontaneously hypertensive rats (SHR) does not lower blood pressure. The magnesium supplementation, however, does blunt the vasoconstrictive response to acutely infused angiotensin II. This, too, is in contrast to calcium in this animal model where chronic calcium loading significantly reduces blood pressure. In humans, short-term administration of magnesium has been associated with a reduction in blood pressure in hypertensive patients with higher ionized calcium values and high renin levels. The failure of chronic magnesium supplementation to lower the SHR's blood pressure may, in part, reflect concurrent alterations in calcium and phosphate balance induced by these diets.

Sodium

Sodium metabolism appears to be an additional ionic cofactor important in mediating calcium and parathyroid hormone's cardiovascular actions. Increased sodium ingestion in humans predicts a better blood pressure response to oral calcium administration. The lower plasma renin values are, that is, the greater one's urinary sodium excretion, the more likely a positive blood pressure response to calcium administration will occur.

Na-K-ATPase activity has been implicated as a primary membrane defect in human hypertension. In a carefully characterized group of hypertensive and normal persons, membrane Na-K-ATPase activity did not differ between the two groups. However, an increase in Na-K-ATPase activity during calcium supplementation was predictive of a beneficial blood pressure response. Those individuals who lower their blood pressure more on oral calcium have exhibited a greater increase in Na-K-ATPase activity. This suggests an effect of oral calcium loading on Na-K-ATPase activity that has been identified as being reduced in selected hypertensive subjects.

Consistent with these observations is the animal's antihypertensive response to oral calcium when sodium status is modified concurrently. Both spontaneously hypertensive rats (SHR) and their genetic control, the Wistar-Kyoto rat (WKY), lower their blood pressures to a greater degree when provided with supplemental dietary sodium. These observations are consistent with population studies that indicate that higher sodium intakes are associated with lower mean arterial pressures in the United States. Conversely, reduced dietary sodium intake patterns are associated with higher blood pressures. This is a relation that is similar to that observed between lower calcium intake and higher blood pressure in adult Americans.

Parathyroid Hormone

Cardiovascular Effect

The calcium-regulating hormone, PTH, has acute vasodilating properties in laboratory animals. PTH's rapid reduction in blood pressure in both normotensive and hypertensive animals is independent of the animal's endogenous PTH status. The acute blood pressure reduction is observed in both PTH-intact and PTX SHRs and WKYs. The vasodilating effect of PTH is dependent upon the animal's calcium and sodium status. Calcium- and sodium-loaded animals experience a greater reduction in blood pressure than do calcium- and sodium-restricted animals.

Blood Pressure Response to Parathyroidectomy

The induction of a hypoparathyroid state in laboratory animals is associated with an increase in mean arterial pressure. This only occurs if adequate calcium repletion is achieved. Parathyroidectomized rats also experience an antihypertensive response to oral calcium loading, though the magnitude of the blood pressure reduction may be diminished.

Modifiers of PTH's Cardiovascular Effects

PTH antagonizes the vasoconstrictor response to endogenous compounds such as norepinephrine and AII. The administration of the calcium-binding protein (calmodulin) inhibitor, trifluoperazine (stelazine), will blunt the antihypertensive effect of PTH in the spontaneously hypertensive rat.

PTH exerts a direct vasodilating action on the vascular smooth muscle cell. This induction of smooth muscle relaxation is dependent, in part, upon induction of prostaglandin-related metabolic pathways. The incubation of vascular tissue with PTH is associated with a decrease in vascular smooth muscle cyclic AMP content. Similar to the animal observations, this in vitro effect of PTH on cyclic AMP, when the peptide is incubated with vascular smooth muscle cells, is also inhibited by the calmodulin antagonist trifluoperazine (stelazine).

Other Calcium-regulating Hormones

Vitamin D metabolism is also modified in humans and experimental animals with high blood pressure. Lower vitamin D levels are associated with higher arterial pressures in both humans and animals. Correction of vitamin D levels in short-term studies of humans results in modest improvements in blood pressure control.

Calcitonin levels, in contrast, are elevated in human hypertension. Patients treated with calcium and experiencing a reduction in blood pressure also have lower circulating calcitonin levels. The acute effect of calcitonin on blood pressure in animals in unknown.

Renin, while not considered a calcium-regulating hormone, has an important interface with calcium metabolism and human hypertension. A decreased calcium status, as manifested by reduced ionized calcium values, and an increased PTH level are associated with suppression of the renin axis. The administration of calcium with a concurrent improvement in blood pressure is associated with the normalization of a patient's renin status. In contrast, the greater the degree of renin suppression that occurs with sodium loading, the greater the adverse impact on calcium metabolism and greater the degree of blood pressure increase observed. These observations suggest that "salt-sensitive" hypertension is, in part, a reflection of impaired calcium homeostasis. Correction of the calcium metabolism, rather than reduction in sodium intake, is associated with the optimal blood pressure response.

Implications for Therapy

Diuretics

Thiazide diuretic drugs have a well-established impact on calcium metabolism. While these drugs lower urinary calcium excretion, recent observations have documented that intestinal calcium absorption is probably decreased reciprocally by chronic thiazide administration. This does not rule out a modest and undetectable increase in calcium accumulation in osseous and nonosseous tissue. In contrast, furosemide increases urinary calcium excretion. Current data indicate that intestinal absorption of calcium is increased in furosemide-treated patients. These two diuretics have opposing effects upon urinary calcium excretion and intestinal absorption of the cation. The possibility that thiazide's chronic antihypertensive effects are related to improvement of human calcium balance remains unproven. It is an intriguing possibility, particularly in light of thiazides' greater efficacy compared to that of furosemide.

Calcium Antagonists

The introduction of calcium antagonists has added to the pharmacologic therapy of hypertensive patients, particularly the elderly and those with marked increases in systolic levels. The calcium antagonists lower blood pressure by a direct vasodilating action. This is, in a large part, secondary to the ability of these compounds to reduce calcium entry into vascular smooth muscle cells, thereby reducing the vasoconstrictive response. Data presented suggest that the calcium antagonist nifedipine is maximally effective in the calcium-depleted animal. This observation is consistent with the finding that calcium depletion enhances membrane permeability to the cation and thereby increase smooth muscle tone and resistance.

Diet

The observation that dietary calcium is decreased in humans with high blood pressure and the recent documentation that provision of additional calcium in the diet to a level within the recommendations of the National Academy of Science has obvious therapeutic implications. The protection of calcium intake and calcium metabolism should be a goal of both physicians and patients involved in the treatment of human hypertension. It is possible that correction of deficient calcium intake will, in part, ameliorate the "salt-sensitive" hypertensive population if the observations presented in this workshop are correct. In addition, other vasodilating antihypertensive agents may be more effective when there is improved calcium intake. This would include compounds whose modes of action share common pathways with that of PTH, a potent vasodilator whose action is calcium dependent.

Summary

This Workshop provided current insights into the roles of calcium, phosphorus, and PTH in blood pressure regulation. The basis for this Workshop represents a body of research that spans less than 5 years of reported investigations. There is an emerging, and substantive body of data that indicates that divalent ion metabolism, and hormones related to these ions, are critical factors in the pathogenesis and therapy of human hypertension. Protection of calcium balance appears to lower blood pressure. Factors that adversely impact upon calcium status are associated with an increase in blood pressure. Hormones associated with protection of calcium homeostasis have associated blood-pressure-lowering effects, whereas hormones associated with decreased calcium mobilization or availability are associated with a pressor response. By implication, these collected observations will impact upon our understanding of the pathogenesis of not only essential hypertension but also secondary forms of hypertension, such as that associated with end-stage renal disease. Future observations will also improve the pharmacologic and nonpharmacologic therapy of this most common of human medical disorders in developed societies.

Role of Sodium and Other Dietary Factors in Hypertension

Herbert G. Langford

The number of special meetings, seminars, reviews, editorials, and favorable references about the role of diet in the genesis and management of hypertension has recently exceeded by far the number of studies on which the conclusions are based. I propose to review the studies that seem to give the most pivotal information on this field. More time will then be devoted to outlining deficiencies in our knowledge and discussing how much of our present patient management can be based on hard, available evidence.

Obesity and Hypertension

All cross-sectional studies show a linear correlation between weight and hypertension. This correlation is not explained by any artifact attributable to the method of measurement. It may be a major cause of the socioeconomic gradient of blood pressure, for obesity normally increases as the socioeconomic scale is descended. The correlation is probably with obesity and not with body mass.

I find it embarrassing that we have no clear idea of how obesity produces hypertension. The explanation currently in vogue is that the elevated insulin of the obese is causing an increased tubular reabsorption of sodium. This explanation requires assuming that the kidney does not share the insulin resistance found in the peripheral tissues in obesity. An alternate explanation was favored by Lewis Dahl. He felt that fat people ate more, including more sodium, and that the sodium was the cause of the hypertension. Our studies superficially support Dahl's assumption. In teenage girls, salt excretion is positively correlated with body weight. However, most of the correlation of weight and blood pressure is independent of the contribution of sodium. In

This manuscript was presented as part of a Symposium on *Controversies in the Therapy of Hypertension.*

other words, the correlation between weight and blood pressure remains almost as strong when the contribution of sodium is removed statistically [1].

Recent studies have examined the blood pressure consequences of weight loss. Tuck and Maxwell [2] studied grand obese patients who were put on a very low-calorie diet and either 70 or 150 mEq of sodium a day. The early fall in blood pressure was greater with the 70-mEq diet, but after some weeks the blood pressure fall was the same in the two groups. The study, as valuable as it is, had an inadvertent imperfection. The investigators had put the participants on "high sodium" (that is, 150 mEq per day) designed to replicate the assumed sodium intake. This amount of sodium was chosen because the investigators' experience was that most individuals took in about that much sodium. These participants were taking considerably more sodium than that, along with the large number of calories that they were consuming. Therefore, both diets were restricted in sodium. However, it made no difference whether it was rigidly restricted or only moderately restricted as far as the long-term blood pressure loss was concerned, and therefore it seems reasonable to think that the weight loss was the major factor contributing to blood pressure fall.

The studies of Reisin et al were very valuable in separating the effect of weight from the effect of salt [3]. They studied obese hypertensive patients on antihypertensive medication. The antihypertensive medication was continued. There was a mean weight loss of 10.5 kg in the weight reduction group, accompanied by a blood pressure fall of 37.4/23.3 mm Hg. This compared to a fall of 6.9/2.5 mm Hg in the conventional therapy group. The differences were highly significant. Moreover, there was no difference in the sodium excretion of the weight reduction group at the end of the study and the control group. Unfortunately, they did not have baseline sodium excretions or frequent determinations of sodium excretion during the study.

My colleagues and I have just completed a study on the effect of weight loss on the return of hypertension in patients who had been treated for 5 years in the Hypertension Detection and Follow-up Program, and whose medication was discontinued. The diet was designed to keep sodium intake unchanged, and was successful in doing this. The mean weight loss was slightly less than 5 kg by the end of the year. Despite this modest change in weight, there was a highly significant decrease in the rate of return of hypertension, compared to a group who stopped their medication and did not have any dietary modification [4].

I conclude from these epidemiologic and therapeutic studies that obesity, by unknown routes, causes or accentuates hypertension, and the correction of obesity aids in the control of hypertension.

Sodium Intake and Hypertension

The fact that there are half-a-dozen tribes living in isolated places who have very low salt intakes and low blood pressures is one of the major rocks upon which the "salt hypothesis" is based. The high blood pressure of the

Japanese is not quite as unequivocal, but I think it should be accepted in general. There have been two specific comparisons of Far Eastern people and participants from the Western world that were controlled for age, disease, and, in part, for weight. Koreans put out daily about 100 mEq of sodium more than Belgians did. Their blood pressure was significantly, but not markedly, higher compared to the Belgians [5]. A paper devoted to circadian rhythms happened to have a comparison of blood pressure and 24-hour sodium excretion between Japanese girls and girls from Minneapolis approximately the same age. Again, there was a difference of about 100 mEq in the daily sodium excretion, with the Japanese of course excreting the larger amount. Blood pressure was only a few millimeters higher in the Japanese, but the difference was significant [6]. We can use these two extremes to imply that a sodium intake of 250 mEq per 24 hours will raise blood pressure higher than that found in Western countries, and that a sodium intake of 50 mEq or less will mark a group with lower blood pressures than those found in the Western world. There are alternate explanations for these differences, which will be discussed later. However, for the moment, we will accept the implications and go on to ask the question as to whether the blood pressure response of the population will be a straight line between 50 and 250 mEq/day.

Sodium Restriction in the Hypertensive Patient

The best evidence that the shape of the curve relating sodium intake and blood pressure is not flat between 50 and 250 mEq/day is found in the small but carefully done study of MacGregor et al on sodium restriction in the untreated hypertensive patient [7]. Using a placebo control and a crossover design, they showed quite clearly that a reduction of sodium intake from approximately 150 to 70 mEq/day was associated with a significant fall in blood pressure. The patients did not reach normal blood pressure, but I submit this must be considered as evidence that at least a part of their blood pressure elevation was "salt-sensitive" and that they were taking too much sodium.

Individual Differences in Sodium Sensitivity

One of the first workers in the field, F. M. Allen, introduced the idea of differing sensitivities to sodium in different patients. Dahl bred two strains of rats differing in their blood pressure response to sodium loading. There are now several studies that corroborate in humans this hypothesis based on rats. Kawasaki showed a range of blood pressure responses to reductions of sodium intake to 10 mEq per 24 hours [8]. He spoke of salt-sensitive and salt-resistant individuals. However, the data show an essentially continuous range of response. Piettenen found a significant correlation between sodium excretion and blood pressure in individuals whose first-degree relatives were hypertensive, but not in individuals whose first-degree relatives were normotensive. We studied teenage black girls in Jackson, Mississippi, and found no appreciable significant correlation between sodium excretion and blood pressure. Ten years later, we restudied these patients. Sixteen of them had been diagnosed as hypertensive by their physicians and put on antihypertensive medication. When we reinspected their data, we found that there was a significant correlation between sodium excretion and blood pressure ($r = 0.7$; $P = 0.05$) in the hypertensive girls, which had been hidden by the lack of a correlation between sodium excretion and blood pressure in the entire cohort [9].

I would sum up the information that I have recounted above to indicate the following:

1. Marked differences of sodium intake between populations will be accompanied by statistically significant differences in blood pressure.
2. Most hypertensive individuals are taking too much sodium, and their blood pressure will be lowered by moderate sodium restriction.
3. Within the presently normotensive population, there is probably a salt-sensitive subset who will become hypertensive in the future if they eat a standard amount of sodium found in the American diet.

Sodium Intake in the Treated Hypertensive Patient

Fallis and Ford compared the blood pressure drop and negative potassium balance of hypertensive individuals on 100 mEq of sodium and 100 g of hydrochlorothiazide with the same individuals on 50 mEq of sodium and receiving 50 mg of hydrochlorothiazide per day. The patients dropped to the same blood pressure level on the two regimes, but the resultant negative potassium balance and hypokalemia was much less on the lower sodium intake with the lower thiazide dose [10]. Ram and Kaplan have repeated and extended those studies and fully confirmed the concept. Owens and Brackett showed how a low-sodium intake increased the blood-pressure-lowering effect of propranolol [11], and Gavras et al showed how sodium restriction increased the hypotensive response to converting enzyme inhibition [12]. Sodium restriction may be more important in the treated hypertensive than as sole therapy for the mild hypertensive where its efficacy may be rather limited.

Other Nutritional Factors Affecting Blood Pressure

There is now considerable evidence that a low intake of potassium may be as important as a high intake of sodium in the genesis of hypertension. I have reviewed this information recently [13]. It may be summarized as follows:

1. We found a significant correlation between the Na/K ratio in the urine and blood pressure, but no correlation between blood pressure and sodium excretion in the entire population studied.

2. Walker found a significant negative correlation between sodium excretion and blood pressure, with no contribution at all from sodium to the equation.
3. Five studies have shown that the much higher blood pressure in blacks in the United States is accompanied by a significantly lower potassium excretion.
4. Potassium partially blocks the blood-pressure-raising effects of sodium.
5. Increased potassium intake lowers blood pressure in hypertensive individuals and probably in normotensive individuals.

In addition, there are other dietary factors that may well be involved in blood pressure homeostasis. Two studies suggest that chloride is necessary for the blood-pressure-raising effects of sodium. Manipulation of the fatty content of the diet, with increased unsaturated fats and decreased saturated fats, is said to lower blood pressure. The results are not clear enough to say which of the two dietary moves is the important one. Calcium is said to lower blood pressure, and now magnesium is being considered as a possible candidate.

Studies on the dietary management of hypertension are appropriately increasing. What practical guidelines can be given at this time?

1. The treated hypertensive should follow a moderately restricted sodium intake. I have not developed the theme, but it is probably necessary to measure sodium output to determine whether the patient is adequately restricting his sodium intake.

2. Obese hypertensive patients should lose weight. Weight loss usually requires a well-planned program. If there is not a nearby hospital-based nutritional program using psychological principles, consider referring your patients to commercial organizations such as Weight Watchers®.

3. The use of sodium restriction as sole therapy for mild hypertensives has excellent theoretical and some limited experimental backing. However, its efficacy and feasibility are completely untested, and it should be prescribed and followed like any other experimental procedure, with careful follow-up examinations to determine compliance and effectiveness, and willingness to switch to more established means of therapy if continued success is not achieved.

4. There is considerable evidence that potassium may be almost as important as sodium in the genesis of hypertension, with a high potassium intake serving to neutralize partially the blood-pressure-raising effects of sodium. In addition, the effects of calcium, magnesium, chloride, and fats need greater study, and replication of some of the published experiments.

Acknowledgment. This work was supported by NIH grant R01 HL24369.

References

1. WATSON RL, LANGFORD HG, ABERNETHY J, BARNES TY, WATSON MJ: Urinary electrolytes, body weight, and blood pressure: Pooled cross-sectional results among four groups of adolescent females. *Hypertension* 2(Part 2):193–198, 1980

2. TUCK ML, SOWERS J, DORNFELD L, KLEDZIK G, MAXWELL M: The effect of weight reduction on blood pressure, plasma renin activity, and plasma aldosterone levels in obese patients. *N Engl J Med* 304:930–933, 1981

3. REISIN E, ABEL R, MODAN M, SILVERBERG DS, ELIAHOU HE, MODAN MB: Effect of weight loss without salt restriction on the reduction of blood pressure in overweight hypertensive patients. *N Engl J Med* 298:1–6, 1978

4. LANGFORD HG, BLAUFOX D, OBERMAN A, HAWKINS M, SMOLLER S, CUTTER G, for the DISH Investigative Group: Effect of dietary change on the return of hypertension after withdrawal of prolonged antihypertensive therapy (*abstract*). *Clin Res* 32: April, 1984

5. KESTELOOT H, PARK CC, LEE CS, JOOSENS JV: Abstracts of the American Heart Association. *Circulation* 45:3, 1977

6. KAWASAKI I, UENO M, UEZONO K, MATSUOKA M, OMAE T, HALBERG F, WENDT H, TAGGETT-ANDERSON MA, HAUS E: Differences and similarities among circadian characteristics of plasma renin activity in healthy young women in Japan and the United States. *Am J Med* 68:91–96, 1980

7. MACGREGOR GA, BEST FE, CAM JM, MARKANDU ND, ELDER DM, SAGNELLA GA, SQUIRES M: Double-blind randomised crossover trial of moderate sodium restriction in essential hypertension. *Lancet* 1:351–355, 1982

8. KAWASAKI T, KUMAMOTO K, FUKIYAMA K, NODA Y, TAKISHITA S, OMAE T: Individual renin-aldosterone responses of clinically healthy young Japanese men to dietary sodium and posture. *Jpn Heart J* 5:631–642, 1979

9. LANGFORD HG, WATSON RL: Close correlation between blood pressure and sodium excretion in hypertensives (*abstract*). Circulation 66(suppl II):II–105, 1982

10. FALLIS N, FORD RV: Electrolyte excretion and hypotensive response. *JAMA* 176:581–584, 1961

11. OWENS CJ, BRACKETT NC JR: Role of sodium intake in the antihypertensive effect of propranolol. *South Med J* 71:43–46, 1978

12. GAVRAS H, BRUNNER HR, LARAGH JH, SEALEY JE, GAVRAS I, VUKOVITCH RA: An angiotensin converting enzyme inhibitor to identify and treat vasoconstrictor and volume factors in hypertensive patients. *N Engl J Med* 291:817–821, 1974

13. LANGFORD HG: Dietary potassium and hypertension: Epidemiologic data. *Ann Intern Med* 98(Part 2):770–772, 1983

Hypertension in the Elderly

Robert C. Tarazi

Discussions of hypertension in elderly patients are dominated frequently by questions about isolated systolic hypertension. Although legitimate, these questions address only part of the problem and, thus, sometimes distort the approach to one of the important and frequent diseases of the elderly [1]. Hypertension in patients over 60 years of age is not limited to isolated elevations of systolic pressure; it is just as apt to be diastolic as systolic and more frequently both. The risk of cardiovascular disease increases with elevations in either the diastolic or systolic level, often more steeply with the latter [2]. The epidemiological characteristics of hypertension and its risks in the over 60 years age group have been defined in several excellent reviews [2–4]. These aspects will, therefore, not be reviewed again here; the following discussion will deal mainly with some of the pathophysiologic characterics of hypertension in the elderly and their therapeutic implications.

There are two reasons for this approach: (a) the risks associated with hypertension in the elderly have been demonstrated clearly in many studies from many parts of the world [4–7], and (b) the evidence gathered by the Hypertension Detection and Follow-up Program (HDFP) and other studies have shown convincingly the efficacy of treatment for diastolic hypertension in that age group [1]. Although there is no similar proof of efficacy of treatment in patients with pure systolic hypertension, the correlation between systolic pressure and risk from cardiovascular disease [2] would argue in favor of treatment if it were not for the difficulties and side effects of the treatment. The controversy raised concerning hypertension in the elderly does not question the risks or advisability of treatment as much as its safety in that high-risk population.

This question is best addressed, in my opinion, by careful consideration of the pathophysiologic mechanisms involved in hypertension in the elderly and utilization of this knowledge in the choice of safe and effective therapy.

This manuscript was presented as part of a Symposium on *Controversies in the Therapy of Hypertension.*

Pathophysiologic Considerations

Hypertension is the result of the interaction of different pressor mechanisms with the various types of hypertension differing from each other not by the presence of a single pressor factor but rather by a difference in which these factors are integrated. Age is one such variable that affects many of these physiologic mechanisms. There is no age at which hypertension suddenly becomes qualitatively different but some characteristics which influence the response to treatment gradually assume greater importance. One example is the gradual reduction in compliance of the aorta and large vessels with age; since compliance is one factor that determines arterial pressure, loss of this buffering capability will influence the characteristics of the hypertension and the response to therapy [8]. Although reduced aortic compliance is more frequent in older patients, it occurs in younger subjects and has the same consequences.

Other important changes occurring with age include the gradual reduction in beta-adrenergic receptors in the heart and blood vessels [9, 10] and changes in liver and kidney function that alter excretion rates of various antihypertensive agents [1]. The reduction in beta-receptors would enhance the vasoconstrictor effect of alpha-adrenergic stimuli and might alter response to alpha-blocking agents. A diminished excretion rate of drugs could enhance their hypotensive potential and risk of adverse side-effects.

Relation Between Systolic and Diastolic Blood Pressure Levels

Wiggers [11] long ago defined the relation between the diastolic pressure and vascular compliance when he pointed out that distensibility is reduced as diastolic blood pressure (DBP) increases, with pulse pressure (all else being equal) increasing with the development of hypertension (Fig. 1). The implication is that the loss of elasticity of these large vessels (windkessel) leads to a steeper slope of the relation between systolic blood pressure (SBP) and DBP, its maximum manifestation occurring in isolated systolic hypertension due to aortic sclerosis. Thus a larger drop of SBP must be expected with an equal reduction of DBP during treatment of these patients (Fig. 2). This can lead to greater risk of side effects and the need for reduced dosage of drugs and a much more patient approach to blood pressure control in the elderly.

A second hemodynamic consideration is the direct relation of systolic pressure, not diastolic pressure, in determining afterload [12]. The systolic level is the pressure variable used to define ventricular afterload, hence its importance for patients with reduced cardiac function or potential heart disease. Indications for antihypertensive therapy based exclusively on diastolic pressure miss the importance of SBP in patients with systolic hypertension or cardiac disease. Similar arguments could be advanced for the traumatizing effect of increased systolic pressure on diseased arteries with the consequent risk of strokes [2].

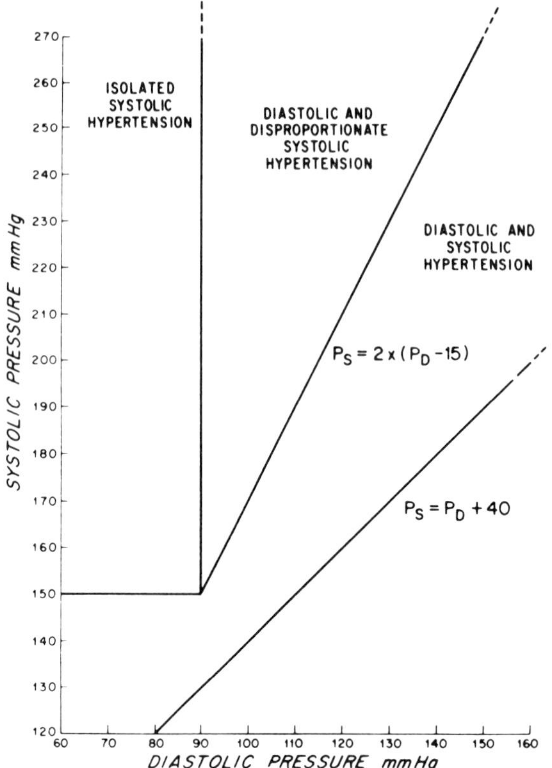

Fig. 1. The relationship between diastolic (P_D) and systolic (P_S) blood pressure would have been given by the first line ($P_S = P_D + 40$) if aortic distensibility remained the same whatever the P_D level. However, since distensibility is reduced as diastolic blood pressure increases, systolic pressure rises relatively more than the diastolic, as given by the equation of the second line. Inappropriate systolic elevations for the level of diastolic pressure can cover the whole spectrum from $P_S > 2 \times (P_D - 15)$ to isolated systolic elevations [32].

Hemodynamic Patterns

An increase in total peripheral resistance remains the hemodynamic hallmark of established hypertension in either young or older subjects [13]. Plasma volume is commonly reduced, sometimes markedly, in older patients [14, 15]. Cardiac output remains normal, although more frequently reduced in older patients [13, 14] with the combination of a small stroke volume and high pulse pressure suggesting reduced aortic distensibility (vide infra). There are exceptions with some elderly patients presenting with hyperkinetic circulation despite long-standing hypertension; in these patients sympatholytic or beta-blocking drugs are more useful [16].

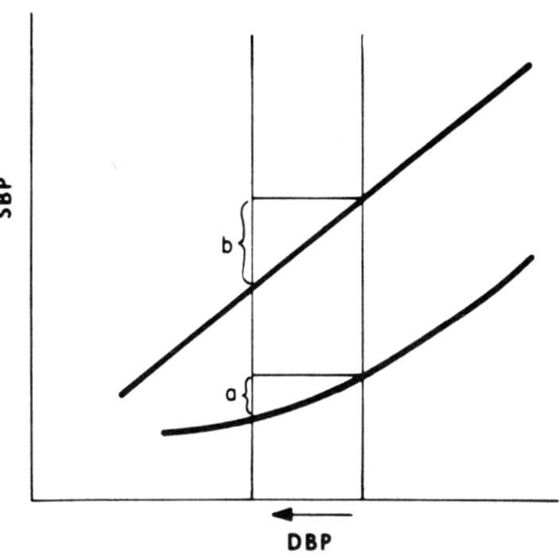

Fig. 2. The steeper slope of the relation between systolic blood pressure (*SBP*) and diastolic blood pressure (*DBP*) (see Fig. 1) signifies that one should expect a greater drop of *SBP* in patients with inappropriate systolic hypertension ($b > a$) for the same reduction in diastolic pressure.

Aortic Compliance and Arterial Dynamics

Arterial compliance reflects the visco-elastic properties of the walls of the large arteries, and determines the effectiveness of their role in buffering the wide fluctuations in pressure generated by the heart (windkessel effect) [11]. Although there is a general tendency for arterial compliance to diminish with age and for hypertension in the elderly to be associated with aortic rigidity, there are enough exceptions to make an investigation needed in problem cases [8].

Many indexes have been proposed to determine aortic compliance in man [8, 17, 18]. The ratio of pulse pressure to stroke volume (PP/SV, mm Hg rise in pressure per ml of ejected blood) is an easy approximation of systemic arterial compliance (SAC). More precise mathematical derivations derive from the slope of fall in intraarterial pressure during diastole [18, 19] (Fig. 3). In our experience and that of others, there has been a close correlation in most older patients between the PP/SV ratio and the index derived from pulse pressure tracings. In younger patients, however, there are many excep-

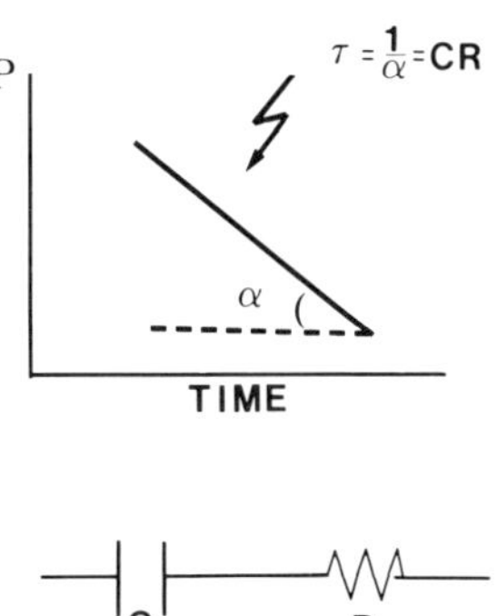

Fig. 3. The fall in arterial pressure from the dicrotic notch until the beginning of the next cardiac cycle is exponential and can be likened to a simple model linking in series a capcitance element (*C*) with a resistive element (*R*). Arterial compliance can therefore, be calculated from the slope of the diastolic part of the pulse and from simultaneously determined total peripheral resistance. (The method has been validated in man by Safar et al [18].)

tions. The difference is explained by the dependence of systolic BP on both aortic distensibility and the velocity of ventricular ejection of blood. When the elevation of SBP is related to a reduction in aortic compliance, the two indices agree, but when ventricular ejection is rapid, SBP may be high even though SAC is normal or reduced slightly (Table 1).

The work of Safar, Simon and their colleagues [18, 20, 21] has helped characterize the role of the larger arteries in hypertension, which has value in the choice of antihypertension therapy. They showed that the effects of different vasodilators on small arterioles (resistance vessels) are *not* similar to their effects on the large arteries, either in degree, direction or time course [22]. Those that produce arterial as well as arteriolar dilation may be more suitable for patients with vascular disease.

Neurohumoral Factors

One of the significant features in circulatory homeostasis with age is the gradual reduction in baroceptor sensitivity that develops both in normotensive and hypertensive subjects [23]. The early clinical observations of Appenzeller et al, who reported blunting or even absence of the arterial pressure rebound in older patients after a Valsalva maneuver, were further extended and quantified by studies of heart rate response to variations in blood pressure. Baroceptor sensitivity was defined by slope of the relation between RR interval and SBP; the reflex bradycardia expected from increases in arterial pressure was reduced with advancing ages in normotensive subjects [24]. The reduction in baroceptor sensitivity may help explain the high incidence in older subjects of marked drops in SBP ($>$ 20 mm Hg) after one minute of quiet standing [25]. At all ages, baroceptor sensitivity was lower in hypertensive than in normotensive subjects. It is obvious that complaints of hypotension and dizziness will be more frequent when antihypertensive therapy is initiated in patients over 60 years. The combined effects of age, hypertension, and occasionally sedatives, which depress baroceptor sensitivity further [26], have patients living at the edge of baroceptor compensation. The practical implications are that they should be warned against sudden standing-up, straining, etc.,

Table 1. Ventricular ejection and aortic compliance[a]

Subject	$<$ 35 years (Control)	$>$ 35 years (Control)
PP/SV, mm Hg/ml	1.54[b] (0.94)	1.89[b] (1.31)
SAC, ml/mm Hg	2.45 (2.67)	1.41[b] (2.18)

[a] It's apparent from these data (derived from Simon et al [21, 22]) that estimates of aortic distensibility based on the ratio of pulse pressure to stroke volume (PP/SV) [8] were abnormal in both young and older patients with systolic hypertension—while estimates of systemic arterial compliance (SAC) based on the peripheral pulse method [17] were abnormal only in older subjects. The difference in results between the two indexes is related probably to the influence of velocity of ventricular ejection (see text).

[b] Significantly different from control of same age group.

and physicians should avoid drugs that interfere with the baroceptor mechanism.

Despite low plasma volume, older patients often have low plasma renin activity [27]. This feature has been used to explain their sensitivity to diuretic agents [28] and more recently the enhanced antihypertensive efficacy of calcium entry blockers in this age group [29, 30]. It is not yet completely clear whether this increased sensitivity is causally related to the low plasma renin activity, low plasma volume, or diminished baroceptor reflexes, but stresses the need to begin treatment with small doses of whatever antihypertensive drug is being used.

Therapeutic Implications

The concepts summarized in the preceding paragraphs suggest that a subdivision of hypertension into systolic versus diastolic, or into hypertension of the old versus hypertension in the adult, imposes arbitrary definitions that are not always warranted or useful. Blood pressure as well as age are continuous variables, so that "set" or "definite" numerical limits are always arbitrary and the rate at which blood pressure increases with age varies from one individual to another.

It is more useful, in my opinion, to emphasize the pathophysiologic changes occurring with age and adjust accordingly the therapeutic approach. The controversy about treatment of hypertension in the elderly cannot be answered in statistical terms; it must be resolved by a pathophysiologic approach, which would make antihypertensive therapy safer.

1. Careful analysis of blood pressure measurements is essential in the elderly, particularly the stability of hypertension, its reality (falsely high readings are more frequent in older patients because of the difficulty to compress arteries) [31], the response to posture (to define baroceptor adequacy), and appropriateness of systolic to diastolic blood pressure levels. An inappropriate systolic elevation ($>$ than $2 \times [DBP - 15]$) [32] suggests reduced aortic compliance in the absence of aortic insufficiency, arterio-venous aneurysm, thyrotoxicosis or an evident hyperkinetic circulation.

2. Elderly patients are not immune to secondary hypertension, and may be at greater risk of atherosclerotic renal artery stenosis. However, extensive diagnostic work-up is not recommended unless abrupt exacerbation of a previously stable hypertension or a de novo onset after age 55 raises the level of suspicion; then, secondary causes should be sought.

3. Drugs that interfere with baroceptor reflexes should be avoided if at all possible because of the borderline "baroceptor compensation" of older patients.

4. The initial doses and subsequent increments of any antihypertensive agent selected should be quite small (half of the usual adult dose) because of the many factors that enhance their hypotensive effect in older patients. These include low plasma volume, impaired mechanisms of cardiovascular homeostasis, reduced excretion rate of some drugs, and greater sensitivity

to sympatholytics and α-blockers because of enhanced sympathetic vasoconstriction tone.

There are many published discussions of antihypertensive drugs for older patients such as the excellent summary by Kirkendall and Hammond [1]. A rapidly evolving field is the direct study of the effect of different vasodilators on arterial dynamics as opposed to their arteriolar [22] or venous effect [33]. The results may help decide on a balanced vasodilator that would not unduly stimulate the heart, increase cardiac rate or output, or induce drowsiness or orthostatic hypotension.

To the extent that general rules can be summarized in a few sentences and be helpful, one might suggest that antihypertensive therapy in older patients could begin—if indicated—with small doses of a diuretic to which later small doses of an adequate vasodilator could be added later. Hydralazine has been suggested because it does not interfere with baroceptor reflexes and can be well tolerated; however, it could induce or worsen angina pectoris [1]. The hemodynamic pattern produced by converting enzyme inhibitors and most calcium entry blockers appears favorable; the latter can serve more than one purpose if the hypertensive patient also suffers from some form of arterial insufficiency, peripheral or coronary.

Summary

Hypertension in patients over 60 years is associated with a greater risk of cardiovascular complications, whether the hypertension is diastolic, purely systolic, or diastolic with inappropriate systolic elevations of pressure. The benefits from prudent and effective therapy have been demonstrated in different trials but definite proof that therapy is beneficial for patients with isolated systolic hypertension is not yet available. Yet definite concerns still remain about the frequency of side effects or fear of vascular accidents during antihypertensive treatment in older patients. Hypertension in the elderly is not a qualitatively different disease from hypertension in adults, but it does have some pathophysiologic features that lead to enhanced response to antihypertensive drugs. These include reduced compliance of the aorta and large vessels, low plasma volume, greater alpha-adrenergic tone and impaired baroceptor sensitivity. Careful attention to these features, the use of small doses (half the usual) of antihypertensive drugs, and avoidance of drugs that interfere with baroceptor mechanisms, all help minimize the side effects, improve compliance, and allow more effective blood pressure control.

References

1. KIRKENDALL WM, HAMMOND JJ: Hypertension in the elderly. *Arch Intern Med* 140:1155–1161, 1980
2. KANNEL WB: Role of blood pressure in cardiovascular morbidity and mortality. *Prog Cardiovasc Dis* 17:5–24, 1974

3. HYPERTENSION DETECTION AND FOLLOW-UP PROGRAM COOPERATIVE GROUP: Five-year findings of the Hypertension Detection and Follow-up Program: I. Reduction in mortality of persons with high blood pressure, including mild hypertension. *JAMA* 242:2562–2571, 1979

4. HYPERTENSION DETECTION AND FOLLOW-UP PROGRAM COOPERATIVE GROUP: Five-year findings of the Hypertension Detection and Follow-up Program. II. Mortality by race, sex and age. *JAMA* 242:2572–2577, 1979

5. KANNEL WB: Some lessons in cardiovascular epidemiology from Frahmigham. *Am J Cardiol* 37:269–282, 1976

6. KURAMOTO K, MATSUSHITA S, KUWAJIMA I: The pathogenetic role and treatment of elderly hypertension. *Japn Circ J* 45:833–843, 1981

7. KANNEL WB, WOLF PA, MCGEE DL, DAWBER TR, MCNAMARA P, CASTELLI WP: Systolic blood pressure, arterial rigidity and risk of stroke. *JAMA* 245:1225–1232, 1981

8. TARAZI RC, MAGRINI F, DUSTAN HP: The role of aortic distensibility in hypertension, in *Recent Advances in Hypertension,* edited by MILLIEZ P, SAFAR M, Reims-France, Boehringer Ingelheim, 1975, pp. 133–142

9. AMER SM, GOMOLL AW, PERHUCH JL JR, FERGUSON HC, MCKINNEY GR: Aberrations of cyclic nucleotide metabolism in the hearts and vessels of hypertensive rats. *Proc National Acad Sci* 71:4930–4934, 1974

10. BAKER SP, POTTER LT: Cardiac β-adrenoceptors during normal growth of male and female rats. *Brit J Pharmacol* 68:65–70, 1980

11. WIGGERS CJ: Circulatory dynamics, in *Physiologic Studies, Modern Medical Monographs,* New York, Grune and Stratton, 1952

12. TARAZI RC, LEVY MN: Cardiac responses to increased afterload. *Hypertension* 4 (Suppl II):II8-18, 1982

13. TARAZI RC: The hemodynamics of hypertension, Chapter 2, in *Hypertension, 2nd Edition,* edited by GENEST J, KUCHEL O, HAMET P, CANTIN M, New York, McGraw-Hill, 1983, pp. 15–42

14. ADAMAPOULOS PN, CHRYSANTHALKOPOULIS SG, FROHLICH ED: Systolic hypertension: Non-homogenous diseases. *Am J Cardiol* 36:697–701, 1975

15. MESSERLI FH, SUNDGAARD-RIISE K, VENTURA HO, DUNN FG, GLADE LB, FROHLICH ED: Essential hypertension in the elderly: Haemodynamics, intravascular volume, plasma renin activity, and circulating catecholamine levels. *Lancet* 2: 983–986, 1983

16. IBRAHIM MM, TARAZI RC, DUSTAN HP, BRAVO EL, GIFFORD RW JR: Hyperkinetic heart in severe hypertension: A separate clinical hemodynamic entity. *Am J Cardiol* 35:667–674, 1975

17. ABBOUD FM, HOUSTON JH: The effects of aging and degenerative vascular diseases on the measurement of arterial rigidity in man. *J Clin Invest* 40:933–939, 1981

18. SIMON, AC, SAFAR ME, LEVENSON JA, LONDON GM, LEVY BI, CHAU NP: An evaluation of large arteries compliance in man. *Am J Physiol* 237:H550–H554, 1979

19. RANDALL OS, ESLER MD, BULLOCH GF, MAISEL AS, ELLIS CN, ZWEIFLER AJ, JULIUS S: Relationship of age and blood pressure to baroreflex sensitivity and arterial compliance in man. *Clin Sci Mol Med* 51(Suppl 3):357s–360s, 1976

20. LEVENSON J, CHELLY J, PAYEN D, SIMON A, SAFAR M: Vaso-dilating antihypertensive drugs: effect on arterial compliance, a preliminary report, in *Les Alpha-Bloquants: Pharmacologie Experimentale et Clinique,* Symposium International Paris, Paris, Masson, 1981, pp. 271–276

21. SIMON AC, SAFAR MA, LEVENSON GA, KEHDER AM, LEVY BI: Systolic hypertension. Hemodynamic mechanism and choice of antihypertensive therapy. *Am J Cardiol* 44:505–511, 1979

22. Simon AC, Levenson JA, Bouthier J, Maarek B, Safar ME: Effects of acute and chronic angiotensin converting enzyme inhibition on the human hypertensive large arteries. *J Cardiovasc Pharm* (in press, 1984)
23. Sleight P: Reflex control of the heart. *Am J Cardiol* 44:889–894, 1979
24. Gribbin B, Pickering TG, Sleight P, Peto R: Effect of age and high blood pressure on baroreflex sensitivity in man. *Circ Res* 29:424–431, 1971
25. Caird FI, Andrews GR, Kennedy RD: Effect of posture on blood pressure in the elderly. *Br Heart J* 35:527–530, 1973
26. Tarazi RC, Fouad FM: Circulatory dynamics in progressive autonomic failure, Chapter 7, in *Autonomic Failure: A Textbook of Clinical Disorders of the Autonomic Nervous System,* edited by Bannister R, Oxford, Oxford University Press, 1983, pp. 96–113
27. Birkenhager WH, Schalekamp MADH, Krauss XH, Kolsters G, Schalekamp-Kuyken MPA, Kroon BJM, Teulings FAG: Systemic and renal haemodynamics, body fluids and renin in benign essential hypertension with special reference to natural history. *Eur J Clin Invest* 2:115–122, 1972
28. Niarchos AP, Laragh JH: Effects of diuretic therapy in low-, normal-, and high-renin isolated systolic systemic hypertension. *Am J Cardiol* 53:797–801, 1984
29. Buhler FR, Hulthen L, Kiowski W, Müller FB, Bolli P: The place of the calcium antagonist verapamil in antihypertensive therapy. *J Cardiovasc Pharm* 4:S350–S357, 1982
30. Fouad FM, Pedrinelli R, Bravo EL, Abi-Samra F, Textor SC, Tarazi RC: Clinical and systemic hemodynamic effects of nitrendipine. *Clin Pharm Ther* 35:768–775, 1984
31. Tarazi RC, Dustan HP, Bravo EL, Niarchos AP: Vasodilating drugs: Contracting haemodynamic effects. *Clin Sci Mol Med* 51(Suppl 3):575–578, 1976
32. Koch-Weser J: Correlation of pathophysiology and pharmacology in primary hypertension. *Am J Cardiol* 32:499–510, 1973

Mechanisms of Action and Use of Newer Antihypertensive Agents

Chairpersons: David B. Case and Norman M. Kaplan
Discussants: Trefor O. Morgan, Richard de Zeeuw, Michael Weber, Keishi Abe, and Peter Weidmann

New drugs and techniques for the management of hypertension have been introduced. This Workshop focused on the mechanisms of actions and the clinical views on several major types of newer agents and techniques.

Morgan considered the issue of nondrug therapies. He noted that even though many practitioners institute treatment of hypertension routinely with drugs, there is an increasing trend, particularly in patients with mild hypertension, to try nondrug therapies before embarking on a long-term course of drug therapy. Paramount in the consideration of the use of drugs is their immediate and long-term safety as it relates to the potential benefit in terms of additional life span. With few exceptions the nonpharmacologic treatments are considered relatively safe and are generally deployed before and during conventional drug therapy.

The principal nondrug therapies include diet, stress management, and control of obesity.

There is preliminary evidence that regular and vigorous exercise can reduce blood pressure acutely in some patients with mild to moderate hypertension. Many questions remain unanswered with respect to the value of moderate and nonregular vigorous exercise. Moreover, it is difficult to eliminate a hypotensive contribution by the numerous, potentially important factors that often become operative in individuals who undertake vigorous athletic or exercise programs. These would include weight reduction, change in salt intake, modification of fat, sodium, and alcohol intake, and use of other drugs.

Techniques for dealing with stress as an issue in hypertension are only moderately successful, although there seems to be evidence that acute stress may raise blood pressure. Whether or not chronic stress can continuously raise blood pressure in essential hypertension or the removal of stress lower the pressure remains unanswered, despite popular opinion. As with many other techniques involving drug and nondrug therapies, more refined tech-

---

This narrative is the summary of a Workshop of the same title.

niques such as 24-hr blood pressure monitoring will be helpful in determining the value of these techniques.

There has been a major emphasis directed toward dietary changes as primary treatment of hypertension: decreased caloric intake and weight reduction, reduction of sodium and saturated fats, increased intake of potassium, magnesium, calcium, and fiber, and other dietary substances. There seems to be general agreement that weight reduction in obese individuals is useful, although only a few studies have shown dramatic results. Considerable emphasis has recently been placed on reduction of alcohol intake based on findings from both Australian and American studies of chronic, drug-resistant hypertension. Reducing alcohol intake from excess, however, has only a limited application in the general treatment of hypertension.

Perhaps the greatest interest in dietary changes has been in sodium intake. About 80% of studies recently reviewed indicated that blood pressure was lower on low salt intake. Interestingly, eight well-conducted studies did not show that decreased sodium intake reduced blood pressure. There is good evidence that reduced sodium intake has a similar antihypertensive effect as continuous diuretic therapy.

There are other considerations that involve reduced sodium intake. Rises in plasma renin activity induced by low sodium intake may counteract the antihypertensive response from volume depletion. In addition, the chloride ion may play an important role in blood pressure homeostasis since repletion of sodium in the form of sodium bicarbonate to individuals who have been depleted of sodium chloride did not restore blood pressure to control levels. There is support for the idea that potassium chloride may prevent the rise in blood pressure induced by increases in sodium chloride. The bulk of the evidence suggests that sodium restriction may be more effective in elderly patients than in the younger because of the relative reactive rises in the renin-angiotensin system.

Diuretics and their use was next presented by de Zeeuw. He said that newer diuretics offer the possibility of effective control of blood pressure through fluid/volume reduction but with the potential of adverse metabolic derangements. The common complications of diuretics include hyperuricemia, hypokalemia, hyperglycemia, hypercalcemia, hyperkalemia, hypovolemia, and azotemia. In addition, there has been concern that in studies using diuretic therapy, there does not seem to be a significant reduction in death from coronary heart diseases or essential hypertension. Moreover, there is increasing concern about the frequency of ventricular ectopy related to diuretic-induced hypokalemia and hypomagnesemia raised by a number of studies in the United States and by the Medical Research Council trial in Great Britain.

To reduce the sideeffects of thiazide-type diuretics, various investigators have suggested reducing the diuretic dose, increasing potassium in diet and in the form of supplements, and modifying the amount of sodium in the diet. Combining thiazide with potassium-sparing diuretics or with other drugs capable of conserving potassium has gained popularity. Recent studies in Europe support the use of the potassium-sparing diuretics such as triamterene or amiloride with thiazide, which attenuate but do not completely prevent hypokalemia. The combination of thiazide diuretics with converting enzyme inhibitors, which block the reactive hyperreninemia and hyperaldosteronemia, also prevents hypokalemia as well as reduces the diuretic doses needed to achieve good blood pressure control.

A number of new diuretics have been developed that have similar effectiveness and side-effect profiles as the well-established ones. Both muzolimine and mefruside are similar in action and structure to thiazides. Indamide, also a sulfonamide diuretic, has been reported to cause minimal perturbation of potassium and lipid disturbances. Although not classically diuretic in the traditional sense, converting enzyme inhibitors may in certain cases induce a natriuresis through their blockade of the effects of angiotensin II on tubular sodium handling and aldosterone secretion.

Adrenergic inhibitors were considered by Weber who noted that there has been growing interest and enthusiasm for the use of both alpha and beta blockers as single agents in the treatment of hypertension. There is general agreement that beta adrenergic blockers can be used effectively in large numbers of hypertensive patients but may be selectively more effective in white patients than black. Beta blockers also appear to be preferentially effective in younger as compared to older subjects. The differences in drug responses to beta adrenergic blockade on one hand and to diuretics on the other indicate a heterogeneity of mechanisms responsible for maintaining elevated blood pressure. Moreover, it is unlikely that any given single agent will be effective in all individuals.

Recent evidence suggests that different types of adrenergic inhibitors may combine well. For example, in one recent study by Stokes, the addition of prazosin, a peripheral postsynaptic alpha blocker, reduced blood pressure additionally when added to the regimen of individuals receiving chronic beta adrenergic blockade with propranolol. These findings and those of others have led to the development of combined alpha/beta blockers such as labetolol, which is currently under investigation in the United States. Not all combinations, however, of adrenergic inhibitors are necessarily additive. For example, a recent study by Weber and colleagues indicated that clonidine, a central alpha agonist, and prazosin were not additive.

The use of adrenergic inhibitors as single agents without causing sodium retention, as has previously been thought, has been shown recently using clonidine and prazosin essential hypertension. Thus, both clonidine and prazosin may be used as single agents in certain hypertensive patients without having their effects be attenuated by induced sodium and water retention.

New delivery systems are being developed to enhance compliance and ensure smooth effective delivery of medications. For example, clonidine has been recently developed for transdermal delivery through patch application on the chest. A single patch lasts approximately one week and delivers a steady plasma concentration, in contrast to the irregular levels that have been measured during intermittent oral dosing. Bockhorst and his colleagues in Europe have demonstrated that substitution of the transdermal clonidine for the oral form produces the same blood pressure control at lower plasma concentrations and thereby reduced side effects such as dry mouth and drowsiness.

Considerable attention has now recently focused on the metabolic consequences of antihypertensive therapy since not only diuretics but also the beta blockers may produce small but adverse changes in blood lipid profiles. Peripheral-acting alpha-adrenergic blockers such as prazosin may have an advantage in this respect since they appear to slightly decrease total cholesterol concentrations while simultaneously increasing the levels of the beneficial high density lipoprotein fractions. This same effect has been seen with central alpha agonists as well and may be directly related to eventual alpha-adrenergic blockade.

A final consideration has been raised by the use of adrenergic inhibitors in the regression of left ventricular hypertrophy in hypertension. Studies using echocardiography, a technique sensitive in detecting enlargement of left ventricular dimensions, have demonstrated that beta adrenergic blockade (as with atenolol) may significantly reduce left ventricular mass. Drayer and colleagues demonstrated that although hydrochlorothiazide reduced blood pressure, it did not reduce left ventricular mass until alpha methyl dopa was added to the regimen. Direct vasodilators alone in both experimental animals and in man do not appear to reduce left ventricular mass. Altogether the data suggests a specific adrenergic effect in facilitating left ventricular hypertrophy, which may be blocked by adrenergic inhibitors.

Abe discussed inhibitors of the renin-angiotensin system. Two kinds of pharmacologic inhibitors of the renin-angiotensin system are available: (1) angiotensin II analogues; (2) others designed to block the enzyme responsible for the conversion of angiotensin I to II. Clinical studies with angiotensin analogues showed that their hypotensive effects occurred in hypertensive patients with relatively high plasma renin activity, while a pressor response was induced in patients with relatively low plasma renin activity due to intrinsic agonist activity. Angiotensin analogues have limited clinical utility in the treatment of hypertension because of their lack of oral activity.

A series of orally active converting enzyme inhibitors, including captopril, enalopril, and a Japanese compound SA446, are potent inhibitors of the angiotensin I converting enzyme. The biological activity of enalopril is approximately 10 times greater than that of SA446 and greater than 5 times more potent than that of captopril. Captopril is rapidly and extensively absorbed from the gastrointestinal tract and has a quick onset of action within 15 minutes after oral ingestion. In contrast, enalopril is absorbed more slowly, requires hydrolysis for activity, and has a prolonged duration of action. The main hypotensive mechanism of these drugs is due to inhibition of the renin-angiotensin system by means of a decrement in angiotensin II formation. For this reason, these inhibitors are preferentially effective in patients with high plasma renin activity. However, all three of these converting enzyme inhibitors also have reduced blood pressure, albeit modestly, in some low renin hypertensive patients, often in association with a modest natriuresis and increase in the urinary excretion of kinins and metabolism of prostaglandin E. These latter results indicate that enhanced kinin and prostaglandin activity may contribute to the hypotensive effects in this group of patients with lower plasma renin activity. Recent evidence suggests that the prostaglandin inhibitor indomethacin blocks the action of captopril and low-renin essential hypertension, but does not in the normal-renin group.

Initial clinical trials with relatively high doses of captopril have revealed marked antihypertensive efficacy yet occasional adverse effects including rash (9%), loss of taste (7%), and rare instances of leukopenia and proteinuria. In contrast, clinical trials using low doses of captopril have proved to be equally effective in the treatment of mild to moderate essential hypertension at higher doses without serious side effects. Clinical trials with the nonconverting enzyme inhibitor enalopril indicate efficacy at least equal to captopril with a low incidence of adverse effects.

Calcium entry blockers were discussed by Weidmann. There are three available calcium entry blockers, which differ structurally and also in their influence on the cardiac pacemaker, vasodilating potential, and their effects on the sympathetic nervous system and plasma renin activity. All three drugs, nifedipine, verapamil, and diltiazem, share in common the ability to block the slow channel entry of calcium into the cell and thus prevent availability of calcium from the electromechanical contractile process. Nifedipine, at one end of the spectrum, appears to have the greatest vasodilator action with a minimum of activity on the cardiac pacemaker. Verapamil, on the other end, has significantly more activity on the cardiac pacemaker and less action as a vasodilator. Diltiazem has intermediate properties. Nifedipine, diltiazem, and verapamil, given either as acute single doses or over treatment periods beyond six months, have lowered blood pressure in patients with mild to moderate hypertension by about 10 to 20%. Blood pressure is largely unchanged by calcium entry blockers in normotensive subjects. Blood pressure responses to calcium entry blockers appear to be age related: more effective in older patients than in younger ones. Nifedipine and verapamil may produce ankle swelling in a small fraction of patients but this is generally not associated with weight gain and positive sodium and water balance. Combinations of calcium entry blockers with thiazide diuretics, with or without beta blockers, methyldopa, or reserpine, may enhance the antihypertensive action of these drugs in essential hypertension.

Although each of these drugs acts to block slow channel calcium entry into cells, there appears to be a wide range of different physiologic effects. Plasma renin activity, norepinephrine and heart rate increase consistently following nifedipine either in single doses or in long-term administration while very little changes are observed after institution of equihypotensive doses of verapamil. Monotherapy with calcium entry blockers can effectively control hypertension associated with type II diabetes mellitus or in primary hyperaldosteronism. Oral or sublingual nifedipine has been shown to be effective in the emergency antihypertensive treatment of certain life-threatening conditions associated with very high levels of blood pressure. Nifedipine, when given sublingually, may act within minutes reaching a peak effect within 30 minutes, an effect lasting up to 4 hours. Time release formulations of nifedipine, soon to be released, will maintain vasodilation for up to 10 hours. The side-effect profile of calcium entry blockers is acceptable and seems to be relatively free of alterations in potassium or carbohydrate metabolism. However, currently available preparation of nifedipine, verapamil, and diltiazem are short acting and thus require multiple doses per day. Finally, recent studies indicate that calcium entry blockers may have beneficial effects in improving regional blood flow.

An Analysis for and Against Treatment of Mild Hypertension

Nemat O. Borhani

The general subject of controversies in the therapy of hypertension is, perhaps, a misnomer. The positive association between an elevated blood pressure and subsequent mortality on the one hand, and the efficacy of therapy in reducing the mortality associated with severe hypertension on the other, are firmly established [1–3]. If there is a controversy, it seems to be in the choice of determining the level of blood pressure that requires therapy [4–6] and not on the issue of treatment itself.

There are many who believe that a sustained elevation of diastolic blood pressure above 90 mm Hg must be treated. Others set the level of blood pressure requiring treatment at a higher level than 90 mm Hg; hence, the controversy. Unfortunately, this seemingly benign debate is more profound than a passing academic interest. The lives of thousands of people are at stake [7]. Therefore, the issue deserves attention and must be considered with utmost scientific objectivity.

To address this important issue objectively, we need a definition of the so-called less severe hypertension. The adjective *mild* commonly used to describe this dreadful disease is, perhaps, unwarranted. There is nothing mild about elevated blood pressure, at any level. Hypertension is a "silent killer" in any of its forms or degrees. Arterial blood pressure is a quantifiable biological characteristic. The adverse effects of elevated blood pressure, both systolic and diastolic, are related proportionally to the degree of elevation [1, 2].

If we must classify hypertension in different categories to denote the degree of blood pressure elevation, an appropriate and meaningful index would be to use the actual level of blood pressure. For example, the distribution of diastolic blood pressure (DBP) can be divided into several strata as follows:

Stratum I: 90 to 104 mm Hg
Stratum II: 105 to 114 mm Hg
Stratum III: 115 mm Hg and above

This manuscript was presented as part of a Symposium on *Controversies in the Therapy of Hypertension.*

The phrase *stratum I hypertension* can be used, therefore, to define the clinical entity of the so-called less severe hypertension (that is, a DBP in the range of 90 to 104 mm Hg).

Magnitude of the Problem of Stratum I Hypertension

Approximately 72% of all men and women whose DBP is consistently above 90 mm Hg are in stratum I. Although the positive, and graded, association between the level of blood pressure (both systolic and diastolic) and mortality is known, it is noteworthy that an elevated blood pressure, including stratum I hypertension, is one of the established and recognized major risk factors for coronary heart disease (along with hyperlipidemia and cigarette smoking), and it is the single most important risk factor for stroke [1, 2]. Two important and subtle points relevant to the problem of stratum I hypertension are not universally appreciated. One is that chronic elevation of blood pressure, left untreated, causes injury to the endothelial surface of the arterial wall, increasing permeability to lipids and other noxious substances and leading both to platelet aggregation and to infiltration of lipids into the subendothelial tissue. Eventually, both processes will lead to the formation of atherosclerosis, with its known unfortunate clinical and pathological consequences, for instance, sudden death or acute myocardial infarction. This unfortunate vicious cycle resulting from atherosclerosis starts with a persistent elevation of blood pressure, even in its lowest substratum of stratum I (a DBP of 90 to 94 mm Hg). Epidemiologic and actuarial data indicate that the association between blood pressure and risk of coronary heart disease is a continuous one, which begins with even a DBP of less than 80 mm Hg [1, 2]. Results of the U.S. Pooling Project indicate that during a follow-up period of more than 8 years, the age-adjusted rates for coronary heart disease mortality, nonfatal myocardial infarction, and death from all causes were progressively higher for each stratum of DBP above 80 mm Hg than for those with levels below 80 mm Hg [2]. Further, the incidence of premature atherosclerosis, and its subsequent mortality and morbidity, increases with the level of blood pressure regardless of presence, or absence, of other risk factors [2]. Thus, the contention that elevated blood pressure in its lowest substratum is not a significant risk factor of immediate concern [8] is not correct; it is indeed misleading.

The second point is the numerical expression of the magnitude of risk of hypertension. Generally, there are two specific terms that denote the degree of association between a risk factor (for example, high blood pressure) and the incidence of an event (for example, mortality). One term is *relative risk* (RR). It means the proportion of those with a risk factor (for example, hypertension) who succumb to the event (for example, mortality) to those who do not have the risk factor but do succumb to the event nevertheless (that is, the ratio of age-adjusted mortality rate among those with a DBP above 80 mm Hg to the rate in those with a DBP below 80 mm Hg). The relative risk of mortality, and morbidity, increases proportionally with the level of blood pressure. But this important epidemiologic index does not portray true magnitude of hypertension in the community, especially that of stratum I. Nor is it a good measure of the impact of treatment and control of hypertension on the health of the community. The other term, which is perhaps more relevant than the first term, is *attributable risk* (AR). This refers to the excess number of deaths in a community caused by the risk factor under consideration, for example, hypertension. In other words, the absolute excess risk is the difference in risk between those with a DBP above 80 mm Hg and those below that level. Attributable risk is the measure that indicates the anticipated quantitative effect of treatment and control of hypertension. The magnitude of the problem of stratum I hypertension, and the impact of its control, is best appreciated when attributable risk is used as an index and not relative risk. The attributable risk of mortality from hypertension is always highest in its lowest strata. The reason for this is that blood pressure distribution in a given population is in itself asymmetrical, with the highest number of people in the lowest strata of hypertensive level. In other words, even when the absolute number of deaths associated with hypertension may be very low in its lowest stratum, the large number of people who are in that stratum and, therefore at risk, would make the excess number of deaths in that stratum the largest. It is estimated that each year 40 to 45% of excess deaths (that is, the attributable risk) attributed to hypertension in any community is borne by those in stratum I hypertension (that is, a DBP of 90 to 104 mm Hg) [9]. This means that if we could successfully treat 100% of those hypertensive persons who are in the high strata of hypertension (a DBP of 100 mm Hg and above)—which in itself is an impossible task—we would still be left with 40 to 45% of excess deaths in our communities owing to untreated hypertension. Further, untreated stratum I hypertension perpetuates the danger of progression toward severe hypertension and its concomitant complications, such as left ventricular hypertrophy (LVH) or coronary artery disease, hence, increasing the probability of final catastrophic events such as sudden death or acute myocardial infarction. The proportion of myocardial infarctions that are silent (unrecognized) are much higher among hypertensive persons than among normotensive persons, with a 5-fold to 7-fold risk ratio. In the Framingham study, among hypertensive women, 66% of acute myocardial infarctions were unrecognized, compared to only 25% among normotensives. Corresponding figures for men were 40% for the hypertensive group compared to 25% for the normotensive group [10]. Thus, not only does hypertension predispose individuals to acute myocardial infarction, but when the infarction occurs, it is more likely to be silent or atypical, increasing the probability of going unnoticed and leading to premature mortality or sudden death. Finally, from a strictly scientific point of view, the positive association between the level of blood pressure and diseases such as myocardial infarction and stroke is *strong, continuous, temporal, consistent, independent, predictive,* and *coherent* (that is, the epidemiologic findings are in agreement with those from clinical, postmortem, and animal experimental research). In addition, reasonable pathogenic mechanisms for this observed association have been delineated. Based on these criteria, therefore, this association is considered as a "cause-and-effect" relationship; elevated blood pressure is both a necessary and a sufficient cause for the adverse effects associated with it.

Evidence on the Efficacy of Treatment

The Veterans Administration study on the efficacy of drug treatment of hypertension in the prevention of mortality and morbidity is still a classic and, indeed, a landmark study [11]. It was the first randomized, double-blind, controlled, drug–placebo clinical trial providing evidence on the efficacy of drug treatment in the prevention of mortality and morbidity. The VA study provided conclusive evidence on the efficacy of drug treatment for men with baseline DBPs of 105 to 114 mm Hg and 115 to 129 mm Hg. In regard to the efficacy of treatment for DBP in the range of 90 to 104 mm Hg, the study reported a 35% reduction in morbid events among the drug-treated men compared to the placebo-treated group. However, owing to the small sample size of men in this stratum, a small number of events, and a short follow-up period, this difference was not statistically significant. Unfortunately, this lack of statistical significance at a nominal level of $P = 0.05$ has been erroneously interpreted as "no difference." This is not correct. Nevertheless, the VA study has made a significant contribution to our understanding of treatment for hypertension. Following the completion of the VA study, a series of clinical trials were conducted to answer questions left unanswered by the results of the VA study. Among these, the Hypertension Detection and Follow-Up Program (HDFP), the Australian Therapeutic Trial in Mild Hypertension, the Oslo study, and the USPHS Hospitals study provide the best evidence on the efficacy of treatment in stratum I hypertension [12–15]. The USPHS Hospitals and the Oslo studies [14, 15] were modest in sample size and had a relatively small number of morbid events, especially for coronary heart disease end-points. The discussion of the evidence on the efficacy of treatment of stratum I hypertension will be limited, therefore, to the other two major trials [12, 13], using most recent HDFP data for illustration.

Much has been written about the design and methods of both the HDFP and the Australian studies. Suffice to say that the latter was a placebo–drug controlled trial, whereas in the former, participants were randomized into stepped-care (SC) groups (those who received a rigorous drug treatment in the HDFP centers) and referred-care (RC) groups (those who were referred to their usual source of care for treatment). The Australian study randomized 3427 white men and women, aged 30 to 69 years, with baseline DBPs of 90 to 109 mm Hg, 75% of whom were in stratum I (DBP, 90 to 104 mm Hg). The average follow-up period was 4 years. Patients were randomized into a drug-treated group (a SC regimen) and a placebo-treated group. At the end of the study, the investigators reported a significant reduction in mortality (all causes, cardiovascular diseases, and stroke) and morbidity (that is, nonfatal trial end-points) in the actively treated group, compared to placebo [13].

The HDFP randomized 10,940 men and women, black and white, aged 30 to 60 years, with baseline DBPs of 90 mm Hg and above (72% of those randomized were in stratum I hypertension). Since the HDFP design did not use placebo, its critics have argued that the HDFP compared "one treated group with another treated group and that there was no 'scientifically pure' control" [6]. This argument has been answered convincingly by in-depth analyses of HDFP data. These analyses demonstrate that the percentage of HDFP participants who were at or below the desired blood pressure at the end of the study was much higher in SC than the RC groups (64% vs. 43%). The average DBP among those in stratum I at the end of the study was 83.4 mm Hg in SC and 87.8 mm Hg in RC. Also, well over half of the excess deaths among the RC group in the HDFP study was attributed to differences in factors related to proper treatment of high blood pressure alone [16].

Data presented in Table 1 show a 5-year mortality (per 100) from all causes (that is, total mortality) among HDFP participants in stratum I. The percent reduction in mortality in favor of SC was 20.3% for the entire stratum ($P < 0.01$). Relative reductions in 5-year mortality in favor of SC were 21.9%, 23.1%, and 13.8%, respectively, in each substratum of stratum I [12].

The greatest benefit of SC treatment in the HDFP was realized among those participants in stratum I who did not have any evidence of target organ damage at baseline (that is, no history of myocardial infarction, intermittent claudication or stroke, serum creatinine above 1.7 mg/dl, or left ventricular hypertrophy). These results are presented in Table 2. Among this particular subgroup of the HDFP population, the 5-year mortality was reduced in favor of SC by 28.6% in stratum I as a whole ($P < 0.01$). In its lowest substratum, a DBP of 90 to 94 mm Hg, the reduction in mortality in favor of SC was 34% [12].

Similarly in favor of SC, there was an impressive reduction in the incidence of fatal and nonfatal stroke [17], fatal and nonfatal myocardial infarction, and angina pectoris [18]. These results are summarized in Table 3.

The 5-year incidence of fatal coronary heart disease (ICDA 410–414, 9th revision) and nonfatal myocardial infarction (that is, the first coronary event) was reduced among the SC group, compared to the RC group, in all race-sex categories. Overall, the percent reduction in the incidence of first coronary

Table 1. Five-year life table mortality rate (per 100) among HDFP participants with stratum I hypertension[a]

DBP strata (mm Hg)	With stepped care (SC)			With referred care			Percent reduction in favor of SC
	Sample size	No. of deaths	Rate per 100	Sample size	No. of deaths	Rate per 100	
Stratum I							
90 to 104	3903	231	5.9	3922	291	7.4	20.3[b]
Substrata							
90 to 94	1474	84	5.7	1467	107	7.3	21.9
95 to 99	1390	69	5.0	1341	87	6.5	23.1
100 to 104	1039	78	7.5	1114	97	8.7	13.8

[a] Stratum I hypertension refers to a diastolic blood pressure (DBP) of 90 to 104 mm Hg. Stepped care refers to a rigorous drug treatment in HDFP centers; referred care, to the care provided by the patient's usual source of treatment
[b] $P < 0.01$.

Table 2. Five-year life table mortality rate (per 100) among HDFP participants with stratum I hypertension but free of end-organ damage and not on antihypertensive treatment at baseline[a]

DBP strata (mm Hg)	With stepped care (SC)			With referred care			Percent reduction in favor of SC
	Sample size	No. of deaths	Rate per 100	Sample size	No. of deaths	Rate per 100	
Stratum I							
90 to 104	2619	106	4.0	2703	151	5.6	28.6[b]
Substrata							
90 to 94	1022	36	3.5	1023	54	5.3	34.0
95 to 99	932	39	4.2	913	53	5.8	27.6
100 to 104	665	31	4.7	767	44	5.8	19.0

[a] Stratum I hypertension refers to a diastolic blood pressure (DBP) of 90 to 104 mm Hg.
[b] $P < 0.01$.

event was 12.1% in favor of SC (Table 3). Not shown in the table is the finding that although the percent reduction in favor of SC was slightly higher in men than in women, the difference between the two sexes was not significant [18]. Similarly, there was no difference in reduction of incidence of first coronary event between whites and blacks. When these data were analyzed by age groups, the most dramatic finding was a significant reduction (26.1%) in the incidence of first coronary event in the 30- to 40-year age group, in favor of SC. Further, the 5-year incidence of de novo angina pectoris was lower in SC, compared with RC, by 15.2% [18]. These findings strongly suggest that among those with persistently elevated DBP in the range of 90 to 104 mm Hg, there is a very high likelihood of developing stroke, coronary heart disease, or angina pectoris in the presence of untreated hypertension, and that when hypertension is treated these individuals demonstrate a definite benefit in favor of treatment.

Data presented in Figure 1 depict the 5-year incidence rate of progression and regression of left ventricular hypertrophy (LVH) among the two groups

Table 3. Five-year incidence of morbid events among HDFP participants with stratum I hypertension[a]

Morbid Events	With stepped care (SC)			With referred care			Percent reduction in favor of SC
	Sample size	No. of events	Rate per 100	Sample size	No. of events	Rate per 100	
Fatal and nonfatal myocardial infarction	3553	307	8.7	3558	355	9.9	12.1[b]
Fatal and nonfatal stroke	3903	59	1.5	3922	87	2.2	31.8[b]
Angina pectoris	3635	241	6.7	3649	291	7.9	15.2[b]

[a] Stratum I hypertension refers to a diastolic blood pressure (DBP) of 90 to 104 mm Hg.
[b] $P < 0.05$.

of participants in the HDFP. The incidence rate of progression from a normal ECG pattern to a tall R wave was 3.9% in the SC group and 4.2% in the RC group, a difference of 7.1% in favor of SC. By far the most dramatic finding was the rate of progression from a tall R wave to a frank LVH: 4.7% in SC and 7.6% in RC, a difference of 38.2% in favor of SC. Overall, the 5-year incidence of LVH was lower in SC than in RC in both men and women [19].

Also, presented in Figure 1 are data on the rate of regression of an abnormal ECG pattern presented at baseline. The 5-year incidence of regression from a tall R wave to normal was 53.4% in SC and 43.3% in RC, a difference of 23.3% in favor of the SC. Similarly, the rate of regression from a frank LVH to a tall R wave was greater in SC than in RC, 21.4% in SC and 14.2% in RC, a difference of 51.0% in favor of SC.

Similarly, when the cardiothoracic ratio (CTR) on chest x-ray was used as an index of cardiomegaly (CTR $\geq$ 0.50), the incidence of cardiomegaly was higher in RC than in SC. Conversely, the rate of regression from cardiomegaly to normal, using CTR as an index, was higher in SC than RC [19].

These data indicate that SC drug treatment of stratum I hypertension aimed at reducing the elevated DBP and maintaining it at goal level will reduce the incidence of left ventricular hypertrophy, one of the known major sequelae of untreated hypertension. Further, among those patients who have already developed left ventricular hypertrophy, rigorous treatment will cause regression of this abnormality. In other words, left ventricular hypertrophy associated with hypertension in stratum I (DBP of 90 to 104 mm Hg) seems reversible with treatment. The argument that the outcome of HDFP in favor of stepped-care was due to good medical care and not necessarily the treatment

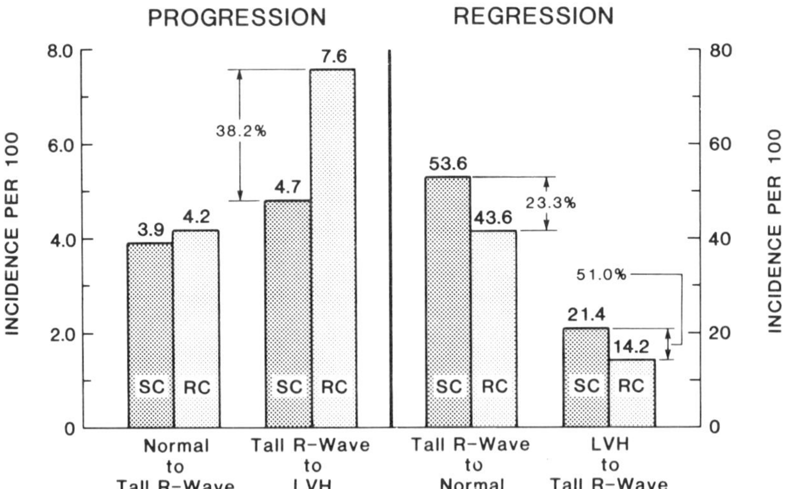

Fig. 1. Adjusted five-year incidence rate of changes in ECG pattern from baseline, in HDFP stratum I (DBP 90 to 104 mm Hg).

of hypertension itself is inconsistent with these data. Good quality medical care does not halt progression of left ventricular hypertrophy (LVH) in hypertensive patients; a good control of high blood pressure does.

It should be pointed out that although the difference in total mortality between SC and RC in young HDFP participants (age group, 30 to 49 years) was not statistically significant, the incidence of LVH was reduced significantly in favor of SC in this particular age group. Further, the HDFP data have demonstrated that any evidence of LVH in stratum I hypertension carries a very high risk of mortality. Therefore, it is necessary to emphasize the fact that in our attempt to control stratum I hypertension as a force of mortality and morbidity, we should be concerned with young individuals with stratum I hypertension as well as those who are beyond the age of 50 years.

Argument Against Treatment

There are two conceptual arguments used frequently by opponents of the use of treatment for hypertension in its lowest substratum of stratum I (DBP of 90 to 94 mm Hg). Some prefer 90 mm Hg as the limit for treatment, whereas others prefer 95 mm Hg. Today, very few argue that the limit of DBP requiring treatment should be 100 mm Hg, as was the case one or two years ago [8].

One of the conceptual arguments against treatment of hypertension in the DBP range of 90 to 94 mm Hg is the potential side effects of antihypertensive drugs. Since, by tradition, the majority of patients in the lowest substratum of stratum I hypertension will be on step-1 antihypertensive drug, which traditionally has been an oral diuretic (for example, chlorthalidone or thiazides), discussion on the evidence of any side effect or adverse effect will be limited to these drugs. By far, the most troublesome report is the one in which the use of these diuretics is related to elevated levels of serum lipids, especially LDL-cholesterol [20], and the possibility of an adverse effect of treatment in the presence of resting ECG abnormalities at baseline in this particular subgroup of hypertensive population [21].

A recent report of the Multiple Risk Factor Intervention Trial (MRFIT) implied a possible adverse effect of thiazide diuretics for stratum I hypertension in the presence of resting ECG abnormalities [21]. These findings for this particular subgroup of patients may be due to random variation (i.e., chance alone) resulting from the analysis of subgroups with a small sample size and an even smaller number of events. In view of the difficulties in interpreting findings of subgroup analyses in a study like MRFIT, in which the sample size and the power of the study was based on the primary endpoint (that is, coronary heart disease mortality) among a total cohort population, it is impossible to draw any definitive conclusion from these results. Nevertheless, it seems prudent to heed the implicit suggestion that there may be an adverse effect associated with the rigorous treatment of hypertension in the DBP range of 90 to 94 mm Hg when the patient exhibits minor

ECG abnormalities such as a tall R wave. In other words, a question of possible adverse effect has been posed, albeit implicitly, and must be considered. Unfortunately, this important clinical question cannot be adequately answered based on available data, including the results of a further analysis that was conducted on the HDFP data [22].

Immediately after the publication of MRFIT data, a further analysis of HDFP data was undertaken to determine whether the MRFIT findings could be replicated in a MRFIT-like cohort of the HDFP population. This analysis of HDFP data revealed that 5-year mortality rates from coronary heart disease (CHD), total cardiovascular diseases (CVD), and all-cause mortality were consistently lower in SC than in RC for all age-sex-race subgroups in stratum I (DBP, 90 to 104 mm Hg) participants free of resting ECG abnormalities at baseline. Interestingly, for those who did have evidence of resting ECG abnormalities at baseline, all-cause mortality rates and total cardiovascular disease mortality rates were also lower in SC than RC, a finding that is not consistent with the MRFIT results [21, 22]. Only for CHD mortality were the rates for SC slightly and insignificantly higher than those for the RC among those with resting ECG abnormalities at baseline. Further, this was the case only in all women and white men but not for black men. It should be pointed out, however, that none of the differences in rates observed between SC and RC in these analyses were significant at a nominal level of $P = 0.05$. Thus, the observed difference between SC and RC in CHD mortality among those with resting ECG abnormalities could be due to chance alone. The problem of interpreting these data, and the MRFIT results, was further complicated by a death rate lower than had been expected in the usual-care group in MRFIT, and by the fact that in the HDFP both the SC and RC groups with resting ECG abnormalities at baseline experienced a much higher mortality rate than those without resting ECG abnormalities at baseline, which was not the case in MRFIT. In MRFIT, the usual-care group with resting ECG abnormalities at baseline experienced a lower mortality rate than those without such abnormalities [21]. It is logical to assume that if the mortality experience of the usual-care group of men in MRFIT had been as expected, and if the HDFP results had prevailed in MRFIT, there would have been perhaps little or no excess CHD mortality for the special-intervention hypertensive men with resting ECG abnormalities at baseline. In any event, and despite all of these speculations, the MRFIT experience clearly indicated that nutritional counseling, in regard to both calorie balance and diet composition, could avoid the possible adverse effects of oral diuretics or other antihypertensive drugs on levels of serum lipids. Also, it is perhaps noteworthy that for the "bottom line" end-point (that is, the total mortality) HDFP, unlike MRFIT, showed a favorable outcome of SC treatment compared to RC in its specific "MRFIT-like" subgroup with resting ECG abnormalities at baseline [22]. Thus, it seems that the sobering decision for treatment of stratum I hypertension should not be based on reports of possible adverse effects, the validity or repeatability of which cannot be determined with certainty. Nevertheless, the challenge posed by these data must not be ignored either. As a whole, there is enough evidence favoring drug treatment of stratum I hypertension. When necessary, treatment should be augmented with proper nutritional counseling.

The other conceptual question raised against treatment is the issue of "yield" in terms of benefits versus "risk," for lifelong drug therapy for a large segment of the population [5]. This argument, although of great concern, dismisses two important issues. One is the fact that individuals in stratum I hypertension are very rarely free of other major risk factors (for example, hyperlipidemia and cigarette smoking). Thus, any calculation of benefits versus "risk" of treatment should consider the strong interaction among these risk factors and their additive effects in the presence of hypertension. The second point is the issue of attributable risk (that is, the excess deaths from hypertension) discussed earlier. The very high prevalence of hypertension in stratum I exposes a great majority of people at risk; very few of them are free of other risk factors. Thus, even though the yield of treatment may be small in terms of absolute numbers, the relative reduction in mortality resulting from an appropriate treatment of hypertension in this population subgroup, multiplied by the large number of people in that subgroup, would result in a significant number of lives saved [7]. In the HDFP, relative reduction in 5-year mortality among participants in stratum I was 20.3% in favor of SC. A simple projection of this figure to the total number of hypertensive persons in the country who are in stratum I will put the number of lives saved by treatment at more than hundreds of thousands each year. Is this a small yield?

It is sometimes argued that those in stratum I hypertension are "at relatively little risk" from their elevated blood pressure [8]. This is not true. The HDFP data on the progression of the ECG pattern from a tall R wave toward frank LVH convincingly demonstrate that the risk is real in all substrata of stratum I, especially in individuals under the age of 40 years [19].

Unfortunately, most arguments against treatment of hypertension in the lowest substrata of stratum I are based on either a misinterpretation of the HDFP results (or similar studies) or a misunderstanding of the reports of these studies. For example, it is claimed that "the results of the HDFP show that the percentage of the patient population saved by more intensive therapy was similar for those with and for those without target organ damage at entry into the trial" [8]. This statement seems to be based on a misinterpretation of the published HDFP data [12]. The published HDFP data clearly indicate that the greatest reduction in 5-year mortality in favor of SC (34%) was in those who had no evidence of end-organ damage at entry [12], whereas among those with end-organ damage at entry, the relative reduction in 5-year mortality in favor of SC was only 7.1%, a great difference, indeed, from 34.1%.

Conclusion and Summary

Hypertension in its lowest stratum (a DBP of 90 to 94 mm Hg) is just as bad as it is in its severe forms. The association between blood pressure level and mortality is graded and continuous in nature and increases proportionally with the level of blood pressure, both systolic and diastolic.

The results of recent clinical and community-based trials on the efficacy of treatment clearly indicate the benefit of rigorous treatment. Further, based on the available scientific evidence, rigorous treatment of hypertension is most beneficial when administered before end-organ damage occurs.

In addition, treatment of stratum I hypertension prevents progression to severe hypertension, which occurs frequently among those in whom hypertension is left untreated or is inadequately treated. As to the practical implications of the recent data reported by MRFIT in regarding those with stratum I hypertension who exhibit abnormalities on their resting ECG, it is important to emphasize that, for the "bottom line" end-point (total mortality), the HDFP data, unlike MRFIT, yielded results indicating a favorable outcome for SC treatment compared to RC, in its specific "MRFIT-like" cohort.

Patients with stratum I hypertension (a DBP of 90 to 104 mm Hg) who develop major end-organ damage (for example, LVH) carry a great risk of mortality and morbidity, even when they receive rigorous antihypertensive therapy. These patients need optimal medical care; their high blood pressure must be lowered by the safest means possible. Of course nutritional counseling, in regard to both calorie balance and diet composition, is useful and must be done routinely to avoid possible adverse effects of antihypertensive drugs (for example, hyperlipidemia). However, nonpharmacological modes of treatment should not be continued as a substitute when the DBP remains above 90 mm Hg.

References

1. BUILD AND BLOOD PRESSURE STUDY, New York, Society of Actuaries, 1979, vol. 1
2. POOLING PROJECT RESEARCH GROUP: Relationship of blood pressure, serum cholesterol, smoking habit and ECG abnormalities to incidence of major coronary events. *J Chronic Dis* 31:201–306, 1978
3. VETERANS ADMINISTRATION COOPERATIVE STUDY GROUP ON ANTIHYPERTENSIVE AGENTS: Effects of treatment on morbidity in hypertension: Results in patients with diastolic blood pressure averaging 115 through 129 mm Hg. *JAMA* 202:1028–1034, 1967
4. MCALISTER NH: Should we treat mild hypertension? *JAMA* 365:379–382, 1983
5. PICKERING TG: Treatment of mild hypertension and the reduction of cardiovascular mortality: The 'of-or-by' dilemma. *JAMA* 249:399–400, 1983
6. FREIS ED: Should mild hypertension be treated? *N Engl J Med* 307:306–309, 1982
7. GIFFORD RW, BORHANI NO, KRISHAN I, MOSER M, LEVY RI, SCHOENBERGER JA: The dilemma of "mild" hypertension, another viewpoint of treatment. *JAMA* 250:3171–3173, 1983
8. KAPLAN NM: Therapy of mild hypertension: An overview. *Am J Cardiol* 53:2A–8A, 1984
9. THE HDFP COOPERATIVE GROUP: A progress report. *Circ Res* 40(Suppl I):I-107–I-109, 1977
10. KANNEL WB, ABBOTT RD, DANNENBERG AL: Unrecognized myocardial infarction and hypertension: The Framingham Study (*abstract*). *CVD Newsletter* 35 (SC-84–E-35):28, 1984
11. VETERANS ADMINISTRATION COOPERATIVE STUDY GROUP ON ANTIHYPERTENSIVE AGENTS: Effects of treatment on morbidity in hypertension: Results in pa-

tients with diastolic blood pressure averaging 90 through 114 mm Hg. *JAMA* 213:1143–1152, 1970

12. THE HDFP COOPERATIVE GROUP: The effect of treatment on mortality in "mild" hypertension. *N Engl J Med* 307:976–980, 1982

13. Report of the Management Committee on the Australian therapeutic trial in mild hypertension. *Lancet* 1:261–267, 1980

14. HELGELAND A: Treatment of mild hypertension: A five-year controlled drug trial. *Am J Med* 69:725–732, 1980

15. SMITH WM: Treatment of mild hypertension: Results of a ten-year intervention trial. *Circ Res* 40(Suppl I):I-98–I-105, 1977

16. HARDY JH, HAWKINS CM: The impact of selected indices of antihypertensive treatment on all-cause mortality. *Am J Epidemiol* 117:566–574, 1983

17. THE HDFP COOPERATIVE GROUP: Reduction in stroke incidence among persons with high blood pressure. *JAMA* 247:633–638, 1983

18. THE HDFP COOPERATIVE GROUP: Effect of stepped care treatment on the incidence of myocardial infarction and angina pectoris: Five-year findings of the HDFP. *Hypertension* 6(Suppl 1):I-198–I-206, 1984

19. THE HDFP COOPERATIVE GROUP: Regression of left ventricular hypertrophy with antihypertensive therapy (*abstract*). *Circulation* 64(Suppl IV):322, 1981

20. GRIMM R, LEON A, HUNNINGBAKE D: Effect of thiazide diuretics on plasma lipids in mildly hypertensive patients. *Ann Intern Med* 94:7–11, 1981

21. MULTIPLE RISK FACTOR INTERVENTION TRIAL RESEARCH GROUP: Risk factor changes and mortality results. *JAMA* 248:1465–1477, 1982

22. HYPERTENSION DETECTION AND FOLLOW-UP PROGRAM COOPERATIVE GROUP: The effect of antihypertensive drug treatment on mortality in the presence of resting ECG abnormalities at baseline: The HDFP Experience. *Circulation,* in press

Phosphate Depletion

Clinical Spectrum of Phosphate Depletion and Its Effects on Urinary Acidification

Sandra Sabatini

The body contains 23 moles of phosphate, approximately 80% of which is in bone and 9% in skeletal muscle. The intracellular concentration of phosphate is approximately 100 mmoles/liter. The bulk of intracellular phosphate is organic in the form of intermediary carbohydrates, lipids, and protein. A small fraction is inorganic, and is of pivotal importance in serving as the source of adenosine triphosphate (ATP) [1].

A normal adult ingests one gram of phosphorus daily. Approximately 90% is excreted into the urine while the remainder appears in the feces [2, 3]. Plasma phosphate concentrations in children vary between 4.0 and 7.1 mg/dl while in the adult normal concentrations average 3.0 to 4.5 mg/dl (1.7 to 2.6 mEq/liter). Renal excretion of phosphate is regulated by glomerular filtration and tubular reabsorption. There is some evidence that tubular secretion of phosphate occurs; although this is of minor importance in the overall regulation of the plasma phosphate concentration [4–7].

There are a wide variety of pathophysiologic states associated with hypophosphatemia (Table 1). Hypophosphatemia does not necessarily mean phosphate depletion. In fact, severe deficiency may be present in the face of normal or elevated plasma phosphate concentrations. This dichotomy is likely the result of cellular shifts from muscle and bone, tissues which contain large quantities of phosphate. When dietary phosphate is reduced to 100 mg/day or less, negative balance occurs and fecal phosphate excretion exceeds that in urine. In females, the plasma serum phosphate concentration may fall to values as low as 1.0 mg/dl, while the plasma phosphate concentration tends to stay within normal limits in males. This reduction occurs early in females (within 3 weeks), and it is not related to an increase in parathyroid hormone activity [8].

Respiratory alkalosis may cause a marked decrease in the plasma phosphate concentration. This decrease is associated with a fall in urinary phosphate

This manuscript was presented as part of a Symposium on *Renal and Vascular Consequences of Phosphate Depletion.*

Table 1. Pathophysiologic states associated with hypophosphatemia[a]

Moderate hypophosphatemia (plasma levels 1.0 to 2.5 mg/dl)
Starvation, dietary restriction
Gastrectomy, bile salt deficiency
Vitamin D deficiency
Laxative abuse, beryllium, iron administration, calcium carbonate
Hemodialysis
Hormone excess (parathyroid hormone, insulin, glucagon, epinephrine, gastrin, corticosteroids, androgens)
Volume expansion
Administration of glucose, fructose, lactate, bicarbonate and glycerol
Osteomalacia
Pregnancy
Hypomagnesemia
Diuretic therapy
Renal tubular defects
Recovery from hypothermia
Salicylate intoxication
Severe hypophosphatemia (plasma levels <1.0 mg/dl)
Respiratory alkalosis
Alcohol withdrawal
Hyperalimentation, "Nutrional Recovery Syndrome"
Recovery from severe burns
Phosphate binders

[a] Adapted from [9,10].

excretion. While this may be due solely to cellular shifts, the fall in plasma phosphate concentration may also be due to stimulation of glycolysis and increased utilization of ATP as a consequence of intracellular alkalosis.

Perhaps the most life threatening causes of phosphate depletion occur during alcohol withdrawal, hyperalimentation, and recovery from diabetes mellitus or severe third degree burns (see [9, 10] for review). For example, patients with severe third degree burns retain large quantities of salt and water. As recovery progresses, the retained salt and water are mobilized and subsequently excreted into the urine. In the face of this diuresis, a substantial loss of phosphate may occur. This loss occurs in combination with tissue anabolic processes in which cellular repair is utilizing large quantities of phosphate. The nutritional recovery syndrome seen during refeeding of patients with severe protein malnutrition was first recognized in World War II when prisoners of war were released from camps in Europe, Japan, and the South Pacific [11–13]. Refeeding of these people, particularly with simple carbohydrates, was followed by the appearance of edema, ascites, hydrothorax, and death. While it was well recognized that a thiamine deficiency was present, it appears that phosphate depletion was the cause of death.

In diabetes mellitus, particularly in association with ketoacidosis, there is an increased excretion of phosphate into the urine. Initial losses of phosphate were reported to range up to 400 mmoles, values now thought to be underestimated. With insulin administration, the plasma phosphate concentration falls markedly, secondary to an insulin-induced shift of phosphate inside the cells along with glucose and potassium. This intracellular shift of phosphate, coupled with poor dietary intake, is probably the mechanism for the hypophosphatemia seen in the alcoholic. Hypophosphatemia is generally seen on the second or third hospital day and it may be profound if not repaired. Additionally, patients with diabetes mellitus and alcoholism may also have magnesium deficiency. A characteristic finding in magnesium deficiency is an increase in phosphate excretion. Alcoholic patients may also have hypercalcemia. Taken together, these electrolyte abnormalities could lead to severe phosphate depletion [9].

Aluminum-containing antacids, beryllium, and iron will bind both dietary phosphate and secreted fecal phosphate, consequently producing a negative phosphate balance [14]. The serum phosphate concentration falls approximately 10% to that of normal; however, with prolonged administration of phosphate-binders, a negative phosphate balance of 200 to 300 mg/day is achieved eventually. The combination of phosphate-binders plus dietary phosphate restriction (to less than 400 mg/day) will produce severe hypophosphatemia with serum phosphate concentration below 1.0 mg/100 ml within two weeks. This is associated with weakness, debility, and bone pain [15].

The main consequences of severe phosphate depletion appear to be: erythrocyte, leukocyte, and platelet dysfunction, central nervous system and cardiovascular abnormalities, and rhabdomyolysis. The latter, in addition to causing acute renal failure, could also be the cause of the severe congestive heart failure that has been reported in phosphate depleted animals [16–31]. The clinical characteristics and biochemical mechanisms of phosphate depletion are given in Table 2.

Phosphate deprivation (or depletion) may cause a wide range of changes in renal function. There may be alterations in glomerular filtration rate, disorders of tubular transport and alterations in renal metabolism. These effects are summarized in Table 3.

Mechanisms of Acidification

Proximal Tubule Bicarbonate Reabsorption

Most of the filtered bicarbonate is reabsorbed in the proximal tubule. The proximal tubule is a high capacitance, low pH gradient system that reabsorbs 80 to 90% of filtered bicarbonate by sodium for hydrogen exchange. The remaining 10 to 20% is reabsorbed in the distal nephron, a low capacitance, high pH gradient system [33]. Bicarbonate does not appear in the urine under most conditions. Many factors control proximal bicarbonate reabsorption, the most important of which is changes of extracellular fluid volume (see [33–37] for reviews). Expansion of extracellular volume depresses bicarbonate absorption in the proximal tubule. Bicarbonate reabsorption is related inversely to body potassium stores such that hyperkalemia depresses bicarbonate reabsorption. This inverse relationship is independent of the state of

Table 2. Consequences of severe phosphate depletion

Clinical characteristics	Biochemical mechanisms	Reference
Erythrocyte dysfunction	↓ ATP content, ↓ 2-3 DPG[a]	[16–18]
(hemolysis, ↓ O$_2$ carrying	↓ Utilization of glucose	[18]
capacity, polychromasia,	↑ Glyceraldehyde-3-phosphate	[18]
microspherocytosis, ↓ cell	↑ Dihydroxyacetone phosphate	[18]
viability)	↓ O$_2$ carrying capacity	[16, 19, 20]
Leukocyte dysfunction	↓ ATP content	[21]
(bacterial and fungal infections)	Impaired phagocytosis and	
	bacteriocidal activity	[22–24]
	Impaired phosphoinosotide	
	synthesis	[24–26]
Platelet dysfunction	↓ ATP content (modest)	
(? microvascular hemorrhage)	Thrombocytopenia	
	Marrow megakaryoctosis	[26, 27]
	↓ Platelet survival	
	Impaired clot retraction	
Central nervous system disorders	±↓ Brain ATP content	[28]
(irritability, ataxia, paresthe-	Diffuse EEG slowing	[18]
sias, dysarthria, seizures,	↓ 2-3 DPG	
muscular weakness, coma)	↓ O$_2$ carrying capacity	[18]
Rhabdomyolysis	↓ ATP content	
(weakness, myalgias necrosis,	↓ Resting membrane potential	[9]
acute renal failure, congestive	±↓ Cell potassium	[9, 25]
heart failure)	↑ Cell sodium and H$_2$O	[9, 31, 32]

[a] 2-3 diphosphoglycerate.

extracellular fluid volume. Bicarbonate reabsorption is enhanced by an increase of arterial P_{CO_2}. This effect is believed to be caused by a change of intracellular pH. Since carbon dioxide diffuses readily across cell membranes, a rise in the arterial P_{CO_2} is probably accompanied by a parallel rise of the intracellular carbon dioxide tension. A rise in intracellular P_{CO_2} would increase the intracellular hydrogen ion concentration. This effect would increase sodium-for-hydrogen exchange and enhance bicarbonate reabsorption sec-

Table 3. Renal effects of phosphate depletion[a]

Decreased glomerular filtration rate	Hypercalciuria
Decreased bicarbonate Tm and glucose Tm	Hypermagnesuria
Decreased proximal sodium reabsorption without natriuresis	Hypophosphaturia
Decreased titratable acid excretion	Decreased response to parathyroid hormone and volume expansion
Decreased intracellular hydrogen ion concentration	Decreased gluconeogenesis
	Increased 1-25 vitamin D$_3$
Decreased renal content of phosphorus and ATP	Decreased/normal cyclic-AMP excretion

[a] Adapted from [32].

ondarily. Bicarbonate reabsorption is decreased by pharmacologic doses of parathyroid hormone. Hypercalcemia and vitamin D increase bicarbonate reabsorption. Since the effect of hypercalcemia is also seen in thyroparathyroidectomized animals, it appears that its mechanism of action is independent of any effect of parathyroid hormone [38]. Phosphate depletion can cause a decrease in proximal bicarbonate reabsorption.

Distal Nephron Acidification

Ammonium Excretion

Ammonia is a weak base that is freely diffusable across all cell membranes. It is produced locally within both the proximal and distal nephron. At the inner mitochondrial membrane, glutamine, normally present in cytosol, is converted to glutamate, liberating one ammonia molecule. Glutamate is converted subsequently to alpha-ketoglutarate, thus liberating a second molecule of ammonia. The mitochondrial pathway is under the influence of glutaminase I, a phosphate-dependent enzyme [39–41]. A reduction of tissue phosphate may thus decrease glutaminase I activity, consequently decreasing ammonia production by the kidney.

The pK of the ammonia-ammonium buffer is 9.15; at a physiologic pH virtually all of the ammonia is present in ionized form. It is thought that ammonium is trapped in the tubule lumen and excreted subsequently as ammonium chloride or ammonium sulfate. More recently, Goldstein, Claiborne, and Evans [42] have shown that the gills of fish are permeable to the ionized form of the molecule (ammonium). This appears to be true for other transporting membranes as well [43, 44]. While direct measurements are required to define these observations precisely, it appears that our prior view of nonionic diffusion as the sole or principal transport mechanism for ammonia may need to be reconsidered.

Ammonium excretion is influenced by two major factors: urine pH and acid-base status. An acute reduction of urine pH allows more ammonia to be trapped as the ammonium ion. This effect is believed to be due to the change in ammonia distribution. Chronic states of acidosis stimulate glutamine utilization directly, thus leading to increased ammonium excretion. While the adaptive enhancement of ammonium excretion requires several days, the magnitude of enhancement may be considerable. In chronic metabolic acidosis, ammonium excretion may increase from negligible levels to 200 mEq/liter per day.

Titratable Acid Excretion, Distal Delivery, and Urine P_{CO_2}

Unlike ammonium excretion, titratable acid excretion is relatively fixed in both animals and man. Under normal conditions, titratable acid in man is 10 to 40 mEq/day and is present in the urine in the form of weak acid anions. Most of these anions are in the form of phosphate, although uric acid, creatinine and other organic acids may be present in small quantities.

The delivery of buffer to the distal nephron is decreased in hypophosphatemic states, regardless of the cause of hypophosphatemia (that is, cellular shifts or phosphate depletion). Acid-base homeostatis is then influenced by the distal delivery of phosphate. This influence may be assessed by direct measurement of urine titratable acid or the ability of the urine to generate CO_2 tension. In a maximally alkaline urine, the ability to generate CO_2 tension has been used by many laboratories as an index of distal urinary acidification [34, 45–47]. This is based on the premise that, in the face of adequate distal delivery of buffer (bicarbonate, phosphate, and so forth), proton secretion by the terminal nephron will combine with a buffer such as bicarbonate to form carbonic acid. The acid formed will then decompose at a slower rate to generate water and CO_2. A rise in CO_2 tension is indicative of normal distal acidification.

In the case of phosphate delivery to the terminal nephron, proton secretion would result in the formation:

$$H^+ + HPO_4^= \underset{}{\overset{pK\ 6.8}{\rightleftharpoons}} H_2PO_4^-$$
$$\downarrow\uparrow$$
$$H^+ \quad + HCO_3^-$$
$$\Big\downarrow\Big\uparrow \quad pK\ 6.1$$
$$H_2CO_3 \rightleftharpoons H_2O + CO_2$$

As this is in equilibrium at pH 6.8, one hydrogen of the monovalent phosphate may dissociate in the lumen resulting in the formation of a free proton. The proton is free to combine with bicarbonate, which will then form carbonic acid and dissociate to water and CO_2 in the lower urinary tract.

It is obvious that phosphate will not contribute to urinary CO_2 tension in an alkaline urine; whereas the anionic form of buffer is present ($H_2PO_4^-$) in an acid urine, there will be no bicarbonate present to titrate to CO_2. At a urine pH near 6.8, however, the ability to increase the urine CO_2 tension is dependent directly on the urinary phosphate concentration. Normal subjects with low urinary phosphate concentration will not increase the urine CO_2 tension (to 40 mm Hg higher than blood) even though the mechanism for distal acidification is intact [48].

Effect of Phosphate Depletion on Glomerular Filtration Rate and Proximal Acidification

Glomerular Filtration Rate (GFR)

In some studies in man, dog, and rat, phosphate depletion causes a fall in GFR, which returns to control values following repletion in some species [49, 50, 62]. While the mechanism for the decrease in GFR is not completely known, several possibilities exist. Chronic hypercalciuria or transient hypercalcemia may be associated with deposition of calcium in the kidney. Both have been reported in phosphate depletion [15, 49–52] and could cause renal insufficiency. However, histologic evaluation of the kidneys from dogs subjected to phosphate depletion is totally normal, as is the calcium content of cortex and medulla [49]. Thus, it is unlikely that this is the cause of the reduction in GFR noted in dogs and humans. A second possibility is that of a decrease in cardiac output. If cardiac performance declines, as has been shown by several investigators, GFR may be expected to fall secondarily [53, 54].

Proximal Bicarbonate Reabsorption

Hyperchloremic metabolic acidosis has been reported in a variety of species with severe hypophosphatemia, including dogs with phosphate depletion and patients with parathyroid hormone (PTH) excess, cachexia, and those receiving parenteral nutrition [9, 55, 56]. In animals, the effect of phosphate depletion on proximal bicarbonate reabsorption is complex; it may be species related.

Gold et al [56] demonstrated that prolonged phosphate depletion in dogs (40 to 139 days), induced by the ingestion of a phosphate deficient diet and the administration of aluminum-containing phosphate-binders, caused a significant fall in the plasma bicarbonate concentration. The fall in plasma bicarbonate concentration from 24.5 to 21.0 mEq/liter was related directly to the level of the fall in serum phosphate concentration. In this study, GFR did not change as compared to controls. Bicarbonate titration curves in these animals revealed that phosphate depletion was associated with a fall in bicarbonate Tm at all levels of filtered bicarbonate. The threshold for the appearance of bicarbonate in the urine was reduced in all phosphate depleted animals. Thus, there was not only a decreased Tm for bicarbonate, but also a small leak of bicarbonate into the urine at every level of filtered load. These results suggest that prolonged phosphate depletion may be associated with proximal renal tubular acidosis.

Further indirect evidence for a proximal tubular leak comes from the data of Gold, Massry, and Friedler [57] in which a defect in glucose transport was noted in phosphate depleted dogs (decreased glucose Tm). The plasma phosphate concentration was 0.5 mg/dl and, in contrast to the previous study, the GFR fell substantially in some of the animals. Harter et al [58] were unable to show a decrease in the glucose Tm with diet-induced phosphate depletion; however, the glucose Tm did decrease when parathyroid hormone was infused. It is possible that the infusion of parathyroid hormone caused a more profound hypophosphatemia, thus uncovering a proximal defect for glucose.

Schmidt [59] also studied bicarbonate reabsorption in three groups of dogs. The first were controls, the second were phosphate-depleted (dietary depletion only), and the third were phosphate-depleted dogs subjected to parathyroidectomy. The dogs in each group were maintained on their respective diets up to 14 weeks prior to the study. In the phosphate-depleted dogs, regardless of whether the parathyroid glands were intact or not, bicarbonate titration curves were identical to those seen in control animals. In contrast to the observations of Gold et al [56], these investigators were unable to show a relationship between the plasma phosphate and bicarbonate concentrations. Plasma pH and P_{CO_2} were the same as controls. In this study, however, there was a marked decrease in the GFR of the phosphate-depleted animals as compared to controls (69 vs. 111 ml/min, respectively), indicating the probable presence of some degree of extracellular fluid volume contraction. Volume contraction could stimulate proximal bicarbonate reabsorption independent of any effect of phosphate depletion.

Kurtz and Hsu [60] studied the effect of phosphate depletion on the threshold for bicarbonaturia in female rats. After one month of phosphate depletion (dietary deprivation), the animals had a normal acid-base status. Following bicarbonate infusion, bicarbonaturia occurred at a plasma bicarbonate of 25 mEq/liter, a value identical to that seen in the control group. The bicarbonate infusion was performed after 3 days of acid loading, and it is possible that the stimulation of proton secretion by the distal nephron could have masked an effect on proximal tubular acidification. In male rats, Emmett et al (61) found marked bicarbonaturia after 18 days of phosphate depletion (18 μEq/hr) and lesser, though significant bicarbonaturia (4 μEq/hr) after 45 days of phosphate depletion. In both of these studies arterial pH, P_{CO_2}, and bicarbonate concentration were normal.

We studied the effect of phosphate depletion on proximal bicarbonate reabsorption in pair-fed male rats [62]. After 30 or 60 days of phosphate depletion, proximal bicarbonate reabsorption was identical to that of control animals. Arterial pH, P_{CO_2} and bicarbonate concentration were likewise normal, despite the fact that the urine pH was higher in phosphate-depleted animals.

In humans, the effects of phosphate depletion on proximal bicarbonate reabsorption are not clear. Kohaut et al (63) studied eleven malnourished infants. These infants presented with a mean plasma bicarbonate of 12.8 mEq/liter. While a bicarbonate titration curve was not performed, Kohaut et al (63) suggested that a proximal tubular defect for bicarbonate absorption may have been present because of the large quantities of bicarbonate that were required by these infants. Three of the infants were restudied after the partial correction of phosphate depletion; significant bicarbonaturia was found at a plasma HCO_3 of 16.6 mEq/liter (in infants the normal renal threshold for bicarbonate is in a range from 21.5 to 24 mmoles/liter).

In summary, in rats and humans there is no direct evidence that a proximal tubular leak for bicarbonate occurs with phosphate depletion, although there is suggestive indirect evidence that such may be the case in malnourished infants. In the dog, a proximal bicarbonate leak occurs in profound phosphate depletion (dietary deprivation plus phosphate binders). Dietary deprivation alone does not appear to be sufficiently severe to unmask this effect. While the mechanism for the proximal tubular bicarbonate defect seen in some studies is not known, it may be due to intracellular alkalosis of the proximal tubule cells. Gold et al [56] estimated that the intracellular pH of skeletal muscle was 7.02 following phosphate depletion, a value significantly higher than that in controls [6, 86].

Effect of Phosphate Depletion on Distal Acidification

There is considerable evidence in many species that distal acidification is affected by phosphate depletion. Klahr, Tripathy, and Lotero [64] reported that there was a marked decrease in urine titratable acid and ammonia excretion in seven malnourished humans, although acid-base homeostasis was normal. When these patients were subjected to standard ammonium chloride loading, a marked decrease in the plasma bicarbonate concentration was observed. The plasma bicarbonate concentration was 16.1 mEq/liter before protein repletion. After repletion, when submitted to the same ammonium chloride load, the plasma bicarbonate concentration was 20.3 mEq/liter. In this study, both titratable acid and ammonium excretion were decreased in the protein depleted state. Similarly, in acidotic malnourished infants, Kohaut et al [63] found a marked decrease in net acid excretion to approximately one-third of normal. Titratable acid was 7- to 10-fold lower in malnourished infants, and ammonium excretion was 50% of control values. With phosphate infusion or two days of phosphate supplementation, net acid excretion in these malnourished infants rose to normal values. In the rat, following 18 days of dietary phosphate deprivation, Emmett et al [61] found a marked decrease in net acid excretion, which was due to a decrease in titratable acid and ammonia excretion.

We further assessed distal acidification in the rat following one and two months of dietary phosphate depletion [62]. The results of these studies are compared with controls that were phosphate depleted for only 3 days. In both experimental groups (1 and 2 months), the plasma bicarbonate concentration and GFR were the same as the control animals in response to NH_4Cl. Urine pH, however, was significantly higher under baseline conditions in phosphate depleted animals than were their pair fed litter mates. In these studies plasma phosphate was 1.7 mEq/liter as compared to controls, which had a plasma phosphate of 3.5 mEq/liter. Following ammonium chloride loading both groups of phosphate depleted rats had a higher urine pH and a lower titratable acid excretion when compared to controls. Ammonium excretion was significantly lower than controls only following long-term phosphate depletion (60 days). During sodium sulfate administration, a potent stimulus to distal acidification, the urine pH of phosphate depleted animals (60 days) was significantly higher than that of controls. At comparable levels of urine pH and acidemia, ammonium excretion was significantly lower in the phosphate depleted rats. These data suggest that phosphate deprivation is associated with a distal acidification defect. The defect is characterized by a decrease in titratable acid excretion and impaired ammonium excretion. The decrease in titratable acid is due to the decrease in distal phosphate delivery. The decrease in ammonium excretion may be due to decreased production secondary to a fall in specific activity of the phosphate-dependent glutaminase I and intracellular alkalosis.

Effect of Phosphate Depletion on Extrarenal Buffering

While there are obvious species differences in the response of urinary acidification to phosphate depletion, most of the available evidence suggests that the arterial pH, P_{CO_2}, and plasma bicarbonate concentration are essentially within normal limits. Despite this, a defect in either proximal or distal tubular acidification has been noted. It has been suggested that the normal arterial pH, P_{CO_2}, and plasma bicarbonate concentration are due to an enhanced extrarenal buffering providing bicarbonate to buffer body stores. Infants, in whom there are marked profound rates of muscular and skeletal growth, develop a severe acidemia when malnourished and phosphate depleted [63]. This indirectly suggests that extrarenal buffer stores are important in preserving acid-base homeostasis in the phosphate-depleted state.

Several studies have examined extrarenal buffering in phosphate-depleted animals and the results are consistent [61, 62, 65, 66]. For example, in the nephrectomized animal following sixty days of phosphate deprivation, the infusion of a constant acid load causes a lesser fall in plasma pH and plasma bicarbonate concentration than in control nephrectomized animals. When colchicine or diphosphonates are administered, agents that prevent the release of buffer from bone, phosphate-depleted animals behave as controls developing a profound acidemia [65]. That is, the plasma pH and bicarbonate concentration fall to a level indistinguishable from that of controls. While these results suggest that extrarenal buffering is primarily due to the release of bicarbonate or carbonates from bone, it is possible that the liver and muscle also contribute to extrarenal buffering. Both acute and chronic hyperparathyroidism have been shown to enhance extrarenal buffering [65]. The precise mechanism whereby phosphate deprivation enhances extrarenal buffering is not known. It is unlikely, however, that the effect of phosphate depletion on extrarenal buffering is mediated by enhanced parathyroid hormone activity. In studies of humans and animals, phosphate depletion is associated with low levels of immunoreactive parathyroid hormone and the glands appear hypoplastic when they are examined morphologically [8]. Vitamin D enhances extrarenal buffering in the normal animal [65, 66]. This hormone is increased in phosphate depletion and may contribute substantially to the maintenance of normal acid-base status due to its effect on extrarenal buffering.

Conclusions

In summary, the effects of phosphate depletion on acid-base homeostasis are complex. There appears to be a defect in proximal tubular acidification in some species. There also appears to be an acidification defect in the distal nephron. While the precise mechanism of the distal defect is not characterized completely, it appears to be due to a decrease in the buffer content of urine (titratable acid) and a defect in ammonia excretion (or production). Extrarenal buffering contributes in a major way to the overall maintenance of arterial pH. This effect on extrarenal buffering is not due to an increase in the activity of parathyroid hormone; instead, it may be related to an increase in $1,25(OH_2)D_3$.

The mechanism whereby $1,25(OH)_2D_3$ increases in phosphate depletion is not known [67]. It has been suggested that the depletion of cellular phosphate is the stimulus, although cultured chick kidney cells do not increase vitamin D in the presence of low phosphate despite the fact that an increase occurs following PTH [68, 69]. Gray, Garthwaite, and Phillips [70] have shown recently that hypophysectomy in phosphate-depleted rats prevents the rise in vitamin D. This effect appears to be due to the permissive role of both T_3 and growth hormone on vitamin D metabolism. This effect is seen as early as 4 days after phosphate depletion [70, 71].

Certain parts of the nephron, particularly the cortex, may be more sensitive to the lack of phosphate in the presence of glucose. Brazy et al [72] have shown impaired oxidative metabolism in isolated proximal convoluted tubules when incubated with luminal glucose in the absence of phosphate. The Crabtree effect thus depletes intracellular ATP as it is used for intracellular phosphorylation. This effect is not seen in proximal straight tubules. Whether the Crabtree effect occurs in other parts of the nephron (that is, the cortical collecting duct) is not known.

Recent studies with ^{31}P nuclear magnetic resonance have shown that the cytosolic levels of free inorganic phosphate and adenosine nucleotides are probably a log unit lower than those estimated by conventional extraction methods [73]. Free inorganic phosphate in the whole kidney is estimated to be 100 μM by this technique. Changes in this fraction are probably key to the maintenance of normal renal function. The unique manner in which this fraction changes and its response to hormones during phosphate depletion are not yet understood.

Acknowledgments. This work was supported in part by the National Institutes of Health grant AM20170 and Chicago Heart Association Grant No. 83–41.

References

1. KREBS H: Rate limiting factors in cell respiration, in *Ciba Foundation Symposium on the Regulation of Cell Metabolism,* Boston, Little Brown and Co, pp 1–10, 1959
2. DAUM K, TUTTLE WW, WEBER A, SCHUMACHER M, SALZANO J: Calcium and phosphorus utilization in older man, *J Am Diet Assoc* 31:149–151, 1955
3. LEICHSENRING JM, NORRIS LM, LAMISON SA, WILSON ED, PATTON MB: The effect of level of intake on calcium and phosphorus metabolism in college women. J Nutr 45:407–411, 1951

4. PITTS RF: *Physiology of the Kidney and Body Fluids,* second edition, Chicago, Yearbook Publishers, 1968

5. KNOX FG, SCHNEIDER EG, WILLIS LR, STRANDHOY JW, OTT CE: Site and control of phosphate reabsorption by the kidney. *Kidney Int* 3:347–353, 1973

6. HAAS JA, BERNDT T, KNOX FG: Nephron heterogeneity of phosphate reabsorption. *Am J Physiol* 234:F287-F290, 1978

7. BIJOVET OLM: The importance of the kidneys in PO_4 homeostasis, in *Phosphate Metabolism in Kidney and Bone,* edited by AVIOLI LV, BORDIER PN, FLEISCH H, MASSRY SG, SLATOPOLSKY E, Paris, Noruelle Imprimerie Fournie, p 421, 1976

8. DOMINGUEZ JH, GRAY RW, LEMANN J JR: Dietary phosphate deprivation in women and men. Effects on mineral and acid balances, parathyroid hormone and the metabolism of 25-OH-vitamin D. *J Clin Endocrinol Metab* 43:1056-1068, 1976

9. KNOCHEL J: The pathophysiology and clinical characteristics of severe hypophosphatemia. *Arch Intern Med* 137:203–220, 1977

10. AGUS ZS, GOLDFARB S, WASSERSTEIN A: Disorders of calcium acid phosphate balance, in *The Kidney,* edited by BRENNER BM, RECTOR FC, Philadelphia, WB Saunders & Co, pp 940–1022, 1981

11. MOLLISON PL: Observations on cases of starvation at Belsen. *Br Med J* 1:4–8, 1946

12. BROZEK J, CHAPMAN CB, KEYS A: Drastic food restriction. *JAMA* 137:1569–1574, 1948

13. SCHNITKER MA, MATTMAN PE, BLISS TL: A clinical study of malnutrition in Japanese prisoners of war. *Ann Intern Med* 35:69–96, 1951

14. COX GJ, DODDS ML, WIGMAN HB, MURPHY FJ: The effects of high doses of aluminum and iron on phosphorus metabolism. *J Biol Chem* 92:11–12, 1931

15. LOTZ M, ZISMAN E, BARTTER FC: Evidence for a phosphate depletion syndrome in man. *N Engl J Med* 278:409–415, 1968

16. LICHTMAN MA, MILLER DR, FREEMAN RB: Erythrocyte adenosine triphosphate depletion during hypophosphatemia in an uremic subject. *N Engl J Med* 280:240–244, 1969

17. LICHTMAN MA, MILLER DR, COHEN J, WATERHOUSE C: Reduced red cell glycolysis, 2,3-diphosphoglycerate and adenosine triphosphate concentration, and increased hemoglobin oxygen affinity caused by hypophosphatemia. *Ann Intern Med* 74:562–568, 1971

18. NAKAO K, WADA T, KAMIYANA T: A direct relationship of adenosine triphosphate level and in vivo viability of erythrocytes. *Nature* 194:877–878, 1962

19. TRAVIS SF, SUGERMAN HJ, RUBERG RL, DUDRICK SJ, DELAVORIA-PAPADAPOULOS M, MILLER LD, OSKI FA: Alterations of red cell glycolytic intermediates and oxygen transport as a consequence of hypophosphatemia in patients receiving intravenous hyperalimentation. *N Engl J Med* 285:763–768, 1971

20. BENESCH R, BENESCH RE: Intracellular organic phosphates as regulators of oxygen release by hemoglobin. *Biochem Biophys Res Commun* 26:162–174, 1967

21. LENFANT C, TORRANCE JF, WOODSON RD, JACOBS P, FINCH CA: Role of organic phosphate in the adaptation of man to hypoxia. *Fed Proc* 29:1115–1117, 1970

22. CRADDOCK PR, YAWATA Y, VAN SANTEN L, GILLERSTADT S, SILVIS S, JACOB HS: Acquired phagocyte dysfunction: A complication of the hypophosphatemia of parenteral hyperalimentation. *N Engl J Med* 290:1403–1407, 1974

23. GARNER CB, HEUBNER PF, O'DELL BL: Dietary phosphorus and salmonellosis in guinea pigs (*abstract*). *Fed Proc* 26:799, 1967

24. TATSUMI N, SHIBATA N, OKAMURA Y: Actin and myosin A from leukocytes. *Biochem Biophys Acta* 305:433–444, 1973

25. LICHTMAN MA: Hypophosphatemia during hyperalimentation. *N Engl J Med* 290:1432–1433, 1974
26. TOU JS, STJERNHOLM RL: Stimulation of the incorporation of ^{32}Pi and myo(2–3H)inositol into the phosphoinositides in polymorphonuclear leukocytes during phagocytes. *Arch Biochem Biophys* 160:487–494, 1974
27. YAWATA Y, HEBBEL RP, SILVIS S, HORNE R, JACOB HS: Blood cell abnormalities complicating the hypophosphatemia of hyperalimentation: Erythrocytes and platelet ATP deficiency associated with hemolytic anemia and bleeding in hyperalimented dogs. *J Lab Clin Med* 84:643–653, 1974
28. YAWATA Y, CRADDOCK P, HEBBEL R: Hyperalimentation hypophosphatemia: Hematologic and neurologic dysfunction due to ATP depletion (*abstract*). *Clin Res* 31:729, 1973
29. JACOB HS: Severe hypophosphatemia: A previously ignored cause of cellular dysfunction. *West J Med* 122:501–502, 1975
30. PERKOFF GT, HARDY P, VELEZ-GARZIA E: Reversible acute muscular syndrome in chronic alcoholism. *N Engl J Med* 274:1277–1285, 1966
31. KLINKERFUSS G, BLEISCH V, DIOSO MM: A spectrum of myopathy associated with alcoholism. II. Light and electron microscopic observations. *Ann Intern Med* 67:493–510, 1967
32. MASSRY SG: Effect of phosphate depletion on renal function and metabolism. *Proc Internat Cong Nephrol* 7:625–633, 1978
33. SABATINI S: Acidosis of chronic renal failure. *Med Clin N Amer* 67:845–858, 1983
34. SABATINI S, ARRUDA JAL, KURTZMAN NA: Disorders of acid-base balance. *Med Clin N Amer* 62:1223–1235, 1978
35. WARNOCK DJ, RECTOR FC: Renal acidification mechanisms, in *The Kidney*, edited by BRENNER BM, RECTOR FC, Philadelphia, WB Saunders & Co, p 440, 1981
36. SIEGFRIED D, KUMAR R, ARRUDA J, KURTZMAN NA: Influence of vitamin D on bicarbonate reabsorption, in *Phosphate Metabolism*, edited by MASSRY SG, RITZ E, New York, Plenum Press, pp 395–404, 1978
37. ARRUDA JAL, KURTZMAN NA: Metabolic alkalosis and acidosis. *Clin Nephrol* 7:201, 1977
38. HULTER HN, SEBASTIAN A, TOTO RD, BANNER EL, ILNICKI LP: Renal and systemic acid-base effects of chronic administration of hypercalcemia producing agents: Calciferol, PTH and intravenous calcium. *Kidney Int* 21:445–458, 1982
39. KALRA J, BROSNAN JT: The subcellular localization of glutaminase isoenzymes in rat kidney cortex. *J Biol Chem* 249:3255, 1974
40. KALRA J, BROSNAN JT: The localization of phosphate-independent glutaminase in brush border of rat kidney cortex. *Canad J Biochem* 2:762, 1974
41. KOVACEVIC Z: Distribution of glutaminase isoenzymes in kidney cells. *Biochem Biophys Acta* 334:199, 1974
42. GOLDSTEIN L, CLAIBORNE JB, EVANS DE: Ammonia excretion by the gills of two marine teleost fish: Importance of NH_4^+ permeance. *J Exp Zool,* (in press, 1984)
43. ROOS A, BORON WF: Intracellular pH. *Physiol Reviews* 61:297, 1981
44. GOOD DW, KNEPPER MA, BURG MB: Ammonia and bicarbonate transport by thick ascending limb of rat kidney (*abstract*). *Proc Am Soc Nephrol,* Wash DC, 1983, p 138A
45. ARRUDA JAL, NASCIMENTO L, MEHTA PK, RADEMACHER DR, SEHY JT, WESTENFELDER C, KURTZMAN NA: The critical importance of urinary concentrating ability in the generation of urinary carbon dioxide tension. *J Clin Invest* 60:922–935, 1977

46. BATLLE DC, KURTZMAN NA: Distal renal tubular acidosis with intact capacity to lower urine pH. *Am J Med* 72:751–759, 1982

47. KURTZMAN NA, ARRUDA JAL: Phosphate and acid-base homeostasis, in *Phosphate and Minerals in Health and Disease,* edited by MASSRY SG, RITZ E, *Adv Exper Med* 128:187–196, 1980

48. ARRUDA JAL, NASCIMENTO L, MEHTA PK, KURTZMAN NA: Factors influencing the formation of urinary carbon dioxide tension. *Kidney Int* 11:307–317, 1977

49. COBURN JW, MASSRY SG: Changes in serum and urinary calcium during phosphate depletion: Studies on mechanisms. *J Clin Invest* 49:1073–1087, 1970

50. KREUSSER WJ, KUROKAWA K, AZNAR E, MASSRY SG: Phosphate depletion: Effect on renal inorganic phosphorus and adenine nucleotides, urinary phosphate and calcium, and calcium balance. *Mineral Elect Metab* 1:30–42, 1978

51. CUISINIER-GLEIZES P, THOMASSET M, SAINTENY-DEBOVE I, MATHIEU H: Phosphorus deficiency, parathyroid hormone, and bone resorption in the growing rat. *Calcif Tiss Res* 20:235–249, 1976

52. GOLDFARB S, WESTBY GR, GOLDBERG M, AGUS ZS: Renal tubular effects of chronic phosphate depletion. *J Clin Invest* 59:770–779, 1977

53. O'CONNOR LR, WHEELER WS, BETHUNE JE: Effect of hypophosphatemia on myocardial performance in man. *N Engl J Med* 297:901–903, 1977

54. FULLER RJ, NICHOLS WW, BRENNER BJ, PETERSON JC: Effects of phosphorus depletion on left ventricular energy generation, in *Homeostasis of Phosphate and Other Minerals,* edited by MASSRY SG, RITZ E, RAPADO A, New York, Plenum Publishing Co, 1978, vol 103, pp 395–400

55. WEINSIER RL, KRUMDIECK CL: Death resulting from overzealous total parenteral nutrition: The refeeding syndrome revisited. *Am J Clin Nutr* 34:393–399, 1980

56. GOLD LW, MASSRY SG, ARIEFF A, COBURN JW: Renal bicarbonate wasting during phosphate depletion: A possible cause of altered acid-base homeostasis in hyperparathyroidism. *J Clin Invest* 52:2556–2562, 1973

57. GOLD LW, MASSRY SG, FRIEDLER RM: Effect of phosphate depletion on renal tubular reabsorption of glucose. *J Lab Clin Med* 89:554–559, 1977

58. HARTER HR, MERCADO A, RUTHERFORD WE, RODRIGUEZ H, SLATOPOLSKY E, KLAHR S: Effect of phosphate depletion and parathyroid hormone on renal glucose reabsorption. *Am J Physiol* 227:1422–1427, 1974

59. SCHMIDT RW: Effects of phosphate depletion on acid-base status in dogs. *Metabolism* 27:943–952

60. KURTZ TW, HSU CH: Impaired distal nephron acidification in chronically phosphate depleted rats. *Pflügers Arch* 377:229–234, 1978

61. EMMETT M, GOLDFARB S, AGUS ZS, NARINS RG: The pathophysiology of acid-base changes in chronically phosphate-depleted rats: Bone-kidney interactions. *J Clin Invest* 59:291–298, 1977

62. ARRUDA JAL, JULKA NK, RUBINSTEIN H, SABATINI S, KURTZMAN NA: Distal acidification defect induced by phosphate deprivation. *Metabolism* 29:826–836, 1980

63. KOHAUT EC, KLISH WJ, BEACHLER CW, HILL LL: Reduced renal acid excretion in malnutrition: A result of phosphate depletion. *Am J Clin Nutr* 30:861–867, 1977

64. KLAHR S, TRIPATHY K, LOTERO H: Renal regulation of acid-base balance in malnourished man. *Am J Med* 48:325–331, 1970

65. ARRUDA JAL, ALLA V, RUBINSTEIN H, CRUZ-SOTO M, SABATINI S, BATLLE DC, KURTZMAN NA: Parathyroid hormone and extrarenal buffering. *Am J Physiol* 239:G533–538, 1980

66. ARRUDA JAL, ALLA V, RUBENSTEIN H, CRUZ-SOTO M, SABATINI S, BATLLE DC, KURTZMAN NA: Metabolic and hormonal factors influencing extrarenal buffering of an acute acid load. *Mineral Elect Metab* 8:36–42, 1982
67. GRAY RW: Dietary phosphate deprivation increases 1,25(OH)$_2$-vitamin D$_3$ synthesis in rat kidney (abstract). *Fed Proc* 40:899, 1981
68. TANAKA Y, DELUCA HF: The control of 25-hydroxyvitamin D metabolism by inorganic phosphorus. *Arch Biochem Biophys* 154:566–574, 1973
69. TRECHSEL U, BONJOUR JP, FLEISCH H: Regulation of the metabolism of 25-hydroxyvitamin D$_3$ in primary cultures of chick kidney cells. *J Clin Invest* 64:206–217, 1979
70. GRAY RW, GARTHWAITE TL, PHILLIPS LS: Growth hormone and triiodothyronine permit an increase in plasma 1,25(OH)$_2$D concentrations in response to dietary phosphate deprivation in hypophysectomized rats. *Calcif Tiss Int* 35:100–106, 1983
71. GRAY RW: Control of plasma 1,25(OH)$_2$-vitamin D concentrations by calcium and phosphorus in the rat: Effects of hypophysectomy. *Calcif Tiss Int* 33:485–488, 1981
72. BRAZY PC, GULLAN SR, MANDEL LJ, DENNIS VW: Metabolic requirement for inorganic phosphate by the rabbit proximal tubule: Evidence for a Crabtree effect. *J Clin Invest* 70:53–62, 1982
73. BALABAN RS: The application of nuclear magnetic resonance to the study of cellular physiology. *Am J Physiol* 246:C10–C19, 1984

Effect of Phosphate Depletion on Renal Tubular Transport

Zalman S. Agus and Renée E. Garrick

Removal of phosphate from one's diet has immediate and striking effects on a variety of tubular functions. There are alterations in the transport of sodium, calcium, phosphate, magnesium, glucose, and bicarbonate. These effects occur at different sites within the nephron, and they presumably cannot be ascribed to a single effect of modifying phosphate balance. While cellular mechanisms are not yet completely understood, the use of phosphate depletion as a model for investigating the cellular regulation of transepithelial solute transport has provided important information. In this review, we will summarize the currently available information on the effects and sites of action of phosphate depletion and will discuss the cellular mechanisms that are potentially responsible for the observed alterations in ion transport.

Phosphate Transport

With reduction of dietary phosphate intake, urinary phosphate excretion falls. This change, which occurs in the presence and absence of parathyroid hormone (PTH) [1, 2], takes place quickly; in humans, it can be demonstrated within 24 hr [3]. Recent studies, in fact, have been able to show increased phosphate uptake in brushborder membrane vesicles taken from rats exposed to dietary phosphate restriction for only 4 hr [4]. Although the serum phosphate concentration can fall quickly in rats, studies in humans and dogs have shown that the change in urinary excretion precedes any measurable fall in filtered load, which implies an increase in fractional reabsorption. Phosphate infusion studies in phosphate-depleted rats have provided further evidence that hypophosphatemia per se is not the sole mechanism responsible for the marked reduction in urinary excretion. In these studies [1, 2], despite

This manuscript was presented as part of a Symposium on *Renal and Vascular Consequences of Phosphate Depletion.*

markedly acute elevations of the filtered load of phosphate, urinary phosphate excretion failed to increase appreciably.

Although phosphate depletion does result in suppression of PTH secretion, the decrease in circulating PTH levels also is not the sole mechanism responsible for the antiphosphaturia. Thus, infusion of PTH into phosphate-depleted rats results in only trivial increases in phosphate excretion [5, 6], although urinary cyclic AMP excretion increases to values comparable to those present in control rats. Regardless of the mechanism responsible for the transduction of changes in dietary phosphate intake into altered phosphate transport, it seems to be intrinsic to the renal tubule. Tubule segments from the rabbit and brushborder membrane vesicles isolated from phosphate-depleted rats demonstrate enhanced phosphate transport and sodium-dependent phosphate uptake, respectively, when placed in serum from normal animals or media containing normal concentrations of phosphate [7, 8].

The site of this adaptive process has been evaluated with a number of techniques. Phosphate transport occurs throughout the nephron, with the exception of the components of the loop of Henle [9]. The late proximal convoluted tubule, the pars recta, and the distal convoluted tubule all exhibit PTH-sensitive phosphate absorption [10]. There is also a small component of phosphate transport in the cortical collecting tubule (CCT), but this appears to be a purely passive phenomenon driven by electrochemical gradients and is not sensitive to hormonal modulation [11]. Micropuncture and in vitro perfusion studies in the dog, rat, and rabbit (examining animals with varying degrees of phosphate depletion) have shown increased phosphate transport in virtually all of the transporting segments [7, 12, 13]. For reasons that are not clear, the adaptive response to dietary phosphate restriction appears to be greater in the proximal tubules of superficial nephrons than of deep nephrons [13].

As noted above, the changes in phosphate transport observed during phosphate depletion appear to be intrinsic to the renal tubule. In the proximal tubule, current evidence indicates that these changes are expressed at the membrane level. As discussed above, sodium-dependent phosphate uptake in brushborder membrane vesicles from phosphate-depleted animals is increased, compared to vesicles from animals fed a normal dietary phosphate intake. Current concepts concerning phosphate transport in the proximal tubule suggest that it is a two-component process [14]. The uptake across the brushborder membrane is active, as it occurs against a negative intracellular potential in the absence of a significant concentration gradient [15]. However, uptake in vesicle studies is linked to sodium transport and is markedly enhanced by the addition of sodium to the media. Therefore, it is thought that phosphate transport is secondarily active and represents a sodium-phosphate carrier mechanism that is driven by the electrochemical gradient favoring sodium entry across the brushborder membranes. This favorable sodium gradient is created by Na-K-ATPase activity in the basolateral membrane. The phosphate that enters the cell can interact with mitochondrial pools and intermediary metabolism, thus serving as a substrate for adenosine triphosphate (ATP) synthesis. Phosphate liberated by degradative processes enters the cell pool and the cytosolic phosphate concentration as well, as the favorable electrical gradient appears to be responsible for the movement of phosphate across the basolateral membrane. This exit process, which is sodium-independent, may involve another carrier mechanism [16] and possibly a facilitated diffusion.

Alterations in phosphate transport produced by dietary depletion could be theoretically due to changes in sodium transport and gradients and affinity or modification of the carrier, as well as to changes in intermediary metabolism and/or the intracellular concentration of phosphate or phosphorylated compounds. The enhanced phosphate uptake that is observed in brushborder membrane vesicles prepared from phosphate-depleted animals is specific for sodium-dependent phosphate transport (that is, sodium-dependent glucose and amino acid uptake are not affected). Thus, it seems likely that the process involves modification of either the carrier density, the carrier affinity, or the rate of carrier translocation. Recent studies by Cheng et al [17] that evaluate phosphate uptake by brushborder membrane vesicles from rabbits fed a low-phosphate diet demonstrated an increased V_{max} with no change in affinity for phosphate. In addition, dietary adaptation was associated with an alteration in the pH dependency of the transport system. Viewed together, these observations suggest that the adaptive process involves both an intrinsic change in the carrier and an increased rate of translocation, rather than a change in the number of carrier sites.

The administration of actinomycin D, which is an inhibitor of protein synthesis at the transcription level, did not prevent the adaptive changes in membrane uptake associated with acute phosphate depletion [4]. However, in a separate study, brushborder membrane adaptation to more prolonged phosphate depletion was sensitive to the effects of actinomycin D [18]. Thus, it is possible that new protein synthesis may be necessary for the maintenance of the membrane changes associated with phosphate depletion. Recent studies have identified a proteolipid, phosphorin, which has been extracted from rabbit kidney brushborder membranes. Phosphorin has been shown to bind inorganic phosphate with high affinity and specificity, and thus may be involved in the uptake process [19–21].

Hypotheses and factors that are currently being evaluated [22, 23] as possible modifiers of the carrier and its rate of translocation include gluconeogenesis, NAD, adenosine diphosphate-ribosylation, and changes in membrane fluidity. Preliminary studies have shown a selective decrease in brushborder membrane cholesterol, as compared with the basolateral membrane [24]. Further studies are required to determine if this change alters the membrane fluidity or the lipid microenvironment of the phosphate carrier.

In summary, the renal tubule adapts quickly to changes in dietary phosphate intake by increasing the rate of phosphate transport in proximal and distal segments. The mechanism of this adaptation is independent of changes in filtered load and PTH; in the proximal tubule, it can be localized to the brushborder membrane. It seems likely that further investigation will uncover a carrier protein that is modified by cellular or membrane events dependent on phosphate balance. In addition to defining the mechanism of phosphate adaptation, these studies will provide important information regarding both the transport process of phosphate and proximal tubular function.

Calcium Transport

Hypercalciuria has been observed as a prominent manifestation of dietary phosphate depletion in every species studied. The effect is immediate, occurs within 24 hr, and is dramatic, with urinary excretion rates increasing 3- to 20-fold. As phosphate depletion alters bone dynamics producing net resorption and also stimulates gut calcium absorption presumably by increasing circulating $1,25(OH)_2D_3$ levels, it might be expected that an increase in filtered load of calcium could play a role in increasing calcium excretion. This could occur by a direct effect of filtered load, by effects of hypercalcemia (which inhibits calcium transport in the thick ascending limb), and by suppression of PTH (which stimulates calcium transport in distal portions of the nephron).

Recent studies have corroborated and extended the original hypothesis of Coburn and Massry [25] that in addition to the effects of a higher filtered load and PTH suppression, a specific renal tubular defect in calcium transport is produced by phosphate depletion. Thus, in the face of phosphate depletion, hypercalciuria is present despite a reduction of the filtered load; and, an increase in calcium excretion occurs with phosphate depletion in parathyroidectomized animals. Furthermore, chronic replacement of thyroparathyroidectomized phosphate-depleted animals with exogenous PTH does not reduce calcium excretion to normal levels [26].

Micropuncture studies in the rat and the dog have demonstrated reduced calcium transport in various portions of the nephron, compared to control animals [27, 28]. Three pieces of information viewed together suggest that it is the distal or terminal portions of the nephron that exhibit a specific effect of dietary phosphate content on tubular calcium transport. First, the currently available data suggest that calcium transport in the proximal convoluted tubule and the thick ascending limb can be accounted for primarily by passive forces generated by sodium transport. If this is the case, it is not necessary to postulate transcellular movement that requires active extrusion from the cell, which could be modified by intracellular events associated with phosphate depletion. The distal segments (distal convoluted tubule and connecting tubule) prior to the collecting tubule exhibit hormone-sensitive active calcium transport. Second, micropuncture studies in the dog demonstrated reduced transport of sodium and calcium in the proximal tubule, as well as reduced calcium transport in the distal nephron [27]. Acute intravenous (i.v.) infusion of phosphate immediately corrected the hypercalciuria, but the proximal defect persisted. Thus, it would seem likely that altered transport of calcium from the proximal convoluted tubule may be secondary to altered sodium transport, but it is not the source of the increased urinary calcium excretion. Rather, the distal portion of the nephron, where calcium transport is discrete from sodium, is the site of a direct calcium transport defect in phosphate depletion. Finally, phosphate infusions in parathyroidectomized rats acutely reduced urinary calcium excretion and stimulated calcium reabsorption in the terminal nephron (that is, beyond the late distal tubule puncture site), and it had no effect on the proximal tubule, loop of Henle, or distal convoluted tubule [28]. Thiazides, which stimulate calcium transport in the distal convoluted tubule, blunt the calciuria of phosphate-deficient rats; however, it has not been established whether this effect takes place at the same site as phosphate depletion [29].

The cellular mechanism by which dietary phosphate intake modulates active calcium transport is unknown. Moreover, our knowledge in this area is hampered by the technical difficulties that complicate the study of the distal or terminal nephron segments, and also by our lack of information concerning mechanisms of calcium transport. In view of both the electrochemical gradient opposing paracellular diffusion from the lumen and the low-calcium permeability of the distal convoluted tubule and early cortical collecting duct, calcium movement in this region is most likely transcellular [30]. Calcium entry probably is a function of apical cell membrane permeability, and its transcellular movement may be related to the presence of vitamin D-dependent calcium-binding protein. As the interior of the cell is electronegative and cytosolic calcium concentration probably is extremely low (10^{-7} M), the extrusion of calcium across the basolateral membrane occurs against a very large electrochemical gradient. Membrane transport processes that may regulate calcium exit have been identified in other tissues and include Ca-Mg-ATPase and coupled Na-Ca exchange. The role of any, or all, of these factors remain to be elucidated in active transepithelial calcium transport and the effect of dietary phosphate depletion on membrane permeability to calcium and/or Ca-Mg-ATPase activity.

Magnesium Transport

Phosphate depletion induces an increase in urinary magnesium excretion in all species studied; however, in contrast to phosphate and calcium, the degree of magnesuria varies from species to species. Thus, in humans and dogs, the changes are moderate, but marked magnesuria in the rat occurs sufficiently to induce a strikingly negative net balance and leads to significant hypomagnesemia [31, 32]. As with calcium and phosphate, these changes occur rapidly, with excretion in the rat increasing 3-fold within 24 hr. As urinary excretion increases despite a significant decrease in serum magnesium and filtered load, there is a significant decrease in net tubular reabsorption. Moreover, since magnesuria occurs in rats subjected to thyroparathyroidectomy (TPTX) and phosphate depletion, it is not simply a function of PTH suppression.

The site and mechanism of the alterations in magnesium transport produced by dietary phosphate depletion are poorly understood. Micropuncture studies in the phosphate-depleted dog suggest that the site of altered transport is between the proximal convoluted tubule and the distal tubule puncture site [33]. As the bulk of filtered magnesium is reabsorbed in the thick ascending limb, this would seem to be a potential site. However, magnesium transport in this site can be accounted for by passive forces [34]; thus, it is difficult to attribute the magnesuria to an effect of phosphate depletion on cellular events. Microperfusion studies in vivo have suggested an interaction between calcium and magnesium at the basolateral membrane in this intermediate segment of the nephron [35]. Therefore, it is possible that changes in ionized calcium concentration in phosphate-depleted animals could influence magnesium transport in this segment. However, these interactive changes could not be demonstrated in in vitro perfusion studies of the rabbit cortical thick ascending limb [34]. Thus, it is not clear whether this interaction occurs in the medullary segment or whether there are important species differences or differences between the in vivo and in vitro situations that alter magnesium transport.

Glucose and Bicarbonate Transport

Clearance studies in the dog have indicated that phosphate depletion results in a rather marked depression of the Tm of glucose [36]. It is not clear whether this represents a specific defect in cellular glucose uptake or is related to the decreased sodium transport observed in the proximal tubule of the dog [27]. There is an interaction between glucose and phosphate proximal tubular transport, to a degree that increasing glucose transport interferes with phosphate transport and that inhibition of glucose uptake with phlorizin is associated with increased phosphate transport [37–39]. Studies with vesicles suggest that the interaction is not competition for a carrier, but rather may reflect the effects of the various solutes on the transmembrane electrochemical sodium gradient [40]. However, defects in sodium-dependent glucose transport have not been demonstrable in brushborder membrane vesicles from phosphate-depleted animals. Therefore, it is possible that the in vivo glucose transport changes observed in severely depleted animals reflected a defect in sodium transport (discussed below) that is not apparent in brushborder membranes.

Both proximal [41, 42] and distal [43] acidifying defects have been reported in phosphate depletion. The distal acidifying defects are discussed elsewhere in this section. Initial studies suggested that hypophosphatemia in dogs reduced both the Tm for bicarbonate and the serum bicarbonate [41]. Subsequent studies [42] demonstrated that while proximal bicarbonate wasting could be detected in phosphate-depleted rats, the direct effects of hypophosphatemia on bone resorption and carbonate release tended to offset the decline in serum bicarbonate. Thus, nonspecific inhibition of bone resorption by colchicine led to a fall in the serum bicarbonate, and it unmasked the renal bicarbonate wasting. Conversely, bilateral nephrectomy left the bone mineral dissolution unbalanced, and it resulted in a rise in serum bicarbonate levels. Other, more recent studies have been unable to consistently demonstrate a significant proximal defect in bicarbonate handling [44–46]. However, most studies overall would agree that the alterations in renal bicarbonate handling present in phosphate depletion have only small effects on the serum bicarbonate due to the direct effect of phosphate depletion on bone dissolution.

Sodium Transport

Micropuncture studies in the dog and in the rat have suggested the presence of reduced sodium transport in the proximal tubules of chronically phosphate-depleted animals [27, 28]. Urinary sodium excretion in these preparations was not increased, implying that the increased load of sodium delivered out of the proximal tubule was reabsorbed in the middle or distal portions of the nephron. Support for this thesis is provided by studies in the isolated perfused rat kidney and by clearance studies in the dog. The isolated perfused kidney is a preparation exhibiting increased urinary sodium excretion as a consequence of impaired distal nephron function. Kidneys isolated from phosphate-depleted rats were significantly more natriuretic than kidneys from control rats, implying an increase in delivery [47]. Similarly, phosphate-depleted dogs did not exhibit increased urinary sodium excretion under baseline conditions; however, during volume expansion with saline, a significantly greater fraction of filtered sodium was excreted in the phosphate-depleted dogs than in comparably expanded normal animals [48].

The defect in sodium transport observed in phosphate depletion may represent a direct, specific effect of phosphate depletion that is very similar to the alterations seen in the renal handling of calcium and phosphate. Alternatively, the sodium transport defect may be an expression of altered cellular metabolism, which could occur in severe or chronic phosphate depletion secondary to reductions in intracellular stores of adenosine triphosphate and inorganic phosphate. Although a definitive statement is not yet possible, several lines of evidence favor the latter thesis. It has been observed in the phosphate-depleted dog that the defect in proximal tubule sodium transport—unlike the defect in calcium excretion—is not corrected by acute phosphate repletion, but it is corrected by chronic replacement [27]. Second, a defect in sodium transport is not observed in brushborder membrane vesicles prepared from phosphate-depleted animals, suggesting that the membrane transport mechanisms are intact [8, 17]. In addition, although total adenosine triphosphate content has been shown to be reduced in isolated cortical tubules prepared from phosphate-depleted rats [49], the specific activity of basolateral Na-K-ATPase (assessed by the addition of exogenous adenosine triphosphate) has been shown to be normal [24]. Finally, perfusion studies on isolated, proximal convoluted tubules have demonstrated that wide, acute variations in the bath or perfusate phosphate concentrations have no effect on the transport of water and sodium [50]. However, if the entire dissection and perfusion procedure is performed in phosphate-free media, sodium transport by the proximal convoluted tubule is markedly reduced [51]. That this change could be prevented either by glycolytic inhibitors or by the addition of transported—but nonmetabolized—glucose substitutes suggests that the imposed limitation of inorganic phosphate availability interfered with oxidative metabolism; therefore, it secondarily affected tubular transport. It is interesting to note that in this same study, proximal straight tubule transport was unaffected by phosphate-free dissection and perfusion. Thus, one may speculate that these later tubular segments, which have different metabolic requirements than the more proximal segments, are less sensitive to the effects of phosphate depletion. This reasoning may be invoked to explain the observation that the sodium rejected by the proximal tubules (in the setting of phosphate depletion) is reabsorbed by more distal nephron sites, thereby obviating a net urinary loss of sodium.

Viewed together, these observations support the notion that severe or chronic phosphate depletion may lead to alterations in cellular metabolism. Within this context, the defect in sodium transport potentially represents a somewhat secondary phenomenon that may stem from alterations in the cellular metabolic machinery (induced by phosphate depletion), rather than from a direct and specific effect of phosphate depletion at the level of the cellular membrane. Extrapolation of this hypothesis would suggest that the defects in glucose and bicarbonate transport noted in vivo are at least partly secondary to the defects in sodium transport. Indeed, the inability to demonstrate abnormalities in sodium-dependent glucose uptake in brushborder membrane vesicles prepared from phosphate-depleted animals further supports this concept. Finally, as discussed above, the defect in proximal tubule calcium transport (a nephron segment in which calcium and phosphate transport are closely linked) is not repaired by acute phosphate infusion; thus, this too is most likely related to a nonspecific defect in cellular function induced by phosphate depletion. However, the defect in distal calcium reabsorption, which is independent of sodium reabsorption and can be corrected by acute phosphate infusion, presumably stems from other distinct alterations induced by phosphate depletion.

Summary

Renal tubular function is appreciably altered subsequent to dietary phosphate deprivation. Changes are observed in the transport of a variety of solutes, including sodium, calcium, magnesium, phosphate, bicarbonate, and glucose. There are several mechanisms that contribute to these alterations. Phosphate depletion results in systemic changes in PTH and $1,25(OH)_2D_3$ levels, which alter calcium and phosphate transport. In addition, there appear to be specific tubular effects in the proximal tubule, where phosphate uptake at the brushborder membrane is increased, possibly due to changes in the membrane lipid content or distribution. Specific changes also occur in the distal nephron, which are also possibly related to changes in membrane permeability that modulate calcium and possibly magnesium transport. These changes are acute and are rapidly reversible with phosphate infusion. With more severe and/or chronic phosphate depletion, changes in proximal tubule function become apparent. These are not as readily reversible, and they may represent limitations on transport imposed by reductions in availability of high-energy phosphate compounds, as suggested in other tissues. These effects, which may also affect bicarbonate and glucose transport, are not necessarily expressed in the final urine because of the capacity of more resistant distal segments to reabsorb the increased delivered load. However, in addition to understanding the manifestations of the phosphate depletion syndrome, it seems clear that further study of this experimental model will provide important new insights into the cellular mechanisms responsible for the regulation of transport and for the cellular factors regulating mineral homeostasis.

References

1. STEELE TH, DELUCA HF: Influence of dietary phosphorus on renal phosphate reabsorption in the parathyroidectomized rat. *J Clin Invest* 57:867–874, 1976
2. TROEHLER U, BONJOUR JP, FLEISCH H: Inorganic phosphate homeostasis: Renal adaptation to the dietary intake in intact and thyroparathyroidectomized rats. *J Clin Invest* 57:264–273, 1976
3. DOMINGUEZ JH, GRAY RW, LEMANN J JR: Dietary phosphate deprivation in women and men: Effects on mineral and acid balance, parathyroid hormone and the metabolism of 24-OH vitamin D. *J Clin Endocrinol Metab* 43:1056–1068, 1976
4. LEVINE BS, CROOKS PW, KATZ JA, KUROKAWA K, COBURN JW: Early events during renal adaptation to low dietary phosphorus (*abstract*). *Kidney Int* 25:148, 1984
5. STEELE TH, UNDERWOOD JL, STROMBERG BA, LARMORE CA: Renal resistance to parathyroid hormone during phosphorus deprivation. *J Clin Invest* 58:1461–1464, 1976
6. BONJOUR JP, TROEHLER U, PRESTON C, FLEISCH H: Parathyroid hormone and renal handling of phosphate: Effect of dietary phosphate and diphosphonates. *Am J Physiol* 234:F497–505, 1978
7. BRAZY PC, MCKEOWN JW, HARRIS RH, DENNIS VW: Comparative effects of dietary phosphate, unilateral nephrectomy, and parathyroid hormone on phosphate transport by the rabbit proximal tubule. *Kidney Int* 17:788–800, 1980
8. STOLL R, KINNE R, MURER H: Effect of dietary phosphate intake on phosphate transport by isolated rat renal brush border vesicles. *Biochem J* 180:465–470, 1979
9. HARAMATI A, KNOX FG: Is phosphate reabsorped by the distal nephron. *Min Electr Metab* 6:165–173, 1981
10. PASTORIZA-MUNOZ E, COLINDRES RE, LASSITER WS, LECHENE E: Effect of parathyroid hormone on phosphate reabsorption in rat distal convolution. *Am J Physiol* 235:F321–330, 1978
11. SHAREGHI GR, AGUS ZS: Phosphate transport in the light segment of the rabbit cortical collecting tubule. *Am J Physiol* 242:F379–384, 1982
12. WEN SF, BOYNAR JW JR, STOLL RW: Effect of phosphate deprivation on renal phosphate transport in the dog. *Am J Physiol* 234(Suppl 3):F199–206, 1978
13. HARAMATI A, HAAS JA, KNOX FG: Adaptation of deep and superficial nephrons to changes in dietary phosphate intake. *Am J Physiol* 244:F265–269, 1983
14. KNOX FG, HARAMATI A: Renal handling of phosphate, in *Divalent Ion Homeostasis, Contemporary Issues in Nephrology* (vol 11), edited by BRENNER BN, STEIN JH, New York, Churchill Livingstone, 1983, pp 33–51
15. FREEMAN D, BARTLETT S, RADDA G, ROSS B: Energetics of sodium transport in the kidney, saturation transfer ^{31}P-NMR. *Biochem Biophys Acta* 762:325–336, 1983
16. SCHWAB SJ, HAMMERMAN MR: Mechanisms of phosphate exit across basolateral membrane of the renal proximal tubular cell (*abstract*). *Clin Res* 32:535A, 1984
17. CHENG L, LIANG CT, SACKTOR B: Phosphate uptake by renal membrane vesicles of rabbits adapted to high and low phosphorus diets. *Am J Physiol* 245:F175–180, 1983
18. DOUSA TP, KEMPSON SA, SHAH SV: Adaptive changes in renal cortical brush border membranes. *Adv Exp Med Biol* 128:69–76, 1980
19. KESSLER RJ, DUKE AV, FANESTIL DD: Divalent alkali metal requirement for phosphate binding by a renal brush border protein (*abstract*). *Kidney Int* 25:146, 1984

20. KESSLER RJ, VAUGHN DA, FANESTIL DD: Phosphate-binding proteolipid from brush border. *J Biol Chem* 257:14311–14317, 1982
21. SCHALI C, KESSLER RJ, FANESTIL DD: Co-purification of the renal phosphate transporter with phosphorin, a Pi binding proteolipid (*abstract*). *Kidney Int* 25:153, 1984
22. DOUSA TP, KEMPSON SA: Regulation of brush border membrane transport of phosphate. *Min Electr Metab* 7:113–121, 1982
23. HAMMERMAN MR, CORPUS VM, MORRISSEY JJ: NAD-induced inhibition of phosphate transport in canine renal brush-border membranes. Mediation through a process other than or in addition to NAD$^+$ hydrolysis. *Biochim Biophys Acta* 732:110–116, 1983
24. MOLITORIS BA, ALFREY AC, SIMON FR: The role of altered proximal tubule brush border membrane cholesterol content in the regulation of phosphate transport (*abstract*). *Kidney Int* 25:150, 1984
25. COBURN JW, MASSRY SG: Changes in serum and urinary calcium during phosphate depletion: Studies on mechanisms. *J Clin Invest* 49:1073–1087, 1970
26. GRABIE M, LAU K, AGUS ZS, GOLDBERG M, GOLDFARB S: Role of parathyroid hormone in the hypercalciuria of chronic phosphate depletion. *Min Electr Metab* 1:279–287, 1978
27. GOLDFARB S, WESTBY GR, GOLDBERG M, AGUS ZS: Renal tubular effects of chronic phosphate depletion. *J Clin Invest* 59:770–779, 1977
28. LAU YK, AGUS ZS, GOLDBERG M, GOLDFARB S: Renal tubular sites of altered calcium transport in phosphate depleted rats. *J Clin Invest* 64:1681–1687, 1979
29. MEYER-SABELLEK W, BRAUTBAR N, MOSER S, MONTCALM A, MASSRY SG: Effect of thiazides on the hypercalciuria of phosphate depletion. *J Lab Clin Med* 96:830–837, 1980
30. COSTANZO LS, WINDHAGER EE: Calcium and sodium transport by the distal convoluted tubule of the rat. *Am J Physiol* 235:F492–506, 1978
31. KREUSSER WJ, KUROKAWA K, AZNAR E, SACHTJEN E, MASSRY SG: Effect of phosphate depletion on magnesium homeostasis in rats. *J Clin Invest* 61:573–581, 1978
32. BRAUTBAR N, LEE DBN, COBURN JW, KLEEMAN CR: Dietary magnesium in experimental phosphate depletion: Bone and soft tissue mineral changes. *Am J Physiol* 237:E152–162, 1979
33. WONG NL, QUAMME GA, O'CALLAGHAN TJ, SUTTON RA, DIRKS JH: Renal tubular transport in phosphate depletion: a micropuncture study. *Can J Physiol Pharmacol* 58:1063–1071, 1980
34. SHAREGHI GR, AGUS ZS: Magnesium transport in the cortical thick ascending limb of Henle's loop of the rabbit. *J Clin Invest* 69:759–769, 1982
35. QUAMME GA: Effect of hypercalcemia on renal tubular handling of calcium and magnesium. *Can J Physiol Pharmacol* 60:1275–1280, 1982
36. GOLD LW, MASSRY SG, FRIEDLER RM: Effect of phosphate depletion on renal tubular reabsorption of glucose. *J Lab Clin Med* 89:554–559, 1977
37. CORMAN B, TOUVAY C, POUJOL P, DE ROUFFIGNAC C: Glucose mediated inhibition of phosphate reabsorption in rat kidney. *Am J Physiol* 235:F430–439, 1978
38. DENNIS VW, BRAZY PC: Sodium, phosphate, glucose, bicarbonate, and alanine interactions in the isolated proximal convoluted tubule of the rabbit kidney. *J Clin Invest* 62:387–397, 1978
39. NUSSBAUM P, DEFRONZO R, LAU K, GOLDBERG M, AGUS ZS, GOLDFARB S: Interactions of insulin, phlorizin, and PTH on renal tubular phosphate transport (*abstract*). *Clin Res* 26:472, 1978
40. BARRETT PQ, ARONSON PS: Glucose and alanine inhibition of phosphate transport in renal microvillus membrane vesicles. *Am J Physiol* 242:F126–131, 1982

41. GOLD LW, MASSRY SG, ARIEFF AI, COBURN JW: Renal bicarbonate wasting during phosphate depletion: A possible cause of altered acid base homeostasis in hyperparathyroidism. *J Clin Invest* 52:2556–2562, 1973
42. EMMETT M, GOLDFARB S, AGUS ZS, NARINS RG: The pathophysiology of acid-base changes in chronically phosphate-depleted rats: Bone-kidney interactions. *J Clin Invest* 59:291–298, 1977
43. ARRUDA JAL, JULKA NK, RUBINSTEIN H, SABATINI S, KURTZMAN NA: Distal acidification defect induced by phosphate deprivation. *Metabolism* 29:826–836, 1980
44. SCHMIDT RW: Effects of phosphate depletion on acid-base status in dogs. *Metabolism* 27:943–952, 1978
45. KURTZ TW, HSU CH: Impaired distal acidification in chronically phosphate depleted rats. *Pflügers Arch* 377:229–239, 1978
46. STEELE TH: Impaired bicarbonate reabsorption in the phosphate depleted rat. *Min Electr Metab* 2:74, 1979
47. STEELE TH: Effect of phosphorus depletion on the renal transport of phosphate. *Adv Exp Med Biol* 103:343–355, 1978
48. MASSRY SG: Effect of phosphate depletion on renal tubular transport, in *Phosphate Metabolism Kidney and Bone,* edited by AVIOLI L, BORDIER P, FLEISCH H, MASSRY S, SLATOPOLSKY E, Paris, Nouvelle Imprimerie Fournie, 1978, pp 25–34
49. KREUSSER WJ, DESCOEUDRES C, ODA Y, MASSRY SG, KUROKAWA K: Effect of phosphate depletion on renal gluconeogenesis. *Min Electr Metab* 3:312–322, 1980
50. MCKINNEY TD, MYERS P: Effect of calcium and phosphate on bicarbonate and fluid transport by proximal tubules in vitro. *Kidney Int* 21:433–438, 1982
51. BRAZY PC, GULLANS SR, MANDEL LJ, DENNIS VW: Metabolic requirement for inorganic phosphate by rabbit proximal tubule: Evidence for a Crabtree effect. *J Clin Invest* 70:53–62, 1982

Phosphate Depletion and Renal Cell Metabolism

Kiyoshi Kurokawa

Adenosine triphosphate (ATP) is the major energy-coupling mechanism between the energy-producing and the energy-consuming systems in the cells. In a variety of diseased states, alterations in adenine nucleotide metabolism have been implicated in their pathogenesis. There are a few experimental model systems in which one can alter adenine nucleotide metabolism through different mechanisms and can examine the role of adenine nucleotides in cellular functions. These are listed in Table 1. Since a major portion of ATP is synthesized from adenosine diphosphate (ADP) and inorganic phosphate (Pi) by oxidative phosphorylation in mitochondria, a deficiency of Pi will impair ATP generation. Thus, various organ dysfunctions described in phosphate depletion have been attributed to a fall in the availability of energy-rich phosphate compounds such as ATP.

The effects of phosphate depletion, brought about principally by dietary phosphate restriction, on the metabolism of ATP and other phosphate compounds in various organ systems have been extensively studied in the last decade. In red blood cells, leukocytes, and platelets, relationships between a fall in plasma Pi, a fall in tissue Pi, a decrease in tissue ATP, and some forms of cellular dysfunction have been clearly demonstrated [1].

In phosphate depletion, there develops a variety of renal tubular dysfunctions, including altered tubular reabsorption of Pi, calcium, sodium bicarbonate, and glucose [2]. Some of these tubular dysfunctions may be due to a fall in ATP since tubular transport of these substances may depend on energy, the source of which could be ATP. In addition, changes in tubule cell metabolism may appear in response to phosphate depletion. It has been shown that gluconeogenesis may be suppressed [3] and that 25-OH-D$_3$-1α-hydroxylase (1α-OHase) may be activated with increased conversion of 25-hydroxycholecalciferol (25-OH-D$_3$) to 1,25-dihydroxycholecalciferol (1,25[OH]$_2$D$_3$) [4].

This manuscript was presented as part of a Symposium on *Renal and Vascular Consequences of Phosphate Depletion.*

Table 1. Models to induce changes in adenine nucleotides

1. Deficiency of inorganic phosphate
   a. Dietary phosphate restriction
2. Trapping of excess inorganic phosphate (with AMP deamination)
   a. Fructose or glycerol load
   b. 2-Deoxyglucose load
3. Interference with oxidative generation of ATP
   a. Temporary or permanent ligation of blood supply
   b. Injection of uncouplers of oxidative phosphorylation
4. Trapping of adenosine moiety as S-adenosyl derivative
   a. Ethionine in rat and guinea pig—mainly liver
   b. Methionine in guinea pig—liver

These metabolic changes may be caused by a fall in tissue Pi levels and ATP.

Energy Metabolism

The time course of phosphate depletion in growing rats [5] revealed that during week 1 of dietary phosphate restriction, there was little change in tissue Pi and ATP content in the kidney whereas plasma Pi fell rapidly. Kidney Pi decreased at week 2, whereas ATP started to fall only after week 6 of the diet. Thus, there seems to be no direct correlation between plasma Pi, tissue Pi, and ATP during the 8 weeks of low-phosphate diet. In contrast, there is a good correlation between these parameters in erythrocytes in phosphate depletion [1]. This is probably due to the lack of intracellular phosphate-storing organelles, mitochondria, in erythrocytes and also due to the fact that Pi diffuses passively across the red cell membrane. In the kidney, however, a large portion of phosphate can be stored in mitochondria; thus, only prolonged phosphate depletion may result in significant depletion of the intracellular phosphate store. Because of its abundance within the cells, it may require a certain time for cell Pi to decrease to a rate-limiting level for ATP generation in mitochondria where the synthesis of ATP from ADP and Pi takes place. This may explain the time lag between a fall in tissue Pi and ATP. It may also suggest that only after 6 weeks of low-P diet with severe phosphate depletion, intramitochondrial Pi might fall below the critical level for oxidative phosphorylation.

Other factors may be operative in the kidney to prevent a fall in cell Pi during phosphate depletion. One possible factor is an altered vitamin D metabolism. It has been shown that vitamin D may play an important role in extracellular and intracellular phosphate homeostasis through its action on intestine, bone, and kidney [6]. It is thought that the phosphate-mobilizing action of vitamin D is primarily due to its active metabolite, $1,25(OH)_2D_3$. It is possible that high plasma $1,25(OH)_2D_3$ levels in phosphate depletion may enhance Pi uptake into the tubule cells, thus helping to maintain cellular

Pi and ATP against the low plasma Pi concentration. Stated in another way, at any given extracellular Pi concentration in response to dietary phosphate restriction, an elevated $1,25(OH)_2D_3$ may facilitate entry of Pi into cells and maintain cell ATP levels; thus, it is only with severe phosphate depletion that tubule cell Pi and ATP may fall.

Another factor that may help the kidney preserve its function in the face of phosphate depletion is the unique structure of the tubules in providing polarity to the cell. Thus, extracellular Pi may enter tubule cells across two distinct membranes: the brushborder and the basolateral membranes [7]. In response to dietary phosphate restriction, proximal tubules avidly reabsorb filtered Pi, so that little Pi appears in the urine. Indeed, the virtual absence of Pi in the urine is the most sensitive and early sign of phosphate depletion. The nearly complete Pi reabsorption in the presence of very low Pi in the plasma, and thus in the glomerular filtrate, suggests the presence of highly effective Pi-reabsorptive mechanisms across the brushborder membrane. Kinetic analyses of Pi transport of isolated brushborder membrane vesicles [8] have shown the presence of Pi transport coupled with that of sodium ions with the Km of approximately 0.1 mM or 0.3 mg/dl; levels of plasma Pi encountered in severe phosphate depletion. Studies using isolated proximal tubule cells suggest that the major fraction of Pi entering the cells does so across the brushborder membrane in a sodium-dependent manner. It is possible therefore that the renal tubule cells may be supplied with sufficient quantities of Pi from the tubular lumen even in the presence of very low ambient Pi concentrations. In this regard, a recent study by Brazy et al [9] is of considerable interest. They showed that oxidative metabolism of isolated perfused proximal convoluted tubules may be impaired when perfused with a perfusate containing glucose, but without Pi. Their data suggests the presence of the Crabtree effect in proximal convoluted tubules. Thus, the intracellular Pi may deplete rapidly upon glucose entry (which will consume cell Pi for phosphorylation reactions) from the tubular lumen in the absence of Pi in the luminal perfusate, resulting in ATP depletion. Since physiologic concentration of Pi was present in the bath medium, their observations suggest that the availability of Pi from basolateral membranes is limited and that cell Pi is primarily supplied from the lumen in the proximal convoluted tubules. This Crabtree effect was not observed in the proximal straight tubules, suggesting that the permeability of basolateral membranes to Pi may be different in proximal convoluted and straight tubules and that the supply of Pi from the lumen plays a critical role in maintaining the cellular Pi concentration in the proximal convoluted tubules.

The pattern of changes in adenine nucleotides in the kidney during experimental phosphate depletion may be different from that observed in the other conditions listed in Table 1. In acute ischemia, there is a rapid fall in ATP with reciprocal rises in ADP and AMP in the kidney [10]. The fall in ATP in the kidney is very rapid, reaching to 25% of normal levels at 30 sec of ischemia.

Intracellular Pi depletion occurs in response to fructose loading. In this model, trapping of excess Pi by fructose injection causes an immediate fall in ATP with concomitant, but transient, rises in ADP and adenosine monophosphate (AMP) and thus a fall in the energy charge [11]. Following this initial event, ADP and AMP fall, and the energy charge returns toward normal despite a sustained low ATP level. This "adaptive" change in adenine nucleotide metabolism to restore the energy charge with further reduction of total adenylate pool may be of importance for the maintenance of cell integrity under such stressful conditions. This fall in AMP occurs because of the stimulation of AMP deaminase and 5′-nucleotidase to cleave the accumulated AMP [12]. It has been shown that AMP deaminase is inhibited by both ATP and Pi, and 5′-nucleotidase is suppressed by ATP under normal conditions. A fall in ATP and/or Pi deinhibits these enzyme activities, resulting in the degradation of AMP and the production of inosine monophosphate and adenosine. Inosine monophosphate is a potent inhibitor of fructose-1-phosphate aldolase; the enzyme that catalyzes the clearance of fructose-1-phosphate. Inosine monophosphate and adenosine are further metabolized to inosine by 5′-nucleotidase and adenosine deaminase, respectively, and inosine will then be metabolized to uric acid, the level of which rises in plasma and in urine after a fructose load. Thus, after a fructose load, there is a net loss of adenine nucleotide, primarily in liver and kidney. It has been suggested that these biochemical changes in fructose loading observed in rats occur in patients with hereditary fructose intolerance; a condition with defective fructose-1-phosphate aldolase in liver, kidney, and possibly gut, and part of the symptoms of this disorder may be due to ATP deficiency in these organs. In response to fructose ingestion, these patients demonstrate a complex dysfunction of the renal tubule resembling Fanconi syndrome [13]. Such proximal tubular dysfunction may be related to ATP deficiency brought about by Pi depletion. Indeed, there is a good correlation between renal ATP and Pi content in response to fructose loading in the rat [14]. Moreover, an administration of Pi just prior to fructose loading can prevent a fall in ATP in the kidney [14].

Another change in adenine nucleotide metabolism in the kidney in the experimental phosphate depletion model is a fall in the equilibrium constant (Keq) of adenylate kinase, which coincides with a fall in ATP. The change in Keq of adenylate kinase may be related to abnormal extracellular and intracellular distribution of magnesium; a key ion for the regulation of this enzyme. Thus, it is likely that an alteration in cellular magnesium may occur in phosphate depletion. Indeed, hypomagnesemia, with a negative magnesium balance that is due to an excess urinary Mg loss, develops during phosphate depletion in rats [15]. Hypomagnesemia and hypermagnesuria are also noted during phosphate depletion in humans [16]. Consequently, there may occur a decrease in cytosolic magnesium, which comprises a portion of the total cellular magnesium. Since adenylate kinase is localized primarily in cytosol, a change in the cytosolic magnesium ionic concentration will affect the Keq of adenylate kinase significantly and may affect the integrity of cellular functions. It is of interest that the maintenance of serum magnesium concentration during phosphate depletion by oral magnesium supplementation can prevent a fall in the Keq of adenylate kinase, though it is ineffective on the fall in tissue Pi and ATP [17]. This supports the possibility that magnesium deficiency plays a pathogenic role in changing the Keq of the enzyme in phosphate depletion. The significance of this altered Keq of adenylate kinase on biochemical and physiologic functions of the kidney needs further study.

Renal Gluconeogenesis

An ability to produce glucose from noncarbohydrate precursors, gluconeogenesis, is unique to the kidney and the liver. Renal gluconeogenesis is localized only in the proximal tubules and is regulated by a variety of hormonal and ionic perturbations. Thus, it has been shown that renal gluconeogenesis is stimulated in metabolic acidosis and in response to parathyroid hormone (PTH), catecholamines, angiotensin II, and glucocorticoid. In response to a low-phosphate diet, the glucose production rates (measured in vitro using separated proximal tubules) were reduced within 3 days [3]. This reduction in gluconeogenesis was accompanied by detectable decreases in both tubular Pi and ATP content and was corrected, not by the in vitro addition of Pi in the incubation medium, but by the in vivo supplementation of phosphate to the diet. These in vitro data of reduced Pi and ATP in separated tubules may seem at variance from the data that showed normal Pi and ATP in the kidney in vivo as discussed earlier. It is possible, however, that separated proximal tubules in vitro with their lumens collapsed may depend on their supply of Pi primarily on the bath, whereas proximal tubules in vivo gain Pi from the lumen.

Activation of 25(OH)D$_3$-1α-Hydroxylase

It has been well established that 1α-OHase in the kidney is tightly regulated and that PTH is the major stimulator of the enzyme [6]. Recent studies using microdissected tubules nevertheless revealed the presence of two distinct 1α-OHase systems in the mammalian kidney [18]: one is present in the proximal convoluted tubules and stimulated by parathyroid hormone (PTH) via cyclic AMP, and thus activated in vitamin D deficiency; the other being present in proximal straight tubules, being insensitive to PTH and cyclic AMP, and selectively stimulated by calcitonin via cyclic AMP-independent mechanism. The mechanism by which calcitonin stimulates 1α-OHase is not known.

It has been well documented that the production of 1,25(OH)$_2$D$_3$ is increased in response to a low dietary phosphate intake owing to the activation of 1α-OHase [4, 6]. The cellular mechanism underlying the activation of 1α-OHase in the kidney in response to phosphate depletion is not known. It has been thought that the 1α-OHase may be stimulated by a decrease in the renal tubular cell Pi concentration. However, as discussed, there are no data to support the decrease in renal tissue Pi within a few days of low dietary phosphate intake when marked rises in plasma 1,25(OH)$_2$D$_3$ and activation of 1α-OHase are observed. In response to low dietary phosphate, one of the early events that takes place in the proximal tubule is an avid Pi reabsorption [2]. This can be easily detected within 24 hr of low-phosphate diet and is accompanied by an enhanced Pi uptake by isolated brushborder membrane vesicles in vitro [8]. Although the exact nature of this renal tubular adaptation to low-phosphate intake has not been clarified, it is conceivable that some alterations in Pi concentrations in proximal tubules or in some critical areas of tubule cells may be important for this activation of 1α-OHase. In this regards, it is of interest to note that both PTH and calcitonin are phosphaturic and that Pi uptake across the brushborder membrane is suppressed by PTH. It is possible that as a consequence of inhibition of Pi uptake by the brushborder membrane, tubule cell Pi concentrations may fall in response to these peptide hormones and may participate in the stimulation of 1α-OHase by these hormones. Such a mechanism may be involved in the stimulation of 1α-OHase by calcitonin, which is independent of cyclic AMP. Thus, a fall in cell Pi in some critical areas within the proximal tubular cells may be regulatory for 1α-OHase activation in response to phosphate depletion, calcitonin, and perhaps PTH.

A recent study has demonstrated that prostaglandin E$_2$ (PGE$_2$) is yet another hormone capable of stimulating 1α-OHase. Its administration into the abdominal aorta just above renal arteries stimulated 1α-OHase in the rat [19]. However, the magnitude of maximum stimulation of 1α-OHase by PGE$_2$ was less than those by PTH and calcitonin. Unpublished observations by Ogata et al showed that when administered together with PTH or calcitonin, PGE$_2$ had no effect on the PTH-stimulated 1α-OHase, but that it inhibited the effect of calcitonin to stimulate 1α-OHase to the level observed by PGE$_2$ alone. Since PTH and calcitonin stimulate 1α-OHase in the proximal convoluted and straight tubules, respectively [18], these data suggest that both PTH and PGE$_2$ stimulate 1α-OHase in the proximal convoluted tubules and that PGE$_2$ inhibits specifically calcitonin-sensitive 1α-OHase in the proximal straight tubules while stimulating the enzyme in the proximal convoluted tubules. Moreover, they showed that PGE$_2$ had no effect on PTH-stimulated phosphaturia, but inhibited calcitonin-stimulated phosphaturia. PGE$_2$ itself had little phosphaturic effect. These data indicate that PGE$_2$ can abolish the action of calcitonin in the proximal tubules to stimulate 1α-OHase and to inhibit Pi reabsorption, and they suggest the possible causal relationships between tubular Pi reabsorption and 1α-OHase activity. However, a recent micropuncture study by Berndt and Knox [20] suggest that PTH inhibits Pi reabsorption both in the proximal convoluted and straight tubules, whereas calcitonin inhibits it in the proximal convolution and not in the straight portion. Then, it seems that PGE$_2$ abolishes the effects of calcitonin in the proximal convoluted tubules to inhibit Pi reabsorption and in the proximal straight tubules to stimulate 1α-OHase. Thus, these data rather suggest that there may not be any causal relationship between Pi transport and 1α-OHase activity in the proximal tubules in response to calcitonin or PTH.

Conclusion and Future Perspective

Measurements of ATP and Pi at a steady state do not provide information on the turnover of this nucleotide and high-energy Pi. Considering the facts that Pi is necessary for the formation of ATP and that magnesium is a cofactor for most of the ATP-catalyzing enzymes (such as kinases, ATPases), it is conceivable that in phosphate depletion, both ATP synthesis and utilization are impaired owing to a lack of Pi and owing to a fall in magnesium ions, respectively. Certainly, the evaluation of ATP and Pi turnover will provide further insight into the altered energy metabolism in phosphate depletion. Recent development in nuclear magnetic resonance (NMR) in biomedical research will be of great importance in this area of research. With phosphorus NMR, it has become possible to determine noninvasively the dynamic changes in relatively free adenine nucleotides and Pi in cytosol. Available data with phosphorus NMR suggest that the concentrations of free Pi and ADP in the kidney may be much lower than expected and about only one-tenth of the values estimated from conventional extraction methods [21]. These data suggest that the free Pi concentration may be in a range of 0.1 mM instead of the 1 to 3 mM measured by conventional chemical determinations. If this is the case, it becomes apparent that many reactions involving Pi, such as the generation of ATP, may be critically controlled by the concentration of Pi in the cell. Such a postulate may explain the rapid appearance of the Crabtree effect in the proximal tubule and the dependency of proximal tubules upon the supply of Pi from the tubular lumen. The unique property of proximal convoluted tubules, which depend primarily upon luminal Pi for the supply of cell Pi, is of importance in the consideration of the pathophysiology of tubular dysfunction and altered cell metabolism in phosphate depletion. Further studies to elucidate cell metabolism and its regulation in individual nephron segments will certainly add new insights into our understanding of the coupling mechanism between cell metabolism and function in the kidney.

Acknowledgments. Supported by the Veterans Administration and in part by a grant from the National Institutes of Health (AM21351).

References

1. KNOCHEL JP: The pathophysiology and clinical characteristics of severe hypophosphatemia. *Arch Intern Med* 137:203–220, 1977
2. AGUS Z: Effect of phosphate depletion on renal hemodynamics and tubular transport. *9th International Congress of Nephrology,* June 11–15, 1984, Los Angeles
3. KREUSSER WJ, DESCOEUDRES C, ODA Y, MASSRY SG, KUROKAWA K: Effect of phosphate depletion on renal gluconeogenesis. *Mineral Electrolyte Metab* 3:312–322, 1980

4. TANAKA Y, DELUCA HF: The control of 25-hydroxyvitamin D metabolism by inorganic phosphorus. *Arch Biochem Biophys* 154:566–574, 1973

5. KREUSSER WJ, KUROKAWA K, AZNAR E, MASSRY SG: Phosphate depletion. Effect on renal inorganic phosphorus and adenine nucleotides, urinary phosphate and calcium, and calcium balance. *Mineral Electrolyte Metab* 1:30–42, 1978

6. NORMAN AW: *Vitamin D: The Calcium Homeostatic Steroid Hormone.* New York, Academic Press, 1979

7. DENNIS VW, BRAZY PC: Divalent anion transport in isolated renal tubules. *Kidney Int* 22:498–506, 1982

8. DOUSA TP, KEMPSON SA, SHAH SV: Adaptive changes in renal cortical brush border membrane, in *Phosphate and Mineral in Health and Disease,* edited by MASSRY SG, RITZ E, KAHN H, New York, Plenum Publishing Co, 1980, pp 69–76

9. BRAZY PC, GULLANS SR, MANDEL LJ, DENNIS VW: Metabolic requirement for inorganic phosphate by the rabbit proximal tubule: Evidence for a Crabtree effect. *J Clin Invest* 82:53–62, 1982

10. HEMS DA, BROSNAN JT: Effects of ischaemia on content of metabolites in rat liver and kidney in vivo. *Biochem J* 120:105–111, 1970

11. BURCH HB, LOWRY OH, MEINHARDT L, MAX P JR, CHYU KJ: Effect of fructose, dihydroxyacetone, glycerol and glucose on metabolites and related compounds in liver and kidney. *J Biol Chem* 245:2092–2102, 1970

12. WOODS HF, EGGLESTON LV, KREBS HA: The cause of hepatic accumulation of fructose-l-phosphate on fructose loading. *Biochem J* 119:501–510, 1970

13. MORRIS RC JR: An experimental renal acidification defect in patients with hereditary fructose intolerance: II. Its distinction from classic renal tubular acidosis; its resemblance to the renal acidification defect associated with the Fanconi syndrome of children with cystinosis. *J Clin Invest* 47:1648–1663, 1968

14. MORRIS CR JR, NIGON K, REED EB: Evidence that the severity of depletion of inorganic phosphate determines the severity of the disturbance of adenine nucleotide metabolism in the liver and renal cortex of the fructose-loaded rat. *J Clin Invest* 61:209–220, 1978

15. KREUSSER WJ, KUROKAWA K, AZNAR E, SACHTJEN E, MASSRY SG: Effect of phosphate depletion on magnesium homeostasis in rats. *J Clin Invest* 61:573–581, 1978

16. DOMINGUEZ JH, GRAY RW, LEMANN J JR: Dietary phosphate deprivation in women and men: Effects on mineral and acid balances, parathyroid hormone and the metabolism of 25-OH-vitamin D. *J Clin Endocrinol Metab* 43:1056–1068, 1976

17. KUROKAWA K, KREUSSER WJ, MASSRY SG: Phosphate depletion and adenine nucleotide metabolism in kidney and liver. *Adv Exper Med Biol* 103:327–341, 1978

18. KAWASHIMA H, KUROKAWA K: Unique hormonal regulation of vitamin D metabolism in the mammalian kidney. *Mineral Electr Metab* 9:227–235, 1983

19. YAMADA M, MATSUMOTO T, TAKAHASHI H, SUDA T, OGATA E: Stimulatory effect of prostaglandin E_2 on $1\alpha,25$-dihydroxyvitamin D_3 synthesis in rats. *Biochem J* 216:237–240, 1983

20. BERNDT TJ, KNOX FG: Proximal tubule site of inhibition of phosphate reabsorption by calcitonin. *Am J Physiol* (in press, 1984)

21. BALABAN RS: The application of nuclear magnetic resonance to the study of cellular physiology. *Am J Physiol* 246:C10–C19, 1984

Mechanisms of Myocardial Injury in Phosphate Depletion

Nachman Brautbar

Interest in the metabolic consequences of phosphate depletion, in recent years, has demonstrated that the functional integrity of almost every organ is affected. This is not surprising, since two basic disturbances occur during prolonged phosphate depletion. First, there is a decrease in the adenosine triphosphate content of the cell and a reduction in the availability of energy-rich phosphate compounds [1, 2]. Second, there is a decrease in 2,3-diphosphoglycerates in the red blood cells, and this abnormality increases the affinity for oxygen; therefore, tissue hypoxia may ensue [2, 3].

A major clinical finding in patients with chronic phosphate depletion is myopathy, which is consistent with muscle pain and muscle weakness. Fuller et al [4] have studied the effects of phosphate depletion on skeletal muscle, and they found decreased phosphorus contents in the skeletal muscle of dogs following prolonged phosphate depletion. The levels of adenosine triphosphate and inorganic phosphorus were not evaluated. These abnormalities were reversed following phosphate repletion. O'Connor, Wheeler, and Bethune [5] evaluated the effect of phosphate depletion on cardiac function in seven patients. They found that stroke work was reduced, but returned to normal after phosphate administration. The authors showed that with correction of the hypophosphatemia, left ventricular stroke volume improved and pulmonary artery wedge pressure decreased. Fuller et al [6] studied cardiac function in dogs before and during phosphate depletion. During phosphate depletion, the stroke volume, maximum ascending aortic blood flow, and maximum left-ventricular time rate of change of pressure decreased significantly; all of these changes disappeared on phosphate repletion. These studies did not evaluate changes in myocardial phosphate, adenosine triphosphate, or creatine phosphate. In all of the above studies, the mechanisms for cellular injury have not been elucidated.

Work from our laboratory has examined the effects of experimental phos-

This manuscript was presented as part of a Symposium on *Renal and Vascular Consequences of Phosphate Depletion.*

phorus depletion on cellular bioenergetics [7], carbohydrate metabolism [8], phospholipid synthesis [9], and fatty acid oxidation [9] in the heart and skeletal muscles. This review will examine the mechanism for myocardial cellular injury in phosphate depletion.

The contractile properties of the heart are the result of the interaction of a complex system of intracellular filaments that lay longitudinally in the cell and consist of alternating arrays of thick and thin filaments. The process of contraction requires energy in the form of high-energy terminal phosphate grouping of adenosine triphosphate (ATP). Alongside the myofibrils lay the mitochondria, which are the intracellular site of ATP production. The mitochondrion is a compartment separated from the cytosol by a membrane that has an inner membrane and an outer membrane. The mitochondrial membrane is permeable to some ions and metabolites, and is less so to others; therefore, an active mechanism for maintaining intramitochondrial concentration of ions, pH, and electric potential is necessary. This energy is derived from the degradation and synthesis of mitochondrial ATP. The ATP produced via oxidative phosphorylation is not able to diffuse effectively from the mitochondrial space to the myofibrils or sarcoplasmic reticulum. Therefore, a mechanism for overcoming this is provided by the creatine phosphate shuttle [10] shown in Figure 1.

The current concept of cellular bioenergetics is based on microcompartmentation and the ability to use spedivid enzymes in energy production, transport, and usage. Three steps are recognized: (1) Energy production—energy is produced in the mitochondria via oxidative phosphorylation in the form of ATP. (2) Energy transport—the energy in the form of ATP is converted to diffusible energy in the form of creatine phosphate. This step is catalyzed via the mitochondrial isoenzymes of creatine kinase. The creatine phosphate then diffuses to the various cellular sites, such as the sarcoplasmic reticulum or myofibril [10, 12]. (3) Energy in the form of creatine phosphate is used at the myofibrillar site via the myofibrillar isoenzymes of creatine kinase [10, 11]. The adenosine diphosphate released after muscle contraction is rephosphorylated to ATP, and creatine is released to diffuse back to the mitochondrial site for rephosphorylation. Thus, creatine and the creatine kinase isoenzymes form a shuttle: the creatine phosphate shuttle [10].

The sarcoplasmic reticulum and sarcolemmal membrane play a major role in keeping the cell membrane system and its compartments intact. We have examined, in this study, aerobic and anaerobic energy production, cellular bioenergetics, and the biochemical integrity of the cell membrane.

Methods

Sprague-Dawley rats, weighing 150 to 200 g, were studied after 4, 8, and 12 weeks of selective phosphorus depletion produced by dietary phosphorus restriction. The animals were fed rat chow containing 0.025% phosphorus. Another group of weight- and age-matched, pair-fed rats received diets containing 0.35% phosphorus, and they served as controls. On the day of the experiments, rats were anesthetized, intubated, and respirated.

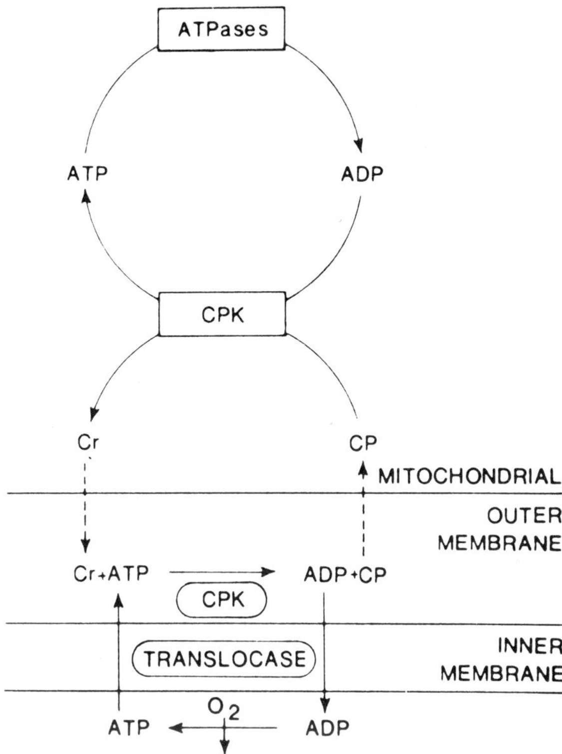

Fig. 1. The creatine phosphate shuttle (*CPK,* creatine phosphokinase; *Cr,* creatine; *CP,* creatine phosphate). (Reproduced with permission, Mahler [18])

Aerobic Energy Production

A biopsy specimen was taken from the left ventricle by using freeze-clamping liquid nitrogen techniques [7], and blood was collected for the measurement of serum inorganic phosphorus. The myocardial samples were then analyzed for high-energy nucleotides, as described previously [7].

Mitochondria and myofibrils were isolated by using standard methods from our laboratory described previously [7, 8]. The substrate oxidation ratio and ADP/O ratios were determined polarographically by means of a Clark oxygen electrode (Gilson Electronics, Middleton, Wisconsin).

Anaerobic Energy and Carbohydrates

Liquid nitrogen myocardial biopsy specimens were examined for glycogen by using enzymatic methods [8], and glucose-6-phosphate was estimated using the Bessman ashomatic analyzer.

Biochemical Integrity of Cellular Membrane-Phospholipid and Lipid Synthesis

Phospholipid Precursors

Samples also were processed for evaluation of acid-extractable phospholipid precursors and glycerol, as well as for acid-extractable tissue phospholipids. Myocardial samples were extracted with acid as described above, and the following phospholipid precursors were examined by using the Bessman ashomatic phosphorus analyzer: phosphocholine (PC), phosphoethanolamine (GPE), and cytidine triphosphate (CTP). Glycerol phosphate was measured by using enzymatic methods [9].

Fatty Acid Oxidation

Mitochondria were isolated as described above, and fatty acid oxidation was measured by using the Clark electrode.

Long-chain Fatty Acids

The activated fatty acid, palmytoil coenzyme-A, was purchased from Sigma (Sigma Biochemicals, St. Louis, Missouri), and 50 μl of 2 mM carnitine and 30 μl of 0.1 mM palmytoil coenzyme-A were added consecutively to the incubation chamber; oxygen consumption was recorded.

Short-chain Fatty Acids

Beta-hydroxybutyric acid was obtained from Sigma Biochemicals. The same medium was used for short-chain fatty acids; 100 μl mitochondria were added to the incubation oxygraph vessel and 50 μl of 0.4 mM of beta-hydroxybutyric acid was added. This acid was used to examine short-chain fatty acid oxidation.

Results

Bioenergetics

Aerobic Energy Production

The effects of various durations of phosphate depletion are shown in Table 1, such as on the serum concentration of phosphorus and body weight, and on the intracellular concentration of inorganic phosphorus, adenine nucleotides, and creatine phosphate and creatine of myocardium. Dietary phosphate

Table 1. Effect of 4, 8, and 12 weeks (wk) of dietary phosphate restriction on the concentration of serum phosphorus intracellular concentration of inorganic phosphorus, adenine nucleotide, and creatine phosphate in the myocardium

| | | Serum phosphorus mg/dl | Intracellular concentration (μmoles/g protein) | | | | | Phosphorylation potential $M - 1$ |
			Inorganic phosphorus	ATP	ADP	AMP	Creatine phosphate	
Control	$N = 8$	8.5 ± 0.1	28.0 ± 3.5	23.2 ± 1.6	6.0 ± 0.7	1.2 ± 0.1	33.0 ± 1.0	1400 ± 195
4-wk PD	$N = 8$	5.8 ± 0.5[a]	13.6 ± 1.4[a]	23.8 ± 1.4	6.3 ± 0.3	0.8 ± 0.1	28.7 ± 1.5	3128 ± 295[a]
Control	$N = 4$	9.2 ± 0.7	25.6 ± 1.8	22.3 ± 3.2	5.2 ± 1.0	1.1 ± 0.5	30.6 ± 1.8	1654 ± 260
8-wk PD	$N = 6$	4.5 ± 0.3[a]	13.2 ± 1.5[a]	20.1 ± 4.4	6.5 ± 0.9	1.0 ± 0.1	21.0 ± 1.9[a]	2380 ± 315[a]
Control	$N = 4$	7.6 ± 0.3	32.0 ± 2.5	27.0 ± 1.1	7.9 ± 0.6	1.3 ± 0.3	32.3 ± 1.3	1071 ± 210
12-wk PD	$N = 7$	3.4 ± 0.1[a]	10.9 ± 1.0[a]	14.6 ± 1.3[a]	4.8 ± 0.3[a]	0.9 ± 0.1	21.7 ± 2.1[a]	3290 ± 610[a]

Data are presented as mean $\pm$ *SEM*.

[a] Indicates significant difference from control at $P < 0.01$.

PD, phosphate depletion; ATP, adenosine triphosphate; ADP, adenosine diphosphate; and AMP, adenosine monophosphate.

restriction was associated with a significant ($P < 0.01$) and marked decrement in serum concentration of phosphorus, with the levels being lowest after 12 weeks of phosphate depletion. A significant ($P < 0.01$) reduction in the myocardial concentration of inorganic phosphorus was evident after 4 weeks of phosphate depletion, and it remained low thereafter. There was a significant ($P < 0.01$) and direct correlation between serum levels of phosphorus and the concentration of inorganic phosphorus in the myocardium.

The myocardial concentrations of adenosine triphosphate and adenosine diphosphate in phosphate-depleted rats were significantly ($P < 0.01$) lower than those in control animals only after 12 weeks of phosphate depletion. There was no correlation between the concentrations of these nucleotides and the serum levels of phosphorus or the cellular concentration of inorganic phosphorus. Phosphorylation potential was significantly increased at 4 weeks of phosphate depletion, and it remained elevated throughout the study (Table 1).

The myocardial concentration of creatine phosphate displayed a decrease after 4 weeks of phosphate depletion, but the decrements were statistically significant ($P < 0.01$) after 8 and 12 weeks. There were significant ($P < 0.01$) and direct correlations between the myocardial concentration of creatine phosphate and both myocardial inorganic phosphorus and serum levels of phosphorus (Fig. 2).

The effects of phosphate depletion on mitochondrial function are shown in Figure 2. Oxygen consumption per unit time was significantly ($P < 0.05$) reduced both after 8 weeks (94.0 ± 10.0 nmoles versus 65.0 ± 4.0 nmoles oxygen/mg protein/min) and 12 weeks (114.0 ± 9.2 nmoles versus 82.0 ± 8.0

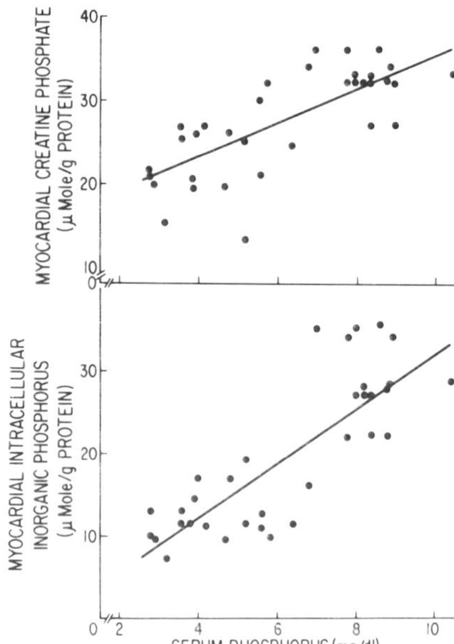

Fig. 2. Correlations between myocardial cellular creatine phosphate (*upper panel*), inorganic phosphorus (*lower panel*), and serum phosphorus during 4, 8, and 12 wk of phosphate depletion. *Upper panel:* $y = 1.99x + 5.35$; $r = 0.72$; $P < 0.01$. *Lower panel:* $y = 3.29x - 0.98$; $r = 0.80$; $P < 0.01$.

nmoles oxygen/mg protein/min) of phosphate depletion. The energy charge was unchanged in all stages of phosphate depletion, and the phosphorylation potential was calculated according to:

$$[ATP]/[ATP][P_i]$$

This was elevated significantly at 4 weeks of phosphate depletion, and it remained elevated throughout the study (Table 1).

Mitochondrial Energy Transport

The activity of creatine phosphokinase was significantly reduced after 4 weeks of phosphate depletion (1.7 ± 0.12 IU/mg versus 0.50 ± 0.10 IU/mg protein), and it fell even further after 12 weeks of phosphate depletion. The addition of creatine to state 4-respiring mitochondria significantly enhanced oxygen consumption in mitochondria from control, but not from phosphate-depleted animals, as expressed by the ratio of oxygen consumption with and without creatine.

Myofibrillar Energy Usage

There also was a significant and marked decline in the activity of myofibrillar creatine phosphokinase, which became apparent within 4 weeks of phosphate depletion and remained reduced throughout the study.

Total extractable creatine phosphokinase after 4 weeks of phosphate depletion was 2.9 ± 0.5 IU/mg protein, which is a value significantly lower ($P < 0.01$) than normal (10.0 ± 0.9 IU/mg protein). There was a significant direct correlation ($P < 0.01$) between total extractable creatine phosphokinase and serum phosphorus concentrations ($y = 1.7x - 2.3$, $r = 0.73$, $N = 10$; y, total extractable creatine phosphokinase, and x, serum inorganic phosphorus).

Carbohydrate Metabolism and Anaerobic Energy Production

The effects of phosphate depletion on carbohydrate pathways of the myocardium are given in Table 2. A decrease in glucose-6-phosphate concentration, which represents mainly glucose-6-phosphate, became evident at 8 weeks of phosphate depletion (1.5 ± 0.33 μmoles/g versus 3.8 ± 0.6 μmoles/g protein), and it remained low thereafter ($P < 0.01$). Glycogen content was also significantly reduced both at 8 weeks (22.0 ± 2.9 μg/mg versus 61.6 ± 1.8 μg/mg protein, $P < 0.01$) and at 12 weeks ($32.0 < 3.1$ μg/mg versus 63.0 ± 4.4 μg/mg protein, $P < 0.05$) of phosphate depletion. There was a highly significant correlation between cellular inorganic phosphorus and glucose-6-phosphate content ($P < 0.01$).

Table 2. Effects of phosphate depletion on myocardial cellular phospholipid metabolism and carbohydrate pathways[a]

	Glycerol P (μmole/g protein)	Glucose 6-P (μmole/g protein)	Glycogen (μg/mg protein)	CTP (nmol/g protein)
NP 4 wk	325.0 ± 36.0	5.0 ± 0.9	62.0 ± 9.0	330 ± 40
LP 4 wk	270.0 ± 46.0[c]	5.2 ± 0.5	—	340 ± 23
8 to 12 wk NP	405.0 ± 51.0	3.8 ± 0.6	62.2 ± 3.1	403 ± 41
8 to 12 wk LP	119.0 ± 12.0[b]	1.35 ± 0.2[b]	27.0 ± 3.0[b]	288 ± 31[b]

[a] Results are expressed as mean ± SEM of 8 to 12 rats.

[b] $P < 0.01$.

[c] $P < 0.05$.

NP, normal phosphate diet; LP, low-phosphate diet; Glycerol P, glycerol phosphate; Glucose 6-P, glucose-6-phosphate; and CTP, cytidine triphosphate.

Biochemical Integrity of Cellular Membrane-Phospholipid Synthesis and Fatty Acid Oxidation

The changes in acid-extractable phospholipid precursors are shown in Figure 3. At 4 weeks, the levels of glycerol phosphoethanolamine and glycerol phosphocholine (1.5 ± 0.33 μmoles/g protein) were significantly ($P < 0.01$) lower than in control rats (2.6 ± 0.130 μmoles/g protein), and they remained low at 8 and 12 weeks. By contrast, the levels of phosphocholine and phosphoethanolamine were reduced only at 4 weeks (1.1 ± 0.06 μmole/g versus 2.0 ± 0.21 μmole/g protein). There was a marked fall in the concentration of cytidine triphosphate and glycerol phosphate in phosphate depletion (Table 2). The changes in glycerol phosphate were highly correlated with the changes in cellular inorganic phosphorus.

After 8 to 12 weeks of phosphate depletion, there was a significant fall

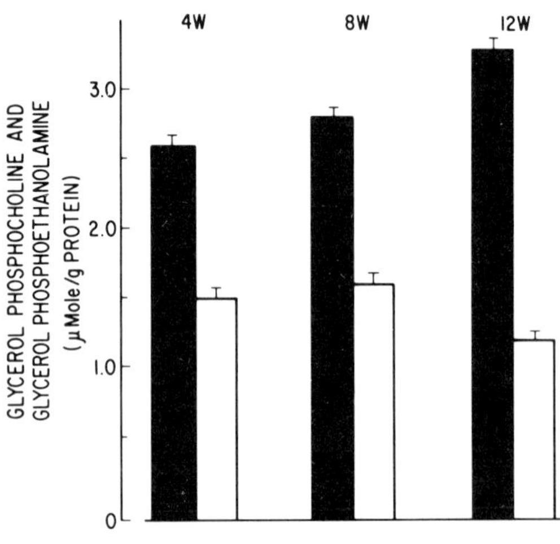

Fig. 3. Changes in acid-extractable, water-soluble phospholipids (glycerol phosphocholine and glycerol phosphoethanolamine) in phosphate-depleted (*open bars*) and control rats (*closed bars*), during 4, 8, and 12 wk of phosphate depletion. Results represent the mean ± SEM of six to eight rats.

in the content of phosphatidylcholine from $57.2 \pm 1.6\%$ to $29.3 \pm 4.1\%$ phospholipid phosphorus $(P < 0.01)$, and phosphatidylethanolamine from $39.2 \pm 3.0\%$ to $24.0 \pm 4.0\%$ phospholipid phosphorus $(P < 0.05)$. The ratio of phosphatidylcholine to phosphatidylethanolamine was significantly altered with phosphate depletion from 1.58 ± 0.05 to 1.25 ± 0.09 $(P < 0.01)$. No changes were observed in phosphatidylinositol and diphosphatidylglycerol. There was also a significant fall in total phospholipid phosphorus from 8700 ± 680 nmoles/g to 5900 ± 570 nmoles/g protein $(P < 0.01)$.

Mitochondrial oxidation of long-chain fatty acids was markedly reduced in 8 to 12 weeks of phosphate depletion. Mitochondria from phosphate-depleted rats demonstrated a marked reduction in the ability to oxidize long-chain-activated fatty acids $(89.7 \pm 11.3$ versus 37.2 ± 4.1 nmoles O_2/mg protein/min, $P < 0.01)$. Respiratory control rate and ADP:O ratios were not different, indicating intact-coupled mitochondria.

To further evaluate whether the impaired fatty acid oxidation is the result of reduced mitochondrial acetylcarnitine transferase activity, we examined short-chain fatty acid oxidation. There was a marked reduction in the ability of mitochondria from phosphate-depleted rats to oxidize short-chain fatty acids as well $(38.35 \pm 2.11$ versus 9.30 ± 3.12 nmoles O_2/mg protein/min, $P < 0.01)$.

Discussion

The results of our study show that dietary phosphate restriction is associated with impairments in myocardial cellular bioenergetics, aerobic and anaerobic energy metabolism, and the biochemical integrity of the cellular membrane.

There were reductions in the cellular concentrations of inorganic phosphorus, ATP and adenosine diphosphate, acid-extractable phospholipid precursors, hexose-6-phosphate, and glycogen. In addition, the concentrations of creatine and creatine phosphate and the activity of mitochondrial myofibrillar and total extractable creatine phosphokinase were also reduced.

The decrease in the concentration of inorganic phosphorus of the myocardium is (at least partly) due to the marked fall in the concentration of inorganic phosphorus in serum; indeed, there was a direct and significant correlation between these two parameters. The demonstration in our study that creatine phosphate of the rat myocardium is reduced during phosphate depletion indicates that the transfer of energy from the mitochondria to the contractile apparatus (the creatine phosphate energy shuttle) is impaired.

The changes in cellular inorganic phosphorus may influence the cell via several mechanisms.

Phosphorylation State of the Cell-ATP

The supply of inorganic phosphorus in the cytosol plays a major regulatory role in mitochondrial respiration, glycolysis, and oxidative ATP synthesis.

The relationship between energy-supplying and energy-using processes in the intact cell is the net energy state of the cell; it is represented by the phosphorylation potential, which is the ratio of cytosolic $ATP/ADP \times P_i$. From this equation, it is clear that any condition that will increase the ratio will signal the mitochondria, and also will slow respiration and oxidative phosphorylation. Indeed, the phosphorylation potential in the phosphate-depleted rats was markedly elevated; mitochondrial respiration and oxygen consumption were reduced. Therefore, it is possible to suggest a mechanism by which the extremely sensitive phosphorylation potential is immediately altered by the changes in cytosolic-inorganic phosphorus.

Adenine Nucleotide Pool—Adenosine Monophosphate Deaminase Deinhibition

Cytosolic-inorganic phosphorus content is an important regulator of the overall adenine nucleotide pool size. A marked reduction in intracellular phosphorus content results in accelerated degradation of adenosine monophosphate via the deinhibition of adenosine monophosphate deaminase, and (in turn) a reduction in the total adenine nucleotide pool. This mechanism may play a role in cell injury, only in situations where hypophosphatemia develops rapidly, and where there is intracellular "trapping" of free inorganic phosphorus, such as acute hyperalimentation or fructose administration. Indeed, our data do not support such a mechanism, since adenosine monophosphate and IMP levels in phosphate depletion were not different from those of normal controls.

The decrease in the concentration of creatine phosphate occurred after 8 weeks of phosphate depletion; it was preceded by reduced activity of mitochondrial creatine phosphokinase. These observations suggest that the alteration in the activity of this enzyme is (at least partly) responsible for the reduction in the content of creatine phosphate.

The activity of mitochondrial creatine phosphokinase, as well as that of the myofibrils, was markedly reduced. Thus, it appears that phosphate depletion affects the activity of these isoenzymes present at various locations in the myocardial cells. The decrease in intracellular concentration of inorganic phosphorus could be a critical factor that regulates the activity of the enzyme, either via enzyme synthesis or its phosphorylation. Therefore, a decrease in intracellular concentration of inorganic phosphorus could result in reduced activity of the enzyme. Indeed, the changes in cellular creatine phosphokinase activity were correlated with the reduction in serum phosphorus levels. This— and the observation that creatine phosphate levels were correlated with the myocardial-inorganic phosphorus—suggest that inorganic phosphorus may regulate creatine phosphokinase activity. The reduction in the activity of the creatine phosphokinase isoenzymes may play a critical role in the cardiomyopathy of phosphate depletion.

The fall in glucose-6-phosphate concentration and the reduced levels of glycogen are compatible with reduced glycolysis, glucose phosphorylation, and reduced glycogen synthesis. Indeed, decreased glucose uptake, as well as insulin resistance, have been reported in both hypophosphatemic patients [13] and rats [14]. Increased glucose-6-phosphate use also could be present and could contribute to its reduced cellular content. Our data do not support or refute this possibility. However, the metabolic pathway of glucose-6-phosphate is facilitated by phosphofructokinase. This enzyme is sensitive to the cellular concentration of inorganic phosphorus, and it is inhibited when the latter is low. It is reasonable to suggest that in phosphate depletion, the activity of this enzyme is reduced; therefore, increased use of glucose-6-phosphate does not occur.

The reduced cellular levels of glycogen are consistent with impaired glucose phosphorylation and glycogen synthesis; however, the possibility of increased glycogen breakdown cannot be ruled out. Indeed, Horl et al [15] have reported both decreased glycogen synthesis and increased glycogen breakdown in the myocardium of phosphate-depleted rabbits.

Most of the energy for myocardial contraction is derived from the oxidation of fatty acids. The finding of reduced oxidation of both long- and short-chain fatty acids suggests the presence of impairments at various steps of the mitochondrial processes that are responsible for the oxidation of fatty acids. The transport and oxidation of long-chain fatty acids requires intact activity of acetylcarnitine transferase of the outer and inner mitochondrial membrane, adequate carnitine content, and sufficient acetyl-CoA [16, 17]. Therefore, a defect in any of these steps could account for the reduced oxidation of long-chain fatty acids. By contrast, short-chain fatty acids enter mitochondria freely and independently of the activity of the acetylcarnitine transferase or carnitine [17]. Therefore, impaired oxidation of short-chain fatty acids should indicate depletion of acetyl-CoA. The observation that CoA synthesis requires ATP for its synthesis—and that the levels of the latter are reduced in phosphate depletion—is compatible with the notion of an intra-mitochondrial impairment in fatty acid oxidation. Such a derangement also could be responsible for the impaired oxidation of the long-chain fatty acids.

Several lines of evidence suggest an abnormality of cell membrane integrity in phosphate depletion. The derangement in cell membrane integrity may be due to abnormalities in phospholipid biosynthesis. Indeed, findings of reduced phosphatidylcholine (PC), phosphatidylethanolamine (PE), and total phospholipid phosphorus in the myocardium of phosphate-depleted rats demonstrate impaired biochemical integrity of the cell membrane. Furthermore, the observation of altered ratios of PC:PE is compatible with altered membrane phospholipid abnormality and possibly with function.

Since all of the abnormalities described in our study were preceded by a fall in cellular-inorganic phosphorus and creatine phosphokinase isoenzymes, we propose the following cellular mechanism for mediating the skeletal myopathy of phosphate depletion (Fig. 4).

Prolonged hypophosphatemia causes a reduction in intracellular-inorganic phosphorus stores; this, in turn, reduces the activity of the creatine phosphokinase isoenzymes. Since creatine phosphokinase plays a major regulatory role in mitochondrial respiration, energy transport, and myofibrillar energy use,

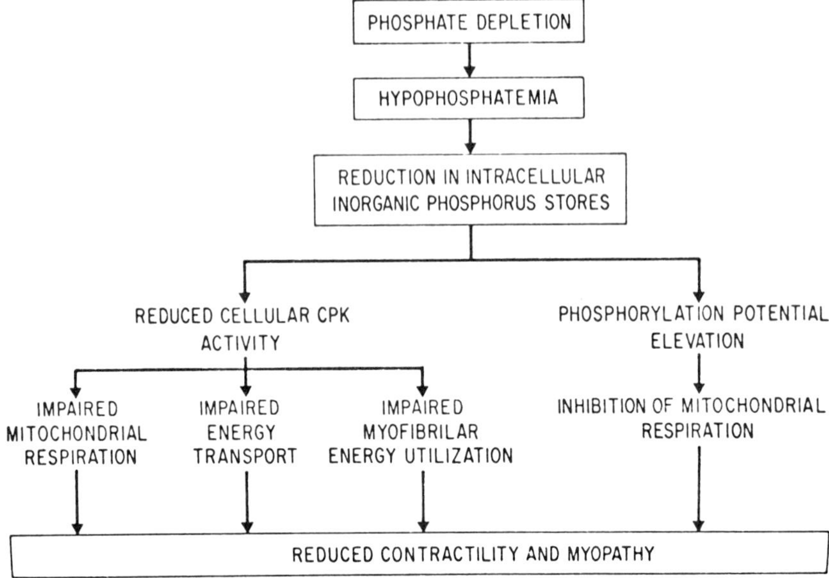

Fig. 4. Proposed chain of events leading to both intracellular phosphorus store depletion and cellular injury in phosphate depletion.

phosphate depletion would result in impairment of all these steps. The reduction in creatine phosphokinase activity also impairs phospholipid synthesis; and, in turn, cellular membrane functional integrity will be impaired.

Since phosphate depletion is not an isolated metabolic abnormality and is associated with hypomagnesemia and hypercalcemia, it is not possible to rule out some effects of intracellular magnesium depletion or calcium overload, in addition to the reduction of intracellular-inorganic phosphorus stores.

References

1. LICHTMAN MA, MILLDER DR, et al: Reduced red cell glycolysis, 2,3-diphosphoglycerate and adenosine triphosphate concentration, and increased hemoglobin oxygen affinity caused by hypophosphatemia. *Ann Intern Med* 74:562–568, 1971
2. JACOB HS, YAWATA Y, et al: Hyperalimentation hypophosphatemia: Hematologic-neurologic dysfunction due to ATP depletion. *Trans Assoc Am Phys* 86:143–153, 1973
3. BUNN HF, JANDL JH: Control of hemoglobin function within the red cell. *N Engl J Med* 282:1414–1421, 1970
4. FULLER TJ, CARTER NW, et al: Reversible changes of the muscle cell in experimental phosphorus deficiency. *J Clin Invest* 57:1019–1024, 1976
5. O'CONNOR LR, WHELLER WS, BETHUNE JE: Effect of hypophosphatemia on myocardial performance in men. *N Engl J Med* 294:901–904, 1977
6. FULLER TJ, NICHOLS WW, BRENNER BJ, PETERSON JC: Reversible depression

in myocardial performance in dogs with experimental phosphorus deficiency. *J Clin Invest* 62:1194–1200, 1978

7. BRAUTBAR N, BACZYNSKI R, CARPENTER C, MOSER S, GEIGER P, FINANDER P, MASSRY SG: Impaired energy metabolism in rat myocardium during phosphate depletion. *Am J Physiol* 242:F669–F704, 1982

8. BRAUTBAR N, CARPENTER C, BACZYNSKI R, KOHEN R, MASSRY S: Impaired energy metabolism in skeletal muscle during phosphate depletion. *Kidney Int* 24:53–57, 1983

9. BRAUTBAR N, TABERNERO-ROMO J, COATS J, MASSRY S: Effects of phosphate depletion on lipid metabolism. *Kidney Int* 26:18–23, 1984

10. BESSMAN S, GEIGER PJ: Transport of energy in muscle: the phosphoryl creatine shuttle. *Science* 211:448–452, 1981

11. SAKS V, LIPIN N, SHARNOV V, CHAGOV E: The localization of the MM isoenzyme of creatine kinase on the surface membrane of myocardial cells and its functional coupling to ouabain inhibited (Na,K) ATPase. *Biochim Biophys Acta* 465:550–558, 1977

12. BESSMAN S, GEIGER P, YANG WC, ERICKSON-VIITANEN S: Intimate coupling of creatine phosphokinase and myofibrillar adenosinetriphosphatase. *Biochem Biophys Res Comm* 96(31):1414–1420, 1980

13. DEFRONZO RA, LANG R: Hypophosphatemia and glucose intolerance: Evidence for tissue insensitivity to insulin. *N Engl J Med* 303:1259–1263, 1980

14. DAVIS JL, LEWIS SB, SCHULTZ TA, KAPLAN RA, WALLIN JD: Acute and chronic phosphate depletion as a modulator of glucose uptake in rat skeletal muscle. *Life Sci* 24:629–632, 1979

15. HORL WH, KREUSSER W, HEIDLAND A, RITZ E: Abnormalities of glycogen metabolism in cardiomyopathy of phosphorus depletion, in *Phosphate and Minerals in Health and Disease,* edited by MASSRY SG, RITZ E, JAHN H, New York, Plenum Press, 1980, pp 343–350

16. HOPPEL CL: Carnitine palmityl transferase and transport of fatty acids, in *The Enzymes of Biological Membranes* (vol 2), edited by MARTONOSI A, New York, Plenum Press, 1976, pp 119–143

17. BRASS EP, HOPPEL CL: Carnitine metabolism in the fasting rat. *J Biol Chem* 253:2688–2693, 1978

18. MAHLER M: Progressive loss of mitochondrial creatine phosphokinase activity in muscular dystrophy. *Biochem Biophys Res Comm* 88:895–906, 1979

Pathogenesis and Consequences of Chronic Renal Failure

Mechanisms of Progression of Renal Disease

Barry M. Brenner and Timothy W. Meyer

It is now clear that in addition to the extent and severity of the primary renal disease, a number of other factors may also influence the rate of progression to end-stage renal failure. Poorly controlled hypertension, urinary tract infection, obstruction, and intrarenal deposition of calcium and urate salts all are well-known examples. More often, however, disorders associated with mild, but permanent, nephron injury progress even when these commonly sought risk factors are excluded—as evidenced by inexorable and near-linear declines in time plots of glomerular filtration rate (GFR) or reciprocal serum creatinine concentration [1, 2]. These observations suggest that after a certain point, reduction in the functioning nephron number leads to failure of the remaining units. Hope of interrupting this process has stimulated investigation into the mechanism(s) responsible for injury to functioning nephrons in kidneys damaged by disease. Recent experimental evidence suggests that progressive loss of these residual nephron units may be a predictable consequence of the glomerular hemodynamic response to widespread renal injury.

Glomerular Hyperperfusion and the Progression of Experimental Renal Disease

The most simple model of reduced nephron number is provided by surgical nephrectomy. As is well known, a reduction of renal mass induces an increase in the single-nephron glomerular filtration rate (SNGFR) of remnant nephrons [3]. Vascular resistance is reduced in both afferent and efferent arterioles, thus allowing an increase in single-nephron glomerular plasma flow rate [4]. Furthermore, the reduction in afferent arteriolar resistance is proportionately greater than the reduction in efferent arteriolar resistance, so that the average glomerular transcapillary hydraulic pressure gradient is increased. Together,

This manuscript was presented as a State-of-the-Art lecture of the same title.

the increases in capillary plasma flow and hydraulic pressure account for the elevation in GFR of remnant nephrons. The magnitude of the increase in remnant nephron GFR, and of the underlying reductions in arteriolar resistance, correlates closely with the amount of renal mass that has been ablated. Thus, in the rat, removal of 80% of the renal mass results in an increase in remnant nephron GFR to more than twice that of normal, while the increment averages 40 to 50% with uninephrectomy [4].

Increased filtration by remnant nephrons generally has been regarded as "adaptive," since it partially offsets the loss of function that would otherwise follow nephrectomy. However, a growing body of evidence suggests that the hemodynamic changes that cause remnant nephron hyperfiltration eventually prove injurious to residual glomeruli. Chanutin and Ferris [5], 50 years ago, showed that removal of three-fourths of the renal mass in rats led to a syndrome of proteinuria and to progressive glomerular sclerosis, ultimately resulting in uremic death. Shimamura and Morrison [6] profiled the development of pathologic changes in initially normal remnant glomeruli following an approximately 85% renal ablation. Early glomerular hypertrophy was accompanied at 3 months by ultrastructural changes, including vacuolization of epithelial cells and "fusion" of epithelial cell foot processes. At 6 months, there was notable expansion of the mesangium, along with focal areas of denudation of endothelial and epithelial cells from the glomerular basement membrane (GBM). Progressive mesangial expansion and collapse of capillary lumina eventually resulted in the appearance of focal and segmental glomerular sclerosis.

Focal sclerosing lesions of remnant glomeruli are typically segmental in their early phase. With time, the prevalence of sclerotic lesions increases, and global sclerosis is observed. In rats, the pace of injury to remnant glomeruli, like the magnitude of remnant glomerular hemodynamic changes, increases in proportion to the loss of renal mass [6–8]. Uninephrectomy, which results in a modest increase in glomerular capillary hydraulic pressure and a 40 to 50% increase in glomerular capillary plasma flow rate, is associated with moderate acceleration of the glomerular sclerosis normally seen in aging rats with two kidneys [9]. However, following a 90 to 95% nephrectomy, increases in glomerular capillary pressures and flows are more dramatic; and, glomerular morphologic changes can be detected within 2 weeks of the ablation procedure [8].

Evidence that increased capillary pressures and flows initiate glomerular injury has been obtained from these studies of extensive renal ablation. Severe restriction of dietary protein intake, which lowers GFR in intact animals [10], was used to blunt adaptive hyperfiltration following reduction of renal mass [8]. In animals fed a 6% protein diet, capillary flows and pressures were maintained at/or near normal values following renal ablation; therefore, the average value of the SNGFR in the remnant kidney was restricted to 38 ± 6 nl/min. This was markedly lower than the average SNGFR of 62 ± 6 nl/min found in rats that had undergone a similar degree of ablation, but had been fed standard laboratory chow containing 24% protein. Limitation of glomerular hyperfiltration and prevention of glomerular capillary hypertension and hyperperfusion by protein restriction were associated with preservation of glomerular structure. Within 2 weeks following ablation, remnant kidneys of animals fed standard chow showed protein reabsorption droplets in glomerular epithelial cells, attenuation of epithelial cell bodies, and focal fusion of foot processes. These epithelial cell changes were associated with lifting of endothelial cells from the inner aspect of the GBM and with increases in mesangial area. Glomerular morphologic abnormalities were much less extensive in remnant kidneys of protein-restricted rats. In addition, proteinuria was limited in protein-restricted rats, which suggests preservation of the glomerular permselectivity barrier. More recent studies have shown that dietary protein restriction also lowers remnant kidney GFR and retards development of proteinuria and glomerular sclerosis in rats subjected to less extensive renal ablation [11–13]. The beneficial effects of protein restriction have been demonstrated not only in these functional and morphologic studies, but in other studies showing that reduction of protein intake increases the lifespan of rats subjected to renal ablation [14].

Increased glomerular pressures and flows have been observed not only following surgical nephrectomy, but in various experimental models of diffuse renal disease [15]. The ability of remnant glomeruli during injury to respond to reductions in renal mass was initially demonstrated in animals with unilateral renal disease. Removal of the normal kidney promptly induced hyperfiltration in residual functioning nephrons of the diseased kidney [16]. Hyperfiltration has since been shown to occur when the number of functioning nephrons is reduced by advancing disease, rather than by nephrectomy. As with hyperfunctioning glomeruli of remnant kidneys, hyperperfused residual glomeruli of diseased kidneys presumably may be damaged by increased capillary pressures and flows. Support for this concept has been provided by Azar et al [17, 18], who demonstrated that premature glomerular sclerosis is associated with elevated glomerular capillary pressures and flows in "post-salt" hypertensive rats. An association between glomerular capillary hypertension and hyperperfusion and glomerular pathology also has been established in "DOCA-salt" hypertensive rats by Dworkin et al [19].

Studies of protein restriction in "DOCA-salt" hypertension appear to confirm the importance of glomerular hemodynamic changes in the initiation of glomerular pathology. In DOCA-salt-treated rats, as in rats subjected to extensive renal ablation, protein restriction lowers glomerular capillary pressures and flows, limits proteinuria, and lessens the extent of glomerular morphologic changes [19]. Variation of dietary protein content has not been studied extensively in other disease models, but protein restriction has been shown to retard both the progression of nephrotoxic serum nephritis in rats [20–22] and the lupus-like nephropathy of the NZB/NZW strain mouse [23]. While the effects of protein restriction could be due to suppression of immune responsiveness, other manipulations affecting the progression of experimental disease suggest the importance of altered glomerular hemodynamic parameters. Thus, uninephrectomy worsens histopathology and increases mortality in the NZB/NZW mouse [24] and in rabbits given nephrotoxic serum [25]. Presumably, an increase in capillary pressures and flows induced by nephrectomy accelerates glomerular destruction. Other maneuvers that increase glomerular capillary pressures and flows likewise magnify pathologic changes in experimental glomerular disease. Heymann nephritis can be aggravated by DOCA-salt treatment [26], while in Dahl rats, experimental immune complex disease becomes more severe when glomerular capillary hydraulic pressure is raised above control levels by salt-feeding [27]. Likewise, when a clip is placed round one renal artery ("two-kidney" Goldblatt hypertension), glomerular capillary pressures and flows are higher in the unclipped kidney than in the clipped kidney. As might be expected, when unilateral clip hypertension is superimposed on nephrotoxic serum nephritis, lesions are more severe in the unclipped kidney than in the clipped kidney [28].

The Progression of Human Renal Disease

Viewed together, the experimental studies described above suggest that increased glomerular capillary pressures and flows initiate glomerular injury when the nephron number is reduced; and, they accelerate glomerular injury following other insults to the kidney. Studies in humans, although necessarily less direct, also support the view that hyperperfused nephrons ultimately fail. Morphologic studies in human renal disease have demonstrated hypertrophy (presumably reflecting hyperperfusion and hyperfiltration) of those nephrons least damaged by disease [29]. Clinical studies have demonstrated a progressive loss of renal function that is associated with increasing glomerular sclerosis in patients whose initiating disease process has remitted spontaneously or has been controlled therapeutically. Patients with bilateral cortical necrosis may temporarily recover stable, although reduced, renal function before proceeding to end-stage renal failure [30]. Recovery of renal function frequently is incomplete in acute renal failure of other etiologies; and, in some of these cases, progressive loss of renal function also follows initial recovery [31]. Patients with vesicoureteric reflux who have developed significant impairment of renal function and glomerular disease manifested by proteinuria, may progress to renal failure despite control of systemic hypertension, prevention of urinary tract infection, and surgical correction of the reflux [32]. Likewise, patients with analgesic nephropathy (sometimes believed to exhibit stable renal insufficiency) often progress to renal failure despite discontinuation of analgesic medications [33]. Progressive glomerular sclerosis in the absence of continuing immunologic injury has been demonstrated in certain patients after initial recovery from acute poststreptococcal glomerulonephritis [34]. Moreover, in an analogy with animal experiments illustrating the effects of renal artery constriction on experimental nephritis, patients with coincident glomerulonephritis and renal artery stenosis have been shown to have less severe glomerulonephritic lesions in the hypofunctioning kidney that is "protected" by the arterial stenosis [35–37]. Hemodynamic factors also might explain the observation that pregnancy—which raises glomerular filtration and renal blood flow rates in normal women—frequently accelerates loss of renal function in women with pre-existing renal disease [38].

These studies are consistent with the hypothesis that progressive glomerular injury in humans is hemodynamically mediated (Table 1). A number of impor-

Table 1. Possible hemodynamic glomerulopathies in humans

Oligomeganephronia	Poorly controlled hypertension
Unilateral agenesis/segmental hypoplasia	Diabetes mellitus
Loss of renal mass (parenchymal injury, surgery, cortical necrosis)	Sickle cell disease
	Familial dysautonomia

tant clinical questions are suggested by this hypothesis. First, how much renal mass must be lost in humans to induce progressive glomerular disease in the absence of ongoing renal injury? An increased incidence of focal and segmental glomerular sclerosis has been reported in patients with unilateral renal agenesis [39, 40]; however, it is possible that the solitary kidneys of these patients are congenitally abnormal, like the kidneys of patients with bilateral reduction in nephron number (oligomegonephronia [41]). Recent reports of patients who were followed from 10 to 20 years after nephrectomy for transplant donation suggest an increased incidence of mild hypertension and proteinuria, but no major reduction in the GFR during this time period [42, 43]. Longer term follow-up studies of patients who have had one kidney removed for trauma or localized tumor, and of patients who have had uninephrectomy and partial resection of the other kidney for bilateral tumor, are required to establish the consequences of reducing the nephron number in humans. There is reason to believe that the renal graft recipient may also be at risk for hemodynamically mediated renal injury. Two reports have appeared that describe the delayed occurrence of de novo focal and segmental glomerular sclerosis in recipients of grafts from monozygotic twins—circumstances in which immunologically mediated "chronic rejection" can be ruled out with certainty [44, 45]. Therefore, whether similar events contribute to delayed loss of renal function in allograft recipients must be explored, especially since glucocorticoid therapy—by enhancing renal vasodilation—may increase the tendency toward hemodynamically mediated glomerulopathy in these patients.

A second question is whether increased glomerular capillary pressures and flows can initiate progressive glomerular disease when the number of functioning nephrons is normal. Normal subjects show a progressive decline in glomerular filtration and renal blood flow rates after the third decade; values in the eighth decade are only one-half to two-thirds of those measured in young adults [46, 47]. Progressive loss of renal function with aging is associated with sclerosis of an increasing portion of the total glomerular population [48]. We have recently suggested that age-related glomerular sclerosis is caused by sustained elevations in glomerular capillary pressures and flows that are associated with current dietary practices; in particular, with ad libitum intake of protein-rich foods [49]. Certain disease processes may increase further the hemodynamic burden of an initially normal glomerular population. Patients with sickle cell anemia have markedly increased glomerular filtration and renal plasma flow rates during the first decade of life; but, by the third decade, renal function is reduced [50]. Sickle cell nephropathy usually is attributed to medullary and papillary ischemia, but glomerular sclerotic lesions occur often, accompanied by notable proteinuria [51]. We hypothesize that sustained glomerular hyperperfusion early in life contributes to later development of glomerular pathology. The GFR also is increased in juvenile-onset diabetic patients at the time of diagnosis and throughout the first decade of the disease [52]. Equivalent hyperfiltration in rats with experimental diabetes has been shown to be due to elevations in glomerular capillary pressures and flows similar to those seen in the remnant kidney [53]. These observations have prompted the suggestion that glomerular hyperperfusion in diabetes initiates a cycle of glomerular injury that causes exaggerated glomerular hemodynamic changes and leads, in turn, to accelerated glomerular destruction [54]. Why renal failure ultimately develops in only about one-half of juvenile diabetic patients is unknown; studies remain to be performed correlating the magnitude of early hyperfiltration in juvenile diabetic subjects with later development of diabetic nephropathy. Early glomerular sclerosis in familial dysautonomia, occasionally severe enough to cause renal insufficiency, likewise could be related to glomerular hemodynamic abnormalities in this disorder [55].

A third question concerns the role of hyperperfusion of individual glomerular capillary loops in progressive glomerular disease. Hyperperfusion of capillary segments may occur not only when perfusion of structurally normal glomeruli is increased, but also when glomerular blood flow is channelled through a reduced number of capillary loops. A reduction in the number of glomerular capillary loops—so-called glomerular "simplification"—has been observed in DOCA-salt hypertension, and it may contribute to accelerated glomerular sclerosis in this condition [56]. Likewise, a reduction in the number of capillary channels could contribute to progressive glomerular sclerosis following recovery from acute glomerulonephritis. Ongoing glomerular damage reflected by proteinuria appears to occur in these patients when the total nephron number is reduced by less than 50%; that is, with a lesser reduction in the nephron number than would result from uninephrectomy [57]. However, the role of glomerular simplification in this process remains to be established.

Alternative Explanations of the Progressive Nature of Renal Disease

Factors other than glomerular capillary hypertension and hyperperfusion have been considered to account for progressive glomerular sclerosis, both following surgical nephrectomy and in diffuse renal disease (Table 2). Early investigators believed that systemic hypertension induced by renal ablation was responsible for pathologic changes in the remnant kidney [59]. However, subsequent studies showed that these glomerular sclerotic changes were poorly correlated with elevations in systemic blood pressure [58]. Moreover, while early glomerular sclerosis occurs in "postsalt" and "DOCA-salt" hypertensive rats, it is not prominent in spontaneously hypertensive rats (SHRs), which have equally elevated systemic pressures—but more normal glomerular capil-

Table 2. Risk factors for chronic renal failure

Persistent activity of underlying renal disease	Other factors promoting sustained elevations in glomerular pressures/flows
Commonly sought amplifiers	High-protein diet
Uncontrolled hypertension	Diabetes mellitus
Obstruction/reflux	Severe anemia
Infection	Chronic renal vasodilator therapy (for example, steroids)
Analgesics or other nephrotoxins	
Calcium or urate deposits	Pregnancy
Marked reduction in nephron number	Diastolic blood pressure > 70 mm Hg
	Persistent nephrotic-range proteinuria

lary pressures and flows [60]. Early proteinuria and sclerosis in this strain are confined to juxtamedullary glomeruli, which have higher filtration rates and presumably higher pressures and/or flows than those of the outer cortex [61, 62]. These studies suggest that systemic hypertension is associated with accelerated glomerular sclerosis only when transmitted to the glomerular capillary network. They further suggest that antihypertensive therapy directed toward lowering glomerular capillary pressure, as well as systemic blood pressure, should preserve renal function when the nephron number is reduced. This hypothesis is supported by the recent demonstration that treatment with an angiotensin I-converting enzyme inhibitor lowers arterial and glomerular capillary blood pressures and limits glomerular injury in rats following surgical ablation of a renal mass [63]. Less effective control of glomerular capillary hypertension may explain the observation of continuing glomerular injury, despite normalization of systemic blood pressure with a different antihypertensive regimen in a prior study of rats subjected to a similar degree of renal ablation [7].

Alfrey et al have suggested that deposition of calcium salts in the renal interstitium causes progressive loss of renal function in rats with remnant kidneys [64] or NSN [65]. This suggestion was supported by the demonstration that restriction of phosphorus intake preserved renal function, prolonged the lifespan, and reduced ultimate renal tissue calcium content in both groups. Excess calcification in animals maintained on normal chow, which was confined largely to the tubules and interstitium, was considered to be due to an increase in the calcium-phosphorus product, an increase in the single-nephron inorganic phosphate load, and/or an increase in the level of parathormone. However, later studies by this group revealed that parathyroid ablation does not protect against progressive loss of renal function in nephrotoxic serum nephritis [66]. Moreover, in these studies, marked interstitial pathology, proteinuria, and functional deterioration were shown to precede any increase in renal calcium content. Therefore, the efficacy of phosphate restriction in preventing these manifestations of progressive disease must not depend entirely on inhibition of intrarenal calcification. Moreover, rats with nephrotoxic serum nephritis that developed terminal uremia while maintained on standard phosphate intake, in one study, had elevations of kidney calcium content up to only three times that of normal; this suggests that the earlier finding of a 20-fold elevation in kidney calcium content, in remnant kidney animals maintained on standard phosphorus intake, was due largely to calcification of scar tissue [64, 65]. Finally, the degree of phosphate restriction that was shown to preserve renal function in rats with remnant kidneys or nephrotoxic serum nephritis was stringent enough both to reduce plasma phosphate levels below normal and to reduce kidney weight in the nephritic animals. Viewed together, these studies suggest that the well-documented protective effect of phosphate restriction may not have been related to prevention of intrarenal deposition of calcium salts, but to some other effect of phosphate deprivation—possibly including reduction of the GFR [67] or suppression of immune responsiveness.

The presence of immunoglobulins (particularly IgM) in diseased glomeruli of remnant kidneys has raised the possibility that an immune response directed against renal antigens could cause progressive loss of kidney function following renal ablation. However, immune complexes have not been noted in damaged glomeruli of remnant kidneys. Furthermore, when part of one kidney is infarcted and the contralateral kidney is left intact rather than excised, accelerated glomerular damage does not occur [7, 68].

It also has been recently suggested that progression of chronic renal disease may be mediated by abnormalities of lipid metabolism [69]. According to this view, levels of circulating lipids are increased in response to initial renal injury. Various lipid fractions, primarily low-density lipoproteins, are hypothesized to cause further progressive damage to the GBM and to mesangial structures. To the best of our knowledge, current evidence favoring the nephrotoxicity of circulating lipids is slim. Hyperlipidemia in early renal insufficiency is most clearly related to both nephrotic proteinuria and hypoalbuminemia. However, rates of decline in renal function are poorly related to rates of protein excretion. In patients without primary renal disease, hyperlipidemia is not usually associated with early loss of renal function, although a rare familial syndrome of lecithin:cholesterol acyltransferase deficiency—characterized by an abnormal low-density lipoprotein fraction and chronic anemia—does lead to renal failure in adults [70].

Therapies Aimed at Interrupting the Progression of Renal Disease

If elevated glomerular capillary pressures and flows cause progressive glomerular sclerosis in patients with renal insufficiency, therapies aimed at an initial reduction in glomerular perfusion may be required to preserve long-term renal function. An obvious possible therapy is restriction of dietary protein intake, which is implemented early in the course of intrinsic renal disease. Promising results have recently been presented suggesting that protein restriction indeed slows the progression of a variety of renal disorders [71–74]. Other therapies directed toward limiting glomerular capillary pressures and flows may ultimately prove to be more effective or more palatable than protein restriction. The mechanisms responsible for the reduction in afferent arteriolar resistance, which causes hyperfiltration when the nephron number is reduced, are as yet unknown. Elucidation of these mechanisms obviously is important to the design of therapeutic interventions aimed at preventing glomerular hyperperfusion and hyperfiltration.

It is conceivable that injury to hyperfiltering remnant glomeruli can be prevented by means other than reducing capillary pressures and flows. In this regard, it is worth considering how elevated pressures and flows damage the glomerulus. One possible mechanism is mechanical injury to the glomerular endothelium. Denudation of endothelial cells from the GBM has been noted following extensive renal ablation [8]. Endothelial damage, in turn, may result in exposure of circulating plasma proteins to basement membrane constituents, thereby precipitating intracapillary coagulation. Capillary thrombosis has been demonstrated in glomeruli of remnant kidneys following renal ablation in rats; and, heparin therapy has been shown to retard the progression of glomerular disease in this model [7, 75, 76]. Administration of drugs that inhibit thromboxane synthesis and impair platelet aggregation also has been shown to limit glomerular injury following renal ablation [77]. Of note, heparin and thromboxane synthesis inhibitors also appear to lower blood pressure in rats with remnant kidneys. Therefore, it is possible that the efficacy of these agents is due not only to their anticoagulant properties, but perhaps to some as yet undefined effects on intrarenal hemodynamics.

Increased capillary pressures and flows also may damage the glomerulus by promoting increased movement of macromolecules through the glomerular capillary wall and into the glomerular mesangium. Rats subjected to high-grade nephrectomy eventually excrete several hundred mg/d of protein, as compared to approximately 10 mg/d in control animals [5]. Studies employing tracer macromolecules have shown that proteinuria in remnant nephrons results from defects in both the charge- and size-selective properties of the glomerular capillary wall [78, 79]. It is not clear whether passage alone of macromolecules through the capillary wall and into the urinary space aggravates glomerular injury. However, damage to the filtration barrier has been associated with increased deposition of tracer macromolecules into the mesangium, both in the remnant kidney [79] and in other disease models [80]. An increase in mesangial "trafficking" of macromolecules, in turn, may promote increases in the mesangial matrix area and cellularity, leading eventually to glomerular sclerosis [80, 81].

A great deal clearly remains to be learned about the mechanisms responsible for progressive glomerular injury when the nephron number is reduced. Exciting, but as yet unexplained, recent findings include observations that increasing dietary intake of the prostaglandin precursor, linoleic acid, preserves renal function in remnant kidney rats [82], while inhibition of prostaglandin synthesis retards development of proteinuria and glomerular sclerosis in aging rats with intact kidneys [83]. It is hoped that further experimental studies relating both nutritional and pharmacologic maneuvers to glomerular function ultimately will enable us to prevent progressive loss of renal function in patients whose kidneys have been damaged by disease.

Summary

The adverse consequences of reduction in the nephron number have recently been the subject of intense study. Remnant nephrons of partially nephrectomized animals undergo an increase in single-nephron glomerular filtration rate (SNGFR), which is the result of increases in glomerular capillary plasma flow and hydraulic pressure. Maintenance of these hemodynamic alterations is associated with progressive sclerosis of remnant glomeruli. Glomerular injury also has been associated with increased capillary pressures and flows in rats with systemic hypertension and experimental diabetes. These observations suggest that intraglomerular hypertension and hyperperfusion cause progressive glomerular damage. In accord with this hypothesis, dietary protein restriction (which lowers glomerular capillary pressures and flows) has been shown to limit the harmful morphologic effects of renal ablation, nephrotoxic serum nephritis, diabetes mellitus, and systemic hypertension.

Studies in humans with a wide variety of renal disorders are consistent with the view that progressive glomerular destruction is mediated by local hemodynamic factors. Two broad categories of patients may be at risk from this proposed mechanism: those with chronic reduction in the number of functioning nephron units (for example, acquired primary renal disease, congenital renal hypoplasia, or surgical renal ablation) and those with primary renal vasodilation (for example, diabetes mellitus or sickle cell disease).

These experimental and clinical findings suggest that hemodynamically mediated glomerular injury may constitute a "final common pathway" with sufficient destructive potential to lead to end-stage renal failure, irrespective of the original cause of altered renal function. Accordingly, if this hypothesis is proven to be correct, it will necessitate that therapy for renal insufficiency be directed toward control of glomerular hypertension and hyperperfusion. One obvious therapeutic maneuver is to restrict protein intake early in the course of renal insufficiency. Clinical studies are also needed to evaluate the efficacy of strict glycemic control in diabetes patients and to assess the potential benefits of aggressive hypotensive therapy in patients with all forms of renal disease; the latter, to reduce diastolic blood pressure to levels below those now generally regarded as acceptable.

References

1. MITCH WE, WALSER M, BUFFINGTON GA, LEMANN J JR: A simple method for estimating progression of chronic renal failure. *Lancet* 2:1326–1328, 1976
2. RUTHERFORD WE, BLONDIN J, MILLER JP, GREENWALT AS, VAVRA JD: Chronic progressive renal disease: rate of change of serum creatinine. *Kidney Int* 11:62–70, 1977
3. HAYSLETT JP: Functional adaptation to reduction in renal mass. *Physiol Rev* 59:137–164, 1979
4. DEEN WM, MADDOX DA, ROBERTSON CR, BRENNER BM: Dynamics of glomerular ultrafiltration in the rat. VII. Response to reduced renal mass. *Am J Physiol* 227:556–562, 1974

5. CHANUTIN A, FERRIS EB: Experimental renal insufficiency produced by partial nephrectomy. I. Control diet. *Arch Intern Med* 49:767–787, 1932

6. SHIMAMURA T, MORRISON AB: A progressive glomerulosclerosis occurring in partial five-sixths nephrectomized rats. *Am J Pathol* 79:95–101, 1975

7. PURKERSON ML, HOFFSTEN PE, KLAHR S: Pathogenesis of the glomerulopathy associated with renal infarction in rats. *Kidney Int* 9:407–417, 1976

8. HOSTETTER TH, OLSON JL, RENNKE HG, VENKATACHALAM MA, BRENNER BM: Hyperfiltration in remnant nephrons: a potentially adverse response to renal ablation. *Am J Physiol* 241:F85–F93, 1981

9. STRIKER GE, NAGLE RB, KOHNEN PW, SMUCKLER EA: Response to unilateral nephrectomy in old rats. *Arch Pathol* 87:439–442, 1969

10. ICHIKAWA I, PURKERSON ML, KLAHR S, TROY JL, MARTINEZ-MALDONADO M, BRENNER BM: Mechanism of reduced glomerular filtration rate in chronic malnutrition. *J Clin Invest* 65:982–988, 1980

11. MEYER TW, HOSTETTER TH, RENNKE HG, NODDIN JL, BRENNER BM: Preservation of renal structure and function by long term protein restriction in rats with reduced nephron mass (*abstract*). *Kidney Int* 23:218, 1983

12. MADDEN MA, ZIMMERMAN SW: Protein restriction and renal function in the uremic rat (*abstract*). *Kidney Int* 23:217, 1983

13. EL-NAHAS AM, PARASKEVAKOU H, ZOOB S, REES AJ, EVANS DJ: Effect of dietary protein restriction on the development of renal failure after subtotal nephrectomy in rats. *Clin Sci* 65:399–406, 1983

14. KLEINKNECHT C, SALUSKY I, BROYER M, GUBLER M-C: Effect of various protein diets on growth, renal function, and survival of uremic rats. *Kidney Int* 15:534–541, 1979

15. HOSTETTER TH, BRENNER BM: Glomerular adaptations to renal injury, in *Contemporary Issues in Nephrology: Chronic Renal Failure* (vol 7), edited by BRENNER BM, STEIN JH, New York, Churchill Livingstone, 1981, pp 1–27

16. LUBOWITZ H, PURKERSON ML, SUGITA M, BRICKER NS: GFR per nephron and per kidney in chronically diseased (pyelonephritic) kidney of the rat. *Am J Physiol* 217:853–857, 1969

17. AZAR S, JOHNSON MA, HERTEL B, TOBIAN L: Single-nephron pressures, flows and resistances in hypertensive kidneys with nephrosclerosis. *Kidney Int* 12:28–40, 1977

18. AZAR S, JOHNSON MA, IWAI J, BRUNO L, TOBIAN L: Single-nephron dynamics in "post-salt" rats with chronic hypertension. *J Lab Clin Med* 91:156–166, 1978

19. DWORKIN LD, HOSTETTER TH, RENNKE HG, BRENNER BM: Hemodynamic basis for glomerular injury in rats with mineralocorticoid-induced hypertension. *J Clin Invest* in press

20. FARR LE, SMADEL JE: The effect of dietary protein on the course of nephrotoxic nephritis in rats. *J Exp Med* 70:615–627, 1939

21. NEUGARTEN J, FEINER HD, SCHACHT RG, BALDWIN DS: Amelioration of experimental glomerulonephritis by dietary protein restriction. *Kidney Int* 24:595–601, 1983

22. EL-NAHAS AM, ZOOB S, EVANS DJ, REES AJ: Modification of the course of nephrotoxic nephritis by diet (*abstract*). *Kidney Int* 22:219, 1982

23. FRIEND PS, FERNANDES G, GOOD RA, MICHAEL AF, YUNIS EJ: Dietary restrictions early and late: effects on the nephropathy of the NZB/NZW mouse. *Lab Invest* 38:629–632, 1978

24. BEYER MM, STEINBERG AD, NICASTRI AD, FRIEDMAN EA: Unilateral nephrectomy: effect on survival in NZB/NZW mice. *Science* 198:511–513, 1977

25. TEODURU CV, SAIFER A, FRANKEL H: Conditioning factors influencing evolution of experimental glomerulonephritis in rabbits. *Am J Physiol* 196:457–460, 1959

26. TIKKANEN I, FYHRQUIST F, MIETTINEN A, TÖRNROTH T: Autologous immune complex nephritis and DOCA-NaCl load: a new model of hypertension. *Acta Path Microbiol Scand* 88:241–250, 1980

27. RAIJ L, AZAR S, KEANE WF: Role of hypertension and mesangial injury in progressive glomerular damage (*abstract*). *Proc Am Soc Nephrol* 15:126A, 1982

28. NEUGARTEN J, FEINER HD, SCHACHT RG, GALLO GR, BALDWIN DS: Aggravation of experimental glomerulonephritis by superimposed clip hypertension. *Kidney Int* 22:257–263, 1982

29. GOTTSCHALK CW: Function of the chronically diseased kidney: The adaptive nephron. *Circ Res* 28(Suppl 1):1–13, 1971

30. KLEINKNECHT D, GRÜNFELD J-P, GOMEZ PC, MOREAU J-F, GARCIA-TORRES R: Diagnostic procedures and long-term prognosis in bilateral renal cortical necrosis. *Kidney Int* 4:390–400, 1973

31. FINN WF: Recovery from acute renal failure, in *Acute Renal Failure,* edited by BRENNER BM, LAZARUS JM, Philadelphia, WB Saunders & Co, 1983

32. TORRES VE, VELOSA JA, HOLLEY KE, KELALIS PP, STICKLER GB, KURTZ SB: The progression of vesicoureteral reflux. *Ann Intern Med* 92:776–784, 1980

33. KINCAID-SMITH P: Analgesic abuse and the kidney. *Kidney Int* 17:250–260, 1980

34. BALDWIN DA: Poststreptococcal glomerulonephritis: a progressive disease? *Am J Med* 62:1–11, 1977

35. PALMER JH, EVERSOLE SL, STAMEY TA: Unilateral glomerulonephritis. *Am J Med* 40:816–822, 1966

36. DIKMAN SH, STRAUSS L, BERMAN LJ, TAYLOR NS, CHURG J: Unilateral glomerulonephritis. *Arch Pathol Lab Med* 100:480–483, 1976

37. GODIN M, FILLASTRE J-P, DUCASTELLE T, HEMET J, MORERE P, NOUVET G: Sarcoidosis: retroperitoneal fibrosis, renal artery involvement, and unilateral focal glomerulosclerosis. *Arch Intern Med* 140:1240–1242, 1980

38. KINCAID-SMITH P: *The Kidney, a Clinico-Pathological Study.* Oxford, Blackwell Scientific Publications, 1975, pp 222–239

39. KIPROV DD, COLVIN RB, MCCLUSKEY RT: Focal and segmental glomerulosclerosis and proteinuria associated with unilateral renal agenesis. *Lab Invest* 46:275–281, 1982

40. BAUMELOW A, MEHAMHA H, CHATELAIN C, LEGRAIN M: Aspects cliniques du syndrome dit de reduction nephronique. *Seminaires d'Uronephrologie* 10:94–109, 1984

41. ELEMA JD: Is one kidney sufficient (*abstract*)? *Kidney Int* 9:308, 1976

42. HAKIM RM, GOLDSZER RC, BRENNER BM: Hypertension and proteinuria: Long term sequelae of uninephrectomy in humans. *Kidney Int* 25:930–936, 1984

43. DELANO BG, LAZAR IL, FRIEDMAN EA: Hypertension, a late consequence of kidney donation (*abstract*). *Kidney Int* 23:168, 1983

44. DAMMIN GJ: Transplantation in the 1950s. *Transpl Proc* 13:16–23, 1981

45. RIVOLTA E, PONTICELLI C, IMBASCIATI E, VEGETO A: De novo focal glomerular sclerosis in an identical twin renal transplant recipient. *Transplantation* 35:328–331, 1983

46. DAVIES DF, SHOCK NW: Age changes in glomerular filtration rate, effective renal plasma flow, and tubular excretory capacity in adult males. *J Clin Invest* 29:496–507, 1950

47. ROWE JW, ANDRES R, TOBIN JD, NORRIS AH, SHOCK NW: The effect of age on creatinine clearance in man: a cross sectional and longitudinal study. *J Gerontol* 31:155–163, 1976

48. KAPPEL B, OLSEN S: Cortical interstitial tissue and sclerosed glomeruli in the normal human kidney, related to age and sex. *Virchows Arch (Pathol Anat)* 387:271–277, 1980

49. BRENNER BM, MEYER TW, HOSTETTER TH: Dietary protein intake and the progressive nature of kidney disease. *N Engl J Med* 307:652–659, 1982

50. ETTELDORF JN, SMITH JS, TUTTLE AH, DIGGS LW: Renal hemodynamic studies in adults with sickle cell anemia. *Am J Med* 18:243–248, 1955

51. ALFREY AC: The renal response to vascular injury, in *The Kidney* (2nd ed), edited by BRENNER BM, RECTOR FC JR, Philadelphia, WB Saunders & Co, 1981, pp 1668–1718

52. MOGENSEN CE: Renal function changes in diabetes. *Diabetes* 25:872–879, 1976

53. HOSTETTER TH, TROY JL, BRENNER BM: Glomerular hemodynamics in experimental diabetes. *Kidney Int* 19:410–415, 1981

54. HOSTETTER TH, RENNKE GH, BRENNER BM: The case for intrarenal hypertension in the initiation and progression of diabetic and other glomerulopathies. *Am J Med* 72:375–380, 1982

55. PEARSON J, GALLO G, GLUCK M, AXELROD F: Renal disease in familial dysautonomia. *Kidney Int* 17:102–112, 1980

56. HILL GS, HEPTINSTALL RH: Steroid-induced hypertension in the rat. *Am J Pathol* 52:1–23, 1968

57. GALLO GR, FEINER HD, STEELE JM, SCHACHT RG, GLUCK MC, BALDWIN DS: Role of intrarenal vascular sclerosis in progression of poststreptococcal glomerulonephritis. *Clin Nephrol* 13:49–57, 1980

58. WOOD JE JR, ETHRIDGE C: Hypertension with arteriolar changes in the albino rat following subtotal nephrectomy. *Proc Soc Exp Biol Med* 30:1039–1041, 1933

59. KOLETSKY S: Role of salt and renal mass in experimental hypertension. *AMA Arch Pathol* 68:11–22, 1959

60. ARENDSHORST WJ, BEIERWALTES WH: Renal and nephron hemodynamics in spontaneously hypertensive rats. *Am J Physiol* 236:F246–251, 1979

61. FELD LG, VANLIEW JB, GALASKE RG, BOYLAN JW: Selectivity of renal injury and progression in the spontaneously hypertensive rat. *Kidney Int* 12:332–343, 1977

62. BANK N, ALLERMAN L, AYNEDJIAN HS: Selective JM nephron hyperfiltration in SHR rats with reduced renal mass (*abstract*). *Kidney Int* 23:211, 1983

63. ANDERSON S, MEYER TW, DEGRAPHENREID R, RENNKE HG, BRENNER BM: Control of glomerular hypertension preserves glomerular structure and function in rats with renal ablation (*abstract*). *Clin Res* (in press, 1984)

64. IBELS LS, ALFREY AC, HAUT L, HUFFER WE: Preservation of function in experimental renal disease by dietary restriction of phosphate. *N Engl J Med* 298:122–126, 1978

65. KARLINSKY ML, HAUT L, BUDDINGTON B, SCHRIER NA, ALFREY AC: Preservation of renal function in experimental glomerulonephritis. *Kidney Int* 17:293–302, 1982

66. TOMFORD RC, KARLINSKY ML, BUDDINGTON B, ALFREY AC: Effect of thyroparathyroidectomy and parathyroidectomy on renal function and the nephrotic syndrome in rat nephrotoxic serum nephritis. *J Clin Invest* 68:655–664, 1981

67. CARTER HR, MERADO A, RUTHERFORD WE, RODRIGUEZ H, SLATOPOLSKY E, KLAHR S: Effects of phosphate depletion and parathyroid hormone on glucose reabsorption. *Am J Physiol* 227:1422–1427, 1974

68. WHITE FN, GROLLMAN A: Autoimmune factors associated with infarction of the kidney. *Nephron* 1:93–102, 1964

69. MOOREHEAD JF, EL-NAHAS M, CHAN MK, VARGHESE Z: Lipid nephrotoxicity in chronic progressive glomerular and tubulo-interstitial disease. *Lancet* ii:1309–1311, 1982

70. GJONE E, BLOMHOFF JP, SKARBONK AJ: Possible association between an abnor-

mal low density lipoprotein and nephropathy in lecithin: cholesterol acyltransferase deficiency. *Clinica Chimica Acta* 54:11–18, 1974

71. MASCHIO G, OLDRIZZI L, TESSITURE N, D'ANGELO A, VALVO E, LUPO A, LOSCHIAVO C, FABRIS A, GAMMARO L, RUGLO C, PANZETTA G: Effects of dietary protein and phosphorus restriction on the progression of early renal failure. *Kidney Int* 22:371–376, 1982

72. GIORDANO C: Protein restriction in chronic renal failure. *Kidney Int* 22:401–408, 1982

73. MITCH WE, STEINMAN TI, WALSER M: The effect of protein restriction plus ketoacids on progression of chronic renal failure (*abstract*). *Clin Res* 31:437A, 1983

74. MITCH WE: Nutritional therapy in the progression of chronic renal insufficiency. *Ann Rev Med* 35:249–264, 1984

75. PURKERSON ML, JOIST JH, GREENBERG JM, KAY D, HOFFSTEN PE, KLAHR S: Inhibition of anticoagulant drugs of the progressive hypertension and uremia associated with renal infarction in rats. *Thrombosis Res* 26:227–240, 1982

76. OLSON JL: Role of heparin as a protective agent following reduction of renal mass. *Kidney Int* 25:376–382, 1984

77. PURKERSON ML, VALDES A, YATES J, MORRISON A, KLAHR S: Inhibition of thromboxane synthesis prevents progressive renal disease in rats with 5/6 nephrectomy (*abstract*). *Kidney Int* 25:251, 1984

78. ROBSON AM, MOR J, ROOT ER, JAGER BV, et al: Mechanism of proteinuria in nonglomerular disease. *Kidney Int* 16:416–429, 1979

79. OLSON JL, HOSTETTER TH, RENNKE HG, BRENNER BM, VENKATACHALAM MA: Altered glomerular permselectivity and progressive sclerosis following extreme ablation of renal mass. *Kidney Int* 22:112–126, 1982

80. STERZEL RB, LOVETT DH, STEIN HD, KASHGARIAN M: The mesangium and glomerulonephritis. *Klin Wochenschr* 60:1077–1105, 1982

81. MICHAEL AF, KEANE WF, RAIJ L, VERNIER RL, MAUER SM: The glomerular mesangium. *Kidney Int* 17:141–154, 1980

82. BARCELLI UO, WEISS M, POLLAK VE: Effects of a dietary prostaglandin precursor on the progression of experimentally induced chronic renal failure. *J Lab Clin Med* 100:786–797, 1982

83. VANRENTERGHEM Y, ROELS L, VANDAMME B, MICHIELSEN P: Influence of indomethacin treatment on the spontaneous glomerulosclerosis of the rat. (*abstract*). *Kidney Int* 16:659, 1979

Pathogenesis of Uremia

Eberhard Ritz

The chore of reviewing the pathogenesis of uremia is challenging and frustrating at the same time. One is confronted with a striking paradox: the discoveries of acute and chronic hemodialysis by Haas [1], Kolff and Berk [2], and Scribner et al [3] have put at our disposal highly efficacious treatment modalities, the success of which has exceeded predictions; but the striking advances in treatment have not been matched by equally dramatic advances in our understanding of the pathophysiology of uremia. In view of the rudimentary information available, the most rewarding way to proceed will be to retrace the main lines of thought of past nephrologists in their endeavor to understand uremia. Following the precept of August Comte, "to understand a science one must know its history."

Initially, uremia was exclusively understood as an excretory failure; however, recent developments emphasize the role of renal biosynthetic failure (including failure of endocrine secretion) and regulatory failure (disruption of homeostatically useful hormonal feedback control systems). Although "excretory failure" is more relevant for the understanding of acute renal failure, the concepts of biosynthetic and regulatory failure have over-riding importance in the evaluation of the more chronic multiorgan disturbances of chronic uremia. The recognition of the deleterious effects of homeostatically useful but excessive hormonal responses, as in the "trade-off theory" of Bricker [4], represents a major conceptual breakthrough. According to Kuhn [5], it is the introduction in science of such new revolutionary concepts and paradigms that allows not only more profound understanding of known phenomena but also provides the rationale for innovative experimentation.

This manuscript was presented as a State-of-the-Art lecture of the same title.

Substances Involved in the Acute Toxicity of Excretory Failure

The relation of shrunken kidneys to oliguria and dropsy was recognized by Saliceto in his *Liber in Scientia Medicinali* (1476), in which he stated "Signa duritiei in renibus sunt, quid minoratur quantitas urinae, . . . et incipit venter inflari post tempus et fit hydropicus secundum dies" ["Signs of shrunken kidneys are oliguria, . . . delayed appearance of ascites and edema formation"]. In contrast to the early recognition of the kidney's role in fluid excretion, more sophisticated chemical methodology was required for Prévost and Dumas' (1821) recognition that an elevated urea concentration in the blood was associated with the intoxication syndrome developing in nephrectomized or ureter-ligated dogs [6]. Despite continuing discussion over 150 years, the role, if any, urea plays in the genesis of the uremic syndrome has not been finally settled upon. The neurotoxic features of uremia cannot be reproduced in animals by infusion of urea, and patients with acute renal failure in whom urea concentrations are maintained by the addition of urea to the dialysate clinically improve despite no change of blood urea concentration [7]. Furthermore, the remarkable tolerance of some species (for example, marine elasmobranch fish and lung fish) to high blood concentrations of urea led Smith [8] to the conclusion that "urea, the most diffusable and non-toxic nitrogeneous substance known" has through a process of natural selection become the chief metabolic waste product of nitrogen metabolism [9].

Acute infusion studies may not be relevant if, as pointed out by Leiter [10], "the time element . . . is as important as the high concentration." Volhard [11] first proposed that urea may act in concert with other substances ("Summationswirkung"), for which some experimental evidence has been adduced [12, 13].

The discrepancy between low toxicity of urea and clinical evidence of "toxicity" in uremia led Frerichs (1851) to postulate that urea in the blood of uremic patients was converted to ammonia [14]. Although this view was later disproved, the general concept of delayed toxicity resulting from a urea reaction product may be valid. When concentrations of urea above 500 mg/dl were maintained in the extracellular fluid of nephrectomized dogs by means of intermittent peritoneal lavage, some symptoms encountered in uremia (weakness, hypothermia, anorexia, nausea, vomiting, and bloody diarrhea) were reproduced. One possible explanation is provided by the observation of Gilboe and Javid [15], who proposed that similar symptoms can be elicited with either urea or potassium isocyanate in bilaterally nephrectomized dogs. Isocyanate is in thermodynamic equilibrium with urea, and the concentrations used in the experiment were comparable to the expected concentration in a 1% aqueous solution of urea at 37°C in vitro [16]. The authors proposed that nonenzymatic nucleophilic addition would link isocyanate with N-terminal and epsilon-amino groups. Such carbamylation of the N-terminal amino groups of the alpha- and beta-chains of hemoglobin, proportional to concentration of blood urea, was reported by Flückiger et al [17], as well as carbamylation of plasma proteins by Oimomi et al [18]. Cyanate was found to interfere

with binding of drugs by albumin [19], which was implied to be a cause of
the decreased acidic drug binding in uremia [20]; however, other observations
are difficult to reconcile with this conclusion [21]. This evidence of protein
carbamylation in uremia is of interest in view of reports that neurotoxicity
with polyneuropathy develops in patients who are chronically exposed to
sodium cyanate for treatment of sickle cell disease [22]. In experimental
studies, incorporation of ^{14}C-cyanate into brain proteins has been demonstrated both in vivo and in vitro [23]. Interference of such carbamylation
with neurobehavioral function is suggested by the observation of a parallel
relation between brain protein carbamylation and memory [24]. Furthermore,
rodents exposed to cyanate show decreased motor activity and drowsiness
[25], and injection of small doses of sodium cyanate into rats and rabbits
is followed by drowsiness and hypothermia [26]. Surprisingly, the possibility
carbamylation-related neurotoxicity has not been eliminated by studies of
other brain proteins in uremic animals for carbamylation of free amino groups
has not been carried out.

Clinical trials suggest a relation of neurobehavioral changes [27] and morbidity [28] to urea. However, the complexity of the clinical situation and
the possibility of some other low-molecular weight water-soluble substance
varying in parallel with urea preclude conclusions with respect to underlying
mechanisms. Whether urea or one of the innumerable other water-soluble
substances removed by dialysis is responsible for the acute neurotoxicity has
not been resolved and remains a challenge for nephrological investigation.

Concepts concerning the mechanisms by which "toxins" in uremic serum
alter cell metabolism include the demonstration by Renner and Heintz [29,
30] that oxygen consumption as well as utilization of CoA-dependent substrates (for example, pyruvate, alpha-keto-glutarate, acetoacetate) are diminished when brain or kidney slices are exposed to serum of uremic patients.
However, in patients with renal failure, oxygen consumption is normal or
only moderately decreased, and tissue ATP levels measured with freeze clamp-
ing [31] or NMR (unpublished) are not decreased in experimental uremia.
The high rate of acetate metabolism in dialysis patients argues against a
major role of inhibition of CoA-dependent steps in uremic patients [32].
Other abnormalities in tissue preparations elicited by serum of uremic patients
include inhibition of glucose uptake and utilization at the level of phosphofructokinase in rat diaphragm and enhanced gluconeogenesis in liver slices [33].
Uremic serum, or fractions thereof, also inhibits cell proliferation in various
test systems [34].

Although earlier explanations of such metabolic derangements focused
on enzyme inhibition by urea [35] or other low-molecular weight substances
[30], such explanations appear inadequate today. More complex interference
at higher levels of the organization of cell metabolism must be considered;
examples are interference with ion transport across plasma membranes [36],
transmembrane substrate transport [37], membrane phospholipid and arachidonate metabolism [38], interference with intracellular signal nucleotides such
as calmodulin [39], or possible transcription-translation abnormalities.

The concept that peptides in the "middle-molecular weight" range (300
to 2000 daltons) play a role in the toxicity of uremia has recently generated

much interest. The concept was based on the belief that neuropathy was less frequent in peritoneal dialysis compared to hemodialysis patients. This was taken to reflect better clearance of substances with molecular weights higher than urea through the peritoneal membrane. The clinical response to variations in dialysis technique to test this hypothesis has been equivocal or negative [40].

No convincing evidence has been presented that material in the middle-molecular size range reproduces major facets of uremia in vivo or in vitro. One approach has been to use appropriate separation techniques based on the principle of size exclusion (for example, membrane filtration, gel chromatography, ion-exchange chromatography, or HPLC) to separate the substances of the respective molecular-weight range in the serum of dialyzed patients. This approach has yielded equivocal results [41]. Another approach has been to identify and isolate from serum, dialysate, or ultrafiltrate a chemically defined substance that would reproduce facets of the uremic syndrome in appropriate test systems. Such identification meets formidable analytical problems including interactions of amino acid side chains and gel matrix influencing elution volume, and low-molecular weight substances that comigrate and contaminate "mid-molecular" peptidic fractions. Although the hypothetical "middle-molecules" were first thought to be oligopeptides, some of the substances subsequently identified were not peptides, notably the peak 7c identified by Bergström [41], which was identified as a double conjugate of o-hydroxybenzoic acid with glucuronic acid and glycin and has a mol wt of 371 daltons [42]. The unpredictability of such studies is illustrated by the work of Bovermann et al [43], who isolated a hexapeptide from dialysate of uremic patients by fractionation on Sephadex G-15, reverse-phase gel, and absorption chromatography. The identity of the fully synthetic hexapeptide with the original substance was established by ^{1}H- and ^{13}C-NMR spectroscopy, but the substance had no toxic activity in several test systems. Abiko et al [44, 45] were more successful. They isolated from plasma of uremic patients two oligopeptides, one of which corresponded to positions 13–19 of human beta-2-microglobulin. With fully synthetic peptides, they were able to imitate the effects of uremic serum on several in vitro test systems (for example, SRBC rosettes, lymphocyte transformation using PHA, and Con A). With a synthetic pentapeptide sequence of Abiko's material [44], which interfered with in vitro lymphocyte function [46], we were unable to demonstrate actions on the behavior or cardiovascular functions when administered by intracerebral injection into instrumented conscious rats (unpublished observations). The number of publications on middle molecules has plummeted in the past 2 years—silent evidence of the lack of significant progress in the pursuit of the hypothesis.

If we are unable to identify the toxins responsible for uremia, we can at least hypothesize what would be the characteristics of a "toxin." It has been proposed that such a substance must conform to "Koch's postulates" [47]: its blood level should be elevated in uremia, it must cause symptoms similar to uremia, such symptoms must be alleviated by reduction in its blood levels, and symptoms must be reproduced in experimental animals. Since there might well be a multiplicity of "toxins" with different characteristics, different time courses in their pharmacodynamic action, and interaction of toxicities, such a postulate may be restrictive.

Biosynthetic (Including Endocrine) Failure

Whereas hemodialysis abrogates the acute, mainly neurobehavioral, manifestations of uremic toxicity, patients treated by chronic hemodialysis continue to manifest numerous metabolic derangements (anemia, hyperlipidemia, endocrine disturbances, and so on) that are reversed by renal transplantation. Such derangements are related, at least in part, to failure of the biosynthetic and endocrine functions of the kidney. In recent years, the role of the kidney as an endocrine organ has found increasing attention. Its secretions include renin, prostaglandins, kinins, an active principle involved in the complex erythropoietin system, and $1,25(OH)_2$ vitamin D_3 (calcitriol). This discussion will focus on the potential consequences of a deficiency of this latter compound in the uremic organism.

Circulating calcitriol is known to be decreased in uremia and has been thought to cause the known abnormalities of calcium metabolism. However, it is now recognized that calcitriol receptors are present in many tissues that are not involved directly in the control of calcium metabolism; for example, pituitary cells, mammary gland, placenta, melanoma cells, a variety of tumor cell lines, and testes [48]. This latter finding is of note, since it has been demonstrated previously that the cyclic AMP response to luteinizing hormone (LH) is defective in testes [49] and ovaries [50] of acutely or chronically uremic rats. Such demonstration of LH resistance would explain the observation of hypergonadotropic hypogonadism in uremic patients. The abnormality in experimental animals is reversed by administration of calcitriol in vivo [50]. Recently, calcitriol receptors have been demonstrated in circulating monocytes (presumed osteoclast precursor cells) [51, 52], which is of note in view of the recent recognition of the action of calcitriol on myeloblast/monocyte maturation [53] and myc-oncogen mRNA synthesis in transformed blast cell lines [54]. Calcitriol receptors have also been demonstrated in the basal cell layer of the epidermis [55].

Regulatory Failure: Disruption of Hormonal Control Systems

Much progress has been made in recent years concerning the endocrine disturbances of uremia. It has been due primarily to the availability of highly sophisticated and sensitive methodologies.

Loss of functioning nephrons may cause the following endocrine disturbances [56, 57]: (a) hormone oversecretion because of disruption of hormonal control systems (for example, hypothetical natriuretic hormone, PTH); (b) disturbed renal (or extrarenal) catabolism of polypeptide hormones (for example, insulin, C-peptide, PTH); (c) circulation of multiple molecular forms of hormones with varied or no biological activity (for example, glucagon); (d) end-organ resistance at the receptor or postreceptor level (for example, beta-adrenergic agonists, insulin, PTH); (e) accumulation of hormones with opposing actions. Whereas all of these disturbances have been documented adequately [56], the following discussion will focus on the first derangement.

In principle, uremia may disrupt hormonal feedback systems by a signal that leads to a continued excess concentration of circulating hormones that may compromise the function of organs other than the classic target organ. The evolution of this concept is the combined work of Platt [58] and Bricker [4] on the astonishing ability of the diseased kidney to maintain orderly sodium balance despite a loss of functioning nephrons. Sodium intake in the presence of diminished nephron mass requires more aggressive natriuresis per nephron for the organism to remain in sodium balance. It was proposed that such adaptation was mediated by a circulating inhibitor of sodium transport, which would induce abnormalities in extrarenal systems. According to this view, the uremic "toxin" would not be a retained substance, but rather a circulating hormone.

The evidence for such hypothetical natriuretic factor (or factors) has become increasingly strong in recent years [59]. However, because chemical identification of the active principle (or principles) is still lacking, all data currently available are tenuous and potentially subject to revision. The powerful tools of molecular biology should settle this issue very soon.

The "trade-off" concept, however, has proved eminently fertile as a paradigm to understand disturbances in other endocrine feedback systems. One example that has recently gained much interest is parathyroid hormone (PTH) secretion. Massry [60] proposed that some features of the uremic syndrome, unrelated to the classic hormonal actions of PTH, were caused by the high concentration of PTH in uremia. It is curious that this hormone, which under normal circumstances is involved in the maintenance of normocalcemia and skeletal homeostasis, might be deleterious and cause widespread multiorgan damage. One possible explanation for this paradox is provided by the fact that PTH increases the cellular calcium content [61]. This phenomenon might provide a powerful amplification mechanism for cell damage. Under various circumstances (hypoxemia, ischemia, agonist stimulation, and so on) cells may become unable to maintain calcium balance, which may cause mitochondrial dysfunction [62] and cell death [63]. The paramount importance of calcium in this sequence is demonstrated by the efficacy of calcium entry blockers to prevent cell damage [63].

Apart from cell death, a multitude of cell functions can be affected by calcium [64]. An incomplete list of its actions include excitation contraction coupling, excitation secretion coupling, membrane stability, cell contractility, assembly/disassembly of microtubules, modulation of plasma membrane receptors, mediation of endocytosis, and control of gap junction function. Two systems have been recognized to mediate such calcium-dependent actions: calmodulin [39] and calcium and phospholipid-dependent C-kinase [65].

It is known that PTH receptors are present not only on the classical target organs—renal [66] and bone cells [67]—but also on other cells; for example, lymphocytes [68]. There may be important differences between these renal and bone receptors [69].

The postreceptor effects of PTH are mediated through two different pathways. PTH stimulates cell membrane cyclic AMP, which generates an increase in cytoplasmic cyclic AMP [69] with activation of cyclic AMP-dependent protein kinase. However, an increase in cellular cyclic AMP concentration cannot explain all PTH-induced cellular events. Dziak and Stern [70] dissociated the effects of cyclic AMP and PTH on increased permeability of bone cell membranes to calcium. Recent work of Herrmann-Erlee et al [71] gives suggestive evidence for two different types of PTH receptors on bone cells: one regulating calcium influx and the other governing adenylate cyclase activity. Based on differences in response to PTH analogues, they concluded that these receptors are different with respect to their affinities toward the agonist and antagonist. Such cyclic AMP-independent actions raise the issue of the mechanism by which a cyclic AMP-independent ionophoric increase of calcium uptake is effected. The phosphatidate-phosphoinositide cycle has been shown to be a messenger system in the action of many hormones and neurotransmitters [72]. Recently, Meltzer et al [73] demonstrated cyclic AMP-independent stimulation of ^{32}Pi-incorporation into phosphatidyl-inositol esters, and phosphatidic acid was associated with a net increase of the actual tissue level of these phospholipids. This effect of PTH corresponds to a known mechanism of action of many other hormones; that is, that a phospholipid-derived ionophore, possibly phosphatidic acid, mediates transmembrane transport of calcium. The exact nature of the subsequent steps and the potential participation of a calcium phospholipid-dependent protein kinase [74] have not been defined.

Two recent observations are pertinent to explain previously puzzling observations on the action of PTH. Based on indirect evidence using PTH analogues in their bone culture system, Herrman-Erlee et al [75] postulated that the domains that activate the two hypothetical PTH receptors on bone cells are localized in the N-terminal segment for the adenylate cyclase and in the middle-carboxyterminal segment for the calcium ionophoric action. This may explain previous differences of the actions of intact vs. aminoterminal PTH fragments on erythropoiesis [76]. A further previously puzzling finding might also be explained in the light of recent evidence. Bogin et al demonstrated stimulation of brain microsomal Na-K-ATPase in vitro [77] and inhibition of mitochondrial respiration and phosphorylation in myocardial mitochondria by PTH. It was difficult to envisage how a polypeptide hormone could cross the plasma membrane [79]. However, recent findings of Arnaud et al [80], obtained with the use of the recycling inhibitor monensin, provided evidence that bone cell receptors undergo a cycle of internalization and reinsertion into the plasma membrane, thus indicating a mechanism by which intact PTH may reach the interior of the cell.

Table 1 gives an incomplete list of the features of uremia for which an action of PTH has been implied or demonstrated.

In the genesis of the anemia of renal failure, both diminished erythropoiesis and shortened erythrocyte half-life due to an extracorpuscular factor have been demonstrated. A role of PTH in both of these abnormalities is conceiv-

Table 1. Features of uremia with possible involvement of PTH

PTH-dependent increase of brain calcium, EEG changes, and decreased motor nerve conduction velocity	Carbohydrate intolerance via impaired insulin secretion
Decrease of erythropoiesis and shortened erythrocyte survival	Hyperlipidemia
Leukocyte dysfunction	Hypercatabolism and negative protein balance
Platelet dysfunction	Myopathy
Myocardiopathy	Sexual dysfunction

able. Aurbach, Mallete, and Patten [82] and Mallete, Bilezikian, and Heath [83] found the anemia in patients with primary hyperparathyroidism was reversed by parathyroidectomy. In patients with secondary hyperparathyroidism, improvement of anemia or reduction of blood transfusion requirements was reported [84–86] after parathyroidectomy. The intact (1–84) PTH, but not the 1,34-aminoterminal fragment of PTH, had an effect on erythroid burst-forming units (BFU-E) in mouse bone marrow cultures [76]. This effect of PTH was antagonized by the addition of erythropoietin to the media. The dual roles of PTH and erythropoietin may explain the moderate or absent anemia in patients with primary hyperparathyroidism and the variable relation between PTH and hematocrit in patients with advanced secondary hyperparathyroidism. A biphasic in vitro effect of PTH on RNA and heme synthesis by embryonic mouse liver erythroid precursors was reported by Levi et al [87], who found stimulation of RNA synthesis at low and inhibition at high PTH concentrations [88]. However, the effect of PTH on erythropoiesis is complex; some investigators [89] have noted overall marrow hypoplasia and reduction of the erythroid population after parathyroidectomy only in animals that were kept hypocalcemic by calcium-deficient diets.

The in vitro actions of PTH on erythropoiesis [76] were confirmed by the in vivo observations described in Figure 1 [90]. In rats with nutritionally induced secondary hyperparathyroidism, the incorporation of an isotope of iron into red blood cells was decreased both under basal conditions and after stimulation with hemorrhage. Conversely, parathyroidectomy increased the isotope's incorporation independent of plasma calcium and $1,25(OH)_2$ vitamin D_3 status. An action on red blood cell survival is suggested by the observation of a dose-dependent increase of osmotic fragility of human erythrocytes upon incubation with intact (1–84) PTH and the (1–34) PTH fragment [91]. The action of PTH on osmotic fragility was dependent on calcium as shown by partial blockade of the effect by verapamil, but it was independent of Na-K-ATPase and glycolysis. Such calcium-dependent action was not mediated by cyclic AMP, since dibutyryl cyclic AMP had no effect on osmotic fragility. One reasonable concept to explain these observations would be calcium-dependent actions on the cytoskeleton or membrane fluidity.

A role of PTH has also been implicated in disturbed myocardial function in uremia. On the basis of the molecular mechanism of action of PTH just described, one would predict a positive inotropic and chronotropic action of PTH. However, one might anticipate a potential risk of high-energy phos-

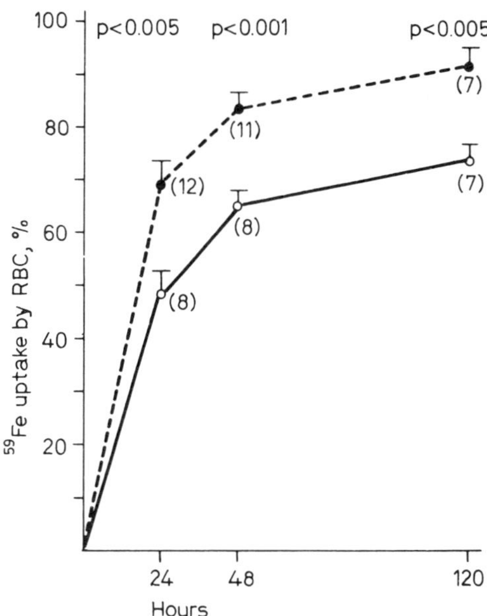

Fig. 1. Inhibition of ^{59}Fe uptake by red blood cells in rats with secondary hyperparathyroidism induced by a low calcium diet (*solid line*) and control rats (*broken line*). ^{59}Fe uptake was studied after bone marrow stimulation by hemorrhage (time 0). The figure demonstrates the reduced isotope turnover in hyperparathyroid rats. (Reprinted with permission of *Eur J Bio Chem* 130:303–308, 1983)

phate exhaustion from mitochondrial calcium overload as seen in other forms of cardiac necrosis [63]. A positive chronotropic effect of PTH on myocardial cell cultures was observed by Bogin, Massry, and Harary [92], which was independent of adrenergic agonists, but required calcium and was accompanied by a rise in cyclic AMP. An augmentation of the contractile force of papillary muscle by PTH was observed by Kahot et al [93], thus confirming indirect evidence [94] that PTH antagonized the depressor effect of propranolol on the contractile force of the auricles.

The potentially deleterious effects of PTH on myocardial function were illustrated by the early work of Lehr [95], who found that the cardiac lesions in rats after bilateral nephrectomy were prevented by parathyroidectomy. A PTH-dependent increase of myocardial calcium content in uremic dogs has been demonstrated [96], which may explain the observation of a dose-dependent PTH-induced shortening of myocardial cell survival in tissue culture [92]. Such reduced myocardial cell survival is understood readily in view of the finding that PTH interferes with myocardial mitochondrial function [78]. These effects again depend on the presence of calcium.

PTH may also play a role in the genesis of the hyperlipidemia of renal failure. PTH has various actions on lipid metabolism [97], although conflicting observations on serum lipids have been made in primary hyperparathyroidism. Ljunghall, Lithell, and Wide [98] found type IV hyperlipoproteinemia in a large proportion of patients with primary hyperparathyroidism; postoperatively, peak insulin levels decreased and serum lipids became normal without a change of adipose tissue lipoprotein lipase. On the other hand, other authors [90, 100] reported low cholesterol and triglyceride levels in patients with primary hyperparathyroidism and a postoperative rise of both cholesterol and triglycerides after parathyroid adenoma surgery.

In patients with secondary hyperparathyroidism, De Moor et al [99] found no change of serum lipids after parathyroidectomy, and some authors even reported an inverse correlation between iPTH and serum triglycerides [101]. However, in uremic rats, parathyroidectomy (associated with hypocalcemia) decreased the elevated triglyceride, cholesterol, and phospholipid values [102]. This observation complements the studies of Cantin [103], who showed that removal of the parathyroid glands partially inhibited the rise in blood lipids observed after bilateral nephrectomy and that administration of parathyroid extract to parathyroidectomized rats restored hyperlipidemia.

These effects of PTH on the lipidemia of uremia are in agreement with recent findings of Lacour [104] in rats with secondary hyperparathyroidism induced by a calcium-poor diet. Such hyperparathyroidism caused a significant increase in serum cholesterol and triglyceride concentration and a decrease in the clearance rate of infused lipids. Conversely, parathyroidectomized rats had decreased serum cholesterol and triglyceride concentrations and had a significant increase in postheparin lipolytic activity. Although these findings document a PTH dependence of VLDL clearance, other observations point to PTH stimulation of adipose tissue hormone-sensitive lipase activity in animals [105, 106] and humans [107]. PTH is known to activate adipose tissue lipase of human adults [108, 109]. The sensitivity of lipolysis to PTH stimulation is shown by the observation that injection of a bolus of PTH in fasted dogs causes an increase in serum glycerol and serum free fatty acids prior to, and even in the absence of, a change in serum calcium [110].

The foregoing actions of PTH on anemia, myocardiopathy, and hyperlipidemia are examples where a role of PTH may be postulated in some abnormalities of uremia.

Vascular disease is such a prominent feature in uremic patients that a final comment on the potential role of PTH in the genesis of hypertension [111] and hypertension-induced vascular lesions [112] appears appropriate, although a role of PTH in the development of these features in uremia has not been established. Acutely, PTH has a vasodilatory action on the renal, celiac, and coronary vasculature and thus lowers the mean arterial blood pressure [111]. However, it has a paradoxical effect on the development of hypertension in various experimental models; for example, in DOCA-salt hypertension [112] or the hypertension of spontaneously hypertensive rats (Fig. 2). The chronic permissive action of PTH may be related to its calcium ionophoric action, providing calcium for the vascular smooth muscle contractile apparatus. Such a chronic effect of PTH may, on the one hand, explain the high prevalence of hypertension in patients with primary hyperparathyroidism [113] and might conceivably contribute to hypertension in chronic renal failure. Of even greater importance, the old observations of Lehr and Martin [114] and the more recent findings of Nickerson [112] suggest a role for PTH in the genesis of vascular lesions in renal and mineralocorticoid hypertension. This action may also be related to the ionophoric action of PTH, since calcium overload is an important feature of vessel wall necrosis [63]. While it would be premature to comment on potential implications in

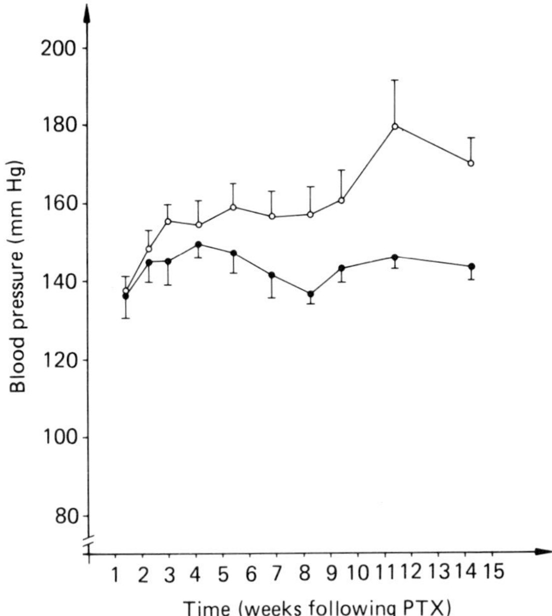

Fig. 2. Weanling spontaneously hypertensive rats (*SHR*) either totally parathyroidectomized (*PTX*) (●—●) or sham operated (○—○) (*N* = 12 per group). PTX rats received a high-calcium diet, which restored serum calcium to normal. Systolic blood pressure (*ordinate*) was measured by the tail cuff method, with rats lightly anesthetized with ether. Values represent the mean ± SD., (Reprinted with permission of *Mineral Electrolyte Metab* [90])

uremic patients, this problem is certainly a fertile area for future investigations.

The recognition of the involvement of PTH in the genesis of multiorgan damage of uremia [60, 81] is not only of interest for our understanding of pathogenesis, but also has important clinical implications. Development of secondary hyperparathyroidism can be prevented by the timely prophylactic intervention with dietary phosphate restriction and the administration of calcitriol.

Acknowledgments. The help of Prof. Dengler in Bonn and Prof. Ganten in Heidelberg in providing the synthetic pentapeptide and carrying out the rat experiment mentioned in the text is acknowledged. I also thank Drs. Kreusser, Mann, Merke, and Rambausek for permitting a perusal of experimental data, in part unpublished.

References

1. HAAS G: Versuche der Blutauswaschung am Lebenden mit Hilfe der Dialyse. *Klin Wochenschr* 4:13–14, 1925

2. KOLFF WJ, BERK TJ: The artificial kidney: A dialyser with great area. *Acta Med Scand* 117:121–134, 1944

3. SCRIBNER BH, BURI R, CANER JEZ, HEGSTROM R, BURNELL JM: The treatment of chronic uremia by means of intermittent hemodialysis: A preliminary report. *Trans ASAIO* 6:114, 1960

4. BRICKER NS: On the pathogenesis of the uremic state: An exposition of the "trade-off hypothesis." *N Engl J Med* 286:1093–1099, 1982

5. KUHN TS: *The Structure of Scientific Revolutions* (2nd ed). Chicago, University of Chicago Press, 1970

6. PRÉVOST JL, DUMAS JA: Examen du sang et de son action dans les divers phénomènes de la vie: Lu a la Société de Physique et Histoire Naturelle de Genève, le 15 novembre 1821. *Ann Chim Phys* 23:90–104, 1823

7. MERRILL JP, LEGRAIN M, HOIGNE R: Observations on the role of urea in uremia (*abstract*). *Am J Med* 14:519–520, 1953

8. SMITH HW: *From Fish to Philosopher: The Story of Our Internal Environment* (2nd ed). Summit, New Jersey, CIBA, 1959, p 252

9. JOHNSON WJ: Does elevated blood urea participate in the pathogenesis of the uremic syndrome? *Semin Nephrol* 3:265–271, 1983

10. LEITER L: Observations on the relation of urea to uremia. *Arch Intern Med* 28:331–354, 1921

11. VOLHARD F: *Handbuch der Inneren Medizin: 2. Auflage.* Berlin, Springer, p 780

12. LASCELLES PT, TAYLOR WH: The effect upon tissue respiration in vitro of metabolites which accumulate in uraemic coma. *Clin Sci* 31:403–413, 1966

13. SCHEUER J, STEZOSKI SW: The effect of uremic compounds on cardiac function and metabolism. *J Mol Cell Cardiol* 5:287–300, 1973

14. FRERICHS T: *Die Bright'sche Nierenkrankheit und deren Behandlung: Eine Monographie.* Braunschweig, F Vieweg u Sohn, 1851

15. GILBOE DD, JAVID MJ: Breakdown products of urea and uremic syndrome. *Proc Soc Exp Biol Med* 115:633–637, 1964

16. HAGEL P, GERDING JJT, FIEGGEN W, BLOEMENDAL H: Cyanate formation in solutions of urea: I. Calculation of cyanate concentrations at different temperature and pH. *Biochem Biophys Acta* 243:366–373, 1971

17. FLÜCKIGER R, HARMON W, MEIER W, LOO S, GABBAY KH: Hemoglobin carbamylation in uremia. *N Engl J Med* 304:823–827, 1981

18. OIMOMI M, ISHIKAWA K, KAWASAKI T, KUBOTA S, YOSHIMURA Y, BABA S: Plasma carbamylated protein in renal failure. *N Engl J Med* 308:655–656, 1983

19. BACHMANN K, VALENTOVIC M, SHAPIRO R: A possible role for cyanate in the albumin binding defect of uremia. *Biochem Pharmacol* 29:1598–1601, 1980

20. ERILL S, CALVO R, CARLOS R: Plasma protein carbamylation and decreased acidic drug protein binding in uremia. *Clin Pharmacol Ther* 27:612–618, 1980

21. LICHTENWALNER D, SUH B, LORBER B, RUDNICK MR, CRAIG WA: Partial purification and characterization of the drug-binding defect inducer in uremia. *J Lab Clin Med* 97:72–81, 1981

22. PETERSON CM, TSAIRIS P, OHNISHI A: Sodium cyanate induced polyneuropathy in patients with sickle-cell disease. *Ann Intern Med* 81:152–158, 1974

23. FANDO J, GRISOLIA S: Carbamylation of brain proteins with cyanate in vitro and in vivo. *Eur J Biochem* 47:389–396, 1974

24. CRIST RD, GRISOLIA S, BETTIS CJ, GRISOLIA J: Carbamoylation of proteins following administration to rats of carbamoyl phosphate and cyanate and effects on memory. *Eur J Biochem* 32:109–116, 1973

25. CRIST RD, PARELLADA PP: Central nervous system toxic manifestations of sodium cyanate. *Physiol Chem Phys* 6:371–374, 1974
26. BIRCH KM, SCHUTZ F: Actions of cyanate. *Br J Pharmacol* 1:186, 1946
27. TESCHAN PE, GINN HE, BOURNE JR, WARD JW, SCHAFFER JD: A prospective study of reduced dialysis. *ASAIO* 6:108–122, 1983
28. HARTER HR: Review of significant findings from the national cooperative dialysis study and recommendations. *Kidney Int* 23:S107–S112, 1983
29. HEINTZ R, RENNER D: Über Hemmwirkungen des Serums von Kranken mit hepatorenalem Syndrom und mit chronischer Urämie auf Sauerstoffverbrauch und Kohlenhydratstoffwechsel von Nieren- und Hirngewebe der Ratte. *Klin Wochenschr* 43:1167–1173, 1965
30. RENNER D, HEINTZ R: Untersuchungen des Zellstoffwechsels im Serum von Kranken mit Urämie. *Klin Wochenschr* 44:1204–1209, 1966
31. RITZ E: Myopathy of uremia. *Proc 6th Int Workshop on Phosphate and Other Minerals, Verona, June 24–26, 1983,* New York, Plenum (in press, 1984)
32. LEWIS EJ, TOLCHIN N, ROBERT JL: Estimation of the metabolic controversion of acetate to bicarbonate during hemodialysis. *Kidney Int* 18:551–555, 1980
33. DZURIK R: *Uraemia: The Pathophysiology of Carbohydrate Metabolism.* Bratislava, Publishing House of the Slovak Academy of Sciences, 1973
34. GUTMAN RA, HUANG AT: Inhibitor of marrow thymidine incorporation from sera of patients with uremia. *Kidney Int* 18:715–724, 1980
35. GIORDANO C, BLOOM J, MERRILL JP: Effects of urea on physiologic systems: I. Studies on monoamine oxidase activity. *J Lab Clin Med* 59:396–400, 1962
36. COTTON J, WOODARD TA, CARTER N, KNOCHEL JP: Resting skeletal muscle membrane potential as an index of uremic toxicity. *J Clin Invest* 63:501, 1979
37. MATTHEWS C, HEIMBERG KW, RITZ E, AGONISTINI B, FRITZSCHE J, HASSELBACH W: Effect of 1,25-dihydroxycholecalciferol on impaired calcium transport by the sarcoplasmic reticulum in experimental uremia. *Kidney Int* 11:227–235, 1977
38. EATIN AG, GORDILL SG, COUAUX JL: Metabolism of nephrectomized dogs. *Am J Med Sci* 194:214–230, 1937
39. RITZ E: Role of intracellular calcium and calmodulin in cellular metabolism: Possible implications for renal failure. *Kidney Int* 24(Suppl 16):S161–S166, 1983
40. KESHAVIAH P, KJELLSTRAND CM: Middle molecules: Do they exist? Are they toxic? *Semin Nephrol* 3:297–307, 1983
41. BERGSTROM J, FÜRST P: Uremic middle molecules. *Clin Nephrol* 5:143–152, 1976
42. ZIMMERMAN L, JORNVALL H, BERGSTROM J: Characterization of a double conjugate in uremic body fluids: Glucuronidated o-hydroxybenzoyglycine. *FEBS Lett* 129:237–240, 1981
43. BOVERMANN G, RAUTENSTRAUCH H, SEYBOLD G, JUNG G: Isolierung, Strukturaufklärung und Synthese eines Hexapeptids aus dem Hämodialysat urämischer Patienten. *Hoppe-Seylers Z Physiol Chem* 363:1187–1202, 1982
44. ABIKO T, KUMIKAWA M, SEKINO H: Inhibition effect of rosette formation between human lymphocytes and sheep erythrocytes by specific heptapeptide isolated from uremic fluid and its analogs. *Biochem Biophys Res Commun* 86:945–952, 1979
45. ABIKO T, KUMIKAWA M, DAZAI S, TAKAHASHI H, ISHIZAKI M, SEKINO H: Studies of uremic toxins: Structure-activity correlation in H-Asp(Gly)-OH. *Biochem Biophys Res Commun* 82:707–715, 1978

46. NIESE D, DREβEN P, HIESTER E, GILSDORF K, SCHMIDT RE: Immundefizienz bei Urämiepatienten: ein synthetisches Pentapeptid aus der Mittelmolekülfraktion von Urämikerplasma beeinfluβt die Lymphozytenfunktion in vitro. *Verh Dtsch Ges Inn Med* 89:169, 1983

47. MASSRY SG, KOPPLE JD: Uremic toxins: What are they? How are they identified? *Semin Nephrol* 3:263–264, 1983

48. MERKE J, KREUSSER W, BIER B, RITZ E: Demonstration and characterization of a testicular receptor for 1,25-dihydroxycholecalciferol in the rat. *Eur J Biochem* 130:303–308, 1983

49. KREUSSER W, SPIEGELBERG U, RITZ E: Chapter in *Vitamin D: Basic Research and its Clinical Application,* edited by NORMAN AW, Berlin, New York, Walter de Gruyter, 1979, pp 763–765

50. KREUSSER W, MADER H, HAAG W-D, RITZ E: Diminished response of ovarian cAMP to luteinizing hormone in experimental uremia. *Kidney Int* 22:272–279, 1982

51. PROVVEDINI DM, TSOUKAS CD, DEFTOS LJ, MANOLAGAS SC: 1,25-dihydroxy-vitamin D_3 receptors in human leucocytes. *Science* 221:1181–1183, 1983

52. MERKE J, RITZ E: Demonstration and characterization of 1,25-dihydroxyvitamin D_3 receptors in human mononuclear blood cells. *Biochem Biophys Res Commun* (in press, 1984)

53. BAR-SHAVIT Z, NOFF D, EDELSTEIN S, MEYER M, SHIBOLEIT S, COLDMAN R: 1,25-dihydroxyvitamin D_3 and the regulation of macrophage function. *Calcif Tissue Res* 33:673–676, 1981

54. REITSMA PH, ROTHBERG PG, ASTRIN SM, TRIAL J, BAR-SHAVIT, HAL A, TEITELBAUM SL: Regulation of myc gene expression in HL 60 leukemia cells by a vitamin D metabolite. *Nature* 306:492–494, 1983

55. MERKE J, SCHWITTAY D, FÜRSTENBERGER G, MARKS F, RITZ E: Skin as a target organ for 1,25(OH)$_2$D$_3$: Implications for skin changes in uremia? *IX Int Congr Nephrol,* Los Angeles, June 1984, Abst CA 37

56. EMMANOUEL DS, LINDHEIMER MD, KATZ AI: Pathogenesis of endocrine abnormalities in uremia. *Endocrinol Rev* 1:28–44, 1980

57. RABKIN R, KITAJI J: Renal metabolism of peptide hormones. *Mineral Electrol Metab* 9:212–226, 1983

58. PLATT R: Structural and functional adaptation in renal failure. *Br Med J* 1:1313–1317, 1372–1377, 1952

59. DE WARDENER HE, CLARKSON EM: The natriuretic hormone: Recent developments. *Clin Sci* 63:415–420, 1982

60. MASSRY SG: Is parathyroid hormone a uremic toxin? *Nephron* 19:125–130, 1977

61. BORLE A: Control, modulation and regulation of cell calcium. *Rev Physiol Biochem Pharmacol* 90:14–152, 1981

62. CARAFOLI E: The regulation of intracellular calcium. *Adv Exp Biol Med* 151:461–472, 1982

63. FLECKENSTEIN A, DORING JH, LEDER D: The significance of high energy phosphate exhaustion in the etiology of isoproterenol-induced cardiac necrosis and its prevention by iproveratil, compound D600 or prenylamine. *Int Symposium on Drugs and Metabolism of Myocardium and Striated Muscle,* 1969, pp 11–22

64. RASMUSSEN H: Calcium as intracellular messenger in hormone actions. *Adv Exp Biol Med* 151:473–491, 1982

65. TAKAI Y, KAIBUCHI K, MATSUBARA T, SANO K, YU B, NISHIZUKA Y: Two transmembrane control mechanisms for protein phosphorylation in bidirectional regulation of cell functions, in *Calmodulin and Intracellular Ca^{++} Receptors,*

edited by KAKIUCHI S, KIDAKA H, MEANS J, New York and London, Plenum Press, 1982, p 333

66. NUSSBAUM SR, RÖSENBLATT M, POTTS JT JR: Parathyroid hormone: Renal receptor interaction. *J Biol Chem* 255:10183–10187, 1980

67. RIZZOLI RE, SOMERMAN M, MURRAY TM, AURBACH GD: Binding of radioiodinated parathyroid hormone to cloned bone cells. *Endocrinology* 113:1832–1838, 1983

68. YAMMAMOTO I, POTTS JT JR, SEGRE GV: Circulating bovine lymphocytes contain receptors for parathyroid hormone. *J Clin Invest* 71:404–407, 1983

69. NISSENSON RA: Functional properties of parathyroid hormone receptors. *Mineral Electrolyte Metab* 8:151–158, 1982

70. DZIAK R, STERN PH: Calcium transport in isolated bone cells: III. Effects of parathyroid hormone and cyclic 3',5'-cAMP. *Endocrinology* 97:1281–1287, 1975

71. HERRMANN-ERLEE, MPM, NIJWEIDE PJ, VAN DER MEER JM, OOMS MAC: Action of bPTH and bPTH fragments on embryonic bone in vitro: Dissociation of the cyclic AMP and bone resorbing response. *Calcif Tiss Res* 35:70–77, 1983

72. FARESE RV: The phosphatidate-phosphoinositide cycle: An intracellular messenger system in the action of hormones and neurotransmitters. *Metabolism* 32:628–641, 1983

73. MELTZER V, WEINREB S, BELLORIN-FONT E, HRUSKA KA: Parathyroid hormone stimulation of renal phosphoinositide metabolism is a cyclic nucleotide-independent effect. *Biochim Biophys Acta* 712:258–267, 1982

74. LÖWIK CWGM, VAN ZEELAND JK, HERRMANN-ERLEE MPM: Effect of PTH-fragments on ornithine descarboxylase activity in isolated chicken osteoblasts, measured with an in situ assay. *VIII Int Conf Calcium Regulating Hormones,* Kyoto, Osaka, Kobe, Tokyo, and Niigata, Japan, October 1983, abst E-15

75. HERRMANN-ERLEE MPM, VAN DER MEER JM, LÖWIK CWGM: A new concept for the role of cAMP and Ca in PTH-stimulated bone resorption. *VIII Int Conf Calcium Regulating Hormones ("The Parathyroid Conferenes"),* Kobe, Japan, October, 1983, Abst P-52

76. MEYTES D, BOGIN E, MA A, DUKES PP, MASSRY SG: Effects of parathyroid hormone on erythropoiesis. *J Clin Invest* 67:1263–1269, 1981

77. BOGIN E, SACHTJEN E, BRISTOL C, MASSRY SG: Parathyroid hormone and brain microsomal Na-K-ATPase. *Mineral Elect Metab* 3:104–108, 1980

78. BOGIN E, LEVI J, HARARY I, MASSRY SG: Effects of parathyroid hormone on oxidative phosphorylation of heart mitochondria. *Mineral Elect Metab* 7:151–156, 1982

79. NORDQUIST RE, PALMIERI GMA: Intracellular localization of parathyroid hormone in the kidney. *Endocrinology* 95:229–237, 1974

80. ARNAUD C, NISSENSON R, TEITELBAUM A, SILCE C, KUGAI N: Parathyroid hormone receptor-adenylate cyclase interaction in kidney and bone. *VIII Int Conf Calcium Regulating Hormones,* Kyoto, Osaka, Kobe, Tokyo, Niigata, October 1983, abst E 1

81. MASSRY SG: The toxic effects of parathyroid hormone in uremia. *Semin Nephrol* 3:308–330, 1983

82. AURBACH GD, MALLETE LE, PATTEN BM: Hyperparathyroidism: Recent studies. *Ann Intern Med* 79:566–581, 1973

83. MALLETE LA, BILEZIKIAN JP, HEATH DA: Primary hyperparathyroidism: Clinical and biochemical features. *Medicine* 53:127–146, 1974

84. BETTER OS, SHASHA SM, WINAVER J, CHAIMOVITZ C: Improvement in the anemia of hemodialysis patients following parathyroidectomy (*abstract*). *Kidney Int* 10:487, 1976

85. SHASHA SM, BETTER OS, WINAVER J, CHAIMOVITZ C, BARZILAI A, ERLIK

D: Improvement in the anemia of hymodialyzed patients following subtotal parathyroidectomy: Evidence for the role of secondary hyperparathyroidism in the etiology of the anemia of chronic renal failure. *Isr J Med Sci* 14:328–332, 1978

86. ZINGRAFF J, DRUEKE T, MARIE P, MAN NK, JÜNGERS P, BORDIER P: Anemia and secondary hyperparathyroidism. *Arch Intern Med* 138:1650–1652, 1978

87. LEVI J, BESSLER H, HIRSCH I, DJALDETTI M: Increased RNA and heme synthesis in mouse erythroid precursors by parathyroid hormone. *Acta Haematol* 61:125–129, 1979

88. ZEVIN D, LEVI J, BRESSLER H, DJALDETTI M: Effect of parathyroid and 1,25(OH)₂ vitamin D₃ on RNA and heme synthesis by erythroid precursors. *Mineral Electrolyte Metab* 6:125–126, 1981

89. RIXON RH, WHITFIELD JF: Hypoplasia of the bone marrow in rats following removal of the parathyroid glands. *J Cell Physiol* 79:343–352, 1972

90. BASILE C, LACOUR B, DRÜEKE T, BOFFA G-A, FUNCK-BRENTANO J-L: Parathyroid function and erythrocyte production in rat. *Mineral Electrolyte Metab* 7:197–206, 1982

91. BOGIN E, MASSRY SG, LEVI J, DJALDETTI M, BRISTOL G, SMITH J: Effects of parathyroid hormone on osmotic fragility of human erythrocytes. *J Clin Invest* 69:1017–1025, 1982

92. BOGIN E, MASSRY SG, HARARY I: Effect of parathyroid hormone on heart cells. *J Clin Invest* 67:1215–1227, 1981

93. KATHO Y, KLEIN KL, KAPLAN RA, SANBORN WG, KUROKAWA K: Parathyroid hormone has a positive inotropic action in the heart. *Endocrinology* 109:2252–2254, 1981

94. LHOSTE F, DRÜEKE T, LARUS S, BOISSIER JR: Cardiac interaction between parathyroid hormone, β-adrenoreceptor, and verapamil in the guinea pig in vitro. *Clin Exp Pharmacol Physiol* 7:377–385, 1967

95. LEHR D: The role of certain electrolytes and hormones in disseminated myocardial necrosis, in *Cardiovascular Disease,* edited by BAZUSZ E, Basel, S Karger, 1966, vol 1, p 248

96. KRAIKIPANITCH S, LINDEMAN RD, YOENICE AA, BAXTER RK, JAYGROD CC, BLUE MM: Effect of azotemia and myocardial accumulation of calcium. *Mineral Electrolyte Metab* 1:12–20, 1978

97. RITZ E, HEUCK CC, BOLAND R: Phosphate, calcium and lipid metabolism. *Adv Exp Biol Med* 128:197–209, 1980

98. LJUNGHALL S, LITHELL H, WIDE L: Hyperlipoproteinemia type IV and hyperinsulinemia in primary hyperparathyroidism: Effect of parathyroidectomy. *Acta Endocrinol* 89:580–589, 1978

99. DE MOOR P, CREYTTENS G, BOUILLON R, JOOSSENS JV: Results obtained in 75 patients operated upon for hyperparathyroidism: Low cholesterol levels in overt primary hyperparathyroidism. *Ann Endocrinol* 34:616, 1973

100. CHRISTENSEN T, EINARSON K: Serum lipids before and after parathyroidectomy in patients with primary hyperparathyroidism. *Clin Chim Acta* 78:411, 1977

101. BRUNZELL JD, GOLDBERG AP: Hormonal regulation of human adipose tissue lipoprotein lipase, in *Atherosclerosis IV,* edited by SCHETTLER G, et al, Berlin, Springer, 1977, p 336

102. BASILE C, LACOUR B, DRÜEKE T: Parathyroidectomy and lipid abnormalities in the rat. *Bari Semin Nephrol,* March 29–31, 1984, abst 9

103. CANTIN M: Kidney, parathyroid and lipemia. *Lab Invest* 14:1691, 1965

104. LACOUR B, BASILE C, DRÜEKE T, FUNCK-BRENTANO J-L: Parathyroid function and lipid metabolism in the rat. *Mineral Electrolyte Metab* 7:157–165, 1982

105. WERNER S, LÖW H: Stimulation of lipolysis and calcium accumulation by parathyroid hormone in rat adipose tissue in vitro after adrenalectomy and administra-

tion of high doses of cortisone acetate. *Hormone Metab Res* 5:192–296, 1973
106. GOZARIU L, FORSTER K, FAULHABER JD, MINNE H, ZIEGLER R: Parathyroid hormone and calcitonin: Influences upon lipolysis of human adipose tissue. *Hormone Metab Res* 6:243–245, 1974
107. SINHA TK, THAJCHAYAPONG P, QUEENER SF, ALLEN DO, BELL NH: On the lipolytic action of parathyroid hormone in man. *Metabolism* 25:251–260, 1976
108. KATHER H, SIMON B: Human fat cell adenylate cyclase: Responsiveness towards catecholamines, peptide hormones and prostaglandins, in *Lipoprotein Metabolism and Endocrine Regulation,* edited by HESSEL LW, KRAUS HMJ, Amsterdam, Elsevier, 1979, p 189
109. KATHER H, SIMON B: Adenylate cyclase of human fat cell ghosts, stimulation of enzyme activity by parathyroid hormone. *J Clin Invest* 59:730–732, 1977
110. HALLBERG D, WERNER S: Circulatory and lipolytic effects of parathyroid hormone. *Hormone Metab Res* 9:424, 1977
111. RAMBAUSEK M, RITZ E, RASCHER W, KREUSSER W, MANN JFE, KREYE V, MEHLS O: Vascular effects of parathyroid hormone. *Adv Exp Biol Med* 15:617–632, 1982
112. NICKERSON PA, CONRAN RM: Parathyroidectomy ameliorates vascular lesions induced by deoxycorticosterone in the rat. *Am J Pathol* 105:185–190, 1981
113. CHRISTENSSON T, HELLSTRÖM K, WENGLE B: Blood pressure in subjects with hypercalcemia and primary hyperparathyroidism detected in a health screening program. *Eur J Clin Invest* 7:109–113, 1977
114. LEHR D, MARTIN CR: Prevention of severe cardiovascular and smooth muscle necrosis in the rat by thyroparathyroidectomy. *Endocrinology* 59:273–288, 1956

Endocrine and Metabolic Abnormalities

Regulation of Parathyroid Gland Activity

Joel F. Habener

The secondary hyperparathyroidism and ensuing osteodystrophy that frequently develops as a consequence of chronic renal failure has continued to constitute a formidable clinical problem for nephrologists who care for such patients. Renal osteodystrophy is a complex metabolic process involving disorders of not only parathyroid hormone secretion, but also of the metabolism of vitamin D, phosphate excretion, and probably the effects of the accumulation of unknown metabolites that are not properly excreted by the failing kidney. Eventual success in the amelioration and prevention of renal osteodystrophy will require an understanding of the normal physiologic interrelationships between parathyroid hormone, vitamin D, calcium, and phosphorus.

Although the precise cellular mechanisms by which calcium regulates the activity of the parathyroid gland remain unknown, investigations carried out over the past several years have provided some insights into the cellular levels through which calcium regulates the expression of the parathyroid hormone gene in normal, hyperplastic, and neoplastic parathyroid tissues [1–3]. The purpose of this discussion is to provide evidence that, in the short term (minutes to hours), the primary site in the cell of the regulation of parathyroid hormone production by calcium is that of the intracellular turnover, or degradation, of parathyroid hormone. Subsequently, over the longer term (weeks to months), a persistent lowered concentration of the serum ionized calcium acts primarily as a mitogen resulting in hyperplasia of the parathyroid glands. The marked hyperplasia of the parathyroid glands that takes place particularly in the secondary hyperparathyroidism of chronic renal failure appears to amplify a component of parathyroid hormone secretion that is insensitive to changes in extracellular calcium concentrations; this component also exists in the cells of normal-sized parathyroid glands. In addition, as an accompaniment to, or possibly a consequence of the hyperplasia, the parathyroid cells appear to become less sensitive to the suppression

This manuscript was presented as part of a Symposium on *Parathyroid Hormone and Vitamin D in Uremia.*

of hormone secretion by extracellular calcium. This so-called set-point error in the sensing of extracellular concentrations of calcium by the gland, coupled with the exaggerated hormone secretion by the enlarged parathyroid glands that is not suppressible by calcium, leads to a state of chronic hyperparathyroidism.

The Structure of Preproparathyroid Hormone

Analyses of the structure of the major parathyroid cell protein resulting from cell-free synthesis programmed by parathyroid gland messenger RNA [4], as well as by analyses of the gene-encoding parathyroid hormone [5], has revealed that parathyroid hormone is encoded in a precursor, preproparathyroid hormone (Fig. 1). Preproparathyroid hormone consists of parathyroid

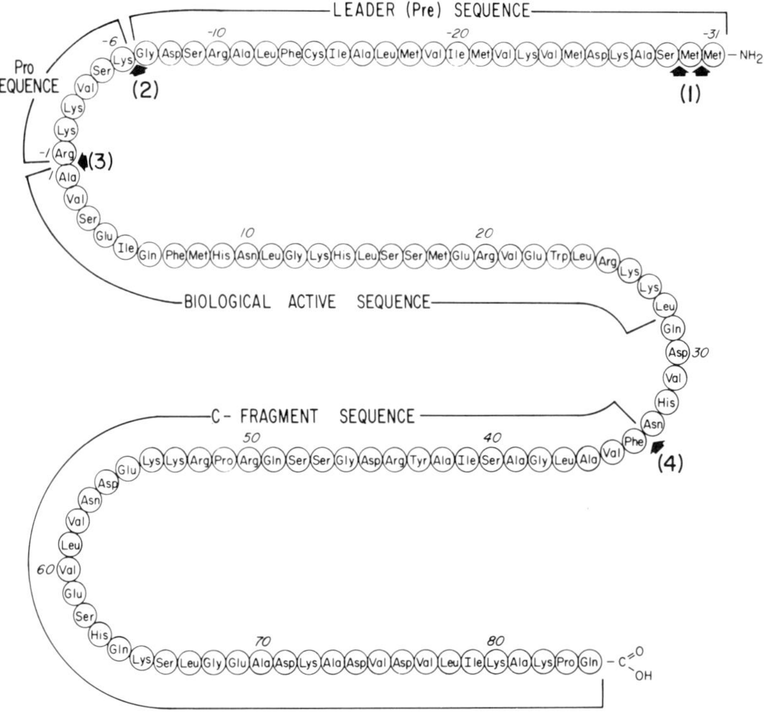

Fig. 1. Structures of bovine preproparathyroid hormone. The amino acid sequence was determined by automated Edman degradation on the product of parathyroid mRNA translation in a wheat germ cell-free system [4]. *Arrows* indicate cleavage sites cleaved by processing enzymes in the parathyroid gland and in the liver after secretion of the hormone. The biologically active region of the molecule is flanked by sequences not required for activity on target organ receptors.

hormone with an amino-terminal extension that contains a signal sequence necessary for the intracellular translocation of the precursor into the secretory pathway, and a short hexapeptide prosequence of unknown function. The preprohormone is sequentially processed by a series of proteolytic cleavages in the parathyroid cell leading to the formation of parathyroid hormone, which is the major hormonal product stored and secreted from the parathyroid gland (Fig. 2). Additional cleavages of parathyroid hormone occur both within and outside the gland after its secretion and during passage through the liver and possibly the kidney [6]. The cleavage of parathyroid hormone leads to the formation of an amino-terminal, biologically active fragment and a carboxy-terminal fragment that has no known biologic activity, but which constitutes the major form of circulating immunoreactive hormone both in normal individuals and in patients with primary and secondary hyperparathyroidism [6]. Because the carboxy-terminal fragment of parathyroid hormone is cleared by the kidneys, concentrations of the fragment in the circulation become particularly high in patients with renal failure.

Regulation of Parathyroid Hormone Secretion and Synthesis

An understanding of the defects in the regulation of parathyroid hormone production that occur in primary and secondary hyperparathyroidism requires

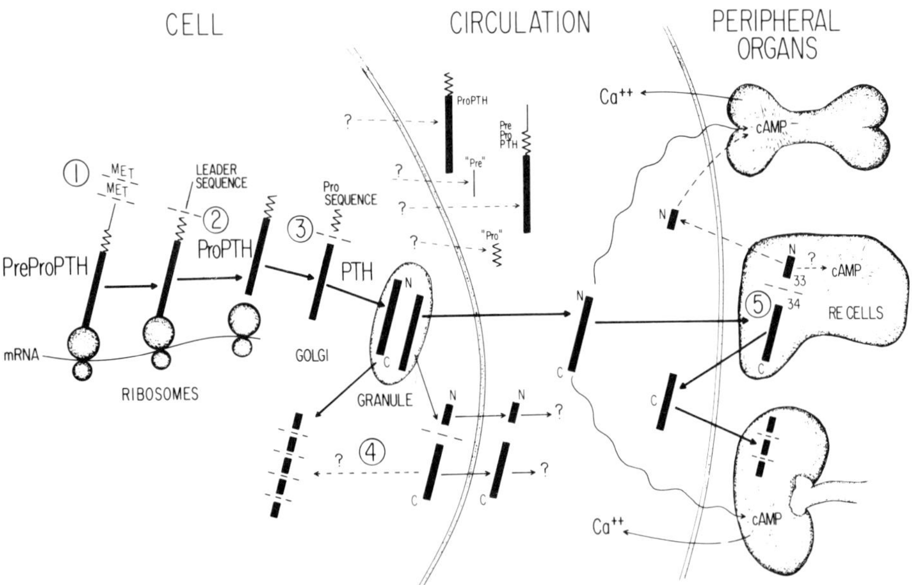

Fig. 2. Schema showing extensive co- and post-translational processing in the biosynthesis and metabolism of parathyroid hormone [6].

a fundamental understanding of the mechanisms by which extracellular calcium, and other factors, regulate both the secretion and the biosynthesis of the hormone. Over the past several years, studies of the regulation of the secretion and synthesis of parathyroid hormone utilizing parathyroid gland slices [7, 8] and preparations of dispersed cells [9] have provided some insights, albeit incomplete, into the mechanisms by which calcium regulates the activity of the parathyroid gland. Lowered concentrations of extracellular calcium markedly increase the secretion of parathyroid hormone and an additional protein, parathyroid secretory protein [10], from parathyroid gland slices or dispersed cells in vitro (Fig. 3). Partial sequence analysis of the parathyroid secretory protein by Cohn and his coworkers [11] indicates that the secretory protein is closely related in structure to chromogranin A: the ubiquitous protein found in multiple different secretory cells and originally discovered in the adrenal medulla. Factors other than calcium that regulate the secretion of parathyroid hormone include magnesium, which is similar in its regulatory effects to calcium except that it is approximately one-third as potent on a molar basis, catecholamines, and possibly metabolites of vitamin D (see [6] and the chapter by Slatopolsky, Martin, Morrissey, and Hruska in this volume).

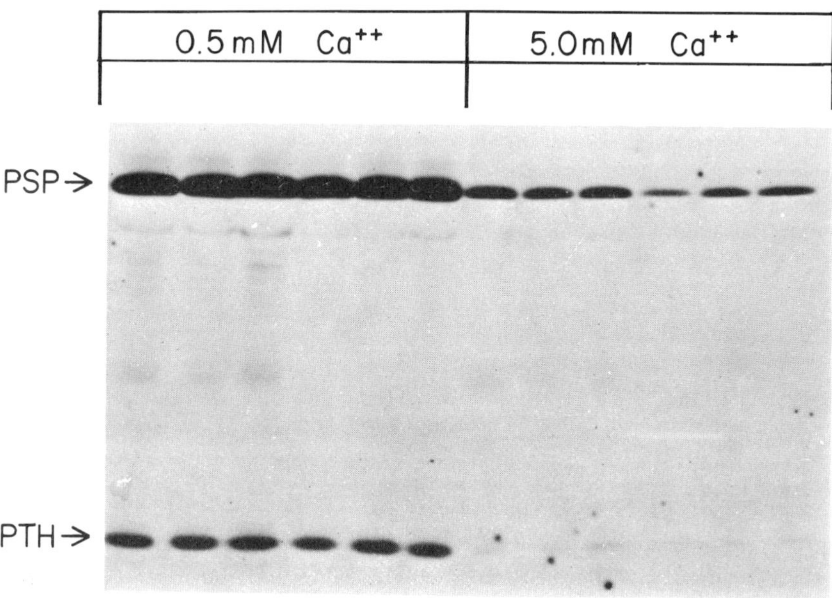

Fig. 3. Effect of extracellular calcium on the secretion of PTH and PSP [12]. Bovine parathyroid gland slices were incubated for 5 hr at 37°C in medium containing Ca^{++} at the indicated concentrations and [³H]- methionine (100 Ci/ml). Equal amounts of medium were removed and subjected to SDS-polyacrylamide gel electrophoresis. The gel was impregnated with En³Hance (New England Nuclear), dried, and exposed to Kodak SB-5 film (Eastman Kodak, Rochester, NY). The bands corresponding to PSP and PTH on the autofluorogram were scanned densitometrically to quantify relative PTH and PSP secretion. *Each lane* represents a separate incubation.

Although changes in extracellular fluid concentrations of calcium have pronounced effects on the release of parathyroid hormone, numerous studies of the effects of calcium on hormone biosynthesis in vitro, at least over periods of 6 to 8 hr of study, have shown very little, if any, effect (Fig. 4) [7, 12]. Only small differences in the amounts of proparathyroid hormones synthesized are observed during a short pulse-labeling (5 to 20 min) of parathyroid gland slices incubated in the presence of high compared to low concentrations of calcium. Such short pulse-labeling experiments provide an index of the rates of messenger RNA translation and/or the endogenous levels of messenger RNA encoding the preproparathyroid hormone. A further distinction between purely translational effects of calcium and effects on levels of parathyroid hormone messenger RNA were obtained by direct measurements of messenger

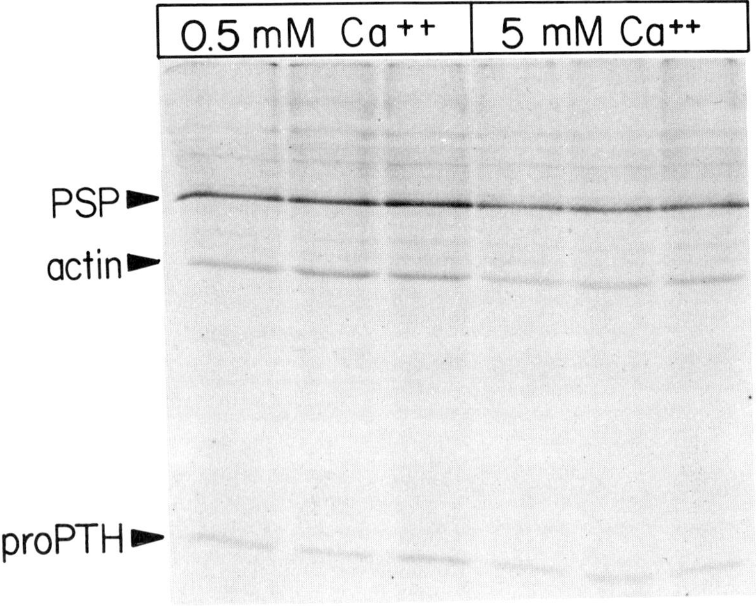

Fig. 4. Effect of extracellular calcium on synthesis of pro-PTH and PSP by intact parathyroid cells [12]. Bovine parathyroid gland slices were incubated for 5 hr at 37°C in medium containing the indicated concentrations of Ca++ and [³H]-methionine. At the end of the incubation, the slices were pulsed for 20 min with [³⁵S]-methionine (100 Ci/ml). The tissue slices were extracted with urea-acid, and equal volumes of each extract were subjected to SDS-polyacrylamide gel electrophoresis. The dried gel was exposed to Kodak SB-5 film, and the autoradiogram was scanned densitometrically to quantitate amounts of labeled protein in individual bands. Each lane of the autoradiogram represents a separate incubation. The *upper arrow* indicates the parathyroid secretory protein band, and the *lower arrow* represents the band containing pro-PTH.

RNA utilizing recombinant cDNA probes prepared from cloned gene sequences encoding the preproparathyroid hormone (Fig. 5) [12]. These hybridization analyses show that incubations of parathyroid gland slices, in either conditions of high or low concentrations of calcium, have no effect on the total cellular content of parathyroid hormone messenger RNA. An intriguing but unexplained additional finding was that incubation in conditions of high calcium leads to an approximately 3-fold increase in the amounts of Poly A$^+$ parathyroid hormone messenger RNA [12]. Inasmuch as the parathyroid

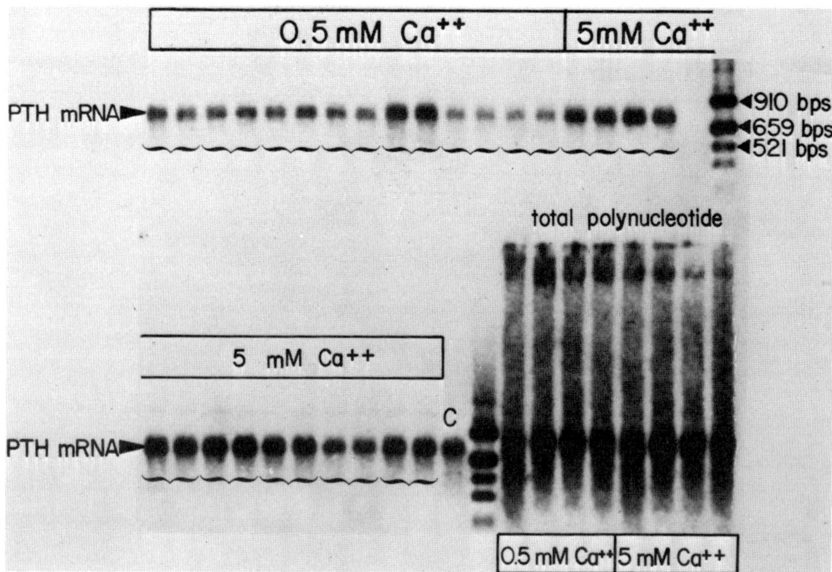

Fig. 5. Effect of the concentration of extracellular calcium on cellular levels of poly (A)-rich and total PTH mRNA [12]. Bovine parathyroid slices were incubated for 7 hr at 37°C in medium containing the indicated concentrations of Ca^{++} (seven samples at each concentration of Ca^{++}). Total polynucleotide was extracted from the tissue slices, and equal volumes were used to prepare poly (A)-rich RNA. Total polynucleotide and poly(A)-rich RNA were then assayed for hybridizable PTH mRNA with the radiodensitometric hybridization assay. The autoradiogram of the RNA blot shown was overexposed to improve photographic reproduction. A shorter exposure was used for densitometric analysis and PTH mRNA quantitation. The autoradiogram represents the blot from a single agarose gel on which 40 samples were fractionated simultaneously in 2 rows (11 cm apart) of 20 lanes each. Each of the 14 poly (A)-rich RNA samples (7 high Ca^{++} and 7 low Ca^{++}) was assayed in duplicate, whereas total polynucleotide samples were assayed once each, and only 8 of the 14 total polynucleotide assays are represented in the autoradiogram shown. An assay of all 14 samples were performed separately (not shown). pBR322 fragments, whose size in base pairs (bps) is indicated, were electrophoresed along with the PTH mRNA-containing samples. Note that the PTH mRNA bands center at an estimated length of 750 bases, but span a range of over 200 bps, most likely as a result of heterogeneity of the poly(A) extension of PTH mRNA. *Lane C* contains a sample previously assayed for PTH mRNA to control for proper assay conditions.

hormone messenger RNA that is poly A$^+$, as defined by its hybridization
to oligodT cellulose, constitutes only 10 to 30% of the total parathyroid
hormone messenger RNA, it represents a subgroup of the total messenger
RNA population. This paradoxical increase in Poly A$^+$ parathyroid messenger
RNA in response to high calcium, which suppresses parathyroid hormone
secretion, remains unexplained but may come about as a consequence of
relative differences in the lengths of the Poly (A) tracts of parathyroid hormone
messenger RNA in conditions of incubation of gland slices in the presence
of high as compared to low calcium concentrations.

A large number of studies of the regulation of parathyroid hormone biosynthesis and secretion in vitro by not only our laboratory, but the laboratories
of Cohn [13, 14] and Brown [15, 16], are summarized in Figure 6. The
regulation of the production of parathyroid hormone over the short term

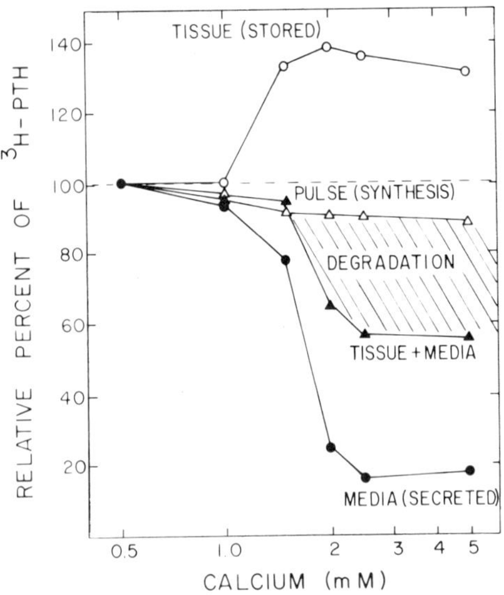

Fig. 6. Effect of extracellular calcium concentrations on synthesis ($\triangle$), secretion ($\bullet$),
and storage ($\bigcirc$) of PTH. The calcium-dependent degradation of PTH ($\blacktriangle$) is also
shown. Slices of parathyroid glands were incubated in vitro for 4 hr in MEM media
containing [³H]-leucine and various concentrations of calcium. Amounts of ³H-labelled
PTH were determined by polyacrylamide gel electrophoresis of extracts of tissue
($\bigcirc$) and media ($\bullet$) at the end of the incubation as described previously [7]. Rates of
PTH synthesis ($\triangle$) were determined by preincubating tissue slices for 3 hr in various
concentrations of calcium and then adding [³H]-leucine for an additional 35 min of
incubation (*pulse*-label). Extracts of tissues were analyzed for their content of ³H-
labelled Pro-PTH and PTH by gel electrophoresis. In the higher concentrations of
calcium, up to 40% of the [³H]-PTH is neither secreted from nor stored in the
tissue, but, instead, is degraded within the tissue (*shaded area*). Data are expressed
as % of [³H]-PTH in extracts from tissues and media incubated at lowest concentration
of calcium (0.5 mM-calcium = 100% [³H]-PTH).

(minutes to hours) takes place primarily at the level of the intracellular turnover of parathyroid hormone. There is little, if any, regulation at the level of translation or at the level of the steady-state concentrations of parathyroid hormone messenger RNA. Over the longer term (days to weeks), the predominant cellular mechanism utilized to increase the production of parathyroid hormone appears to be that of cellular hyperplasia or an increase in the number of parathyroid hormone-producing cells. By unknown cellular mechanisms, chronic stimulation of the parathyroid gland by hypocalcemia results in a proliferation of the parathyroid cells. This proliferation of the parathyroid gland is particularly noteworthy under circumstances of chronic renal failure in which prolonged hypocalcemia leads to increases in the parathyroid gland mass of up to 100- to 1000-fold above normal. A normal parathyroid gland weighs approximately 30 mg and it is not unusual in secondary hyperparathyroidism to find hyperplastic glands weighing several grams. It should be noted, however, that the information on the regulation of parathyroid hormone production obtained thus far has been derived from studies carried out with parathyroid tissue in vitro over relatively short periods of investigation. It is possible that under in vitro conditions, regulatory mechanisms that normally operate in vivo cannot function and thereby escape detection with the experimental methods applied. However, preliminary studies of the levels of parathyroid hormone messenger RNA in the parathyroid glands obtained from rats, rendered hypocalcemic for periods of up to 6 weeks, showed increased levels of messenger RNA compared to the control or normocalcemic rats (Heinrich et al, unpublished observations). However, the increased levels of RNA parallel the 3- to 4-fold increase in parathyroid gland mass and similar increases in levels of circulating parathyroid hormone. These observations in vivo are consistent with those obtained in studies in vitro in that, on a per cell basis, there does not appear to be any marked changes in the cellular levels of parathyroid hormone messenger RNA in response to the extracellular concentrations of calcium.

Consideration of the Glandular Defect in the Production of Parathyroid Hormone That Occurs in Primary Hyperparathyroidism

At least two cellular mechanisms appear to be operative in the development of the excess production of parathyroid hormone characteristic of both primary and secondary hyperparathyroidism. As alluded to earlier, a component of parathyroid hormone secretion appears to be insensitive to regulation by calcium (Fig. 6). Low levels of parathyroid hormone secretion persist despite exposure of the gland to prolonged hypercalcemia. This continued secretion of a small fraction of the parathyroid hormone has been observed in studies in vitro as well as those in vivo. Measurements of the parathyroid hormone levels in the effluent blood from parathyroid glands in calves made hypercalcemic by prolonged calcium infusions for several days demonstrated a continued secretion of parathyroid hormone in the effluent blood at levels above those in the arterial blood (Fig. 7) [17]. Thus, an expansion of the parathyroid gland mass that occurs in secondary hyperparathyroidism as well as in primary hyperparathyroidism results in an exaggeration of the total production of hormone by the gland despite persistent hypercalcemia. This calcium-insensitive, nonsuppressible secretion of parathyroid hormone, characteristic of normal parathyroid cells, becomes pathogenetic in the face of an increased parathyroid gland mass. In addition to the excess of secreted parathyroid hormone that is not suppressible by calcium, a second cellular defect appears to accompany increased parathyroid hormone mass, and that defect is a blunting of the sensitivity of the parathyroid cell to extracellular levels of calcium (Fig. 8) [16, 18]. This so-called set-point error in the sensing of the calcium by the parathyroid cell results in a requirement of higher-than-normal levels of calcium to suppress the calcium-regulated release of parathyroid hormone at a given increment. The basis for the alteration of the responsivity of the parathyroid gland to calcium that occurs in enlarged parathyroid glands is

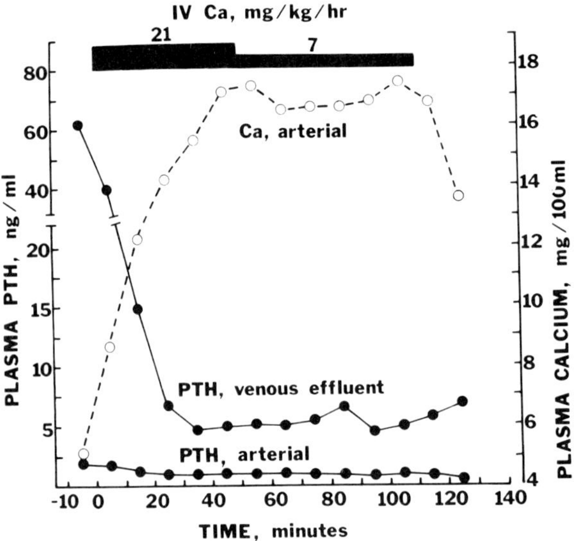

Fig. 7. Incomplete suppression of parathyroid secretion in a calf during hypercalcemia [17]. Parathyroid effluent blood was collected during general anesthesia by surgical cannulation of the vein draining a superior parathyroid gland. Arterial and venous blood samples were collected concurrently by continuous flow for 10-min intervals. Immunoreactive parathyroid hormone concentration was measured using antiserum GP-133. The initial hypocalcemia was induced by intravenous infusion of NA_2EDTA. The rapid increase in arterial concentration of calcium was accompanied by a sharp decline in parathyroid secretion (blood flow through the gland remained relatively constant while the hormone concentration declined). The persistence of a significant arteriovenous difference in concentration of immunoreactivity despite hypercalcemia demonstrates an inability of calcium to completely suppress secretion.

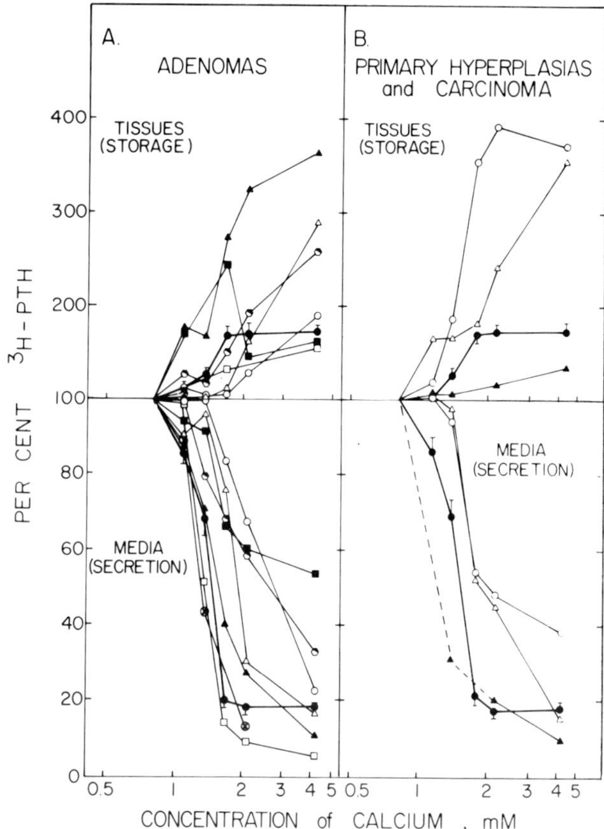

Fig. 8. Effects of extracellular calcium concentrations on the release of PTH into media (*lower panel*) and on the content of PTH in tissues (*upper panel*) during incubation of parathyroid tissues for 4 hr with [^{3}H]-leucine. Amounts of [^{3}H]-PTH were determined by polyacrylamide gel electrophoresis for each point. Results are expressed as percent of the value for maximum release of hormone at 0.5 mM of calcium. **a** Parathyroid adenomas (human): □, no. 1; ■, no. 2; ▲, no 3; △, no. 4; ◑, no. 5; ○, no. 6. Normal parathyroid glands for comparison: ●, bovine; ⊕, human. **b** Chief-cell hyperplasia (human): ○, no. 1, and △, no. 2. Carcinoma of the parathyroid gland, ▲.

unknown. The change in the set-point of the gland to calcium could be a consequence of the hyperplastic or neoplastic process or may simply accompany it by unknown mechanisms. Thus, at least two cellular defects appear to be involved in the excess production of parathyroid hormone in primary and secondary hyperparathyroidism (Fig. 9). These two defects are: (1) an increase in a component of parathyroid hormone secretion that is not suppressible by calcium and that is exaggerated by the increased parathyroid hormone mass, and (2) a change in the set-point of the sensitivity of the para-

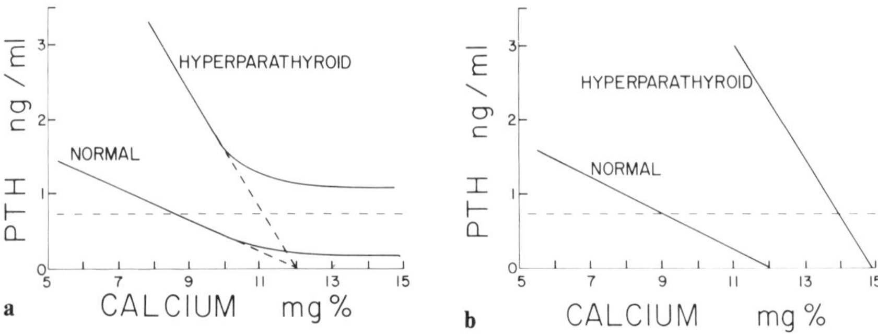

Fig. 9. a Diagram of an alternative hypothesis to explain secretory defect in primary hyperparathyroidism. Hypothesis requires that a small amount of hormone secretion persists despite elevated calcium. In the normal parathyroid, this secretion is small and insignificant. In hyperparathyroidism, greatly increased tissue mass leads to persistent secretion of hormone above normal range (*horizontal dashed line*). Note slopes of both normal and hyperparathyroid extrapolate to same calcium value (12 mg/dl). **b** Diagram hypothesis of set-point error to explain physiological mechanism of abnormality in control of hormone secretion in primary hyperparathyroidism. *Ordinate* represents plasma parathyroid hormone concentration, and *abscissa,* plasma calcium. Hyperparathyroid individuals show steeper slopes of response, owing to large mass of tissue. Complete suppression of hormone output occurs at abnormally high calcium concentration. *Horizontal dashed line* represents upper limit of normal PTH concentration.

thyroid cell to extracellular calcium resulting in a requirement for greater than normal concentrations of calcium to suppress the calcium-regulated component of the secretion of parathyroid hormone.

Directions for the Future Investigation of the Regulation of the Parathyroid Gland

Further understanding of the cellular molecular mechanisms involved in the development of hyperparathyroidism will require an understanding of: (1) mechanisms by which prolonged hypocalcemia leads to division and growth of parathyroid cells; that is, the mechanism by which lowered extracellular calcium acts as a mitogen for the parathyroid gland (Fig. 10). It is clear that this mitogenic action of hypocalcemia is a unique property of the parathyroid cells inasmuch as prolonged hypocalcemia is not known to lead to hyperplasia of other glandular tissues. (2) An understanding of the processes that lead to alteration of the responses of the calcium-sensing apparatus of the parathyroid cell to extracellular levels of calcium. In this regard, it should be noted that the parathyroid gland is somewhat paradoxical with respect to secretory cells. Increased levels of extracellular calcium generally lead to increased secretion in hormone-secreting cells other than those of the parathyroid gland. Studies by Shoback et al [16], utilizing Quin-2 fluorescent probes that can detect and measure levels of intracellular, ionized calcium, have

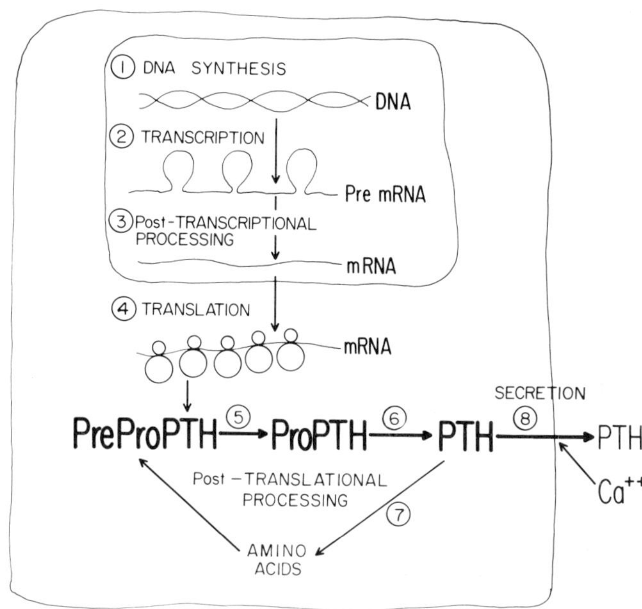

Fig. 10. Diagram of parathyroid cell depicting hypothetical steps in the formation of parathyroid hormone that may be regulated. Evidence is discussed in this chapter that regulation occurs at steps *1, 7,* and *8.*

shown that increased extracellular concentrations of calcium both suppress parathyroid hormone secretion and lead to increased concentrations of ionized (free) calcium in the cytosol. The free cytosolic calcium appears to originate from calcium stores that are bound within subcellular organelles such as the endoplasmic reticulum and mitochondria. Shoback et al [16] have also shown that in hyperplastic parathyroid glands, the set-point error in the regulation of parathyroid hormone secretion is also reflected in parallel changes in free cytosolic calcium.

Thus, when the processes involved in the regulation of parathyroid hormone secretion in both normal and hyperplastic parathyroid glands are understood at a molecular level, they should provide insights into the cellular role of calcium in the regulation of intracellular protein transport, exocytosis, and the coupling of extracellular signals to secretory processes.

Acknowledgments. I thank Gerhard Heinrich, Henry Kronenberg, and John Potts, Jr. who participated in many of these studies.

References

1. HABENER JF, POTTS JT JR: Parathyroid physiology and primary hyperparathyroidism, in *Metabolic Bone Disease,* edited by AVIOLI LV, KRANE SM, New York, Academic Press, 1978, pp 1–147

2. HABENER JF: Regulation of parathyroid hormone secretion and biosynthesis. *Ann Rev Physiol* 43:211–223, 1981
3. HABENER JF, POTTS JT JR: Clinical features of primary hyperparathyroidism, in *Endocrinology,* edited by DeGROOT LJ, CAHILL GF JR, MARTINI L, NELSON DH, ODELL WD, POTTS JT JR, STEINBERGER E, WINEGRAD AI, New York, Grune and Stratton, 1979, pp 693–701
4. HABENER JF, ROSENBLATT M, KEMPER B, KRONENBERG H, RICH A, POTTS JT JR: Pre-proparathyroid hormone: Amino acid sequence, chemical synthesis, and some biological studies of the precursor region. *Proc Natl Acad Sci USA* 75:2616–2620, 1978
5. HEINRICH G, KRONENBERG HM, POTTS JT JR, HABENER JF: Gene encoding parathyroid hormone: Nucleotide sequence of the rat gene and deduced amino acid sequence of rat pre-proparathyroid hormone. *J Biol Chem* 259:3320–3329, 1984
6. HABENER JF, ROSENBLATT M, POTTS JT JR: Parathyroid hormone: Biochemical aspects of biosynthesis, secretion, action and metabolism. *Physiol Rev* (in press, 1984)
7. HABENER JF, KEMPER B, POTTS JT JR: Calcium-dependent intracellular degradation of parathyroid hormone: A possible mechanism for the regulation of hormone stores. *Endocrinology* 97:431–441, 1975
8. COHN DV, HAMILTON JW: Newer aspects of parathyroid chemistry and physiology. *The Cornell Veterinarian* 66:1–37, 1976
9. BROWN EM, HURWITZ S, AURBACH GD: Preparation of viable isolated bovine parathyroid cells. *Endocrinology* 99:1582–1595, 1976
10. KEMPER B, HABENER JF, RICH A, POTTS JT JR: Calcium-dependent intracellular degradation of parathyroid hormone: A possible mechanism for the regulation of hormone stores. *Endocrinology* 97:431–441, 1975
11. COHN DV, ZANGERLE R, FISCHER-COLBRIE R, CHU LLH, ELTING JJ, HAMILTON JW, WINKLER H: Similarity of secretory protein I from parathyroid gland to chromogranin A from adrenal medulla. *Proc Natl Acad Sci USA* 79:6056–6059, 1982
12. HEINRICH G, KRONENBERG HM, POTTS JT JR, HABENER JF: Parathyroid hormone messenger ribonucleic acid: Effects of calcium on cellular regulation in vitro. *Endocrinology* 112:449–458, 1983
13. HAMILTON JW, SPIERTO FW, MACGREGOR RR, COHN DV: Studies on the biosynthesis in vitro of parathyroid hormone. *J Biol Chem* 240:3224–3233, 1971
14. MORRISSEY JJ, COHN DV: Regulation of secretion of parathormone and secretory protein-I from separate intracellular pools by calcium, dibutyryl cyclic amp and (1)-isoproterenol. *J Cell Biol* 82:93–102, 1979
15. BROWN EM, GARDNER DG, WINDECK RA, AURBACH GD: Relationship of intracellular 3′, 5′-adenosine monophosphate accumulation to parathyroid hormone release from dispersed bovine parathyroid cells. *Endocrinology* 103:2323–2330, 1978
16. SHOBACK DM, THATCHER J, LEOMBRUNO R, BROWN EM: Relationship between parathyroid hormone secretion and cytosolic calcium concentration in dispersed bovine parathyroid cells. *Proc Natl Acad Sci USA* 81:3113–3117, 1984
17. MAYER GP, HABENER JF, POTTS JT JR: Parathyroid hormone secretion in vivo: Demonstration of a calcium-independent, non-suppressible component of secretion. *J Clin Invest* 57:678–683, 1976
18. HABENER JF: Responsiveness of neoplastic and hyperplastic human parathyroid tissue to calcium in vitro. *J Clin Invest* 62:436–450, 1978

The Status of Parathyroid Hormone Measurements in Humans

Jan A. Fischer, Ulrich Binswanger, Walter Born, Maximilian A. Dambacher, and Fritz A. Tschopp

For diagnostic and clinical purposes, circulating parathyroid hormone (PTH) has thus far been generally estimated via radioimmunoassay (RIA). Recently, measurements of adenylate cyclase activity and a cytochemical bioassay based on the activation of renal glucose-6-phosphate dehydrogenase have been introduced into clinical medicine [1–6]. The cytochemical bioassay is the only method for detecting bioactive PTH in unextracted peripheral plasma from normal subjects [2, 3]. Alternatively, presumably bioactive PTH can be recognized in serum from normal subjects after immunoextraction and gel permeation chromatography [6–8]. The methods for extraction and separation of peptides are not yet precise; and, losses due to adsorption of PTH to glass and gels are considerable and are not entirely predictable. Recoveries of radioiodinated bovine PTH-(1–84), added to human plasma samples during the extractions, range from 30 to 70%; they may not entirely reflect the yield of the rather low amounts of endogenous PTH encountered in normal subjects. Taking these limitations into account, the concentration of intact human PTH-(1–84) in the plasma of normal subjects is of the order of 10 pg/ml or 10^{-12} M, both in the cytochemical bioassay [2, 3] and following gel filtration and analysis of an immunoreactive peak coeluting with intact PTH-(1–84) (Fig. 1) [7]. At this stage, precise measurements of absolute PTH concentrations in normal subjects are still questionable. This is critically reflected in all of the RIAs reported thus far, in which basal PTH levels in normal subjects are partly due to nonspecific inhibition of the immunologic reaction by plasma proteins, salts, or other interfering substances. This is especially true in so-called N-RIA, which supposedly measure predominantly intact PTH and NH_2-terminal PTH fragments. Nonetheless, N-RIA are very useful—not so much for the measurement of absolute PTH levels, but for the evaluation of secretory responses and treatment effects in both normal subjects and hyperparathyroid patients [9–14].

This manuscript was presented as part of a Symposium on *Parathyroid Hormone and Vitamin D in Uremia.*

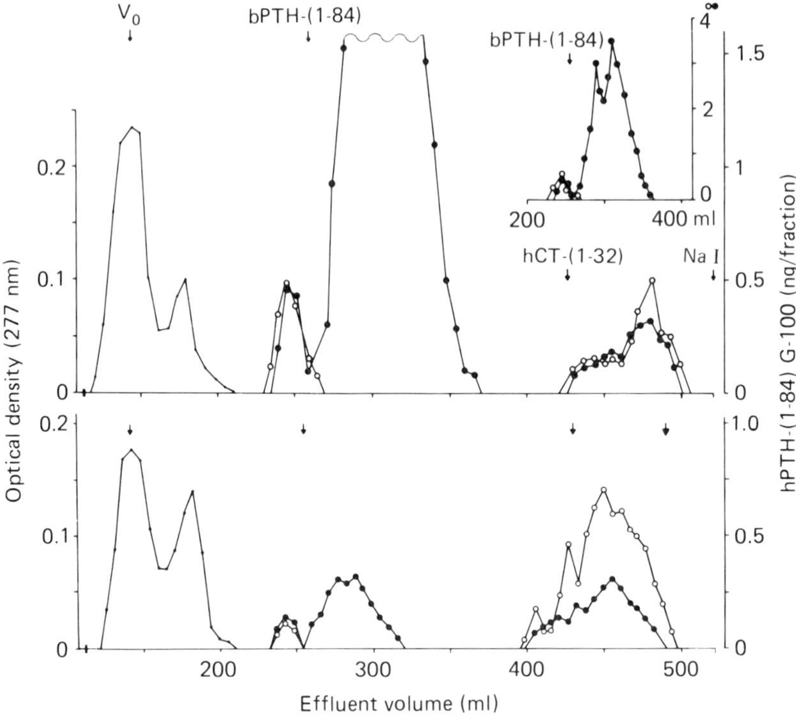

Fig. 1. Characterization of immunoreactive PTH in serum from a patient with chronic renal insufficiency (*top panel*) and from a normal subject (*bottom panel*) via chromatography on Bio-Gel P-150. [¹³¹I]bovine PTH-(1–84) [*bPTH-(1–84)*] and human calcitonin-(1–32) [*hCT-(1–32)*] were added as calibrating substances to 10-ml samples of serum (for details [7]). Optical density readings at 277 nm (●); PTH was analyzed with "N-RIA" (○), and "C-RIA" (●). (After Fischer et al [59])

In this chapter, we intend to summarize biologic measurements of circulating PTH and to emphasize the present "state of the art" of establishing RIAs for measuring PTH for diagnostic and clinical purposes. We shall conclude with an outlook related to the development of improved methodology for the study of physiologic changes of PTH in normal subjects and in disorders unrelated to hyperfunctioning parathyroid glands.

Bioassay

Ideally, the true biologic responses of circulating PTH (hypercalcemia and phosphaturia) should be quantified [15]. Unfortunately, this is impossible, since the sensitivity of the classic in vivo bioassays of PTH is several orders of magnitude too low to be physiologically and diagnostically useful. In vitro assays can be more sensitive than in vivo bioassays. However, the results obtained do not necessarily represent biologic effects recognized in vivo. The only clinically useful enzymatic assays are based on the stimulation of renal glucose-6-phosphate dehydrogenase and adenylate cyclase activity [1–6].

The cytochemical bioassay measures the activation of glucose-6-phosphate dehydrogenase of PTH via microdensitometry in distal tubule cells of segments of guinea pig kidneys [1]. Intact PTH-(1–84) is measured between 0.005 to 5 pg/ml. The predominant peak recognized on gel permeation chromatography of plasma in patients with hyperparathyroidism and normal renal function coelutes with PTH-(1–84) [2, and unpublished observations]. Moreover, fragments are detected in uremic secondary hyperparathyroidism [2]. Much like the rapid (within min) disappearance of immunoreactive intact PTH following parathyroidectomy [12, 16], PTH measured in the cytochemical bioassay had initial half-lives of disappearance ranging from 0.7 to 7.6 min [17]. The cytochemical bioassay is a research tool that is not generally available.

The measurement of adenylate cyclase activity is more simple. Besides intact PTH, a 4500 to 5000 molecular weight fragment has been detected in the serum of patients with primary hyperparathyroidism [4]. The sensitivity has been improved by the addition of 5′-guanylimidodiphosphate, and PTH has been measured in both the venous parathyroid effluent and some peripheral sera of patients with renal hyperparathyroidism [5]. Recently, immunoextraction has been introduced for estimating PTH in normal subjects [6].

Besides serum calcium and PTH measurements, the amount of cyclic AMP excreted in the urine has been established as a diagnostic tool—provided that it is related to the clearance of creatinine (C_{cr}) [18]. In terms of a biologic response, the urinary excretion of cyclic AMP—a cellular mediator of renal effects of PTH—reflects the integrated activity of PTH rather well; however, it should not necessarily be equated with a biologic effect. Conceptually, therefore, the measurement is useful for diagnostic purposes; in this context, it can be treated much like an RIA, measuring the biologic activity of PTH indirectly.

Radioimmunoassay

Berson and Yalow [19] were the first (in 1966) to report PTH measurement in the plasma of patients with hyperparathyroidism. Moreover, they recognized immunochemical heterogeneity of circulating PTH and suspected, as a cause, both metabolic alterations of the hormone and the presence of several immunoreactive components in the circulation [20]. These were subsequently discovered in cultured parathyroid explants and plasma [21–23].

Methods for measuring immunoreactive PTH in human serum or plasma have been extensively covered since Arnaud et al [24] described the first clinically useful heterologous RIA in 1971. In 1974, we reported the feasibility of generating antibodies to a crude extract of human parathyroid tumors (0.5 to 1% pure), using about 25 μg PTH injected into three goats [25]. The detailed methodology and the composition of chemicals used in RIAs recently have been summarized [26]. In the past, essential reagents, such as pure PTH used for radioiodination and suitable antibodies for the hormone, have been difficult to generate or obtain; this has now changed. At present, almost any laboratory has the possibility for developing a diagnostically valid RIA along the lines discussed in some detail here.

Radioactive Ligands

Both commercially available synthetic human PTH-(1–84) and its fragments and purified bovine PTH-(1–84) are used as radioiodinated peptides. Unfortunately, asparatate was substituted for asparagine in position 76 of human PTH-(1–84) and -[Tyr^{52}](52–84) because of an error in the initial amino acid sequence analysis [27]. In our hands, incorporation of radioactive iodine into the intact human [Asp^{76}]PTH-(1–84) was low (15 to 20%), and the ligand was not suitable in an RIA system described in Figure 2. Possibly, a [Tyr]human PTH analog not yet available may yield a higher specific activity. Several synthetic human PTH fragments can be tested in a systematic way, together with antibodies to PTH to yield a diagnostically useful RIA (see below). The workhorse of many RIAs still is radioiodinated-extracted bovine PTH.

Immunization

In the past, heterologous RIAs have proven to be excellent for the diagnosis of hyperparathyroidism [24]. However, diagnostically useful cross-reacting antibodies that detect human PTH have only exceptionally been raised, whereas homologous antisera can be readily generated [3, 6, 7, 9, 11–14, 16, 25, 26, 28–37].

We have extracted peptides that coelute with intact PTH-(1–84) and its fragments on both gel permeation and high-pressure liquid chromatography (HPLC), with a yield of 1 to 4 mg PTH/100 g human parathyroid tumors. The amount of crude extract (1 to 4% pure) obtained from 100 g parathyroid tumors is sufficient for the successful immunization of four to eight goats, rabbits, guinea pigs, or chickens by using previously described procedures [25]. We prefer to use goats, since we have been uniformly successful in raising antibodies in large quantities in every animal that was immunized. Antibodies to synthetic human PTH fragments, by definition, recognize unique antigenic determinants of the intact PTH-(1–84) molecule. Since a large fraction of circulating PTH consists of COOH-terminal PTH fragments (Fig. 1), it might be assumed that antibodies to synthetic PTH fragments are more useful than to extracted PTH. In our experience, this is not necessarily the case, because the structure of circulating PTH fragments remains to be elucidated; therefore, an ideal PTH has not yet been constructed. Crude extracts of human parathyroid tumors are likely to contain important endogenous PTH fragments, although some of them will be in small amounts.

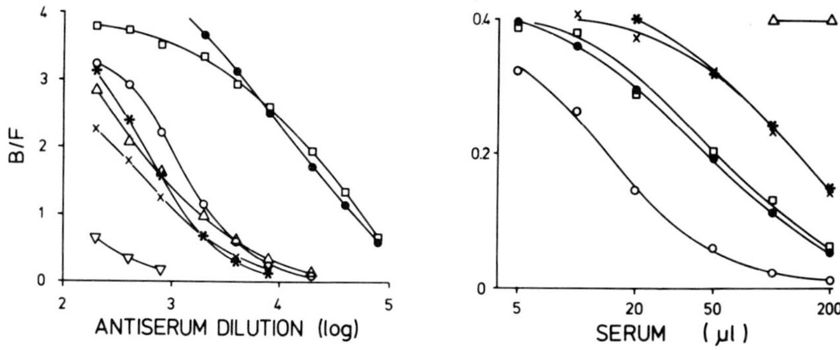

Fig. 2. Quantitative and qualitative properties of antibodies to a crude extract of human parathyroid tumors. Specific binding of [^{131}I]human PTH-[Asp^{76}](1–84) (●), -(1–34) (▽), -(1–44) (△), -[Tyr^{27}](27–48) (□), -[Tyr^{43}](43–68) (○), -[Tyr^{52},Asp^{76}](52–84) (x), and bovine PTH-(1–84) (*) (*left panel*). Inhibition of specific binding of the radioactive ligands by serum from patients with primary hyperparathyroidism (*right panel*). (After Tschopp et al [34])

Immunodilution curves of intact PTH-(1–84) and of natural and synthetic PTH fragments differ widely. Conformational properties of antigenic recognition sites probably are not the same when an identical structure is analyzed as a fragment or is contained within the sequence of the intact hormone [25]. Therefore, we prefer to immunize with extracted endogenous PTH, but we use synthetic human PTH peptides as radioactive ligands to obtain optimal sensitivity and specificity for measuring circulating PTH in humans.

Characterization of Antibodies and Immunoreactive PTH Components in Human Sera

Figure 2 illustrates quantitative and qualitative properties of antibodies, raised in a goat, to a crude extract of human parathyroid tumors [34]. The antiserum dilution, yielding 50% binding (ratio of antibody-bound [^{131}I]PTH and free [^{131}I]PTH [B:F] = 1), was determined with various PTH peptides. In this case, the antibodies recognized intact human PTH-[Asp^{76}](1–84) and the human PTH-[Tyr^{27}](27–48) fragment best followed next by human PTH-[Tyr^{43}](43–68), -(1–44), -[Tyr^{52},Asp^{76}](52–84), and bovine PTH-(1–84). Binding to human PTH-(1–34) was negligible. Since the polyclonal antibodies are not recognized to any great extent by the NH$_2$-terminal PTH-(1–34) fragment, they presumably are directed to antigenic determinants localized in the middle of and the COOH-terminal region of the intact human PTH-(1–84) molecule.

Qualitative properties of the antibodies that have been generated and their potential usefulness for radioimmunologic measurements of circulating PTH have been examined through immunodilution curves of pooled serum from patients with primary hyperparathyroidism. The optimal B:F for both sensitivity and precision ranges from 0.3 to 0.5, which equals 23 to 33% specific binding of radioactive ligands to antibodies. In this case, we have used B:F of 0.4. With [^{131}I]human PTH-[Tyr^{43}](43–68), 50% inhibition of the immunologic reaction was obtained with 15 μl hyperparathyroid serum, whereas 50 μl were required with [^{131}I]human PTH-[Asp^{76}](1–84) and -[Tyr^{27}](27–48). Circulating PTH was only minimally detected with both radioiodinated human PTH-[Tyr^{52}, Asp^{76}](52–84) and intact bovine PTH; it was not recognized with [^{131}I]human PTH-(1–44). Even though the antibodies were recognized at rather high dilution by radiolabeled intact human PTH, this RIA system was not sensitive enough for the measurement of circulating PTH in a considerable fraction of normal subjects. On the other hand, a sensitive RIA was established with relatively low titer antibodies and the use of radioiodinated human PTH-[Tyr^{42}](43–68). A related ligand has been successfully used in recently developed RIAs [29, 30].

Using gel permeation chromatography of serum from normal subjects and from patients with hyperparathyroidism, the antibodies recognize predominantly COOH-terminal PTH fragments besides a peak coeluting with intact PTH-(1–84) (Fig. 1) [7]. In terms of PTH components that were detected (using peptide separation methodology) and diagnostic and clinical implications, there appears to be no clear difference between C-RIA and midregion-RIA. C-RIA, according to the definition in this report, are directed to antigenic sites localized in the middle and COOH-terminal parts of the intact PTH-(1–84) molecule, and they recognize predominantly natural fragments from the same regions.

The N-RIA are supposed to predominantly recognize a peak coeluting with intact PTH-(1–84) and NH$_2$-terminal PTH fragments. The term "intact PTH RIA" is misleading, because additional components are always detected on gel permeation and HPLC (Fig. 1) [8, 10, 14, 25, 32, and unpublished observations]. If NH$_2$-terminal PTH fragments are indeed present in the circulation, the amounts are very low [2, 4, 8, 10, 25, 32]. The PTH peaks eluting in the vicinity of the salt peak on gel permeation chromatography are detected with some N-RIA and C-RIA (Fig. 1) [7]. The components are also present in serum from hypoparathyroid patients; therefore, they may be unrelated to the secretion and metabolism of PTH and may be caused by salts eluting in the same column-effluent fractions. A useful homologous PTH-(1–34) RIA that measures secretory responses in normal subjects has recently been developed [9]. As with the cytochemical bioassay (but using more convenient methodology), N-RIA detect minute-to-minute changes in serum PTH levels in normal subjects and hyperparathyroid patients [9, 13, 14].

Standards

Relatively close results have been obtained both with purified human PTH-(1–84) and with a crude extract of human parathyroid tumors distributed among 29 laboratories by the National Institute for Biological Standards and Control in London. This was not the case with tissue-culture PTH and plasma diafiltrate, which yield a wide range of values based on nonparallel immunodilution curves with respect to purified PTH [36]. Since COOH-terminal PTH fragments are most often recognized with the presently available diagnostically useful RIAs, this result is not unexpected. Therefore, it is mandatory that immunodilution curves from unknown serum or plasma samples yield parallel displacement curves with the standard used, regardless of the absolute values obtained. The use of pooled human hyperparathyroid serum, plasma diafiltrate from a patient with chronic renal failure, tissue-culture medium of human parathyroid tumors in primary culture, purified human tumor extracts, and synthetic PTH peptides as standards have all been documented with parallel displacement curves to hyperparathyroid plasma and serum and to column-effluent fractions [7, 12, 24, 25, 28, 37, 38]. Unknown samples are analyzed in several dilutions to ascertain parallel inhibition curves comparable to the standards used. For practical purposes, duplicate or multiple determinations are less meaningful and are not required.

The PTH measurements obtained in different laboratories can only be compared if the same reagents are used [39]. Even then, the precision obtained in a study of 21 participating investigators was poor in some laboratories.

Normal Levels

The PTH values of unextracted serum estimated in N-RIA that was developed with extracted PTH as antigen usually are one order of magnitude higher than the levels of intact PTH-(1–84) recognized with peptide separation methodology and the cytochemical bioassay [2, 3, 7, 11, 14, 32]. Normal values are somewhat lower after immunoextraction of serum [6]. The antibodies recognize considerable amounts of nonidentified fragments besides intact PTH-(1–84), especially in peripheral serum of patients with renal failure. The normal values reported also are partly due to nonspecific inhibition of the immunologic reaction by plasma or serum that is present in up to 46% of concentrations during incubations in the RIA. In homologous human PTH-(1–34) RIAs, a synthetic fragment is used as a standard and the results obtained are not measured against native PTH [9, 12, 13, 28].

So-called "normal" serum or plasma levels of PTH in both N-RIA and C-RIA are primarily used to discriminate normal subjects from hyperparathyroid patients with raised serum levels of immunoreactive PTH. Indeed, the degree of overlap between PTH levels in normal subjects and patients with primary hyperparathyroidism should not exceed 10% [24, 40, 41].

Interpretation of RIA Results

Predominant circulating PTH peptides are immunoreactive (4000 to 7000 molecular weight) COOH-terminal breakdown products of the hormone that are biologically inactive, as measured in both the cytochemical and renal adenylate cyclase bioassays [2, 4]. Similar, if not identical, fragments are secreted by the parathyroid glands; however, they are also generated after

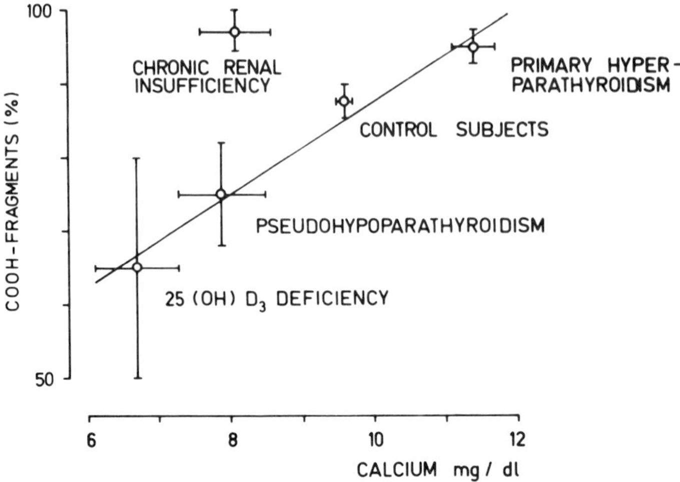

Fig. 3. Fractional levels (with SEM) of COOH-terminal PTH fragments as a function of calcium in the serum of control subjects and hyperparathyroid patients. Concentrations of intact PTH-(1–84) and COOH-terminal fragments were measured after gel permeation chromatography on Bio-Gel P-150 (see Fig. 1 and [7]) in patients with nutritional 25-hydroxyvitamin D-deficiency ($N = 6$), pseudohypoparathyroidism ($N = 9$), primary hyperparathyroidism ($N = 8$), and chronic renal insufficiency ($N = 10$); and, in control subjects ($N = 5$).

intravenous (i.v.) administration of PTH into cows, as well as during perfusions of the liver and the kidneys with exogenous bovine PTH-(1–84) [42–45]. COOH-terminal fragments are secreted by the parathyroid glands in proportionally larger amounts at high- than at low-extracellular calcium concentrations [46, 47]. Similarly, the proportion of COOH-terminal fragments in peripheral serum is related to the calcium concentration, provided that the renal function is normal (Fig. 3) [7]. As a result, the levels of COOH-terminal fragments are higher in patients with hypercalcemia and primary hyperparathyroidism than in patients with secondary hyperparathyroidism due to vitamin D deficiency or pseudohypoparathyroidism (Fig. 4). Since the metabolic clearance rate of exogenously administered intact PTH-(1–84) in dogs is the same at low- and at high-serum calcium concentrations [48], the biologically inactive fragments are most likely secreted by the parathyroid glands in a calcium-dependent manner concomitant with an inhibition of PTH secretion.

Rates of disappearance of PTH after parathyroidectomy or exogenous administration of PTH in humans are prolonged in patients with end-stage renal disease (ESRD) failure [20, 49, 50]. COOH-terminal PTH fragments mainly are catabolized by the kidneys, and they accumulate in the circulation of patients with chronic renal failure (Fig. 1). As a result, absolute levels and fractional amounts of the fragments are particularly high in patients with chronic renal failure who are on hemodialysis (Figs. 3, 4) [7].

Subtle increases in levels of PTH in C-RIA in persons of advanced age

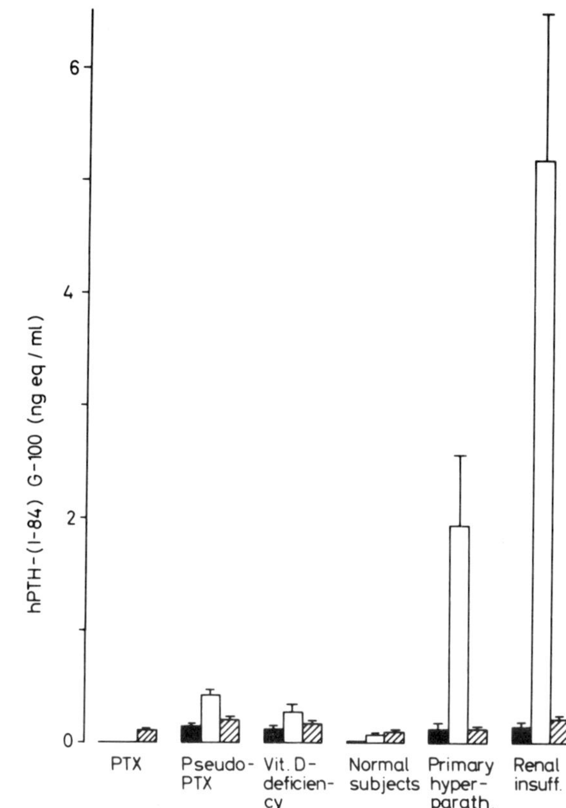

Fig. 4. Levels (with SEM) of intact PTH-(1–84) (■), COOH-terminal PTH fragments with 4000–7000 mol wt (□), and less than 4000 (▨), all measured after gel permeation chromatography on Bio-Gel P-150 (see Fig. 1 and [7]). The PTX ($N = 5$) are patients with hypoparathyroidism following parathyroidectomy; the other subjects are mentioned in Figure 3.

are partly caused by accumulation of biologically inactive fragments with deteriorating renal function, and they may not be due to hyperfunctioning parathyroid glands [35, 51–55]. However, poor nutritional intake of calcium and vitamin D may cause secondary hyperparathyroidism in the elderly [56].

Comparison of N-RIA and C-RIA

Arnaud et al [57] pointed out that the overlap of PTH measurements in normal subjects and hyperparathyroid patients was smaller with C-RIA than N-RIA; the later was particularly suitable for monitoring rapid changes in PTH secretion. A better recognition of raised PTH levels in C-RIA than in N-RIA, although generally true, is not always perceived [58, 59]. Serum levels of intact PTH-(1–84) estimated radioimmunologically after gel permeation chromatography are about 10 pg/ml in normal subjects [7], whereas those measured by N-RIA in unextracted serum usually are at least one order of magnitude higher. COOH-terminal fragments are present in higher absolute amounts than intact PTH. Therefore, serum levels of normal subjects estimated in C-RIA are less likely (than in N-RIA) to be due to nonspecific inhibition of the immunologic reaction. As a consequence, the sensitivity required to measure actual circulating levels of PTH in normal subjects is more likely to be achieved with C-RIA than with N-RIA. Moreover, the late eluting peaks prominently recognized in serum from normal subjects, but also in patients with hypoparathyroidism, probably are biologically inactive; however, they represent the highest fractional amounts of serum PTH levels estimated in a N-RIA in normal subjects (Fig. 1).

Dynamic changes in parathyroid secretory function can be better evaluated with N-RIA than with C-RIA. Rates of disappearance of PTH after parathyroidectomy were much faster when estimated in N-RIA than in C-RIA [16]. In response to calcium infusions, more marked suppression of PTH levels was observed in peripheral serum from patients with end-stage renal failure within 1 hr with N-RIA than with C-RIA [10, 13]. On gel filtration analysis of the venous parathyroid effluent, the levels of intact PTH-(1–84) were suppressed in response to 10-min calcium infusions, whereas the secretion of COOH-terminal fragments was inhibited more slowly [14]. This finding is in contrast with results obtained with the exogenous administration of bovine PTH-(1–84) in calves, in whom the rate of disappearance of intact PTH was only slightly faster than the COOH-terminal fragments that were generated [43]. Besides suppressing the release of PTH-(1–84), calcium may also enhance the conversion of intact PTH into COOH-terminal biologically inactive fragments, thus counterbalancing the hypercalcemic effects of the hormone [46, 47]. During long-term treatment of chronic renal failure patients with 1,25-dihydroxyvitamin D_3, PTH returned toward the normal range with increasing serum calcium concentrations. Mean PTH levels decreased by 34% ($P < 0.05$) when measured in a N-RIA, but only by 13% ($P > 0.1$) in a C-RIA [11]. Clearly, N-RIAs are more suitable than C-RIA for monitoring acute secretory changes of PTH and treatment effects.

Conclusions and Outlook

Circulating PTH is measured both with in vitro bioassays (stimulation of adenylate cyclase and glucose-6-phosphate dehydrogenase activity) and radioimmunology. Biologically active intact PTH-(1–84) is recognized in plasma from hyperparathyroid patients on gel permeation chromatography, in combination with the adenylate cyclase, and in the cytochemical bioassays [2, 4]. Biologically active NH_2-terminal PTH fragments probably are present in smaller relative amounts. The concentration of circulating PTH in the cytochemical bioassay in normal subjects is about 10 pg/ml [1–3]. The levels are somewhat higher in immunoextracted serum analyzed in the adenylate cyclase assay [6]. The throughput, especially of the cytochemical bioassay, is low and the assay requires considerable skill on the part of the investigator. The amounts of immunoreactive PTH in a peak that coelutes with intact PTH-(1–84) on gel permeation chromatography also are about 10 pg/ml [7]. The methodology is tedious and requires 50 to 100 ml of plasma to be extracted. Immunoreactive PTH levels in unextracted human plasma or serum from normal subjects usually are one order of magnitude higher, even in N-RIA presumed to recognize predominantly biologically active PTH. They are partly due to nonspecific inhibition of the immunologic reaction by proteins and salts that are present in plasma incubated up to a 46% concentration in several otherwise diagnostically useful RIAs. The PTH responses to hypocalcemia and hypercalcemia can be assessed in normal subjects in a qualitative manner. Quantitative changes in the levels of intact PTH-(1–84) have not yet been investigated by using peptide separation methodology in combination with RIAs or bioassays. To assess physiologic changes of PTH both in normal subjects and in disorders unrelated to hyperfunctioning parathyroid glands, extraction of PTH from plasma probably is mandatory, since none of the available RIAs and the adenylate cyclase assay permit PTH-(1–84) to be analyzed directly in normal subjects.

The levels of both intact PTH-(1–84) and the 4000 to 7000 molecular weight COOH-terminal fragments are raised in the plasma and serum of patients with hyperparathyroidism. Predominant components are the biologically inactive COOH-terminal PTH fragments. In view of the higher amounts of COOH-terminal fragments present in relation to intact PTH-(1–84), the fragments are more easily detected radioimmunologically. Therefore, C-RIA serve rather well to discriminate serum levels of PTH in both normal subjects and patients with hypercalcemia and tumors unrelated to the parathyroid glands from those patients with hyperparathyroidism. Following parathyroidectomy, or in response to calcium infusions, the levels of intact PTH are lowered within minutes, whereas COOH-terminal PTH fragments remain in the circulation longer. Rapid secretory changes and suppression of PTH levels within minutes can be assessed rather well in hyperparathyroid patients by using N-RIA, but not C-RIA. COOH-terminal PTH fragments are mainly catabolized by the kidneys, and they accumulate in the circulation of elderly subjects and in patients with end-stage renal failure. It is obvious that N-RIAs, which do not recognize the 4000 to 7000 molecular weight COOH-terminal fragments to any great extent, may be more suitable than C-RIAs for monitoring secretory changes; for example, in response to treatment with D vitamins in patients with chronic renal insufficiency.

Acknowledgments. This work was supported by the Swiss National Science Foundation grants 3.813-0.81 and 3.932-0.82, the Kanton Zürich, and the Schweizerische Verein Balgrist.

References

1. CHAYEN J: Parathyroid hormone, in *The Cytochemical Bioassay of Polypeptide Hormones,* Berlin, Springer-Verlag, 1980, pp 156–165
2. GOLTZMAN D, HENDERSON B, LOVERIDGE N: Cytochemical bioassay of parathyroid hormone. Characteristics of the assay and analysis of circulating hormonal forms. *J Clin Invest* 65:1309–1317, 1980
3. NAGANT DE DEUXCHAISNES C, FISCHER JA, DAMBACHER MA, DEVOGELAER

JP, ARBER CE, ZANELLI JM, PARSONS JA, LOVERIDGE N, BITENSKY L, CHAYEN
J: Dissociation of parathyroid hormone bioactivity and immunoreactivity in pseudohypoparathyroidism type I. *J Clin Endocrinol Metab* 53:1105–1109, 1981
4. CANTERBURY JM, LEVEY GS, REISS E: Activation of renal cortical adenylate
cyclase by circulating immunoreactive parathyroid hormone fragments. *J Clin
Invest* 52:524–527, 1973
5. NISSENSON RA, ABBOTT SR, TEITELBAUM AP, CLARK OH, ARNAUD CD: Endogenous biologically active human parathyroid hormone: Measurement by a
guanyl nucleotide-amplified renal adenylate cyclase assay. *J Clin Endocrinol Metab*
52:840–846, 1981
6. LINDALL AW, ELTING J, ELLS J, ROOS BA: Estimation of biologically active
intact parathyroid hormone in normal and hyperparathyroid sera by sequential
N-terminal immunoextraction and midregion radioimmunoassay. *J Clin Endocrinol Metab* 57:1007–1014, 1983
7. DAMBACHER MA, FISCHER JA, HUNZIKER WH, BORN W, MORAN J, ROTH
HR, DEVIN EE, GLORIEUX FH: Distribution of circulating immunoreactive components of parathyroid hormone in normal subjects and in patients with primary
and secondary hyperparathyroidism: The role of the kidney and of the serum
calcium concentration. *Clin Sci* 57:435–443, 1979
8. ROOS BA, LINDALL AW, ARON DC, ORF JW, YOON M, HUBER MB, PENSKY
J, ELLS J, LAMBERT PW: Detection and characterization of small midregion
parathyroid hormone fragment(s) in normal and hyperparathyroid glands and
sera by immunoextraction and region-specific radioimmunoassays. *J Clin Endocrinol Metab* 53:709–721, 1981
9. SEGRE GV: Amino-terminal radioimmunoassays for human parathyroid hormone,
in *Clinical Disorders of Bone and Mineral Metabolism,* edited by FRAME B, POTTS
JT JR, Amsterdam, Excerpta Medica, 1983, pp 14–17
10. GOLDSMITH RS, FURSZYFER J, JOHNSON WJ, FOURNIER AE, SIZEMORE GW,
ARNAUD CD: Etiology of hyperparathyroidism and bone disease during chronic
hemodialysis. *J Clin Invest* 52:173–180, 1973
11. BINSWANGER U, FISCHER JA, ISELIN H, OSWALD N, KEUSCH G, FREI D,
WILLIMANN P: 1,25-dihydroxycholecalciferol treatment of clinically asymptomatic renal osteodystrophy. *Min Electr Metab* 2:103–115, 1979
12. PAPAPOULOS SE, MANNING RM, HENDY GN, LEWIN IG, O'RIORDAN JLH:
Studies of circulating parathyroid hormone in man using a homologous amino-
terminal specific immunoradiometric assay. *Clin Endocrinol* 13:57–67, 1980
13. ADAMI S, MUIRHEAD N, MANNING RM, GLEED JH, PAPAPOULOS SE, SANDLER
LM, CATTO GRD, O'RIORDAN JLH: Control of secretion of parathyroid hormone
in secondary hyperparathyroidism. *Clin Endocrinol* 16:463–473, 1982
14. BORN W, DAMBACHER MA, MEYRIER A, ARDAILLOU R, FISCHER JA: Parathyroid suppressibility in hyperparathyroidism due to chronic renal failure: Studies
with autotransplanted parathyroid tissue. *Clin Endocrinol* 17:333–343, 1982
15. FISCHER JA: Parathyroid hormone, in *Disorders of Mineral Metabolism,* edited
by BRONNER F, COBURN JW, New York, Academic Press, 1982, pp 271–358
16. MANNING RM, ADAMI S, PAPAPOULOS SE, GLEED JH, HENDY GN, ROSEN-
BLATT M, O'RIORDAN JLH: A carboxy-terminal specific assay for human parathyroid hormone. *Clin Endocrinol* 15:439–449, 1981
17. GOLTZMAN D, GOMOLIN H, DELEAN A, WEXLER M, MEAKINS JL: Discordant
disappearance of bioactive and immunoreactive parathyroid hormone after parathyroidectomy. *J Clin Endocrinol Metab* 58:70–75, 1984
18. BROADUS AE: Nephrogenous cyclic AMP. *Rec Progr Horm Res* 37:667–695,
1981
19. BERSON SA, YALOW RS: Parathyroid hormone in plasma in adenomatous hyperparathyroidism, uremia, and bronchogenic carcinoma. *Science* 154:907–909, 1966

20. BERSON SA, YALOW RS: Immunochemical heterogeneity of parathyroid hormone in plasma. *J Clin Endocrinol Metab* 28:1037–1047, 1968
21. SHERWOOD LM, RODMAN JS, LUNDBERG WB: Evidence for a precursor to circulating parathyroid hormone. *Proc Natl Acad Sci USA* 67:1631–1638, 1970
22. ARNAUD CD, SIZEMORE GW, OLDHAM SB, FISCHER JA, TSAO HS, LITTLEDIKE ET: Human parathyroid hormone: Glandular and secreted molecular species. *Am J Med* 50:630–638, 1971
23. HABENER JF, POWELL D, MURRAY TM, MAYER GP, POTTS JT JR: Parathyroid hormone: Secretion and metabolism in vivo. *Proc Natl Acad Sci USA* 68:2986–2991, 1971
24. ARNAUD CD, TSAO HS, LITTLEDIKE T: Radioimmunoassay of human parathyroid hormone in serum. *J Clin Invest* 50:21–34, 1971
25. FISCHER JA, BINSWANGER U, DIETRICH FM: Human parathyroid hormone. Immunological characterization of antibodies against a glandular extract and the synthetic amino-terminal fragments 1–12 and 1–34 and their use in the determination of immunoreactive hormone in human sera. *J Clin Invest* 54:1382–1394, 1974
26. BIKLE DD (editor): *Assay of Calcium-Regulating Hormones,* New York, Springer-Verlag, 1983, pp 151–227
27. HENDY GN, KRONENBERG HM, POTTS JT JR, RICH A: Nucleotide sequence of cloned cDNAs encoding human preproparathyroid. *Proc Natl Acad Sci USA* 78:7365–7396, 1981
28. DESPLAN C, JULLIENNE A, MOUKHTAR MS, MILHAUD G: Sensitive assay for biologically active fragment of human parathyroid hormone. *Lancet* 2:198–199, 1977
29. ATKINSON MJ, NIEPEL B, JUEPPNER H, BUTZ R, CASARETTO M, ZAHN H, HEHRMANN R, HESCH RD: Homologous radioimmunoassay for human mid-regional parathyroid hormone. *J Endocrinol Invest* 4:363–366, 1981
30. MARX SJ, SHARP ME, KRUDY A, ROSENBLATT M, MALLETTE LE: Radioimmunoassay for the middle region of human parathyroid hormone: studies with a radioiodinated synthetic peptide. *J Clin Endocrinol Metab* 53:76–84, 1981
31. MALLETTE LE, TUMA SN, BERGER RE, KIRKLAND JL: Radioimmunoassay for the middle region of human parathyroid hormone using an homologous antiserum with a carboxy-terminal fragment of bovine parathyroid hormone as radioligand. *J Clin Endocrinol Metab* 54:1017–1024, 1982
32. DI BELLA FP, HAWKER CD: Parathyrin (parathyroid hormone): Radioimmunoassays for intact and carboxyl-terminal moieties. *Clin Chem* 28:226–235, 1982
33. HITZLER W, SCHMIDT-GAYK H, SPIROPOULOS P, RAUE F, HUEFNER M: Homologous radioimmunoassay for human parathyrin (residues 53–84). *Clin Chem* 28:1749–1753, 1982
34. TSCHOPP FA, DAMBACHER MA, FISCHER JA: The contribution of synthetic human parathyroid hormone and of its fragments to parathyroid hormone measurements, in *Clinical Disorders of Bone and Mineral Metabolism,* edited by FRAME B, POTTS JT JR, Amsterdam, Excerpta Medica, 1983, pp 18–19
35. BINSWANGER U: 1,25 dihydroxycholecalciferol in patients with renal failure: The case against its prophylactic use, in *Controversies in Nephrology and Hypertension,* edited by NARINS RG, New York, Churchill Livingstone, 1984 (in press)
36. ZANELLI JM, GAINES-DAS RE: The first international reference preparation of human parathyroid hormone for immunoassay: characterization and calibration by international collaborative study. *J Clin Endocrinol Metab* 57:462–469, 1983
37. STREIBL W, MINNE H, RAUE F, ZIEGLER R: Radioimmunoassay for human parathyroid hormone for differentiation between patients with hypoparathyroidism, hyperparathyroidism and normals. *Horm Metab Res* 11:375–376, 1979
38. STOEGMANN W, FISCHER JA: Pseudohypoparathyroidism: Disappearance of the

resistance to parathyroid extract during treatment with vitamin D. *Am J Med* 59:140–144, 1975

39. MINNE HW: Quality control in parathyroid hormone radioimmunoassays: A multicentre study performed by the European Parathyroid Hormone Study Group. *Europ J Clin Invest* 14:16–23, 1984

40. RAISZ LG, YAJNIK CH, BOCKMAN RS, BOWER BF: Comparison of commercially available parathyroid hormone immunoassays in the differential diagnosis of hypercalcemia due to primary hyperparathyroidism or malignancy. *Ann Intern Med* 91:739–740, 1979

41. GOROG RH, HAKIM MK, THOMPSON NW, RIGG GA, McCANN DS: Radioimmunoassay of serum parathyrin: comparison of five commercial kits. *Clin Chem* 28:87–91, 1982

42. FLUECK JA, DI BELLA FP, EDIS AJ, KEHRWALD JM, ARNAUD CD: Immunoheterogeneity of parathyroid hormone in venous effluent serum from hyperfunctioning parathyroid glands. *J Clin Invest* 60:1367–1375, 1977

43. HUNZIKER W, BLUM JW, FISCHER JA: Plasma kinetics of exogenous bovine parathyroid hormone in calves. *Pflügers Arch* 371:185–192, 1977

44. CANTERBURY JM, BRICKER LA, LEVEY GS, KOZLOVSKIS PL, RUIZ E, ZULL JE, REISS E: Metabolism of bovine parathyroid hormone. Immunological and biological characteristics of fragments generated by liver perfusion. *J Clin Invest* 55:1245–1253, 1975

45. HRUSKA KA, MARTIN K, MENNES P, GREENWALT A, ANDERSON C, KLAHR S, SLATOPOLSKY E: Degradation of parathyroid hormone and fragment production by the isolated perfused dog kidney. *J Clin Invest* 60:501–510, 1977

46. HANLEY DA, TAKATSUKI K, SULTAN JM, SCHNEIDER AB, SHERWOOD LM: Direct release of parathyroid hormone fragments from functioning bovine parathyroid glands in vitro. *J Clin Invest* 62:1247–1254, 1978

47. MAYER GP, KEATON JA, HURST JG, HABENER JF: Effects of plasma calcium concentration on the relative proportion of hormone and carboxyl fragments in parathyroid venous blood. *Endocrinology* 104:1778–1784, 1979

48. FOX J, SCOTT M, NISSENSON RA, HEATH H III: Effect of plasma calcium concentration on the metabolic clearance rate of parathyroid hormone in the dog. *J Lab Clin Med* 102:70–77, 1983

49. FREITAG J, MARTIN KJ, HRUSKA KA, ANDERSON C, CONRADES M, LADENSON J, KLAHR S, SLATOPOLSKY E: Impaired parathyroid hormone metabolism in patients with chronic renal failure. *N Engl J Med* 298:29–32, 1978

50. MELICK RA, MARTIN TJ: Parathyroid hormone metabolism in man: Effect of nephrectomy. *Clin Sci* 37:667–674, 1969

51. WISKE PS, EPSTEIN S, BELL NH, QUEENER SF, EDMUNDSON J, JOHNSTON CC JR: Increases in immunoreactive parathyroid hormone with age. *N Engl J Med* 300:1419–1421, 1979

52. GALLAGHER JC, RIGGS BL, JERPBAK CM, ARNAUD CD: The effect of age on serum immunoreactive parathyroid hormone in normal and osteoporotic women. *J Lab Clin Med* 95:373–385, 1980

53. DELMAS PD, STENNER D, WAHNER HW, MANN KG, RIGGS BL: Increase in serum bone γ-carboxyglutamic acid protein with aging in women: Implications for the mechanism of age-related bone loss. *J Clin Invest* 71:1316–1321, 1983

54. FRANCIS RM, PEACOCK M, STORER JH, DAVIES AEJ, BROWN WB, NORDIN BEC: Calcium malabsorption in the elderly: The effect of treatment with oral 25-hydroxyvitamin D_3. *Europ J Clin Invest* 13:391–396, 1983

55. MARCUS R, MADVIG P, YOUNG G: Age-related changes in parathyroid hormone and parathyroid hormone action in normal humans. *J Clin Endocrinol Metab* 58:223–230, 1984

56. PETERSEN MM, BRIGGS RS, ASHBY MA, REID RI, HALL MR, WOOD PJ, CLAYTON BE: Parathyroid hormone and 25-hydroxyvitamin D concentrations in sick and normal elderly people. *Br Med J* 287:521–523, 1983
57. ARNAUD CD, GOLDSMITH RS, BORDIER PJ, SIZEMORE GW, LARSEN JA, GILKINSON J: Influence of immunoheterogeneity of circulating parathyroid hormone on results of radioimmunoassays of serum in man. *Am J Med* 56:785–793, 1974
58. MARTIN KJ, HRUSKA K, FREITAG J, BELLORIN-FONT E, KLAHR S, SLATOPOLSKY E: Clinical utility of radioimmunoassays for parathyroid hormone. *Min Electr Metab* 3:283–290, 1980
59. FISCHER JA, DAMBACHER MA, BORN W, BINSWANGER U: Circulating parathyroid hormone components and interpretation of radioimmunoassay results in normal subjects and in hyperparathyroid patients. *Adv Nephrol* 11:91–204, 1982

Parathyroid Hormone: Alterations in Chronic Renal Failure

Eduardo Slatopolsky, Kevin J. Martin, Jeremiah J. Morrissey, and Keith A. Hruska

In the last 10 years, investigators have made great progress in the understanding of calcium homeostasis in living organisms. The regulation of calcium metabolism in the body involves precise control of the level of ionized calcium in the blood and maintenance of a normal skeleton. The regulation of calcium homeostasis depends on two closely inter-related hormonal systems: parathyroid hormone (PTH) and vitamin D. This chapter will focus primarily on PTH, which is the hormone responsible for the control of ionized calcium on a minute-to-minute basis. Parathyroid hormone exerts important effects on kidney and bone, and it indirectly affects the intestine. With the development of region-specific radioimmunoassays that can determine not only the intact PTH molecule (PTH 1–84), but also amino-(N) and carboxy-(C) terminal fragments of the PTH molecule, investigators have greatly advanced their understanding of the peripheral metabolism of PTH. The remarkable relationship between PTH and the kidney is clearly demonstrated in patients with renal insufficiency. Secondary hyperparathyroidism is a universal finding in patients with renal insufficiency. Chief cell hyperplasia of the parathyroid glands and high levels of immunoreactive parathyroid hormone (i-PTH) are among the earliest alterations of mineral metabolism in patients with chronic renal failure. Significant elevations of i-PTH in serum have been reported in patients with only slightly abnormal renal function (glomerular filtration rate [GFR] 60 to 80 ml/min).

Although many factors are responsible for regulation of the secretion of PTH, it appears that in patients with renal insufficiency, the most important factor for the development of secondary hyperparathyroidism is a reduction in the serum-ionized calcium. Factors that may contribute to hypocalcemia and to the development of secondary hyperparathyroidism in renal insufficiency include: (1) retention of phosphorus, (2) altered vitamin D metabolism, (3) skeletal resistance to the calcemic action of PTH, (4) altered set point

This manuscript was presented as part of a Symposium on *Parathyroid Hormone and Vitamin D in Uremia.*

for calcium-regulated PTH release, and (5) impaired degradation of PTH. Moreover, the high levels of circulating immunoassayable PTH not only may produce the well-known changes in the skeleton characterized by osteitis fibrosa, but they also may affect other organs. The aim of this chapter is to review the secretion, metabolism, and radioimmunoassay of PTH in health and renal disease.

Synthesis, Structure, and Secretion of Parathyroid Hormone

Parathyroid hormone is a single-chain protein of 84 amino acids [1]. The hormone is initially synthesized in the rough endoplasmic reticulum of the parathyroid chief cell as the 115-amino acid precursor, pre-pro-PTH [2]. This precursor is converted within seconds of synthesis to another hormone precursor, pro-PTH, which contains 90 amino acids [3]. The pro-PTH, in turn, is converted to PTH 1–84 by proteolytic cleavage at/or in the vicinity of the Golgi region of the cell [3, 4]. This conversion occurs approximately 15 min after biosynthesis of the original pre-pro-PTH and about 5 min prior to hormone secretion.

The concentration of the calcium ion in the extracellular space is the primary factor that controls the secretion of PTH [5, 6]. Hypocalcemia is the most potent stimulus for the secretion of PTH. Conversely, hypercalcemia suppresses PTH secretion. However, the secretion of PTH is not completely suppressed during hypercalcemia, and a basal rate of secretion of the hormone persists [7, 8]. In addition to a decrease in hormone secretion, an increase in calcium decreases parathyroid cell cyclic adenosine monophosphate (cyclic AMP) levels [9, 10] or adenylate cyclase activity of isolated parathyroid membranes [11–15]. A complicating issue of parathyroid research is whether the increase in extracellular calcium primarily affects cellular cyclic AMP levels, which subsequently affects hormone secretion, or whether this calcium-mediated parathyroid function is an epiphenomenon to hormone secretion.

The concentration of magnesium ions also influences, through an inverse relationship, the secretion of PTH [6, 16]. Physiologically, however, severe hypomagnesemia has been found to inhibit hormone secretion and to be more clinically relevant than suppression of PTH by hypermagnesemia [17–21].

There is increasing evidence that a variety of agents, other than calcium, may secondarily modify PTH secretion by affecting the cyclic AMP level of parathyroid cells [9, 22].

A number of studies have suggested that the majority of calcium-regulated PTH that is secreted is obtained from a recently synthesized pool of protein that is not in rapid equilibrium with the bulk of the hormone stored in the cell [10, 23–26]. Beta agonist-stimulated hormone secretion, which is cyclic AMP mediated, will take place in the presence of a protein synthesis inhibitor, suggesting that this occurs from a pool of previously synthesized older protein [27]. Phenomenologically, stimulation of hormone secretion by hypocalcemia—as opposed to stimulation by agents that operate through cyclic AMP—appear to occur through different mechanisms [10, 28, 29]. Studies describing the manner in which calcium and cyclic AMP-mediated secretagogues affect PTH secretion suggest that there are two cellular pools of hormone available for secretion (Fig. 1). Ionized calcium affects the secretion from both a newly synthesized and an older pool of hormone [23]. Agents that influence cellular cyclic AMP levels, on the other hand, seem to affect secretion from an older pool of stored hormone [23]. The net amount of hormone secreted from each pool is not precisely known.

Calcium is an inhibitor of the adenylate cyclase activity of isolated parathyroid membranes [11–15]. Membranes prepared from hyperplastic glands are less susceptible to the inhibition of enzyme activity by calcium than are membranes prepared from normal human parathyroid tissue [14]. This suggests that the "set point for calcium" (the calcium ion concentration causing a 50% decrease in overall hormone secretion) for inhibiting parathyroid adenylate cyclase is elevated above normal in hyperfunctioning human parathyroid glands. The magnesium ion concentration also influences the ability of calcium to inhibit the adenylate cyclase of membranes derived from both normal and hyperplastic parathyroid glands [14]. An increase in the magnesium concentration led to an increase in the set point for calcium to inhibit the generation of cyclic AMP. These results have been qualitatively confirmed in another laboratory [15]. Since calcium-mediated changes in cellular cyclic

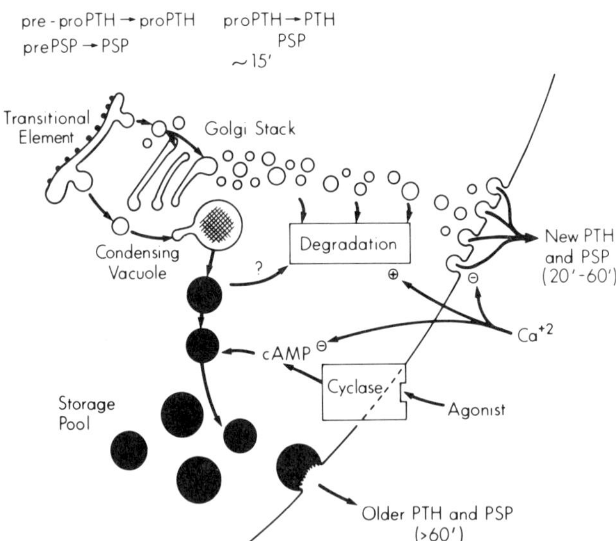

Fig. 1. Cellular pathways in the parathyroid cell for the secretion of PTH. Calcium primarily affects the secretion of newly synthesized PTH, while agents that influence cellular cyclic AMP levels affect the secretion of stored (older) hormone. This diagram summarizes aspects of hormone secretion. (From [2–4, 9, 10, 23, 25])

AMP cannot account for all the calcium-induced changes in hormone secretion, it is suggested that the elevated calcium set point for inhibition of adenylate cyclase is a general manifestation of the hyperplastic state.

In addition to the altered set point for the inhibition by calcium ofparathyroid adenylate cyclase in membranes obtained from hyperfunctioning human glands, there is an altered set point for calcium in the inhibition of hormone secretion [30–34]. The accumulated data obtained for collagenase-dispersed human parathyroid cells indicates a set point in normal cells of 0.97 ± 0.04 mM calcium ion; while in adenoma, primary hyperplasia, and secondary hyperplasia, the set point was found to be increased to 1.26 ± 0.13 mM, 1.09 ± 0.15 mM, and 1.17 ± 0.19 mM calcium ion, respectively [34]. Not only is the set point for calcium, with respect to hormone secretion, elevated in cells obtained from hyperplastic parathyroid tissue, but also the degree of responsiveness across the calcium-sensitive range is altered. The degree of suppression of hormone secretion with increasing calcium apparently is lower for cells obtained from all types of hyperplastic glands than for cells from normal glands [34]. Thus, several factors can lead to elevated serum PTH levels in humans. These include an increase in tissue mass through cell hypertrophy and/or hyperplasia, an increase in the set point for calcium to inhibit hormone secretion, and a change in the degree of suppression by calcium throughout the calcium-sensitive range (that is, the slope of the suppression line). These factors are diagramatically illustrated in Figure 2. The relative secretion rate of parathyroid hormone from a normal gland and a gland that has doubled in size is depicted in Figure 2A. The individual cells of the enlarged gland (Fig. 2) have retained both a normal set point for calcium and their normal sharp responsiveness to calcium to suppress secretion. In this case, serum hormone levels will be increased by an amount that is proportional to the increase in tissue mass at any calcium ion concentration; that is, provided there are no changes in the peripheral metabolism of the hormone. While each cell is operating in an essentially normal manner,

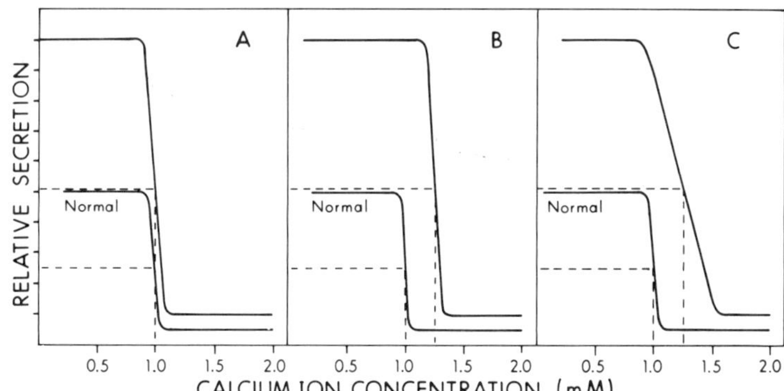

Fig. 2. Diagramatic representation of factors contributing to abnormal PTH secretion. For description, see the text. (From Morrissey et al, in *Proc 6th Int Workshop on Phosphate and Other Minerals,* Verona, Italy, 1983)

the increase in the number of cells causes the hyperparathyroidism. Since there is a nonsuppressible component to hormone secretion, there will be increased circulating hormones even in severe hypercalcemia. In Figure 2B, in addition to an increase in tissue mass, there also is depicted the relative secretion rate when the set point for suppression is increased from the normal 1.0 to 1.25 mM calcium. The slope of the calcium suppression remains normal. In this situation, the hyperparathyroidism is a product of both the increase in tissue mass and the lack of suppression by calcium in the normocalcemic range. The serum PTH levels are then greater than the proportionate increase in tissue mass. In Figure 2C, not only an increase in tissue mass and an increase in the calcium set point are depicted, but also less responsiveness of individual cells to calcium. Alternately, the change in slope-to-calcium sensitivity could be the result of autonomous drifting of the calcium set point of individual cells in the tissue mass, with the majority of cells adopting a set point higher than normal. From a summation of the available data obtained in vitro [34], the secretion of PTH from hyperplastic human parathyroid cells approximates the diagramatic representation in Figure 2C.

Potential Regulation of Parathyroid Hormone by Vitamin D Metabolites

Treatment of dialysis patients with a 1,25-dihydroxyvitamin D preparation given i.v. was found to decrease radioimmunoassayable serum PTH levels before this decrease in PTH could be attributed to an increase in serum-ionized calcium [35].

We selected 20 patients with hypocalcemia who were maintained on chronic hemodialysis. In the control part of the studies, blood was obtained before dialysis three times per week for a period of 3 weeks. In the treatment period, 1,25-dihydroxy D_3 was given intravenously at the end of each dialysis for a period of 8 weeks. The starting dose was 0.5 μg, and it was gradually increased to a maximum of 4.0 μg per treatment. Finally, a second post-treatment control period was continued for an additional 3 weeks. Blood samples were obtained for total and ionized calcium, magnesium, and phosphorus. The PTH was measured with our chicken antibody CH9. This antibody recognizes the C terminal, middle region, and the intact PTH molecule.

The mean serum calcium increased from 8.5 to 9.4 mg/100 ml, with a peak response of 10.9 mg/100 ml during 1,25-dihydroxy D_3 administration. In the post-treatment period, serum calcium decreased to a mean of 9.0 mg/100 ml. In general, there was a tendency for serum phosphorus to increase during 1,25-dihydroxy D_3 administration. Magnesium, on the other hand, remained fairly constant during the entire study in all patients. Every single patient had a substantial decrease in the levels of PTH during 1,25-dihydroxy D_3 treatment; the mean decrement was 70%. After 1,25-dihydroxy D_3 was discontinued, PTH increased in every single patient (Fig. 3). After 3 weeks of treatment, there was a gradual rise in the levels of ionized calcium. Concomitantly, there was a significant decrease in the levels of i-PTH. However, it

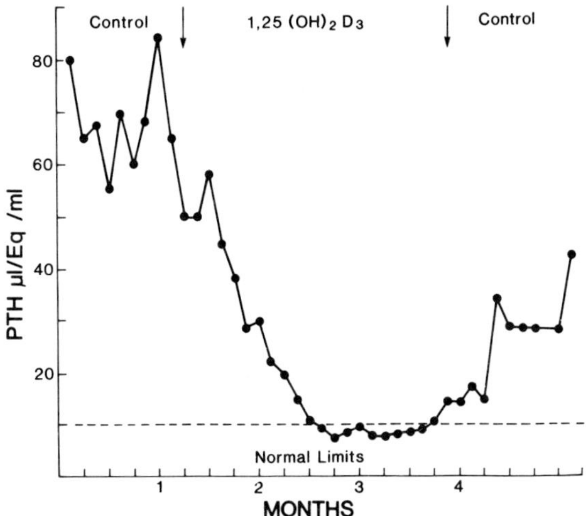

Fig. 3. The effects of 1,25(OH)₂D₃ on i-PTH in a uremic patient. During control studies, i-PTH was increased 6- to 8-fold above baseline. During the administration of IV 1,25(OH)₂D₃, the levels of serum i-PTH returned to normal. After 1,25(OH)₂D₃ was discontinued, i-PTH again increased 3- to 4-fold above normal. (Reproduced from Slatopolsky et al, in *Clinical Disorders of Bone and Mineral Metabolism,* edited by Frame B, Potts JT Jr, Amsterdam, Excerpta Medica, 1983)

would seem that early in the administration of 1,25-dihydroxy D₃, before there was any significant increase in ionized calcium, there already was a decrease in the levels of i-PTH.

Thus, the present studies demonstrate that 1,25(OH)₂D₃ has remarkable suppressive effects on the release of PTH. It is likely that the effects are mainly due to elevation in serum calcium to the upper limits of normal. However, it would seem that in addition to the calcemic effect, 1,25-dihydroxy D₃ per se modified the secretion of PTH. It is known that parathyroid glands obtained from uremic patients have a shift in the set point for calcium, requiring a higher concentration of ionized calcium than normal parathyroid glands for the suppression of PTH release. These studies raise the possibility that 1,25-dihydroxy D₃ may affect the regulation of PTH secretion by making the parathyroid gland more sensitive to calcium. Obviously, further studies are necessary to clarify this point.

Peripheral Metabolism of Parathyroid Hormone

Hruska et al [36] demonstrated in vivo that the kidney plays a key role in the metabolism of PTH. The half-life of carboxy-terminal immunoreactive PTH was prolonged in dogs with chronic renal failure. Further studies were performed to characterize the role of the peritubular uptake and GFR in the renal handling of PTH. Martin et al [37] demonstrated that both GFR and peritubular uptake are important mechanisms for the renal uptake of PTH. The degradation of carboxy-terminal fragments of PTH is dependent exclusively on glomerular filtration and tubular reabsorption, whereas peritubular uptake can only be demonstrated for biologically active intact 1–84 or its biologically active fragment, syn b-PTH 1–34.

The liver also plays a critical role in the degradation of PTH. Studies in the dog by Martin et al [38] indicated that the hepatic uptake of i-PTH is selective for intact hormone; and, this organ does not remove either carboxy-terminal or amino-terminal fragments from the circulation. Within 2 min after a bolus injection of intact PTH, the liver demonstrates an arteriovenous difference for i-PTH of roughly 35%. However, after 20 min, when intact PTH is no longer present in blood, the liver ceases to remove any fragments from the circulation. Moreover, when the synthetic 1–34 fragment has been injected in vivo into dogs, the liver has again failed to demonstrate any uptake of this fragment. Since the kidney accounts for roughly 45% of the metabolic clearance rate for the amino-terminal fragment of PTH, the major portion is left to be accounted for by extrarenal sites. Since bone is an important target organ for PTH, studies were designed to examine the possibility that the skeleton may represent the extrarenal site of metabolism for the synthetic amino-terminal PTH fragments.

Using an experimental model in which the canine tibia is isolated and perfused in vitro, Martin et al [39] clearly demonstrated that the isolated perfused bone has an arteriovenous difference of 35% for the synthetic b-PTH 1–34. However, when similar studies were performed during infusion of the native hormone (b-PTH 1–84), no significant uptake was observed. In addition, when oxidized (biologically inactive) synthetic biologic 1–34 was used, no arteriovenous difference was observed. These studies in bone suggest that in the dog, the skeleton is the major site of metabolism of the amino-terminal PTH fragment synthetic bovine 1–34.

In summary, PTH is secreted from the parathyroid glands predominantly in the intact form. However, there is evidence that PTH fragments can also be secreted from the glands. Intact PTH is degraded by the liver and kidney, resulting in the production of amino- and carboxy-terminal fragments. The carboxy-terminal fragments are further metabolized by the kidney via a process of glomerular filtration and tubular reabsorption. The amino-terminal fragments, in addition to intact PTH, also act on the peritubular side of the renal tubular cells, and they mediate the biologic effect of PTH in the kidney. These studies suggest that the peripheral metabolism of PTH may be necessary for the biologic effect of PTH on bone. The fact that the liver removes only intact hormone and that the kidney is responsible for the removal of amino- and carboxy-terminal fragments offers an explanation for the high levels of carboxy-terminal i-PTH seen in patients with chronic renal failure. In primary hyperparathyroidism, the liver and the kidney degrade the hormone, and the carboxy-terminal fragments are removed by the intact kidney. In advanced renal insufficiency, the native hormone (1–84) is degraded by the liver; however, in the absence of renal function, there is an accumulation of carboxy-terminal fragments. Patients with advanced renal failure may have detectable levels of PTH up to 2 weeks after parathyroidectomy, if the antibody that is used detects carboxy-terminal fragments. On the other hand, 24 hr after a successful renal transplant, the circulating levels of carboxy-terminal i-PTH decreases by 80% [40].

Measurements of Parathyroid Hormone in Primary and Secondary Hyperparathyroidism

Antisera produced against PTH tend to have antigenic determinants directed toward limited regions of the PTH molecule. In the past, if an assay used an antiserum that reacted with PTH 1–34, it was designated an amino (N)-terminal assay; and, if there was no interaction with PTH 1–34, the assay was designated a carboxy (C)-terminal assay. In recent years, with the availability of several synthetic and enzymatically produced fragments of PTH, a more precise definition is possible of the region of the PTH molecule that reacts with an antiserum.

Antisera directed toward the N-terminal region of PTH will recognize intact hormone, as well as N-terminal fragments. Antisera directed toward the C-terminal region of PTH will recognize both intact PTH and any hormone fragments containing the C-terminal sequence of the molecule. In addition, it is now increasingly recognized that some anti-PTH sera may react with a middle region of the PTH molecule; thus, they would recognize intact PTH, as well as fragments of the hormone containing the midregion sequence. As mentioned earlier, many assays have previously been termed C-terminal assays simply because they did not contain recognition sites for the N-terminal region of the molecule. It is now more appropriate to subdivide these assays into those that recognize the midregion and/or the C-terminal region of PTH (Fig. 4).

Since the structural requirements for the biologic activity of PTH reside within the first 34 amino acids of the molecule, it might seem that N-terminal assays would be the most useful for clinical purposes. Actually, the experience of several investigators has shown that this is not necessarily the case; the N-terminal assays generally provide variable discrimination between normal and hyperparathyroid subjects (Table 1). The clinical usefulness of such assays can be somewhat improved by analyzing the results of i-PTH together with the levels of serum calcium.

However, the reason for the marked variation in the results obtained by using N-terminal assays remains unclear. One possible explanation is that since the plasma half-lives of intact hormone and N-terminal fragments are very short, the steady-state value of PTH in peripheral plasma would only be consistently elevated in primary hyperparathyroidism if the secretion of intact PTH is constant. There is evidence that the secretion of PTH may, in fact, be episodic; this accordingly may partly account for the variable results of N-terminal PTH assays.

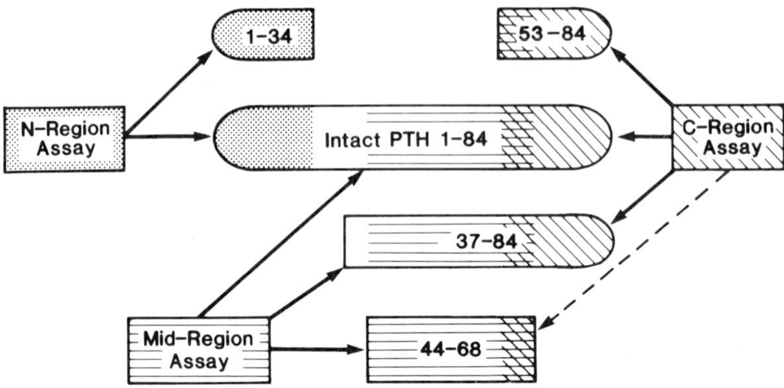

Fig. 4. Diagramatic representation of the recognition sites on PTH for different PTH antisera. For complete description, see the text. (From Martin et al: Parathyroid hormone, in *Renal Osteodystrophy,* edited by Catto GRD, Coburn J, The Hague, The Netherlands, Martinus Nifhoff Publishers, in press.

In the diagnosis of primary hyperparathyroidism, clinical experience has shown, in most instances, that assays directed toward the C-terminal and/ or midregion of the molecule provide better discrimination between states of normal and abnormal parathyroid function. These assays measure both the intact hormone and the major circulating species of i-PTH (fragments from the middle and C-terminal regions of the PTH molecule).

There is evidence that these biologically inactive fragments depend exclusively on the process of glomerular filtration for their removal from plasma. Thus, in patients with chronic renal failure, marked accumulations of C-terminal PTH fragments are seen. The levels of i-PTH obtained in patients with chronic renal disease may not be analogous to those seen in patients with primary hyperparathyroidism and normal renal function. In spite of this, it has been shown that the results of assays directed toward the middle and/or C-terminal regions correlate extremely well with evidence of the biologic effects of PTH on bone in patients with renal failure.

Serial determination of i-PTH, with an assay directed toward the middle and C-terminal portion of PTH, have provided a reliable index of the progression and/or improvement of secondary hyperparathyroidism in patients with chronic renal failure.

In conclusion, PTH radioimmunoassays directed toward the C-terminal and middle regions of PTH have been shown to be the most sensitive for detection and evaluation of hyperparathyroidism, as well as for the initial assessment and continued monitoring of patients with renal osteodystrophy. N-terminal PTH assays may be useful adjuncts to the C-terminal and midregion assays in certain situations, such as selective venous catheterization.

Acknowledgments. This work was supported by grants AM–009976, AM–07126, and RR–00036 from the National Institutes of Health.

Table 1. PTH radioimmunoassays in primary hyperparathyroidism

Authors	Antiserum	Percent absolute elevated values in 1° HPT
Antisera with recognition sites within amino acid sequence 1–34 of PTH		
Silverman and Yalow		
J Clin Invest 52:1958, 1973	C329	25
Arnaud et al		
Am J Med 56:785, 1974	CH14M	60
Woo and Singer		
Clin Chim Acta 54:161, 1974	AS211/32	86
Sparks		
Bio Sci Bull, 1900	AS211/32	33
Papapoulos et al		
Clin Endocr 13:57, 1980	G36	80
Potts et al		
Nichols Institute, 1982	CK67	80
Antisera with recognition sites within amino acid sequence 37–84 of PTH		
Reiss and Canterbury		
Proc Soc Exp Bio Med 128:501, 1968	CH824	100
Arnaud et al		
Am J Med 56:785, 1974	GPIM[a]	90
Slatopolsky et al		
Contr Issues Nephrol 4:169, 1976	CH9[a]	96
Freaney et al		
Ir J Med Sci 150:6, 1981	CH9[a]	96
Silverman and Yalow		
J Clin Invest 52:1958, 1973	273	94
Conaway and Anast		
J Lab Clin Med 83:129, 1974	GPO-6	96
DiBella et al		
Clin Chem 24:451, 1978	GPFM	96
Roos et al		
J Clin Endocrinol Metab 53:709, 1981	C9[a]	81
Roos et al		
J Clin Endocrinol Metab 53:709, 1981	C29	81
Kao et al		
Clin Chem 28:69, 1982	GP235	82
Marx et al		
J Clin Endocrinol Metab 53:76, 1981	G5[a]	90
Simon and Cuan		
Clin Chem 26:1672, 1980	CIS	41
Potts		
Nichols Institute brochure No. 0-60-1029, 1979	Anti-PTH-1	87
Antisera with recognition sites within the amino terminal and carboxy terminal region of PTH		
Potts et al		
Am J Med 50:639, 1971	GP1	50
Nichols Institute, cited by Broadus et al		
J Clin Invest 60:771, 1977	GP101	73

From MARTIN K, SLATOPOLSKY E, CLARK S, et al: Parathyroid hormone: Chemistry, physiology, and metabolism. Comparative utility of different PTH assays. *Smith Kline Clinical Confirmations* 2:1–12, 1982. Used with permission.
[a] Major reactivity with amino acid sequence 44–68 of PTH.
Abbreviations: 1° HPT = primary hyperparathyroidism.

References

1. KEUTMANN HT, SAUER MM, HENDRY GN, et al: Complete amino-acid sequence of human parathyroid hormone. *Biochemistry* 17:5723–5729, 1978

2. HABENER JF, POTTS JT JR, RICH A: Pre-proparathyroid hormone: Evidence for an early biosynthetic precursor of proparathyroid hormone. *J Biol Chem* 251:3893–3899, 1976

3. HABENER JF, ROSENBLATT M, KEMPER B, et al: Pre-proparathyroid hormone: Amino acid sequence, chemical synthesis, and some biological studies of the precursor region. *Proc Natl Acad Sci USA* 75:2616–2620, 1978

4. CHU LL, MACGREGOR RR, HAMILTON JW, et al: Conversion of proparathyroid hormone to parathyroid hormone: The use of amines as specific inhibitors. *Endocrinology* 95:1431–1438, 1974

5. SHERWOOD LM, MAYER GP, RAMBERG CF, et al: Regulation of parathyroid hormone secretion: Proportional control by calcium, lack of effect of phosphate. *Endocrinology* 83:1043–1051, 1968

6. SHERWOOD LM, HERRMAN I, BARRETT CA: Parathyroid hormone secretion *in vitro:* Regulation by calcium and magnesium ions. *Nature* 225:1056–1057, 1970

7. GITTES RF, RADDIE IC: Experimental hyperparathyroidism from multiple isologous parathyroid transplants: Homeostatic effect of simultaneous thyroid transplants. *Endocrinology* 78:1015–1022, 1966

8. MAYER GP, HABENER JF, POTTS JT JR: Parathyroid hormone secretion *in vivo.* Demonstration of a calcium-independent non-suppressible component of secretion. *J Clin Invest* 57:678–683, 1976

9. BROWN EM, GARDNER DG, WINDECK RA, et al: Relationship of intracellular 3',5'-adenosine monophosphate accumulation to parathyroid hormone release from dispersed bovine parathyroid cells. *Endocrinology* 103:2323–2333, 1978

10. MORRISSEY JJ, COHN DV: Regulation of secretion of parathormone and secretory protein-I from separate intracellular pools by calcium, dibutyryl cyclic AMP, and (1)-isoproterenol. *J Cell Biol* 82:93–102, 1979

11. DUFRESNE LR, GITELMAN HJ: A possible role of adenyl cyclase in the regulation of parathyroid activity by calcium, in *Calcium, Parathyroid Hormone and the Calcitonins,* edited by TALMADGE RV, MUNSON PL, Amsterdam, Excerpta Medica Foundation, 1972, pp 202–206

12. MATSUZAKI S, DUMONT JE: Effect of calcium ion on horse parathyroid gland adenyl cyclase. *Biochim Biophys Acta* 284:227–234, 1972

13. RODRIGUEZ JH, MORRISON A, SLATOPOLSKY E, et al: Adenyl cyclase of human parathyroid glands. *J Clin Endocrinol Metab* 47:319–325, 1978

14. BELLORIN-FONT E, MARTIN KJ, FREITAG JJ, et al: Altered adenylate cyclase kinetics in hyperfunctioning human parathyroid glands. *J Clin Endocrinol Metab* 52:499–507, 1981

15. ONTJES DA, MAHAFFEE DD, WELLS SA: Adenylate cyclase activity in human parathyroid tissues: Reduced sensitivity to suppression by calcium in parathyroid adenomas as compared with normal glands from normocalcemic-subjects or noninvolved glands from hyperparathyroid subjects. *Metabolism* 30:406–411, 1981

16. BUCKLE RM, CARE AD, COOPER CW, et al: The influence of plasma magnesium concentration on parathyroid hormone secretion. *J Endocrinol* 42:529–534, 1968

17. HABENER JF, POTTS JT JR: Relative effectiveness of magnesium and calcium on the secretion and biosynthesis of parathyroid hormone *in vitro. Endocrinology* 98:197–202, 1976

18. ANAST CS, MOHR JM, KAPLAN SL, et al: Evidence for parathyroid failure during magnesium deficiency. *Science* 177:606–608, 1972

19. SUH SM, TASHJIAN AH JR, MATSUO N, et al: Pathogenesis of hypocalcemia

in primary hypomagnesemia: Normal end-organ responsiveness to parathyroid hormone impaired parathyroid gland function. *J Clin Invest* 52:153–160, 1973

20. CHASE LR, SLATOPOLSKY E: Secretion and metabolic efficiency of parathyroid hormone in patients with severe hypomagnesemia. *J Clin Endocrinol Metab* 38:363–371, 1974

21. LEVI J, MASSRY SG, COBURN JW, et al: Hypocalcemia in magnesium-depleted dogs: Evidence for reduced responsiveness to parathyroid hormone and relative failure of parathyroid gland function. *Metabolism* 23:323–335, 1974

22. HEATH H: Biogenic amines and the secretion of parathyroid hormone and calcitonin. *Endocr Rev* 1:319–338, 1980

23. MORRISSEY JJ, COHN DV: Secretion and degradation of parathormone as a function of intracellular maturation of hormone pools. *J Cell Biol* 83:521–528, 1979

24. MACGREGOR RR, CHU LLH, HAMILTON JW, et al: Studies on the subcellular localization of parathyroid hormone in the bovine parathyroid gland: Separation of newly synthesized from mature forms. *Endocrinology* 93:1387–1397, 1973

25. MACGREGOR RR, HAMILTON JW, COHN DV: The by-pass of tissue hormone stores during the secretion of newly synthesized parathyroid hormone. *Endocrinology* 97:178–188, 1975

26. BROWN EM, THATCHER JC: Adenosine 3′,5′-monophosphate (cAMP)-dependent protein kinase and the regulation of parathyroid hormone release by divalent cations and agents elevating cellular cAMP in dispersed bovine parathyroid cells. *Endocrinology* 110:1374–1380, 1982

27. HANLEY DA, TAKATSUKI K, BIRNBAUMER ME, et al: *In vitro* perfusion for the study of parathyroid hormone secretion: Effects of extracellular calcium concentration and beta-adrenergic regulation on bovine parathyroid hormone secretion *in vitro. Calcif Tiss Int* 32:19–27, 1980

28. BROWN EM: Relationship of 3′,5′-adenosine monophosphate accumulation to parathyroid hormone release in dispersed cells from pathological human parathyroid tissue. *J Clin Endocrinol Metab* 52:961–968, 1981

29. BLUM JW, FISHER JA, HUNZIKER WH, et al: Parathyroid hormone response to catecholamines and to changes of extracellular calcium in cows. *J Clin Invest* 61:1113–1122, 1978

30. HABENER JF: Responsiveness of neoplastic and hyperplastic parathyroid tissue to calcium *in vitro. J Clin Invest* 62:436–450, 1978

31. BROWN EM, BRENNAN MF, HURWITZ S, et al: Dispersed cells prepared from human parathyroid glands: Distinct calcium sensitivity of adenomas vs. primary hyperplasia. *J Clin Endocrinol Metab* 46:267–275, 1978

32. BROWN EM: Set-point for calcium: Its role in normal and abnormal parathyroid secretion, in *Hormonal Control of Calcium Metabolism,* edited by COHN DV, TALMAGE RV, MATTHEWS JL, Amsterdam, Excerpta Medica 1981, pp 35–44

33. BROWN EM, WILSON RE, EASTMAN RC, et al: Abnormal regulation of parathyroid hormone release by calcium in secondary hyperparathyroidism due to chronic renal failure. *J Clin Endocrinol Metab* 54:172–179, 1982

34. BROWN EM: Four-parameter model of the sigmoidal relationship between parathyroid hormone release and extracellular calcium concentration in normal and abnormal parathyroid tissue. *J Clin Endocrinol Metab* 56:572–581, 1983

35. SLATOPOLSKY E, WEERTS C, THIELAN B, GALCERAN T, MARTIN K: Suppression of secondary hyperparathyroidism by 1,25(OH)$_2$D$_3$, in *Clinical Disorders of Bone and Mineral Metabolism,* edited by FRAME B, POTTS J, Amsterdam, Excerpta Medica, 1983, p 267

36. HRUSKA KA, KOPELMAN R, RUTHERFORD WE, KLAHR S, SLATOPOLSKY E: Metabolism of parathyroid hormone in the dog. The role of the kidney and the effects of chronic renal disease. *J Clin Invest* 56:39–48, 1975

37. MARTIN KJ, HRUSKA KA, LEWIS J, ANDERSON C, SLATOPOLSKY E: Renal

handling of parathyroid hormone. Role of peritubular uptake and glomerular filtration. *J Clin Invest* 60:808–814, 1977

38. MARTIN K, HRUSKA K, GREENWALT A, SLATOPOLSKY E: Selective uptake of intact parathyroid hormone by the liver. Differences between hepatic and renal uptake. *J Clin Invest* 58:781–788, 1976

39. MARTIN KJ, FREITAG JJ, CONRADES MB, HRUSKA K, KLAHR S, SLATOPOLSKY E: Selective uptake of the synthetic amino terminal fragment of parathyroid hormone (syn b-PTH 1–34) by isolated perfused bone. *J Clin Invest* 62:256–261, 1978

40. FREITAG J, MARTIN KJ, HRUSKA KA, ANDERSON C, CONRADES M, LADENSON J, KLAHR S, SLATOPOLSKY E: Impaired parathyroid hormone metabolism in chronic renal failure. *N Engl J Med* 298:29–31, 1978

Vitamin D and Kidney Disease

Jacob Lemann, Jr., Richard W. Gray, and Adel B. Korkor

The classic biologic effects of vitamin D are to stimulate intestinal calcium absorption and to heal rickets, which is the bone disease of vitamin D deficiency in children. In the nineteenth century, it was observed that children with kidney disease may exhibit rickets. Almost 50 years ago, Liu and Chu demonstrated that patients with chronic renal failure exhibit reduced intestinal calcium absorption despite a normal dietary calcium intake. This defect was not corrected by the administration of physiologic doses of vitamin D, but it was corrected by the administration of dihydrotachysterol [1]. Subsequent studies of bone have shown that patients with chronic renal disease also exhibit a wide range of skeletal abnormalities that are collectively termed renal osteodystrophy. When the availability of radiolabeled vitamin D permitted study of vitamin D metabolism, the critical role of the kidney in the formation of $1,25\text{-}(OH)_2\text{-}D_3$ became apparent [2, 3]. Subsequent studies have shown that $1,25\text{-}(OH)_2\text{-}D_3$ is the most potent metabolite of the vitamin with respect to the stimulation of intestinal calcium absorption [2, 3]. Although the existence of a direct effect of vitamin D to stimulate bone formation remains controversial, $1,25\text{-}(OH)_2\text{-}D_3$ does stimulate bone resorption [4]. It is the purpose of this review to consider the abnormalities of vitamin D metabolism that are associated with kidney disease, the mechanisms for these abnormalities and their consequences, and the therapeutic use of vitamin D metabolites in renal osteodystrophy.

Vitamin D Metabolism in Health

Table 1 summarizes the plasma levels, plasma half-life, body stores, and daily turnover rates of the major vitamin D metabolites in health [5]. Previta-

This manuscript was presented as part of a Symposium on *Parathyroid Hormone and Vitamin D in Uremia.*

Table 1. Plasma concentrations, plasma half-lives, and estimated body stores and daily production rates of major vitamin D metabolites in health

Metabolite	Plasma concentration (per liter)	Half-life in plasma	Body stores (nmoles)	Daily Production (nmoles)
Vitamin D	5 nmoles	<1 d	170	100
25-OH-D	60 nmoles	25 d	1000	50
24,25-$(OH)_2$-D	4 nmoles	7 hr	?	48
1,25-$(OH)_2$-D	80 pmoles	<6 hr	1	1.4

min D_3 is synthesized in the skin from 7-dehydrocholesterol under the influence of ultraviolet light, and it is then thermally converted to vitamin D_3 (cholecalciferol) [6]. Thus, vitamin D may be considered a cutaneous prehormone. Vitamin D_3 is also present in some foods, including milk, eggs, liver, some fish, and fish oils. Some foods in the United States, especially milk and dry cereals, are fortified with vitamin D_3 or vitamin D_2 (ergocalciferol), which is derived from irradiated plant sterols. Vitamin D is transported in the circulation by vitamin D-binding protein (DBP), which is a α-globulin that has a molecular weight of about 53,000 daltons. Each molecule of DBP has one binding site for vitamin D metabolites, and the normal serum concentration of DBP is about 8×10^{-6} moles/liter (400 mg/liter), so that a large excess binding capacity is normally present in the serum [7, 8]. Vitamin D is converted by the liver to 25-OH-D (calcifidiol), which is the principal circulating and storage metabolite of vitamin D (Table 1). 25-OH-D undergoes an enterohepatic circulation. There appears to be little regulation of hepatic 25-OH-D synthesis, since administration of large amounts of vitamin D results in marked elevation of serum 25-OH-D concentrations [9]. Consequently, serum 25-OH-D concentrations provide the best available assessment of body stores of vitamin D. 25-OH-D appears to be the precursor of all other known vitamin D metabolites. The 1α-hydroxylation of 25-OH-D_3 in the kidney results in the formation of 1,25-$(OH)_2$-D_3 (calcitriol), the hormonal form of the vitamin. The kidney and other tissues also convert 25-OH-D to 24,25-$(OH)_2$-D_3. An array of other metabolites of 25-OH-D_3 are also known, but nearly all of these appear to be biologically inactive. 1,25-$(OH)_2$-D_3 and 24,-25-$(OH)_2$-D_3 also circulate largely bound to DBP.

Vitamin D Nutrition and Kidney Disease

Serum 25-OH-D concentrations in health largely reflect sun exposure and cutaneous synthesis of vitamin D [10–12]. Some patients with chronic kidney disease exhibit reduced serum 25-OH-D concentrations [13–19]. It seems likely that these patients, because of their illness, are likely to be less active, thus receiving less sun exposure. However, there does not appear to be any intrinsic abnormality in cutaneous vitamin D synthesis in uremia, since dialysis patients have been observed to spontaneously exhibit higher serum 25-OH-D levels in summer compared to late winter [18]. To the extent that patients with established renal disease are treated by dietary protein restriction [20], a reduced intake of milk, eggs, cheese and fish would also reduce serum 25-OH-D levels. There is no evidence of impaired hepatic conversion of vitamin D_3 to 25-OH-D_3 in renal failure [21]. Urinary excretion of 25-OH-D is increased in proportion to the magnitude of proteinuria among patients with glomerular disease [22, 23], presumably because of increased urinary losses of DBP. Speculatively, the loss of DBP into the urine does not significantly alter the serum concentration of unbound (free) 25-OH-D, which may be most important in determining its further metabolic and biologic effects [24]. Urinary losses of 25-OH-D theoretically could result in vitamin D deficiency, if the demands for vitamin D were increased; for example, during growth or if sun exposure were limited. Although histologic evidence of osteomalacia has been observed among patients with the nephrotic syndrome [25], this observation is not a consistent one [26]. Moreover, there is no evidence that symptomatic renal osteodystrophy occurs more frequently among nephrotic patients with progressive kidney disease. There is no evidence for accelerated 25-OH-D catabolism in patients with kidney disease, other than the urinary losses found in nephrotic patients. In fact, the serum half-life of 25-OH-D_3 is prolonged to about 44 days in anephric patients, compared to about 22 days in healthy subjects [27]. Thus, vitamin D deficiency probably is no more common among patients with kidney disease than among patients who have other chronic diseases.

Serum 1,25-$(OH)_2$-D in Health

In health, as summarized in Tables 1 and 2, serum 1,25-$(OH)_2$-D concentrations determined in many laboratories average about 85 pmoles/liter (35

Table 2. Some representative reports of serum or plasma 1,25-$(OH)_2$-D concentrations in healthy adults

Author	Year	Reference number	Number of subjects	Mean serum or plasma 1,25-$(OH)_2$-D (pmoles/liter)	Mean ± 2 SD or range (pmoles/liter)
Hughes et al	1976	28	78	79	50–108
Eisman et al	1976	29	20	70	27–113
Lambert et al	1978	30	59	83	37–129
Gray et al	1979	31	97	89	39–139
Taylor et al	1979	32	30	78	14–157
Clemens et al	1979	33	26	98	53–142
Lund et al	1979	34	65	80	28–190
Mason et al	1980	35	47	86	29–168
Bishop et al	1980	36	57	101	48–154
Bouillion et al	1980	37	54	91	33–149
Yamaoka et al	1981	38	37	88	29–168

pg/ml), but range from about 35 to (about) 150 pmoles/liter [28–38]. Serum 1,25-(OH)$_2$-D concentrations appear to reflect renal synthesis of the hormone [39]. The wide variation in serum 1,25-(OH)$_2$-D levels is likely, in part, to be related to the analytically difficult measurement of 1,25-(OH)$_2$-D; but, more importantly, it may be related to biologic factors known to influence serum 1,25-(OH)$_2$-D levels, including dietary calcium intake [40], caloric intake [41], and growth [42, 43].

As shown in Figure 1, net intestinal calcium absorption, which is determined by the balance technique, varies directly with prevailing serum 1,25-(OH)$_2$-D concentrations over a wide range of dietary calcium intake in healthy adults [44, 45]. Intestinal calcium absorption, which is expressed as a percentage of intake, or the fractional absorption of radiolabeled calcium [46], is also dependent on prevailing serum 1,25-(OH)$_2$-D levels, but it is less importantly influenced by the level of dietary calcium intake. Thus, it is apparent that when serum 1,25-(OH)$_2$-D levels vary over the normal range of 35 to 150 pmoles/liter, absolute net intestinal calcium absorption, which determines the supply of calcium to the body, is critically dependent on the dietary content of calcium.

When renal function is normal, the regulation of serum 1,25-(OH)$_2$-D

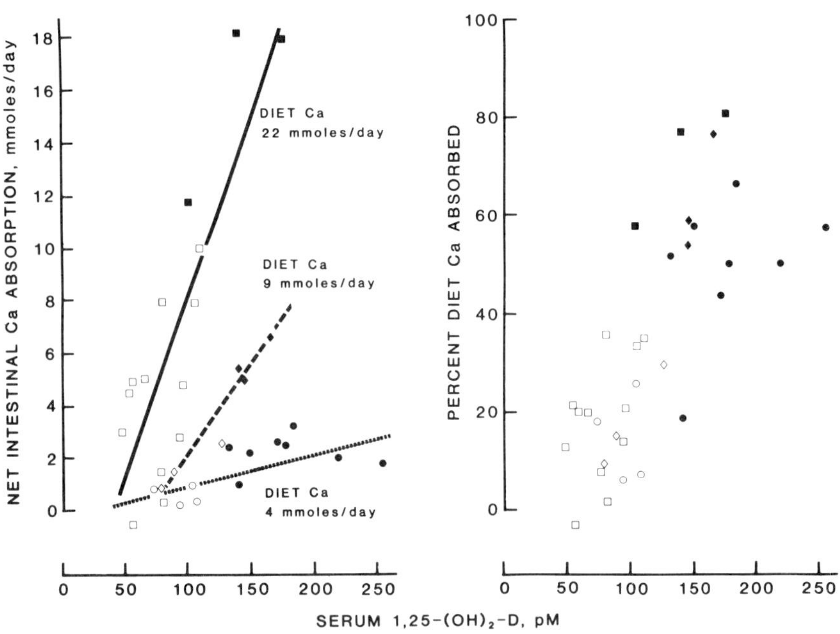

Fig. 1. Relationships between absolute intestinal calcium (*Ca*) absorption (*left panel*), percent of dietary Ca absorbed (*right panel*), and prevailing serum 1,25-(OH)$_2$-D concentrations in healthy men eating diets providing either 4, 9, or 22 mmoles Ca/d alone (*open symbols*), or while also taking calcitriol (*closed symbols*). (Adapted and extended from [44, 45])

levels appear to be dependent on the level of parathyroid hormone (PTH) secretion, since 1,25-(OH)$_2$-D levels: (1) are low among patients with hypoparathyroidism or normal subjects who eat high-calcium diets [40] and rise in response to PTH—either exogenously administered [48, 49] or endogenously secreted in primary hyperparathyroidism [47, 50], or (2) in response to the ingestion of a low-calcium diet [40] or induced hypocalcemia [51]. Serum 1,25-(OH)$_2$-D levels also rise in response to dietary phosphate deprivation [52–54]. Even when dietary phosphate intake is normal, serum 1,25-(OH)$_2$-D levels also vary inversely with serum phosphate concentrations, because the serum phosphate concentration rises with limitation of caloric intake [41]. Serum 1,25-(OH)$_2$-D concentrations are increased during growth in children, but the mechanism for this effect is not yet known. Although the kidney appears to be the principal—if not the sole—source of 1,25-(OH)$_2$-D in health, extrarenal production of 1,25-(OH)$_2$-D occurs during pregnancy in the placenta [55].

1,25-(OH)$_2$-D in Kidney Disease

Since the kidney is the principal source of 1,25-(OH)$_2$-D, serum concentrations fall as renal failure becomes more severe both among adults (Fig. 2) [29, 31, 32, 44, 45, 52, 56–65] and children (Fig. 3) [42, 66–68] with kidney disease. Although 1,25-(OH)$_2$-D concentrations usually are analytically undetectable among anephric hemodialysis patients and very low or undetectable among hemodialysis patients with kidneys [29, 31, 32, 58, 64, 65], there have been reports of low concentrations in anephric patients [61, 62]. In another report [69], the anephric patient had sarcoidosis, and it has recently been reported that the sarcoid granulomas may be capable of producing 1,25-(OH)$_2$-D [70]. We have recently observed another anephric patient with sarcoidosis who exhibited an increased serum concentration of 1,25-(OH)$_2$-D. Patients with kidney disease and lymphomas also may exhibit elevated 1,25-(OH)$_2$-D concentrations [71]. However, most reports of low (but measurable) 1,25-(OH)$_2$-D levels in anephric patients have indicated that the patients had no other significant illnesses. Among these patients, serum 1,25-(OH)$_2$-D levels do not increase after administration of 25-OH-D$_3$ [62]. Since cultured bone cells have been shown to produce 1,25-(OH)$_2$-D$_3$ [72], it is possible that the skeleton is the source of the small residual serum 1,25-(OH)$_2$-D concentrations observed among anephric subjects. In any event, the data in Figures 2 and 3 emphasize that the kidneys are the major source of 1,25-(OH)$_2$-D. As shown in Figure 2, among adults with kidney disease, serum 1,25-(OH)$_2$-D concentrations appear to be maintained mostly within the normal range until the glomerular filtration rate (GFR) falls to less than one-half of normal; however, even some of these patients may have somewhat lower than normal serum 1,25-(OH)$_2$-D concentrations. Among children with kidney disease (Fig. 3), serum 1,25-(OH)$_2$-D concentrations may also be low, with mild renal failure. This decrease presumably reflects impaired renal synthesis of 1,25-(OH)$_2$-D as the functioning kidney mass is reduced, but

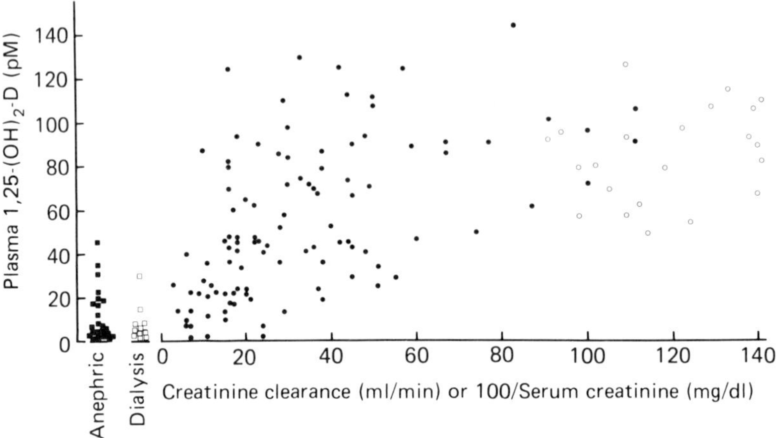

Fig. 2. Serum or plasma 1,25-(OH)$_2$-D concentrations in relation to creatinine clearance, ml/min or 100/serum creatinine—mg/dl in healthy adults (○), and in adult patients with chronic kidney disease (●)—as well as in patients with kidneys on hemodialysis (□) or anephric patients on hemodialysis (■). (Adapted from [29, 31, 32, 44, 45, 52, 56–65])

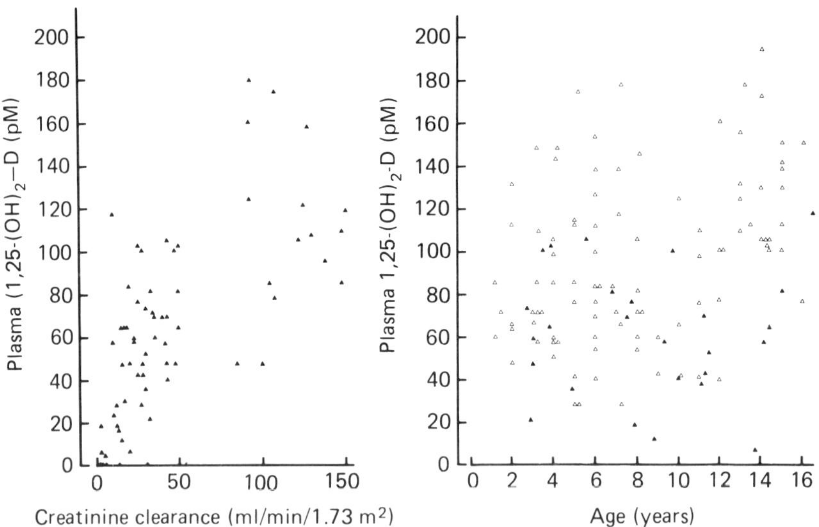

Fig. 3. Serum or plasma 1,25-(OH)$_2$-D concentrations in relation to C_{cr}, ml/min/ 1.73 m^2 (*left panel*) or age (*right panel*) in healthy children (△), or in children with kidney disease (▲). (Adapted from [42, 66–68])

the mechanism is not yet completely clear. It has been suggested that serum
1,25-(OH)$_2$-D concentrations fall earlier in the course of tubulointerstitial
kidney disease, as compared to glomerular disease [66]. Some studies have
suggested that the maintenance of normal serum 1,25-(OH)$_2$-D concentrations, until GFR is reduced to about one-half of normal or less, is the consequence of the earlier development of secondary hyperparathyroidism [56];
this, in turn, is related to phosphate retention [73]. However, even if this
sequence were correct, a normal serum 1,25-(OH)$_2$-D concentration with
even a mild degree of renal failure would be inappropriately low in relation
to the degree of hyperparathyroidism. On the other hand, more recent studies
have shown that serum 1,25-(OH)$_2$-D concentrations are low among patients
with kidney disease, even when GFR is still 50% of normal (when secondary
hyperparathyroidism is also evident) and despite somewhat reduced (not elevated) serum phosphate concentrations [63, 74]. Since there are other reports
of low serum phosphate concentrations in early renal failure, these observations further emphasize the possibility of impaired renal 1,25-(OH)$_2$-D synthesis in early renal disease. Dietary phosphate restriction in early renal disease
in children is accompanied by an increase in serum 1,25-(OH)$_2$-D concentrations and a decrease in the degree of hyperparathyroidism [74]. Restoration
of normal serum 1,25-(OH)$_2$-D concentrations in adults with early renal failure (creatinine clearances, 40 to 90 ml/min), via the administration of calcitriol, appears to be accompanied by lesser degrees of hyperparathyroidism
based on a fall in urinary cyclic AMP/GFR [63]. Although unconfirmed,
these preliminary observations suggest that a decline in renal 1,25-(OH)$_2$-D
synthesis early in the course of renal failure may be a factor in the pathogenesis
of secondary hyperparathyroidism, since the cytosolic receptor for 1,25-
(OH)$_2$-D is present in the parathyroids [75] and 1,25-(OH)$_2$-D suppresses
PTH secretion via cultured parathyroid glands [76]. Although controversial,
fractional intestinal calcium absorption also may be maintained close to the
normal range with mild degrees of renal failure [77], which would be consistent
with maintenance of a normal serum 1,25-(OH)$_2$-D concentration. However,
it should be re-emphasized that whether serum 1,25-(OH)$_2$-D concentrations
are within the normal range or slightly reduced, the dietary supply of calcium
would appear to be crucial with respect to net absorption of calcium in
early renal disease (Fig. 1). Clearly, additional simultaneous measurements
of renal function, serum 1,25-(OH)$_2$-D concentrations, and intestinal calcium
absorption are needed in patients with early renal insufficiency who are eating
diets that provide normal quantities of calcium and who have never taken
aluminum-containing antacids (see below).

24,25-(OH)$_2$-D in Kidney Disease

In health serum, 24,25-(OH)$_2$-D levels are directly correlated to precursor
25-OH-D concentrations [78–80]. Although extrarenal 24,25-(OH)$_2$-D$_3$ synthesis occurs in humans [27, 81], the kidney appears to be the major site
of 24,25-(OH)$_2$-D$_3$ production, since serum 24,25-(OH)$_2$-D concentrations

fall as renal failure progresses [32, 82]. The possible biologic effects of 24,25-$(OH)_2$-D remain controversial [75]. The administration of 24,25-$(OH)_2$-D_3 both to normal subjects and to anephric patients was shown initially to increase intestinal calcium absorption and to promote calcium retention [83], but subsequent studies failed to confirm such an effect [84]. 24,25-$(OH)_2$-D_3 administration was also reported to reduce PTH secretion in dogs with experimental renal failure [85, 86]. However, further studies once again have shown that the chronic administration of 24,25-$(OH)_2$-D_3 fails to either lower serum PTH or modify the bone histology of dogs with experimental renal failure [87]. Moreover, 24,25-$(OH)_2$-D_3 did not directly inhibit PTH secretion by cultured parathyroid glands [76].

Other early studies showed that vitamin D_3 or 25-OH-D_3 or the combination of 1,25-$(OH)_2$-D_3 and 24,25-$(OH)_2$-D_3 were required to completely heal the bones of patients with nutritional vitamin D deficiency and osteomalacia; whereas, 1,25-$(OH)_2$-D_3 alone did not completely correct the impairment of mineralization or the accompanying secondary hyperparathyroidism [88]. However, more recent reports indicated that the administration of 1,25-$(OH)_2$-D_3 alone was capable of completely healing the bone disease of vitamin D deficiency [89]. Moreover, treatment of vitamin D-deficient animals with 24,24-difluoro-25-OH-D_3, which is a compound that cannot undergo 24-hydroxylation, completely corrects the skeletal abnormalities in vitamin D-deficient animals [90]. In other studies of dialysis patients with osteomalacia, the administration of 24,25-$(OH)_2$-D_3 alone had no effect on the bone disease [91]. However, in comparison to 1,25-$(OH)_2$-D_3 alone, the combination of 24,25-$(OH)_2$-D_3 and 1,25-$(OH)_2$-D_3 appeared to enhance healing [91]. Further evidence that 24,25-$(OH)_2$-D_3 may exert an effect on bone is provided by the observation that only a combination of 24,25-$(OH)_2$-D_3 and 1,25-$(OH)_2$-D_3—but not 1,25-$(OH)_2$-D_3 alone—completely corrected the blunted calcemic response to PTH in acutely uremic animals [92]. In animals, either 24,25-$(OH)_2$-D_3 [75] or perhaps some other metabolite [93] appears to be essential for a completely normal life cycle. Clearly, further controlled studies are needed to clarify the role and effects of 24,25-$(OH)_2$-D_3 in renal failure in both adults and children.

The Therapeutic Use of Vitamin D Metabolites in Renal Osteodystrophy

Current studies indicate the existence of several skeletal disorders in patients with chronic renal failure. Osteitis fibrosa is found among untreated patients with hyperphosphatemia, normal or low serum calcium levels, and marked elevation of serum PTH concentrations. This lesion is accompanied both by accelerated bone resorption and by mineralization, but the former predominates. Other patients exhibit osteoid excess and reduced bone formation in addition to osteitis fibrosa—the mixed lesion. Still other patients exhibit only excess osteoid and decreased bone mineralization, with little or no evidence of increased bone resorption (pure osteomalacia) [94]. In the last several years, the latter lesion has been found to be associated with the deposition of aluminum at the site of osteoid mineralization [95, 96]. These patients also exhibit less severe secondary hyperparathyroidism in relation to their degree of renal failure. The aluminum apparently is absorbed from drinking water, from antacids given to limit intestinal phosphate absorption, and from dialysate [97–99]. Iron also may be deposited with aluminum at the mineralization front and may contribute to the development of pure osteomalacia in patients who have received multiple transfusions [100]. The precise mechanism by which aluminum affects bone, or even whether it affects bone, remains controversial. Aluminum administration to vitamin D-replete normal dogs is accompanied by the development of osteomalacia with aluminum deposition at the mineralization front; however, serum $1,25\text{-}(OH)_2\text{-}D$ concentrations also fall [101, 102]. Moreover, aluminum appears to inhibit bone mineralization in cultured embryonic bone [103]. On the other hand, administration of aluminum to vitamin D-deficient dogs with osteomalacia caused greater accumulation of aluminum in bone at the mineralization front; but, this aluminum did not prevent subsequent healing of osteomalacia in response to vitamin D repletion [104].

The therapeutic goal in the use of vitamin D metabolites in the treatment of renal bone disease is to stimulate intestinal calcium absorption [105], to elevate serum calcium levels, to suppress PTH secretion [73, 106], to inhibit bone resorption, and to promote bone mineralization.

Since serum $1,25\text{-}(OH)_2\text{-}D$ concentrations appear to be maintained within or slightly below the normal range in early renal failure (Figs. 2, 3), it would appear that the use of vitamin D metabolites should presently be reserved for patients with more advanced renal insufficiency. With only mild renal failure, calcium supplements provided as calcium carbonate, calcium lactate, or calcium gluconate (not as calcium and phosphate in milk or cheese) should be provided in addition to restriction of dietary phosphate; especially, since dietary surveys have shown that patients with renal failure eat diets providing less than normal quantities of calcium [107]. It is to be hoped that a substitute for aluminum-containing antacids will soon become available because of the difficulty in limiting dietary phosphate intake and because of the possible toxicity of aluminum.

Among patients with advanced renal failure or patients on dialysis with osteitis fibrosa, $1,25\text{-}(OH)_2\text{-}D_3$ administration [108–111] as well as the administration of $25\text{-}OH\text{-}D_3$ [112, 113], $1\alpha\text{-}OH\text{-}D_3$ [114–118], or dihydrotachysterol [119] have been shown to augment intestinal calcium absorption, elevate serum calcium concentrations, suppress serum PTH and alkaline phosphatase activities, and improve both histologic and radiographic evidence of osteitis fibrosa. The studies employing $1,25\text{-}(OH)_2\text{-}D_3$ have used doses of calcitriol ranging from 0.25 to 2.0 $\mu g/d$ (0.6 to 4.8 nmoles/d). Double-blind placebo-controlled trials of calcitriol in asymptomatic dialysis patients have provided similar results [120, 121]. The administration of calcitriol to adult patients with pure osteomalacia often has resulted in the rapid development of hypercalcemia during both the administration of only small doses of calcitriol and a failure to alter the abnormal histopathology of bone [122]. The mechanism for the failure of $1,25\text{-}(OH)_2\text{-}D_3$ in providing therapeutic benefit is not yet certain, but it may be related to the accumulation of aluminum in bone.

The use of 1,25-(OH)$_2$-D$_3$ in advanced renal failure requires careful and frequent monitoring of serum calcium and phosphate concentrations because of the risks of hypercalcemia, hyperphosphatemia, and the potential development or worsening of soft tissue calcification. When 1,25-(OH)$_2$-D$_3$ was given to patients with renal disease who had creatinine clearances ranging from 5 to 35 ml/min at a dose of 0.5 to 1 μg(1.2 to 2.4 nmoles)/d, there appeared to be more rapid progression of renal failure that was partly reversible [123]. However, in a more recent report, administration of 1,25-(OH)$_2$-D$_3$ in a dose of 0.5 to 1.0 μg(1.2 to 2.4 nmoles)/d to patients with creatinine clearances between 15 to 55 ml/min did not adversely affect renal function, while either healing or markedly improving histologic evidence of bone disease [124]. Among children with renal failure, treatment with 1,25-(OH)$_2$-D$_3$ clearly improves evidence of bone disease and accelerates growth [125, 126].

Therefore, it is evident that control of serum phosphate concentrations, provision of an adequate calcium intake, and the judicious use of 1,25-(OH)$_2$-D$_3$ or an analog are beneficial in both the management and possibly the prevention of uremic hyperparathyroid bone disease. However, the role and use of vitamin D metabolites in the pathogenesis and therapy for other types of uremic bone disease remain to be clarified, especially in relation to the possible toxic effects of aluminum on the skeleton.

References

1. LIU SH, CHU HI: Studies of calcium and phosphorus metabolism with special reference to pathogenesis and effects of dihydrotachysterol (A.T. 10) and iron. *Medicine* 22:103–161, 1943
2. DELUCA HF: Recent advances in the metabolism of vitamin D. *Ann Rev Physiol* 43:199–209, 1981
3. NORMAN AW (editor): *Vitamin D: Molecular Biology and Clinical Nutrition.* New York, Marcel Dekker, 1980
4. STERN PH: The D vitamins and bone. *Pharmacol Rev* 32:47–80, 1980
5. LEMANN J JR, GRAY RW: Vitamin D metabolism and the kidney, in *Renal Endocrinology,* edited by DUNN MJ, Baltimore, Williams & Wilkins, 1983, chap 4, pp 114–141
6. HOLICK MF: The cutaneous photosynthesis of pre-vitamin D$_3$: A unique photoendocrine system. *J Invest Derm* 76:51–58, 1981
7. HADDAD JG JR, WALGATE J: 25-hydroxyvitamin D transport in human plasma. Isolation and partial characterization of calcifidiol-binding protein. *J Biol Chem* 251:4803–4809, 1976
8. BOUILLON R, VAN BAELEN H: The transport of vitamin D, in *Vitamin D: Basic Research and its Clinical Application,* edited by NORMAN AW et al, Berlin, Walter DeGruyter, 1979, pp 137–143
9. FARRINGTON K, SKINNER RK, VARGHESE Z, MOREHEAD JF: Hepatic metabolism of vitamin D in chronic renal failure (*letter*). *Lancet* 1:321, 1979
10. POSKITT EMG, COLE TJ, LAWSON DE: Diet, sunlight and 25-hydroxyvitamin D in healthy children and adults. *Br Med J* 1:221–223, 1979
11. STRYD RP, GILBERTSON TJ, BRUNDEN MN: A seasonal variation study of

25-hydroxyvitamin D_3 serum levels in normal humans. *J Clin Endocrinol Metab* 48:771–775, 1979

12. DEVGUN MS, PATERSON CR, JOHNSON BE, COHEN C: Vitamin D nutrition in relation to season and occupation. *Am J Clin Nutr* 34:1501–1504, 1981

13. BAYARD F, BEC PH, LOUNET JP: Measurement of plasma 25-hydroxycholecalciferol in man. *Eur J Clin Invest* 2:195–198, 1972

14. BAYARD F, BEC PH, TONTHAT H, LOUNET JP: Plasma 25-hydroxycholecalciferol in chronic renal failure. *Eur J Clin Invest* 3:447–450, 1973

15. OFFERMAN G, VON HERRATH D, SHAFFER K: Serum 25-hydroxycholecalciferol in uremia. *Nephron* 13:269–277, 1974

16. LETTERI J, ROGINSKY M, MOO F, SCIPIONE R, ELLIS K, COHN S: The relationship between calcified tissue mass and plasma 25-hydroxycholecalciferol in chronic renal failure, in *Vitamin D and Problems Related to Uremic Bone Disease,* edited by NORMAN AW, SCHAEFER K, COBURN JW, DeLUCA HF, FRASER D, GRIGOLEIT HG, VON HERRATH D, Berlin, Walter deGruyter, 1975, p 303.

17. COOK DB, PIERIDES AM, SHANNON G: Seasonal variation of serum 25-hydroxyvitamin D in patients with chronic renal failure treated by regular haemodialysis. *Clin Chem Acta* 76:251–258, 1977

18. PIETREK J, KOKOT F: Serum 25-hydroxyvitamin D in patients with chronic renal disease. *Eur J Clin Invest* 7:283–287, 1977

19. EASTWOOD JB, DALY A, CARTER GD, ALAGHBAND-ZADEH J, DEWARDENER HE: Plasma 25-hydroxyvitamin D in normal subjects and patients with terminal renal failure on maintenance haemodialysis and after transplantation. *Clin Sci* 57:473–476, 1979

20. BRENNER BM, MEYER TM, HOSTETTER TH: Dietary protein intake and the progressive nature of kidney disease. *N Engl J Med* 307:652–658, 1982

21. AVIOLI LV, BIRGE S, LEE SW, SLATOPOLSKY E: The metabolic fate of vitamin $D_3^{-3}H$ in chronic renal failure. *J Clin Invest* 47:2239–2252, 1968

22. SATO KA, GRAY RW, LEMANN J JR: Urinary excretion of 25-hydroxyvitamin D in health and the nephrotic syndrome. *J Lab Clin Med* 99:325–330, 1982

23. LAMBERT PW, DEOREO PB, FU IY, KAETZEL BM, VON AHN K, HOLLIS BW, ROOS BA: Urinary and plasma vitamin D_3 metabolites in the nephrotic syndrome. *Metab Bone Dis Rel Res* 4:7–15, 1982

24. BOUILLON R, VAN ASSCHE FA, VAN BAELEN H, HEYNS W, DEMOOR P: Influence of the vitamin D-binding protein on the serum concentrations of 1,25-dihydroxyvitamin D_3. Significance of the free 1,25-dihydroxyvitamin D_3 concentration. *J Clin Invest* 67:589–596, 1981

25. MALLUCHE HH, GOLDSTEIN DA, MASSRY SG: Osteomalacia and hyperparathyroid bone disease in patients with nephrotic syndrome. *J Clin Invest* 63:494–500, 1979

26. KORKOR AB, SCHWARTZ J, BERGFELD M, TEITELBAUM S, AVIOLI LV, SLATOPOLSKY E: Absence of metabolic bone disease in adult patients with the nephrotic syndrome and normal renal function. *J Clin Endocrinol Metab* 56:496–500, 1983

27. GRAY RW, WEBER HP, DOMINGUEZ JD, LEMANN J JR: The metabolism of vitamin D_3 and 25-hydroxyvitamin D_3 in normal and anephric humans. *J Clin Endocrinol Metab* 39:1045–1056, 1974

28. HUGHES MR, BAYLINK DJ, JONES PG, HAUSSLER MR: Radioligand receptor assay for 25-hydroxyvitamin D_2/D_3 and 1α-dihydroxyvitamin D_2/D_3. *J Clin Invest* 58:61–70, 1976

29. EISMAN JA, HAMSTRA AJ, KREAM BE, DELUCA HF: 1,25-dihydroxyvitamin D in biological fluids: a simplified and sensitive assay. *Science* 193:1021–1023, 1976

30. LAMBERT PW, TOFT DO, HODGSON SF, LINDMARK EA, WITRAK BJ, ROOS BA: An improved method for the measurement of 1,25-(OH)$_2$-D$_3$ in human plasma. *Endocr Res Commun* 5:293–310, 1978

31. GRAY RW, LEMANN J JR, ADAMS ND: The regulation of plasma 1,25-(OH)$_2$-D concentrations in healthy adults, in *Vitamin D: Basic Research and its Clinical Application,* edited by NORMAN AW, SCHAEFER K, VON HERRATH D, GRIGOLEIT HG, COBURN JW, DELUCA HF, MAWER EB, SUDA T, Berlin, Walter de Gruyter, 1979, pp 545–551

32. TAYLOR CM, JANN J, ST JOHN J, WALLACE JE, MAWER EB: 1,25-dihydroxycholecalciferol in human serum and its relationships with other metabolites of vitamin D$_3$. *Clin Chim Acta* 96:1–8, 1979

33. CLEMENS TL, HENDY GN, PAPAPOULOS SE, FREHER LJ, CARE AD, O'RIORDAN JLH: Measurement of 1,25-dihydroxycholecalciferol in man by radioimmunoassay. *Clin Endocrinol* 11:225–234, 1979

34. LUND B, LUND B, SORENSEN OH: Measurement ofcirculating 1,25-dihydroxyvitamin D in man. Changes in serum concentrations during treatment with 1α-hydroxycholecalciferol. Acta *Endocrinologica* 91:338–350, 1979

35. MASON RS, LISSNER D, GRUNSTEIN HS, POSEN S: A simplified assay for dihydroxylated vitamin D metabolites in human serum: application to hyper- and hypovitaminosis D. *Clin Chem* 26:444–450, 1980

36. BISHOP JE, NORMAN AW, COBURN JW, ROBERTS PA, HENRY HL: Studies of the metabolism of calciferol XVI: Determination of the concentration of 25-hydroxyvitamin D, 24,25-dihydroxyvitamin D and 1,25-dihydroxyvitamin D in a single 2 ml plasma sample. *Min Electr Metab* 3:181–189, 1980

37. BOUILLION R, DEMOOR P, BAGGIOLINI EG, USKOKOVIC MR: A radioimmunoassay for 1,25-dihydroxycholecalciferol. *Clin Chem* 26:562–567, 1980

38. YAMAOKA K, SEINO Y, ISHIDA M, ISHII T, SHIMOTSUJI T, TANAKA Y, KUROSE H, MATSUDA S, SATOMURA K, YABUUCHI H: Effect of dibutyryl adenoise 3′,5′-monophosphate administration on plasma concentrations of 1,25-dihydroxyvitamin D in pseudohypoparathyroidism type I. *J Clin Endocrinol Metab* 53:1096–1100, 1981

39. MAIERHOFER WJ, GRAY RW, ADAMS ND, SMITH GA, LEMANN J JR: Synthesis and metabolic clearance of 1,25-dihydroxyvitamin D as determinants of serum concentrations: A comparison of two methods. *J Clin Endocrinol Metab* 53:472–475, 1981

40. ADAMS ND, GRAY RW, LEMANN J JR: The effects of oral CaCO$_3$ loading and dietary calcium deprivation on plasma 1,25-dihydroxyvitamin D concentrations in healthy adults. *J Clin Endocrinol Metab* 48:1008–1016, 1979

41. LEMANN J JR, GRAY RW, MAIERHOFER WJ, ADAMS ND: Effects of weight loss on serum 1,25-(OH)$_2$-vitamin D concentrations in adults: A preliminary report. *Calcif Tissue Int,* in press, 1984

42. CHESNEY RW, ROSEN JF, HAMSTRA A, DELUCA HF: Serum 1,25-dihydroxyvitamin D concentrations in normal children and in vitamin D disorders. *Am J Dis Child* 134:135–139, 1980

43. SEINO Y, SHIMOTSUJI K, YAMAOKA K, ISHIDA M, ISHII T, MATSUDA S, IKEHARA C, YABUUCHI H, DOKOH S: Plasma 1,25-dihydroxyvitamin D concentrations in cords, newborns, infants, and children. *Calcif Tissue Int* 30:1–3, 1980

44. MAIERHOFER WJ, GRAY RW, CHEUNG HS, LEMANN J JR: Bone resorption stimulated by elevated serum 1,25-(OH)$_2$-vitamin D concentrations in healthy men. *Kidney Int* 24:555–560, 1983

45. MAIERHOFFER WJ, LEMANN J JR, GRAY RW, CHEUNG HS: Dietary calcium protects bone when serum 1,25-(OH)$_2$-vitamin D concentrations are elevated (*abstract*). *Kidney Int* 25:148, 1984

46. KAPLAN RO, HAUSSLER MR, DEFTOS LJ, BONE H, PAK CYC: The role of 1α,25-dihydroxyvitamin D in mediation of intestinal hyperabsorption of calcium in primary hyperparathyroidism and absorptive hypercalciuria. *J Clin Invest* 59:767–770, 1977

47. HAUSSLER MR, BAYLINK DJ, HUGHES MR, BRUMBAUGH PF, WERGEDAL JE, SHEN FH, NIELSEN RL, COUNTS SJ, BURSAC KM, McCAIN TA: The assay of 1α,25-dihydroxyvitamin D_3: physiologic and pathologic modulation of circulating hormone levels. *Clin Endocrinol* 5(Suppl):151–165, 1976

48. EISMAN JA, WARK JD, PRINCE RL, MOSELEY JM: Modulation of plasma 1,25-dihydroxyvitamin D in man by stimulation and suppression tests. *Lancet* 2:931–933, 1979

49. KRAUT JA, GORDON EM, RANSOM JC, HORST R, SLATOPOLSKY E, COBURN JW, KUROKOWA K: Effect of chronic metabolic acidosis on vitamin D metabolism in humans. *Kidney Int* 24:644–648, 1983

50. BROADUS AE, HORST RL, LANG R, LITTLEDIKE ET, RASMUSSEN H: The importance of circulating 1,25-dihydroxyvitamin D in the pathogenesis of hypercalciuria and renal-stone formation in primary hyperparathyroidism. *N Engl J Med* 302:421–426, 1980

51. BILEZIKIAN JP, CANFIELD RE, JACOBS TP, POLAY JS, D'AMATO AP, EISMAN JP, DeLUCA HF: Response of 1α,25-dihydroxyvitamin D_3 to hypocalcemia in human subjects. *N Engl J Med* 299:437–441, 1978

52. MAIERHOFER WJ, GRAY RW, LEMANN J JR: Phosphate deprivation increases serum 1,25-(OH)-vitamin D concentrations in healthy men. *Kidney Int* 25:571–575, 1984

53. LUFKIN EG, KUMAR R, HEATH H III: Hyperphosphatemic tumoral calcinosis: Effects of phosphate depletion on vitamin D metabolism, and of acute hypocalcemia on parathyroid hormone secretion and action. *J Clin Endocrinol Metab* 56:1319–1322, 1983

54. INSOGNA KL, BROADUS AE, GERTNER JM: Impaired phosphorus conservation and 1,25-dihydroxyvitamin D generation during phosphorus deprivation in familial hypophosphatemic rickets. *J Clin Invest* 71:1562–1569, 1983

55. WHITSETT JA, HO M, TSANG RC, NORMAN EJ, ADAMS KG: Synthesis of 1,25-dihydroxyvitamin D_3 by human placenta in vitro. *J Clin Endocrinol Metab* 53:484–488, 1981

56. SLATOPOLSKY E, GRAY RW, ADAMS ND, LEWIS J, HRUSKA K, MARTIN K, KLAHR S, DeLUCA H, LEMANN J JR: The pathogenesis of secondary hyperparathyroidism in early renal failure, in *Vitamin D: Basic Research and its Clinical Application,* edited by NORMAN AW, SCHAEFER K, VON HERRATH D, GRIGOLEIT HG, COBURN JW, DeLUCA HF, MAWER EB, SUDA T, Berlin, Walter de Gruyter, 1979, pp 1209–1215

57. JUTTMANN JR, BUURMAN CJ, DE KAM E, VISSER TJ, BIRKENHAGER JC: Serum concentrations of metabolites of vitamin D in patients with chronic renal failure (CRF). Consequences for the treatment with 1-α-hydroxy-derivatives. *Clin Endocrinol* 14:225–236, 1981

58. MASON RS, LISSNER D, WILKINSON M, POSEN S: Vitamin D metabolites and their relationship to azotaemic osteodystrophy. *Clin Endocrinol* 13:375–385, 1980

59. CHRISTIANSEN C, CHRISTENSEN MS, MELSEN F, RODBRO P, DeLUCA HF: Mineral metabolism in chronic renal failure with special reference to serum concentrations of 1,25-$(OH)_2$-D and 24,25-$(OH)_2$-D. *Clin Nephrol* 15:18–22, 1981

60. CHEUNG AK, MANOLAGAS SC, CATHERWOOD BD, MOSELY CA JR, MITAS JA II, BLANTZ RC, DEFTOS LJ: Determinants of serum 1,25-$(OH)_2$D levels in renal disease. *Kidney Int* 24:104–109, 1983

61. LAMBERT PW, STERN PH, AVIOLI RC, BRACKETT NC, TURNER RT, GREENE

A, Fu IY: Evidence for extrarenal production of 1α,25-dihydroxyvitamin D in man. *J Clin Invest* 69:722–725, 1982

62. ZERWEKH JE, MCPHAUL JJ JR, PARKER TF, PAK CYC: Extra-renal production of 24,25-dihydroxyvitamin D in chronic renal failure during 25 hydroxyvitamin D₃ therapy. *Kidney Int* 23:401–406, 1983

63. WILSON L, FELSENFELD A, DREZNER M, KUROKAWA K, LLACH F: Divalent ion metabolism, 1,25-dihydroxyvitamin D, parathyroid hormone and cyclic AMP in early renal failure (*abstract*). *Kidney Int* 25:254, 1984

64. SHEPARD BM, HORST RL, HAMSTRA AJ, DELUCA HF: Determination of vitamin D and its metabolites in plasma from normal and anephric man. *Biochem J* 182:55–69, 1979

65. LUND B, FRIEDBERG M, LUND B, MOSZKOWICZ M, NIELSEN SP, SORENSEN OH: Serum 1,25-dihydroxycholecalciferol in anephric, haemodialyzed and kidney-transplanted patients. *Nephron* 25:30–33, 1980

66. CHESNEY RW, HAMSTRA AJ, MAZEES RB, ROSE P, DELUCA HF: Circulating vitamin D metabolite concentrations in childhood renal diseases. *Kidney Int* 21:65–69, 1982

67. PORTALE AA, BOOTH BE, TSAI HC, MORRIS RC JR: Reduced plasma concentration of 1,25-dihydroxyvitamin D in children with moderate renal insufficiency. *Kidney Int* 21:627–632, 1982

68. TAYLOR A, NORMAN ME: Interrelationship of serum 25-dihydroxyvitamin D₃ and 1,25-dihydroxyvitamin D in juvenile renal osteodystrophy after therapy with 25-hydroxyvitamin D₃. *Metab Bone Dis Rel Res* 4:255–261, 1982

69. BARBOUR GL, COBURN JW, SLATOPOLSKY E, NORMAN AW, HORST RL: Hypercalcemia in an anephric patient with sarcoidosis: evidence for extrarenal generation of 1,25-dihydroxyvitamin D. *N Engl J Med* 305:440–443, 1981

70. MASON RS, FRANKEL T, CHAN Y-L, LISSNER D, POSEN S: Vitamin D conversion by sarcoid lymph node homogenate. *Ann Intern Med* 100:59–61, 1984

71. BRESLAU NA, MCGUIRE JL, ZERWEKH JE, FRENKEL EP, PAK CYC: Hypercalcemia associated with increased calcitriol levels in three patients with lymphoma. *Ann Intern Med* 100:1–7, 1984

72. TURNER RT, PUZAS JE, FORTE MD, LESTER GE, GRAY TK, HOWARD GA, BAYLINK DJ: In vitro synthesis of 1α,25-dihydroxycholecalciferol and 24,25-dihydroxycholecalciferol by isolated calvarial cells. *Proc Natl Acad Sci USA* 77:5720–5724, 1980

73. SLATOPOLSKY E, CAGLAR S, PENNELL JD, TAGGART DD, CANTERBURY JM, REISS E, BRICKER NS: On the pathogenesis of secondary hyperparathyroidism during chronic experimental renal insufficiency in the dog. *J Clin Invest* 50:492–499, 1971

74. PORTALE AA, BOOTH BE, HALLORAN BP, MORRIS RL JR: Effect of phosphate restriction and supplementation of dietary phosphate on plasma 1,25-(OH)₂-D and serum iPTH in children with moderate renal insufficiency (*abstract*). *Kidney Int* 23:108, 1983

75. NORMAN AW, ROTH J, ORCI L: The vitamin D endocrine system: Steroid metabolism, hormone receptors and biological response (calcium binding protein). *Endocrine Rev* 3:331–366, 1982

76. DIETEL M, DORN G, MONTZ R, ALTENAHR E: Influence of vitamin D₃, 1,25-dihydroxyvitamin D₃ and 24,25-dihydroxyvitamin D₃ on parathyroid hormone secretion, adenosine 3',5'-monophosphate release and ultrastructure of parathyroid glands in organ culture. *Endocrinology* 105:237–245, 1979

77. MALLUCHE HH, WERNER E, RITZ E: Intestinal absorption of calcium and wholebody calcium retention in incipient and advanced renal failure. *Min Electr Metab* 1:263–270, 1978

78. HADDAD JG, MIN C, MENDELSOHN M, SLATOPOLSKY E, HAHN TJ: Competitive protein-binding radioassay of 24,25-dihydroxyvitamin D in sera from normal and anephric subjects. *Arch Biochem Biophys* 182:390–395, 1977
79. TAYLOR CM: The measurement of 24,25-dihydroxycholecalciferol in human serum, in *Vitamin D: Biochemical, Chemical and Clinical Aspects Related to Calcium Metabolism,* edited by NORMAN AW, SCHAEFER K, COBURN JW, DeLUCA HF, FRASER D, GRIGOLEIT HG, VON HERRATH D, Berlin, Walter de Gruyter, 1977, p 541
80. CALDAS AE, GRAY RW, LEMANN J JR: The simultaneous measurement of vitamin D metabolites in plasma: Studies in healthy adults and in patients with calcium nephrolithiasis. *J Lab Clin Med* 91:840–849, 1978
81. HORST RW, LITTLEDIKE ET, GRAY RW, NAPOLI JL: Impaired 24,25-(OH)$_2$-D production in anephric man and pig. *J Clin Invest* 67:274–280, 1980
82. WEISMAN Y, LUM GM, REITER EO, GILBOA N, KNOX GR, ROOT AW: Serum concentrations of 24,25-(OH)$_2$-D in uremic children: A reflection of renal function. *J Pediatr* 94:190–193, 1979
83. KANIS JA, HEYNEN G, RUSSELL RGG, SMITH R, WALTON RJ, WARNER GT: Biological effects of 24,25-dihydroxycholecalciferol in man, in *Vitamin D: Biochemical, Chemical and Clinical Aspects Related to Calcium Metabolism,* edited by NORMAN AW, SCHAEFER K, COBURN JW, DeLUCA HF, FRASER D, GRIGOLEIT HG, VON HERRATH D, Berlin, Walter de Gruyter, 1977, pp 793–795
84. PIERIDES AM, ALJAMA P, KERR DNS, SCOTT M, NORMAN AW: Effect of 1α-hydroxycholecalciferol, 1,25-dihydroxycholecalciferol, 3 deoxy-1α-hydroxycholecalciferol, 24^R, 25-dihydroxycholecalciferol and successful renal transplantation on calcium absorption in haemodialysis patients. *Nephron* 20:203–211, 1978
85. CANTERBURY JM, LERMAN S, CLAFLIN AJ, HENRY H, NORMAN A, REISS E: Inhibition of parathyroid hormone secretion by 25-hydroxycholecalciferol and 24,25-dihydroxycholecalciferol in the dog. *J Clin Invest* 61:1375–1383, 1978
86. CANTERBURY JM, GAVELLAS G, BOURGOIGNIE J, REISS E: Metabolic consequences of oral administration of 24,25-dihydroxycholecalciferol to uremic dogs. *J Clin Invest* 65:571–576, 1980
87. OLGAARD K, SCHWARTZ J, FINCO D, ABELAEZ M, TEITELBAUM S, KLAHR S, SLATOPOLSKY E: Long term treatment with 24,25-(OH)$_2$-D$_3$ in uremic dogs: Effect of PTH and the skeleton. *Calcif Tissue Int* 33:340, 1981
88. BORDIER P, RASMUSSEN H, MARIE P, MIRAVET L, GUERIS J, RYCKWAERT A: Vitamin D metabolites and bone mineralization in man. *J Clin Endocrinol Metab* 46:284–294, 1978
89. PAPAPOULOS SE, CLEMENS TL, FRAHER LJ, GLEED J, O'RIORDAN JL: Metabolites of vitamin D in human vitamin D deficiency: effect of vitamin D$_3$ or 1,25-dihydroxycholecalciferol. *Lancet* 2:612–615, 1980
90. PARFITT AM, MATHEWS CHE, BROMMAGE R, JARNAGIN K, DeLUCA HF: Calcitriol but no other metabolite of vitamin D is essential for normal bone growth and development in the rat. *J Clin Invest* 73:576–586, 1984
91. HODSMAN AB, WONG EGC, SHERRARD DJ, BRICKMAN AS, LEE DBN, SINGER FR, NORMAN AW, COBURN JW: Preliminary trials with 24,25-dihydroxyvitamin D$_3$ in dialysis osteomalacia. *Am J Med* 74:407–414, 1983
92. MASSRY SG, TUMA S, DUA S, GOLDSTEIN DA: Reversal of skeletal resistance to parathyroid hormone in uremia by vitamin D metabolites. *J Lab Clin Med* 94:152–157, 1979
93. HART LE, DeLUCA HF: Defective development in embryos from hens fed 1,25-(OH)$_2$-D$_3$ as their sole source of vitamin D (*abstract*). *Fed Proc* 43:985, 1984
94. TEITELBAUM SL: Pathology of uremic bone disease, in *Divalent Ion Homeostasis,*

Contemporary Issues in Nephrology (Vol II), edited by BRENNER BM, STEIN JH, New York, Churchill Livingstone, 1983, chap 8

95. COURNOT-WITMER G, ZINGRAFF J, PLACHOT JJ, ESCAIG F, LEFEVRE R, BOUMATI P, BOURDEAU A, GARABEDIAN M, GALLE P, BOURDON R, DRUEKE T, BALSAN S: Aluminum localization in bone from hemodialyzed patients: Relationship to matrix mineralization. *Kidney Int* 20:375–385, 1981

96. OTT SM, MALONEY NA, COBURN JW, ALFREY AC, SHERRARD DJ: The prevalence of bone aluminum deposition in renal osteodystrophy and its relation to the response to calcitriol therapy. *N Engl J Med* 307:709–713, 1982

97. PARKINSON IS, WARD MK, FEEST TG, FAWCETT RWP, KERR DNS: Fracturing dialysis osteodystrophy and dialysis encephalopathy. An epidemiological survey. *Lancet* 1:406–409, 1979

98. KAEHNY WD, HEGG AP, ALFRED AC: Gastrointestinal absorption of aluminum from aluminum-containing antacids. *N Engl J Med* 296:1389–1390, 1977

99. RECKER RR, BLOTCKY AJ, LEFFLER JA, RACK EP: Evidence for aluminum absorption from the gastrointestinal tract and bone deposition by aluminum carbonate ingestion with normal renal function. *J Lab Clin Med* 90:810–815, 1977

100. PIERCE-MYLI M, PIERIDES A: Iron and aluminum osteomalacia during hemodialysis: A new syndrome (*abstract*). *Kidney Int* 25:151, 1984

101. HENRY DA, GOODMAN WG, NUDELMAN RK, DIDOMENICO NC, ALFREY AC, SLATOPOLSKY TM, STANLEY TM, COBURN JW: Parenteral aluminum administration in the dog: I. Plasma kinetics, tissue levels, calcium metabolism and parathyroid hormone. *Kidney Int* 25:362–369, 1984

102. GOODMAN WG, HENRY DA, HORST R, NUDELMAN RK, ALFREY AC, COBURN JW: Parental aluminum administration in the dog: II. Induction of osteomalacia and effect on vitamin D metabolism. *Kidney Int* 25:370–375, 1984

103. LIU CC, HOWARD GA: Effects of aluminum onbone in vitro (*abstract*). *Clin Res* 32:50A, 1984

104. QUARLES LD, DENNIS VW, GITELMAN HJ, HARRELSON J, DREZNER MK: Aluminum deposition in bone: An epiphenomenon of the osteomalacic state (*abstract*). *Clin Res* 32:522A, 1984

105. BRICKMAN AS, COBURN JW, FRIEDMAN GR, OKAMURA WH, MASSRY SG, NORMAN AW: Comparison of the effects of 1-alpha-hydroxyvitamin D_3 and 1,25-dihydroxyvitamin D_3 in man. *J Clin Invest* 57:1540–1547, 1976

106. SLATOPOLSKY E: Suppression of secondary hyperparathyroidism by 1,25-$(OH)_2$-D_3, in *Clinical Disorders of Bone and Mineral Metabolism*, edited by FRAME B, POTTS JT JR, Amsterdam, Excerpta Medica, 1983

107. COBURN JW, KOPPEL MH, BRICKMAN AS, MASSRY SG: Study of intestinal absorption of calcium in patients with renal failure. *Kidney Int* 3:264–272, 1973

108. BRICKMAN AS, SHERRARD DJ, JOWSEY J, SINGER FR, BAYLINK DJ, MALONEY N, MASSRY SG, NORMAN AW, COBURN JW: 1,25-dihydroxycholecalciferol. Effect on skeletal losses and plasma parathyroid hormone in uremic osteodystrophy. *Arch Intern Med* 134:883–888, 1974

109. PRIOR JC, CAMERON EC, BALLON HS, LIRENMAN DS, MORIARTY MV, PRICE JDE: Experience with 1,25-dihydroxycholecalciferol therapy in undergoing hemodialysis patients with progressive vitamin D_2-treated osteodystrophy. *Am J Med* 67:583–589, 1979

110. GOLDSTEIN GA, MALLUCHE HM, MASSRY SG: Management of renal osteodystrophy with 1,25-$(OH)_2$-D_3. Effects of clinical, radiographic and biochemical parameters. *Min Electr Metab* 2:35–47, 1979

111. MALLUCHE HH, GOLDSTEIN A, MASSRY SG: Management of renal osteodystrophy with 1,25-$(OH)_2$-D_3. Effects of histopathology of bone: Evidence for healing of osteomalacia. *Min Electr Metab* 2:48–55, 1979

112. BORDIER PJ, MARIE PJ, ARNAUD CD: Evolution of renal osteodystrophy: Correlation of bone histomorphometry and serum mineral and immunoreactive parathyroid hormone values before and after treatment with calcium carbonate or 25-hydroxycholecalciferol. *Kidney Int* 7:S102–S112, 1975

113. TEITELBAUM SL, BONE JM, STEIN PM, GILDEN JJ, BATES M, BOISSEAU C, AVIOLI LV: Calcifediol in chronic renal insufficiency. *JAMA* 235:164–167, 1976

114. ELLIS HA, PIERIDES AM, FEEST TG, WARD MK, KERR DNS: Histopathology of renal osteodystrophywith particular reference to the effects of 1α-hydroxyvitamin D₃, in patients treated by long-term haemodialysis. *Clin Endocrinol* 7:S31–S38, 1977

115. MELSEN F, NIELSEN HE, CHRISTENSEN MS: Bone histomorphometry in patients with chronic renal failure: effect of 1α-hydroxyvitamin D₃. *Clin Endocrinol* 7:S39–S44, 1977

116. BALSAN S, GUERIS J, LEVY D, GARABEDIAN M, GUILLOZO H, BROYER M: Suppressive effect of 1α-hydroxyvitamin D₃ on the hyperparathyroidism of children on maintenance hemodialysis. *Metab Bone Dis Rel Res* 1:15–21, 1978

117. KANIS JA, CUNDY T, EARNSHAW M, HENDERSON RG, HEYNEN G, NAIK R, RUSSELL RGG, SMITH R, WOODS CG: Treatment of renal bone disease with 1α-hydroxylated derivatives of vitamin D₃. *Q J Med* 190:289–322, 1979

118. SHARMAN VL, BROWNJOHN AM, GOODWIN FJ, HATELY W, MANNING RM, O'RIORDAN JHL, PAPAPOULOS SE, MARSH FP: Long-term experience of alfacalcidol in renal osteodystrophy. *Q J Med* 203:271–278, 1982

119. CORDY PE, MILLS DM: The early detection and treatment of renal osteodystrophy. *Min Electr Metab* 5:311–320, 1981

120. MEMMOS DE, EASTWOOD JB, TALNER LB, GOWER PE, CURTIS JR, PHILLIPS ME, CARTER GD, ALAGHBAND-ZADEH J, ROBERTS AP, DE WARDENER HE: Double-blind trial or oral 1,25-dihydroxyvitamin D₃ versus placebo in asymptomatic hyperparathyroidism in patients receiving maintenance haemodialysis. *Br Med J* 282:1919–1924, 1981

121. COBURN JW, DIDOMENICO NL, BRYCE GF, BUSSETT LW, SHUPIEN EG, WONG EG, MILLER RB, BENNETT CM, GOLD RH, MALLON JP, MILLER ON, CHUNG PC: Prospective, double-blind trial with calcitriol in the prophylaxis of the bone disease in asymptomatic-dialysis patients, in *Vitamin D: Chemical, Biochemical and Clinical Endocrinology of Calcium Metabolism,* edited by NORMAN AW, SCHAEFER K, VON HERRATH D, GRIGOLEIT HG, COBURN JW, DELUCA HF, MAWER EB, SUDA T, Berlin, Walter de Gruyter, 1982

122. HODSMAN AB, SHERRARD DJ, WONG EGC, BRICKMAN AS, LEE DBN, ALFREY AC, SINGER FR, NORMAN AW, COBURN JW: Vitamin-D-resistant osteomalacia in hemodialysis patients lacking secondary hyperparathyroidism. *Ann Intern Med* 94:629–637, 1981

123. CHRISTIANSEN C, RODBRO P, CHRISTENSEN MS, HARTNACK B: Is 1,25-dihydroxycholecalciferol harmful to renal function in patients with chronic renal failure? *Clin Endocrinol* 15:229–236, 1981

124. MASSRY SG, GRABER H, RIZVI AS, SHERMAN D, GOLDSTEIN DA, LETTERI JM: Use of 1,25-(OH)₂-D₃ in the treatment of renal osteodystrophy in patients with moderate renal failure, in *Clinical Disorders of Bone and Mineral Metabolism,* edited by FRAME B, POTTS JT JR, Amsterdam, Excerpta Medica, 1983

125. CHESNEY RW, HAMSTRA A, JAX DK, MAZEES RB, DELUCA HF: Influence of long-term oral 1,25-dihydroxyvitamin D₃ in childhood renal osteodystrophy. *Contrib Nephrol* 18:55–71, 1980

126. CHAN JCH, KOTROFT MB, LANDWEHR DM: Effects of 1,25-dihydroxyvitamin D₃ on renal function, mineral balance and growth in children with severe chronic renal failure. *Pediatrics* 68:559–571, 1981

Endocrine and Metabolic Abnormalities in Acute Renal Failure

Garabed Eknoyan

Acute renal failure (ARF), as it was described originally, was conceived mainly as the failure of the kidney to excrete waste products. With the emergence of renal physiology and nephrology as independent disciplines following the Second World War, there came definitions for the processes by which the kidney, in addition to excreting waste products, maintains the normal volume and composition of body fluids. As a result, the original concept of ARF, as a disturbance in the elimination of waste products, was expanded to include those disturbances attributable to the kidney's failure to regulate the volume and composition of body fluids. The more recent appreciation of the endocrine functions of the kidney [1] further expanded the perturbances of ARF to include those that are due to the kidneys' failure to regulate the normal endocrine and metabolic balances of the body [2, 3].

The kidney as a target organ of circulating hormones, such as antidiuretic hormone (ADH), aldosterone, and parathyroid hormone (PTH), has long been recognized. This list has now been expanded to include angiotensin, 1,25-dihydroxycholecalciferol $(1,25[OH]_2D_3)$, prostaglandins, catecholamines, thyroid hormone, calcitonin, natriuretic hormone, and insulin [1]. It has also become evident that the kidney itself elaborates hormones with a distant site of action, such as $1,25(OH)_2D_3$, erythropoietin, prostaglandins, renin, and kinins [1]; and that together with the liver, the kidney is a principal site for the metabolic clearance of hormones, principally the polypeptides such as PTH, ADH, insulin, growth hormone, glucagon, prolactin, angiotensin, calcitonin, and various gastrointestinal hormones [4, 5].

Renal failure will therefore result in an elevation of the circulating level of some hormones and a decrease in the level of others. On a broader scale, the development of the uremic environment itself may not only affect hormone secretion, synthesis, and feedback mechanisms, but in addition will alter the end-organ responsiveness to specific hormones. The profound impact that

This manuscript was presented as part of a Symposium on *Endocrine and Metabolic Abnormalities in Renal Diseases.*

this complex series of endocrine and metabolic changes exerts on the function of various organ systems has come to be appreciated as responsible for much of the clinical symptomatology of the uremic syndrome of patients with chronic renal failure. In fact, much of the data on the endocrine disturbances that develop in renal failure has been generated from studies in patients with chronic renal failure. Studies in acute renal failure have been limited by the very nature of the disease process itself, which is potentially reversible and invariably limited in duration, and by the severity of the underlying primary diseases that cause ARF. Nonetheless, the endocrine and metabolic changes that do occur in ARF have been receiving attention mainly through the work of Kokot and his colleagues in Katowice, Poland, and Massry and his coworkers in Los Angeles. As a result, it is now clear that the acute failure of renal function involves the breakdown of the three pivotal functions of the kidney: as an excretory organ, resulting in the accumulation of waste products; as a regulatory organ, causing abnormalities in the volume and composition of body fluids; and as an endocrine organ, leading to derangements of endocrine and metabolic balance. Insight into these endocrine and metabolic abnormalities is essential to an understanding of the pathophysiology of ARF and, on occasion, to the management of some patients.

As a rule, endocrine changes that develop in ARF mimic those of chronic renal failure, which have been defined better [2, 3]. In general, there appears to be little clinical consequence from most of these alterations in ARF, for with recovery from ARF, the endocrine function normalizes. The exception to this generality is the disturbances in PTH and insulin that sometimes result in serious clinical consequences and affect the well-being of patients with ARF. It is not unexpected, then, that the two metabolic and endocrine abnormalities that have attracted the most attention are disturbances in divalent ion metabolism and carbohydrate metabolism, together with the disturbances of their attendant controlling hormones. These will be considered first and in some detail in this review. The abnormalities that develop in the remainder of the endocrine system, which usually are of lesser clinical importance, will be considered subsequently and more briefly.

Divalent Ion Metabolism, PTH, 1,25(OH)$_2$D$_3$, and Calcitonin

Some degree of elevation in the serum phosphorus concentration almost invariably develops in patients with ARF [6]. This is due, in part, to the inability of the failing kidney to excrete phosphorus adequately, and, in part, to the increased release of intracellular phosphorus. The latter is usually due to cellular injury, but may occur in the absence of cell insult because of the coexistent acidosis, which promotes the exit of phosphorus from normal cells [7]. The increment in serum phosphorus that is due to the kidney's inability to excrete it and to the presence of acidosis is usually modest, and the serum concentration of phosphate rarely exceeds 8 mg/dl [6]. However, concentrations of phosphate greater than 8 mg/dl will develop when excessive loads of phosphate, either endogenous or exogenous, are presented to the failing kidney [8, 9]. The source of endogenous phosphorus is extensive tissue injury or rhabdomyolysis. The exogenous source is the phosphate administered in hyperalimentation solutions for the management of some patients with ARF.

As a rule, some degree of hypocalcemia will occur in most patients with ARF. This is an early development—present during the first 24 to 48 hr of oliguric ARF—that persists through the diuretic phase, albeit at a relatively more modest degree than during the oliguric phase, and returns to normal after the recovery of normal renal function [6]. In the study of Massry et al [6], the mean values of total serum calcium ranged from 6.3 ± 0.56 to 8.3 ± 0.21 mg/dl, although lower values have been observed in ARF patients with rhabdomyolysis and acute pancreatitis [9]. The fractions of protein-bound and ionized calcium in these patients are not different from normal, such that the decrements in the calcium concentration will be reflected as a decrease in both moieties of serum calcium [6].

The hypocalcemia of ARF is multifactorial in origin. Whereas hypocalcemia may be observed with low, normal, or elevated serum phosphorus concentrations [6], it is most severe in patients with rhabdomyolysis [8–10]. The serum phosphate of this latter group of patients is sufficiently high to result in a physiochemical interaction with calcium and the consequent deposition of calcium salts in necrotic tissue. Calcification of the injured muscles have been documented in these patients [11] and demonstrated experimentally in the dog [12]. It is important to remember though that even in the absence of cellular injury, the cellular content of calcium is elevated in ARF [13]. Thus, whereas there is no relationship between the concentrations of serum calcium and phosphorus, phosphate retention, particularly if severe, may contribute to the hypocalcemia and will certainly aggravate the degree of hypocalcemia [14]. Any attempt to correct the hypocalcemia of these patients, even if profound and symptomatic, must be tempered by the imminent and potential danger of the tissue deposition of calcium phosphate and the futility of the effort as the serum calcium drops immediately after cessation of calcium infusion. As noted earlier, even in the absence of cellular injury the cellular content of calcium is elevated in ARF; an event that can be aggravated by exogenous loads of calcium [9, 13].

The severe hypocalcemia in patients with pancreatitis is also related to the deposition of calcium in necrotic tissue, but in addition it is due to low circulating levels of PTH [15]. The low levels of circulating PTH in these patients, however, are an exception; elevated levels of circulating PTH is the rule in all other forms of ARF [2, 6, 8, 16]. In fact, the presence of elevated serum levels of PTH are necessary for the deposition of calcium in injured as well as normal tissue that occurs with ARF. In dogs studied 3.5 days after ureteral ligation, the increase in muscle calcium content could be prevented by prior parathyroidectomy, whereas the administration of parathyroid extract increased the muscle calcium of these animals to a level similar to that in uremic animals [17].

The circulating levels of PTH become elevated within hours after the onset of ARF [18, 19], and continue to increase throughout the oliguric and diuretic phases of ARF [6, 16]. This, in the main, is a normal response of the parathyroid gland to the hypocalcemia. The serum PTH levels are inversely related to the concentration of serum calcium of patients with ARF, and fall in response to the infusion of calcium or the addition of calcium to the dialysate of hemodialyzed patients [6]. Another factor that contributes to the elevated PTH levels is the reduction in the metabolic clearance rate (MCR) of the hormone in renal failure [3–5]. PTH is released from the parathyroid gland as an 84 amino acid single-chain polypeptide. In the circulation, it is present in its intact form: the biologically active amino-terminal fragment (residues 53–84) and the inactive carboxy-terminal fragment (residues 1–34) [20]. The normal kidney is the principal organ responsible for the metabolic clearance of PTH; it is responsible for the clearance of 31% of the intact hormone, 45% of the active amino-terminal fragment, and the majority of the inactive carboxy-terminal fragment. In renal failure, the metabolic clearance rate of PTH is decreased not only because of the loss of the contribution of the failing kidney to its clearance, but also because its extrarenal degradation in the liver is depressed because of the coexistent effect of uremia. Thus, the elevated levels of circulating PTH in ARF result from its increased secretion at a time when the body's capabilities to degrade it are reduced.

The apparently paradoxical coexistence of hypocalcemia in the presence of elevated levels of PTH in patients with ARF led Massry et al [6] to suggest that there was a skeletal resistance to the calcemic action of PTH in patients with ARF, a proposal that was substantiated by their experimental and clinical studies [6, 21]. In studies of 10 patients with ARF, the infusion of parathyroid extract did not result in a rise in serum calcium during the oliguric and diuretic phases of ARF. Following recovery from ARF, the same infusion of PTH resulted in an increase in serum calcium by 1.4 $\pm$ 0.14 mg/dl, a value identical to that of normal controls in whom calcium increased by 1.3 $\pm$ 0.14 mg/dl [6]. The resistance to PTH is due, at least in part, to the low levels of $1,25(OH)_2D_3$ [21].

Low circulating levels of $1,25(OH)_2D_3$ have been demonstrated in patients with ARF and rhabdomyolysis [10]. This has been attributed to the severe hyperphosphatemia and marked increase in PTH levels of these patients, both of which suppress the production of $1,25(OH)_2D_3$ by the kidney [10, 14]. Additional factors that would suppress its production would be the limited ability of the injured kidney to hydroxylate $25(OH)D_3$ to its more active form, the presence of metabolic acidosis, and the reduced levels of circulating $25(OH)D_3$. The induction of acute metabolic acidosis by ammonium chloride to dogs results in defective hydroxylation of $25(OH)D_3$ to $1,25(OH)_2D_3$ [22]. Pietrek, Kokot, and Kuska have shown low circulating levels of $25(OH)D_3$ in patients with ARF [23], although others have reported normal values [10]. In any case, the low levels of $1,25(OH)_2D_3$ could contribute to the hypocalcemia because of the resultant reduced calcium absorption from the gut and impaired skeletal response to the circulating PTH.

The serum levels of calcitonin are elevated in ARF, being higher in the oliguric than the polyuric phase of ARF [2, 23]. The response of calcitonin to calcium administration remains normal, however. The infusion of 1.6 ml of a 10% solution of calcium gluconate per kilogram of body wt over 4 hr has been shown to result in increments of calcitonin that are not different from normal [24]. Increased secretion of calcitonin, decreased degradation of the hormone by the failing kidney, or production of abnormal but immunologically reactive fragments of the hormone may all contribute to the hypercalcitoninemia of ARF [2–4, 23].

Unlike the frequent presence of hypocalcemia early in ARF, less common is the periodic development of hypercalcemia in the diuretic or recovery phase of ARF. Save for rare exceptions, this seems to be a problem in patients with severe muscle damage, one-third of whom have been estimated to develop hypercalcemia [8, 10, 24]. Explanations offered for the hypercalcemia in this setting have included secondary hyperparathyroidism, changes in vitamin D metabolism, and mobilization of calcium from previous deposits of calcium salts in damaged muscle tissue [8, 10, 24]. The latter mechanism appears to be the primary cause for the hypercalcemia, with a contributory role played by the increased levels of $1,25(OH)_2D_3$, the higher levels of PTH relative to the existing serum calcium, and the low phosphate concentrations that develop in these patients during the diuretic and recovery phases of their disease.

Carbohydrate Metabolism, Insulin, Glucagon, Growth Hormone

Carbohydrate intolerance, insulin resistance, and elevated levels of insulin, glucagon, and growth hormone develop early in the course of ARF of most patients [2, 3].

The fasting blood sugar and the peak glucose concentrations attained after a glucose load are normal in patients with ARF. It is the decline in blood glucose following the challenge that is abnormal in these patients [2, 25]. In a group of 14 patients with ARF of diverse etiologies studied by Kokot and Kuska [25], after the i.v. infusion of glucose (0.5 g/kg of body wt), the mean glucose concentrations were not different from that of 8 control subjects at 0 and 10 min, but they remained significantly higher than normal at 40 min (210 vs. 130 mg/dl) and 60 min (180 vs. 90 mg/dl). The basal immunoreactive insulin level was normal in these patients, but showed an excessive response to IV glucose, attaining values that were significantly higher than normal at 20 min and remaining abnormally elevated throughout the 60-min duration of the study. There was no correlation between these abnormalities in glucose utilization and insulin clearance and those of the plasma potassium and bicarbonate concentrations. The response to exogenous insulin administration was also abnormal in these patients. At 30 min after the injection of insulin (0.1 U/kg of body wt), the mean value of blood glucose in normals (about 40 mg/dl) was significantly lower than that reached in patients with ARF (about 60 mg/dl). The mean level of immunoreactive growth hormone (GH) at 0, 30, 60, and 120 min after insulin administration was significantly higher in the ARF patients than in the controls. These results are similar to those obtained in experimental models of ARF. Bilaterally nephrectomized rats display glucose intolerance, have higher levels of insulin and growth hormone, and higher insulin/glucose ratios than do sham-operated control animals [26].

The carbohydrate intolerance of ARF despite elevated levels of insulin and the lower decrement in blood glucose in response to insulin indicate a decreased peripheral sensitivity to insulin. The elevated basal levels of GH and the exaggerated insulin-induced release of GH indicate that GH, a known antagonist of insulin effect, plays a role in the resistance in insulin. The resistance to insulin appears to reside primarily at the site of action of insulin on skeletal muscle. In a study of bilaterally nephrectomized rats, glucose uptake mediated by insulin was significantly reduced in the skeletal muscles, whereas hepatic sensitivity to insulin was normal [27]. In fact, glucose production in the isolated perfused liver of these animals was greater than normal. In summary, then, the carbohydrate intolerance of ARF, which is seldom enough to warrant antihyperglycemic therapy, appears to be primarily the consequence of an acquired, but transient, resistance to the peripheral action of insulin owing, at least in part, to the elevated levels of GH.

Whether the elevated levels of glucagon play a role in the carbohydrate intolerance of ARF is less certain. In a study of isolated perfused livers from bilaterally nephrectomized rats, the hepatic production of glucose in response to glucagon infusion was not different from that of control rats [27], although it increased sharply in response to dibutyryl cyclic AMP [28], indicating some degree of altered responsiveness to glucagon in ARF. This is in contrast to results from chronic renal failure patients, in whom glucose response to glucagon infusion is increased [29]. The precise role of the elevated glucagon levels and the response of the liver to glucagon in the overall altered carbohydrate metabolism of ARF is at the moment uncertain.

The elevated levels of insulin, GH, and glucagon in ARF are due, in the main, to the failure of the diseased kidney in its function of degrading polypeptide hormones [2–5]. Both the liver and the kidney play an important role in the metabolism of insulin. About half the insulin released from the pancreas into the portal circulation is extracted by the liver. Of the insulin reaching the systemic circulation, some 30 to 40% is removed by the kidney, while the rest is metabolized in the liver and muscles. Of the small amounts of proinsulin normally reaching the systemic circulation, more than 55% is cleared by the kidney. About 70% of the C-peptide, cleaved from proinsulin during insulin formation, is metabolized by the kidney. In renal failure, the metabolism of all three peptides (insulin, proinsulin, C-peptide) is decreased, and the half-life of insulin is prolonged. The role of the kidney in the metabolism of insulin is enhanced in diabetic patients receiving insulin, because the exogenously administered hormone is absorbed directly into the systemic circulation, thereby circumventing the first-pass metabolic effect of the liver. This will necessitate a reduction in dosage or discontinuation of insulin in diabetic patients who develop ARF.

The kidney accounts for 50 to 70% of the metabolic clearance of GH. Somatomedins, the growth-promoting fractions of GH released by the liver, are also degraded principally by the kidney [4, 5]. The basal levels of GH and its response to exogenous insulin are increased in patients with ARF. Thus, the elevated levels of GH are due to its increased secretion and decreased degradation.

One-third of the metabolic clearance rate of glucagon is due to its degradation by the kidney. In chronic renal failure, the levels of circulating active glucagon and its response to a protein test meal are normal in patients with ARF, but elevated in rats with acute bilateral ureteral ligation [2, 30].

Thyroid Hormone Metabolism

The major pathway of thyroid hormone metabolism (75%) is by deiodination, with the remainder being either conjugated, deaminated, or decarboxylated. The liver is the major site of metabolism. The kidney participates in the metabolism of thyroid hormones to a lesser extent, principally by deamination and decarboxylation. Renal conversion of thyroxine T_4 to triiodothyronine (T_3) and reverse triiodothyroxine (rT_3) also occurs [3, 4]. The kidney is the most important route of inorganic iodide excretion, and in renal failure the plasma levels of inorganic iodide are elevated [3].

Abnormalities in thyroid function tests develop shortly after the onset of ARF [31]. Since any critical illness may result in disturbances of thyroid function tests [32], Kaptein et al [31] evaluated thyroid hormone indices in 12 patients with ARF, but without other systemic illnesses and compared the results to those obtained in 22 patients with critical illnesses, 16 of whom had ARF and 6 had normal renal function. In the group with ARF alone, the serum levels of total T_4 and T_3 were decreased. However, there was no abnormality in the level of free T_4, of the T_3 uptake ratios, and of the baseline level of thyroid-stimulating hormone (TSH). The concentrations of total rT_3 were also normal, but the levels of free rT_3 were elevated. Thus, overall thyroid function was normal, but the binding of T_4 and rT_3 to their carrier proteins was reduced. The 16 patients with ARF and a coexistent critical illness differed only to the extent that the total T_4 and T_3 levels were lower and the T_3 uptake ratio was elevated. As in the group with ARF alone, total rT_3 levels were normal but free rT_3 values were elevated. The group with critical illness alone differed only in that total rT_3 concentrations were elevated. These results indicate that, with the exception of normal total rT_3 levels, the alterations of thyroid hormone indices in ARF are similar to those of other nonthyroidal critical illnesses; the so-called "euthyroid sick" [32].

The TSH response to the i.v. injection of 500 μg of thyrotropin-releasing hormone (TRP), evaluated in 5 patients, was blunted during the oliguric phase of ARF, but normalized with recovery of renal function, indicating a mild reversible pituitary inhibition during early ARF [31].

Hypothalamic-Pituitary-Gonadal Axis

The available information on the hypothalamic-pituitary-gonadal (HPG) axis in ARF comes from the studies by Kokot Mleczko, and Pazera [33] and

Levitan et al [34]. Both studies were limited to male patients with ARF, because of the obvious difficulty in the logistics of such studies in female patients with ARF. There are no data on sexual function in ARF (that is, spermatogenesis in males and ovulatory cycle in females). Nevertheless, the available data from male patients demonstrate that abnormalities in testicular function and HPG axis develop early in ARF and are to a great extent similar to those that occur in chronic renal failure; there is evidence of reversibility of the disturbances early in the polyuric phase of ARF and of total normalization of function after recovery from renal failure [33, 34].

In the 20 patients with ARF studied by Levitan et al [34], during the oliguric phase the serum levels of follicle-stimulating hormone (FSH) and total and free testosterone levels were markedly reduced, those of the sex hormone-binding globulin and luteinizing hormone (LH) were normal, whereas those of prolactin were elevated. During the diuretic phase, the levels of FSH and testosterone remained markedly depressed, but those of prolactin fell to within normal limits. The response of LH and FSH to gonadotropin-releasing hormones (GnRH) and of prolactin to TRH were abnormal. The initial response of LH to GnRH and of prolactin to TRH was normal; however, the serum levels of both hormones remained elevated and did not return to normal during the 4-hr duration of follow-up examination. The response of FSH to GnRH was blunted, with no increase in FSH in 3 of the 6 patients studied. After recovery of renal function, all values and responses to the tropic hormones returned to normal.

In the study of 26 patients with ARF, Kokot et al [33] also reported low levels of testosterone and high levels of prolactin. However, in contrast to the study of Levitan et al [34], they reported significantly elevated levels of LH; a finding similar to those observed in chronic renal failure and more in keeping with the low levels of testosterone and the decreased contribution of the failing kidney to the degradation of LH [3, 4]. In addition, the levels of FSH in their patients were normal rather than reduced as reported by Levitan et al [34]. In chronic renal failure, the FSH levels are elevated; a finding that is in keeping with the azoospermia characteristic of this state and the reduced contribution of diseased kidney to the biogradation of FSH [3, 4]. A reduction in the level of FSH in ARF would therefore be unexpected, whereas a normal level of FSH may reflect on the short duration of the renal failure in this condition. The reason for the discrepancy of the results in LH and FSH levels between these two studies is not evident, but may be due either to differences in technique or severity of the illness between the two groups of patients studied [33, 34].

The elevated levels of prolactin are due to its reduced metabolic clearance rate and increased production. The kidneys are the major site of removal of prolactin, with a reported 16% decrease in the renal arteriovenous levels of the hormone in the normal kidney [4, 35]. In the rat, the kidneys account for about 70% of the overall prolactin metabolism, and ARF results in a significant decrease in its clearance rate [35]. The increased secretion of prolactin may be due to the secondary hyperparathyroidism of ARF. A direct and significant correlation between the serum prolactin and PTH levels has been demonstrated in patients with ARF [34]. Administration of PTH or a rise in the circulating levels of PTH has been shown to be associated with a rise in prolactin in normal persons [36]. Dysfunction of the hypothalamo-hypophyseal regulation of prolactin in ARF, possibly caused by the PTH-induced increased intracellular calcium at these sites, has been suggested as the mechanism for the hyperprolactinemia [34].

Pituitary-Adrenal Axis

The liver is the major site of cortisol and aldosterone metabolism; the kidneys account for only 10% of the metabolic clearance rate of the intact hormones, but are the principal site for the excretion of their hepatic metabolites [4].

In one study of patients with ARF, the basal level of cortisol was reported as normal or only slightly elevated [30]. The infusion of adrenocorticotropic hormone (ACTH) in these patients resulted in a normal or slightly exaggerated response of the adrenal glands, indicating a normal pituitary-adrenal feedback. In another study [37], both the free and glucuronide fractions of the 17-hydroxycorticosteroids were significantly elevated in 11 patients with ARF, but neither was significantly altered in 7 patients with chronic renal failure. Given the severe stress situation that characterizes most patients with ARF, elevated cortisol levels are to be expected.

The levels of plasma renin activity (PRA), immunoreactive angiotensin, and aldosterone are elevated in patients with ARF [2, 38]. The physiologic relation between PRA and aldosterone appears to be abnormal in ARF, with the levels of aldosterone attained for a given PRA being significantly lower than normal. The normal aldosterone to PRA ratio of 4.0 to 4.9 is reduced to less than 1.0 in ARF. The changes in aldosterone level appear to be independent of the extracellular fluid volume and the plasma potassium level of patients with ARF, but display a negative correlation with their plasma sodium concentration [2].

Antidiuretic Hormone

The kidney accounts for 30 to 50% of the metabolic clearance rate of antidi-uretic hormone (ADH), with a capacity to do so over a wide range of levels of the hormone [4]. In patients with ARF, the basal level of ADH is elevated and its response to morphine administration exaggerated [30]. The changes in ADH levels show no correlation to changes in plasma osmolality. The increased ADH levels may be due to the reduced renal degradation by the diseased kidney and the increased secretion from the posterior pituitary, either in response to the elevated PRA or because of "uremic" changes in the pituitary function.

Gastrointestinal Hormones

The gastrointestinal hormones are polypeptides, and the normal kidney con-tributes significantly to their biodegradation [4, 5]. In renal failure, the basal levels of gastrin, secretin, cholecystokinin, and gastric inhibitory polypeptide are elevated [3, 4, 39]. The response to a test meal or calcium administration, where examined, has been normal in patients with ARF, indicating reduced renal degradation by the diseased kidney as the cause of the high basal levels [30].

Erythropoietin

The presence of some degree of anemia is the rule in patients with ARF. Although the anemia is usually multifactorial in origin, the decreased erythropoiesis, appearing several days after the onset of the oliguric phase and persisting well after the recovery of renal function, appears to be the major cause.

Although the precise role of the kidney in the production and metabolism of erythropoietin is still uncertain, it is now well documented that the kidney is the principal site of erythropoietin production in adults [40]. After nephrectomy, the erythropoietin response to hypoxia is impaired in animals [41] and drops significantly in humans [42]. Convincing evidence has been presented that the anemia of chronic renal failure is due to the inadequate production of erythropoietin by the diseased kidney and the impaired response of the erythron due to the "uremic environment" [43]. Conceivably, a similar mechanism could also account for the decreased erythropoiesis of ARF, but it remains to be established.

In summary, it is quite clear that most, if not all, of the endocrine system appears to be adversely influenced by ARF. With recovery of renal function, all noted endocrine abnormalities return to normal, with no evidence of residual long-term detrimental consequences. Although several of the derangements of endocrine function that develop appear to exert no adverse effect on the course of ARF or the well-being of the patient with ARF, others appear to result in significant metabolic effects that deserve special attention and appropriate therapy.

References

1. MASSRY SG (editor): Kidney and hormones. *Nephron* 15:161–408, 1975
2. KOKOT F, KUSKA J: The endocrine system in patients with acute renal failure. *Kidney Int* 10:S26–S31, 1976
3. EMMANOUEL DS, LINDHEIMER MD, KATZ AI: Endocrine function in renal failure, in *The Systemic Consequences of Renal Failure*, edited by EKNOYAN G, KNOCHEL JP, New York, Grune & Stratton, 1984, pp 177–231
4. RABKIN R, KITAJI J: Renal metabolism of peptide hormones. *Mineral Electrolyte Metab* 9:212–226, 1983
5. ARDAILLOU R, PAILLARD F: Metabolism of polypeptide hormones by the kidney. *Adv Nephrol* 9:247–269, 1980
6. MASSRY SG, ARIEFF AI, COBURN JW, PALMIERI G, KLEEMAN CR: Divalent ion metabolism in patients with acute renal failure: Studies on the mechanism of hypocalcemia. *Kidney Int* 5:437–445, 1974

7. KNOCHEL JP: The pathophysiology and clinical characteristics of severe hypophosphatemia. *Arch Intern Med* 137:203–220, 1977
8. TORRENTE A, BERL T, COHN PD, KAWAMOTO E, HERTZ P, SCHREIER RW: Hypercalcemia of acute renal failure: Clinical significance and pathogenesis. *Am J Med* 61:119–123, 1976
9. KNOCHEL JP: Rhabdomyolysis and myoglobinuria. *Sem Nephrol* 1:75–86, 1981
10. LLACH F, FELSENFELD AJ, HAUSSLER MR: The pathophysiology of altered calcium metabolism in rhabdomyolysis-induced acute renal failure. *N Engl J Med* 305:117–122, 1981
11. AKMAL M, GOLDSTEIN DA, TELFER N, WILKINSON E, MASSRY SG: Resolution of muscle calcification in rhabdomyolysis and acute renal failure. *Ann Intern Med* 89:928–930, 1978
12. MERONEY WH, ARNEY GK, SEGAR WE, BALCH HH: The acute calcification of traumatized muscle, with particular reference to acute post-traumatic renal insufficiency. *J Clin Invest* 36:825–832, 1957
13. ARIEFF AI, MASSRY SG: Calcium metabolism of brain in acute renal failure. *J Clin Invest* 53:387–392, 1974
14. SOMERVILLE PJ, KAYE M: Evidence that resistance to the calcemic action of parathyroid hormone in rats with acute uremia is caused by phosphate retention. *Kidney Int* 16:552–560, 1979
15. ROBERTSON GM, MOORE EW, SWITZ DM, SIZEMORE GW, ESTEP HL: Inadequate parathyroid response in acute pancreatitis. *N Engl J Med* 294:512–516, 1976
16. KOVITHAVONGS T, BECKER FO, ING TS: Parathyroid hyperfunction in acute renal failure. *Nephron* 9:349–355, 1972
17. GUISADO R, ARIEFF AI, MASSRY SG: Muscle water and electrolytes in uremia and the effects of hemodialysis. *J Lab Clin Med* 89:322–331, 1977
18. JASTAK JT, MORRISON AB, RAISZ LG: Effect of renal insufficiency on parathyroid gland and calcium homeostasis. *Am J Physiol* 215:84–89, 1968
19. TUMA S, MALLETTE LE: Hypercalcemia after nephrectomy in the dog: Role of the kidneys and parathyroid glands. *J Lab Clin Med* 102:213–219, 1983
20. MARTIN KJ, HRUSKA KA, FREITAG JJ, KLAHR S, SLATOPOLSKY E: The peripheral metabolism of parathyroid hormone. *N Engl J Med* 301:1092–1098, 1979
21. MASSRY SG, STEIN R, GARTY J, ARIEFF AI, COBURN JW, NORMAN AW, FRIEDLER RM: Skeletal resistance to the calcemic action of parathyroid hormone in uremia: Role of 1,25(OH)$_2$D$_3$. *Kidney Int* 9:467–474, 1976
22. LEE SW, RUSSEL J, AVIOLI LV: 25-hydroxycholecalciferol to 1,25 dihydroxycholecalciferol: Conversion impaired by systemic metabolic acidosis. *Science* 195:994–996, 1977
23. PIETREK J, KOKOT F, KUSKA J: Serum 25-hydroxyvitamin D and parathyroid hormone in patients with acute renal failure. *Kidney Int* 13:178–185, 1978
24. KOKOT F, KUSKA J, SLEDZINSKI Z, PIETREK J, BACZYNSKI R: Serum calcitonin levels in patients with acute renal failure. *Mineral Electrolyte Metab* 4:43-48, 1980
25. KOKOT F, KUSKA J: Influence of extracorporeal dialysis on glucose utilization and insulin secretion in patients with acute renal failure. *Eur J Clin Invest* 3:105:111, 1973
26. NITZAN M, METZGER BE, WILBER JF: Effects of acute uremia on metabolic fuels and hormones in the rat. *Isr J Med Sci* 8:771, 1972
27. MONDON CE, DOLKAS CB, REAVEN GM: The site of insulin resistance in acute uremia. *Diabetes* 27:571–576, 1978
28. MONDON CE, REAVEN GM: Evaluation of enhanced glucagon sensitivity as the

cause of glucose intolerance in acutely uremic rats. *Am J Clin Nutr* 33:1456–1460, 1980

29. SHERWIN RS, BASTL C, FINKELSTEIN FO, FISHER M, BLACK H, HENDLER R, FELIG P: Influence of uremia and hemodialysis on the turnover and metabolic effects of glucagon. *J Clin Invest* 57:722–731, 1976

30. KOKOT F: Function of endocrine organs in patients with acute renal failure, in *Acute Renal Failure,* edited by ELIAHOU HE, London, England, John Libbey & Co, Ltd, 1982, pp 288–293

31. KAPTEIN EM, LEVITAN D, FEINSTEIN EI, NICOLOFF JT, MASSRY SG: Alteration of thyroid hormone indices in acute renal failure and in acute critical illness with and without acute renal failure. *Am J Nephrol* 1:138–141, 1981

32. UTIGER RD: Decreased extrathyroidal triiodothyronine production in nonthyroidal illness: Benefit or harm? *Am J Med* 69:807–810, 1980

33. KOKOT F, MLECZKO Z, PAZERA A: Parathyroid hormone, prolactin, and function of the pituitary-gonadal axis in male patients with acute renal failure. *Kidney Int* 21:84–89, 1982

34. LEVITAN D, MOSER SA, GOLDSTEIN DA, KLETZKY OA, LOBO RA, MASSRY SG: Disturbances in the hypothalamo-pituitary-gonadal axis in male patients with acute renal failure. *Am J Nephrol* 4:99–106, 1984

35. EMMANOUEL DS, FANG VS, KATZ AI: Prolactin metabolism in the rat: Role of the kidney in degradation of the hormone. *Am J Physiol* 240:F437–F445, 1981

36. ISAAC R, MERCERON RE, CAILLENS G, RAYMOND JP, ARDAILLOU R: Effect of parathyroid hormone on plasma prolactin in man. *J Clin Endocrinol Metab* 47:18–23, 1978

37. BLAIR AJ, MORGEN RO, BECK JC: The plasma 17-hydroxycorticosteroid levels in acute and chronic renal failure. *Can J Biochem Physiol* 39:1617–1624, 1961

38. KOKOT F, KUSKA J: Plasma renin activity in acute renal insufficiency. *Nephron* 6:115–127, 1969

39. HANSKY J: Effect of renal failure on gastrointestinal hormones. *World J Surg* 3:463–467, 1979

40. FISHER JW: Control of erythropoietin production. *Proc Soc Exp Biol Med* 173:289–305, 1983

41. JACOBSON LO, GOLDWASSER E, FRIED W, PLZAK L: Role of the kidney in erythropoiesis. *Nature* 179:633–634, 1957

42. REGE AB, BROOKINS J, FISHER JW: A radioimmunoassay for erythropoietin: Serum levels in normal human subjects and patients with hemopoietic disorders. *J Lab Clin Med* 100:829–843, 1982

43. FRIED W: Hematologic abnormalities in chronic renal failure. *Semin Nephrol* 1:176–187, 1981.

Insulin, Glucose, Amino Acid, and Lipid Metabolism in Chronic Renal Insufficiency

Ralph A. DeFronzo, Anders Alvestrand, and Douglas J. Smith

It has been shown that patients with chronic renal insufficiency have abnormal insulin degradation, tissue sensitivity to insulin, and insulin secretion. In the following discussion, the pathophysiologic implications of these disturbances will be reviewed.

Insulin Metabolism and the Kidney

The kidney plays an important role in the regulation of many low-molecular weight proteins, including insulin [1]. Normally, the renal arteriovenous insulin concentration difference is approximately 30 to 40% [2, 3] and the renal clearance of insulin is about 200 ml/min in humans [1]. From these data one can estimate that approximately six to eight units per day are degraded by the kidney. This accounts for the removal of about 25% of the daily pancreatic secretion of insulin. Since the normal glomerular filtration rate (120 ml/min) is less than the renal clearance of insulin (200 ml/min), peritubular insulin uptake must be responsible for a significant portion of the renal removal. Both luminal and peritubular uptake have been shown to play important roles in the renal metabolism of insulin [4–6].

The impairment in insulin degradation has important clinical relevance. In humans, the metabolic clearance rate of insulin changes little until the glomerular filtration rate (GFR) has decreased to about 40 ml/min, and marked prolongation of the half-life of insulin does not occur until the GFR has fallen to less than 15 to 20 ml/min [1, 3]. This decrease in insulin degradation is largely responsible for the decreased insulin requirements observed in diabetic subjects who develop chronic renal failure [7–9]. Unless the insulin dosage is appropriately reduced, symptomatic hypoglycemia may ensue [10–

This manuscript was presented as part of a Symposium on *Endocrine and Metabolic Abnormalities in Renal Diseases.*

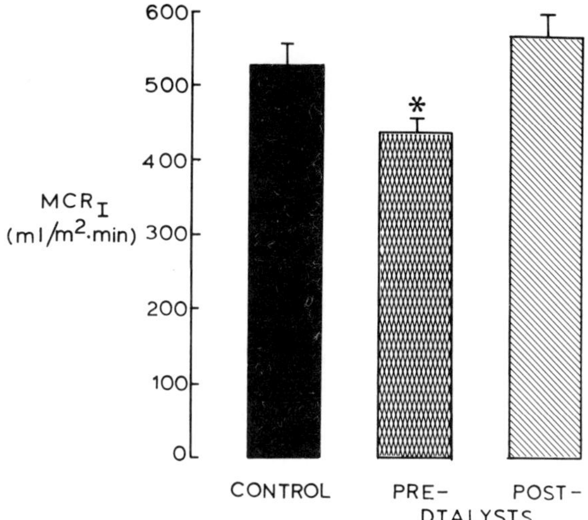

Fig. 1. The metabolic clearance rate (MCR) of insulin in control and uremic subjects before and after 10 wk of thrice weekly hemodialysis. Uremia was associated with a decrease in the MCR of insulin. The MCR was normalized postdialysis.

12]. A similar phenomenon may underlie the hypoglycemia observed in nondiabetic patients with advanced renal insufficiency [13].

Impaired hepatic degradation of insulin also contributes to the prolonged half-life of insulin observed in uremia. Employing the euglycemic insulin clamp technique, DeFronzo et al [14] have shown that the metabolic clearance rate of insulin is prolonged in patients with advanced renal failure (Fig. 1). However, following standard hemodialysis, the metabolic clearance was returned to normal. Since renal function did not improve during the period of dialysis, the increase in insulin clearance must have resulted from enhanced insulin degradation by nonrenal tissues, liver, and muscle [15]. These results indicate that as renal insufficiency develops, there is an accumulation of uremic toxin(s), which inhibit the insulin-degradative systems. Dialysis enhances the clearance of insulin by removing the uremic toxin(s).

Glucose Metabolism in Uremia

Impaired glucose metabolism in chronic renal insufficiency is evidenced by mild fasting hyperglycemia and an abnormal oral or intravenous (i.v.) glucose tolerance test. Recently, the pathogenetic mechanism(s) responsible for the disturbance in glucose metabolism have been delineated. Table 1 lists the clinically relevant aspects of altered glucose metabolism in uremic patients.

The plasma insulin response to glucose administration has been reported to be quite varied in uremic patients [16–18]. The early insulin response

Table 1. Features of glucose metabolism in uremia

Fasting hyperglycemia	Reduced peripheral sensitivity to insulin action
Normal or mild elevation in the fasting blood glucose	Reduced degradation of insulin
Spontaneous hypoglycemia	Decreased requirement for insulin by the patients with diabetes mellitus and uremia
Hyperinsulinemia	
Normal, increased, or decreased insulin secretion in response to glucose load	

following oral and i.v. glucose has been found to be normal, increased, or decreased. By contrast, the late insulin response is increased uniformly. These results suggest that insulin secretion may be impaired in some uremic patients. Results from the i.v. glucose tolerance test (IVGTT) [16] suggest the presence of two distinct groups of uremic patients: (1) one with normal glucose tolerance and an increased plasma insulin response, and (2) a second group with impaired glucose metabolism and either a diminished or "normal" plasma insulin response. These observations can be explained as follows. Tissue insensitivity to insulin is present in essentially all uremic subjects [14]. The normal pancreatic response to this tissue insensitivity to insulin is to augment its secretion of insulin in an attempt to overcome the insulin resistance. This would correspond to the first group of uremic subjects described above, who have normal glucose utilization and an augmented plasma insulin response. However, if a significant inhibition of insulin secretion were superimposed on a state of insulin antagonism, glucose tolerance would become overtly impaired. This would conform to the second group of chronically uremic subjects. Such an interaction between tissue sensitivity to insulin and beta-cell sensitivity to glucose would explain the seemingly discrepant results reported in the literature regarding the plasma insulin response to glucose administration. Using the hyperglycemic and euglycemic insulin clamp techniques, we have attempted to quantitate the relative contributions of impaired insulin secretion versus insulin resistance in the genesis of the glucose intolerance that is observed in patients with chronic renal failure [14].

Insulin Secretion

During the hyperglycemic clamp technique, the plasma glucose concentration is raised acutely and maintained at 125 mg/dl above the fasting level. Under these steady-state conditions of constant hyperglycemia, the total amount of glucose infused—after correction for urinary glucose losses—provides a measure of the total amount of glucose taken up and metabolized (M) by the entire body. The plasma insulin response (I) yields an index of the pancreatic response to hyperglycemia. The M/I ratio yields a measure of the body's sensitivity to the endogenously secreted insulin. These results are summarized in Figure 2.

The typical biphasic plasma insulin response was observed with an early

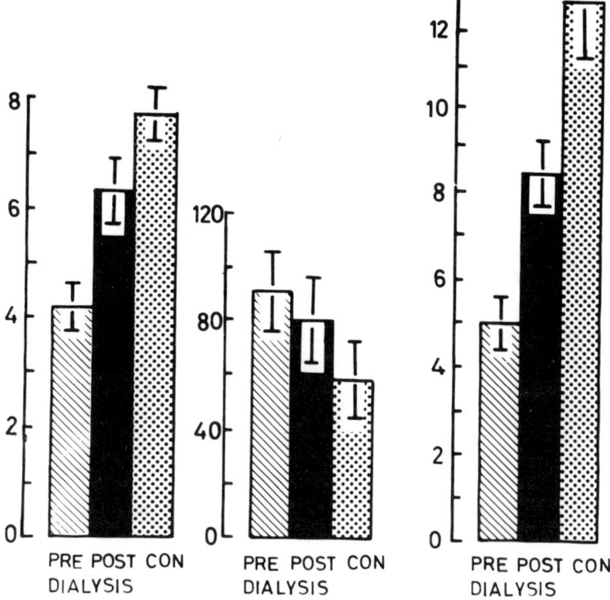

Fig. 2. Summary of glucose metabolism (mg/kg/min) (*left panel*), plasma insulin response to glucose (μU/ml) (*center panel*), and tissue sensitivity to insulin (*M/I* ratio in mg/kg/min per μU/ml $\times$ 100) (*right panel*) in control (*CON*) and uremic subjects pre- and postdialysis during the hyperglycemic clamp study. All values represent the mean $\pm$ SEM.

burst of insulin release within the first 10 minutes, followed by a gradually increasing phase of insulin secretion that lasted until the end of the study. No difference in the early (0 to 10 min) plasma insulin response was observed between uremic and control subjects. However, the late insulin response (10 to 120 min) was significantly greater in the uremic group. Following 10 weeks of hemodialysis, three times weekly, the late plasma insulin response was diminished and was no longer significantly greater than in the control group. As can be seen in Figure 1, the decline in plasma insulin response postdialysis was primarily the result of an increased metabolic clearance rate of insulin. The change in insulin secretion, inferred from the posthepatic systemic delivery rate (mean plasma insulin response $\times$ MCR [metabolic clearance rate] of insulin), was variable. In most patients, insulin secretion was increased, indicating that uremia exerted an inhibitory effect on the beta cell. In some patients, however, insulin secretion declined postdialysis, suggesting that impaired insulin action represented the primary disturbance. Thus, dialysis restored tissue sensitivity toward normal levels, and glucose metabolism improved. Consequently, a diminished need for insulin was present.

The amount of glucose metabolized by the uremic patients during the hyperglycemia was significantly lower (4.2 $\pm$ 0.4 mg/kg body weight/min) than in normal subjects (7.7 $\pm$ 0.4 mg/kg/min) (Fig. 2). Although hemodialysis therapy led to a marked improvement in glucose metabolism, it did not completely return it to normal. Predialysis, the body's sensitivity to insulin (M/I ratio) was markedly diminished in uremic subjects (Fig. 2). Following dialysis, the M/I ratio increased by 80%, but it still remained significantly lower than in controls.

In recent years, much evidence has accumulated to indicate that parathyroid hormone (PTH) is a uremic toxin. To examine its role in the glucose intolerance of uremia, we studied three groups of dogs: controls, 1 7/8 nephrectomized dogs and 1 7/8 nephrectomized dogs who underwent simultaneous parathyroidectomy. Dogs were studied with the hyperglycemic clamp technique before and after 12 weeks of either nephrectomy or combined nephrectomy/parathyroidectomy. The GFR was 10 ± 1 and 13 ± 3 ml/ min in the two nephrectomized groups, respectively. Serum calcium and phosphate concentrations were maintained within the normal range with the administration of calcium supplements and phosphate binders as necessary. In the nephrectomized group, the amount of glucose metabolized during the hyperglycemic clamp study was reduced by 38% (6.6 ± 1.1 versus 10.7 ± 1.1 mg/kg/min), compared to the nephrectomized/parathyroidectomized group. The improvement in glucose utilization in the parathyroidectomized dogs was entirely due to an increase in insulin secretion (143 ± 38 versus 71 ± 10 μU/ml) without any change in insulin sensitivity (M/I ratio $= 9.8 \pm 2.7$ versus 8.9 ± 1.3 mg/kg $\cdot$ min per μU/ml $\times$ 100). Insulin clamp studies performed in the same dogs confirmed that parathyroidectomy did not improve tissue sensitivity to insulin. Compared to controls, nephrectomized dogs were insulin-resistant, and parathyroidectomy did not improve insulin action.

Insulin Resistance

Impaired tissue sensitivity to insulin in uremic individuals is suggested by the following observations: (1) elevated basal insulin concentrations in the face of a normal fasting plasma glucose level, (2) a blunted decline in the plasma glucose concentration following i.v. insulin administration, and (3) a diminished ability of insulin to promote glucose uptake by the human forearm. These abnormalities have been reviewed extensively [16].

To provide a more pure measure of tissue sensitivity to insulin, DeFronzo et al used the euglycemic insulin clamp technique [14]. Briefly, the plasma insulin concentration is raised by 100 μU/ml, and a variable glucose infusion is adjusted to maintain the plasma glucose concentration constant at postabsorptive levels. Under these steady-state conditions of euglycemia, all of the glucose that is infused (M) must be taken up by cells and provides a measure of the body's sensitivity to the infused insulin (Fig. 3). Before dialysis, glucose metabolism was impaired in the uremic group, despite plasma insulin levels that were significantly greater than in controls (Fig. 3). Consequently, the M/I ratio (a measure of tissue sensitivity to insulin) was reduced by approximately 40% in uremic individuals. After dialysis, insulin-mediated glucose

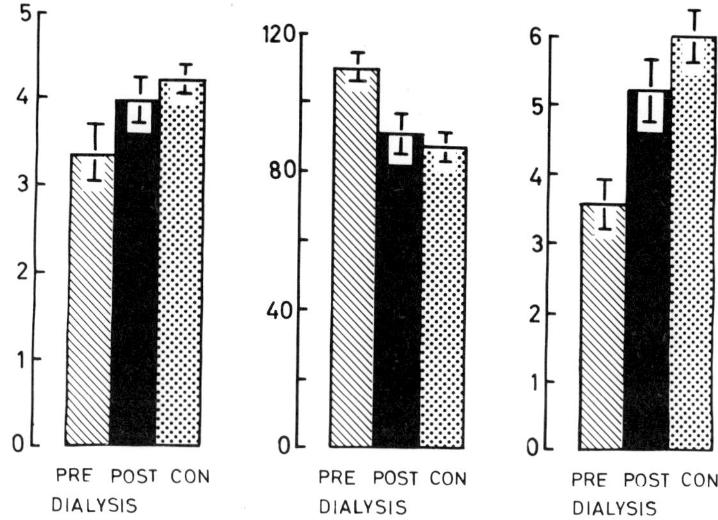

Fig. 3. Summary of glucose metabolism (mg/kg/min) (*left panel*), steady-state (20 to 80 min) plasma insulin concentration (μU/ml) (*center panel*), and tissue sensitivity to insulin (*M/I* ratio in mg/kg/min per μU/ml $\times$ 100) (*right panel*) in control (*CON*) and uremic subjects pre- and postdialysis during the euglycemic insulin clamp. All values represent the mean $\pm$ SEM.

metabolism improved, but it still remained slightly less than in controls (Fig. 3).

Hypothesis

The above observations allow the following formulation (Fig. 4). Insulin resistance is present in the great majority of patients with chronic renal failure, and it is the primary factor responsible for the glucose intolerance of uremia (arrow 1, Fig. 4). Normally, the beta cell would increase its secretion of insulin in an attempt to offset this insulin resistance (arrow 2, Fig. 4). In many subjects, however, uremia also inhibits insulin secretion (arrow 3, Fig. 4). In those individuals in whom uremia impairs both tissue sensitivity to insulin and the beta cell response to glucose, the greatest decline in glucose tolerance develops.

Site of Insulin Resistance

The impairment in insulin-mediated glucose metabolism observed in uremic patients could result from one of three abnormalities: (1) increased basal

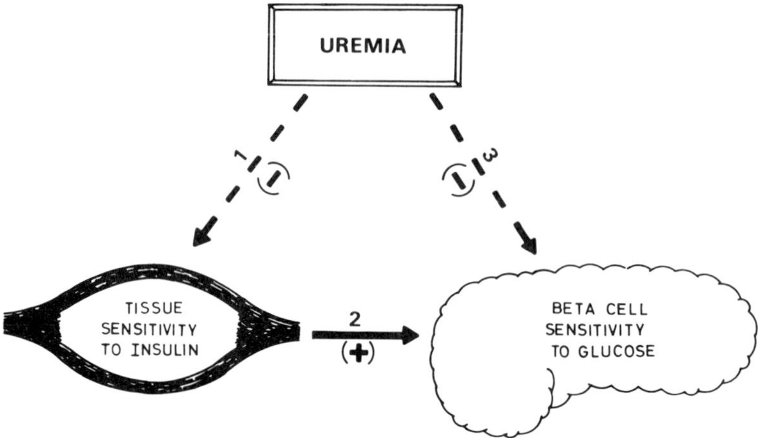

Fig. 4. Effect of uremia on tissue sensitivity to insulin and beta cell sensitivity to glucose. Uremia results in a state of (*1*) peripheral insulin resistance that leads secondarily to (*2*) enhanced insulin secretion. Uremia may also directly (*3*) inhibit insulin secretion. *Interrupted lines* indicate an inhibitory effect of uremia ($-$). *Solid line* represents a stimulatory effect ($+$).

hepatic glucose production that does not suppress normally in response to hyperinsulinemia, (2) decreased hepatic glucose uptake, or (3) diminished glucose uptake by peripheral (muscle and adipose) tissues. Using the insulin clamp technique in combination with both radioisotope (tritiated glucose) turnover methodology and hepatic vein/femoral vein catheterization, we have systematically examined each of these possibilities [14, 17–19]. In uremic subjects, both suppression of hepatic glucose production and splanchnic (hepatic) glucose uptake were found to be normal. By contrast, the ability of insulin to stimulate glucose uptake by leg tissues was markedly impaired. These results indicate that the primary site of insulin resistance in uremic patients resides in the periphery (most likely muscle); and they are consistent with results obtained using the forearm infusion technique [20, 21]. Mondon, Dolkas, and Reaven [22] have published similar results in uremic rats. Following hemodialysis treatment, tissue sensitivity returns toward normal (Figs. 2, 3) and overall glucose tolerance improves [14].

Cellular Mechanism of Insulin Resistance

Recently, the cellular mechanisms contributing to the impairment of insulin action in uremic subjects have been clarified. Insulin, like other peptide hormones, initiates its effects on target tissues by binding to specific receptors on the cell surface. The resulting hormone-receptor interaction triggers a series of membrane and intracellular events that produce characteristic biologic responses. In a general sense, therefore, insulin resistance could develop from either a receptor or a postreceptor defect.

Gambhir et al [23] reported decreased insulin binding to erythrocytes obtained from chronically uremic, nondialyzed subjects. After 1 year of hemodialysis therapy, red blood cell binding increased to values greater than controls [23]. By contrast, insulin binding to adipocytes [24] and hepatocytes [25] obtained from uremic rats has been shown to be normal. We have examined insulin binding to circulating monocytes from uremic subjects and found that this is normal [26]. By inference, our results [26], as well as those of Maloff and Lockwood [24] and Kaufman and Caro [25], would predict that intracellular defects are responsible for the insulin resistance of uremia. Unfortunately, it is not possible in humans to obtain direct measurements of postreceptor events. However, inferences about intracellular abnormalities are possible because of the distinctive dose-response relationship between insulin binding and insulin action [27]. Thus, in circumstances where alterations in insulin binding alone are responsible for the impairment in insulin action, the dose-response curve relating insulin concentration to glucose utilization is shifted to the right; and, the maximal hormone responsiveness is unchanged. By contrast, if a postreceptor abnormality is present, no amount of insulin will produce normal maximal responsiveness. In addition, as in the situation with decreased insulin binding, the dose-response curve may be displaced to the right. Using the insulin clamp technique, Smith and DeFronzo [26] have constructed in vivo dose-response curves relating total body insulin-mediated glucose metabolism to the plasma insulin concentration in both control and chronically uremic subjects. As discussed earlier, monocyte insulin binding was shown to be normal. The whole body in vivo dose-response curve relating glucose metabolism during the insulin clamp to the steady-state plasma insulin concentration displayed a shift to the right and an inability to normalize glucose uptake, even at pharmacologic plasma insulin levels. These results are the predicted functional consequence of a postreceptor defect in insulin action; and, they are consistent with the monocyte binding data, which showed no decrease in either insulin receptor number or affinity. These data are in agreement with those of Maloff and Lockwood [24] and Kaufman and Caro [25], who examined insulin action on adipocytes and hepatocytes, respectively, from chronically uremic rats. They found normal [24] or increased [25] insulin binding, but decreased glucose transport and impaired intracellular glucose metabolism. In the later study [25], ^{125}I-insulin internalization by hepatocytes from uremic rats was normal. By contrast, intracellular insulin degradation was significantly impaired [25].

Clinical Implications of Glucose Intolerance in Uremia: Relationship to Lipid and Protein Metabolism (Fig. 5)

Accelerated atherogenesis is a complication of chronic uremia. Hyperglycemia can lead to the formation of abnormal circulating proteins, such as glycosylated hemoglobin [28]; and, it may *contribute directly to abnormalities in*

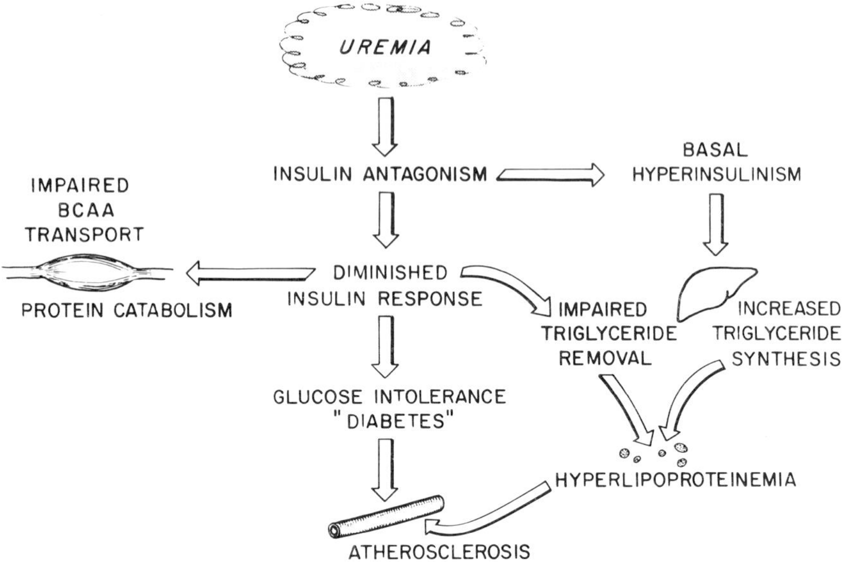

Fig. 5. Inter-relationship between insulin antagonism and disturbances in carbohydrate, lipid, and protein metabolism.

the structural proteins comprising capillary basement membranes in muscle and kidney tissue [29–31]. Thus, the hyperglycemia per se observed in uremic individuals may be partly responsible for the excessive development of atherosclerotic complications.

In addition, resistance to the action of insulin may lead to the development of hypertriglyceridemia via two separate mechanisms (Fig. 5). First, hyperinsulinemia is known to stimulate hepatic triglyceride very low-density lipoprotein (VLDL) synthesis. Second, insulin is the chief regulator of lipoprotein lipase, which is the enzyme regulating triglyceride (VLDL) removal from the circulation. If the insulin resistance affects lipoprotein lipase activity, then impaired triglyceride (VLDL) removal may contribute to the hypertriglyceridemia that is uniformly found in patients with advanced renal insufficiency [32–38]. Using tritiated glycerol, Sanfelippo, Swenson, and Reaven [37] and Cattran et al [35, 36] have documented normal rates of triglyceride synthesis in patients with chronic renal failure. Impaired triglyceride (VLDL) removal was found to be the primary cause of the hypertriglyceridemia in their studies. These findings are in agreement with previous studies demonstrating diminished postheparin-lipolytic activity, which is a measure of lipoprotein lipase activity [32, 33]. Similarly, uremic serum has been shown to inhibit lipoprotein lipase in a rat adipose tissue assay system [34, 39]. Most recently, Caro and Lanza-Jacoby [40] have examined lipid metabolism in hepatocytes isolated from chronically uremic rats. They found that basal and insulin-stimulated lipid synthesis was diminished in uremic animals, and that this was related to decreased activity of the key enzymes (acetyl CoA carboxylase, fatty acid synthetase, citrate cleavage enzyme, malate dehydrogenase, and glucose-6-phosphate dehydrogenase) involved in lipid synthesis. Muscle and adipose tissue lipoprotein lipase were decreased. Several recent studies [41, 42] have suggested that carnitine deficiency may be partly responsible for the hypertriglyceridemia and impaired VLDL clearance. It should be noted, however, that several recent studies using radioisotope turnover techniques and the i.v. fat tolerance test have demonstrated an increased triglyceride production rate [43–45]. Thus, at least in some uremic individuals, both increased synthesis as well as decreased removal of VLDL may contribute to the hypertriglyceridemia. An excellent review of the lipid abnormalities that accompany the uremic state has been published by Henck and Ritz [38].

Another important issue is whether the insulin antagonism observed with respect to glucose utilization also extends to amino acid and protein metabolism (Fig. 5). Branched-chain amino acids, particularly leucine, have been shown to play an important role in the regulation of protein synthesis by muscle [46], and insulin is known to promote net muscle uptake of the branched-chain amino acids. Thus, if the insulin antagonism also involves amino acid transport, a state of intracellular amino acid deficiency might be present; this could be responsible for the muscle wasting that is so commonly encountered in uremic subjects. Previous studies have shown that the plasma levels of all three branched-chain amino acids—valine, leucine, and isoleucine—are uniformly decreased in uremic subjects, while intracellular levels of valine—but not leucine or isoleucine—are reduced [47–49]. To examine the effect of insulin on branched-chain amino acid (BCAA) metabolism, we performed insulin clamp studies ($\triangle$ plasma insulin $= 100\ \mu$U/ml) in chronically uremic subjects (unpublished results). Although insulin-mediated glucose uptake was reduced by 40 to 50%, the decline in plasma BCAA concentration was not impaired. It should be noted that even though insulin-mediated BCAA uptake by human uremic muscle is normal, a significant intracellular defect still may be present; this could impair the incorporation of these amino acids into protein. To examine this question, we measured intracellular amino acid concentrations in quadriceps muscles before and 2 hr after euglycemic hyperinsulinemia (DeFronzo et al, unpublished results). A consistent and similar decline in the intracellular concentration of all amino acids, except alanine, was observed in uremic and control subjects. These results make two important points. First, the combined effect of insulin to enhance amino acid incorporation into protein and to inhibit protein catabolism is quantitatively greater than the ability of insulin to stimulate amino acid transport into the cell. Second, the net effect of insulin to promote amino acid flux into protein is not impaired in uremia. These results demonstrate a clear-cut dissociation between the stimulatory effects of insulin on amino acid, as opposed to glucose metabolism in humans.

It should be noted that the *chronic* effects of uremia on protein and amino acid metabolism may be quite different from the effects of acute uremia. In a recent study, Clark and Mitch [50] demonstrated that acute renal failure in rats was associated with an increased rate of net protein degradation, primarily due to enhanced protein degradation. Whether a similar disturbance in protein metabolism is present in chronic renal failure remains to be established.

Glucagon, Glucose, and Amino Acid Metabolism in Uremia

Glucagon is a small molecular weight protein that is freely filtered by the glomerulus and is reabsorbed and catabolized by the proximal tubular cells [51, 52]. There is also considerable uptake and degradation by the peritubular membrane [51, 52]. In patients with advanced renal insufficiency [53, 54] and in uremic animal models [55], the renal clearance of glucagon is decreased and hyperglucagonemia results. Although proglucagon is primarily responsible for the increased levels of circulating plasma glucagon, there is also a 3-fold elevation in the biologically active 3500-dalton molecular weight glucagon component [56]. The increased plasma glucagon concentration is entirely due to a decrease in the metabolic clearance rate, with glucagon secretion being normal [57]. The primary effect of glucagon is to stimulate hepatic glucose production. Since basal hepatic glucose production is not elevated in uremic subjects and is normally suppressed following hyperinsulinemia, it is unlikely that the hyperglucagonemia plays any role in the glucose intolerance under conditions where plasma insulin levels are elevated. However, Sherwin et al have demonstrated that the plasma glucose response to glucagon is markedly enhanced in uremia, indicating an increased hepatic sensitivity to the hormone [54]. Thus, following protein ingestion—when the plasma glucagon response is high, yet the plasma insulin response is relatively low— excessive stimulation of hepatic glucose output may ensue and may result in glucose intolerance. The elevated glucagon levels also may contribute to the augmented gluconeogenesis from alanine reported by Rubenfeld and Garber [58]. This, in turn, could cause an increased flow of protein nitrogen from peripheral tissues to the liver and could lead to negative nitrogen balance. Recently, we have employed the euglycemic insulin clamp technique in combination with hepatic venous catheterization to examine net splanchnic alanine balance. In uremic subjects, alanine uptake by the splanchnic tissues was increased by 39% compared to controls. These results are consistent with findings of Rubenfeld and Garber [58], and they suggest that gluconeogenesis is enhanced in patients with chronic renal insufficiency. This observation has important clinical implications, since it may explain the muscle wasting and negative nitrogen balance commonly observed in uremic patients. The complete elucidation of such potentially important metabolic disturbances will require further studies. Of particular note to the patient with end-stage renal failure, Sherwin et al [54] have shown that institution of hemodialysis therapy restores hepatic sensitivity to glucagon to normal.

Insulin and Potassium Metabolism

Following the infusion of insulin, the plasma potassium concentration declines due to stimulation of both muscle and hepatic potassium uptake [59]. To examine whether insulin-stimulated potassium uptake is impaired in uremia, we performed insulin clamp studies in combination with combined hepatic/ femoral venous catheterization [60]. The decline in plasma potassium after 2 hr of euglycemic hyperinsulinemia ($\triangle$ plasma insulin concentration = 100 μU/ml) was similar in uremic and control subjects ($\triangle$ plasma potassium concentration = 0.95 ± 0.05 and 0.98 ± 0.10 mEq/liters, respectively). Not surprisingly, the amount of potassium taken up by the leg and splanchnic tissues was similar in both uremic and control subjects. Thus, our studies confirm earlier work published by Westervelt [20, 21].

Summary

Glucose intolerance is characteristic of the uremic state. The impairment in glucose metabolism results from abnormalities in insulin secretion, as well as in insulin action. Excessive PTH levels contribute to the defect in insulin secretion. The insulin resistance primarily results from the inability of insulin to stimulate glucose uptake by peripheral tissues, including muscle. Suppression of hepatic glucose production by insulin, as well as stimulation of hepatic glucose uptake, is not impaired in uremic subjects. At the cellular level, the defect in insulin action appears to result from an intracellular abnormality; insulin binding to its receptor is not diminished. The hypertriglyceridemia of uremia largely results from the inability of insulin to normally inhibit lipoprotein lipase. However, some uremic subjects also demonstrate an increased production rate of VLDL. The amino acid and potassium lowering effects of insulin are not impaired in patients wih chronic renal insufficiency.

References

1. RUBENSTEIN AH, MAKO ME, HOROWITZ DL: Insulin and the kidney. *Nephron* 15:306–326, 1975
2. KATZ AI, RUBENSTEIN AH: Metabolism of proinsulin, insulin, and C-peptide in the rat. *J Clin Invest* 52:1113–1121, 1973
3. RABKIN R, SIMON NM, STEINER S, COLWELL JA: Effect of renal disease on renal uptake and excretion of insulin in man. *N Engl J Med* 282:182–186, 1970
4. MAUDE DL, HANDELSMAN DG, BABU M, GORDON EE: Handling of insulin by the isolated perfused rat kidney. *Am J Physiol* 240:F288–F294, 1981
5. RABKIN R, RUBENSTEIN AH, COLWELL JA: Glomerular filtration and proximal tubular absorption of insulin ^{131}I. *Am J Physiol* 223:1093–1096, 1972
6. RABKIN R, JONES J, KITABCHI AE: Insulin extraction from the renal peritubular circulation in the chicken. *Endocrinology* 101:1828–1833, 1977

7. ZUBROD CG, EVERSOLE SL, DANA GW: Amelioration of diabetes and striking rarity of acidosis in patients with Kimmelstiel-Wilson lesions. *N Engl J Med* 245:518–525, 1951

8. KALLIOMAKI JL, MARKKANEN TK, SOURANDER LB: Correlation between insulin requirement and renal retention in diabetic nephropathy. *Acta Med Scand* 166:423–424, 1960

9. RUNYAN JW, HURWITZ D, ROBBINS SL: Effect of Kimmelstiel-Wilson syndrome on insulin requirements in diabetes. *N Engl J Med* 252:388–391, 1955

10. PIETSMAN SJ, AGARNAL BN: Spontaneous hypoglycemia in end stage renal failure. *Nephron* 19:131–139, 1977

11. RABU M, DOR J, ADAR R, WALDEN R, MOZES M: Spontaneous hypoglycemia in a diabetic patient with renal failure. *Israel J Med Sci* 9:1036–1039, 1973

12. BLOCK MB, RUBENSTEIN AH: Spontaneous hypoglycemia in diabetic patients with renal insufficiency. *JAMA* 213:1863–1866, 1970

13. WHITE MG, KURTZMAN NA: Hypoglycemia in non-diabetics with renal failure (*letter*). *JAMA* 215:117, 1971

14. DEFRONZO RA, TOBIN JD, ROWE JW, ANDRES R: Glucose intolerance in uremia. Quantification of pancreatic beta cell sensitivity to glucose and tissue sensitivity to insulin. *J Clin Invest* 62:425–435, 1978

15. MONDON CE, DOLKAS CB, REAVEN GM: Effect of acute uremia on insulin removal by the isolated perfused rat liver and muscle. *Metabolism* 27:133–142, 1978

16. DEFRONZO RA, ANDRES R, EDGAR P, WALKER WG: Carbohydrate metabolism in uremia: A review. *Medicine* 52:469–481, 1973

17. DEFRONZO RA: Pathogenesis of glucose intolerance in uremia. *Metabolism* 27(Suppl 2):1866–1880, 1978

18. DEFRONZO RA, ALVESTRAND A: Glucose intolerance in uremia: site and mechanism. *Am J Clin Nutr* 33:1438–1445, 1980

19. DEFRONZO RA, ALVESTRAND A, SMITH D, HENDLER R, HENDLER E, WAHREN J: Insulin resistance in uremia. *J Clin Invest* 67:563–568, 1981

20. WESTERVELT FB: Insulin effect in uremia. *J Lab Clin Med* 74:79–84, 1969

21. WESTERVELT FB: Uremia and insulin response. *Arch Intern Med* 126:865–869, 1970

22. MONDON C, DOLKAS C, REAVEN G: The site of insulin resistance in acute uremia. *Diabetes* 27:571–576, 1978

23. GAMBHIR KK, HERURKER SG, CRUZ AC, HOSTEN AO: Insulin receptor defect in diabetic man with chronic renal failure: A comparison of erythrocyte insulin binding in diabetic and non-diabetic patients on maintenance hemodialysis. *Biochem Med* 25:62–73, 1981

24. MALOFF B, LOCKWOOD D: Cellular basis for insulin resistance in chronic uremia. *Am J Physiol* 245:E178–E184, 1983

25. KAUFFMAN JM, CARO JF: Insulin resistance in uremia. Characterization of insulin action, binding, and processing in isolated hepatocytes from chronic uremic rats. *J Clin Invest* 71:698–708, 1983

26. SMITH D, DEFRONZO RA: Insulin resistance in uremia is mediated by postbinding defects. *Kidney Int* 22:54–62, 1982

27. KAHN CR: Membrane receptors for hormones and neurotransmitters. *J Cell Biol* 70:261–286, 1976

28. KOVARIK J, STUMMVOLL HK, GRAF H, MULLER MM: Glucose intolerance and hemoglobin A_I in chronic renal insufficiency. *Nephron* 28:209–212, 1981

29. UITTO J, PEREJDA AJ, GRANT GA, ROWALD EA, KILO C, WILLIAMSON JR: Glycosylation of human glomerular basement membrane collagen. Increased con-

tent of hexose in ketoamine linkage and unaltered hydroxylysine-O-glycosides in patients with diabetes. *Connect Tiss Res* 10:45–54, 1982

30. COHEN MP, WU VY: Identification of specific amino acids in diabetic glomerular basement membrane collagen subject to nonenzymatic glucosylation in vivo. *Biochem Biophys Res Commun* 100:1549–1554, 1981

31. Wahl P, Deppermann D, Deschner W, Fuchs E, Rexroth W: The metabolism of the isolated renal glomerulus and its basement membranes, in *Vascular and Neurological Changes in Early Diabetes,* edited by CAMERINI-DAVALOS RA, COLE HS, New York, Academic Press, 1973, p 85

32. IBELS LS, REARDON MF, NOSTEL PJ: Plasma post-heparin lipolytic activity and triglyceride clearance in uremic and hemodialysis patients and renal allograft recipients. *J Lab Clin Med* 87:648–658, 1976

33. BAGDADE JD: Uremic lipemia: An unrecognized abnormality in triglyceride production and removal. *Ann Intern Med* 126:875–881, 1970

34. MURASE T, CATTRAN DC, RUBENSTEIN B, STEINER G: Inhibition of lipoprotein lipase by uremic plasma, a possible cause of hypertriglyceridemia. *Metabolism* 24:1279–1286, 1975

35. CATTRAN DC, FENTON SSA, WILSON DR, STEINER G: Defective triglyceride removal in lipemia associated with peritoneal dialysis and hemodialysis. *Ann Intern Med* 85:29–33, 1976

36. CATTRAN DC, STEINER G, FENTON SSA, WILSON DR: Hypertriglyceridemia in uremia and the use of triglyceride turnover to define pathogenesis. *Trans Am Soc Art Int Organs* 20:148–152, 1974

37. SANFELIPPO ML, SWENSON RS, REAVEN GM: Reduction of plasma triglyceride by diet in subjects with chronic renal failure. *Kidney Int* 11:54–61, 1977

38. HENCK CC, RITZ E: Hyperlipoproteinemia in renal insufficiency. *Nephron* 25:1–7, 1980

39. BAGDADE JD, SHAFRIR E, WILSON DE: Mechanisms of hyperlipidemia in chronic uremia. *Trans Am Soc Art Int Organs* 22:42–45, 1976

40. CARO JF, LANZA-JACOBY S: Insulin resistance in uremia. Characterization of lipid metabolism in freshly isolated and primary cultures of hepatocytes from chronic uremic rats. *J Clin Invest* 72:882–892, 1983

41. VACHA GM, GIORCELLI G, SILIPRANDI N, CORSI M: Favorable effects of L-carnitine treatment on hypertriglyceridemia in hemodialysis patients: decisive role of low levels of high density lipoprotein-cholesterol. *Am J Clin Nutr* 38:532–540, 1983

42. GUARNIERI GF, RANIERI F, TOIGO G, VASILE A, CIMAN M, RIZZOLI V, MORACCHIELLO M, CAMPANACCI L: Lipid-lowering effect of carnitine in chronically uremic patients treated with maintenance hemodialysis. *Am J Clin Nutr* 33:1489–1492, 1980

43. NORBECK HE: Serum lipoproteins in chronic renal failure. *Acta Med Scand* 649(Suppl):7–49, 1981

44. CRAMP DG, TICKNER TR, BEAL DJ, MOORHEAD JF, WILLS MR: Plasma triglyceride secretion and metabolism in chronic renal failure. *Clin Chim Acta* 76:237–241, 1977

45. VERSCHOOR L, LAMMERS R, BIRKENHAGER JC: Triglyceride turnover in severe chronic non-nephrotic renal failure. *Metabolism* 27:879–884, 1978

46. DEFRONZO RA, FELIG P: Amino acid metabolism in uremia: insights gained from normal and diabetic man. *Am J Clin Nutr* 33:1378–1386, 1980

47. BERGSTRÖM J, FÜRST P, NOREE LO, VINNARS E: Intracellular free amino acids in muscle tissue of patients with chronic uremia: effect of peritoneal dialysis and infusion of essential amino acids. *Clin Sci Mol Med* 54:51–60, 1978

48. ALVESTRAND AP, FÜRST P, BERGSTROM J: Plasma and muscle free amino acid levels: influence of nutrition with amino acids. *Clin Nephrol* 18:297–305, 1982
49. KOPPLE JD, JONES MR: Amino acid metabolism in patients with advanced uremia and in patients undergoing chronic dialysis, in *Advances In Nephrology* (vol 8), Chicago, Year Book Medical Publishers, Inc, 1979, pp 233–268
50. CLARK AS, MITCH WE: Muscle protein turnover and glucose uptake in acutely uremic rats. *J Clin Invest* 72:836–845, 1983
51. MAACH T, JOHNSON V, KAU ST, FIGUEIREDO J, SIGULEM D: Renal filtration, transport, and metabolism of low molecular weight proteins: a review. *Kidney Int* 16:251–270, 1979
52. NATAHARA HT, EVERETT NB, SIMMONS BS, WILLIAMS RH: Metabolism of insulin ^{131}I and glucagon ^{131}I in the kidney of the rat. *Am J Physiol* 192:277–281, 1958
53. BILBREY GL, FALOONA GR, WHITE MG, KNOCHEL JP: Hyperglucagonemia of renal failure. *J Clin Invest* 53:841–847, 1974
54. SHERWIN RS, BASTL C, FINKELSTEIN FO, FISHER M, BLACK H, HENDLER R, FELIG P: Influence of uremia and hemodialysis on the turnover and metabolic effects of glucagon. *J Clin Invest* 57:722–731, 1976
55. BASTL C, FINKELSTEIN FA, SHERWIN RS, HENDLER R, FELIG P, HAYSLETT JP: Renal extraction of glucagon in rats with normal and reduced renal function. *Am J Physiol* 233:F67–F71, 1977
56. EMMANOUEL DS, JASPAN JB, RUBENSTEIN AH, FINK AHH, KATZ AI: Glucagon metabolism in the rat. Contribution of the kidney to the metabolic clearance rate of the hormone. *J Clin Invest* 62:6–13, 1978
57. LEFEBVRE PJ, LUYCKX AS: Effect of acute kidney exclusion by ligation of renal arteries on peripheral plasma glucagon levels and pancreatic glucagon production in the anesthetized dog. *Metab Clin Exp* 24:1169–1176, 1975
58. RUBENFELD S, GARBER AJ: Abnormal carbohydrate metabolism in renal failure. The potential role of accelerated glucose production, increased gluconeogenesis, and impaired glucose disposal. *J Clin Invest* 62:20–28, 1978
59. DEFRONZO RA, FELIG P, FERRANNINI E, WAHREN J: Effect of graded doses of insulin on splanchnic and peripheral potassium metabolism in man. *Am J Physiol* 238:E421–E427, 1980
60. ALVESTRAND A, WAHREN J, SMITH D, DEFRONZO RA: Insulin-mediated potassium uptake is normal in uremia. *Am J Physiol* 246:E174–E180, 1984

Endocrine and Metabolic Abnormalities in the Nephrotic Syndrome: Calcium and Carbohydrate Metabolism

Giuseppe Maschio, Nicola Tessitore, Carmelo Loschiavo, Angela D'Angelo, Ermanno Bonucci, Bjarne Lund, and Birger Lund

Metabolic and endocrine disorders are common in patients with the nephrotic syndrome, even at normal glomerular filtration rate (GFR) values, as a consequence of sustained proteinuria.

Disturbances of calcium metabolism—including hypocalcemia, hypocalciuria, and low concentrations of serum 25-OH-vitamin D_3 (25-HCC)—are constant features in these patients [1–3]; while still controversial the available data on intestinal calcium absorption and circulating concentrations of $1,25(OH)_2D_3$ (1,25-HCC) have been reported to be either normal or reduced in patients with nephrotic syndrome [3, 4–7]. In addition, controversy exists concerning the frequency of bone lesions in patients with nephrotic syndrome and normal GFR [3, 8, 9], and very little is known about the frequency of osteodystrophy in those patients with nephrotic syndrome and renal failure.

Disorders of carbohydrate metabolism frequently may be found in patients with nephrotic syndrome [10–12]. However, no attempt has been made to separate nephrotic patients with normal GFR from those with renal failure—a condition that may impair carbohydrate metabolism [13].

This study was undertaken with the following purposes:

1. To evaluate bone histology and its relationship with calciotropic hormones in two groups of patients with nephrotic syndrome—either with normal or reduced GFR;
2. To compare the bone lesions observed in nephrotic patients and renal failure with those found in patients with renal failure and minimal or no proteinuria; and
3. To evaluate carbohydrate metabolism and its correlations with the histologic lesions (renal biopsy specimen) in a group of patients with nephrotic syndrome and normal renal function.

This manuscript was presented as part of a Symposium on *Endocrine and Metabolic Abnormalities in Renal Diseases.*

Patients and Methods

The study group consisted of 87 patients with nephrotic syndrome (64 males and 23 females, ages 18 to 68 years). The diagnosis of nephrotic syndrome was established on the basis of clinical and laboratory investigations in all patients who had proteinuria in excess of 3.5 g/24 hr and a serum albumin concentration lower than 3 g/100 ml. Of these, 67 had normal renal function (creatinine clearance [C_{cr}] from 81 to 133 ml/min) and 20 had mild renal failure (C_{cr} from 21 to 56 ml/min). None of the patients were taking steroids, diuretics, calcium salts, or vitamin D or its analogs before and during the study. In addition, 55 patients who were matched for age and sex with mild renal failure (C_{cr} from 18 to 58 ml/min) of diverse etiology and minimal or no proteinuria were included in this study.

The GFR was evaluated as the 24-hr creatinine clearance. Serum and urine creatinine and serum albumin concentrations were measured via autoanalyzer. The serum total calcium concentration was evaluated by atomic absorption spectrometry (Perkin-Elmer, model 290), and the ionized calcium was evaluated by specific electrode (Orion SS-20). Serum parathyroid hormone (PTH) (carboxy-terminal fragment) was determined by radioimmunoassay (Sorin Biomedica, Saluggia, Italy). Serum 25-HCC was measured by a competitive protein-binding assay in 28 patients with nephrotic syndrome and in 19 non-nephrotic patients with renal failure. Serum 1,25-HCC wasdetermined by radioimmunoassay based on competitive binding to an intestinal cytosol protein from rachitic chicks [14] in 14 patients with nephrotic syndrome and in 15 non-nephrotic patients with renal failure. Serum 24,25-HCC was measured by radioimmunoassay using rat kidney cytosol [15] in 13 patients with nephrotic syndrome and in 15 non-nephrotic patients with renal failure. Serum vitamin D metabolites were also determined in 12 adult Italian subjects.

Bone biopsy specimens were taken from the iliac crest of both 49 patients with nephrotic syndrome (29 with a normal GFR and 20 patients with renal failure) and 55 patients with early renal failure and minimal or no proteinuria. The specimens were analyzed in nondecalcified sections according to previously described methods [16]. All patients were fully aware of the nature of the investigation and gave their consent for bone biopsy procedures.

In 38 patients with nephrotic syndrome and normal GFR and in 10 control subjects, none of them having evidence or family history of diabetes mellitus, the following metabolic investigations were performed under basal conditions and after an oral glucose tolerance test (OGTT) with 100 g of glucose: (1) blood glucose by autoanalyzer, (2) insulin and growth hormone (GH) secretion rate by double-antibody radioimmunoassay (Sorin, Saluggia, Italy), and (3) plasma cortisol according to Kitabchi and Kitchell [17]. Moreover, a semiquantitative evaluation of total glucose and insulin pools was obtained by planimetric measure of areas delimited by their curves. The insulinogenic index (the ratio between insulin and glucose areas) was also calculated [18].

Renal biopsy specimens were obtained percutaneously from all patients and were examined by light, immunofluorescence, and electron microscopy [19].

Statistical evaluations were performed by using Student's t test for unpaired data and chi-square analysis.

Results

Serum calcium concentrations were low in patients with nephrotic syndrome and normal GFR, and were normal in those patients with early renal failure. The ionized fraction of total serum calcium also was low in approximately 50% of the nephrotic patients with a normal GFR, and it was normal in those patients with renal failure. Serum PTH levels were at the upper limits of normal in nephrotic patients with a normal GFR and were increased in 35% of them; however, they were definitely increased as mean values in patients with renal failure, especially in those patients with nephrotic syndrome who had a longer duration of renal insufficiency (Table 1).

Mean serum 25-HCC values were low in patients with nephrotic syndrome (both with a normal and reduced GFR) and were in the normal range in patients with renal failure and no proteinuria. Nephrotic patients with normal GFR had normal mean values of 1,25-HCC and low borderline levels of 24,25-HCC. In patients with nephrotic syndrome and reduced GFR, both 1,25-HCC and 24,25-HCC levels were reduced when compared with controls,

Table 1. Serum calcium, phosphate, PTH, and albumin concentrations in nephrotic patients with normal or reduced renal function, and in patients with renal failure and no proteinuria[a]

	Patients with NS and normal GFR ($N = 67$)	Patients with NS and renal failure ($N = 20$)	Patients with renal failure ($N = 55$)
Serum total calcium	8.10	8.80	9.50
(mg/dl)	±0.20	0.10	0.10
Serum ionized calcium	2.08	2.18	2.24
(mEq/liter)	±0.12	0.10	0.11
Serum PO_4	3.78	4.10	3.50
(mg/dl)	±0.34	0.20	0.10
Serum i-PTH	2.20	3.30	2.60
(μU/ml)[b]	±0.60	0.85	0.55
Serum albumin	2.16	2.50	3.70
(g/dl)	±0.10	0.10	0.10
Duration of renal	—	1.40	1.00
failure (yrs)	—	0.30	0.40

[a] Values are given as mean ± SD.

[b] Normal range = 0.6 to 2.4; NS = nephrotic syndrome.

Table 2. Serum concentrations of vitamin D metabolites in nephrotic patients with normal or reduced renal function, and in patients with renal failure and no proteinuria[a]

	Patients with NS and normal GFR ($N = 16$)	Patients with NS and renal failure ($N = 12$)	Patients with renal failure ($N = 15$)
Serum 25-HCC (ng/ml)[b]	4.20	8.60	30.02
	±2.60	3.90	4.00
Serum 1,25-HCC (pg/ml)[c]	37.30	4.80	11.50
	±5.20	1.10	2.90
Serum 24,25-HCC (ng/ml)[d]	0.84	0.70	0.60
	±0.16	0.11	0.13

[a] Values are given as mean ± SD; NS = nephrotic syndrome.

[b] Normal range, 12 to 42 ng/ml.

[c] Normal range, 18 to 46 pg/ml.

[d] Normal range, 0.7 to 2.2 ng/ml.

but they were in the same range of those found in patients with renal failure and no proteinuria (Table 2).

In bone biopsy specimens, normal bone was found in 76% of patients with nephrotic syndrome and normal GFR, in 35% of those with nephrotic syndrome and renal failure, and in 53% of those with renal failure and no proteinuria. Isolated osteomalacia was present in 17% of patients with nephrotic syndrome and normal GFR, in 25% of those with nephrotic syndrome and renal failure, and in 34% of those with renal failure and no proteinuria. A mixed lesion (osteomalacia plus increased bone resorption) was found in 7% of patients with nephrotic syndrome and normal GFR, in 40% of those with nephrotic syndrome and renal failure, and in 13% of those with renal failure and no proteinuria (Table 3). A good correlation between the duration

Table 3. Bone histology in patients with nephrotic syndrome (NS) and normal or reduced renal function, and in patients with renal failure and no proteinuria

Percent (%) of patients	Patients with NS and normal GFR ($N = 29$)	Patients with NS and renal failure ($N = 20$)	Patients with renal failure ($N = 55$)
Normal bone	76	35[a]	53
Osteomalacia	17	25	34
Osteomalacia plus hyperparathyroidism	7	40[a]	13[b]

[a] Significantly different from that of patients with nephrotic syndrome and normal GFR (chi-square, 4.6 and 5.8—$P < 0.05$).

[b] Significantly different from that of patients with nephrotic syndrome and renal failure (chi-square, 5.2—$P < 0.05$).

of both associated proteinuria and renal failure and the severity of bone lesions was found in nephrotic patients with reduced GFR. No correlation was observed between bone histology and both PTH and vitamin D metabolites in nephrotic patients with normal GFR; whereas, in patients with renal failure, the presence of defective mineralization was associated with serum 25-HCC levels lower than those found in patients with normal bone histology.

The analysis of the results of OGTT led to the separation of 38 patients with nephrotic syndrome and normal GFR into two groups. Group 1 had 14 patients (36.8%) with a diabetic-like response and group 2 had 24 patients with a normal response. In patients in group 1, blood glucose and plasma insulin concentrations and the glucose and insulin areas were significantly greater than those observed in both controls and patients in group 2. However, the increase in insulin areas was comparable to that of glucose, so that the insulinogenic index was not different from that of controls. In patients in group 2, blood glucose and plasma insulin levels did not differ significantly from controls after OGTT. However, the glucose areas were significantly smaller, so that the insulinogenic index was significantly greater in these patients than in controls.

The basal values of growth hormone (GH) were significantly increased in both groups of patients, compared to controls. At 60 min after OGTT, serum GH levels were significantly higher in patients in group 1 than in both controls and patients in group 2 (Table 4).

No correlation between serum GH levels and serum albumin or proteinuria was observed. Serum cortisol levels were not significantly different in either nephrotic patients or controls.

Virtually all patients with a diabetic-like response to OGTT had histologic evidence of membranous nephropathy or focal glomerular sclerosis. However, there was no strict correlation between the various histologic lesions (minimal

Table 4. Effects of oral glucose tolerance test in patients with nephrotic syndrome (NS) and normal GFR

	Controls ($N = 10$)	Group 1 Patients with NS and diabetic-like response ($N = 14$)	Group 2 Patients with NS and normal response ($N = 24$)
Glucose area (g/min)	17.8	35.2[a]	13.0[b]
	±1.9	3.8	0.9
Insulin area (mU/min)	25.5	48.6[a]	27.9[c]
	±2.4	5.8	2.8
Insulinogenic index	1.43	1.38	2.14[b]
Serum growth hormone	0.4	3.0[a]	0.6
after 60 min (ng/ml)	±0.1	1.0	0.1

Values are given as ± SEM.

[a] Significantly different from controls and group 2.

[b] Significantly different from controls and group 1.

[c] Significantly different from group 1.

change nephropathy, membranous nephropathy, focal glomerular sclerosis, and membranoproliferative glomerulonephritis) and the metabolic abnormalities.

Discussion

Our findings show that a state of vitamin D deficiency and secondary hyperparathyroidism is not a constant feature in patients with nephrotic syndrome and normal GFR. The results obtained by several independent laboratories now support the view that 25-HCC is the only metabolite whose serum concentration is regularly low in nephrotic patients [1–3, 7, 20]. The apparent discrepancy on the serum levels of 1,25-HCC, 24,25-HCC, and PTH raises the possibility that different factors (including corticosteroid treatment, calcium administration, duration and degree of proteinuria, age of patients, and renal function) may affect vitamin D and PTH metabolism in nephrotic patients.

Our findings of normal mean levels of serum 1,25-HCC might be the result, as suggested by Korkor et al [13], of the maintenance of a sufficient level of free 25-HCC in a manner analogous to that of thyroid hormone in the same disease.

Not surprisingly, even more controversial are data on the frequency of bone lesions. Our results show that 24% of nephrotic patients with normal renal function may have bone lesions, which have been found either in none [13] or in all [9] of the reported patients. This apparently low incidence of metabolic bone disease might be explained by the association of low levels of 25-HCC with normal levels of 1,25-HCC in our patients.

The frequency of mineralization defect in our patients with renal failure was unrelated to the presence of proteinuria. On the other hand, patients with persistent proteinuria and early renal failure had a significantly higher frequency of osteoclastic bone disease when compared with a matched group of patients with renal failure and no proteinuria. These morphologic findings might depend on the higher values of serum PTH found in nephrotic patients with renal failure. The longer duration of renal failure in this group of patients might explain the differences in PTH values when compared with patients with renal failure and no proteinuria. However, the observed correlation between the duration of proteinuria and renal failure and the degree of bone involvement suggests that the persistence of the biochemical abnormalities following urinary protein losses is the critical factor in modulating both the magnitude and full development of bone lesions in these patients.

The implications of these findings call for an early treatment with active vitamin D metabolites in all patients with nephrotic syndrome, especially if they are treated with corticosteroids [21].

A condition of "ineffective hyperinsulinism" may be found in nearly 40% of patients with nephrotic syndrome, who may display a diabetic-like response to OGTT, but no significant change in their insulinogenic index. The remaining percentage of nephrotic patients (60%) may display a normal response to OGTT; however, their insulin pool secretion may be excessive when compared to that of glucose, resulting in a condition of "hyperinsulinism." These effects might be the result of increased growth hormone secretion, which is known to stimulate insulin release [22].

The pathogenesis of elevated GH levels in patients with nephrotic syndrome is still unclear [23–25]. In our patients, these elevated values were not correlated with either proteinuria or hypoalbuminemia.

Virtually all patients with a diabetic-like response to OGTT had histologic evidence of membranous nephropathy or focal glomerular sclerosis [26]. In the medical literature, there are conflicting data on this topic. Churg and Ehrenreich [27] observed evidence of diabetic response in approximately 20% of a large group of patients with membranous nephropathy; whereas, in Cameron's [28] series, only 1% of the patients had the same response. Our results only apparently seem to support a potential role for renal histologic lesions in the pathogenesis of altered carbohydrate metabolism in nephrotic syndrome. In fact, since none of the metabolic parameters appeared to be strictly related to the various histologic lesions, the role of renal lesions remains speculative.

References

1. GOLDSTEIN DA, ODA Y, KUROKAWA K, MASSRY SG: Blood levels of 25-hydroxyvitamin D in nephrotic syndrome. Studies in 26 patients. *Ann Intern Med* 87:664–667, 1977
2. BARRAGRY JM, FRANCE MW, CARTER ND, ANTON JA, BEER M, BOUCHER BJ, COHEN RD: Vitamin D metabolism in nephrotic syndrome. *Lancet* 2:629–631, 1977
3. KORKOR A, SCHWARTZ J, BERGFELD M, TEITELBAUM S, AVIOLI L, KLAHR S, SLATOPOLSKY E: Absence of metabolic bone disease in adult patients with the nephrotic syndrome and normal renal function. *J Clin Endocrinol Metab* 56:496–500, 1983
4. LIM P, JACOB E, TOCK EPC, PWEE HS: Calcium and phosphorus metabolism in nephrotic syndrome. *Q J Med* 183:327–338, 1977
5. GOLDSTEIN DA, HALDIMAN B, SHERMAN D, NORMAN AW, MASSRY SG: Vitamin D metabolite and calcium metabolism in patients with nephrotic syndrome and normal renal function. *J Clin Endocrinol Metab* 52:116–121, 1981
6. HALDIMAN B, TRECSEL U: Vitamin D replacement therapy in the nephrotic syndrome (*abstract*). *Kidney Int* 21:905, 1982
7. LAMBERT PW, DEOREO PB, FU IY, KAETZEL K, VON HAN K, HOLLIS BV, ROOS BA: Urinary and plasma vitamin D metabolites in the nephrotic syndrome. *Met Bone Dis Rel Res* 4:7–15, 1982
8. LIM P, JACOB E, TOCK EPC, PWEE HS: Serum ionized calcium in nephrotic syndrome. *Q J Med* 45:421–426, 1976
9. MALLUCHE HH, GOLDSTEIN DA, MASSRY SG: Osteomalacia and hyperparathyroid bone disease in patients with nephrotic syndrome. *J Clin Invest* 63:494–500, 1979
10. SPITZ IM, RUBENSTEIN AH, BERSOHN I, ABRAHAMS G, LOWY G: Carbohydrate metabolism in renal disease. *Q J Med* 39:201–216, 1970
11. KLEINKNECHT D, LAUDAT MH, STRAUCH G, JUNGERS P, LAUDAT P: Lipopro-

tein and carbohydrate disorders in nephrotic syndrome and uremia. *Rev Eur Et Clin Biol* 17:27–37, 1972

12. RYABOV SI, KOZHEVNIKOV AD: Carbohydrate metabolism in glomerulonephritis. *Nephron* 28:118–123, 1981

13. KALHAN SC, RICANATI ES, TSERG K-Y, SAVIN SM: Glucose turnover in chronic uremia: increased recycling with diminished oxidation of glucose. *Metabolism* 32:1155–1162, 1983

14. LUND B, LUND B, SORENSEN OH: Measurement of circulating 1,25-dihydroxyvitamin D in man. Changes in serum concentration during treatment with 1-alpha-hydroxycholecalciferol. *Acta End* 91:338–350, 1979

15. CHRISTENSEN CK, LUND B, SORENSEN OH, NIELSEN HE, MOSEKILDE L: Reduced 1,25-dihydroxyvitamin D and 24,25-dihydroxyvitamin D in epileptic patients receiving chronic combined anticonvulsant therapy. *Met Bone Dis Rel Res* 3:17–22, 1981

16. MASCHIO G, D'ANGELO A, BONUCCI E, PAGANO F, OSSI E, LUPO A, VALVO E, TESSITORE N, MESSA P: Aspects of calcium metabolism in obstructive nephropathy. A metabolic and bone biopsy investigation. *Nephron* 19:32–43, 1977

17. KITABCHI A, KITCHELL LC: A simplified fluorimetric method for determination of blood cortisol using phase-separating filter paper. *Analyt Biochem* 34:529–535, 1970

18. SELTZER HS, ALLEN WA, HERRON AL, BRENNAN MT: Insulin secretion in response to glycemic stimulus: relation of delayed initial release to carbohydrate intolerance in mild diabetes mellitus. *J Clin Invest* 46:323–330, 1967

19. FARAGGIANA T, PAROLINI C, PREVIATO G, LUPO A: Light and electron microscopic findings in five cases of cryoglobulinemic glomerulonephritis. *Virchows Arch Abt A PathAnat Histol* 384:29–44, 1979

20. TESSITORE N, BONUCCI E, D'ANGELO A, LUND B, CORGNATI A, LUND B, VALVO E, LUPO A, LOSCHIAVO C, FABRIS A, MASCHIO G: Bone histology and calcium metabolism in patients with nephrotic syndrome and normal or reduced renal function. *Nephron* (in press, 1984)

21. ALON U, CHAN JCM: Calcium and vitamin D homeostasis in the nephrotic syndrome: current status. *Nephron* 36:1–4, 1984

22. CHRISTENSEN NJ, ORSKOW H, HANSEN AP: Significance of glucose load in oral glucose tolerance tests. Blood glucose, serum insulin, growth hormone and free fatty acids. *Acta Med Scand* 192:337–342, 1972

23. BECHER DJ, PIMSTONE BL, HANSEN JDL, HENDRICKS S: Serum albumin and growth hormone relationship in kwashiorkor and the nephrotic syndrome. *J Lab Clin Med* 78:865–871, 1971

24. BRIDGMAN JF, SUMMERSKILL J, BUCKLER JMH, HELLMAN B, ROSEN SM: Insulin and growth hormone secretion in the nephrotic syndrome. *Q J Med* 173:115–123, 1975

25. HOFELD FD, REED JW, FORSHAM PH: Growth hormone responses following double pulse oral glucose administration in various clinical states. *J Endocrinol Metab* 40:387–392, 1975

26. LOSCHIAVO C, LUPO A, VALVO E, TESSITORE N, FERRARI S, CORGNATI A, MASCHIO G: Carbohydrate metabolism in patients with nephrotic syndrome and normal renal function. *Nephron* 33:257–261, 1983

27. CHURG JI, EHRENREICH T: Membranous nephropathy in *Glomerulonephritis,* edited by KINCAID-SMITH P, MATHEW TH, BECKER EL, New York, John Wiley & Sons, 1973, p 443

28. CAMERON GS: Pathogenesis and treatment of membranous nephropathy. *Kidney Int* 15:88–103, 1979

Osteodystrophy

Renal Osteodystrophy: General Concepts and Current Issues

Albert Fournier, Philippe Morinière, J. L. Sebert, B. Boudailliez, I. Grégoire, M. Garabédian, J. Guéris, and P. Meunier

It is the purpose of this chapter first to summarize our current understanding of the pathophysiology of renal osteodystrophy and then to consider three controversial points: (1) the indications for treatment with 1-alpha-,hydroxylated vitamin D derivatives in patients without radiologic manifestations of hyperparathyroidism; (2) indications for use of other vitamin D sterols; (3) indications for parathyroidectomy in aluminum-loaded patients.

Pathophysiology of Renal Osteodystrophy

The substitution treatment of terminal uremia introducing a new etiologic factor, pathophysiology of renal osteodystrophy, will be discussed successively before and after the beginning of dialysis therapy.

Pathophysiology of Renal Osteodystrophy Before Dialysis

Based on biopsy data, renal osteodystrophy is present in about 90% of uremic patients beginning hemodialysis [1, 2]. Then, it is always characterized by increased osteoclastic resorption and fibrosis due to excessive secretion of parathyroid hormone (PTH), and eventually by an associated defect in mineralization. At this stage, true osteomalacia with increased osteoid width and a decreased mineralization front or mineralization rate occurs with a frequency very different from one region to another; for example, in 6% of patients in Toulouse and 34% of patients in Newcastle-upon-Tyne. Mild histologic evidence of hyperparathyroidism (an excess of woven bone or osteoid surface) also occurs much earlier than the eventual mild mineralization defect (that is, decreased mineralization front or decreased mineralization rate, but with

This manuscript was presented as part of a Symposium on *Renal Osteodystrophy: Recent Advances.*

normal osteoid width); the former occurs at a glomerular filtration rate (GFR) between 40 to 80 ml/min and the latter occurs not before a GFR of 40 ml/min. Soft tissue calcifications sometimes are associated in these bone changes, especially when the hyperparathyroidism is severe.

Pathogenetic Mechanisms of Secondary Hyperparathyroidism in Uremia

These are complex, but may be summarized as follows (Fig. 1).

Phosphate Retention. This is due to GFR reduction and it plays a major role since it always tends to decrease the plasma-ionized calcium, and therefore stimulates PTH secretion indirectly. This latter situation decreases the tubular reabsorption of phosphate and re-establishes phosphate balance and normophosphatemia; this new equilibrium is achieved at the expense of high plasma levels of PTH. This "trade-off" theory of Bricker and Slatopolsky has been questioned regarding the initiation of hyperparathyroidism in early renal failure because hypophosphatemia occasionally can be seen at this stage in fasting patients. However, this is rare, and the phosphate load regularly induces a higher plasma phosphate concentration in uremic patients than in normal subjects, and a well-controlled trial in uremic dogs shows that hyperparathyroidism can be efficiently prevented for 1 year only by a reduction of dietary phosphate proportional to the reduction of GFR. However, a pharmalogic dose of 25-OH-D$_3$ was necessary in this trial to prevent hyperparathyroidism after 18 months of chronic uremia. This leads to a discussion of the second mechanism involving vitamin D.

Altered Vitamin D Metabolism. This also contributes to the stimulation of PTH secretion via three possible mechanisms:

1. By inducing a negative calcium balance;
2. By resetting the level of plasma-ionized calcium necessary to suppress the parathyroid glands; and
3. By inducing a "skeletal resistance" to PTH.

The negative calcium balance of uremia, is due to a combination of the low-calcium diet induced by the usual dietary restriction (milk and meat) prescribed in uremia and the low levels of 1,25(OH)$_2$D$_3$, which generally are observed when the GFR reaches 40 ml/min [1–3]. Decreased formation of 1,25(OH)$_2$D$_3$ in uremic patients is rarely due to decreased plasma levels of 25-OH-D, although the latter is not due specifically to uremia. In fact, the half-life of 25-OH-D$_3$ is increased in uremia, which makes the hypothesis of increased hepatic microsomal enzyme induction by uremia unlikely. However, the plasma concentration of 25-OH-D$_3$ may be low in this condition because of the above-mentioned dietary restriction, sun exposure deficiency, losses in nephrotic urine, and increased catabolism by anticonvulsant hepatic enzymatic induction. However, decreased 1,25(OH)$_2$D$_3$ synthesis is found in uremia despite normal plasma concentrations of 25- OH-D because of

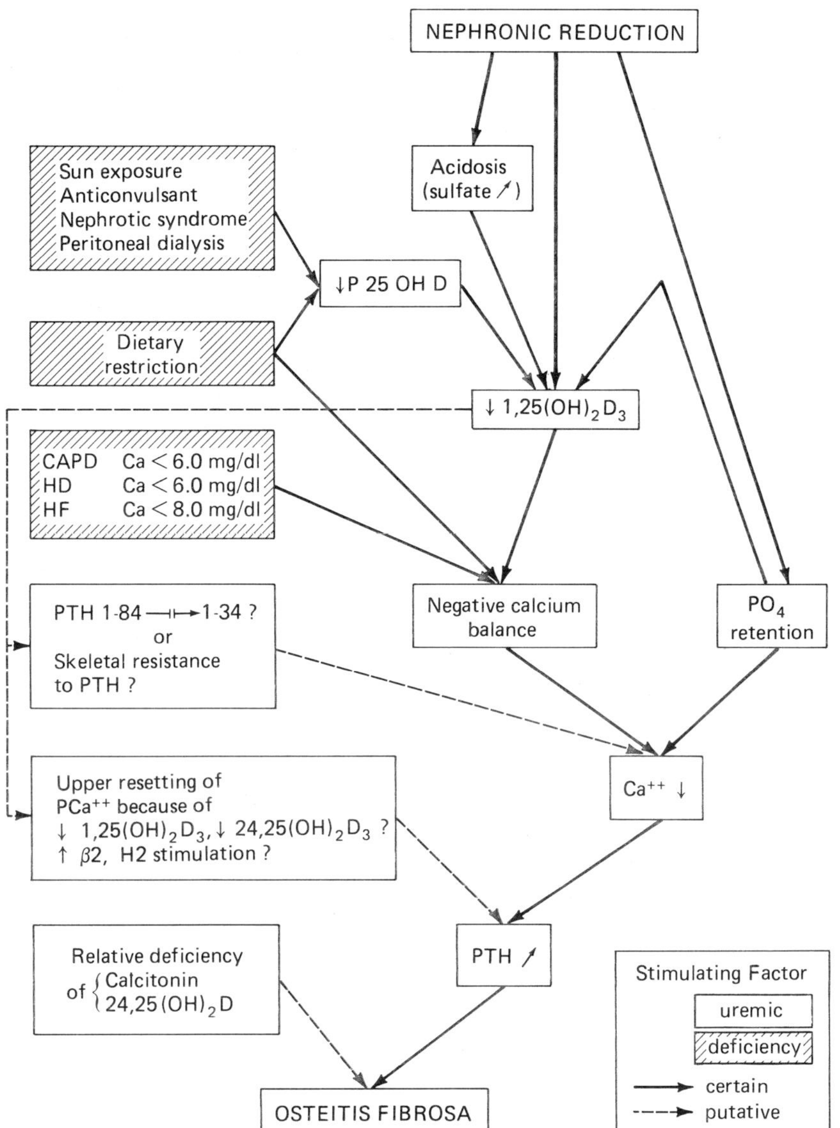

Fig. 1. Schematic outline of the pathogenesis of osteitis fibrosa.

decreased nephron mass and the inhibition of renal 1-hydroxylation secondary to hyperphosphatemia. Chronic acidosis, in contrast to acute acidosis, does not seem to decrease the activity of the 1 α-hydroxylase [3].

The role of 1,25(OH)$_2$D$_3$ deficiency in the upward resetting of the suppressive-ionized calcium levels is still an unproven mechanism [3]. Receptors for 1,25(OH)$_2$D$_3$ have been demonstrated on the parathyroid cells. However, in vitro and in vivo studies have yielded contradictory results as to the existence of a direct suppressive effect of 1,25(OH)$_2$D$_3$ on PTH secretion. The first convincing evidence in humans was given by Madsen [4], who showed a suppressive effect of i.v. 1,25(OH)$_2$D$_3$—while the ionized calcium concentration was kept constant in acutely uremic patients due to peritoneal dialysis with a low-dialysate calcium. More recently, Slatopolsky et al have reported a comparable suppressive effect of i.v. 1,25(OH)$_2$D$_3$ in chronic hemodialysis patients, with plasma PTH decreasing before plasma-ionized calcium increased [5]. However, since 1,25(OH)$_2$D$_3$ may increase the plasma concentration of 24,25(OH)$_2$D$_3$, the observed suppression may have been the result of a direct effect of 24,25(OH)$_2$D$_3$. As a matter of fact, parathyroid receptors for 24,25(OH)$_2$D$_3$ also have been demonstrated (in the chick), and a suppressive effect of 24,25(OH)$_2$D$_3$ has been observed without a concomitant increase of plasma calcium (but rather a decrease) in uremic dogs—provided the diet was rich in calcium [3]. However, it must be pointed out that the plasma concentration of 24,25(OH)$_2$D$_3$ is not always decreased in uremia; it is sometimes normal or even increased [10]. No conclusive data on the suppressive effect of 24,25(OH)$_2$D$_3$ have been reported in uremic patients [7].

"Skeletal resistance" to PTH as a stimulating mechanism of PTH secretion is a pathophysiologic concept that is controversial. It is based on the fact that the calcemic response after injection of parathyroid extract or PTH 1–84 is always decreased in both human patients and animals with acute or chronic uremia [1]. However, recent experimental studies in chronically uremic dogs [8] have shown that prevention of hyperparathyroidism by proportional reduction of dietary phosphate was possible, whereas the skeletal resistance to PTH was still persisting—thus demonstrating the inefficiency of this latter mechanism in the induction of hyperparathyroidism. Furthermore, the decreased calcemic response to PTH 1–84 does not seem to be due to skeletal resistance, but to an impaired metabolism of PTH 1–84 to PTH 1–34, since the calcemic response to an injection of PTH 1–34 is normal [9]. Lack of 1,25(OH)$_2$D$_3$ could be responsible for this deficient metabolism of PTH, since 1,25(OH)$_2$D$_3$ corrected the calcemic response to PTH 1–84 in uremic dogs [9].

Other Modulators of PTH Secretion. Besides ionized calcium, there are other modulators of PTH secretion; namely, ionized magnesium, catecholamines, and histamine. Since serum magnesium tends to rise in renal failure, this ion cannot be involved in the pathogenesis of hyperparathyroidism. Beta receptors have been demonstrated on the parathyroid cells. Although there is no proof that renal failure increases either the number of receptors or the secretion of catecholamines, beta-2 antagonists such as propranolol have been shown to decrease PTH levels [1, 3] in uremic men. H2 receptors also exist on parathyroid glands, but the effect of H2 antagonists such as cimetidine on PTH secretion are inconsistent [1, 3].

Increased Resorption. Besides the effect of increased levels of PTH, the increased bone resorption may be due to a relative lack of calcitonin [3] and to an incapability to increase the levels of $24,25(OH)_2D_3$ to above normal [6].

The Pathogenetic Mechanisms of Renal Osteomalacia

The incidence of true osteomalacia in uremic patients is not as great as that of fibro-osteoclasia; it varies widely from one geographic region to the other. This wide range of incidence suggests that factors other than uremia per se are involved. Among these factors, deficiencies in vitamin D as well as in calcium and phosphate must be stressed [3]. Vitamin D deficiency is not uncommon in uremic patients prior to dialysis because of dietary restrictions (meat and milk). Furthermore, uremic patients are more inclined to stay indoors, and their skin has a decreased capacity to synthetize vitamin D_3 under ultraviolet irradiation, especially in pigmented patients [3]. This explains why plasma concentrations of 25-OH-D often are low in uremic patients in colder countries without industrially fortified food [10]. Usually, vitamin D-deficient osteomalacia in uremic patients can be cured by using physiologic doses of vitamin D_3 or 25-OH-D_3, and their use is as efficient as in nonuremic patients, as shown by Memmos [10].

Besides these various deficiency causes, osteomalacia may be observed in uremic patients who are not yet on dialysis because of intoxication with fluoride (due to the water or certain drugs such as niflumic acid), anticonvulsants, or even aluminum. Four cases of true osteomalacia associated with high plasma aluminum levels and the presence of aluminum at the mineralization front have been reported in relation to oral $Al(OH)_3$ given as a phosphate binder to patients prior to dialysis [11, 12].

Anticonvulsants are known to induce osteomalacia because of decreasing plasma concentrations of 25-OH-D and a direct toxic effect on bone. Since they are widely used, especially in uremic children, their administration may play a role in the osteomalacia observed in these patients [13].

When all of these causes of osteomalacia have been excluded in a given uremic patient, the mechanisms of true renal osteomalacia can be discussed. This presupposes that the plasma concentrations of 25-OH-D, $1,25(OH)_2D$, $24,25(OH)_2D$, PTH, aluminum, and fluoride have been measured simultaneously via a bone biopsy specimen. To our knowledge, no such study has been performed. Nevertheless, many factors are likely to be involved:

1. The negative calcium balance induced by low $1,25(OH)_2D_3$ in combination with the low calcium intake induced by the uremic diet [14];
2. The acidosis especially present in diseases predominantly affecting the medulla [15];
3. The lack of a direct effect of vitamin D metabolites (certainly $1,25[OH]_2D_3$, but perhaps also 25-OH-D_3 and $24,25[OH]_2D_3$) on the osteoblastic and mineralization processes;
4. The increased plasma concentrations of magnesium, which delay the maturation of the osseous crystals [3]; and
5. Low secretion of PTH, since it is remarkable that osteomalacia may be favored by surgical parathyroidectomy [3].

The Pathogenetic Mechanisms of the Metastatic Calcifications

The periarticular calcifications seem to be mainly dependent on the calcium phosphate product and the degree to which PTH levels are elevated. The visceral calcifications also depend on the magnesium load. The vascular ones seem to be independent of the calcium $\times$ phosphorus product, but may be related to age [3].

Pathophysiology of Renal Osteodystrophy During Maintenance Dialysis

Renal osteodystrophy became a major clinical problem in the first decade of the maintenance dialysis era [1]. This development could be a result of: (1) to the imperfect correction of the pathophysiologic mechanisms involved in renal osteodystrophy combined with the longer life expectancy, and/or (2) the addition of new etiologic factors.

Dialysis and Osteitis Fibrosa

As shown in Figure 1 regarding osteitis fibrosa, hemodialysis helps to correct hyperphosphatemia and acidosis, but it may improve the negative calcium balance only when the dialysate calcium is $\geq$ 6.0 mg/dl [16]. The same is true for continuous ambulatory peritoneal dialysis (CAPD) [17]. Although there is no universal agreement, the concentration of 70 mg/dl is now used most widely [3]. In hemodialysis, it generally induces a positive calcium balance of 300 mg per procedure, which counterbalances the negative intestinal calcium balance that has been estimated to be about 1000 mg/wk [3].

In hemofiltration, to get this positive calcium balance per procedure, it is necessary to increase the calcium concentration in the substitution fluid to 8.0 mg/dl or even to 9.0 mg/dl—according to the desired weight loss and the quantity of ultrafiltrate [18].

The CAPD treatment may lead to vitamin D deficiency because of a continued loss of 25-OH-D via binding onto the proteins that enter the peritoneal dialysate [17].

Dialysis and Osteomalacia

As shown in Figure 2, dialysis may improve the osteomalacia because of the better correction of acidosis and the better clearance of uremic inhibitors of calcification (such as pyrophosphate), the decrease of magnesium (Mg) levels (provided that the magnesium concentration in the dialysate is 1 or 0.5 mEq/liter), and (above all) it may make the calcium balance positive with the use of high-dialysate calcium [14]. Corrections of osteomalacia via dialysis have been reported by Nielsen [14] and Bordier; the latter has even reported that anephric patients can have no histologic evidence of osteomala-

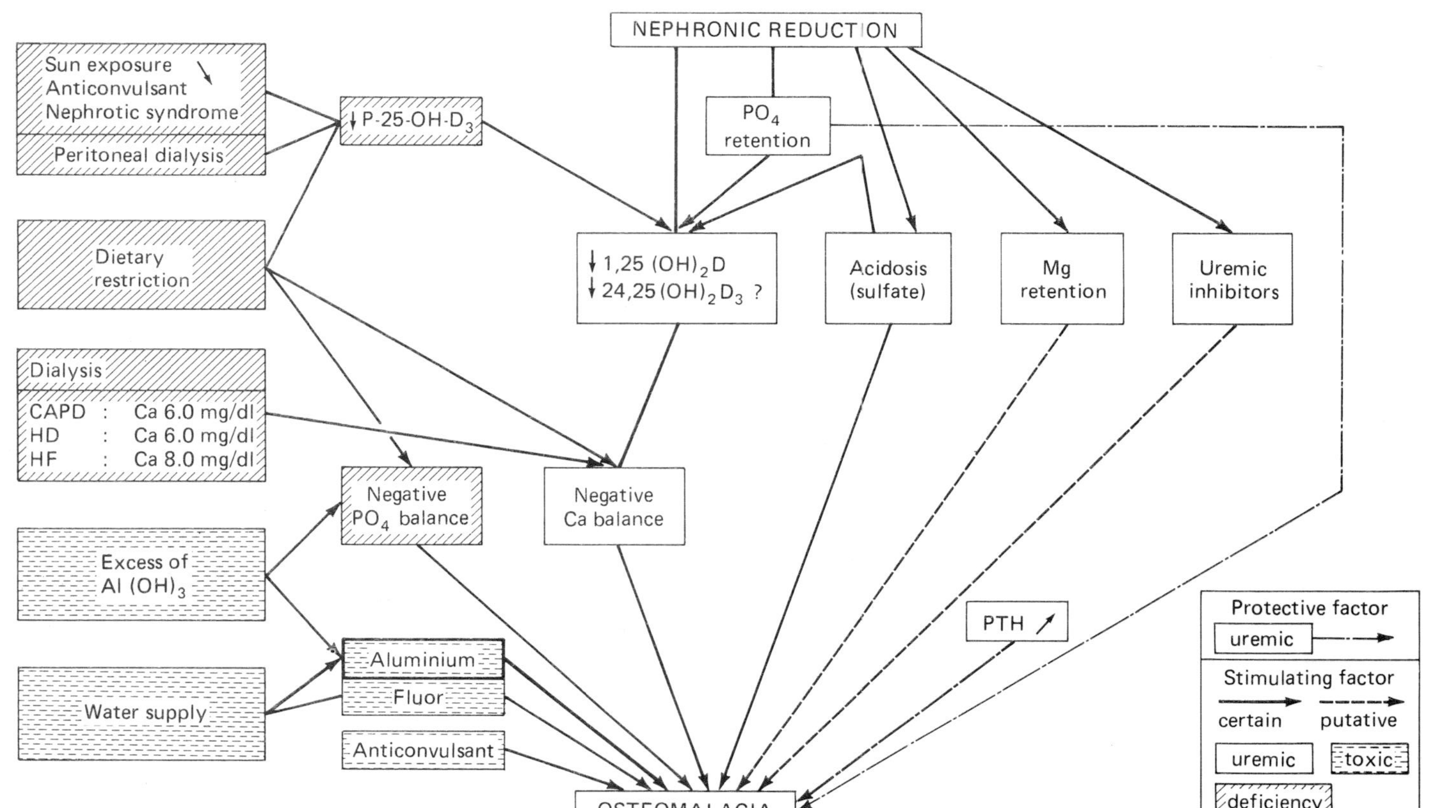

Fig. 2. Schematic outline of pathogenesis of osteomalacia in uremia.

cia [19]. This observation demonstrates that 1,25(OH)$_2$D$_3$ (the levels of which are very low but still detectable in anephric patients because of osteogenic synthesis) does not play a very important direct role on the mineralization process; provided that its deficiency is compensated by the phosphate retention—induced by the renal failure—and by the calcium load, which may be brought on by dialysis or the oral calcium supplement.

However, in certain geographic areas, osteomalacia has been a dramatic and frequent complication of dialysis, because it is painful and leads to multiple fractures; and, above all, because it was associated with an encephalopathy. Circumstantial evidence has suggested that it was due to aluminum intoxication through contaminated water supplies [20]. The recognition of this source of intoxication and the use of a deionizer or reverse osmosis instead of a water softener have led to the disappearance of this disease in the various regions where it was epidemic. Furthermore, animal studies by Ellis [3] proved that aluminum intoxication could indeed lead to osteomalacia.

Besides aluminum, the water supply may be heavily contaminated by fluoride in certain areas and may lead, in a few cases, to fluorosis [3]. However, in one controlled study, fluoridated water at 1 ppm was unable to induce osteomalacia after 1 year [3].

Hodsman has described eight cases of osteomalacia of the same type as that associated with dialysate aluminum intoxication; that is, without increased levels of PTH and alkaline phosphatase, and with decreased osteoblastosis—but not associated with dialysis dementia—and occurring in centers that had low aluminum dialysate. Despite this, aluminum was increased in the plasma and the bone, where it could be found at the interface of mineralized and unmineralized bone. The role of aluminum intoxication by phosphate binders will be discussed by Coburn et al elsewhere in this volume, and Llach et al, also will point to the role of drinking water when it is highly loaded with aluminum.

Indications for 1α-(OH) Vitamin D$_3$ in Renal Osteodystrophy

There are several good theoretic reasons why 1α-hydroxylated vitamin D$_3$ derivatives [that is, 1,25(OH)$_2$ vitamin D$_3$ or calcitriol (Rocaltrol®) or its precursors 1α-OH vitamin D$_3$ (one alpha®)] should be used for the prevention and treatment of renal osteodystrophy in uremic patients; renal 1-α-hydroxylase of 25-OH vitamin D$_3$ is depressed in uremia and leads to low plasma levels of 1,25(OH)$_2$D, usually when the GFR is below 30 ml/min. This may contribute to low-calcium intestinal absorption, to decreased calcemic action of PTH, to a higher set point for PTH suppression by ionized calcium, and to decreased osteoblast activity resulting in decreased formation and mineralization of bone. Thus, administration of 1α-hydroxylated D derivatives should suppress PTH hypersecretion by increasing the plasma calcium concentration and possibly by a direct action on the parathyroid gland; and, it should improve bone formation and mineralization.

However, at the same time, these vitamin D derivatives may have non-beneficial effects. The first one is the increase of intestinal phosphate absorption, which may worsen the hyperphosphatemia when the GFR is reduced and may contribute with hypercalcemia to an acceleration of the reduction of GFR. Fortunately, this has not occurred in the studies by Letteri et al (elsewhere in this Section) of patients with early renal failure (10 to 55 ml/min of GFR) in whom 0.5 to 1 μg/d of 1,25(OH)$_2$D$_3$ without Al(OH)$_3$ did not induce a significant fall of GFR, as in the control group, despite numerous episodes of hypercalcemia. However, earlier experiences with 1,25(OH)$_2$D$_3$ [21] or 1-alpha [22, 23] have shown that the deterioration of renal function could be accelerated, usually in association with an increase of the plasma concentrations of calcium and phosphate—but also without such increases as in studies by Yoshimya with 1-alpha [23]. However, the worsening of hyperphosphatemia usually has been encountered in patients on dialysis when 1-α-OH-D derivatives had normalized plasma alkaline phosphatase and high plasma PTH levels [24]; or, when the patients had only histologic evidence of osteodystrophy without radiologic manifestation [25, 26].

The second nonbeneficial effect of 1-α-OH derivatives is secondary to the former, since worsening of hyperphosphatemia leads to increasing doses of Al(OH)$_3$, which is the most commonly used phosphate binder. The aluminum of these binders may be absorbed, and the aluminum overload [12, 27] of the patients may increase.

Although aluminum overload only induced by phosphate binders has led, up to now, to the report of only 12 cases of clinical osteomalacia (four before dialysis [11, 12] and eight in patients on dialysis [32]), and although none of the 12 patients dialyzed for more than 10 years and exposed only to Al(OH)$_3$ had symptomatic bone disease [33], the bone-toxic effect of aluminum in such a setting is suggested by the negative correlation between bone aluminum and bone formation rate [33, 34].

The risk of aluminum toxicity may be further increased by the fact that plasma aluminum is increased by administration of 1-α-OH vitamin D derivatives. This effect has been demonstrated in the rat by Drueke [28], who observed that plasma aluminum was higher in uremic rats taking Al(OH)$_3$ and 1,25-(OH)$_2$D$_3$ than in uremic rats taking Al(OH)$_3$, but no 1,25(OH)$_2$D$_3$; whereas, their liver aluminum content was lower. In accordance with these observations, Tahiri et al [29] found that in 10 patients on dialysis taking a constant dose of Al(OH)$_3$, the administration of 1 μg of 1-α-OH vitamin D$_3$ increased significantly their plasma aluminum, suggesting increased intestinal absorption and/or decreased tissue storage of aluminum.

Finally, administration of 1-α-OH vitamin D derivatives, even at doses inducing no increase in plasma concentrations of calcium and phosphate, exposes a hazard of vascular calcifications as shown recently by Tvedegaard in the uremic rabbit [30]. An increase of vascular and soft tissue calcifications also have been reported in long-term administration of 1,25(OH)$_2$D$_3$ in dialysis patients, despite efforts to keep the plasma phosphate below 2 mmoles and the plasma calcium below 2.6 mmoles [11]. However, in controlled studies [24, 31], soft tissue calcifications were not more common than in the control group.

The balance between the potential beneficial and hazardous effects of 1α-(OH) vitamin D_3 in uremic patients may vary according to the clinical settings.

In symptomatic osteodystrophy that is not linked to aluminum osteomalacia, both numerous open trials and the controlled trial of Berl obviously have demonstrated the value of $1\text{-}\alpha\text{-OH}$ vitamin D_3 derivatives [3]. As reported in this volume, $1\alpha\text{-OH}$ vitamin D_3 derivatives have no value for treating aluminum osteomalacia that, however, responds to desferrioxamine (a chelating agent of aluminum).

In asymptomatic patients on dialysis, the balance between the beneficial and hazardous effects is not obvious. Three controlled trials [24, 31, 36] have established the effectiveness of the $1\text{-}\alpha\text{-OH}$ vitamin D derivatives versus placebos in preventing the worsening of radiologic subperiosteal resorption, the increase of plasma PTH or alkaline phosphatase, and the decrease of the bone mineral content, all without inducing soft tissue calcifications more than in the control group. However, all of these patients had to take $Al(OH)_3$, often at increasing dosages, to prevent worsening of hyperphosphatemia. Therefore, one may question the ultimate long-term benefit of such a therapeutic approach. Would another approach, in which the normalization of the plasma concentration of calcium and phosphate are achieved only by high doses of calcium carbonate, be more valuable?

In fact, we have shown that high doses of calcium carbonate $(CaCO_3)$ at a mean dose $\pm$ SD of 9 ± 4 g/d could replace $1\text{-}\alpha\text{-OH}$ vitamin D_3 and $Al(OH)_3$, and could maintain normal plasma calcium and acceptable (between 4 to 6 mg/dl) plasma phosphate [37]. Furthermore, we could not demonstrate that at isocalcemic doses, the control of PTH hypersecretion was better with $1\text{-}\alpha\text{-}(OH)D_3$ than that with high doses of $CaCO_3$ [38]. Therefore, we feel that until new nontoxic phosphate binders (such as, possibly, the polymer resin of Schneider [39]) are available, a cheap and pragmatic approach for the control of subradiologic osteodystrophy (histologic evidence only) would be the use of high doses of $CaCO_3$. Because of tolerance and effectiveness problems, their use can solve the problem finally in about 50% of the dialysis population without a greater risk of metastatic calcification than that in the more classic treatment based on $1\text{-}\alpha\text{-OH-}D_3$ and $Al(OH)_3$; provided that close monitoring of the plasma concentrations of calcium and phosphate is performed.

Even when new nontoxic phosphate binders will be available, we feel that trials should be performed comparing high doses of $CaCO_3$ to $1\text{-}\alpha\text{-}(OH)$ vitamin D_3 plus nontoxic phosphate binders, since this approach is more economical.

In patients who are not on dialysis, the study reported in this volume by Letteri in 16 patients is very encouraging for the systematic prophylactic use of $1,25\text{-}(OH)_2D_3$. However, we feel that larger studies are necessary, especially in patients with a GFR between 10 to 30 ml/min—since earlier experiences in patients with this range of GFR have shown that the use of $Al(OH)_3$ was necessary and that (often) the GFR actually declined more rapidly. Comparisons between high doses of $CaCO_3$ and $1\text{-}\alpha\text{-OH}$ vitamin D derivatives also should be tried in these patients.

Indications for use of Vitamin D Sterols Other Than the 1α-Hydroxylated D Derivatives

The indications of vitamin D_2 or vitamin D_3 in renal osteodystrophy are currently limited to the prevention of vitamin deficiency, which is by no means an infrequent situation in uremic patients of colder nonindustrialized countries (with low sun exposure and no vitamin D-fortified industrial foods) because of their dietary restriction in meat and milk. Usually, addition of 400 to 800 IU/d of these sterols suffices. Vitamin D_3 is preferable to vitamin D_2 not because of greater biologic activity, but because metabolites of vitamin D_2 may interfere with the measurement of $24,25(OH)_2$ vitamin D_3 [3].

25-OH vitamin D_3 (Calcifediol, Dedrogyl®) may also be used for the prevention or treatment of vitamin D-deficient osteomalacia in uremic patients. Thus, low or "physiologic" doses (5 μg/d) have been used by Memmos in three uremic patients who were not yet on dialysis (600 to 1000 μmoles/liter of creatininemia) with osteomalacia; and, they cured the abnormality within a few months, as well as in three control patients with pure nutritional osteomalacia (without uremia) [40].

Vitamin D_2 or D_3 has been used at pharmacologic doses (1000 to 3000 μg/d) to treat successfully both renal osteomalacia and secondary hyperparathyroidism. However, since the duration of the hypercalcemia eventually induced may be several months, these pharmacologic doses have been abandoned with the coming of the newer D derivatives with shorter biologic half-lives (0.5 to 1 week for the 1-α-hydroxylated derivatives) [3, 42].

25-OH-D_3 has also been used at pharmacologic doses (50 to 100 μg/d), even in anephric patients to treat efficiently both hyperparathyroidism and osteomalacia. Although the biologic half-life is shorter than that of vitamin D_2 or D_3, it is much longer than that of the 1-α-hydroxylated derivatives. Therefore, its use at these doses may be justified only if special therapeutic effect could be demonstrated for 25-OH-D_3 in comparison to 1-α-hydroxylated D derivatives. To our knowledge, the only study that tries to answer this question is our study comparing isocalcemic doses of 25-OH-D_3 (100 μg/d) to 1-α-OH vitamin D_3 (2 μg/d) in, respectively, six and five patients on chronic hemodialysis. This study showed that the control of the hyperparathyroidism was comparable, but that the mineralization front was better improved by 25-OH-D_3 than by 1-α-OH D_3 despite the fact that the plasma phosphate and (therefore) the plasma calcium phosphate product was significantly more increased by 1-α-OH-D_3. Therefore, these data suggest that 25-OH-D_3 may be preferable to 1-α-OH vitamin D in patients with renal osteomalacia [41].

Dihydrotachysterol (DHT) was used quite successfully to treat severe uremic hyperparathyroidism; and also renal osteomalacia, but with less consistent results at a time when the role of aluminum was underestimated [3, 42]. The doses used were high (200 to 1000 μg/d), but not much higher than the doses used to treat vitamin D-deficiency rickets (200 μg). The reason for the absence of this higher requirement in uremia lies in the fact that the hydroxyl in position 3 is in a pseudo 1-α-hydroxyl configuration because of the 180° rotation of ring A; therefore, no further renal metabolism of DHT is required to make it active after its 25-hydroxylation by the liver. The practical problem in the use of DHT was the instability of its earlier preparation and a longer biologic half-life than that in the 1-α-hydroxylated D derivatives (1 to 3 weeks) [3, 42].

24,25 (OH)$_2$ vitamin D$_3$ was the subject of much interest a few years ago, when Kanis showed that it could stimulate calcium absorption without increasing plasma calcium; in uremic humans, this suggests that it could promote bone formation and mineralization [42]. Furthermore, studies by Canterbury showed that it could suppress PTH hypersecretion in uremic dogs and decrease their plasma calcium, provided their diet was rich in calcium [44]. However, biochemical and histologic studies in uremic men with osteodystrophy [7, 24, 43] did not show a significant effect, either on the osteitis fibrosa or on the mineralization defect. The only consistent effect was the decrease of plasma calcium, which allowed higher doses of 1,-25(OH)$_2$D$_3$ when this was used in combinations. In that case, only improvement of aluminum-induced osteomalacia was observed by Coburn et al [24] in about 50% of the cases, but this improvement was much less impressive than that subsequently observed with desferrioxamine. Therefore, should 24,-25(OH)$_2$ vitamin D$_3$ be totally forgotten in the management of renal osteodystrophy? We do not feel so, since the lack of improvement or even the worsening of hyperparathyroidism observed by Muirhead with 24,25(OH)$_2$D$_3$ alone in patients on dialysis was accompanied by a decrease of plasma calcium; and, these patients were not given high doses of calcium carbonate. By adding 24,25(OH)$_2$D$_3$ to the high doses of CaCO$_3$, one perhaps could increase the tolerance to CaCO$_3$, since this latter treatment often is limited by the occurrence of hypercalcemia.

25,26(OH)$_2$ vitamin D$_3$ has seldom been studied in uremic patients. Two years ago, we showed that at pharmacologic doses (12 μg three times per week) increasing the plasma concentrations 10 times above the normal mean, it had no effect on the plasma concentration of PTH, calcium, phosphate, and alkaline phosphatase. Therefore, 25,26(OH)$_2$ vitamin D$_3$ appears to have no therapeutic potential in renal osteodystrophy.

Indications of Parathyroidectomy

Surgical parathyroidectomy should be performed each time that the medical treatment of uremic hyperparathyroidism, based on 1α-OH vitamin D$_3$ and phosphate binder, is inefficient. That is, when radiologic bone resorption and soft tissue calcifications worsen, while the plasma phosphate cannot be controlled below 6 mg/dl by phosphate binders without inducing plasma aluminum above 100 μg/dl; also, while the plasma calcium is increased at 11 mg/dl or above by CaCO$_3$ and 1-α-OH vitamin D$_3$, and the plasma alkaline phosphatase and plasma PTH continue to increase. In this situation, surgical parathyroidectomy is readily performed, even though the patients rarely have bone pains. On a systematic basis, however, the following causes of hypercalcemia should be previously excluded, such as hypophosphatemia, vitamin D or $CaCO_3$ intoxication, and thiazide and fortuitous association of hypercalcemic diseases (sarcoidosis myeloma, malignancies, immobilization, and so on). Aluminum intoxication especially should be formally excluded, even if alkaline phosphatase and PTH levels are elevated, because Coburn has encountered such cases. Bone pain should alert one to this possibility, and a bone biopsy procedure should be performed each time the picture of overt hyperparathyroidism is not pure or when plasma aluminum or (even better) the desferrioxamine test indicates heavy aluminum overload. A bone biopsy specimen is, in fact, the diagnostic clue for aluminum osteomalacia, when it shows wide osteoid seams and aluminum staining by Aluminon at the interfaces between calcified bone and the osteoid.

Therefore, the description (elsewhere in this volume) by Popovtzer et al of symptomatic and uremic patients who were not improved by parathyroidectomy (PTX) is of interest. The pre-PTX bone and plasma aluminum data of their patients will be crucial for interpretation. As a matter of fact, the pre-PTX symptomatic patients essentially had hyperparathyroidism with high bone turnover. However, there are indications that severe hyperparathyroidism can counteract the depressive effect of aluminum on bone formation [34, 40], and that parathyroidectomy may allow subsequent development of osteomalacia with surface distribution of the aluminum that was previously distributed diffusely throughout the bone [47]. If the aluminum data are available in the pre- and post-PTX symptomatic patients of Popovtzer, and if they show marked aluminum overload in these patients, one may question the opportunity for performing surgical parathyroidectomy without previous aluminum depletion via desferrioxamine. A desferrioxamine test perhaps could be defined to select those patients who will benefit from this depletion treatment before surgical parathyroidectomy. The question then will be: will it be better to perform desferrioxamine treatment before or after surgical parathyroidectomy?

Because of the hazards of aluminum overload by phosphate binders—which are still required in about 50% of our patients despite our endeavor to give exclusively high doses of $CaCO_3$—the problem arises regarding the opportunity to reduce parathyroid mass at an early stage. To select the patients who would not suppress their PTH hypersecretion by long-term treatment with $1,25(OH)_2D_3$ and/or $CaCO_3$ and $Al(OH)_3$, one can perform an acute suppression study of PTH secretion (measured with N-terminal antibody) with an infusion of calcium (4 mg/kg/hr for 4 hr) according to the protocol of Muirhead et al. In fact, these authors have found a good correlation between chronic suppression of PTH secretion with $1,25(OH)_2D_3$ and the acute suppression with calcium infusion [48].

Another complementary approach for the selection of patients for surgical parathyroidectomy is evaluation of the parathyroid mass by high-resolution real-time ultrasonography, since we found a good correlation between the volume measured by ultrasonography and the weight of the parathyroid glands removed by surgery [49].

References

1. FOURNIER A, MORINIERE P, COEVOET B: Prevention and medical treatment of hyperparathyroidism secondary to renal failure, in *Advances in Nephrology,* edited by HAMBURGER, et al, Chicago, Yearbook Medical Publishers, 1982, vol 11, pp 241–276
2. FOURNIER A, SEBERT JL, MORINIERE P, GREGOIRE I, DE FREMONT JF, TAHIRI Y, Dkhissi H: Renal osteodystrophy: pathophysiology and treatment. *Horm Res* (in press, 1984)
3. FOURNIER A, BOUDAILLIEZ B, TOLANI M, ULMANN A: Vitamine D et osteodystrophie rénale in *Vitamine D et Maladiesdes os et du Métabolisme Minéral,* edited by FOURNIER A, GARABEDIAN M, SEBERT JL, MEUNIER P, Paris, Masson 1984, pp 171–246
4. MADSEN S, OLGAARD K, LADGEFOGED J: Suppressive effect of 1.25 $(OH)_2$ vitamin D_3 on circulating parathyroid hormone in acute renal failure. *J Clin Endocrinol Metab* 53:823–827, 1981
5. SLATOPOLSKY E, WEERTS C, THIELAN B, GALCERANT T, MARTIN K: Suppression of secondary hyperparathyroidism by 1.25 $(OH)_2$ vitamin D_3, in *Clinical Disorders of Bone and Mineral Metabolism,* edited by FRAME B, POTTS JT, Amsterdam, Excerpta Medica Int. Congress Series 617, 1983, pp 267–272
6. LAMBREY G, NGUYEN JM, GARABEDIAN M, SEBERT JL, DE FREMONT JF, MARIE P, CAILLENS C, GUERIS J, MEUNIER P, BALSAN S: Possible link between changes in plasma 24,25 dihydroxyvitamin D and healing of bone resorption in dialysis osteodystrophy. *Metab Bone Dis Rel Res* 4:25–30, 1982
7. MUIRHEAD N, ADAMI S, SANDLER M, FRASER RA, CATTO GRD, EDWARD N, O'RIORDAN JLH: Long term effects of 1.25 dihydroxy vitamin D_3 and 24,25 dihydroxy vitamin D_3 in renal osteodystrophy. *Q J Med* (new series) LI:427–444, 1982
8. KAPLAN MA, CANTERBURY JM, GAVELLAS G, JAFFE D, BOURGOIGNIE E, REISS E, BRICKER NS: Interrelations between phosphorus calcium, parathyroid hormone and renal phosphate excretion in response to an oral phosphorus load in normal and uremic dogs. *Kidney Int* 14:207–214, 1978
9. JACOB AI, GAVELLAS G, CANTERBURY JM, BOURGOIGNIE JJ: Calcemic and phosphaturic response to parathyroid hormone in normal and chronically uremic dog. *Kidney Int* 22:21–26, 1982
10. MEMMOS DE, EASTWOOD JB, HARRIS E, O'GRADY A, DE WARDENER HE: Response of uremic osteoid to vitamin D. *Kidney Int* 21(suppl):S-50–S-54, 1982
11. FELSENFELD A, GUTMAN RA, LLACH P, HARRELSON JM: Osteomalacia in chronic renal failure. A syndrome previously reported only with maintenance dialysis. *Am J Nephrol* 2:147–154, 1982
12. ANDREOLI SP, BERGSTEIN JM, SHERRARD DJ: Aluminum intoxication from aluminum containing phosphate binders in children with azotemia not undergoing dialysis. *N Engl J Med* 310:1079–1084, 1984
13. PIERIDES AM, ELLIS HA, WARD M, KERR DNS: Barbiturate and anticonvulsant treatment in relation to osteomalacia with haemodialysis and renal transplantation. *Br Med J* i:190–193, 1976
14. NIELSEN HE, MELSEN F, CHRISTENSEM MS: Interrelationships between calcium phosphorus metabolism, serum parathyroid hormone and bone histomorphometry in non dialyzed and dialyzed patients with chronic renal failure. *Min Electr Metab* 4:113–122, 1980
15. MORA PALMA FJ, ELLIS HA, COOK DB, DEWAR JH, WARD MK, WILKINSON R, KERR DNS: Osteomalacia in patients with chronic renal failure before dialysis or transplantation. *Q J Med* (new series) 52:332–348, 1983

16. FOURNIER AE, ARNAUD CD, JOHNSON WJ, GOLDSMITH RS: Etiology of hyper-parathyroidism and bone disease during chronic hemodialysis. *J Clin Invest* 50:599–605, 1971

17. DE FREMONT JF, BATAILLE P, MORINIERE PH, KACZMARECK P, FIEVET P, FOURNIER A: Metabolic tolerance of continuous ambulatory peritoneal dialysis (C.A.P.D.), in *Advances in Peritoneal Dialysis,* edited by GAHL GM, KESSEL M, NOLPH DK, Berlin, Excerpta Medica, 1981, pp 446–448

18. DE FREMONT JF, MORINIERE PH, PRUNA A, GHEERBRANDT JD, KASSOUF J, ROUSSEL A, GALY CL, FOURNIER A: Long-term evaluation of hemofiltration at home. *Contr Nephrol* 32:119–127, 1982

19. BORDIER PJ, TUN CHOT S, EASTWOOD JB, FOURNIER A, DE WARDENER HE: Lack of histological evidence of vitamin D abnormality in the bones of anephric patients. *Clin Sci* 44:33–41, 1973

20. WARD MK, FEEST TG, PARKINSON IS, ELLIS HM, KERR DNS: Osteomalacic dialytic osteodystrophy: evidence for a water born aetiological agent, probably aluminum. *Lancet* i:841–845, 1978

21. CHRISTIANSEN C, RODBRO P, CHRISTENSEN MC, NAETOFT J, HARTNACK B, ET AL: Deterioration of renal function during treatment of chronic renal failure with 1.25 dihydroxyvitamin D_3. *Lancet* ii:700–703, 1978

22. TOUGGARD L, SORENSEN E, MORTENSEN JB, CHRISTENSEN MS, RODBRO P, SORENSEN AW: Controlled trial of 1-α hydroxycholecalciferol in chronic renal failure. *Lancet* i:1044–1047, 1976

23. NIELSEN HE, ROMER FK, MELSEN F, CHRISTENSEN MS, HANSEN HC: 1-α hydroxyvitamin D_3 treatment of non dialyzed patients with chronic renal failure. Effects of bone, mineral metabolism and kidney function. *Clin Nephrol* 16:359–364, 1976

24. COBURN JW, SHERRARD DJ, OTT SA, DIDOMENICO NC, BRYCE GF, BRICK-MANN AS, MILLER ON, SHUPIEN SA, CHANG PL: Use of active vitamin D sterols in end stage renal failure, in *Clinical Disorders of Bone and Mineral Metabolism,* edited by FRAME B, POTTS JT, Amsterdam, Excerpta Medica Int Congress, series 617, 1983, pp 263–266

25. SEBERT JL, FOURNIER A, GUERIS J, DE FREMONT JF, MARIE P, KUNTZ D, RYCKEWAERT A, MEUNIER P: Limit by hyperphosphatemia of the usefulness of vitamin D metabolites (1α hydroxycholecalciferol and 25 OH cholecalciferol) in the treatment of renal osteodystrophy. *Metab Bone Dis Rel Res* 2:217–222, 1980

26. COEVOET B, MORINIERE PH, SEBERT JL, FOURNIER A: 1.25 $(OH)_2$ D_3 in infrara-diological dialysis osteodystrophy control, in *Hormonal Control of Calcium Metabolism,* edited by TALMAGE RV, MATTHEWS JL, COHN DV, Amsterdam, Excerpta Medica, 1981, p 432

27. TAHIRI Y, MORINIERE PH, FOURNIER A: hyperaluminémie des hémodialysés chroniques. Evaluation du rôle respectif de l'aluminum du dialysat et de la prise orale d'hyxoxide d'alumine. *Néphrologie* 4:129–133, 1983

28. DRUEKE T, LACOUR B, BASILE C, BOURDON R: Oral aluminum intoxication in rats: Role of uremia, parathyroid hormone and vitamin D metabolists. *Nephron* (in press, 1984)

29. TAHIRI Y: 1α (OH) vitamin D increases plasma aluminum in uremic patients taking $Al(OH)_3$ (*abstract*). *International Congress of Nephrology,* Los Angeles, 1984

30. TVEDEGAARD E, LADEFOGED O, NIELSEN M, KRAMSTRUP O: The effect of 1 OH vitamin D_3 and dietary calcium and phosphate on the aortic mineral content in rabbits with mild azotemia. *Nephron* 34:185–191, 1983

31. MEMMOS DE, EASTWOOD J, TALNER, ET AL: Double blind trial of renal 1.25

(OH)$_3$D$_3$ versus placebo in asymptomatic hyperparathyroidism in patients receiving maintenance hemodialysis. *Br Med J* 282:1919–1924, 1981

32. HODSMAN AB, SHERRARD J, WONG EG, ET AL: Vitamin D resistant osteomalacia in hemodialysis patients lacking secondary hyperparathyroidism. *Ann Intern Med* 94:629–637, 1981

33. ANDRESS DL, OTT SM, MILLINER D, MALONEY NA, ENDRES D, COBURN JW, SHERRARD DJ: Diagnosis of aluminum bone disease in long-term dialysis patients using deferoxamine and zero-calcium dialysis (*abstract*). *Kidney Int* 25:139, 1984

34. SEBERT JL, MARIE A, HERVE M, SMADJA A, FOURNIER A: Evaluation by multiple linear regression analysis of the role of aluminum on bone histomorphometry in uremic patients: evidence for a depressive effect on bone formation, in *Bone Histomorphometry*, edited by MELSEN F, 4th International Workshop, Aarhus, June 1984

35. MASSRY SG, GOLDSTEIN DA, MALLUCHE HH: Current status of the use of 1.25 (OH)$_2$ D$_3$ in the management of renal osteodystrophy. *Kidney Int* 18:409–418, 1980

36. SHARMAN VL, ABRAM SML, ADAMI S, ET AL: Controlled trial of 1.25 (OH)$_2$ vitamin D$_3$ in prevention of bone disease in haemodialysis patients. *EDTA Proc* 19:287–292, 1982

37. MORINIERE PH, ROUSSEL A, TAHIRI Y, FOURNIER A: Substitution of aluminum hydroxyde by high doses of calcium carbonate in patients on chronic hemodialysis: disappearance of hyperaluminemia and equal control of hyperparathyroidism. *EDTA Proc* 19:784–787, 1982

38. MORINIERE PH, FOURNIER A, LEFLON A, HERVE M, SEBERT JL, GREGOIRE I, BATAILLE P, GUERIS J: Comparison of 1 α OH vitamin D$_3$ and high doses of calcium carbonate for the control of hyperparathyroidism and hyperaluminemia in patients on maintenance dialysis. *Nephron* (in press, 1984)

39. SCHNEIDER H, KULBE KD, WEBER H, STREICHER E: High effective aluminum free phosphate binder: in vitro and in vivo studies. *Proc Eur Dial Trans Assoc* 20:725–730, 1984

40. MEMMOS DE, EASTWOOD JB, O'GRADY A, DE WARDENER ME: Response of uremic osteoid to vitamin D. *Kidney Int* 21:550–554, 1982

41. FOURNIER A, BORDIER P, GUERIS J, SEBERT JL, MARIE P, FERRIERE C, BEDROSSIAN J, DE LUCA MF: Comparison of 1-α-hydroxy cholecalciferol and 25 hydroxycholecalciferol in the treatment of renal osteodystrophy: greater effect of 25 hydroxycholecalciferol on bone mineralization. *Kidney Int* 15:196–205, 1979

42. KANIS JA, GUILLAN D, CUMMINO DF, RUSSEL RGG: Comparative physiology and pharmacology of the metabolists and analogists of vitamin D, in *Endocrinology of Calcium Metabolism*, edited by PARSONS JA, New York, Raven Press, 1982, pp 321–362

43. EVANS RA, HILL SE, WONG SYP, DUNSTAN CR, NORMAN AW: The use of 24,25 (OH)$_2$ D$_3$ alone and in combination with 1,25 (OH)$_2$ D$_3$ in chronic renal failure, in *Vitamin D, Chemical, Biochemical and Clinical Endocrinology of Calcium Metabolism*, edited by NORMAN AW, Berlin, Walter de Gruyter, 1982, pp 835–840

44. CANTERBURY JM, GAVELLAS G, REISS E: Effect of dietary calcium on the suppressive effects of 24,25 (OH)$_2$ D$_3$ on PTH secretion in hyperparathyroid dogs (*abstract*). *Clin Res* 30:566A, 1982

45. MORINIERE PH, SEBERT JL, SANDLER L, FRAHER L, REDEL J, O'RIORDAN JL, FOURNIER A: Plasma levels and biological effects of 25,26 (OH)$_2$ vitamin D$_3$ in uremic patients, in *Vitamin D, Chemical, Biochemical and Clinical Endocri-*

nology of Calcium Metabolism, edited by NORMAN AW, ET AL, Berlin, Walter de Gruyter, 1982, pp 889–892

46. COURNOT-WITMER G, ZINGRAFF J, PLACHOT JF: Aluminum localization in bone from hemodialyzed patients. Relationship to matrix mineralization. *Kidney Int* 20:375–385, 1981

47. ANDRESS DL, OTT SM, MALONEY NA, SHERRARD DJ: A longitudinal study of bone aluminum accumulative in longterm hemodialysis patients: effect of parathyroidectomy (*abstract*). *Calc Tiss Int* (in press, 1984)

48. MUIRHEAD N, CATTO GRD, EDWARD N, ADAMIS K, MANNING RH, O'RIORDAN JL: Suppression of serum day hyperparathyroidism in uremia: acuteand chronic studies. *Br Med J* 288:177–179, 1984

49. MORINIERE PH, TYAN P, FOURNIER A, DE FREMONT JF, DERAMOND H, RINGOT P, GUERIS J: Exploration par ultrasonographie à haute résolution en temps réel des parathyroides de 60 hémodialysés chroniques. *Néphrologie* 4:135–140, 1983

Prevalence of Various Types of Bone Disease in Dialysis Patients

Francisco Llach, Arnold J. Felsenfeld, Michael D. Coleman, and James A. Pederson

Renal osteodystrophy did not represent a major problem until the advent of maintenance dialysis. In general, the longer that patients remain on maintenance hemodialysis, the more manifested are the complications of renal osteodystrophy.

Several types of bone lesions have been described in hemodialysis patients. These can be divided into osteitis fibrosa, mixed osteitis fibrosa and osteomalacia, low-turnover osteomalacia, and aplastic bone disease. Osteitis fibrosa appears to be the most frequent lesion observed, and it reflects the presence of secondary hyperparathyroidism. Not infrequently, osteitis fibrosa is associated with both increased osteoid volume and a mild decrement in mineralization activity; the so-called mixed lesion.

Low-turnover osteomalacia has been reported as an infrequent bone lesion, and it has been associated with aluminum toxicity [1, 2] (see Coburn et al, in this volume). These patients often present with severe musculoskeletal symptoms, such as bone pain and fractures; and, hypercalcemia usually develops during treatment with vitamin D compounds. The characteristic bone histologic findings are a marked increase in osteoid, minimal cell activity, and the absence of or only minimal endosteal fibrosis. The marked decrease of cell activity, both osteoblastic and osteoclastic, and the absence of endosteal fibrosis differentiates this lesion from osteitis fibrosa. In addition, while patients with osteitis fibrosa exhibit active bone formation (as determined by double tetracycline labeling), patients with low-turnover osteomalacia generally do not form bone during the tetracycline marker period. Finally, marked aluminum deposits are frequently observed at the interface of osteoid and mineralized bone, along the trabecular surface, and at reversal lines. In the majority of reported patients with low-turnover osteomalacia, a high aluminum concentration has been present in the dialysate [3]. Recently, it has been suggested that phosphate binders containing aluminum hydroxide may play an important role in the pathogenesis of the osteomalacia [4].

This manuscript was presented as part of a Symposium on *Renal Osteodystrophy: Recent Advances.*

Aplastic bone disease is considered to be an infrequent entity that is similar to low-turnover osteomalacia; diminished cellular activity, aluminum deposits, and absent bone formation are characteristic histopathologic features. The principal difference from low-turnover osteomalacia is that large osteoid deposits are absent.

The majority of previous studies reporting bone histologic findings have been in symptomatic patients [1, 2]. Thus, less data are available describing the pattern of bone disease in randomly selected patients, regardless of the presence or absence of symptoms. Asymptomatic patients on maintenance hemodialysis were studied by Minnos et al; although bone histology was not evaluated, the radiologic and biochemical data showed that the majority of these patients most likely had osteitis fibrosa, as suggested by high parathyroid hormone (PTH) levels and increased bone resorption radiologically [5]. Another study in 98 asymptomatic dialysis patients has recently been reported by Coburn et al [6]. Again, osteitis fibrosa was the most common lesion, as estimated by radiologic and biochemical criteria.

Prevalence of Osteodystrophy in Chronic Hemodialysis Patients

We have evaluated the prevalence of the several types of bone lesions, as well as the clinical and biochemical findings, in 140 patients on chronic maintenance hemodialysis regardless of the presence or absence of symptoms that are suggestive of renal osteodystrophy. The majority of patients were asymptomatic.

Four dialysis units participated in this study, which included 140 hemodialysis patients ranging in age from 23 to 74 years (mean age 53 $\pm$ 12 years). The criteria for selection of the patients was the willingness of the patient to undergo a bone biopsy procedure. The mean duration of maintenance hemodialysis in these patients was 55 $\pm$ 15 months. Iliac crest biopsy specimens were obtained in all patients. The aluminum concentration of the dialysate water was checked at repeated intervals in the four dialysis units. In three of the dialysis units, the water supply was treated with a reverse osmosis system, and in the other unit with deionization. None of the patients were receiving vitamin D therapy. Serum calcium, phosphate, and alkaline phosphatase were measured by standard techniques. Serum aluminum levels were measured by atomic absorption. Carboxy (C) terminal PTH was determined by a radioimmunoassay, which has been previously published [7].

Bone specimens, after dehydration and defatting, were embedded in methyl methacrylate. Sectioning of the block was accomplished with a Jung model K sledge microtome. For histomorphometric analysis, 5 μ Goldner-stained sections were examined. These 5-μ sections were stained for aluminum by the method of Maloney et al [8]; 15-μ unstained sections were used for analysis of the tetracycline labels. Patients twice received 2 days of tetracycline orally, separated by a 10-day interval prior to the bone biopsy procedure. All histomorphometric analyses were performed with the aid of a Leitz Ortholux II microscope and a Merz-Schenk reticle. Measurement of trabecular bone was made in the following categories: (1) osteoblastic surface, (2) total osteoid surface, (3) osteoclastic resorption, (4) osteoclasts/mm^2, (5) relative osteoid volume, (6) bone volume, and (7) endosteal fibrosis.

The type of bone lesion was categorized according to the following criteria: osteitis fibrosa includes the presence of increased bone resorption, increased osteoblastic activity, endosteal fibrosis, and active mineralization and bone formation, as assessed by the double tetracycline labels (Fig. 1). Low-turnover osteomalacia includes the presence of large acellular osteoid deposits, a relative absence of cell activity, virtual cessation of mineralization and bone formation (as assessed by double tetracycline labeling), and the absence of endosteal fibrosis (Fig. 2). In addition, aluminum deposits usually are present at the interface of osteoid and mineralized bone. Aplastic bone disease includes a normal ratio of osteoid to mineralized bone, decreased cellular activity, absence of endosteal fibrosis (at least $< 0.5\%$), virtual cessation of mineralization and bone formation (as assessed by double tetracycline labeling), and the presence of aluminum deposits.

By these criteria, of the 140 hemodialysis patients, 94 patients are found to have osteitis fibrosa, 36 patients have low-turnover osteomalacia, and 10 patients have aplastic bone disease. The symptomatology of the 140 patients (at the time of the biopsy procedure) with regard to the presence of muscle weakness, bone pain, bone fractures, and pruritus vary according to the type of bone disease. While the frequency of muscle weakness is relatively low in patients with osteitis fibrosa (4%), it is more commonly encountered in patients with low-turnover osteomalacia (26%). Likewise, bone pain is present in only 5% of patients with osteitis fibrosa, in 32% of patients with osteomalacia, and in 25% of patients with aplastic bone disease. Finally, fractures are observed only in 3% of patients with osteitis, in 23% of patients with osteomalacia, and in 17% of patients with aplastic bone disease. Thus, the above incidence of symptoms is low in patients with osteitis fibrosa at the time of the biopsy procedure; an additional 8% developed some of the above-mentioned symptoms during a 2-year follow-up study.

Patients with osteomalacia and aplastic bone disease have a much higher incidence of bone fractures and bone pain not only at the time of the bone biopsy procedure, but also in the follow-up period. Thus, 35% of additional patients with osteomalacia later developed bone fractures, and 38% developed bone pain and muscle weakness. In patients with aplastic bone disease, 58% developed muscle weakness in the follow-up period, 42% developed bone pain, and 17% developed fractures.

The biochemical data of these three groups are shown in Table 1. Patients with osteomalacia have higher serum calcium levels than patients with both aplastic bone disease and osteitis fibrosa. Although the level of serumphosphate is not different between the three groups, patients with osteitis fibrosa have a trend towards higher serum phosphate levels. The mean serum alkaline phosphatase level is significantly higher in patients with osteitis fibrosa than in patients with both osteomalacia and aplastic bone disease. The PTH values of patients with osteitis fibrosa are also higher than those with osteomalacia and aplastic bone disease. The mean serum aluminum concentration of pa-

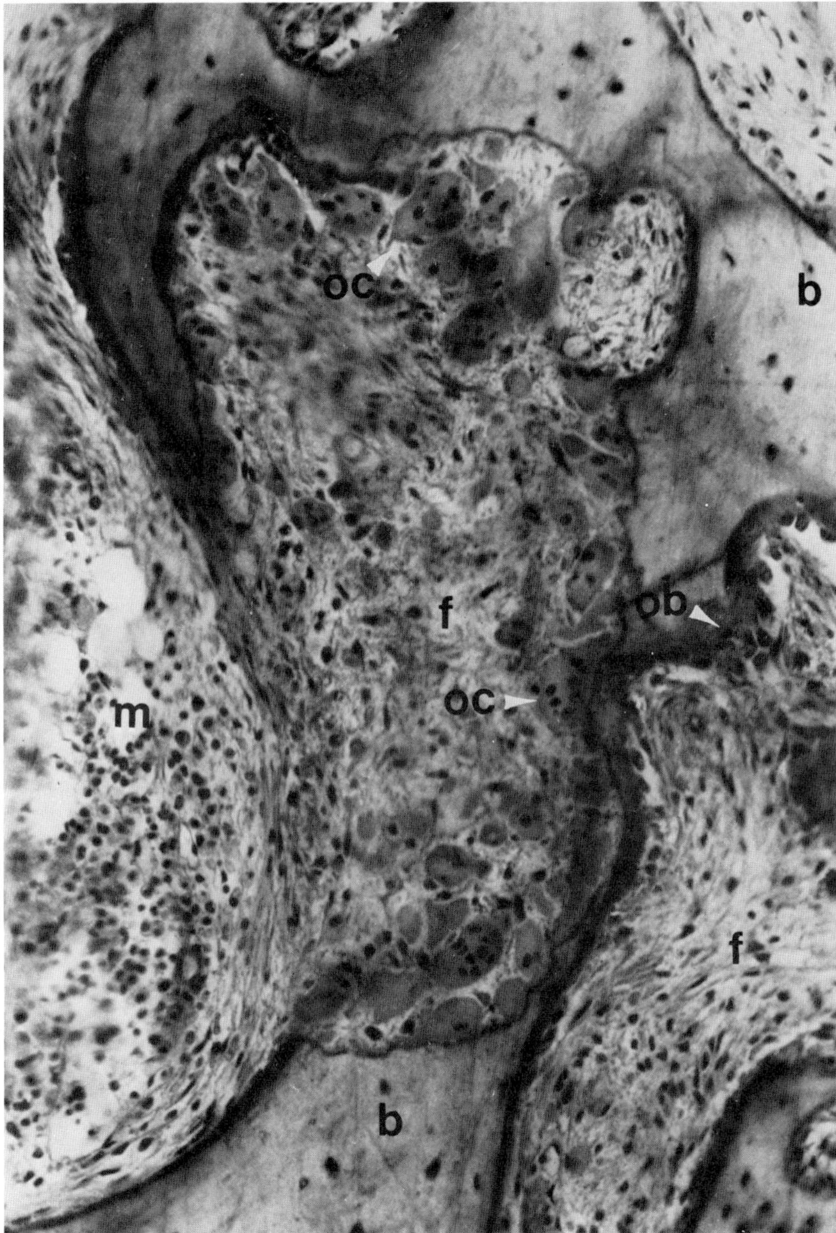

Fig. 1. Bone biopsy specimen of a patient with a lesion that is representative of osteitis fibrosa. Note the presence of cell activity and diffuse fibrosis. (*Ob*, osteoblast; *OC*, osteoclast; *b*, mineralized bone; *f*, endosteal fibrosis; and *m*, marrow space.)

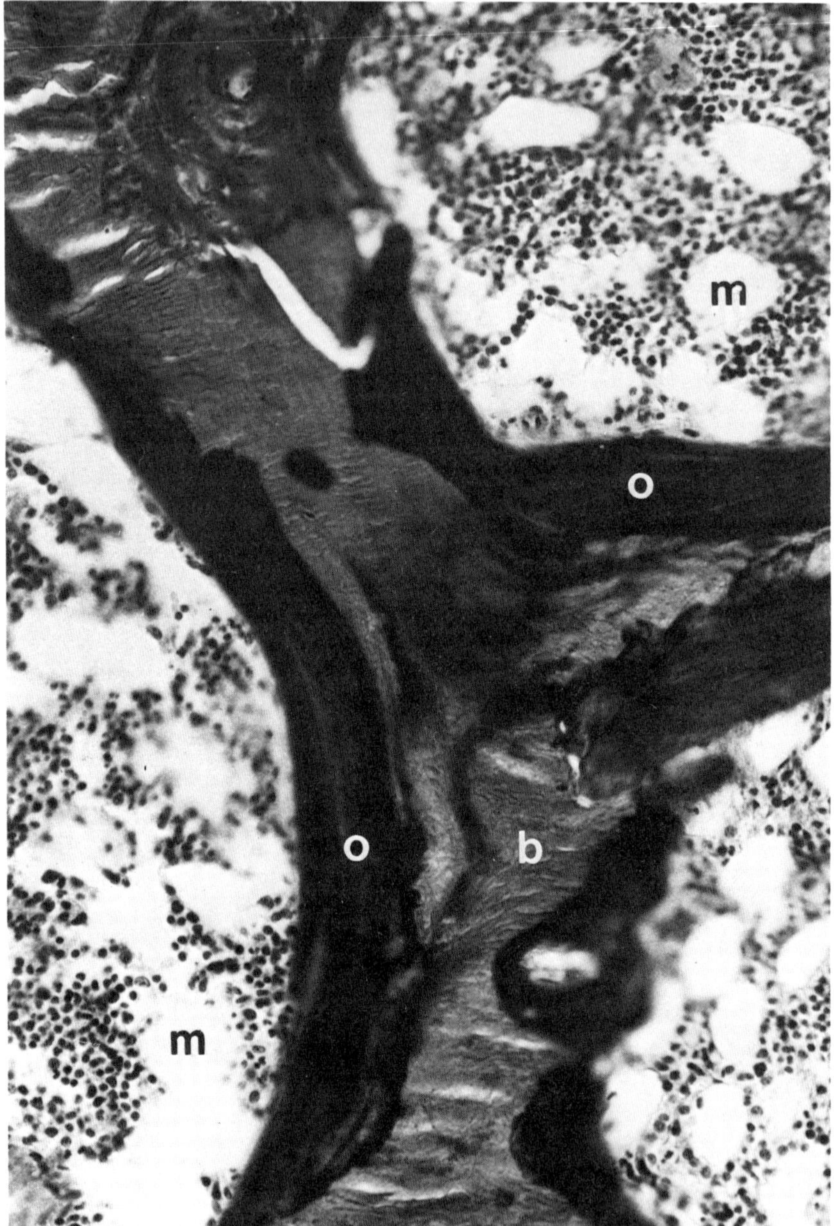

Fig. 2. Bone biopsy specimen of a patient with a lesion that is representative of low-turnover osteomalacia. Note the absence of fibrosis and cell activity. (*O*, osteoid tissue; *b*, mineralized bone; and *m*, mineralized bone.)

Table 1. Biochemical data

	Serum calcium (mg/dl)	Serum phosphate (mg/dl)	Serum alkaline phosphatase (IU)	Serum aluminum (μg/liter)	Plasma PTH (ng/ml)
OF	8.8 ± 1.0[a]	5.8 ± 1.8	192 ± 155	73 ± 51	1.87 ± 0.7[c]
OM	10.0 ± 0.9	4.8 ± 1.7	101 ± 93	199 ± 95[b]	0.95 ± 0.3
ABD	9.3 ± 1.2	4.7 ± 1.1	69 ± 16	158 ± 59[b]	1.10 ± 0.2

OF, osteitis fibrosa; OM, osteomalacia; ABD, aplastic bone disease.

[a] $P < 0.05$ when compared with osteomalacia.

[b] $P < 0.01$ when compared with osteitis fibrosa.

[c] $P < 0.001$ when compared with osteomalacia.

tients with osteitis fibrosa are significantly lower than in patients with osteomalacia and aplastic bone disease.

Bone histomorphometric data of the three groups of patients are displayed in Table 2. By definition, our established diagnostic criteria result in significant differences in histologic parameters between the three groups. Patients with osteitis fibrosa are characterized by an increase in osteoblastic osteoid, osteoclastic resorption, osteoclasts/mm², and endosteal fibrosis.

As already defined, low-turnover osteomalacia is characterized by the complete absence or only a minimal increase in osteoblastic osteoid, osteoclastic resorption, and osteoclasts/mm², and also by the lack of endosteal fibrosis. The typical lesion in these patients is the presence of acellular large osteoid seams. In addition, there is a marked increase in aluminum deposits at the osteoid bone interface and at the surface of trabecular bone.

Patients with aplastic bone disease have histomorphometric features similar to those of patients with osteomalacia. However, patients with aplastic bone disease have a normal ratio of osteoid to mineralized bone. In addition, a lack of cellular activity, an absence of endosteal fibrosis, and aluminum deposits at the osteoid-mineralized bone interface and along the surface of trabecular bone are also observed.

The double tetracycline labeling demonstrates that osteitis fibrosa patients have active mineralization and bone formation, while patients with low-turn-

Table 2. Bone histomorphometric analysis

	OF	OM	ABD
Osteoclastic resorption (%)	7.8 ± 0.6	0.5 ± 0.20	0.5 ± 0.30
Osteoclast (mm²)	2.9 ± 0.3	0.2 ± 0.10	0.2 ± 0.50
Endosteal fibrosis (%)	3.8 ± 0.7	0.07 ± 0.02	0.06 ± 0.03
Osteoblastic surface (%)	11.2 ± 1.4	0.6 ± 0.30	0.8 ± 0.40
Total osteoid surface (%)	51.8 ± 3.0	71.3 ± 19.1	24.1 ± 4.30
Relative osteoid volume (%)	15.2 ± 1.8	21.1 ± 2.30	3.8 ± 0.80
Bone volume (%)	22.4 ± 1.1	19.9 ± 1.20	16.1 ± 1.40

OF, osteitis fibrosa; OM, osteomalacia; and ABD, aplastic bone disease.

over osteomalacia and aplastic bone disease lacked active mineralization and bone formation.

These observations describe, prospectively, the prevalence of bone lesions in a dialysis population from the same geographic region. Osteitis fibrosa is the bone lesion most frequently observed. Low-turnover osteomalacia is present in 24% of the patients, and it is associated with a high incidence of musculoskeletal symptoms. Furthermore, many of these patients often become symptomatic during the follow-up period. Patients with low-turnover osteomalacia (as compared with osteitis fibrosa) have a higher serum calcium, lower plasma PTH, and higher serum aluminum levels. In addition, the presence of bone aluminum deposits is characteristic. Aplastic bone disease is observed in 9% of the patients, and it is manifested clinically in a manner similar to osteomalacia. The biochemical findings, as shown in Table 1, and the clinical course are also similar to osteomalacia.

Only 8% of patients with osteitis fibrosa were symptomatic at the time of the bone biopsy procedure. Few of these patients (8%) developed any symptoms or aggravation of their original symptoms afterward. Hyperphosphatemia, increased serum alkaline phosphatase levels, and high PTH levels reflect the severity of the secondary hyperparathyroidism. As assessed by histomorphometric studies, the severity of the osteoclastic and osteoblastic activity and the endosteal fibrosis varies widely. This is in agreement with previous studies of patients with osteitis fibrosa [9].

The high incidence of osteomalacia is unexpected. This entity recently has been clearly associated with aluminum toxicity [1, 2] (see Coburn et al, in this volume). In this study, a special effort was made to monitor repeatedly the aluminum content in the dialysate water. It was always below 5 μg/liter—a concentration that is within the acceptable range and (by itself) does not explain both the high serum aluminum levels and presence of bone aluminum deposits. It is possible that the aluminum source may not be the dialysate, but the oral ingestion of aluminum. Most of our patients were receiving antacid therapy. An estimate of the amount of antacids that these patients were ingesting, as compared with patients with osteitis fibrosa, does not reveal a significant difference.

Initially, only 32% of the patients with osteomalacia had symptoms. Previous reports have emphasized a low incidence of osteomalacia, with the presence of severe symptoms in all cases [1, 2]. An explanation for this discrepancy may be the fact that most of the patients in the present study undergo bone biopsy procedures at an early stage; at the time, they are asymptomatic. An additional 38% of these patients become symptomatic during the 2-year follow-up. Thus, at the conclusion of the study, 70% of the patients with low-turnover osteomalacia are symptomatic.

The biochemical findings observed in patients with osteomalacia are similar to those published by other investigators [2]. Thus, mild hypercalcemia, a minimal increase in serum alkaline phosphatase level, as well as relatively low plasma levels of PTH are observed. The mean serum aluminum concentration is significantly higher than those of patients with osteitis fibrosa. The bone histomorphometric analysis demonstrates both the characteristic findings of low-turnover osteomalacia large osteoid seams and the lack of, or only minimal, cell activity and endosteal fibrosis. Histologic aluminum deposits are present in significant amounts in all but two patients with low-turnover osteomalacia. Bone mineralization and formation, as assessed by tetracycline labeling, is either completely absent or markedly decreased. The low PTH levels also may suggest the possibility of parathyroid gland aluminum toxicity. We have reported that in patients with aluminum-related osteomalacia, the parathyroid response to hypocalcemia is blunted and the trabecular bone aluminum correlates conversely with the maximum PTH response [10]. Thus, diminished secretion of PTH may be due to a direct effect of aluminum in the parathyroid gland.

Aplastic bone disease has been infrequently reported in patients who are on maintenance hemodialysis. The present study shows an incidence of 9%. Clinically and biochemically, these patients present in a manner similar to those with low-turnover osteomalacia. In addition, the histomorphometric data also are similar; the only major difference is the absence of large osteoid seams. Aluminum deposits are observed in the majority of these patients. Aplastic bone disease may also be a consequence of aluminum toxicity; the data on this point are not conclusive.

The modality of dialytic therapy was changed in seven patients (four with osteitis fibrosa and three with osteomalacia) from maintenance hemodialysis to continuous ambulatory peritoneal dialysis (CAPD). A repeat bone biopsy procedure in all seven patients 1 year later showed (in the patients with osteitis) a worsening of the bone lesion; two out of three patients with osteomalacia changed the bone lesion to osteitis fibrosa [11]. These changes occurred in the absence of any vitamin D or calcium supplement therapy. The worsening of osteitis fibrosa is in agreement with several reports on CAPD patients [12–15]. In general, some patients on CAPD who were not treated with vitamin D metabolites developed biochemical and clinical signs and symptoms indicative of secondary hyperparathyroidism. It is characterized by hypercalcemia, elevated PTH levels, and radiologic evidence of increased subperiosteal resorption [12, 13]. In addition, repeat bone biopsy procedures have shown progression of the osteitis fibrosa [14, 15].

The improvement of osteomalacia after 1 year of CAPD also is in agreement with previous observations [14, 15]. It is possible that a decrease of the aluminum burden, due to both decreased antacid therapy and avoidance of aluminum in the dialysate water, may be responsible for this improvement. In addition, since peritoneal dialysate fluids may not contain aluminum, some removal of aluminum with CAPD may also benefit the patient.

References

1. PLATT MM, GOODE GC, HISLOP JS: Composition of the domestic water supply and the incidence of fractures and encephalopathy in patients on home dialysis. *Br Med J* 2:657–660, 1977
2. COURNOT-WITMER G, ZINGRAFF, J, PLACHOT JJ, ESCAIG F, LEFEVRE R, BOUMATI P, BOURDEAU A, GARABEDIAN M, GALLE P, BOURDON R, DRUEKE T, BALSAN S: Aluminum localization in bone from hemodialysis patients: Relationship to matrix mineralization. *Kidney Int* 20:375–385, 1981

3. PIERIDES AM, EDWARDS WG JR, CULLUM UX JR, MCCALL JT, ELLIS HA: Hemodialysis encephalopathy with osteomalacic fractures and muscle weakness. *Kidney Int* 18:115–124, 1980

4. POGGLITSCH H, KNOPP CH, WAWSCHINEK O, PETEK W: Aluminum intoxication in dialysis patients. *Int J Artif Organs* 5:293–298, 1982

5. MEMMOS DE, EASTWOOD JB, TALNER LB, GOWER PE, CURTIS JR, PHILLIPS ME, CARTER GD, ALAGHBAND-ZADEH J, ROBERTS AP, DEWARDENER HE: Double-blind trial of oral 1,25-dihydroxy-vitamin D_3 versus placebo in asymptomatic hyperparathyroidism in patients receiving maintenance hemodialysis. *Br Med J* 282:1919–1924, 1981

6. COBURN JR, DIDOMENICO NC, BRICE GF, BASSETT LW, SHUPIEN SA, WONG EG, MILLER RB, BENNETT CM, GOLD RH, MALLON JP, MILLER ON, CHANG PC: Prospective double-blind trial with calcitriol in the prophylaxis of bone disease in asymptomatic dialysis patients, in *Vitamin D: Chemical, Biochemical, and Clinical Endocrinology of Calcium Metabolism,* edited by NORMAN AW, SCHAEFER K, VON HERRATH D, GRIGOLEIT HC, Berlin, Walter deGruyter, 1982, p 833

7. LLACH F, FELSENFELD AJ, HAUSSLER MR: The pathophysiology of altered calcium metabolism in rhabdomyolysis-induced acute renal failure. *N Engl J Med* 305:117–123, 1981

8. MALONEY NA, OTT SM, ALFREY AC, MILLER NL, COBURN JW, SHERRARD DJ: Histological quantitation of aluminum in iliac bone from patients with renal failure. *J Lab Clin Med* 99:206–216, 1981

9. HRUSKA KA, TEITELBAUM SL, KOPELMAN R, RICHARDSON CA, MILLER P, DEBMAN J, MARTIN K, SLATOPOLSKY E: The predictability of the histological features of uremic bone disease by non-invasive techniques. *Metab Bone Dis Rel Res* 1:39–44, 1978

10. ANDRESS D, FELSENFELD AJ, VOIGTS A, LLACH F: Parathyroid hormone response to hypocalcemia in hemodialysis patients with osteomalacia. *Kidney Int* 24:364–370, 1983

11. PEDERSON J, FELSENFELD A, VOIGTS A, LLACH F: Effect of CAPD on renal osteodystrophy in unmodified patients moving from hemodialysis to continuous peritoneal dialysis, in *Proc III Int Symp Peritoneal Dial,* June 17–20, 1984, Washington, D.C., in press, 1984

12. KURTZ SB, MCCARTHY JT, KUMAR R: Hypercalcemia in continuous ambulatory peritoneal dialysis patients: Observations on parameters on calcium metabolism, in *Advances in Peritoneal Dialysis,* edited by GAHL GM, KESSEL M, NOLPH KD, Amsterdam, Excerpta Medica, 1981, pp 467–577

13. TIELEMANS C, AUBRY C, DRATWA M: The effect of continuous ambulatory peritoneal dialysis on renal osteodystrophy, in *Advances in Peritoneal Dialysis,* edited by GAHL GM, KESSEL M, NOLPH KD, Amsterdam, Excerpta Medica, 1981, pp 455–460

14. CALDERARO V, OREOPOULOS DG, MEEMA EH, KHANNA R, QUINTON C, CARMICHAEL D: Renal osteodystrophy in patients with continuous ambulatory peritoneal dialysis: A biochemical and radiological study, in *CAPD Update,* edited by MONCRIEF JF, POPOVICH PP, New York, Masson Publishing, Inc., 1981, pp 243–247

15. TEITELBAUM SL, FALLON MD, GEARING BK, DOUGAN CS, DELMEZ JA: The effects of continuous ambulatory peritoneal dialysis on bone histomorphometrics (*abstract*). *Kidney Int* 21:180, 1982

Role of Aluminum Accumulation in Renal Osteodystrophy

Jack W. Coburn, Henry G. Nebeker, Gavril Hercz, Dawn S. Milliner, Susan M. Ott, Dennis L. Andress, Donald J. Sherrard, and Allen C. Alfrey

In 1977, we described a subset of dialysis patients who had symptomatic osteomalacia that was refractory to treatment with 1,25-dihydroxyvitamin D_3 (1,25 $[OH]_2D_3$) despite the rapid appearance of hypercalcemia [1]. These patients lacked features of secondary hyperparathyroidism despite long-standing renal failure. Earlier, Pierides et al [2] had noted that dialysis patients with osteomalacia failed to respond to 1-α-hydroxycholecalciferol, but the osteomalacia was thought to be due to hypophosphatemia, which had not been present in our patients. Thus, we did not relate our observations to their report. From subsequent observations in Newcastle [3–5] and from our results with histochemical staining of bone biopsy samples for aluminum in our patients [6], there is little question that these patients represented the syndrome that we shall term *aluminum-related osteomalacia.* Presently, the weight of evidence is overwhelming that this disorder can be caused by the accumulation of aluminum in bone. Aluminum may act on bone to inhibit matrix synthesis, bone mineralization, or both. This report will summarize the evidence for this. We shall draw in part from our own observations, although parallel and significant observations have been made in the United Kingdom [7], Europe [8], and Australia [9].

Clinical Observations on Refractory Dialysis Osteomalacia

The clinical features of our patients included unrelenting and progressive osteomalacia with severe axial skeletal symptoms of bone pain, muscular weakness, and fractures of the ribs, vertebral bodies, pelvis, and hips. These features often led to severe disability, skeletal deformities, and even death

---

This manuscript was presented as part of a Symposium on *Renal Osteodystrophy: Recent Advances.*

[10]. Serum calcium concentrations were normal or even modestly increased, serum phosphorus concentrations were normal or increased, and the plasma levels of 25(OH)D were not depressed. Some patients developed hypercalcemia spontaneously, and others developed it during the intake of small doses of vitamin D or calcium supplements. On occasion, this led to a parathyroidectomy for suspected secondary hyperparathyroidism. The plasma alkaline phosphatase was normal in the patients reported from the United Kingdom [7], whereas it was generally elevated in our patients [10, 11]. Serum levels of $1,25(OH)_2D_3$ were low, as expected in patients with end-stage renal disease [12]. Serum immunoreactive parathyroid hormone (iPTH) levels were generally lower than those usually noted in dialysis patients [11].

Bone Biopsy Features

When we initially encountered our "sporadic" patients with vitamin-D-refractory osteomalacia, "epidemics" of refractory osteomalacia had been identified in certain areas of England. Reports had linked this "fracturing osteomalacia" to fluoride accumulation [13], phosphate depletion [14], and ultimately to the presence of aluminum in the water used for preparing dialysate [3]. In contrast to the epidemic nature of the cases in England [5] and elsewhere [15, 16], we saw individual patients from widely scattered geographic areas and from dialysis units that used adequate water purification methods [10, 11]. Moreover, most of our patients came from dialysis units with no experience with encephalopathy; a problem commonly associated with the epidemics of this bone disease [4, 15, 16]. Thus, we initially rejected the view that the aluminum content of water was playing a role. However, Dr. H. Ellis subsequently pointed out to us the similarities between our biopsy findings in cases of low-turnover osteomalacia and their findings in Newcastle. We then began to measure the aluminum content of bone by atomic absorption spectroscopy [11] and histochemical staining [17]. With both techniques, there were markedly elevated levels of aluminum in the bone of patients with osteomalacia. Also, the bone aluminum content correlated closely with the degree of osteomalacia [11], and the aluminum stain was largely localized along the mineralization front. Little or no tetracycline incorporation was noted at sites of aluminum staining, and there was a close correlation between bone aluminum content and the bone apposition rate [17].

In uremic patients with osteitis fibrosa, those with mixed components of both osteomalacia and osteitis fibrosa, and in patients with "mild" disease without features of osteitis fibrosa or osteomalacia [18], the bone aluminum content was generally above normal but lower than the values in patients with osteomalacia [11, 17]. Subsequently, a subgroup of patients with "mild" histologic features was identified, but they had fractures and symptoms similar to those seen in patients with osteomalacia [19]. Some of these patients had "patchy" widening of osteoid. Bone formation, as detected by double tetracycline labelling, was absent. A paucity of cellular elements in bone and surface staining for aluminum was noted. This subgroup has been classified as "aplastic" [19]. In several instances, serial bone biopsy samples have shown a change from the aplastic lesion to typical osteomalacia in the same patient, suggesting that the aplastic lesion can precede the development of the typical aluminum-related osteomalacia.

The epidemiologic associations described do not prove cause and effect; it might be argued that aluminum accumulation is merely an epiphenomenon in the development of osteomalacia. However, preliminary anecdotal reports of substantial improvement in symptomatic aluminum-related osteomalacia following the removal of aluminum with the chelating agent desferrioxamine and the demonstration of osteomalacia in animals following aluminum administration provide added support for the pathogenic role of aluminum.

Preliminary evidence suggests that other metals may play a role in the development of osteomalacia, either by themselves or in combination with aluminum. In a preliminary report of a few dialysis patients with osteomalacia, staining of the biopsy samples revealed the deposition of both iron and aluminum at the mineralization front [20]. Other investigators have raised the possibility that other elements, including silicon, sulfur, and iron, may accumulate at the mineralization front and possibly play a role in causing osteomalacia [21, 22].

Role of Parathyroid Hormone

In patients with aluminum-related bone disease, the serum iPTH levels are often lower than expected for patients with renal failure [11]. Moreover, when these patients are exposed to hypocalcemia during dialysis with low-calcium dialysate, the serum iPTH levels fail to show the usual rise [23, 24]. There is experimental evidence that high concentrations of aluminum can inhibit the release of PTH by isolated parathyroid cells [25]. Also, this osteomalacia has appeared following total or subtotal parathyroidectomy [10, 26, 27]. In some cases, the parathyroid surgery may have been done because of hypercalcemia in the face of pre-existing aluminum-related osteomalacia. In other cases, osteitis fibrosa existed prior to parathyroidectomy. Also, we have seen the syndrome appear after a striking reduction of serum iPTH following treatment with the vitamin D sterols $25(OH)D_3$ or $1,25(OH)_2D_3$. In osteitis fibrosa, there may be a diffuse distribution of the aluminum [8], whereas the surface deposition of aluminum may increase following parathyroidectomy [28].

Other observations of uncertain significance are the data that parathyroid hormone can increase the retention or absorption of oral aluminum [29]. It is possible that PTH could increase aluminum absorption and lead to its diffuse distribution in bone because of the higher bone turnover in osteitis fibrosa. After parathyroidectomy, there will be a reduction in iPTH levels and a slowing of bone turnover. The aluminum may then be localized at the mineralization front, with a marked reduction in matrix synthesis and/or mineralization.

Although a striking reduction in PTH activity may predispose to or precipitate the appearance of the syndrome, low PTH levels are not absolutely essential, and we have observed the syndrome in patients with substantially elevated serum iPTH levels. Also, with only modest removal of aluminum with desferrioxamine therapy, the bone histology can change from osteomalacia to osteitis fibrosa, with little or no rise in serum iPTH levels. Further observations are needed to clarify the role that parathyroid hormone plays in protection from this syndrome [30] and to determine how a reduction in PTH may lead to its appearance.

Observations in Aluminum-Loaded Animals

Several studies in experimental animals indicate that parenteral injections of aluminum can produce lesions that are similar to osteomalacia. Ellis, McCarthy, and Herrington [31] have shown that long-term IP injections of aluminum into rats caused impaired mineralization of the epiphyseal cartilage, although lesions of trabecular bone were not described. Subsequent studies demonstrated the development of osteomalacia in aluminum-loaded rats [32–34] and dogs [35]. The observations in rats indicated that a reduction of renal function increased the susceptibility to bone disease following aluminum loading [32, 33]. Moreover, Goodman et al detected impaired mineralization of cortical bone without widening of osteoid in rats with short-term aluminum loading; these findings are analogous to the "aplastic" lesion encountered in dialysis patients [34]. In studies in dogs [35], we noted a distinct increase in the forming surface of bone, a widening of osteoid lamellas, and a decrease in bone apposition rate following aluminum loading. Also, the bone aluminum content correlated with the severity of the osteomalacia. The serum iPTH levels remained normal or increased slightly, but the plasma levels of $1,25(OH)_2D_3$ fell during the repeated injections of aluminum. This decreased ability to generate $1,25(OH)_2D_3$ was associated with a marked increase in kidney content of aluminum; that is, it was greater than in other tissues.

Taken together, these observations in animals clearly indicate that the parenteral administration of aluminum can induce a bone disease that resembles the disease seen in dialysis patients, and with a bone aluminum content similar to the levels observed in uremic patients with osteomalacia. Thus, Koch's postulates seem to be fulfilled with the demonstration that aluminum can produce osteomalacia.

Total Parenteral-Nutrition-Related Bone Disease and Aluminum

Other data collected over this period indicate that low-turnover osteomalacia may arise due to the accumulation of aluminum in certain patients receiving long-term total parenteral nutrition (TPN). These patients, with severe intestinal malfunction but normal or near normal renal function, noted the appearance of bone pain and fractures 1 to 3 years after initiating long-term treatment with TPN and at a time that their nutritional status had improved [36, 37]. Biochemical features included normal to slightly increased serum calcium, normal or increased serum phosphorus, low serum iPTH levels, and low or undetectable serum levels of $1,25(OH)_2D_3$ [36–38]. These patients had substantial hypercalciuria, and their bone biopsy samples revealed reduced numbers of both osteoblasts and osteoclasts with little or no uptake of tetracycline. The bone apposition rate was substantially reduced, and some areas of trabecular bone showed localized widening of osteoid; that is, "patchy osteomalacia." [36]. It was then found that these patients had regularly received substantial quantities of aluminum intravenously in the casein present in the TPN solution [39].

Moreover, balance studies indicated that the patients who had received this aluminum in their TPN solution for several years continued to demonstrate a persistently positive balance for aluminum. Presumably, this led to the slow accumulation of aluminum in bone even in the presence of normal renal function [39]. Also, observations in a patient followed for 5 years after she changed from casein to a solution with free amino acids containing far less aluminum, suggest that several years may be required before the bone aluminum content falls and bone formation rate normalizes [40]. These observations indicate that parenteral aluminum loading can cause osteomalacia in humans with normal renal function. Moreover, such quantities clearly exceed the normal renal excretory capacity. We have also found aluminum concentrations of 400 to 1400 μg/liter in various albumin-replacement solutions, suggesting that there may be other sources of inadvertent aluminum loading.

Sources of Aluminum in Patients with Renal Failure

The initial outbreaks of osteomalacia that were subsequently linked to aluminum occurred in geographic areas with water aluminum in concentrations above 100 μg/liter (3.7 μmoles/liter) [4]. More recently, a high incidence of aluminum-related disease was noted with dialysate aluminum levels near 50 μg/liter [41]. Since the aluminum is 80 to 90% protein-bound in plasma, significant quantities of aluminum can move into the blood from dialysate when the dialysate concentration exceeds the diffusible level in the blood. In our study of patients undergoing hemodialysis with dialysate containing aluminum in concentrations of 30 to 75 μg/liter, the plasma aluminum rose from 165 to 270 $\pm$ 21 μg/liter during a single dialysis, and the rate of aluminum influx during dialysis was 4.8 $\pm$ 0.8 μg/min.

The cartridges that were used for regeneration of dialysate solutions have also been found to be a source of aluminum in isolated instances [42]. Also, there have been instances when the peritoneal dialysate solution has been the source of aluminum [43], although all the samples of the dialysate for continuous ambulatory peritoneal dialysis (CAPD) that we have tested have had aluminum concentrations below 5 to 7 µg/liter [44].

Of even greater concern is the strong probability that there may be slow accumulation of aluminum via its oral absorption. The possible danger of orally absorbed aluminum was initially raised by Berlyne et al [45], although this warning has largely been overlooked. In certain regions of the United States, the water treatment is adequate, but the dietary phosphate intake is higher than in other parts of the world, necessitating the ingestion of large doses of aluminum hydroxide. The sporadic occurrence of aluminum-related bone disease could exist because aluminum is accumulated via oral absorption rather than from dialysate. Several lines of evidence suggest that the continued absorption of aluminum may indeed be important. Studies in normal subjects indicate that small amounts of aluminum are absorbed; thus, urinary aluminum increases from 20 to 30 µg/d to 200 to 400 µg/d after normal individuals ingest aluminum hydroxide in amounts commonly given to dialysis patients [46]. Since the kidney is the principal route for the excretion of aluminum that enters the body, it is apparent that there can be slow accumulation of absorbed aluminum in patients with renal failure. The demonstration of aluminum-related bone disease in patients who have never been treated with dialysis [47–49] provides strong evidence that aluminum is accumulated through routes other than parenteral. Finally, there is a close correlation between plasma aluminum levels, which probably reflect the recent aluminum load, and the quantities of aluminum-containing gels ingested by children under treatment with CAPD [50]; when aluminum-containing compounds are discontinued by dialysis patients, there is a substantial reduction in the plasma aluminum level [51]; an example of this is shown in Figure 1.

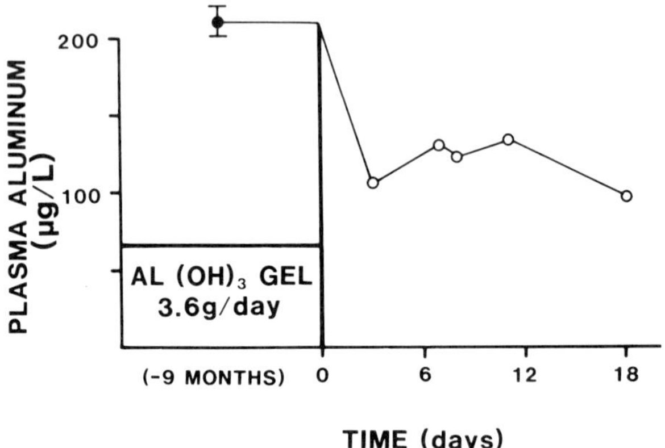

Fig. 1. Serial plasma aluminum concentrations in a CAPD patient whose aluminum hydroxide gel (*Al[OH]₃ gel*) was replaced by calcium carbonate. The plasma concentration prior to replacement represents the mean (± SEM) of 9 determinations for the 5 months he received the aluminum hydroxide gel.

Removal of Aluminum with Desferrioxamine

In dialysis patients, hemodialysis with aluminum-free water leads to the removal of small but insignificant quantities of aluminum, because 80 to 90% of aluminum in plasma is protein-bound. Moreover, long-term dialysis of our aluminum-loaded patients with aluminum-free dialysate has led to little or no improvement [10, 11]. Based on the use of the chelating agent desferrioxamine for iron removal, Ackrill et al [52] gave repeated infusions of desferrioxamine to a patient with aluminum accumulation manifested by osteomalacia and dialysis encephalopathy. The patient showed neurologic improvement and noted remission of his musculoskeletal symptoms.

There are two mechanisms by which desferrioxamine enhances aluminum removal in dialysis patients: First, it can mobilize aluminum from tissue stores; and second, it can increase the aluminum removal during dialysis by raising the fraction of nonprotein-bound aluminum in plasma. Following the infusion of desferrioxamine, 40 mg/kg of body wt, we have noted an increase in plasma aluminum levels, which was more marked in patients with increased aluminum stores on bone biopsy. Indeed, this increment in plasma aluminum following the infusion of desferrioxamine may provide a diagnostic "test" to indicate the magnitude of aluminum accumulation [53]; an example of the change in plasma aluminum following desferrioxamine is shown in Figure 2. In patients with aluminum-related bone disease, hemodialysis following the administration of desferrioxamine leads to a substantial increase in the removal of aluminum. Thus, the aluminum removal during a 4-hr dialysis treatment increased from 50 to 300 μg before desferrioxamine to 4 to 8 mg after its administration [54].

In patients undergoing treatment with CAPD, the aluminum levels in effluent peritoneal dialysate correlated closely with, and were 20 to 25% of, the plasma aluminum levels. The aluminum removal of 100 to 400 μg/d in dialysate of CAPD patients without aluminum-related bone disease is substantially greater than the normal urinary excretion of 20 to 30 μg/d; this observation provides further evidence for the continued oral absorption of aluminum. In a CAPD patient with aluminum-related osteomalacia, treatment with desferrioxamine increased the aluminum removal to 3 mg/d (Fig. 3), and the patient's symptoms substantially improved with repeated treatment [44]. These data clearly indicate that desferrioxamine administration can substantially enhance aluminum removal during various dialysis procedures.

Treatment of Aluminum-Related Osteomalacia

The management of patients with aluminum-related osteomalacia has been difficult [10, 11]. In our initial patients, who were treated in a preliminary trial with 24,25-dihydroxyvitamin D_3 in combination with calcitriol, there was symptomatic improvement and increased bone mineralization [54]. How-

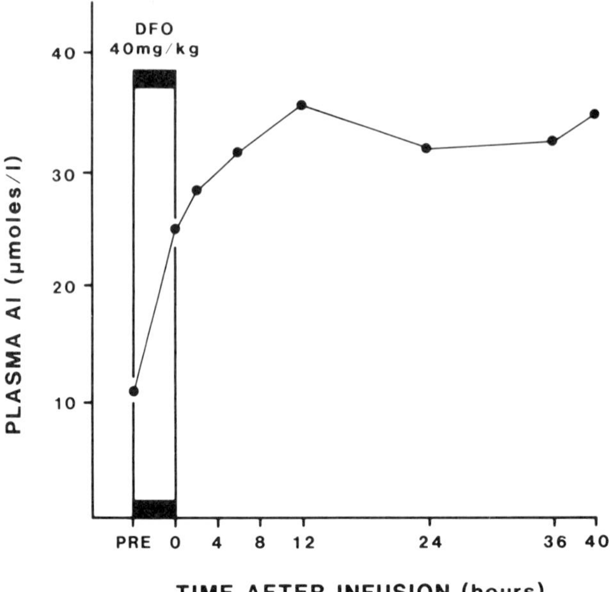

TIME AFTER INFUSION (hours)

Fig. 2. Change in plasma aluminum (*plasma Al*) following the infusion of desferrioxamine (*DFO*), 40 mg/kg, in a hemodialysis patient with aluminum-related bone disease. The "DFO infusion test" was done within 1 to 2 hr after hemodialysis. (Note: 1 μmole/liter = 27 μmg/liter.)

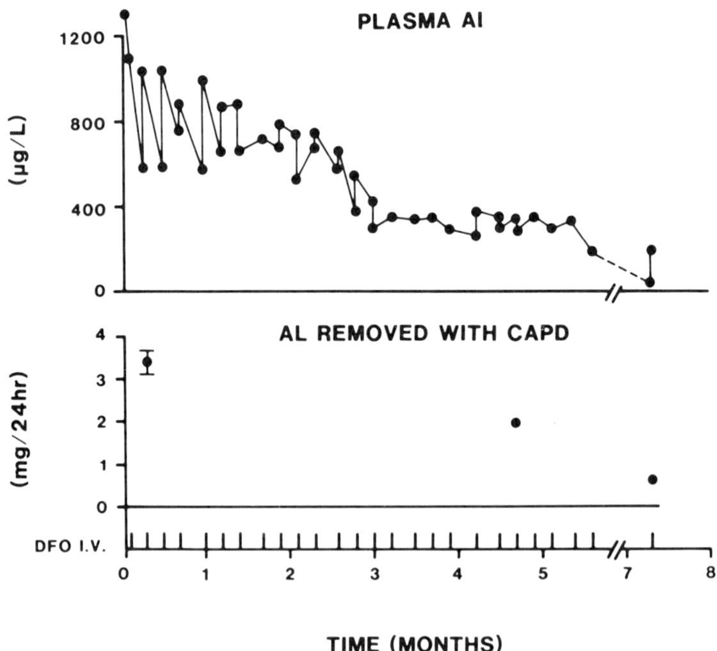

TIME (MONTHS)

Fig. 3. Serial plasma aluminum concentrations in a CAPD patient with aluminum-related osteomalacia who had received weekly infusions of desferrioxamine (*DFO i.v.*) at the times shown. Also, the quantities of aluminum removed in the dialysate are shown (the brackets indicate a mean $\pm$ SEM of daily measurements made during the week after initial treatment with DFO).

ever, as we continued to administer these sterols to additional patients, we noted little or no improvement in many patients [55]. Therefore, we have largely abandoned this therapy in these patients. The mechanism for the improvement observed in some patients remains unclear.

Following the initial report of the use of desferrioxamine for aluminum removal [52], favorable results have been noted in other reports [57, 58]. In our preliminary experience, in which we treated 16 osteomalacic patients with desferrioxamine for 2 months or longer, 15 of them noted clinical improvement, particularly those treated longer than 6 months. Thus, several patients who had been confined to bed or wheelchair were able to walk unassisted, and most patients substantially decreased their use of analgesics. Biochemical changes include a decrease in serum calcium and a transient rise in alkaline phosphatase; observations suggesting increased bone mineralization [59]. Follow-up bone biopsy studies have not yet been completely evaluated. These preliminary results suggest that chelation with desferrioxamine may provide an effective means of managing patients with aluminum-related bone disease, but further studies are clearly indicated.

Prevention of Aluminum-Related Disease

As noted above, many early outbreaks of aluminum-related diseases were associated with the presence of aluminum in water used for the preparation of dialysate. It seems imperative that water supplies be monitored frequently, and that appropriate water treatment methods be used when indicated. It has been the recommendation of the Association for the Advancement of Medical Instrumentation that dialysate aluminum concentrations should be less than 10 μg/liter [60]. Water-softening removes relatively little aluminum; deionizing, however, can be quite effective. Reverse osmosis has been the most effective method, although the water aluminum concentrations should be less than 100 to 200 μg/liter in the water before the reverse osmosis treatment.

The incidence of aluminum-related osteomalacia has decreased in frequency following initiation of water purification; however, certain dialysis patients do develop osteomalacia without exposure to high aluminum levels in dialysate [10, 11]. The source of aluminum in these patients is almost certainly the oral aluminum hydroxide gels, which are used for phosphate binding. A marked reduction of dietary phosphate intake is indicated to reduce the dosage of these gels. In addition, attention should be directed to the development of alternative methods to reduce intestinal phosphate absorption. Calcium carbonate has been shown to be effective in reducing phosphate absorption, although very large doses are required [61]. Also, there are preliminary reports of polymer resins that can bind phosphate effectively [62]. Further trials with these compounds are needed. With adequate treatment of the water used for dialysate and the development of a suitable alternative to the use of aluminum gels as phosphate binders, aluminum-related diseases should largely disappear.

Acknowledgments. This work was supported, in part, by USPHS Grants AM29926 and AM28368, and Research Funds from the Veterans Administration.

References

1. COBURN JW, BRIKMAN AS, SHERRARD DJ, SINGER FR, WONG EGC, BAYLINK DJ, NORMAN AW: Use of 1,25(OH)$_2$-vitamin D$_3$ to separate "types" of renal osteodystrophy, in *Dialysis, Transplantation, Nephrology,* edited by ROBINSON BHB, HAWKINS JB, VEREERSTRACFEN P, Kent, England, Pitman Medical Publishing Co., 1977, vol 14, pp 442–450

2. PIERIDES AM, ELLIS HA, SIMPSON W, DEWAR JH, WARD MK, KERR DNS: Variable response to long-term 1-α cholecalciferol in hemodialysis osteodystrophy. *Lancet* 1:1092–1095, 1976

3. WARD MK, FEEST TG, ELLIS HA, PARKINSON IS, KERR DNS: Osteomalacic dialysis osteodystrophy: Evidence for a water-borne aetiological agent, probably aluminum. *Lancet* 1:841–845, 1978

4. PARKINSON IS, FEEST TG, WARD MK, FAWCETT RWP, KERR DNS: Fracturing dialysis osteodystrophy and dialysis encephalopathy: An epidemiological survey. *Lancet* 1:406–409, 1979

5. ELLIS HA: Aluminum induced osteomalacia in patients with chronic renal failure and in animals. *Nieren Hochendruckkrankheit* 12:198–206, 1983

6. OTT SM, MALONEY NA, COBURN JW, ALFREY AC, SHERRARD DJ: The prevalence of bone aluminum deposition in renal osteodystrophy and its relation to the response to calcitriol therapy. *N Engl J Med* 307:709–713, 1982

7. ALVAREZ-UDE F, FEEST TG, WARD MK, PIERIDES AM, ELLIS HA, PEART KM, SIMPSON W, WEIGHTMAN D, KERR DNS: Hemodialysis bone disease: Correlation between clinical, histologic and other findings. *Kidney Int* 14:68–73, 1978

8. COURNOT-WITMER G, ZINGRAFF J, PIACHOT JJ, ESCAIG F, LEFEVRE R, BOUMATI P, BOURDEAU A, GARABEDIAN M, GALLE P, BOURDON R, DRUECKE T, BALSON S: Aluminum localization in bone from hemodialyzed patients: Relationship to matrix mineralization. *Kidney Int* 20:376–385, 1981

9. BUCHANAN MRC, IHLE BU, DUNN CM: Hemodialysis related osteomalacia: A staining method to demonstrate aluminum. *J Clin Pathol* 34:1352, 1981

10. HODSMAN AB, SHERRARD DJ, WONG EGC, BRICKMAN AS, LEE DBN, ALFREY AC, SINGER FR, NORMAN AW, COBURN JW: Vitamin D-resistant osteomalacia in hemodialysis patients lacking secondary hyperparathyroidism. *Ann Intern Med* 94:629–637, 1981

11. HODSMAN AB, SHERRARD DJ, ALFREY AG, BRICKMAN AS, MILLER A, MALONEY NA, COBURN JW: Bone aluminum and histomorphometric features of renal osteodystrophy. *J Clin Endocrinol Metab* 54:539–546, 1982

12. HAUSSLER MR, MCCAIN TA: Basic and clinical concepts related to vitamin D metabolism and action. *N Engl J Med* 297:974–983, 1041–1050, 1977

13. SIDDIQUI JY, SIMPSON W, ELLIS HA, KERR DN: Fluoride and bone disease in patients on regular haemodialysis. *Proc EDTA* 8:149–160, 1971

14. PIERIDES AM, WARD MK, KERR DNS: Haemodialysis encephalopathy: Possible role of phosphate depletion. *Lancet* 1:1234–1235, 1976

15. FLENDRIG JA, KRUIS H, DAS HA: Aluminium intoxication: The cause of dialysis dementia? *Proc EDTA* 13:355, 1976

16. PIERIDES AM, EDWARDS WG, CULLU UX, MCCALL JT, ELLIS HA: Hemodialysis encephalopathy with osteomalacia fractures and muscle weakness. *Kidney Int* 18:115–124, 1980

17. MALONEY NA, OTT S, ALFREY AC, COBURN JW, SHERRARD DJ: Histologic quantitation of aluminum in iliac bone from patients with renal failure. *J Lab Clin Med* 99:206–216, 1982

18. SHERRARD DJ, COBURN JW, BRICKMAN AS, SINGER FR, MALONEY N: Skeletal response to treatment with 1,25-dihydroxy-vitamin D in renal failure. *Contrib Nephrol* 18:92–97, 1980

19. SHERRARD DJ, OTT SM, MALONEY NA, ANDRESS D, COBURN JW: Uremic osteodystrophy: Classification, cause and treatment, in *Proceedings of The Symposium on Clinical Disorders of Bone and Mineral Metabolism*, edited by FRAME B, POTTS JT, Amsterdam, Excerpta Medica, 1984, pp 254–259

20. PIERCE-MYLI M, PIERIDES A: Iron and aluminum osteomalacia during hemodialysis. *Kidney Int* 25:151, 1984

21. BROWN DJ, HAM F, DAWBORN JK, XIPPEL JM: D-resistant osteomalacia in dialysis patients: Bone collagen and mineral content and treatment with desferrioxamine and calcitriol, in *Vitamin D: Chemical, Biochemical and Clinical Endocrinology of Calcium Metabolism*, edited by NORMAN AW, SCHAEFER K, HERRATH DV, GRIGOLEIT HG, Walter de Gruyter, 1982, pp 873–875

22. BROWN DJ, HAM KN, DAWBORN JK, XIPPEL JM: Treatment of dialysis osteomalacia with desferrioxamine. *Lancet* 2:343–345, 1982

23. KRAUT JA, SHINABERGER JH, SINGER FR, SHERRARD DJ, SAXTON J, MILLER JH, KUROKAWA K, COBURN JW: Parathyroid gland responsiveness to acute hypocalcemia in dialysis osteomalacia. *Kidney Int* 23:725–730, 1983

24. ANDRESS D, FELSENFELD AJ, VOIGTS A, LLACH F: Parathyroid hormone response to hypocalcemia in hemodialysis patients with osteomalacia. *Kidney Int* 24:364–370, 1983

25. MORRISSEY J, ROTHSTEIN M, MAYOR G, SLATOPOLSKY E: Suppression of parathyroid hormone secretion by aluminum. *Kidney Int* 23:699–704, 1983

26. TEITELBAUM SL, BERGFELD MA, FREITAG J, HRUSKA KA, SLATOPOLSKY E: Do parathyroid hormone and 1,25-dihydroxyvitamin D modulate bone formation in uremia? *J Clin Endocrinol Metab* 51:247–251, 1980

27. FELSENFELD AJ, HARRELSON JM, GUTMAN RA, WELLS SA JR, DREZNER MK: Osteomalacia after parathyroidectomy in patients with uremia. *Ann Intern Med* 96:34–39, 1984

28. ANDRESS DL, OTT SM, MALONEY NA, SHERRARD DJ: A longitudinal study of bone aluminum accumulation in long-term hemodialysis patients: Effect of parathyroidectomy (*abstract*). *Calcif Tissue Int* (in press, 1984)

29. MAYOR GH, SPRAGUE SM, HOURANI MR, SANCHEZ TV: Parathyroid hormone-mediated aluminum deposition and egress in the rat. *Kidney Int* 17:40, 1980

30. ELLIS HA: Aluminum and osteomalacia after parathyroidectomy. *Ann Intern Med* 96:533–534, 1982

31. ELLIS HA, MCCARTHY JH, HERRINGTON J: Bone aluminum in hemodialysed patients and in rats injected with aluminum chloride: Relationship to impaired bone mineralization. *J Clin Pathol* 32:832–844, 1979

32. CHAN Y, ALFREY AC, POSEN S, LISSNER D, HILLS E, DUNSTAN CR, EVANS RA: The effect of aluminum on normal and uremic rats: Tissue distribution, vitamin D metabolites and quantitative bone histology. *Calcif Tissue Int* 35:344–351, 1983

33. ROBERTSON JA, FELSENFELD AJ, HAYGOOD CC, WILSON P, CLARKE C, LLACH F: Animal model of aluminum-induced osteomalacia: Role of chronic renal failure. *Kidney Int* 23:327–335, 1983

34. GOODMAN WG, GILLIGAN J, HORST R: Short-term aluminum administration in the rat. *J Clin Invest* 73:171–181, 1984

35. GOODMAN WG, HENRY DA, HORST R, NUDELMAN RK, ALFREY AC, COBURN JW: Parenteral aluminum administration in the dog: II. Induction of osteomalacia and effect on vitamin D metabolism. *Kidney Int* (in press, 1984)
36. KLEIN GL, AMENT ME, BLUESTONE R, NORMAN AW, TARGOFF CM, SHERRARD DJ, YOUNG JH, COBURN JW: Bone disease associated with total parenteral nutrition. *Lancet* 2:1041–1044, 1980
37. SHIKE M, HARRISON JG, STURTRIDGE WT, TAM CS, BOBECNKO PE, JONES G, MURRAY TM, JEEJEEBHOY KN: Metabolic bone disease in patients receiving long-term parenteral nutrition. *Ann Intern Med* 92:343–350, 1980
38. KLEIN GL, HORST G, NORMAN AW, AMENT ME, COBURN JW: Reduced serum levels of 1,25-dihydroxyvitamin D with long-term parenteral nutrition. *Ann Intern Med* 94:638–642, 1981
39. KLEIN GL, OTT SM, ALFREY AC, SHERRARD DJ, HAZLET, MILLER NL, MALONEY NA, BERQUIST WE, AMENT ME, COBURN JW: Aluminum as a factor in the bone disease of long-term parenteral nutrition. *Trans Assoc Am Phys* 95:155–164, 1982
40. OTT SM, MALONEY NA, KLEIN GL, ALFREY AC, AMENT ME, COBURN JW, SHERRARD DJ: Aluminum is associated with low bone formation in patients on chronic parenteral nutrition. *Ann Intern Med* 98:910–914, 1983
41. RICANATI ES, OTT SM, KLEIN KL, ALFREY AC, SHERRARD DJ, COBURN JW: Evaluation of bone in dialysis patients exposed to aluminum in dialysate (*abstract*). *Kidney Int* 21:176, 1982
42. MION C, BRANGER B, ISSAUTIER R, ELLIS HA, RODIER M, SHALDON S: Dialysis fracturing osteomalacia without hyperparathyroidism in patients treated with HCO₃ rinsed redy cartridge. *Trans ASAIO* 27:634–638, 1981
43. CUMMING AD, SIMPSON G, BELL D, COWIE J, WINNEY RJ: Acute aluminum intoxication in patients on continuous ambulatory peritoneal dialysis. *Lancet* 1:103–104, 1982
44. HERCZ G, MILLINER DS, SHINABERGER JH, NISSENSON AR, CUTLER RE, GOODMAN WG, GENTILE DE, KRAUS AP, COBURN JW: Aluminum metabolism and removal during CAPD. *Kidney Int* 25:257, 1984
45. BERLYNE GM, BEN-ARI J, PEST D, WEINBERGER J, STERN M, GILMORE GR, LEVINE R: Hyperaluminaemia from aluminum resins in renal failure. *Lancet* 2:494–496, 1970
46. KAEHNY WD, HEGG AP, ALFREY AC: Gastrointestinal absorption of aluminum from aluminum-containing antacids. *N Engl J Med* 296:1389–1390, 1977
47. FELSENFELD AJ, GUTMAN RA, LLACH F, HARRELSON JM: Osteomalacia in chronic renal failure: A syndrome previously reported only with maintenance dialysis. *Am J Nephrol* 2:147–154, 1982
48. GRISWOLD WR, REINIK V, MIENDORA SA, TRAUNER D, ALFREY AC: Accumulation of aluminum in a non-dialysed uremic child receiving aluminum hydroxide. *Pediatrics* 71:56–58, 1983
49. KAYE M: Oral aluminum toxicity in a non-dialyzed patient with renal failure. *Clin Nephrol* 20:208–211, 1983
50. SALUSKY IB, COBURN JW, PAUNIER L, SHERRARD DJ, FINE RN: Role of aluminum hydroxide in raising serum aluminum levels in children undergoing CAPD. *J Pediatrics* (in press, 1984)
51. LAM M, RICANATI ES, ALFREY AC, COBURN JW: Influence of aluminum-containing antacids on plasma aluminum. *Kidney Int* 23:129, 1983
52. ACKRILL P, RALSTON AJ, DAY JP, HODGE KC: Successful removal of aluminum from patient with dialysis encephalopathy. *Lancet* 2:692–693, 1980
53. MILLINER DS, NEBEKER HG, OTT SM, SHERRARD DJ, ANDRESS DL, ALFREY

AC, Coburn JW: Desferrioxamine infusion test for diagnosis of aluminum osteomalacia. *Kidney Int* 25:149, 1984

54. Hodsman AB, Wong EGC, Sherrard DJ, Brickman AS, Lee DBN, Singer FR, Norman AW, Coburn JW: Preliminary trials with 24,25-dihydroxy-vitamin D₃ in dialysis osteomalacia. *Am J Med* 74:407–414, 1983

55. Ott SM, Recker RR, Coburn JW, Sherrard DJ: Vitamin D therapy in aluminum-related osteomalacia. *Kidney Int* 23:107, 1983

56. Milliner DS, Shinaberger JH, Miller JH, Nissenson A, Coburn JW: Removal of aluminum during hemodialysis: Effect of desferrioxamine. *Kidney Int* (Suppl), in press

57. Ihle BU, Buchanan MRC, Stevens B, Becker GJ, Kincaid-Smith P: The efficacy of various treatment modalities on aluminum associated bone disease. *Proc EDTA* 19:195–201, 1982

58. Ackrill P, Day JP, Garstang FM, Hodge KC, Metcalfe PJ, Benzo Z, Hill K, Ralston AJ, Denton J: Treatment of fracturing renal osteodystrophy by desferrioxamine. *Proc EDTA* 19:203–207, 1982

59. Nebeker HG, Milliner DS, Ott SM, Sherrard DJ, Alfrey AC, Abuelo JG, Wasserstein A, Coburn JW: Aluminum-related osteomalacia: Clinical response to desferrioxamine. *Kidney Int* 25:173, 1984

60. *Standards for Hemodialysis Systems.* Association for the Advancement of Medical Instrumentation, November 1980, p. 11

61. Moriniere Ph, Roussel A, Tahiri Y, et al: Substitution of aluminum hydroxide by high doses of calcium carbonate in patients on chronic haemodialysis: Disappearance of hyperaluminaemia and equal control of hyperparathyroidism. *Proc EDTA* 19:784, 1982

62. Schneider H, Kulbe KD, Weber H, Streicher E: High-effective aluminum free intestinal phosphate binder: in vitro and in vivo studies. *Proc EDTA* 20:725, 1984

Treatment of Renal Osteodystrophy in Chronic Renal Failure

Joseph M. Letteri

Pathogenesis of Renal Osteodystrophy

Renal osteodystrophy is a term generally used to describe a condition that attends the altered mineral metabolism associated with renal disease and is manifested by bone disorder with varying histologic lesions, which are characterized by osteoclastic resorption, fibrosis, and osteomalacia. The pathogenesis of the disorder has been attributed to hyperplasia of the parathyroid glands, alterations in vitamin D metabolism, and the accumulation of toxins or other substances that interfere with bone metabolism and mineralization.

Hyperplasia of the parathyroid glands is almost a constant finding. Mendes et al [1] examined the parathyroid glands in dialysis patients and noted diffuse hyperplasia in 38 glands, diffuse hyperplasia with nodule formation in 62 glands, and pure nodular formation in 30 glands. The average gland weights were 492 ± 93 mg, 730 ± 97 mg, and 1301 ± 203 mg in the three groups of glands. Thus, a tendency towards nodular hyperplasia was associated with increasing gland size. Neff et al [2] noted in that 24 of 37 patients dialyzed over 10 years, parathyroidectomy was required after a median duration of 6.2 years of dialysis. The observation of long-term parathyroid hyperplasia despite normocalcemia raises the important question of why parathyroid hormone (PTH) secretion is not normalized and shut off by normal-ionized calcium in uremia. This may be related to a "noncalcium" suppressible PTH secretory system that is related to exocytosis of secretory granules escaping lyosomal degradation. A "set point error" in hyperplastic glands also may be present, such that higher calcium concentrations are necessary to cause a given inhibition of PTH secretion [3]. Parathyroid gland stimulation in early renal failure, for the most part, is due to hypocalcemia that develops in the course of renal insufficiency and is probably related to phosphate retention and skeletal resistance to the calcemic action of PTH.

Alterations in vitamin D metabolism are present in patients with early

This manuscript was presented as part of a Symposium on *Renal Osteodystrophy: Recent Advances.*

renal failure. These patients display skeletal resistance to the calcemic action of PTH, impaired intestinal calcium absorption, and (in some cases) defective mineralization of osteoid. Thus, a state of relative or absolute vitamin D deficiency exists in these patients. Despite these abnormalities in early renal failure (that is, glomerular filtration rate [GFR] 50 to 75 ml/min), blood levels of $1,25(OH)_2D_3$ usually are normal. Only about 8 to 10% of patients entering a dialysis program with end-stage renal disease (ESRD) have reduced blood levels of $25\text{-}OH\text{-}D_3$.

Liu and Chu [4] suggested that chronic renal failure was associated with a state of vitamin D resistance. The normal levels of $1,25(OH)_2D_3$ in early renal failure that is associated with vitamin D target organ dysfunction support the concept; and, they suggest that azotemia interferes with the action of $1,24(OH)_2D_3$. Alternately, the requirements for $1,25(OH)_2D_3$ may be increased in early renal failure because of the associated secondary hyperparathyroidism both leading to a state of relative vitamin D deficiency and contributing to derangements in mineral metabolism.

Not uncommonly, dialysis patients develop metastatic calcification that is attributable to increased calcium-phosphorus product. However, it should be noted that not all patients with increased calcium-phosphorus product have metastatic calcification, indicating that other factors may be necessary for its development.

Because of the multifaceted origin of the disorder, the goals of a therapeutic program to alleviate or prevent renal osteodystrophy include: (1) preventing or alleviating secondary hyperparathyroidism, and (2) maintaining near-normal blood levels of calcium and phosphorus to heal the defects in the bone and to prevent and reverse soft tissue calcification, as well as the proximal myopathy, pruritus, and bone pain that often attend the uremic state. There is no unified approach to the problem. Overall management includes control of phosphate retention and hyperphosphatemia, dietary calcium supplementation, treatment with vitamin D or one or more of its metabolites, parathyroidectomy, and appropriate dialysate calcium and magnesium concentration in dialysis patients (Table 1).

Table 1. Treatment of renal osteodystrophy

1. Maintain normal serum phosphorus
   Restrict dietary phosphates to less than 1 g/d
   Phosphate-binding antacids
2. Maintain adequate calcium intake
   Calcium carbonate, 1 g/d
   Dialysate calcium concentration, 3.0 to 3.5 mg/dl
3. Vitamin D and related metabolites
   Control of secondary hyperparathyroidism
   Treatment of hypocalcemia
   Prevention of renal-related bone disease
   Improve growth in uremic children
	4. Miscellaneous
	   Water purification to remove aluminum fluoride and to control magnesium and calcium concentration in dialysate
	   Normalize blood pH
	   Normalize serum magnesium
	   Avoid anticonvulsants
	   Chelate aluminum
	5. Parathyroidectomy
	   Overt secondary hyperparathyroid
	   Calciphylaxis

Treatment of Renal Osteodystrophy

Control of Phosphate Retention and Hyperphosphatemia

This may be achieved by dietary restriction, the use of phosphate-binding agents, increased frequency of hemodialysis and/or use of more efficient dialyzers, and inhibition of parathyroid-mediated bone resorption. In early renal failure (GFR 30 to 70 ml/min), reduction of dietary phosphate to 600 to 900 g/d by elimination of dairy products and use of restricted protein diet to 40 g/d (with calcium supplementation) are reported to prevent many of the altered mineral defects in uremia [5]. In advanced renal failure (GFR 2 to 10 ml/min), dietary phosphate retention alone is not adequate to control hyperphosphatemia. Since blood phosphates remain elevated even on severely protein-restricted diets (20 to 40 g/d), other measures are required to maintain serum phosphorus within the normal range. Aluminum containing phosphate-binding antacids are the mainstay of therapy in advanced renal failure. They render the ingested phosphate and the phosphate in saliva, bile, and intestinal juices unabsorbable. A number of compounds are available, and the ones most frequently used are *Alucaps®*, *Amphogel®*, and *Basagel®* concentrate. Care must be taken to avoid both phosphate depletion and hypophosphatemia, which can aggravate bone disease, cause osteomalacia, and contribute to myopathy. In addition, aluminum in the compounds is absorbed by the intestine, and it may accumulate in the tissues, including bone and brain. Aluminum in bone may interfere with the mineralization process and result in low-turnover osteomalacia [6], which is refractory to most therapy [7]. In addition, aluminum may accumulate in the brain and occasionally contribute to dialysis encephalopathy [8]. Despite these potential hazards, the compounds are still recommended. Calcium carbonate has been recommended as a substitute for aluminum-containing phosphate-binding antacids, if taken with meals, to control phosphate absorption and to avoid aluminum accumulation in dialysis patients [9].

The effective control of serum phosphorus with dietary phosphate restriction and phosphate-binding antacids often is associated with an increase in serum calcium, which often is accompanied by a decrease in the blood levels of PTH.

Calcium Supplementation

Malabsorption of calcium and phosphorus in association with low dietary calcium intake may result in negative calcium balance. Clarkson et al [10] and Coburn et al [11] demonstrated that normal amounts of calcium could be absorbed by the intestine of patients with renal failure, when placed on high-calcium intake. Long-term treatment is associated with an increase in blood calcium, a reduction in blood levels of alkaline phosphatase and PTH, and a reduction in osteoclastic-mediated bone resorption. However, mineralization of osteoid is not normalized [12]. The calcium malabsorption appears to occur at a GFR of less than 40 ml/min, and supplementation of the diet with 1.0 to 2.0 g/d of elemental calcium appears to be prudent. Hypercalcemia can be associated with calcium salts administration. It is dangerous to administer large quantities of calcium salts to patients with marked hyperphosphatemia because of the potential hazard of inducing soft tissue calcification. Serum phosphorus should be reduced below 5.5 mg/dl prior to treatment with calcium salts.

Vitamin D_2 and D_3

Dent et al [13] reviewed the treatment of renal osteodystrophy and studied the effects of vitamin D_2, dihydrotachysterol (DHT), and AT-10 (AT10) in 13 patients with renal insufficiency and symptomatic bone disease. Symptomatic improvement, return to normal of the radiologic signs of bone disease, and a lowering to normal of the plasma alkaline phosphatase was noted. Using classic calcium balance techniques, they confirmed that the untreated uremic state closely resembles nutritional vitamin D deficiency. Most patients are in slightly negative calcium balance, with fecal calcium excretion almost equal to the dietary calcium intake and a negligible amount in the urine. Despite this similarity to nutritional rickets, larger quantities of vitamin D_2 or DHT are required in uremia to correct the defect. Lui and Chu [4] noted that more than 10,000 IU/d (0.25 mg) of vitamin D_2 were required to change calcium balance in uremia. Doses as high as 50,000 to 200,000 IU/d (1.25 to 5.0 mg) may be needed to achieve beneficial effects. Long-term therapy with large doses of vitamin D can cause a rise in the serum calcium; and, it may be followed by a decrease in serum levels of alkaline phosphatase and PTH, reduced bone resorption, and amelioration or healing of the bone lesions. Because of the prolonged action of vitamin D and the need for large doses of vitamin D, hypercalcemia is a real and frequent hazard. Hypercalcemia may persist for weeks after discontinuation of therapy; in a hyperphosphatemic patient, it may be associated with a marked rise in the calcium-phosphorus product predisposing to soft tissue calcification. Therapy with vitamin D should not be started prior to normalization of the serum level of phosphorus. After the bones have healed and the alkaline phosphatase has returned to normal, the dose of vitamin D should be reduced to maintenance doses, which may be as low as 0.25 mg/d. When intoxication occurs, vitamin D should be stopped altogether until blood calcium has reverted to normal, and then it can be restarted at a much lower dose.

25 Hydroxyvitamin D_3

This metabolite is an effective therapeutic agent in renal osteodystrophy [15–17]. Although most patients with chronic renal disease do not have low circulating serum levels of $25(OH)_2D_3$, there appears to be a correlation between low blood levels and bone disease in some dialysis patients [16, 17]. Recker et al [15] studied 63 long-term hemodialysis patients treated with $25(OH)_2D_3$. An oral loading dose of 600 μg was given three times during the first week of treatment. Afterwards, a maintenance dose of 200 μg was given three times weekly. Symptoms of bone disease improved in these patients. The serum alkaline phosphatase decreased; this was the best biochemical evidence of improvement. Hypercalcemia occurred, but it was mild and easily reversible in 3 to 7 days by withholding the medication. A decrease in the degree of osteoclastic bone disease and fibrosis, and improvement in bone mineralization has been noted [17–21].

1,25 Dihydroxyvitamin D (Calcitriol)

A relative deficiency of this active metabolite is present in patients with mild and moderate renal failure; and, absolute deficiency exists in these patients with advanced renal failure. Furthermore, the kidney is required to convert the parent vitamin D to the active metabolite. Although therapy with $1,25(OH)_2D_3$ has been beneficial [22–53], it is important to emphasize that most of the beneficial effects could be produced by other vitamin D compounds. The smaller doses of $1,25(OH)_2D_3$ that are needed to achieve beneficial effects and its shorter half-life make it a safer agent than other vitamin D compounds. The high potency of $1,25(OH)_2D_3$ may cause the early appearance of serious side effects, even with small doses. Hypercalcemia and elevations in the calcium-phosphorus product are not uncommon, and close monitoring of patients receiving $1,25(OH)_2D_3$ is mandatory.

The beneficial effects of therapy with $1,25(OH)_2D_3$ include a marked improvement in muscle strength and mobility [22]. In children, an increase in growth velocity has been noted [39]. Bone resorption decrease and complete healing of the bones may occur with prolonged therapy. However, the degree of success in reducing bone resorption is dependent on whether the activity of the parathyroid gland is suppressed. Periosteal fibrosis is markedly reduced, even in patients in whom PTH levels are not reduced during therapy. While the response to osteomalacia has been controversial, the 1-hydroxylated derivatives (1α-OH-D_3 and $1,25[OH]_2D_3$) have been consistently effective in the therapy for uremic hyperparathyroidism. In patients with pure low-turnover osteomalacia, the response to $1,25(OH)_2D_3$ is poor and often associated with hypercalcemia [7]. These patients may respond better to long-term therapy with both $1,25(OH)_2D_3$ and $24,25(OH)_2D_3$ (2.5 to 10 μg/d) [8]. Another group of patients who fail to respond to the 1-hydroxylated derivatives include a heterogeneous population with severe osteitis fibrosa and markedly elevated PTH blood levels. Hypercalcemia develops early in the course of therapy, and parathyroidectomy often is required.

Data on the effect of $1,25(OH)_2D_3$ on the derangements of mineral metabolism in moderate renal failure are limited. Touggard et al [51] studied 12 patients with a GFR between 5 to 25 ml/min and radiographic evidence of renal osteodystrophy. Intestinal calcium absorption improved and PTH levels decreased compared to controls. A decline in renal function was noted in the treated group. Christiansen [52] studied the effects of 1α-OH-D_3 (1 μg) in 18 uremic patients (GFR 20 $\pm$ 15 ml/min) for 6 months. A high incidence of hypercalcemia was noted and was associated with a deterioration of renal function. Massry et al [53] studied 38 patients with moderate renal failure for 1 year (GFR 15 to 55 ml). The placebo-treated patients were characterized by progressive bone disease and elevated PTH levels. GFR decreased 16 ± 3.8%, reflecting the spontaneous progression of renal disease. After 1 year of treatment with 1,25(OH)$_2$D$_3$ (0.8 ± 0.6 μg/d), complete healing of the bone was observed. The PTH blood levels decreased by 38 ± 9%. No change in GFR was noted despite episodes of hypercalcemia in each patient.

Dialysate Composition

Various impurities and trace elements, such as fluoride or aluminum, may contaminate dialysate solutions and cause bone disorders [6, 54–56]. Purification of the water system prior to preparation of dialysate should be performed to eliminate these potential hazards. A syndrome of low-turnover osteomalacia occurs with aluminum intoxication; it is, as noted above, not usually responsive to vitamin D therapy. Use of the chelating agent, desferrioxamine (2 g at the end of each dialysis period), has been associated with an improvement in the clinical picture, with reduction in the incidence of fractures, bone pain, and amelioration of the myopathy [57]. Interestingly, many of these patients after desferrioxamine therapy develop a typical picture of mixed osteitis fibrosis and osteomalacia, suggesting that inhibition of PTH-mediated bone formation may be a major factor in the genesis of the disorder.

Variations in the concentration of calcium in dialysate may affect the course of renal osteodystrophy. The use of a dialysate concentration containing 5.0 to 5.5 mg/dl of calcium is associated with a loss of calcium from the body [58, 59], a progressive increase in alkaline phosphatase, and persistently elevated PTH levels. For this reason, dialysate calcium concentrations of 6.0 to 7.0 mg/dl generally are employed. Higher concentrations of calcium (8.0 mg/dl) in the dialysate are frequently associated with hypercalcemia and enhanced soft tissue calcification.

References

1. MENDES V, JORGETTI V, NEMETH J, LAVERGNE A, LECHARPENTIER Y, DUBOST C, COURTNOT-WITMER C, BOURDON R, BOURDEAU A, ZINGRAFF J, DRÜEKE T: Secondary hyperparathyroidism in chronic hemodialysis patients. *Proc EDTA* 20:731–738, 1983
2. NEFF MS, EISER AR, SLIFKIN RF, BAUM M, BRAEZ A, GUPTAR S, AMARGA E: Patients surviving 10 years of hemodialysis. *Am J Med* 74:996–1003, 1983
3. PARFITT AM: Relationship between parathyroid cell mass and plasma calcium concentration in normal and uremic subjects. *Arch Intern Med* 124:269–278, 1969
4. LIU SH, CHU E: Studies of calcium and phosphorus metabolism with special reference to pathogenesis and effects of dihydrotachysterol (AT 10) and iron. *Medicine* 22:103–161, 1943
5. MASCHIO G, TESSITOME N, ANGELO A, et al: Early dietary phosphorus restriction

and calcium supplementation in the prevention of renal osteodystrophy. *Am J Clin Nutr* 21:1546–1554, 1980

6. DRUEKE T: Dialysis osteomalacia and aluminum intoxication. *Nephron* 26:207–210, 1980

7. OTT SM, MALONEY NA, COBURN JW, ALFREY AC, SHERRARD DJ: The prevalence of bone aluminum deposition in renal osteodystrophy and its relation to the response to calcitriol therapy. *N Engl J Med* 307:709–713, 1982

8. ALFREY AC, HEGG A, MILLER N, BERL T, BERNS A: Interrelationship between calcium and aluminum metabolism in dialyzed uremic patients. *Min Electr Metab* 2:81–87, 1979

9. MORINIERE PH, ROUSSEL A, TAHIRI Y, FOURNIER A: Substitution of aluminum hydroxyde by high doses of calcium carbonate in patients on chronic hemodialysis: disappearance of hyperaluminemia and equal control of hyperparathyroidism. *EDTA Proc* 19:784–787, 1982

10. CLARKSON EM, LUCK VA, HYNSON WV, BAILLEY RR, EASTWOOD JB, WOODHEAD JS, O'RIORDAN JLH, DEWARDENER HE: The effect of aluminum hydroxide on calcium, phosphorus and aluminum content of bone in patients with chronic renal failure. *Clin Sci* 43:519–531, 1972

11. COBURN JW, SLATOPOLSKY E: Vitamin D, parathyroid hormone and renal osteodystrophy, in *The Kidney,* edited by BRENNER BM, RECTOR FC, Philadelphia, WB Saunders & Co, 1981, pp 2213–2303

12. BORDIER P, MARIE P, ARNAUD C: Evolution of renal osteodystrophy: correlation of bone histomorphometry and serum mineral and immunoreactive parathyroid hormone value before and after treatment with calcium carbonate or 25 OH vitamin D_3. *Kidney Int* 2:102–112, 1975

13. DENT CE, HARPER CM, PHILPOT GR: Treatment of renal glomerular osteodystrophy. *Q J Med* 30:1–31, 1961

14. FOURNIER A, BORDIER P, GUERIS J, SEBERT JL, MARIE P, FERRIERE C, BEDROSSIAN J, DE LUCA MF: Comparison of lα hydroxycholecalciferol and 25 hydroxycholecalciferol in the treatment of renal osteodystrophy: greater effect of 25 hydroxycholecalciferol on bone mineralization. *Kidney Int* 15:196–205, 1979

15. RECKER R, SCHOENFELD P, LETTERI J, SLATOPOLSKY E, GOLDSMITH RS, BRICKMAN A: The efficacy of calcifediol in renal osteodystrophy. *Arch Intern Med* 138:857–863, 1978

16. BAYARD F, BEC P, TON THAT H, LOUVET J: Plasma 25 OH cholecalciferol in chronic renal failure. *Eur J Clin Invest* 3:447–450, 1973

17. EASTWOOD JB, BORDIER P, CLARKSON EM, TUN CHOT S, DEWARDENER HE: The contrasting effects on bone histology of vitamin D and of calcium carbonate in the osteomalacia of chronic renal failure. *Clin Sci Mol Med* 47:23–42, 1974

18. TEITELBAUM SL, BONE JM, STEIN PM, GILDEN JJ, BATES M, BOISSEAU VC, AVIOLI LF: Calcifediol in chronic renal insufficiency: skeletal response. *JAMA* 235:164–167, 1976

19. WITMER J, MARGOLIS A, FONTAINE O, FRITSCH J, LENOIR G, BROYER M, BALSAN S: Effects of 25 hydroxycholecalciferol on bone lesions of children with terminal renal failure. *Kidney Int* 10:395–408, 1976

20. FROST HM, GRIFFITH DL, JEE WS, KIMMEL DB, TEITELBAUM S: Histomorphometric changes in trabecular bone of renal failure patients treated with calcifediol. *Metab Bone Dis Rel Res* 2:285–295, 1981

21. ZUCHELLI P, CATIZONE L, CASANOVA S, FABRI L, FUSAROLI M: Therapeutic effects of 25 $(OH)D_3$ and sodium etidronate on renal osteodystrophy. *Min Electr Metab* 7:86–96, 1982

22. GOLDSTEIN DA, MALLUCHE HH, MASSRY SG: Management of renal osteodystrophy with 1,25(OH)$_2$D$_3$. *Min Electr Metab* 2:35, 1979
23. MALLUCHE HH, GOLDSTEIN DA, MASSRY SG: Management of renal osteodystrophy with 1,25 (OH)$_2$D$_3$. II. Effects on histopathology of bone. Evidence of healing of osteomalacia. *Min Electr Metab* 2:48–55, 1979
24. HEALY MD, MALLUCHE HH, GOLDSTEIN DA, MASSRY SG: Effects of long term therapy with calcitriol in patients with moderate renal failure. *Arch Intern Med* 140:1030–1033, 1980
25. HENDERSON RG, RUSSELL RG, LEDINGHAM JGG, SMITH R, OLIVER DO, WALTON RJ, SMALL DG, PRESTON C, WARNER GT, NORMAN AW: Effects of 1,25 dihydroxycholecalciferol on calcium absorption, muscle weakness and bone disease in chronic renal failure. *Lancet* 1:379–384, 1974
26. MASSRY SG, GOLDSTEIN DA, MALLUCHE HH: Current status of the use of 1,25 (OH)$_2$D$_3$ in the management of renal osteodystrophy. *Kidney Int* 18:409–418, 1980
27. MEEMA HE, RABINOVICH S, PIERATOS A, KATIRTZOGLOU A, MURRAY TM, OREOPOULOS DG: The healing effect of 1,25 dihydroxyvitamin D$_3$ on periosteal and intracortical resorption and its failure to prevent progression of endosteal resorption in renal osteodystrophy. *Metab Bone Dis Rel Res* 2:223–231, 1980
28. PIERIDES AM, ELLIS HA, SIMPSON W, DEWAR JH, WARD MK, KERR DNS: Variable response to long term 1α OH D$_3$ in hemodialysis osteodystrophy. *Lancet* ii:1092–1095, 1976
29. NIELSEN HE, ROMER FK, MELSEN F, CHRISTENSEN MS, HANSEN HC: 1α hydroxyvitamin D$_3$ treatment of non dialyzed patients with chronic renal failure. Effects on bone, mineral metabolism and kidney function. *Clin Nephrol* 13:103–108, 1980
30. NIELSEN SP, BINDERUP E, GODSFREDSEN WO: 1α hydroxycholecalciferol: long term treatment of patients with uremic osteodystrophy. *Nephron* 16:359–364, 1976
31. MEMMOS DE, EASTWOOD J, TALNER, et al: Double blind trial of oral 1,25 (OH)D$_3$ versus placebo in asymptomatic hyperparathyroidism in patients receiving maintenance hemodialysis. *Br Med J* 282:1919–1924, 1981
32. PIERIDES AM, KERR DN, ELLIS HA, O'RIORDAN JL, DELUCA HF: 1α OH cholecalciferol in hemodialysis renal osteodystrophy. Adverse effects of anticonvulsant therapy. *Clin Nephrol* 5:189–196, 1976
33. PIERIDES AM, ELLIS HA, SIMPSON W, COOK D, KERR DNS: The effect of 1α OH D$_3$ in predialysis renal bone disease. *Clin Endocr* 7(Suppl):109–116, 1977
34. SCHMITT RL, DAMBACHER MA, GUNCAGA J, OLA H, OMICHI A, JAHN HA: Clinical and biological efficiency of 1,25 (OH)$_2$D$_3$ in chronic dialysis patients with renal osteodystrophy, in *Vitamin D Basic Research and its Clinical Application,* edited by NORMAN AW, Berlin, deGruyter, 1979, pp 807–815
35. SMITH R, WOODS CG: Treatment of renal bone disease with 1α hydroxylated derivatives of vitamin D$_3$. *Q J Med* (new series) XLVIII:289–322, 1979
36. BRICKMAN AS, COBURN JW, SHERRARD J, WONG EG, NORMAN AW, SINGER FR: Clinical effects of 1,25 dihydroxyvitamin D$_3$ in uremic patients with overt osteodystrophy. *Contr Nephrol* 18:29–41, 1980
37. BULLAN M, DELLING G, OFFERMANN G, ZIEGLER R, BENZ G, LUHMANN H, SANCHEZ DE REUTTER A, SEVERIN M: *Renal osteodystrophy in children. Therapy with vitamin D or 1,25 dihydroxycholecalciferol.* Abstract of the XVIth Congress of European Dialysis and Transplant Association, Amsterdam, 1979, p 13

38. CHAN JCM, OLDHAM SB, DELUCA HF: Effectiveness of 1α hydroxyvitamin D_3 in children with renal osteodystrophy associated with hemodialysis. *J Pediatr* 90:820–824, 1977

39. CHAN JCM, DELUCA HF: Growth velocity in a child on prolonged hemodialysis. Beneficial effect of 1α hydroxy vitamin D. *JAMA* 238:2053, 1977

40. CHAN JCM, KODROFF MB, LANDWEHR DM: Effects of 1,25 dihydroxyvitamin D_3 on renal function, mineral balance and growth in children with severe chronic renal failure. *Pediatrics* 68:559–571, 1981

41. BERL T, BERNS AS, HUFFER WT, HAMMILL K, ALFREY AC, ARNAUD CD, SCHRIER RW: 1,25 dihydroxycholecalciferol effects in chronic dialysis. A double blind controlled study. *Ann Intern Med* 88:774–780, 1978

42. SHERRARD D, COBURN JW, BRICKMAN AS, SINGER FR, MALONEY N: Skeletal response to treatment with 1,25 dihydroxyvitamin D in renal failure. *Contr Nephrol* 18:92–97, 1980

43. SHARMAN VL, ABRAM SML, ADAMI S, et al: Controlled trial of 1,25 $(OH)_2$ vitamin D_3 in prevention of bone disease in haemodialysis patients. *EDTA Proc* 19:287–292, 1982

44. SHIMAMATSU K, MAEDA T, HARADA A, et al: 1 year control trial of 1 α OH D_3 in patients on maintenance hemodialysis. *Nephron* 28:70–75, 1981

45. BORDIER P, ZINGRAFF J, GUERIS J, JUNGERS P, MARIE P, PECHET M, RASMUSSEN H: The effect of 1 α $(OH)D_3$ and 1,25 $(OH)_2D_3$ on the bone in patients with renal osteodystrophy. *Am J Med* 64:101–107, 1978

46. LAM M, LLACH F: Effect of 1,25 $(OH)_2D_3$ in patients with early renal failure. *Min Electr Metab* 6:251, 1981

47. SHARMAN VL, BROWNJOHN AM, GOODWIN FJ: Long term experience of alfacalcidol in renal osteodystrophy. *Q J Med* (new series) L1:271–278, 1982

48. SMITH A, WINNEY RJ, STRONG JA, TOTHILL P: Long term effect of dialysate calcium and 1 α OH D_3 on bone calcium content in haemodialysis patients as measured by neutron activation analysis of the forearm. *Nephron* 28:213–217, 1981

49. BINSWANGER U, FISCHER JA, ISELIN H, ISWALD N, KEUSCH C, FREI D, WILLIMAN NP: 1,25 $(OH)_2D_3$ treatment of clinically asymptomatic renal osteodystrophy. *Min Electr Metab* 2:103–115, 1979

50. BALSAN S, GUERIS J, LEVY D, GARABEDIAN M, GUILLOZO H, BROYER M: Suppressive effect of 1α hydroxyvitamin D_3 on the hyperparathyroidism of children on maintenance hemodialysis. *Metab Bonde Dis Rel Res* 1:15–20, 1978

51. TOUGGARD L, SORENSEN E, MORTENSEN JB, CHRISTENSEN MS, RODBRO P, SORENSEN AW: Controlled trial of 1α hydroxycholecalciferol in chronic renal failure. *Lancet* i:1044–1047, 1976

52. CHRISTIANSEN C, RODBRO P, CHRISTENSEN MC, NAESTOFT J, HARTNACK B, et al: Deterioration of renal function during treatment of chronic renal failure with 1,25 dihydroxyvitamin D_3. *Lancet* 2:700–703, 1978

53. MASSRY SG, GRUBER H, ARIF SR, SHERMAN D, GOLDSTEIN DA, LETTERI JM: Use of 1,25$(OH)_2D_3$ in the treatment of renal osteodystrophy in patients with moderate renal failure, in *Clinical Disorders of Bone and Mineral Metabolism,* edited by FRAME R, POTTS J, New York, Excerpta Medica, 1983, pp 260–265

54. MORRISSEY J, ROTHSTEIN M, MAJOR G, SLATOPOLSKY E: Suppression of parathyroid hormone secretion by aluminum. *Kidney Int* 23:699–704, 1983

55. CANN CE, PRUSSIN SG, GORDAN GS: Aluminum uptake by the parathyroid glands. *J Clin Endocrinol Metab* 49:543–545, 1979

56. CANNATA JB, BRIGGS JD, JUNOR BJR, et al: Influence of aluminum on parathyroid hormone levels in hemodialysis patients. *EDTA Proc* 19:244–247, 1982

57. ACKRILL P, DAY JP, GARSTANG FM, et al: Treatment of fracturing renal osteo-dystrophy by desferrioxamine. *EDTA Proc* 19:203–207, 1982
58. BOUILLON B, VERBECKMOES R, DE MOOR P: Influence of dialysate calcium concentration and vitamin D on serum parathyroid hormone during repetitive hemodialysis. *Kidney Int* 7:422–432, 1975
59. DRUEKE T, BORDIER PJ, MAN NK, JUNGERS P, MARIE P: Effect of high dialysate calcium concentration on bone remodeling, serum biochemistry and parathyroid hormone in patients with renal osteodystrophy. *Kidney Int* 11:267–271, 1977

Hematopoietic System

Prostanoid-Related Platelet Abnormalities in Renal Disease

Ariela Benigni, Manuela Livio, and Giuseppe Remuzzi

The abnormalities of platelet function in patients with renal impairment have been the subject of numerous recent studies. Most research in the past 10 years has been stimulated by the discovery that platelets synthetize prostanoids and respond to arachidonic acid (AA) stimulation. Two observations were particularly relevant to this issue; in 1972, Silver et al found that arachidonate metabolites are generated by platelets during blood clotting [1]. Moreover, in 1973, the same investigators discovered that AA is a potent inducer of platelet aggregation in vitro [2]. Since these studies, the potential role of platelet prostanoids in disease conditions has been extensively evaluated.

In this chapter, we report the results obtained by platelet arachidonate metabolism both in patients with renal failure who are on maintenance hemodialysis and in patients with the nephrotic syndrome.

Platelet Arachidonate Metabolism in Renal Failure

Evidence of a qualitative platelet function abnormality exists in uremia; however, despite numerous studies, the precise platelet defect [3–10] that is responsible for the prolonged bleeding time in these patients [11] has not been identified. Beginning with the observation that platelet aggregation and release have been repeatedly, although inconsistently, reported to be abnormal in uremia [12, 13], we studied the capability of uremic platelets to form thromboxane A_2 (TxA_2)—a potent modulator [14] of platelet aggregation that is derived from the metabolism of AA. We first evaluated the formation of thromboxane B_2 (TxB_2), which is the stable breakdown product of TxA_2, in serum obtained after whole-blood clotting in vitro. In these conditions, synthesis and release of platelet thromboxane is stimulated by the thrombin formed during the process of blood coagulation. The formation of TxB_2 in

This manuscript was presented in part of a Symposium on *Prostaglandins and the Kidney.*

serum was found to be significantly reduced in uremic patients, as compared to age- and sex-matched controls [15]. One possible explanation for this difference would simply have been a reduced amount of thrombin formed in vitro, after blood coagulation, in uremic subjects with respect to control subjects. However, failure to correct the abnormal thromboxane generation by adding increasing amounts of thrombin to the system makes this possibility unlikely. Therefore, we oriented our interest towards a possible intrinsic abnormality of platelet AA metabolism in uremia. A possible defect in phospholipase activity—the enzyme that induces the release of AA from membrane phospholipids—appeared unlikely, since the addition of exogenous AA was unable to restore a normal TxB_2 production in our system. Furthermore, a reduced generation of prostaglandin E_2 (PGE_2) in uremic platelets of a similar extent, as observed for TXB_2, argued against a selective defect in the thromboxane synthetase; rather, it suggested a defect in the cyclo-oxygenase enzyme [15]. Additional experiments also indicated that cyclo-oxygenase is normally represented, but is functionally defective, in uremic platelets. Our interpretation is supported further by the observation that a partial acetylation of cyclo-oxygenase with low-dose aspirin reproduced, in normal subjects, the abnormality of TxA_2 formation found in uremia. Further studies are required to establish to what extent the cyclo-oxygenase defect accounts for the abnormal primary hemostasis in uremic patients.

We also investigated the functional properties of TxA_2 receptors in uremic platelets. For this purpose, we studied the aggregation response to an endoperoxide analog, U46619 (which mimics the activity of TxA_2 on platelet membrane), and the capability of the same analog to suppress prostaglandin I_2 (PGI_2) induced elevation in cyclic AMP. Both studies yielded comparable results for uremic and normal platelets, indicating that thromboxane/endoperoxide membrane receptors are normally operating in uremic platelets.

Platelet Arachidonate Metabolism in Nephrotic Syndrome

As opposed to renal failure, a thrombotic tendency in the nephrotic syndrome has been reported and renal vein thrombosis is particularly frequent [16]. Several studies focused on the "hypercoagulable" state of the nephrotic syndrome [17–24]; as far as platelet function is concerned, an enhanced aggregation in response to adenosine-5'-diphosphate (ADP), collagen, and AA has been described in nephrotic patients [25–31]. In 1973, Bang et al [25] demonstrated that the platelet "hyperaggregability" in the nephrotic syndrome was inversely related to the serum albumin concentration. In the same year, a paper by Silver et al [2] reported that albumin regulates platelet function by inhibiting the aggregation response to AA. Our group took advantage of these two studies and showed that the hyperaggregability of nephrotic syndrome platelets was accompanied by an increase in the arachidonate metabolites: malondialdehyde and TxA_2. Experiments performed by mixing washed platelets and plasma from nephrotic and normal individuals, in various combinations, suggested a plasma—rather than a platelet—alteration as being responsible for the exaggerated AA metabolism in nephrotic syndrome platelets. This abnormality was corrected if the albumin concentration of nephrotic plasma was normalized either by adding albumin in vitro or by infusing it into patients. The restoration of normal plasma albumin levels also normalized platelet aggregation in nephrotic syndrome patients [27]. Furthermore, we have been able to demonstrate that both the uptake of ^{14}C-AA and its subsequent conversion to prostaglandins and thromboxane following thrombin stimulation was inversely related to the concentration of albumin. However, it was not possible to establish a simple linear relationship between low concentrations of albumin and increased generation of thromboxane nephrotic syndrome. Therefore, we suspected that the explanation provided by Yoshida et al [26]—that the increased TxA_2 formation in nephrotic syndrome platelet is due to hypoalbuminemia because of the decrease in AA binding—would only partially account for the increased aggregation in response to AA observed in patients with nephrotic syndrome and severe hypoalbuminemia. At that time, the work of Watanabe et al [32] appeared to be of some relevance in identifying an additional mechanism by which albumin might possibly inhibit the abnormal platelet response to AA in nephrotic syndrome. These authors provided evidence that albumin represents the prostaglandin D_2 (PGD_2) synthetizing factor in human platelet-rich plasma (PRP). Prostaglandin D_2 is a potent inhibitor of platelet aggregation, and it has been proposed as a negative feedback modulator of platelet aggregation [33]. Additional evidence for the crucial role of PGD_2 in modulating platelet function came from the observation that a normal subject may be a "responder" or "nonresponder" regarding the inhibition of aggregation of PRP incubated in vitro with a thromboxane synthetase inhibitor [33–35]; this inconstant effect of thromboxane synthetase inhibitors has been related to a different ability to form antiaggregatory PGD_2 [34]. In addition, it has been demonstrated that albumin greatly enhances the ratio between the amount of PGD_2 and PGE_2 formed from cyclic endoperoxides [36, 37]. Therefore, we reasoned that hypoalbuminemia might represent a crucial factor that inhibits the formation of PGD_2 in nephrotic syndrome platelets.

Accordingly, we designed an in vitro study to evaluate the platelet response to an inhibitor of thromboxane synthetase, UK 38,485, in nephrotic syndrome patients. A concentration of UK 38,485, which completely prevented the formation of TxA_2, was unable to inhibit the platelet aggregation in response to AA in all of the 16 patients studied. Normalizing the plasma albumin concentration, we obtained a response to UK 38,485 comparable to what is usually seen in control subjects [33, 34]; 50% of the subjects can be classified as "nonresponders" and 50% as "responders." Furthermore, we performed radio-thin layer chromatography studies of washed control platelets labeled with ^{14}C-AA and resuspended in a medium containing both different amounts of albumin (from 0 to 4 g/dl) and a concentration of UK 38,485, which completely inhibited TxA_2 formation. After thrombin stimulation, platelet PGD_2 formation increased with the albumin concentration (from 2 to 8% of the total radioactivity). Similar results were obtained with washed nephrotic syndrome platelets (from 1.5 to 7%), confirming that hypoalbuminemia in nephrotic syndrome could effectively account for a defective PGD_2 synthesis.

Conclusion

We have found complex abnormalities in AA metabolism in both chronic uremia and nephrotic syndrome. In uremia, a functional defect in the cyclo-oxygenase enzyme accounts for a reduced capability of platelet, from renal failure patients, to form endoperoxides and TxA_2—potent inducers of platelet aggregation. This defect might at least partially explain the hemorrhagic diathesis of these patients, since a similar defect produced by oral low-dose aspirin in normal subjects determines a significant prolongation of their "skin bleeding time." In patients with nephrotic syndrome, at least two major defects have been identified in AA metabolism, with both apparently related to hypoalbuminemia. The decreased plasma albumin content would induce a decrease in AA binding, leading to an exaggerated accumulation of the fatty acid in the platelet membrane. As a consequence, the augmented substrate availability leads to an increased TxA_2 formation in nephrotic syndrome platelets. Moreover, the abnormal platelet response to the platelet thromboxane synthetase inhibitor, UK 38,485, indicates a possible additional defect in AA metabolism by nephrotic syndrome platelets. This abnormality seems to be related to a reduced formation of the antiaggregatory, PGD_2. In nephrotic syndrome, hypoalbuminemia might be a crucial factor in sustaining such an abnormality, since albumin was found to be essential for the conversion of unstable endoperoxides to PGD_2.

Acknowledgments. This work was done in collaboration with Professor Carlo Patrono and Dr. Giovanni de Gaetano to whom we are profoundly indebted. This study was supported by a grant from the National Research Council (CNR) (Program "Tecniche Sostitutive di Funzioni d'Organo"; Progetto Finalizzato "Medicina Preventiva" No. 82.01307.04).

References

1. SILVER MJ, SMITH JB, INGERMAN CM, KOCSIS JJ: Human blood prostaglandins: formation during clotting. *Prostaglandins* 1:429–436, 1972
2. SILVER MJ, SMITH JB, INGERMAN CM, KOCSIS JJ: Arachidonic acid-induced human platelet aggregation and prostaglandin-formation. *Prostaglandins* 4:863–875, 1973
3. LEWIS JH, ZUCKER MB, FERGUSON JH: Bleeding tendency in uremia. *Blood* 11:1073–1076, 1956
4. CASTALDI PA, ROZENBERG MC, STEWART JH: The bleeding disorder of uremia. A qualitative platelet defect. *Lancet* 2:66–69, 1966
5. HOROWITZ HI, COHEN BD, MARTINEZ P, PAPAYOANOU MF: Defective ADP-induced platelet factor 3 activation in uremia. *Blood* 30:331–340, 1967

6. RABINER SF, HRODEK O: Platelet factor 3 in normal subjects and patients with renal failure. *J Clin Invest* 47:901–912, 1967

7. EKNOYAN G, WACKSMAN SJ, GLUECK HI, WILL JJ: Platelet function in renal failure. *N Engl J Med* 280:677–681, 1969

8. STEWART JH, CASTALDI PA: Uraemic bleeding: a reversible platelet defect corrected by dialysis. *Q J Med* (new series) 36:409–423, 1967

9. REMUZZI G, SCHIEPPATI A, MECCA G: Abnormal platelet function in haemodialysed patients: current concepts. *Int J Artif Organs* 2:109–112, 1979

10. SALZMAN EW, NERI LL: Adhesiveness of blood platelets in uremia. *Thromb Diath Haemorrh* 15:89–92, 1966

11. RABINER SF: Uremic bleeding, in *Progress in Hemostasis and Thrombosis,* edited by SPAET TH, New York, Grune & Stratton, 1972, p 233

12. WATHEN R, SMITH M, KESHAVIAH P, CONTY C, SHAPIRO F: Depressed in vitro aggregation of platelets of chronic hemodialysis patients (CHDP): A role for cyclic AMP. *Trans Am Soc Artif Intern Organs* 21:320–328, 1975

13. BENIS J, RIGNEY J, SOSIN A, DEANE N: Enhanced platelet aggregation in chronic renal failure patients receiving hemodialysis treatment. *Trans Am Soc Artif Intern Organs* 23:48–52, 1977

14. HAMBERG M, SVENSSON J, SAMUELSSON B: Thromboxanes: a group of biologically active compounds derived from prostaglandin endoperoxides. *Proc Natl Acad Sci USA* 72:2994–2998, 1975

15. REMUZZI G, BENIGNI A, DODESINI P, SCHIEPPATI A, LIVIO M, DE GAETANO G, DAY JS, SMITH WL, PINCA E, PATRIGNANI P, PATRONO C: Reduced platelet thromboxane formation in uremia. Evidence for a functional cyclooxygenase defect. *J Clin Invest* 71:762–768, 1983

16. LLACH F, ARIEFF AI, MASSRY SG: Renal vein thrombosis and nephrotic syndrome. A prospective study of 36 adult patients. *Ann Intern Med* 83:8–15, 1975

17. KANFER A, KLEINKNECHT D, BROYER M, JOSSO F: Coagulation studies in 45 cases of nephrotic syndrome with uremia. *Thromb Haemost* 24:562–571, 1970

18. KENDALL AG, LOHMANN RC, DOSSETOR JB: Nephrotic syndrome: a hypercoagulable state. *Arch Intern Med* 127:1021–1027, 1971

19. THOMSON C, FORBES CD, PRENTICE CRM, KENNEDY AC: Changes in blood coagulation and fibrinolysis in the nephrotic syndrome. *Q J Med* 43:399–407, 1974

20. ANDRASSY K, RITZ E, BOMMER J: Hypercoagulability in the nephrotic syndrome. *Klin Wochenschr* 58:1029–1036, 1980

21. ADHIKARI M, COOVADIA HM, GREIG HBW, CHRISTENSEN S: Factor VIII-procoagulant activities in children with nephrotic syndrome and post-streptococcal glomerulonephritis. *Nephron* 22:301–305, 1978

22. THOMPSON AR: Factor XII and other hemostatic protein abnormalities in nephrotic syndrome patients. *Thromb Haemost* 48:27–32, 1982

23. TAYLOR FB JR, NILSSON UR, CREECH RH, CARROL ET, BEISSWENGER JG: Coagulolysis: mechanism of formation and lysis of diluted whole blood clots, and application of this assay into study of certain hypercoagulable states. *Ser Haematol* 6:528–548, 1973

24. KAUFFMAN RH, VELTKAMP JJ, VAN TILBURG NH, VAN ES LA: Acquired antithrombin III deficiency and thrombosis in the nephrotic syndrome. *Am J Med* 65:607–613, 1978

25. BANG NU, TRYGSTAD CW, SCHROEDER JE, HEIDENREICH RO, CSISKO BM: Enhanced platelet function in glomerular renal disease. *J Lab Clin Med* 81:651–660, 1973

26. YOSHIDA N, AOKI N: Release of arachidonic acid from human platelets. A key role for the potentiation of platelet aggregability in normal subjects as well as in those with nephrotic syndrome. *Blood* 52:969–977, 1978
27. REMUZZI G, MECCA G, MARCHESI D, LIVIO M, DE GAETANO G, DONATI MB, SILVER MJ: Platelet hyperaggregability and the nephrotic syndrome. *Thromb Res* 16:345–354, 1979
28. STUART MJ, SPITZER RE, NELSON DA, SILLS RH: Nephrotic syndrome: Increased platelet prostaglandin endoperoxide formation, hyperaggregability, and reduced platelet life span. Reversal following remission. *Pediatr Res* 14:1078–1081, 1980
29. TOMURA S, IDA T, KURIYAMA R, CHIDA Y, TAKEUCHI J, MOTOMIYA T, YAMAZAKI H: Activation of platelets in patients with chronic proliferative glomerulonephritis and the nephrotic syndrome. *Clin Nephrol* 17:24–30, 1982
30. JACKSON CA, GREAVES M, PATTERSON AD, BROWN CB, PRESTON FE: Relationship between platelet aggregation thromboxane synthesis, and albumin concentration in nephrotic syndrome. *Br J Haematol* 52:69–77, 1982
31. KUHLMANN U, STEURER J, RHYNER K, VON FELTEN A, BRINER J, SIEGENTHALER W: Platelet aggregation and β-thromboglobulin levels in nephrotic patients with and without thrombosis. *Clin Nephrol* 15:229–235, 1981
32. WATANABE T, NARUMIYA S, SHIMIZU T, HAYAISHI O: Characterization of the biosynthetic pathway of prostaglandin D2 in human platelet-rich-plasma. *J Biol Chem* 257:14847–14853, 1982
33. GRIMM LJ, KNAPP DR, SENATOR D, HALUSHKA PV: Inhibition of platelet thromboxane synthesis by 7-(1-Imidazolyl) heptanoic acid: dissociation from inhibition of aggregation. *Thromb Res* 24:307–317, 1981
34. HEPTINSTALL S, BEVAN J, COCKBILL SR, HANLEY SP, PARRY MJ: Effects of a selective inhibitor of thromboxane synthetase on human blood platelet behaviour. *Thromb Res* 20:219–230, 1980
35. BERTELÉ V, CERLETTI C, SCHIEPPATI A, DI MINNO G, DE GAETANO G: Inhibition of thromboxane synthetase does not necessarily prevent platelet aggregation. *Lancet* 1:1057–1058, 1981
36. HAMBERG M, FREDHOLM BB: Isomerization of prostaglandin H2 into prostaglandin D2 in the presence of serum albumin. *Biochim Biophys Acta* 431:189–193, 1976
37. CHRIST-HAZELHOF E, NUGTEREN DH, VAN DORP DA: Conversions of prostaglandin endoperoxides by glutathione-s-transferases and serum albumins. *Biochim Biophys Acta* 450:450–461, 1976

Gastrointestinal

Intestinal Transport of Minerals in Renal Failure

Chairpersons: David B. N. Lee and Carlo Gennari
Discussants: Zachariah Varghese, Herta C. Spencer,
and Allen C. Alfrey

Calcium and Phosphate Absorption

Physiology

Lee opened the workshop with a discussion of the physiology of calcium and phosphate absorption. He noted that the intestinal mucosa is considered a "leaky epithelium" because the tight junctions that join the cells at the luminal surface are readily permeated by ions and other small solutes. Therefore, calcium (Ca) and inorganic phosphate (P) will cross the intestinal epithelium by moving between cells via the paracellular shunt pathway as well as through the cells. Intestinal absorption of Ca (or P) represents the difference between the flux of this ion in the lumen-to-blood (absorptive) direction and the opposite blood-to-lumen (secretory) direction. To date, there is no convincing evidence to suggest that intestinal secretion of Ca or P is regulated or has any important physiological role in the homeostasis of either of these two molecules.

A major determinant of Ca and P absorption through the shunt pathway is the electrochemical gradients across the intestinal epithelium. Assuming a transepithelial potential difference (PD) of 5 mV (serosal-positive) and an ionized Ca concentration ([Ca]) of 1.25 mM in the extracellular fluid (ECF), the Ussing equation would predict that net diffusion in the absorptive direction will occur when free [Ca] in the lumen exceeds 2.0 mM. Fordtran and Lochlear measured [Ca] in human digesta and found the range to be between 0.5 to 8.5 mM, with the lower value being raised to 3.0 mM when 250 ml of milk were ingested.

The transepithelial PD would favor the diffusional flux of a negatively charged ion such as P in the absorptive direction. Using an average valence of -1.6 for P, and assuming an ECF [P] of 2.4 mM, diffusional absorption

---

This is the Summary of a Workshop by the same title.

of P would occur when luminal [P] exceeds 1.8 mM. When measured under fasting conditions, the gut luminal [P] at all levels of the small intestine in humans is about 2.0 mM. With feeding, one would clearly expect higher luminal [P]. Indeed, the [P] in human fecal fluid as determined by in vivo dialysis was 5.0 mM. Thus, in grown individuals who are in Ca and P balance, absorption of these ions through the paracellular conduit would be expected to satisfy most of the physiological needs.

The transcellular, active absorptive mechanism becomes important under stressful conditions such as rapid growth, pregnancy, or low dietary supply of these minerals. Transcellular transport of solutes across the intestinal epithelium would involve at least three different steps: transport across the luminal membrane, transport through the cytoplasm, and transport across the basolateral membrane of the enterocyte. In terms of Ca and P, energetic considerations would predict a nonenergy-dependent luminal entry for Ca (low cytosolic [Ca] and intracellular electronegativity) and an energy-dependent process for P penetration into the cell. Ca entry does not, while P entry requires sodium (Na). The thermodynamics at the basolateral membrane is opposite to that at the apical membrane. Thus, Ca is actively transported out of the cell while P exits down its electrochemical gradients. Currently, it is believed that at least two "pumps" may participate in the cellular expulsion of Ca: a Na-independent, Ca-ATPase and a Na-dependent, Ca-Na exchange system. Birge and associates have described in addition, a Na-dependent Ca-ATPase. The transcytosolic movement of Ca and P is complex and less well delineated. The regulation of transcellular Ca and P fluxes is mediated through alteration in influx rates at the luminal cell pole. There is now compelling evidence for 1,25-dihydroxyvitamin D (1,25D) as a major regulator for active Ca and P absorption. Although this metabolite causes parallel stimulation in Ca and P absorption in vivo, there is clear evidence to suggest that this hormone acts on separate Ca and P transport mechanisms in the intestine. The separation of these transport mechanisms could account, at least in part, for the differential effect of uremia on Ca and P absorption in human studies (see below). There is now increasing evidence suggesting that 1,25D may not be the only regulator for active absorption of these minerals. Thus, active Ca absorption in duodenum continues even in the most severely vitamin D-deficient young rats. Cross and Peterlik using embryonic chick small intestine have also provided evidence for nonvitamin D-mediated P absorption. Lee and Silis reported that in vitamin D-replete, young adult rats that display spontaneous active Ca absorption, the augmented Ca transport is mediated by a mechanism that is not identical to that mediated by exogenous 1,25D administration.

Finally, although the major focus of 1,25D action on intestinal absorption is thought to occur at the influx step across the apical membrane of the enterocytes, there is now evidence suggesting that more than one mechanism may mediate the action of 1,25D. Thus, we have found that the 1,25D-stimulated Ca absorption consists of a Na-dependent, as well as a Na-independent, component. There also appears to be a heterogeneity in terms of the distribution of these mechanisms in different segments of the intestine. The duodenum has mostly, a Na-dependent mechanism, whereas in the colon a large portion of the 1,25D-responsive, Ca absorptive mechanism is Na-independent.

In summary: (1) Ca and P are absorbed passively through the paracellular pathway and actively through the transcellular pathway. The paracellular pathway may be the major route for the absorption of these minerals under physiological, "nonstressed" conditions. (2) There are separate transport mechanisms for the active absorption of Ca and P and the relative distribution of these "transporters" are different in different intestinal segments. (3) Emerging evidence suggests that the action of 1,25D on intestinal Ca and P absorption may not be limited to the luminal membrane of the enterocytes. Furthermore, in addition to 1,25D, there may be other nonvitamin D factors that are important in the regulation of intestinal absorption of Ca and P.

Calcium and Phosphate Absorption in Uremia

Gennari noted that Ca and P are absorbed from the gut, mainly in the small intestine, by both active and passive mechanisms. The active mechanism is regulated by vitamin D. Despite these common characteristics, the two absorption processess may often be dissociated in different pathologic states characterized by negative effects on bone.

It is well known that Ca and P absorptions are precociously depressed in patients with chronic renal failure (CRF). Gennari has simultaneously measured the intestinal transport of both Ca (radiocalcium) and P (radiophosphate) in 40 patients with different degrees of CRF. The malabsorption of Ca and P correlated significantly with the glomerular filtration rate as assessed by endogenous creatinine renal clearance. An earlier deterioration of Ca absorption was apparent when compared to P absorption with declining renal function. In 16 patients with CRF, with a malabsorption of Ca and P, P absorption remained low after high doses of 25-hydroxycholecalciferol (25D) despite an evident improvement in Ca absorption. In 10 patients with CRF on maintenance hemodialysis, the treatment with pharmacological doses of 1,25D partially corrected Ca malabsorption, inducing a small but not significant increase in P absorption. The mechanism by which the intestinal absorption of Ca and P are depressed in uremia is still unclear. It has been demonstrated that an impaired renal production of 1,25D is the major cause of abnormal Ca metabolism in uremic patients.

The apparent earlier deterioration of Ca compared to P absorption with declining renal function, and the dissociation in recovery from Ca and P malabsorption after treatment with pharmacologic doses of active vitamin D metabolites, suggest the presence of separate regulatory mechanisms in the two transport processes. Gennari's data suggest that the altered metabolism of vitamin D in uremia is mainly responsible for the negative effects seen in the intestinal transport of Ca. On the contrary, in reference to the intestinal transport of P, uremia probably affects a different transport system not dependent on vitamin D.

Calcium and Phosphate Absorption after Renal Transplantation

Varghese considered the post-transplant alterations of calcium and phosphate absorption. Abnormalities of Ca absorption seem to occur earlier in the course of renal failure than abnormalities in P absorption. His studies have shown that Ca absorption improved after successful transplantation, while P absorption remained impaired. P absorption remains inappropriately low despite good renal function. His recent studies also indicate that serum levels of 25D and 24,25D are low, while levels of 1,25D are normal. Since hypophosphatemia stimulates 1-alpha hydroxylase activity, it may be that levels of 1,25D are inappropriately low for the level of serum phosphate. However, the levels of 1,25D seem to be adequate in normalizing Ca absorption. The observations of Varghese suggest that the regulation of P absorption is quite distinct from that of Ca absorption, and the P malabsorption may be an important additional factor contributing to post-transplant hypophosphatemia.

Magnesium Absorption

Spencer led the discussion of magnesium absorption. She noted that the metabolism of magnesium (Mg) had been studied in adult male patients with CRF by determining Mg balances for several weeks under controlled conditions in the Metabolic Research Unit. A strict metabolic routine was followed as outlined in her previous publications. The constant diet that these patients received was a low protein diet, containing 40 to 50 g protein per day, depending on the renal function, and it contained 159 ± 8.7 mg of Mg per day. This diet and complete urine and stool collections were analyzed for Mg by atomic absorption spectroscopy throughout the studies, the duration of which averaged 28 days. The analyzed values for Mg of the diet, urine, and stool formed the basis for calculating metabolic balances. The net absorption of Mg was determined according to the following formula:

$$\text{Net Absorption } (\%) = \frac{\text{Mg Intake} - \text{Fecal Mg}}{\text{Mg Intake}} \times 100$$

Mg balance studies were also carried out in patients with CRF during different Ca intakes, which ranged from 800 to 2000 mg/d. Control studies were carried out in patients with normal renal function, both during matched intakes of Mg of 159 mg/d and during a normal dietary Mg intake averaging 263 mg/d.

Significant differences were found in the intestinal absorption of Mg in patients with CRF compared to the absorption of patients with normal renal function. The average net absorption of Mg of patients with normal renal function was 48.5%, and this was confirmed in studies in which ^{28}Mg was used to determine the absorption of Mg. The ^{28}Mg absorption studies were carried out by giving an oral tracer dose of ^{28}Mg and by determining ^{28}Mg

Table 1. Magnesium balances and magnesium absorption of patients with chronic renal failure

Type of patient	No. of patients	Magnesium (mg/d)				Net absorption of magnesium (%)
		Intake	Urine	Stool	Balance	
Chronic renal failure	8	159	72	130	−43	17
Normal	10	263	142	137	−16	48
Normal	3	159	97	87	−25	46
Normal	3	191	116	92	−17	52

plasma levels and urinary and fecal ^{28}Mg excretions. In contrast to the intestinal absorption of Mg of 48.5% of subjects with normal renal function, patients with CRF had a significantly lower absorption of only 17% of the Mg intake. This difference was due to the significantly higher fecal Mg excretion of patients with CRF, which averaged 82.5% of the Mg intake, compared with an average of 51.5% for control subjects.

The urinary Mg excretion of patients with CRF was significantly lower, 72 ± 5.3 mg/d than the urinary Mg excretion of 97 ± 7.3 mg/d for normal subjects receiving a similar Mg intake. The Mg balances and the net absorption of Mg of a group of patients with CRF and of three groups of patients with normal renal function are shown in Table 1. In interpreting the difference in the intestinal absorption of Mg of patients with CRF and of normals, one has to consider that the intake of Mg of patients with CRF was significantly lower than that of subjects with normal renal function; namely 159 mg/d versus 263 mg/d. Although these Mg intakes differed greatly, the values of the fecal Mg excretion were similar in both populations, resulting in a lower absorption of Mg in the patients with CRF.

Increasing the Ca intake from 200 to 800, 1400, and 2000 mg/d did not change the Mg balance nor the net absorption of Mg of patients with CRF. The higher Ca intakes also had no effect on these parameters of Mg metabolism in subjects with normal renal function. Data of Mg balances and of the net absorption of Mg during different Ca intakes are shown in Table 2. The Mg balance was similar during a Ca intake of 200 mg/d and of 800

Table 2. Magnesium balances and magnesium absorption of patients with chronic renal failure during different calcium intakes

Calcium intake (mg/d)	Magnesium (mg/d)				Net absorption of magnesium (%)
	Intake	Urine	Stool	Balance	
200	150	77	139	−66	7
800	177	62	173	−58	2

mg/d, and the absorption of Mg was very low during both Ca intakes. The details of Mg studies of patients with CRF have been previously published from our Research Unit.

Only a few studies have been carried out on Mg metabolism of patients with chronic renal disease under controlled conditions. In one metabolic balance study of Mg, the urinary Mg excretion was low, the Mg balance was reported to be normal, and the intestinal absorption of Mg was lower than in normals. In another study, the Mg excretions and the intestinal absorption of Mg were reported to be normal in patients with CRF. In an intestinal perfusion study, the jejunal absorption of Mg was significantly lower in patients with CRF than in subjects with normal renal function. In another study, the intestinal absorption of Mg of uremic patients was slightly decreased. Also, in a ^{28}Mg study, the intestinal absorption of four of seven patients with CRF was lower than of subjects with normal renal function. Lack of vitamin D metabolite 1,25D in patients with CRF may contribute to the low absorption of Mg of these patients.

Aluminum Absorption

Alfrey emphasized that aluminum (Al) is plentiful in the environment, but that the lungs, skin, and gastrointestinal tract largely prevent any absorption of this element; the little Al that is absorbed is eliminated rapidly by the kidney. Early studies suggested that 10 to 90 mg of Al was consumed daily as a result of contamination in food sources. However, recent studies using more accurate analytical techniques have shown that these earlier estimates greatly overestimated the amount of dietary Al; probably only 2 to 5 mg of Al is consumed daily with food. If these latter values are correct, water is another potentially important source of Al intake, since municipal water supplies can contain up to 1000 μg/liter because Al is added as a coagulant in the treatment of many water supplies, and there are no water standards for Al. Another potential source of Al is that which could be leached from Al cookware during food preparation. Finally, there are certain plants, including the theaicae (tea family), that are Al accumulators. Thus, it seems possible that individuals drinking large amounts of tea may have even larger oral Al loads. Despite this potentially great variation in Al intake, it would appear that only a very small amount is actually absorbed. This supposition is based on the following findings: Tissue Al levels have been found to be consistently low in previously healthy individuals from a variety of different geographical areas. The only tissue Al content found to increase with aging is lung where the inhaled Al is apparently trapped. It has been estimated that the total body Al burden is less than 40 mg. This suggests that absorbed Al is largely, if not entirely, eliminated from the body.

At the present time the kidney is the only avenue for Al elimination that has been found. Tipton and associates using emission spectroscopy found urine Al levels to be 700 to 1000 μg/d. However, more recent studies using neutron activation analysis and flameless atomic absorption have shown urine Al levels to be much lower. Recker et al using neutron activation analysis reported values of 85.8 $\pm$ 64.9 μg/d, whereas Gorsky et al, Greger and Baier, and Kaehny et al reported values of 55 $\pm$ 16, 36 $\pm$ 4, and 15 $\pm$ 6 μg/d, respectively, by using flameless absorption.

Although it was assumed previously that Al absorption did not occur even with large oral loads of Al given as antacids, more recent studies have shown clearly this is not the case. Recker and associates reported that urinary Al increased from a mean value of 86 to 495 μg/d in five subjects fed 3.8 g of Al daily. Gorsky et al reported an increased urinary Al from 65 to 280 μg/d in patients receiving 2.2 g of Al daily. Similar amounts of Al, as determined by urinary Al excretion, are absorbed from a variety of different Al compounds including aluminum hydroxide, Al carbonate, and dihydroxy Al aminoacetate. Similarly, Greger and Baier found urinary Al to increase from 36 to 129 μg/d in patients given Al as aluminum chloride. The only exception so far described is Al phosphate, which appears to be poorly absorbed because of its insolubility.

Although it is clear that some Al is absorbed from large oral loads of Al, the major question is whether all of the absorbed Al is excreted by the kidney. Balance studies carried out in normal subjects ingesting 1 to 3 g/d of Al show that these individuals are in a positive Al balance of 23 to 313 mg/d. In contrast, balance studies carried out in eight subjects receiving a moderate oral load of Al (125 mg/d) showed that all patients excreted more than 96% of the ingested Al. This latter study would directly correlate with the fact that tissue Al levels have uniformly been found to be low in control subjects. It is possible, however, that when very large oral loads of Al are administered to individuals with normal renal function, some of this Al is retained. However, somewhat contrary to this finding is the fact that urine Al rapidly falls to control values when the oral Al loading is discontinued, suggesting that the absorbed Al has been eliminated.

A number of factors have been suggested to modulate Al absorption from the gastrointestinal tract (Table 3). The solubility of some Al compounds, such as Al hydroxide, depends on the physicochemical conditions of preparation. In one study, the free Al in Al hydroxide was 100 to 1000 times less in the pH range of 6.2 to 8.1 than at pH 4.2. Since Al would have to be in a soluble form for absorption, this would suggest that Al absorption may

Table 3. Factors that may modulate aluminum absorption

Enhanced absorption	Decreased absorption
Aluminum intake	Fluoride
Vitamin D	
Parathyroid hormone	
Gastric acidity	

be somewhat dependent on gastric pH and that absorption may primarily occur in the acid milieu of the stomach and proximal duodenum.

Even though no direct studies have been made, parathyroid hormone (PTH) has been suggested to enhance Al absorption based on the finding that PTH administered to rats undergoing oral Al loading enhances total body Al, as well as preventing its egress following the discontinuance of Al loading. However, at variance with these findings is the fact that neither plasma nor bone Al correlate with PTH levels in uremic patients.

Since vitamin D has been shown to enhance the absorption of a number of elements, including lead, magnesium, strontium, beryllium, barium, zinc cadmium, cesin and cobalt, it has also been suggested that it may increase Al absorption. However, these studies are not conclusive.

A more important modulator of Al absorption may be the fluoride content of the ingested diet and water, since Al has been shown to form tight complexes with fluoride. Spencer et al have shown that Al does decrease fluoride absorption from the gastrointestinal tract, and oral Al has been used to counteract dental fluorosis. Conversely, this might suggest that fluoride may also decrease. Conversely, this might suggest that fluoride may also decrease Al absorption, although this has not been directly studied.

It is unknown how uremia may affect Al absorption. Clarkson et al reported the presence of positive Al balance in 8 uremic patients as did Gorsky et al in control subjects receiving comparable Al loads. However, the validity of such balance studies is more or less in question. Preliminary studies in Alfrey's laboratory have shown that urinary Al excretion is significantly higher in uremic rats following an oral Al load than in control rats given the same amount of Al, thus suggesting that absorption may be enhanced in the uremic state.

Irrespective of whether there is enhanced absorption or reduced ability to excrete Al because of lack of renal function, tissue Al levels are commonly increased in uremic patients. This is especially evident in small uremic children receiving large oral loads of Al-containing, phosphate-binding gels. Because of this finding, it has been suggested that children should not be given more than 50 to 60 mg/kg/d of these Al compounds in efforts to control the serum phosphorus concentration.

Al has been shown to have other effects in the gastrointestinal tract. Besides decreasing fluoride absorption, it also reduces P, strontium, iron, and to a lesser extent, Ca absorption. More recently, Al has been shown to decrease cholesterol absorption. It has been suggested that Al combines with pectin to bind fat to nonabsorbable vegetable fiber preventing its absorption. Finally, Al compounds affect gastrointestinal tract mobility. Al ions inhibit acethycholine-induced contraction of rodent and human gastric smooth muscle, and free Al in the stomach markedly reduces gastric emptying. A well-known complication of Al administration is constipation which probably also results from altered mobility of the gastrointestinal tract.

In summary, although it is apparent that some orally administered Al is absorbed from the gastrointestinal tract, the factors which modulate Al absorption and the region in the gastrointestinal tract where maximum Al absorption occurs have not been well defined.

Zinc Absorption

Spencer acknowledged that a low zinc (Zn) status has been reported in patients with CRF, mostly on the basis of changes in Zn levels in plasma, red blood cells and hair, and in taste and smell. To her knowledge, little if any information is available on the dietary intake of Zn or the excretion or retention of Zn in these patients. Although the dietary protein intake in CRF has been related to the plasma concentrations of Zn, the actual intake of dietary Zn of these patients has not been reported. However, another study reported that the dietary Zn intake of patients with CRF has been shown to be lower than normal, but these intake levels have not been related to plasma concentrations of Zn.

In Spencer's study, complete metabolic balances of Zn were determined under strictly controlled dietary conditions in patients with CRF. These patients did not receive any medications nor did they undergo dialysis. The constant metabolic diet and all urine and fecal collections were analyzed for Zn for several weeks. The diet was a low-protein diet containing 40 to 50 g protein per day depending on the renal status. This diet contained considerably less Zn (5.5 to 8.4 mg/d) than the normal intake of 15 mg/d. The urinary Zn exretion of these patients was relatively low, averaging 0.3 mg/d. However, the fecal Zn excretion was frequently as high or even higher than the dietary Zn intake resulting in a negative Zn balance. The Zn loss in these patients ranged up to 2 mg/d.

With regard to studies of certain parameters of Zn metabolism in CRF, in one study, the plasma levels of Zn were low in patients who were not dialyzed and were severely protein-restricted, while dialyzed uremic patients who received a more liberal protein intake had normal plasma and erythrocyte levels of Zn. Decreased taste acuity and anorexia were observed in chronic dialysis patients, and these symptoms were alleviated by the use of Zn supplements. In dialyzed as well as nondialyzed azotemic patients with CRF, the levels of Zn in plasma, leukocytes, and hair were low, and the concentration of blood ammonia was increased. In a study of tissues of patients with CRF who had expired, the Zn content of hair, heart, liver, and testes was normal, and it was concluded that the decreased concentrations of plasma Zn in CRF may be due to redistribution of Zn rather than to total body deficiency of Zn.

Normal as well as low-normal plasma concentrations of Zn have also been reported. In one of these studies, the plasma concentrations of Zn depended on the type of artificial kidney used. These investigators also reported that in patients who did not undergo hemodialysis, the plasma levels of Zn were only slightly subnormal, while the erythrocyte Zn level was even increased. In another study, the mean serum Zn levels of patients undergoing hemodialysis were in the low-normal range, 77 μg/dl. In animal studies, bilateral ureteral ligation resulted in significant lowering of the plasma level of Zn, showing that the decrease in plasma Zn can occur in uremic rats in the absence of Zn deficiency.

The present study has shown that the negative Zn balance of patients with CRF is due to two factors; namely, to the subnormal dietary intake of Zn due to the low zinc content of the low-protein diet and to the decrease in the intestinal absorption of Zn. The use of Al hydroxide increased the fecal Zn excretion further in some, but not in all, patients studied and resulted in a more negative Zn balance.

Further studies are necessary to determine whether the negative Zn balances observed in CRF are characteristic of this disease or whether a similarly negative Zn balance would be encountered during a comparable low protein (and therefore low dietary) Zn intake in patients with normal renal function.

Evaluation and Management of Kidney Diseases and Renal Failure

Microscopic and Biochemical Analysis of the Urine in the Evaluation of Kidney Disease

Chairpersons: Robert G. Narins and Kenneth F. Fairley
Discussant: Richard A. Zager

When a patient is initially examined for renal disease, the first tests are those done on the urine. A finding of hematuria, which is now easily detectable by dipstick methods, necessitates a major decision by the doctor regarding the necessary line of investigation. The fundamental question is whether the patient should see a urologist or a nephrologist. Microscopic examination of the urine should be used to answer this question. Positive phase contrast microscopy is preferred. Stains can be used, but preferably they should not precipitate Tamm-Horsfall protein and agglutinate red blood cells as do some of the urine stains. There are advantages in counting the formed elements in the urine sediment and expressing the results of cells by unit volume. In centrifuged urine, cells can be counted and casts can be seen in the same specimen. The erythrocytes found in glomerulonephritis are typically different in size and shape, often fragmented, and show very little hemoglobin content. This pattern, the so-called "dysmorphic pattern," is often associated with the presence of casts that may contain erythrocytes. Other features of the urinary deposit in glomerulonephritis are the presence of fat and the phagocytosis of erythrocytes. The erythrocytes from lesions such as tumors have a uniform morphological pattern. Granular or cellular casts imply the presence of renal disease. Such urine samples, in addition to the uniform cells of nonglomerular bleeding, may also contain up to 8000 glomerular red blood cells.

In a double-blind study in which urine microscopy was done on 117 urine samples from patients presenting to the Nephrology Department, the sensitivity of this method of detecting underlying glomerular disease was 99%, with a specificity of 93%. The sensitivity of detecting nonglomerular bleeding was 100% and the specificity was 93%. Only 10 urine samples showed a mixed pattern suggesting dual pathology. A mixed pattern may also be found in a small number of patients with mesangial proliferative glomerulonephritis.

This is the Summary of a Workshop by the same title.

Up to 20% of the erythrocytes in this type of glomerulonephritis may be uniform in appearance. When a cast contains hemoglobin pigment, it is easy to deduce that it was derived from an erythrocyte cast. However, when hemoglobin pigment is not present, phase contrast microscopy makes it much easier to see the red blood cells within the casts. As might be expected, patients with heavy microscopic hematuria have large numbers of red cell casts in a greater percentage of urine samples. Occasionally, in patients with glomerulonephritis and with low urinary erythrocyte counts, red cells may be detected within casts. This is something that is not observed in a normal setting except after extreme exertion.

The urinary red cell count helps to distinguish between the different types of glomerulonephritis. Counts greater than 1,000,000/ml are found in patients with crescentic glomerulonephritis, whereas counts below 100,000/ml are seen in most patients with membranous glomerulonephritis. A small group of patients with membranous glomerulonephritis and associated proliferative changes (e.g., the membranous glomerulonephritis of systemic lupus) may shed high urinary red cell counts. Patients whose biopsy samples showed minimal change glomerulonephritis or focal and segmental hyalinosis and sclerosis usually show low urinary red cell counts.

The assessment of fat in the urine may help to distinguish the type of glomerulonephritis. In membranous glomerulonephritis, for example, the urine may contain large amounts of fat in the form of free fat globules or those contained within epithelial cells; i.e., oval fat bodies. In mesangial proliferative glomerulonephritis, the urine usually contains very little fat except in those patients with impaired renal function and advanced glomerular disease. Erythrophagocytosis by cells in the urine is another sign of glomerular bleeding. The phagocytic cells are renal tubular epithelial cells. These may also be seen within biopsy specimens. A small amount of fat may be seen in any sort of glomerular disease and is also noted in normal subjects after extreme exercise such as running a marathon. Hyaline casts, often in very large numbers, are commonly seen in patients taking diuretics and in this situation have little prognostic or diagnostic significance. Casts in normal people are composed of Tamm-Horsfall protein, whereas in patients with glomerulonephritis they also contain fibrin and complement. In polarized light, starch granules and crystals give a similar appearance to oval fat bodies; i.e., appearing as Maltese crosses. In patients taking diuretics, casts containing many crystals may appear. These disappear when therapy is stopped.

Healthy urine also contains a myriad of proteins of both plasma and urinary tract origin. The Workshop reviewed just how the quantification of selected urinary macromolecules can provide useful information in clinical and experimental approaches to renal disease.

It is clear that the most useful macromolecular determination in urine is that of the total urine protein concentration. Not only is proteinuria a sensitive index of kidney disease, but its quantification can provide useful differential diagnostic and prognostic information. For example, heavy proteinuria (> 3 g/24 hr) is indicative of a glomerulopathy while lesser proteinuria ($\cong$ 1 g/24 hr) is suggestive of tubulointerstitial nephritis. Furthermore, the quantification of proteinuria may convey prognostic information since the rate of progression of selected glomerulopathies may correlate with the amount of excreted protein, and increasing proteinuria in patients with tubulointerstitial nephritis usually implies the development of focal glomerulosclerosis. In recent years, there has been increasing interest in the measurement of microgram quantities of selected proteins by radioimmunoassay (RIA) to detect minor increases in urine protein excretion. The potential utility of these techniques has been demonstrated in a number of studies. For example, Mogensen et al have shown that measurements of albuminuria via RIA in patients with diabetes mellitus, following either exercise or lysine infusion, can offer an early index of underlying diabetic glomerulosclerosis. Viberti et al have further demonstrated the utility of using RIAs for investigative purposes by demonstrating that urine albumin excretion can be reduced by tight glycemic control in patients with early diabetes mellitus, presumably due to improvement in glomerular hemodynamics or a decrease in glomerular permselectivity to protein.

It has also been suggested that qualitative assessments of proteinuria may provide useful information in the evaluation of patients with renal disease. For example, it has long been recognized that patients with tubulopathies excrete a predominance of low molecular weight serum proteins in urine, while patients with a glomerulopathy have a predominance of high molecular weight proteins in urine. However, despite different patterns of protein excretion in patients with differing nephropathies, the techniques of qualitative urinary protein assessments have not gained widespread clinical application largely because these techniques do not lead to specific histologic diagnoses and because many patients exhibit mixed glomerular/tubular proteinuric patterns.

Over the last 10 to 20 years, there has been a substantial interest in the measurement of urinary enzyme excretion in patients with kidney disease. Potential applications of these techniques include the monitoring of patients for impending nephrotoxicity and the diagnosis of specific urogenital disorders. However, despite the fact that studies of urinary enzyme excretion hold promise of providing useful clinical information, a number of practical considerations have limited our ability to use these methods to their full advantage. For example, urinary enzyme excretion does not necessarily reflect clinically relevant renal injury, since increased enzyme excretion can occur in association with such diverse circumstances as exercise, diuresis, or the ingestion of specific drugs. Second, increased enzymuria may result from increased glomerular filtration of circulating enzyme and not from tubular injury. Third, the amount of enzyme excreted in urine may bear little relationship to the severity of renal injury. Further, urine contains a variety of enzyme inhibitors and activators so that an enzyme's concentration, as detected by bioassay, may not reflect its true urinary concentration accurately.

An alternative approach to the diagnosis of acute tubular injury has been explored: the measurement of renal tubular epithelial antigen excretion in urine by radioimmunoassay. The rationale for this approach is that the proximal tubular brushborder is shed into urine in variable amounts with both nephrotoxic and ischemic renal injury. In prospective clinical studies, we have demonstrated that an increased urinary brushborder antigen concentration is a relatively specific marker of acute tubular necrosis. Cumulative experience suggests that abnormal brushborder antigen concentrations in a spot urine sample accurately discriminates 85% of patients with acute tubular necrosis from oliguric patients with prerenal azotemia. It also allows for differentiation between patients with acute tubular necrosis and those with chronic nephropathies. This technique appears to offer promise in the diagnosis of acute tubular necrosis, particularly in those individuals who might otherwise be misdiagnosed on the basis of renal functional data (fractional sodium excretion, urinary osmolality, and so forth).

The Workshop also considered the use of measurements of certain urine solutes in the evaluation of patients with kidney disease. First, insofar as urine sodium is concerned, it was noted that earlier studies had suggested that the fractional excretion of sodium (FE_{Na}) could distinguish clearly between prerenal azotemia and intrinsic parenchymal causes of acute renal failure (ARF). Indeed, a review of published reports up to 1980 indicates that the average FE_{Na} in prerenal azotemia is $0.3 \pm 0.1\%$ and $5.0 \pm 0.5\%$ in patients with established acute tubular necrosis (ATN); very little overlap was observed. However, in clear-cut ATN five recent studies (1980 to 1984) have called attention to the fact that the FE_{Na} has been considerably less than 1.0%. This paradoxical finding has complicated the diagnosis of contrast dye-induced ATN, rhabdomyolysis or the appearance of ATN during the course of various edema-forming states. When vomiting leads to prerenal azotemia, the FE_{Na} often exceeds 1%. In this setting, the gastric generation of HCO_3^- exceeds the renal reabsorptive capacity for bicarbonate. The resultant bicarbonaturia causes natriuresis to occur in the face of extracellular fluid (ECF) volume contraction. Since the tubule efficiently reabsorbs NaCl, the FE_{Cl}^- will be less than 1.0 and therefore reflect the prerenal state more accurately.

Solute excretion: Free-water clearance (C_{H_2O}) and osmolar clearance (C_{Osm}) may be applied effectively to the assessment of polyuric patients and clarification of the patient's need for fluid and electrolyte replacement. Urine volume may be divided into two virtual volumes: the C_{H_2O} and C_{Osm}. The C_{Osm} can be defined as the rate at which urine must be excreted to dilute urinary solute to a concentration equal to that of plasma. Thus, excretion of the normal daily urinary solute load (600 mOsm) in 2 liters of urine will result in the excretion of isotonic urine (300 mOsm/liter). The C_{Osm} will therefore be 2 liters/d. The C_{Osm} may also be calculated using the standard clearance formula: $C_{Osm} = \dfrac{U_{Osm} \times V}{P_{Osm}}$. The C_{H_2O} is calculated indirectly. If a subject's urinary volume is 2 liters with a plasma osmality of 300 mOsm/liter and a urinary osmolality of 150 mOsm/liter, then the C_{H_2O} will be the difference between the urinary volume and the C_{Osm}: $V = C_{Osm} + C_{H_2O}$;

$$2 \text{ liters} = \frac{150 \text{ mOsm/liter} \times 2 \text{ liter}}{300 \text{ mOsm/liter}} \text{ or } C_{H_2O} = 1 \text{ liter}$$

Since polyuria may result from either an increase in C_{H_2O} or C_{Osm}, the differential diagnosis of the polyuric state is best addressed by measuring C_{Osm} and C_{H_2O}.

Osmotic diuresis is characterized physiologically by a C_{Osm} greater than 3 ml/min; $U_{Osm}/P_{Osm} = 1.0 \pm 0.15$. The offending solute can be either an electrolyte: NaCl or Na HCO_3; or a nonelectrolyte: glucosuria, mannitol, or urea. Water diuresis is characterized by a C_{Osm} less than 3 ml/min, a $U_{Osm}/P_{Osm} < 0.7 \pm 0.1$, and it may be caused by suppression of the release of antidiuretic hormone (ADH) or a defect in the renal response to normally secreted hormone. The former circumstance may be caused by polydipsia with physiologic suppression of ADH release or impaired hormone synthesis or release.

The use of C_{Osm} and C_{H_2O} in the clinical setting may be illustrated in the following example: An edematous postoperative man is undergoing a furosemide diuresis. He is unable to take anything orally. His serum electrolyte concentrations are normal while his urinary values are as follows: volume, 2 liters; urine osmolality due to electrolytes, 150 mOsm/liter. How would you replace his urinary losses? He should be allowed to lose isotonic urinary solute, thereby beneficially shrinking his ECF volume, but his C_{H_2O} must be replaced lest progressive hypernatremia ensue. The C_{Osm} is: $\frac{150 \text{ mOsm/L} \times 2 \text{ liters}}{300 \text{ mOsm}} = 1$ liter. Thus, the C_{H_2O} is: 2 liters = 1 liter + C_{H_2O} or 1 liter/d. Thus, this subject should receive 1 liter of water to replace his 2-liter loss of urine. In this way, his serum sodium concentration will remain normal while edema is lost.

Newer Imaging Techniques in Nephrology

Chairpersons: Hedrig Hricak and Zoran L. Barbaric
Discussants: Richard M. Friedenberg, Hooshang Kangarloo, Bruce Hillman, and Bruce L. McClennan

Explosive advances in radiological technology have had a significant impact on the radiological diagnosis of urinary tract disease. This Workshop discussed the newer radiological approaches, some of which are so momentous that we can now diagnose underlying renal disease without an injection of contrast media; information can be obtained on the chemical and physical nature of renal tissue. Furthermore, with the use of computers, minimal differences of tissue density can be enhanced and small vessels can be seen in great detail with no more than very small injections of contrast media. Computed tomography continues to improve until it has now become the standard examination in most hospitals throughout the United States. Diagnostic ultrasound has achieved a high quality and today can be performed with ease. Ultrasonography is rapidly becoming a part of the routine physical examination. By the end of this Workshop, all of us will realize that the advances in radiology have been enormous and that the field is still evolving and progressing with parallel improvements in sensitivity and specificity.

Friedenberg provided a detailed overview on the present and future of renal imaging. He stated that imaging occupies an important place in the diagnosis of abnormalities of the kidney and the genitourinary tract. The technological explosion of the past 10 years has been accompanied by an introduction of new imaging modalities at a rapid pace. Examination of the current status of hospital-based imaging in the United States reveals that there has been an 8% increase in the overall performance of diagnostic procedures between 1973 and 1980; currently, 120 million procedures are being performed yearly, and there has been a 5% decrease in the number of contrast studies performed. In 1980, 4.2 million urograms were carried out in the United States and it is probable that the number will decrease to less than 3 million before the end of the 1980s. The void is being filled by the use of newer procedures, including nuclear radiology, computed tomography, and ultrasonography. Ultrasound is used currently in the triage examination of

This is the Summary of a Workshop by the same title.

the kidney. It can detect the presence and absence of a kidney, hydronephrosis and/or obstruction; it can detect renal masses in the kidney and tell you whether they are solid or cystic, and it can differentiate between the cortical and medullary tissues of the normal kidney and the loss of this distinction in renal failure.

Digital subtraction angiography has also become popular over the past several years. This technique consists of obtaining a first image as a mask image and then a second one with the addition of contrast material. The subtraction of the two images, one from the other, leaves only the residual contrast material to be visualized. If the injection is performed intravenously, the procedure is less invasive than arterial angiography. Digital angiography is well suited for screening examinations, particularly in the evaluation of arterial bypass grafts, donor kidneys, and patients with suspected renovascular hypertension. The problems with digital angiography are those of poor resolution, since the injection on the venous side may overflow into all vascular structures, frequently obscuring proper visualization of the area of interest. The future of digital substraction angiography probably resides in its potential ability to quantify information. This has already been accomplished in areas of the heart where the computer can calculate the ejection fraction and other physiological indexes following the passage of the contrast bolus through the heart. In the near future, we hope to quantify renal blood flow by videodensitometry, thus providing useful information on the status of renal blood flow and the functional significance of a stenotic lesion of the renal artery.

Nuclear magnetic residence has just appeared on the scene. Again, as with ultrasonography, it is a nonradiation emitting technique that has great future potential. It is already recognized as superior to computed tomography in the imaging evaluation of the brain, spine, and pelvis. It is fair to assume that nuclear magnetic resonance will one day become the preferred imaging technique for evaluation of the abdominal organs such as kidney.

The most exciting future development on the horizon is that of tissue characterization. Tissue characterization describes a computerized ability to detect the existence of tissue abnormalities despite the fact that its morphologic appearance is normal. Imaging tools that may be utilized for this purpose include ultrasound, magnetic resonance, spectroscopy, positron-emission tomography, and vascular digital videodensitometry. This will hopefully lead to noninvasive kidney biopsy so that we can detect the actual histological nature of a renal lesion without invasive biopsy. We should be able to detect the degree of interstitial fibrosis in the presence of inflammatory lesions, the presence of abscesses or tumors, etc. Tissue characterization will also provide physiologic information in addition to an anatomical picture of the kidney. The various future means of imaging will include all those mentioned above, and they will be integrated into the computer in such a way that we will be able to extract information from each and thus pool all of our resources to arrive at a probable diagnosis.

Hillman next discussed intravenous digital subtraction angiography (IV-DSA): a relatively new technology that marries the contrast-resolving capacity of image intensification to the image processing capabilities of the digital computer. The result is a technology capable of imaging the major arterial circulation of outpatients with less risk, morbidity, and expense than with conventional film-screen arteriography.

Central catheterization is performed using local anesthesia, percutaneous antecubital puncture, and Seldinger technique and is followed by one to three mechanical injections of contrast material. Typical examinations take 30 to 45 min to perform and patients are released immediately. For renal IV-DSA, arterial images are exposed at one per second; on the initial sequence, delayed images are exposed at 1, 2, and 4 min after injection to depict the renal parenchyma and collecting systems. Subtraction images are obtained via an interactive keyboard, whereby the radiologist bids the computer to subtract precontrast from postcontrast images, then electronically enhances the density of the remaining circulatory structures. Additionally, postprocessing programs such as magnification, filtration, image averaging, and region of interest evaluation may be applied to bring out hidden diagnostic details or evaluate aspects of contrast material transit.

Clinical indications for which Hillman has applied IV-DSA include hypertension, potential renal donor evaluation, investigation of abnormalities in renal allograft recipients, renal masses, unexplained hematuria, and evaluation of the arterial circulation prior to and following invasive therapy. However, 54% of the 240 examinations he has performed have been for the first of these indications; namely, the investigation of possible renovascular hypertension. In this regard, IV-DSA has had a significant impact upon how referring physicians may approach hypertensive patients. The benignity, low expense, and reliability (94% reliable, 93% accurate in proven cases) of IV-DSA has made it a suitable alternative to indiscriminant medical therapy for certain patients. Hillman has shown that, when coupled with percutaneous transluminal angioplasty treatment in identified cases, the IV-DSA approach is economically and medically preferable to medical treatment for moderately and severely hypertensive patients.

Renal transplant patients have embraced the procedure for similar virtues. In 29 patients performed for this indication, there have been no sequelae, and additional hospitalization has been obviated. That 97% of the examinations have been of diagnostic quality and that all proven diagnoses have been accurate has made IV-DSA the preferred examination for referral of suspected transplant vascular abnormalities in our hospital.

Overall, IV-DSA has produced diagnostic quality studies in 94% of cases and has been 92% accurate in the 89 cases where confirmation by conventional arteriography or surgery has been available for comparison. No complications requiring interventional treatment have occurred. Nondiagnostic or indeterminant examinations most frequently are caused by poor cardiac function, resulting in poor concentration of contrast material in the renal arteries. Peristalsing bowel gas—which produces obscuring artifacts following subtraction—and superimposition of multiple renal arteries upon each other have also resulted in suboptimal studies.

IV-DSA, as well as other digital radiographic techniques (for example, digital intra-arterial arteriography, digital interventional procedures, and dual energy subtraction) is still a technology in evolution that must yet find its appropriate role in nephrologic and urologic diagnosis. Still, its virtues of low cost, low risk, low discomfort, and acceptable reliability make IV-DSA a valuable technology for current application to a variety of renal vascular indications.

Barbaric introduced the topic of interventional radiology and emphasized its continuing rapid development. This is perhaps most exemplified by the current management of urinary tract calculi. Instead of classical surgical pyelolithotomy, the percutaneous approach is now favored in most instances. Under fluoroscopic control, a percutaneous nephrostomy tract is established and enlarged to permit a variety of endoscopic instruments to be inserted either in the renal pelvis or ureter. Larger calculi are broken into smaller fragments and extracted. Ureteral calculi are also retrieved using baskets and/or flexible nephroscope. The success rate is well above 80% while significant complications (significant hemorrhage and infection) are around 2%. Percutaneous nephrolithotripsy and percutaneous nephrolithotomy are expected to be the primary method for management of urinary tract calculi for the next several years. It is then likely that they will be replaced and superseded by extracorporal nephrolithrotripsy, where a shock wave propagated through water is concentrated onto the calculus. This mechanical force shatters the calculus into sand, which is then expelled with the urine stream without pain.

Other developments of percutaneous nephrostomy techniques include: (1) internal stent placement; (2) irrigation and dissolution of struvite and uric acid; (3) calculi; (4) dilation of ureteral strictures; and (5) closure of ureteral fistulas.

Intra-arterial embolization other than for renal carcinomas is gaining wider acceptance. Using a variety of embolic material such as ivalon, coils, detachable balloons and alcohol, it is possible to selectively occlude congenital or traumatic arteriovenous fistulas, stop acute hemorrhage, or perform selective or complete internal nephrectomy. For example, in patients with irreversible renal failure and uncontrollable proteinuria, loss of protein can be controlled in this manner. Similarly, patients with successful renal transplants, and difficult-to-control hypertension can benefit from embolization of their native kidneys.

Percutaneous transluminal angioplasty is now a mature technique, and the method of choice for treatment of renal vascular hypertension. The success rate in patients suffering from fibromuscular dysplasia is well above 95%, while simpler types of atherosclerotic disease have 80% positive response. Complication rates are well below surgical approaches.

It is evident that interventional radiology is playing an increasingly important part in the management of patients with a variety of urinary tract diseases. In many instances, it can produce results with greater simplicity, and less suffering to the patient as compared to what surgery could do in the past for identical clinical problems.

Next, the Workshop considered methods of tomographic evaluation of the urinary tract, including ultrasound-computed tomography and magnetic resonance imaging. Ultrasound is increasing in popularity and, in many instances, it is becoming the preferred modality for screening evaluation of the urinary tract.

Kangarloo emphasized that ultrasonography plays a significant role in the evaluation of renal anomalies and pathology in children. Its noninvasive nature, lack of ionizing radiation, and flexibility of the technique allows for rapid evaluation and screening of children suspected of having renal pathology.

Various forms of cystic renal dysplasia can be identified that will assist in predicting a prognosis. Infantile polycystic disease appears as bilateral echogenic masses that are the result of dilated renal tubules. In contrast, in adult polycystic disease, cysts are large enough to be resolved and the sonographic appearance is that of multiple cysts. Multicystic disease is seen as a multiseptated cystic mass (pelvoinfundibular atresia) or a large dilated pelvis with multiple cysts in the periphery without communication (hydronephrotic form of multicystic disease). Renal cystic dysplasia as a result of distal obstructive uropathy is seen either as bilateral fluid-filled masses in the renal fossa without evidence of demonstrable cortex or echogenic kidneys with apparent mild hydronephrosis.

Various forms of urinary tract dilatation can be accurately identified. It is generally possible to identify the location of the obstruction and commonly differentiate between obstructive uropathy and primary megaureter.

Anomalies of renal position (intrathoracic kidney, pelvic kidney, and so forth) are best screened by ultrasonography and, if necessary, confirmed subsequently by other imaging modalities.

One of the most significant roles of ultrasonography is in children with urinary tract infection. Following the comparison of various imaging modalities in children with documented urinary tract infection, we have concluded that ultrasonography and voiding cystourethrography are the screening modalities of choice in the evaluation of children with urinary tract infection. If both ultrasound and voiding cystourethrography are normal, no further diagnostic workup is necessary. However, if ultrasonography is abnormal or inconclusive, further diagnostic imaging is indicated depending on the initial sonographic findings. The use of ultrasonography in this manner permits a reduction of more costly and hazardous procedures requiring ionizing radiation.

The Workshop next considered computed tomography (CT). McClennan noted that, as intravenous urography (IVU) remains the primary screening test for the detection of urinary tract disease, computed tomography (CT) has commanded a (the) major role for definition of renal pathology. Significant progress in CT technology has resulted in the widespread availability of high-resolution fast (sub-5 sec) scanners capable of generating and/or reformatting body section images in multiple planes. Currently accepted indications for renal CT include: (1) evaluation of renal masses; (2) staging renal neoplasia; (3) evaluation of juxtarenal diseases; (4) renal failure; (5) renal and perirenal calcifications; (6) trauma; (7) CT-guided interventional procedures.

Intravenous contrast material is a fundamental requirement for optimal renal CT. It improves both detection and definition of a real or suspected abnormality. Contrast medium-assisted CT provides a gross functional assessment of the kidney and relies on the physiologic phenomena of contrast material excretion. Dynamic CT takes advantage of the same urographic principles related to the appearance of the vascular and tubular nephrogram and the pyelogram. The methods of delivery of contrast material for renal CT are either rapid intravenous bolus injection or intravenous infusion at a variable rate. Direct intra-arterial injections are rarely, if ever, indicated. Rapid (less than 30 sec) bolus injections are by far the best method of contrast administration for renal CT. Infusion techniques are usually reserved for opacification of major vascular structures such as the inferior vena cava, which may be opacified via a foot vein infusion when large, bulky tumors compress or invade it. Small, intravenous injections of 10 to 40 cc of a 50 to 66% solution of water-soluble contrast material are usually sufficient for assessment of renal mass enhancement or renal vascular integrity. Total doses of between 20 and 40 g of iodine given by the multiple bolus techniques are common in renal CT and closely correlates with current urographic practice.

The pharmacokinetics and physiology of contrast medium excretion were reviewed and related to the diagnosis of renal disease by CT. The utility, both real and potential, of the new nonionic and ionic low osmolality contrast media for renal CT were discussed and compared to the conventional ionic hyperosmolar materials regarding nephrotoxicity, efficacy, and patient tolerance.

Last, the Workshop focused on nuclear magnetic resonance, asking whether current interest in this technique is merely fashionable, or whether it is true that it will give rise to the most versatile and powerful imaging modality yet to be seen in medicine. Magnetic resonance does offer certain advantages. It combines the nonionizing and noninvasive advantages of ultrasound with those of CT; mainly its use is not operator-dependent. However, unlike CT, magnetic resonance does not require the use of iodine-containing contrast media for imaging of the abdomen and, particularly, the pelvis. Sources of known CT artifacts do not present a problem. In imaging of the kidney, magnetic resonance offers a unique display of the renal parenchyma with a clear differentiation between the height of the cortex and that of the medulla. In looking at renal allografts, magnetic resonance is very sensitive in the detection of renal fluid collection and the differentiation of hematomas from lymphoceles. It is also useful in the location of an intraperitoneal fluid collection and the evaluation of post-transplant acute renal failure. Even a minimal rejection reaction can be seen clearly by magnetic resonance as a marked change in the normal appearance of the kidney with obscured cortical/medullary differentiation. The most important impact of magnetic resonance will probably be on our ability to differentiate acute immunologic rejection from cyclosporine toxicity. In all patients thus far examined, magnetic resonance depicted acute rejection as an abnormally looking kidney while, in contrast, the kidney remained normal with good cortical/medullary differentiation in cyclosporine toxicity. Further impact of magnetic resonance in nephrology will be its ability to display the vascular system clearly without the use of contrast media. This will be useful in the study of renal tumors, their staging, and the search for vascular involvement.

We are only at the beginning of the era of magnetic resonance; a great impact has been realized already. But, its introduction serves to underscore the fact that there has been an explosive advance in the technology of diagnostic radiology. The advances have been enormous, they are still going on, and we are in the midst of dynamic changes in which the sensitivity and specificity of various modalities are constantly improving.

Are Randomized Trials in Kidney Disease Worthwhile?

Chairpersons: Edmund J. Lewis and Cecil H. Coggins
Discussants: Clark D. West, Adrian Spitzer, Stephen W. Zimmerman,
John Lachin, William Winslade, and Daniel C. Cattran

The Workshop was structured to allow data to be presented from four studies
of the treatment of membranoproliferative glomerulonephritis, including a
discussion of the structure of clinical trials and the results of such trials
(West, Spitzer, Zimmerman, and Cattran). Presentation of these data and
conclusions were followed by an analysis of the principles of the construct
of a clinical trial by Lachin and the ethics of clinical trials by Winslade.

West began the discussion by describing his experience with the treatment
of membranoproliferative glomerulonephritis (MPGN) in 66 children. The
experience is based upon a nonprospective and uncontrolled approach to
the treatment of this disease. The approach is grounded upon his observation
that the clinical course of MPGN in patients who receive alternate-day prednisone therapy for prolonged periods (average follow-up period of 10 years)
is considerably better than historical controls taken from published series
by Habib in Paris, Cameron in London, and Davis in Boston. Thus, for
example, children treated by West had 100% survival of renal function at
6 years and 80% survival at 10 years; both of these statistics are considerably
better than the published data of others. End-stage renal disease had developed
in only 10% of the patients during the period of follow-up and 50% of
patients became free of proteinuria. The major adverse effect of therapy was
growth retardation. Because of the improved survival, and the appearance
of improved proteinuria, hematuria, and histology in patients rebiopsied more
than 2 to 5 years after therapy had begun, West believes that his uncontrolled
observations strongly favor the use of alternate-day prednisone in these patients. An additional point in favor of the effectiveness of prednisone, according to West, was his observation that the slowing of the rate of progression
of renal disease among children receiving long-term prednisone therapy was
often noted to reverse if therapy was stopped. West believes that he cannot,
in good conscience, administer a placebo to a control group. However, a

---

This is the Summary of a Workshop of a similar title.

controlled trial could conceivably be designed by comparing the West approach to an alternative form of therapy that had appeared to be successful elsewhere.

Spitzer represented the International Study of Kidney Diseases in Children. His data derived from a study of MPGN in children in which the effect of prednisone (40 mg/m^2) given every other day was compared to the administration of a lactose placebo. This regimen was given for a period of 5 years. A total of 40 children were assigned to the prednisone group; of these, 23 had type I MPGN. Twenty-eight children were assigned to the placebo group; of these, 14 patients had type I MPGN. Follow-up for a 2 year period was achieved in 16 patients in each group; 8 patients in each group were followed for 4 years. Analysis of this controlled trial revealed that there was a greater degree of maintenance of renal function in those children receiving prednisone as compared to those receiving lactose; this difference almost reaching statistical significance. There was no difference in the degree of proteinuria, and the evaluation of histopathology after 2 years revealed no significant differences with respect to glomerular sclerosis, mesangial hypercellularity, tubular atrophy, or interstitial fibrosis. The major drawback, however, was reflected by the fact that seven children in the prednisone-treated group had to be withdrawn from the trial because of severe hypertension, including encephalopathy. This compared with only two children in the lactose-treated placebo group. Hence, Spitzer concluded that prednisone appeared to be effective in preventing progression of renal dysfunction in type I MPGN in those patients who tolerated such therapy. However, prednisone therapy was associated with significant morbidity, particularly with respect to the onset of severe hypertension, so that the positive effects of prednisone were vitiated considerably by serious side effects.

Zimmerman presented the results of his study in which patients with MPGN were treated with warfarin and dicoumarol. This study employed a crossover design in which patients were assigned to either a placebo control or treatment group for 1 year and then were crossed over to the opposite therapy for the second year of study. Eighteen patients were entered into the study initially. Because patients were withdrawn from the study during the first year, only 13 patients were followed for a complete control and treatment year. During the first year of study, it was found that the loss of renal function was significantly greater in the control group than in the treated group. Only one of eight patients in the anticoagulant-treated group increased the serum creatinine concentration more than 0.2 mg/dl, while 6 of 10 patients in the control group experienced this degree of increase. When all of the groups were analyzed, the patients who received anticoagulants first did better with respect to renal function. Patients treated for 1 year in the control group and then treated with anticoagulants did not appear to show a beneficial effect during the second year of therapy. Hence, anticoagulant therapy did appear to have some beneficial effect. However, significant bleeding complications were encountered. Seven of nine patients had some bleeding abnormality, including a bleeding peptic ulcer, cerebral vascular accident, menorrhagia, and the development of an abdominal wall hematoma. The results of the Zimmerman study showed a potentially beneficial effect of anticoagulant therapy on kidney function; however, the adverse side effects were very significant.

Cattran presented the results of the cooperative study of MPGN carried out in Canada. In this study, dicoumarol, dipyridamole, and cyclosphophamide were compared against a control group receiving no medications. Fifty-nine patients entered the trial; 27 patients were in the treatment group and 32 were in the control group. Analysis of the data at 6, 9, and 12 months failed to reveal any difference in renal function or proteinuria. Some patients in the therapeutic group had significant complications, including leukopenia and bleeding abnormalities. Cattran concluded that there was no significant benefit of anticoagulant-immunosuppressive therapy in the treatment of MPGN.

Lachin reviewed the principles of design for a controlled clinical trial. He emphasized that randomization is the cornerstone of a controlled trial. This means that patients are assigned to therapy on the basis of chance, thus eliminating selection bias. Masking, or blinding, implies that the investigator is not aware of the treatment regimen to which the patient has been assigned. This therefore eliminates bias according to the outcome of the trial. Lachin then further described various aspects of study design and data management that would minimize the entry of bias into a controlled trial. In addition, he indicated that any trial required an estimate of patient entry requirements in order that false-positive and false-negative conclusions are avoided.

Winslade discussed some of the aspects of the ethics of a clinical trial. He indicated that two important factors must be considered as the ethical basis for scientific research in a controlled clinical trial. First, he noted that the investigation must consider the so-called "cost-benefit" approach. That is, the benefits of trial therapy must outweigh the risks. Second, the investigator must reflect upon the value of the patient's personal autonomy when entering into a trial. Hence, the patient should ideally be aware not only of the possible benefits and risks of treatment, but also the alternative benefits and risks from therapies other than those under study. He stressed the critical need for detailed and informed consent in the development of a randomized trial. In addition, he felt that the ethics of the randomized trial were satisfied more easily when one was testing two treatments, both of which were believed to be of possible value, instead of one therapy versus a placebo.

The discussion at the end of these presentations involved questions relative to the ethics and conduct of trials with respect to our present level of ignorance in the treatment of glomerular diseases. Ferris (Louisville, Ky, USA) stated that the editorial boards of medical journals should bear a responsibility for the dissemination of information about treatment that did not include controlled observations. He felt that journals should bear considerable guilt over disseminating inaccurate information derived from uncontrolled studies, and therefore should only accept observations that resulted from controlled trials. Couser (Seattle, Wash, USA) questioned just why practitioners appear to have difficulty accepting the results of controlled clinical trials, even though the observations appear to indicate a clear advantage to one of the groups in the trial. As an example, he spoke of the hesitation on the part of some to use prednisone in the treatment of patients with membranous glomerulone-phritis, despite the results of the Coggins study.

Discussion ensued thereafter on the problems of convincing physicians that the results of controlled trials may not necessarily support past dogma. A quotation taken from the writings of Count Leo Tolstoy seemed appropriate; he wrote: "I know that most men . . . not only those considered clever, but even those who are clever and capable of understanding the most difficult scientific, mathematical, or philosophic problems . . . can seldom discern even the simplest and most obvious truth if it be such as obliges them to admit the falsity of conclusions they have formed, perhaps with much difficulty . . . conclusions of which they are proud, which they have taught to others, and on which they have built their lives."

The deliberations of this Workshop reflected the importance of carrying out clinical trials in order to provide a firm basis for the treatment of glomerular diseases. Presented were examples of uncontrolled experiments (West) that must be undertaken if we are to know what therapies to test. Spitzer demonstrated that a controlled trial could provide information on efficacy; however, his data emphasized the need for adequate patient numbers and the importance for one to consider all outcomes, positive and negative, in the interpretation of any trial. Zimmerman echoed this conclusion and reflected on the problems of small numbers of patients in a cross-over studies. Cattran was able to demonstrate the lack of efficacy in the regimen that he studied, but he too was plagued by small numbers of patients. Nonetheless, his conclusions appeared to be valid at a reasonable confidence level. The studies demonstrated the value and pitfalls of clinical trials and emphasized their need.

Infections

Current Concepts in the Management of Urinary Tract Infections

Chairpersons: A. William Asscher and Jan Winberg
Discussants: M. P. Glauser, Renée Kuytens, Roland Möllby, James A. Roberts, and Kate Verrier-Jones

The management of urinary tract infections (UTI) has two objectives: to minimize morbidity and to prevent kidney damage. Despite the numerous potent antibacterial agents now available, both morbidity and mortality from UTI at all ages are still considerable. Up to 60 per 1000 consultations in primary care centers are on account of symptoms that suggest UTI; namely, frequency and dysuria and loin pain and fever. Chronic pyelonephritis (CPN) remains the second most common cause of end-stage kidney failure, accounting for 17% of the patients treated in European dialysis and transplant units. There are several possible explanations for why therapy fails.

The symptoms of UTI may not be due to bacterial infection. The observation that 50% of the patients with frequency and dysuria do not show "significant" numbers of bacteria in the urine (that is, $>10^5$ organisms/ml of urine) has been used as evidence for the existence of the entity known as abacterial cystitis or the urethral syndrome. Whereas it is true that some patients with frequency and dysuria do show a sterile urine culture, many such patients, particularly those with pyuria, do show lesser numbers of bacteria in the urine. To claim that such findings are not significant shows a basic misunderstanding of the concept of significant bacteriuria. It was introduced as an epidemiological tool for the detection of covert infection and was never intended as an aid to the diagnosis of symptomatic UTI. In symptomatic patients, the presence of pus cells and small numbers of bacteria can be highly significant and their eradication can bring relief of symptoms. Some of the so-called abacterial cystitis is attributable to the abuse of colony counts for the diagnosis of symptomatic UTI. Other reasons for the failure to reduce the morbidity from UTI include a neglect in recognizing the role of bacteria that are not usually regarded as urinary pathogens; for example, staphylococcus epidermidis, CO_2-dependent bacteria, and chlamydial organisms. So-called, abacterial cystitis is also partly attributable to bad history taking; for example, missing the fact that burning and frequency can result from

---

This is the Summary of a Workshop by the same title.

pruritis vulvae and excoriation of the external urethral orifice. Such a diagnosis can also be attributable to incomplete physical examination; for example, missing a urethral carbuncle as the cause of frequency and dysuria. In short, if meticulous attention is paid to history taking, physical examination, urine microscopy, and culture results, the enigma of abacterial cystitis largely vanishes.

A further reason for failure to eliminate morbidity and mortality from UTI could be lack of detection and treatment of covert UTI. In pregnancy, treatment of covert UTI prevents acute pyelonephritis. In the elderly and in patients with impaired defenses or indwelling catheters, treatment of covert UTI may prevent death from gram-negative septicemia. In other age groups, screening and treatment of covert infections have so far failed to prevent symptomatic recurrences. In fact, short courses of treatment such as those that might be used on a large scale are followed by reinfections, which are more often symptomatic than if the original infecting strains were left untreated. This suggests that patients with covert UTI have developed a symbiotic host–parasite relationship. The nature of this relationship is becoming clearer as we learn more about the surface structure of urinary pathogens and its relevance to virulence. Screening for and treatment of covert UTI have also failed to reduce kidney damage, at least after the age of 5 years. There are now numerous prospective studies to confirm this.

The tendency to repeated symptomatic UTI may be genetically determined. Associations between ABO blood groups, secretor status, and blood group P have been described. Because blood group determinants are also found on the periurethral cells, it is possible that a susceptibility to repeated UTI relates to the binding of urinary pathogens to the sugar determinants of the blood groups expressed on the periurethral cells. Of particular interest in this regard is the blood group substance P, whose disaccharide determinant (D-galactose $\frac{1-4}{\alpha}$ galactose) is the attachment site for P-fimbriated *Escherichia coli.* As yet, there are no therapeutic applications for these findings. Women with recurrent UTI still have to rely on long-term low-dose prophylaxis with drugs that have the least effect on the resistance pattern of the bowel flora. In this respect, trimethoprim has proved the most outstanding drug for long-term prophylaxis. In the case of patients in whom the infections are precipitated by sexual intercourse, the prophylaxis need only be used postcoitally. In children, urodynamic abnormality, particularly detrusor/sphincter dyssynergia, have been claimed to predispose to symptomatic UTI, and bladder training has been alleged to bring relief.

The prevention of kidney damage following UTI poses enormous problems. Prospective studies of the natural history of UTI have shown that kidney damage from febrile UTI occurs at a very early age. Experimental studies show that kidney scarring from infection can only be prevented if treatment is started very soon after the initiation of the infection. This, together with the fact that UTI in the young is difficult to diagnose because of the absence of localized symptoms and the difficulty of obtaining uncontaminated urine samples, may explain why infective kidney scars remain so common. The prevalence of infective kidney scars in surveys of apparently healthy schoolgirls has been shown to be up to 1 in 200. The lesson is that the urine must be looked at microscopically and cultured in *all* febrile children who lack localizing symptoms or signs and that treatment must be started *at once* if evidence of infection is found.

There has been a considerable advance in the understanding of the pathogenesis of kidney scarring caused by infection. Until recently, it was suggested that kidney scars can only occur if UTI exists in the presence of severe vesicoureteric reflux (VUR) sufficient to produce intrarenal reflux (IRR). The view is still widely held that this is the reason why kidney scars occur only in the young, since VUR of sufficient severity to cause IRR rarely occurs after the age of 4 because of the maturation of the vesicoureteric junction. There is now also evidence that IRR and kidney scarring can occur in the absence of VUR as a result of high intrapelvic pressure. The pressure is created by paralysis of ureteric peristalsis, which is possibly due to the effect of bacterial endotoxin; IRR caused by whatever mechanism delivers bacteria to the kidney. Certain types of *E. coli* are now known to be especially nephropathogenic. More than 90% of the organisms isolated from children with acute pyelonephritis have been shown to be P-fimbriated strains. These organisms adhere to human, monkey, and possibly mouse urothelium because they bind to the gal-gal receptors on the host cells. It has been suggested that fimbrial adhesion accounts for the ascent of organisms to the kidney in the absence of VUR. One group claims that P-fimbriation is a characteristic of the bacteria present in fresh urine in patients with acute pyelonephritis. Others claim that fresh isolates in patients with acute pyelonephritis lack fimbriae, for the urine, by virtue of its low iron content and high osmolality, is a poor culture medium for the expression of fimbriae. It is thus open for discussion whether P-fimbriae are virulence markers or virulence effectors. Whether the fact that P-fimbriae *E. coli* show nephropathogenicity and the discovery of a simple slide agglutination test for the detection of P-fimbriation will contribute to primary prevention is a matter for future research.

The mechanism of the scarring has also been the subject of a number of recent studies. Their polar location has been related to the configuration of the compound renal papillae that are confined to the upper and lower poles and allow IRR. For a scar to form, an inflammatory reaction has to take place. The interaction between urinary pathogens and inflammatory cells leads to exocytosis of lysosomal enzymes, which produces acute tissue damage followed by scarring. These new concepts of the pathogenesis of kidney scarring open up exciting new avenues of therapy. In experimental models of infective kidney scarring, immunization against P-fimbriae, white cell depletion with colchicine, and superoxide dismutase administration have all been shown to ameliorate kidney scarring.

Long-term follow-up studies have shown that kidney scars established in childhood have three important consequences in later life. They are: rise of blood pressure, which often appears when oral contraception is started or during pregnancy; persistent bacteriuria, which leads to a greater frequency of symptomatic UTI; and progressive kidney impairment with eventual development of end-stage kidney failure. The last of these events is fortunately very rare and affects at most 0.5% of children with kidney scars. The more extensive the initial scarring, the more likely the progression to kidney failure is. The relationship between the isolated scars caused by UTI in childhood and progressive impairment of kidney function is still not clear. Neither continuing VUR nor continuing infection play a part in this progression. Hypertension may contribute, but most important of all is the development of a glomerulopathy. Virtually all children with infective scars who show progressive impairment of kidney function show proteinuria in excess of 1 g/d. This finding supports the view that there must be a glomerular lesion. It has been suggested that hyperfiltration by healthy glomeruli in the non-scarred kidney tissue may lead to proteinuria and focal glomerulosclerosis, which eventually produces kidney failure. Although this is a likely explanation for the glomerular disease, the possibility that immune complex deposition in the glomeruli causes the glomerulopathy cannot be ruled out. Putative antigens in these immune complexes include bacteria and kidney-derived antigens including Tamm-Horsfall protein.

Treatment of Glomerular Diseases

Treatment of Glomerulonephritis Based on Knowledge of Its Pathogenesis

J. Stewart Cameron

Ideally, treatment of any disease should grow naturally from an understanding of the mechanisms that produce the disorder. In practice, this is rarely the case. Progress in treatment proceeds in a crabwise fashion, and the greatest effort has to be devoted to discarding forms of treatment thought to be effective but which have never been tested critically before acceptance. Doctors have always been eager to administer active treatment, whether or not the "treatment" has any basis in a framework of knowledge about the condition, or even empirical observations suggesting an effect on the disease. In this they have been abetted by their patients' belief that for every disease there is a treatment; a delusion also fostered by most medical textbooks. However, we must also admit at the outset that we are as yet relatively incapable of altering the course of most chronic or progressive renal diseases. The principal advances in the management of these disorders have been the treatment of edema by powerful diuretics, the elimination of infection in nephrotic or uremic patients by antibiotics, and the restoration of blood pressure toward normal levels by hypotensive agents.

What are the implications for treatment of our present ideas on the pathogenesis of nephritis [1] (Table 1)? Clearly we cannot yet alter an individual's genetic makeup, but in the future we may be able to alter the phenotypic expression of this makeup in regard to immune responses, although the complexity of control mechanisms governing the response to antigen challenge makes this, for the moment, a daunting task [2]. However, in the spontaneous lupus nephritis of the NZB/NZW mouse, Adelman, Watling, and McDevitt [3] have used anti-Ia (DR) antibody, and Hahn and Ebling [4] anti-idiotype antibody to switch off anti-DNA antibody to minimize nephritis and prolong survival. Obviously to reduce the overall incidence of glomerulonephritis in the world, one effort should be toward improvement of the environment and of nutrition. Although the interaction of malnutrition and the immune response is an extremely complicated one [5], it seems likely that an improve-

---

This manuscript was presented as part of a Symposium on *The Treatment of Glomerulonephritis.*

Table 1. Possible modes of treatment for glomerulonephritis

Aim	Means
Removal of inciting antigen	
From the environment	Public health measures
From the patient	Remove tumors, treat infections, remove infected prostheses
From the plasma	Plasmapheresis
Alter immune balance of patient	
Suppress or remove antibody	Plasmapheresis, immunosuppression, anti-idiotypic antibody
Improve antibody responses	Immunomodulating drugs, anti-idiotypic antibody, nutrition
	Anti-T cell or B cell antibody and DR antibody
Solubilize immune complexes	Add excess antigen; improve complement function; competing cationic protein
Increase reticuloendothelial function	? Plasmapheresis
Inhibit or remove mediators of injury	
Complement	Plasmapheresis, anticomplement drugs
Fibrin	Antithrombin drugs
Kinins	Serine protease inhibitors
Monocytes { Proteases	?
Vasoactive amines	Antiserotonin and antihistamine drugs
Prostaglandins	Cyclo-oxygenase inhibitors } antimonocyte antibody
Platelets { Thromboxane	Thromboxane synthetase inhibitors } antiplatelet drugs
Leukotrienes	Lipoxygenase inhibitors
Lymphokines	?
Inhibit nonimmunologic injury	
Glomerulosclerosis	Dietary restriction of phosphorous, nitrogen, or calories
Hypertension	Hypotensive agents

ment in nutrition worldwide would cut down the incidence of glomerulonephritis.

Antigen Elimination

What about the elimination of the immunizing pathogen? In Europe, we no longer have malaria, cholera, and plague; hepatitis is uncommon, and leprosy has retreated to a few tiny pockets. In the Third World all these, schistosomiasis, filiariasis, and many other infections are common. However, the difficulties of generating hard data in this situation are evident. All the more credit that a mine doctor, Giglioli, working in Guyana between the great wars, should have been able to demonstrate the link between the elimination of *Plasmodium malariae* and a fall in the incidence of the nephrotic syndrome from 2.8% of all admissions to only 0.05% [6].

More data are available on the elimination of antigens from the host, but even here there are only a handful of cases recorded. (The implications of our failure to identify antigens in the majority are discussed later.) The principal evidence comes from persisting postinfectious glomerulonephritis, when the offending organism can be identified and eliminated. Recovery after treatment has been shown for syphilis [7], streptococcal or staphylococcal infection of heart valves [8], and predominantly staphylococcal infection of juguloatrial shunts inserted for hydrocephalus [9]. In the last two groups, recovery of function can be remarkable and unexpected in response to treatment, as in one of our patients who had an infected juguloatrial shunt and who required peritoneal dialysis for mesangiocapillary glomerulonephritis (MCGN). After treatment for the infecting staphylococcus, he achieved a glomerular filtration rate (GFR) of 30 ml/min for a while. Another, with an infected intracardiac synthetic (Dacron™) patch and MCGN, made a complete recovery to normal urine and renal function from severe uremia and a nephrotic syndrome after the prosthesis was removed. Boulton-Jones et al [9] reported a nurse, again with MCGN, requiring peritoneal dialysis. At this point it was discovered that for some years she had been injecting herself with triple toxoid containing pertussis, diphtheria, and tetanus antigens. After she stopped these injections, renal function recovered remarkably, leaving her proteinuria-free and with normal renal function. Beaufils et al [10] reported 11 patients in whom crescentic glomerulonephritis was associated with deep-seated sepsis. Prompt elimination of the infecting organisms led to complete recovery of renal function in four, whereas four of the remaining patients in whom infection could not be controlled died.

Recovery of glomerulonephritis has been reported also in tumor-associated nephrotic syndromes after tumor removal, but it usually occurs in patients with Hodgkin disease and a "minimal change" histology. Lokich, Galvanek, and Moloney [11] reported complete remission, and Froom et al [12] clinical remission with persistence of glomerular deposits, in presumed immune-complex nephritis associated with Hodgkin disease when this condition was treated. Cantrell [13] described remission of a nephrotic syndrome when a carcinoma of the stomach was removed, but the histology of the kidney was not examined. Couser et al [14] reported complete histologic and clinical remission in a patient bearing a carcinoma of the colon after resection of the growth. Tumor antigen was demonstrated in the glomeruli before removal of the tumor, and was absent after. Finally, Barton, Vaziri, and Spear [15] described complete remission of a nephrotic syndrome in a woman with carcinoma of the breast who also had membranous nephropathy, when this was treated by mastectomy and chemotherapy.

Probably, however, the most common form of remission in response to disappearance of infecting antigen is in transient postinfectious glomerulonephritis associated with, for example, typhoid [16], Epstein-Barr virus [17], or hepatitis B [18].

Secondary Autologous Responses

There is, however, one notable exception to the rule that identification of a pathogen, and its successful treatment, leads to remission of the disease: this is *Plasmodium malariae* [19]. A problem in this condition is to know whether parasite antigen remains within the reticuloendothelial system, or in privileged sites such as the renal medulla, in sufficient quantities to continue immunization, even though replicating parasites may have been eliminated from the circulation. However, this failure raises the question whether secondary autologous immune responses may be important in the pathogenesis—and especially the persistence—of glomerulonephritis. If this mechanism is important, it might explain why it has proved so difficult to find antigens in glomeruli and immune complexes; it could be not that they are present in only small amounts, or are masked by immunoglobulins or complement, but that after the initiating events they are no longer present. These secondary immune mechanisms must involve some induction of auto-immunity. It is now well known that such auto-antibody is regularly induced as part of the T-cell independent polyclonal antibody response to many acute and chronic infections [20, 21]—witness the positive antinuclear factor tests, together with other auto-antibodies, in many patients and animals suffering from acute or chronic infections.

Endotoxin, known to induce polyclonal B-cell activation, can induce anti-DNA antibody and kidney-fixing DNA-anti-DNA complexes in mice [22]. We and others [23] have shown that mice infected with malaria develop anti-DNA antibody and anti-DNA complexes, and that immune complexes persist in the kidney after malarial antigens and antimalarial antibody can be demonstrated. Anti-DNA complexes are also present in the kidney in murine *Schistosoma mansoni* infections [24], and in humans. In our laboratory, Adu et al have shown [25] that anti-ssDNA antibody is common in malaria, and in Ghanian patients with apparent idiopathic nephrotic syndrome; moreover, Lewis and Roberts [26] have shown DNA-anti-DNA complexes in idiopathic nephritis, and Williams et al (unpublished) have demonstrated dsDNA and dsDNA complexes to be regularly present in sera specimens from patients with poststreptococcal nephritis, but not pneumococcal pneumonia. There is also evidence of the participation of anti-idiotypic antibodies in glomerular deposits of both mice injected with the polyclonal B cell stimulator lipopolysaccharide [27] and also in rabbits with chronic serum sickness [28]. In addition, there is growing evidence that antibody directed against specific epitopes may recognize these small epitopes in a variety of macromolecules, thus allowing multiple cross-reactions with antigens other than the main immunizing agent [29, 30].

There is also growing evidence that antiglobulins ("rheumatoid factors") are involved in glomerular immune deposits, both in poststreptococcal glomerulonephritis [31, 32] and possibly other idiopathic glomerulonephritides, as well as the classical mixed "essential" cryoglobulinemia [33]. Mixed cryoglobulins also contain anti-idiotypic antibodies [34].

Manipulation of the Immune Response

The implications of this hypothesis for treatment are clear; only modulation of this secondary phase of auto-immunization will make a difference if secondary mechanisms are the most important factor in the persistence and progression of the disease. Although detailed manipulation of the immune response is already possible (for example, by the selective injection of anti-idiotype antibody [4], or of antibody directed against surface antigens of specific subsets of reacting cells [3]), our knowledge is too fragmentary as yet to allow the clinical use of this possibility—for the moment.

Clearly, also, if circulating immune complexes represent only a residue— or even an epiphenomenon in most human glomerulonephritis [1]—then their removal by plasmapheresis or plasma filtration may achieve nothing in terms of direct inhibition of injury, although it might achieve an alteration in immune balance by removal of regulatory immune complexes [35], unloading the reticuloendothelial system [36], or dissociation of complexes on site by removal of circulating free antigen and antibody. However, the technique in its present form is far too blunt and nonspecific to achieve the former. In this model, plasmapheresis might of course achieve something by removal of the separately circulating antigen and antibody going to form in situ or insoluble complexes within the kidney, and of course immunosuppressive regimes could inhibit antibody formation, and thus be as effective—or ineffective—as pictured by the preformed soluble complex model. Pusey and Lockwood review these aspects of treatment in detail elsewhere in this section. I do not propose to deal here either with the nature of specific anti-GBM antibody or with the possible immunomodulation of its production; we now realize that its production is a transient affair in both human disease [37] and animal models, and it is possible that immunomanipulation may soon play a role in its treatment.

However, most forms of human glomerulonephritis seem to relate to the combination of antibody with nonrenal antigen (although a proportion of membranous nephropathy may be the result of fixation of antibody to an intrinsic but discontinuously distributed glomerular capillary wall antigen as in Heymann nephritis—and even here anti-idiotype antibody may play a role [Abrass and Cohen, unpublished observations]. If the induction of nephritis relates to a relative immunoincompetence in clearing foreign antigens, as many believe [38], the patients should benefit from immune stimulation in the direction of a greater and more avid immune response. At the moment, the tools needed to achieve this response are beyond the horizon. Both Bacille Calmette Guerin vaccine (BCG) and the antihelminthic levamisole have been used in a number of situations to stimulate the immune response [39], but their use in glomerulonephritis has been limited, although a few anecdotal reports of levamisole therapy have appeared for systemic lupus erythematosus [40, 41]. A disturbing incidence of agranulocytosis and failure to affect the disease have led to no further trials.

Extracorporeal removal of antibody, perhaps of poor affinity forming the complexes, is another goal that might be attempted if the antigen is known. To date this approach has only been used experimentally to deplete anti-DNA and anti-GBM antibody [42, 43]. Anti-idiotypic antibodies could be removed in the same way.

The use of immunosuppressive drugs is dealt with in the next Section, since it is my belief that any benefit that might have accrued from these drugs is likely to have resulted more from inhibition of inflammatory responses than suppression of immune responses. However, both azathioprine and particularly cyclophosphamide depress both humoral and cell-mediated immune responses in humans [44], and it was for this reason that they were first given to patients with glomerulonephritis. It is well documented that circulating antibody to identifiable antigen (for example, DNA) is suppressed by corticosteroids, azathioprine, and particularly cyclophosphamide (see below).

Finally, there is evidence from experimental nephritis in rabbits [45] and mice [46] that the administration of a huge excess of antigen to animals given bovine serum albumin (BSA) nephritis will elute complexes from the kidney. Not surprisingly, this approach is yet to be applied in humans! The possibility also arises of using competing cationic substances to displace cationic antigen bound to the GBM [47].

Glomerular Injury and its Inhibition

Before we can consider the inhibition of glomerular injury, we must take a brief look at what we know about how that injury comes about. We know a good deal about acute, potentially reversible injury in experimental animals [48, 49], but our need is to understand chronic, irreversible glomerular injury in humans, and in particular the genesis of glomerulosclerosis.

There are numerous humoral and cellular systems capable of inducing inflammation, which are mutually sustaining and interlocked at many points in their function [50]. To some extent, therefore, it is arbitrary to consider them separately. What is certain is that fixed antibody, either combined with glomerular antigen or as an immune aggregate, is capable of entering these multiple pathways at several points, principally through the activity of the Fc part of the molecule.

A number of studies have given a fairly complete picture of the routes of injury in anti-GBM nephritis, both acute and chronic serum sickness, and Heymann nephritis in animals (Table 2). The best studied (but not necessarily the most important) mechanisms of injury have been those involving polymorphonuclear leukocytes and complement [48, 49]. Polymorphs are capable of exerting an influence through the secretion of inflammatory substances and proteases, but are dependent in many situations for their recruitment upon the activation of the complement system, with release of leukotactic proteins and peptides during cleavage of C3 and C5. Complement was, until recently, thought only capable of inducing tissue damage through fixing and attracting polymorphs and monocytes; but recently, the role of C3b in solubilizing immune complexes has been emphasized [51, 52]. Interpretation of the finding of C3 at a site of injury is therefore now complicated, since it

Table 2. Modes of glomerular injury in experimental glomerulonephritis

| | Type of glomerulonephritis | | | |
| | Anti-GBM antibody nephritis | | Acute serum sickness | Heymann or "planted" antigen |
Mediator	Heterologous	Autologous accelerated		
Complement	+++	+	−	+++
Polymorphs	+++	+++	−	−
Monocytes	? −	+++	+++	? −
Fibrin	−	+++	++	? −
Platelets	−	++[a]	++	+ ?
"Other"	+++	?	?	?

[a] Proteinuria only; fibrin-dependent injury is platelet-independent.

may indicate complex dissolution rather than injury. Also, Groggel et al have described a new polymorph-independent function of the C5–9 attack complex of complement; the induction of proteinuria in passive Heymann nephritis and in "planted" antigen nephritis characterized by a membranous nephropathy and subepithelial deposits [53]. If this mechanism operates in humans, it might explain how in human membranous nephropathy there is usually profuse proteinuria in the absence of obvious glomerular proliferation or infiltration.

In human nephritis, we are reasonably sure of the pathogenesis of injury in only one situation: the formation of "crescents" of cells within Bowman's space [48, 49], often found complicating forms of endocapillary nephritis, but also in association with necrotizing glomerulitis/vasculitis and anti-GBM nephritis. The events that have been identified are familiar and include gaps in the capillary basement membrane, leakage of fibrin into the extracapillary space, proliferation of local epithelial cells, and infiltration with monocytes. Unfortunately, we are much less sure of the genesis of chronic endocapillary injury, especially that leading to glomerulosclerosis rather than healing.

Recently, however, two newer candidates for mediators of injury in both experimental and human nephritis have been advanced: monocytes [54] and platelets [55]. Since I have reviewed the role of platelets in glomerulonephritis elsewhere [55] and Donadio will consider the topic in detail elsewhere in this Section, I will not consider them further; but it is worth making a few points about macrophages [54]. These are potent cells that release a large range of products, many of them inflammatory. Their presence in human disease is well documented, above all, in forms of "proliferative" glomerulonephritis; and in animal models of both anti-GBM disease and serum sickness, they have been shown to be essential for the induction of proteinuria. Further, bearing as they do DR antigens, they are a resident population of antigen-presenting cells capable of initiating an immune response, which further adds to the properties of hemodynamics and charge by which the glomerulus is far from being an innocent bystander in immune injury.

Given these many mediators of inflammation listed in Table 2, how can we inhibit them? Corticosteroids, cytotoxic drugs, and anti-inflammatory agents have all been used in the treatment of glomerulonephritis, as have antiplatelet agents and antithrombin drugs. In many instances, these have been used together, in the reasonable but unproven belief that inhibition of several channels of fluid phase or cellular inflammation would produce better results than inhibition of only one.

One major problem with any assessment of treatment regimens is to assure homogeneity of patients. Perhaps only in the case of anti-GBM disease can we achieve this, since all our other histological classifications (membranous nephropathy, mesangiocapillary glomerulonephritis, and so on) merely describe identifiable and consistent patterns of response to injury on the part of the glomerulus, which may (as in the case of membranous nephropathy and in situ complex formation) or may not bear any relation to fundamental pathogenesis; certainly in terms of identifiable antigen-antibody systems we know they are not specific [48].

Corticosteroids

Corticosteroids have been used in proliferative glomerulonephritis, mostly in the belief that they would inhibit particularly cell-released inflammatory substances [54]. Two controlled trials organized by the British Medical Research Council, one of prednisone alone [56] and one of prednisone plus azathioprine [57], failed to show an effect, as did our own small trial of the same combination [58]. Following encouraging reports from McEnery, McAdams, and West on long-term alternate-day prednisone in children with MCGN [59], the International Study of Kidney Disease in Children organized a controlled trial [60]. After 6 years of effort, it is obvious that the regimen (60 mg on alternate days) is by no means free of side effects; unfortunately the number of dropouts from the test group has been large enough more or less to vitiate the trial, although there is a suggestion of benefit for those who were able to continue the treatment.

Corticosteroids have also been used extensively in membranous nephropathy without evident effect; two early trials did not show any difference between control and treated patients [61], but in retrospect did not contain enough patients to answer the question either way. Then, in 1979, the results of the Interhospitals Collaborative Trial in adult nephrotic patients with membranous nephropathy were published [62]. This appeared to demonstrate that only 8 weeks' treatment with 125 mg of prednisone on alternate days was without significant toxicity and diminished the number of patients entering renal failure within the next 4 years. This trial has evoked much discussion. Some of the criticisms relate to the facts that the rate of entry into renal failure of the control group appeared greater than expected; not all eligible patients in all centers were put into the trial, a number of patients relapsed so far that proteinuria was concerned (an unusual pattern in previous experience), and repeat biopsy examinations to assess the incidence of interstitial nephritis from diuretics were not performed. Even so, the results stand, and a similar repeat trial has been under way since December 1981 in the United Kingdom, which now has nearly 100 patients entered in it; the results should be available for presentation at the ISN meeting in 1990.

The detailed treatment of lupus nephritis lies outside this article, but the use of corticosteroids is now standard [63], even though there is no controlled evidence that survival or morbidity is improved. With a single exception [64], all workers' retrospective uncontrolled data suggest that survival of patients with lupus nephritis, especially the more severe forms, has become dramatically superior since steroid treatment was introduced. Whether the addition of cytotoxic agents improves survival and morbidity, or allows lower doses of prednisone to be used is more controversial, although I share the belief of many that this is indeed the case [65]. Here, the heterogeneity of the patients has resulted in no less than six controlled trials failing to answer the question one way or another [66]. In severe lupus nephritis, i.v. methyl-prednisolone in doses of 1 g have been popular since its use was first described in 1974, and Bolton will discuss this topic. Whether equally good results could be obtained by oral or i.v. cytotoxic agents, or brief oral high-dose steroids has never been tested.

Finally, corticosteroids have been used to treat severe proliferative glomerulonephritis with extensive crescent formation. Results using "conventional" oral doses of prednisone, alone or in combination with cytotoxic agents, did not seem to us to show better than the 25 to 30% of improvement to be expected in untreated patients [67], and certainly did not benefit those with anti-GBM disease. However, from an analysis of approximately the same data base, Heaf, Jorgensen, and Nielsen [68] came to the conclusion that cytotoxic agents *did* aid those without oliguria. Bolton reviews the use of i.v. methylprednisolone and his own data elsewhere in this symposium.

Cytotoxic Agents

Turning to cytotoxic agents, I reviewed the controlled trials at the ISN meeting of 1975 in Florence [69]. The only trials that appeared to show a positive result were two short-term trials using cyclophosphamide in proliferative glomerulonephritis assessed at 1 year and 3 months following treatment. However, one semicontrolled trial showed an effect of chlorambucil in diminishing proteinuria, without a change in GFR, in patients with membranous nephropathy [70]. This prompted a recent Italian trial, which used alternate-month treatment with chlorambucil and prednisolone for 6 months. The most recent data in this trial [71] (which is still in progress) demonstrate a highly significant increase in remission rate, degree of proteinuria, and average plasma creatinine at 1 and 2 years. In view of the American results already discussed [62], it is not clear what role, if any, the chlorambucil may have had in this.

Anticoagulants

Anticoagulant drugs (antithrombin agents and antiplatelet drugs) have been used for 15 years, usually in combination with immunosuppressive regimens, and often in the most serious forms of glomerulonephritis characterized by crescent formation. The main justification is the known crucial role of extra-capillary fibrin formation in the genesis of crescents [48, 49] and the protective effects of admittedly toxic amounts of heparin and warfarin in experimental anti-GBM crescentic nephritis (reviewed in [72]). A number of accounts of such treatment in primary glomerulonephritis have been published, and when data from severely affected individuals with the majority of (>60%) of glomeruli showing occluding crescents are examined, renal function is found to be retained, regained, or improved in about 70 to 75% of the patients [72, 73] compared with 25 to 30% in untreated patients. However, in view of the similar results obtained with i.v. methylprednisolone discussed above, the latter has become more popular, including in our own unit.

Anticoagulants (warfarin plus dipyridamole) together with immunosuppressive agents have been used also in severe MCGN without extensive crescent formation, after encouraging anecdotes from Australia [74] and our own unit [66]. In passing, it is worth noting that most of our patients who showed initial improvement [75] went into renal failure subsequently. However, the subsequent Australian trial failed to show any effect over controls, perhaps because of poor recruitment of patients; the regimen used (warfarin, dipyridamole, and cyclophosphamide) did not contain corticosteroids. Likewise, the Toronto trial of the same combination [76] did not show any difference either. Finally, the defibrinating agent ancrod has been advocated recently for both idiopathic [77] and lupus nephritis. Despite this, the general mood is one of scepticism [78]. The hopes here are the preliminary results of Donadio's trial of dipyridamole alone in type I MCGN [79], which he discusses elsewhere in this volume, and the recent results from Zimmerman et al [80].

Finally, Futrakul, Poshyachimda, and Mitraku [81] have reported favorably on anticoagulation (heparin plus dipyridamole) in addition to immunosuppression (prednisone with or without cyclophosphamide) in nephrotic children with focal segmental glomerulosclerosis—the condition, besides MCGN, with the greatest acceleration of platelet turnovers.

Cyclosporin A

Recently, in our laboratory, Neild et al [82] demonstrated that in acute serum sickness nephritis, cyclosporin A (Cy A) would almost abolish the proteinuria of acute serum sickness nephritis, even when administered 4 days after the immunizing injection. How this might be achieved is not clear, since Cy A is not known to have any direct effect on monocytes; presumably, the signal for monocyte accumulation arises from some cell or system that is Cy A-dependent. Cy A has not been used in idiopathic nephritis, but results in nonrenal lupus were disappointing [83], with problems from nephrotoxicity that make the present agent unattractive.

Prostaglandins

Finally, we have to consider what role there may be for antagonists of prostaglandin of various types. Lianos, Andres, and Dunn [84] showed that in anti-GBM nephritis in the rat, not only was the fall of renal blood flow dependent on thromboxane production, but that the proteinuria correlated closely with thromboxane production. Trials of thromboxane synthetase antagonists (such as OKY 046) are only now being performed in nephritis; but Saito, Ideura, and Takeuchi reported recently a beneficial effect of 1-benzylimidazole in serum sickness nephritis [85], and we are currently investigating the effects of OKY 046 in experimental nephritis. How such agents might act is not clear, since both platelets and monocytes produce large amounts of thromboxanes. Ciabattoni et al [86] have demonstrated recently that sulindac lacks the effects on renal prostacyclin synthesis and does not depress the GFR as other prostaglandin synthetase inhibitors do, which makes it an attractive prospect. The possibility of using prostaglandins or prostaglandin analogues as therapeutic agents also holds promise; both spontaneous lupus of NZB/NZW mice and anti-GBM nephritis in rabbits are inhibited by prostaglandins of the E series [87].

Conclusions

What conclusions can we draw from all these attempts at controlled and uncontrolled trials of treatment aimed at the inhibition of glomerular inflammation? It must be admitted that we have failed to identify a group of patients in whom any of our treatments make a dramatic difference, with the possible exceptions of anti-GBM antibody nephritis, if caught before oliguria has set in, and of lupus nephritis. Less dramatic effects are possibly achievable in membranous nephropathy and uncertainly in crescentic nephritis and MCGN. This may be, in part, the result of the inadequate classification of nephritis into histologically similar but fundamentally diverse groups for trial allocation. But the suspicion persists that in the long run, we have made no great impact on the natural evolution of the bulk of primary glomerulonephritis with attempts at inhibiting glomerular inflammation. We may even be making things worse [88]. Certainly, we should not treat with toxic drugs unless we have at least reasonable clinical evidence to support the behavior.

Nonimmunologic Mechanism of Progression

Much interest has been generated recently in the possibility that nonimmunologic mechanisms may operate in most forms of progressive renal disease

[89, 90], including those in which the presumed initiation is through immuno-logical injury. Already, enough information is available to allow a tentative construction of vicious circles, which *could* lead to the perpetuation of damage without further intervention from either primary or secondary immunologic mechanisms. Old observations, substantiated in several recent studies, show that restriction of nitrogen (or phosphorus, or both) will increase survival in experimental nephrotoxic nephritis as well as prolong life after one and five-sixths nephrectomy in rats. Conversely, protein overload shortens life. It is worrying that all these data come from a species in which, without any manipulation of the kidney, dietary restriction prolongs life and spontane-ous focal glomerulosclerosis occurs with age, which can moreover be acceler-ated by protein feeding. Even so, there is evidence (admittedly uncontrolled) that dietary nitrogen restriction will prolong life in renal failure in humans. The first observations came from Kluthe et al [91] using a potato-egg diet, and later from Walser [92] using low-nitrogen diets supplemented by ketoacid analogues of essential amino acids. Others [93–95] have more recently made similar observations using conventional low-nitrogen diets, and particularly in early uremia a similar effect seems to be observed. So far, all the observations can be criticized on technical grounds, and no controlled trials are yet availa-ble.

The protein content of the diet may not be the only aspect that requires consideration. The complexity of the nutritional-immunological relation was noted at the beginning of this article, and in particular the quantity and type of fat in the diet greatly influences the expression of auto-immune disease in several species (reviewed in [96]), possibly through modifying prostaglandin synthesis, although this is by no means certain.

Role of Hypertension and Vascular Disease

What of the role of vascular disease and hypertension? It is well known that many normotensive patients with forms of glomerulonephritis that later prove progressive may show, even early in their disease, quite severe "hyaline" lesions of the afferent arterioles. These lesions are disproportionate to not only the blood pressure, but also the age of the patient [97]. These lesions are common, but infrequently commented upon, and have been observed in early systemic lupus erythematosus, early membranous nephropathy, mes-angiocapillary disease, and particularly focal glomerulosclerosis and IgA ne-phropathy. In our own study of the long-term evolution of membranous nephropathy [98], these lesions predicted a poor prognosis for renal function a decade later with some degree of precision, whereas severity of glomerular change did not. Their nature is quite unknown; in some cases, these vascular "deposits" stain for C3 complement or IgG (or both); in most they are nega-tive.

The intervention of hypertension in a patient with glomerulonephritis is regarded as a bad sign by most nephrologists, although the evidence for this in humans is slender. From studies of morbidity and mortality in patients with essential hypertension, it would be very unlikely to prove otherwise.

Despite this evidence, there have been no clinical trials of mild hypertension in patients with glomerulonephritis as yet, although data from diabetic patients is convincing [99]. Most nephrologists take a low threshold for treating blood pressure in patients with nephritis, and many would regard it as unethical, in view of data from primary essential hypertension, not to treat a group of patients with severe hypertensive glomerulonephritis for trial purposes. Thus, we may never find out from human studies what the clinical impact may be.

What is more interesting is the possibility that hypertension might exacerbate the glomerulonephritis by a mechanism *other* than ischemic glomerulosclerosis. Knowlton, as long ago as 1946 [100], superimposed desoxycorticosterone on nephrotoxic serum nephritis, and noted worsening of the glomerular disease.

How hypertension might induce glomerulosclerosis in a patient already suffering from primary glomerulonephritis is not clear. Several recent investigators have superimposed hypertension on experimental glomerulonephritis and found augmented proteinuria and renal damage [101–104]; this may be the result of glomerular hyperperfusion [105], as in the nephrectomy model, or it may be due to some secondary mechanism directed toward protecting the kidney from the hypertension itself. Of interest are the observations of Dworkin et al [106], who found that in the unilaterally nephrectomized rat with superimposed DOC hypertension, protein restriction independent of salt intake prolonged life and reduced renal damage.

The mechanisms of progression in glomerulonephritis are most likely to be those that apply generally to all forms of progressive renal disease, and some of these are nonimmunological at base. This may explain our relative failure to treat progressive glomerulonephritis by immune suppression or manipulation. By a combination of recent experiment and reinterpretation of older observations, a picture has emerged rapidly of hyperperfusion (or high-pressure perfusion) leading to progressive glomerulosclerosis, with an immediate prospect that late renal failure might be delayed to a certain extent by a reduction in dietary nitrogen, phosphorus, or total solute intake. The role of secondary autologous mechanisms, perhaps controlled via the major histocompatibility locus, seem to be of importance, at least in Western Europe where the majority of cases of glomerulonephritis do not arise from overwhelming infections and parasitemias. However, a search for persistent immunization is always worthwhile, since in the minority of patients in which this mechanism can be demonstrated, the disease may be controllable by removal of the antigenic stimulus, provided this can be achieved!

References

1. CAMERON JS: Glomerulonephritis: Current problems and understanding. *J Lab Clin Med* 99:755–787, 1982
2. NEILSON EG, ZAKHEIM B: T cell regulation, anti-idiotypic immunity and the nephritogenic immune response. *Kidney Int* 24:289–302, 1983
3. ADELMAN NE, WATLING DL, McDEVITT HO: Treatment of (NZB×NZW)F

disease with anti-I-A monoclonal antibodies. *J Exp Med* 158:1350–1355, 1983
4. HAHN BH, EBLING FM: Suppression of murine lupus nephritis by administration of an anti-idiotype antibody to antiDNA. *J Immunol* 132:187–190, 1984
5. GOOD RA: Nutrition and immunity. *J Clin Immunol* 1:3–11, 1981
6. GIGLIOLI G: Malaria and renal disease with special reference to British Guyana: II. The effect of malaria eradication on the incidence of renal disease in British Guiana. *Ann Trop Med Parasitol* 56:225–241, 1962
7. LOSITO A, BUCCARELLI E, MASI-BENEDETTI F, LATO M: Membranous glomerulonephritis in congenital syphilis. *Clin Nephrol* 12:32–37, 1979
8. KIM Y, MICHAEL AF: Chronic bacteremia and nephritis. *Annu Rev Med* 29:319–325, 1978
9. BOULTON-JONES JM, SISSONS JGP, NAISH PF, EVANS DJ, PETERS DK: Self-induced glomerulonephritis. *Br Med J* 3:387–390, 1974
10. BEAUFILS M, MOREL-MAROGER L, SRAER J-D, KANFER A, KOURILSKY O, RICHET G: Acute renal failure of glomerular origin during visceral abscesses. *N Engl J Med* 295:185–189, 1976
11. LOCKICH JJ, GALVANEK EG, MOLONEY WC: Nephrosis of Hodgkin's Disease. An immune complex-induced lesion. *Arch Intern Med* 132:597–600, 1973
12. FROOM DW, FRANKLIN WA, HANO JE, POTTER EV: Immune deposits in Hodgkin's disease with nephrotic syndrome. *Arch Pathol Lab Med* 94:547–553, 1972
13. CANTRELL EG: Nephrotic syndrome cured by removal of gastric carcinoma. *Br Med J* 2:739–740, 1969
14. COUSER WG, WAGONFELD JB, SPARGO BH, LEWIS EJ: Glomerular deposition of tumor antigen in membranous nephropathy associated with colonic carcinoma. *Am J Med* 57:962–970, 1974
15. BARTON CH, VAZIRI ND, SPEAR GS: Nephrotic syndrome associated with adeno-carcinoma of the breast. *Am J Med* 68:308–312, 1980
16. SITPRIJA V, PIPATANAGUL V, BOONPUCKNAVIG V, BOONPUCKNAVIG S: Glomerulitis in typhoid fever. *Ann Intern Med* 81:210–213, 1974
17. LEE S, KJELLSTRAND CM: Renal disease in infectious mononucleosis. *Clin Nephrol* 9:236–240, 1978
18. LEVY M, KLEINKNECHT C: Membranous glomerulonephritis and hepatitis B infection. *Nephron* 26:259–265, 1980
19. KIBUKAMUSOKE JW: *Nephrotic Syndrome of Quartan Malaria.* Bristol, Edward Arnold, 1973
20. MOLLER G, STROM H, AL-BALAGHI S: Role of polyclonal activation in specific immune responses. *Scand J Immunol* 12:177–182, 1980
21. GOODMAN MG: Cellular aspects of polyclonal activation of B lymphocytes. *Immunol Today,* Nov 1980, pp 92–96
22. IZUI S, LAMBERT PH, FOURINE GJ, TURLER H, MIESCHER PA: Features of systemic lupus erythematosus in mice injected with bacterial lipopolysaccharides: Identification of circulating DNA and renal localisation of DNA-anti-DNA complexes. *J Exp Med* 145:1115–1130, 1977
23. POELS LG, VAN NIEKERK CC, JERUSALEM C: Glomerulopathy in mice infected with *plasmodium berghei:* Induction of an auto-immune process. *Isr J Med Sci* 14:651–654, 1978
24. DANNO K, FUKUYAMA K, EPSTEIN WL: Renal deposition of antinuclear antibody in athymic mice infected with *Schistosoma mansoni. Lab Invest* 40:358–363, 1979
25. ADU D, WILLIAMS DG, QUAYKI I, VOLLER A, ANIM-ADDO A, BRUCE TAGOE AA, JOHNSON GD, HOLBOROW EJ: Anti-ssDNA and nuclear antibodies in human malaria. *Clin Exp Immunol* 49:310–316, 1982

26. LEWIS EJ, ROBERTS J: Is auto-immunity a common denominator in immune complex disease? *Lancet* 1:178–180, 1980

27. GOLDMAN M, ROSE LM, HOCHMANN A, LAMBERT PH: Deposition of idiotype anti-idiotype immune complexes in renal glomeruli after polyclonal B-cell activation. *J Exp Med* 133:1385–1399, 1982

28. ZANETTI M, WILSON CB: Participation of auto-anti-idiotypes in immune complex glomerulonephritis in rabbits. *J Immunol* 131:2781–2783, 1983

29. WILLIAMS RC: Antibodies in systemic lupus: Diversity finally simplified. *J Lab Clin Med* 100:161–164, 1982

30. COOKE A, LYDYARD PM, ROITT IM: Mechanisms of auto-immunity: A role for cross-reactive idiotypes. *Immunol Today* 4:170–175, 1983

31. MCINTOSH RW, GARCIA R, RUBIO L, RABIDEAU D, ALLEN JE, CARR RI, RODRIGUEZ-ITURBE B: Evidence for an autologous immune complex pathogenesis mechanism in acute post-streptococcal glomerulonephritis. *Kidney Int* 14:501–510, 1978

32. RODRIGUEZ-ITURBE B, RABIDEAU D, GARCIA R, RUBIO L, MCINTOSH RM: Characterization of the glomerular antibody in acute post-streptococcal glomerulonephritis. *Ann Intern Med* 92:478–481, 1980

33. MAGGIORE Q, BARTOLOMEO F, L'ABBATE A, MISERFARI V, MARTORANO C, CACCAMO A, BARBRANO DI BELGIOJOSO G, TARANTINO A, COLASANTI G: Glomerular localization of circulating antiglobulin activity in essential mixed cryoglobulinemia with glomerulonephritis. *Kidney Int* 21:387–394, 1982

34. GELTNER D, FRANKLIN EC, FRANGIONE B: Anti-idiotype activity in the IGM fractions of mixed cryoglobulins. *J Immunol* 125:1530–1535, 1980

35. THEOPHILOPOULOS AN, DIXON FJ: The biology and detection of immune complexes. *Adv Immunol* 28:89–220, 1979

36. LAWLEY TJ: Immune complexes and reticuloendothelial system function in human disease. *J Invest Dermatol* 74:339–343, 1980

37. LOCKWOOD CM, PETERS DK: Plasma exchange in glomerulonephritis and related vasculitides. *Annu Rev Med* 31:167–179, 1980

38. PETERS DK, LACHMANN PJ: Immunity deficiency in pathogenesis of glomerulonephritis. *Lancet* 1:58–60, 1974

39. EDITORIAL: Immunostimulation. *Lancet* 1:349–350, 1976

40. GORDON BL, YANAGIHARA R: Treatment of systemic lupus erythematosus with the T cell immunopotentiator levamisole: A follow-up report of sixteen cases under treatment for a minimum of four months. *Ann Allergy* 39:227–236, 1977

41. HADIDI T, DECKER JL, EL NAGDY L, SAMY M: Ineffectiveness of levamisole in systemic lupus erythematosus. *Arthritis Rheum* 24:60–63, 1981

42. TERMAN DS, BUFFALOE G, MATTIOZI C, COOK G, TILLQUIST R, SULLIVAN M, AYUS JC: Extracorporeal immunoadsorption: Initial experience in human systemic lupus erythematosus. *Lancet* 2:824–826, 1979

43. TERMAN DS, DURANTE D, BUFFALOE G, MCINTOSH R: Attenuation of canine nephrotoxic glomerulonephritis with an extracorporeal immunoabsorbent. *Scand J Immunol* 6:195–202, 1977

44. REES AJ, LOCKWOOD CM: Immunosuppressive drugs in clinical practice, in *Clinical Aspects of Immunology,* edited by LACHMANN TJ, PETERS DK, Oxford, Blackwell, 1982, pp 507–564

45. WILSON CB, DIXON FJ: The quantitation of acute and chronic serum sickness in the rabbit. *J Exp Med* 134(suppl):7s–18s, 1971

46. HAAKENSTAD AO, STRIKER GE, MANNIK M: Removal of glomerular immune complex deposits by excess antigen in chronic mouse model of immune complex disease. *Lab Invest* 48:323–331, 1983

47. ADLER S, WANG H, COHEN A, BORDER W: Electropharmacologic modulation

of in situ complex formation in experimental membranous nephropathy. *Abst Am Soc Nephrol,* 1981, p 68

48. WILSON CB, DIXON FJ: The renal response to immunological injury, in *The Kidney* (2nd ed), edited by BRENNER BM, RECTOR FC, Philadelphia, Saunders, 1981, pp 1237–1350

49. THOMSON NM, HOLDSWORTH SR, GLASGOW EF, PETERS DK, ATKINS RC: Mechanism of injury in experimental glomerulonephritis, in *Progress in Glomerulonephritis,* edited by KINCAID SMITH P, D'APICE AJF, ATKINS RC, New York, John Wiley & Son, p 51

50. ZIMMERMAN TS: The coagulation mechanisms and the inflammatory response, in *Clinical Immunopathology,* edited by MIESCHER PA, MULLER-EBERHARD HE, New York, Grune & Stratton, 1976, pp 95–115

51. NUSSENZWEIG V: Interaction between complement and immune complexes: Role of complement in containing immune complex damage, in *Immunology 80,* edited by FOUGEREAU M, DAUSSET J, New York, Pergamon Press, 1980, pp 1044–1052

52. SCHIFFERLI JA, MORRIS JM, DASH A, PETERS DK: Complement-mediated solubilisation in patients with systemic lupus erythematosus, nephritis or vasculitis. *Clin Exp Immunol* 46:557–564, 1981

53. GROGGEL GC, ADLER S, RENNKE G, COUSER WG, SALANT DJ: Role of the terminal complement pathway in experimental membranous nephropathy in the rabbit. *J Clin Invest* 72:1948–1957, 1983

54. COTRAN RS (Moderator): The role of monocytes and macrophages in glomerulonephritis. *Proc 8th Int Congr Nephrol, Athens,* Basel, Karger, 1981, pp 853–887

55. CAMERON JS: Platelet involvement in glomerulonephritis. *Annu Rev Med* 35:175–180, 1984

56. BLACK DAK, ROSE G, BREWER DE: Controlled trial of prednisone in adult patients with the nephrotic syndrome. *Br Med J* 3:421–426, 1970

57. MEDICAL RESEARCH COUNCIL: Controlled trial of azathioprine and prednisone in chronic renal disease: Report of a Medical Research Council Working Party. *Br Med J* 2:239–247, 1971

58. SHARPSTONE P, OGG CS, CAMERON JS: Nephrotic syndrome due to primary renal disease in adults: II. A controlled trial of prednisolone and azathioprine. *Br Med J* 2:535–539, 1969

59. MCENERY PT, MCADAMS AJ, WEST CD: Membranoproliferative glomerulonephritis: Improved survival with alternate day prednisone therapy. *Clin Nephrol* 13:117–124, 1980

60. INTERNATIONAL STUDY OF KIDNEY DISEASE IN CHILDREN: Membranoproliferative glomerulonephritis (MPGN): A double blind trial of alternate day prednisone (*abstract*). *Paediatr Res* 17:1000 (abst 140), 1980

61. CAMERON JS: Membranous nephropathy: The treatment dilemma. *Am J Kidney Dis* 1:371–375, 1982

62. COLLABORATIVE STUDY OF THE ADULT IDIOPATHIC NEPHROTIC SYNDROME: A controlled study of short-term prednisone treatment in adults with membranous nephropathy. *N Engl J Med* 301:1301–1306, 1979

63. GINZLER EM, BOKEL AJ, FRIEDMAN EA: The natural history and response to therapy of lupus nephritis. *Annu Rev Med* 31:463–487, 1980

64. ALBERT DA, HADLER NM, ROPES MW: Does corticosteroid therapy affect the survival of patients with systemic lupus erythematosus? *Arthritis Rheum* 22:945–953, 1979

65. ADU D, CAMERON JS: Lupus nephritis, in *Clinics in Rheumatic Diseases,* edited by HUGHES GRV, 1982, vol. 8, no. 1, pp 153–182

66. WAGNER L: Immunosuppressive agents in lupus nephritis: A critical analysis. *Medicine* 55:239–250, 1976
67. NEILD GH, CAMERON JS, OGG CS, TURNER DR, WILLIAMS DG, BROWN CB, CHANTLER C, HICKS J: Rapidly progressive glomerulonephritis with extensive crescent formation. *Q J Med* 52:395–416, 1983
68. HEAF JG, JORGENSEN F, NIELSEN LP: Treatment and prognosis of extracapillary glomerulonephritis. *Nephron* 35:217–224, 1983
69. CAMERON JS: The treatment of severe glomerulonephritis with combined immunosuppression and anticoagulation, in *Proc 6th Int Congr Nephrol, Montreal,* Basel, Karger, 1978, pp 419–424
70. LAGRUE G, BERNARD D, BARIÉTY J, DRUET P, GUEREL J: Traitement par le chlorambucil et l'azathioprine dans les glomerulonéphritis primitives: Resultats d'une étude "controlée." *J d'Urol Néphrol* 9:655–672, 1975
71. PONTICELLI C, ZUCCHELLI P, IMBASCIATI E, CAGNOLI L, POZZI C, GRASSI C, LIMIDO D, PASQUALI S, PASSERIN P, VOLPINI T, LOCATELLI F: Controlled trial of monthly alternated courses of steroid and chlorambucil for idiopathic membranous nephropathy. *Proc EDTA* 19:717–721, 1982
72. CAMERON JS: The treatment of glomerulonephritis with inhibitors of coagulation, in *Glomerulonephritis,* edited by KLUTHE R, VOGT A, BATSFORD S, New York, Wiley, 1977, pp 154–164
73. NAKAMOTO Y, DOHI K, FUJIOKA M, KIDA H, HATTORI N, TAKEUCHI J: Combined anticoagulant and immunosuppressive treatment in rapidly progressive glomerulonephritis (RPGN): A long term follow-up study. *Jpn J Med* 18:210–217, 1979
74. KINCAID-SMITH P: The treatment of chronic mesangiocapillary (membranoproliferative) glomerulonephritis with impaired renal function. *Med J Aust* 2:587–592, 1972
75. CHAPMAN SJ, CAMERON JS, CHANTLER C, TURNER D: Treatment of mesangiocapillary glomerulonephritis in children with combined immunosuppression and anticoagulation. *Arch Dis Child* 55:446–451, 1980
76. CATTRAN DC, CHARRON R, CARDELLA C, ROSCOE J, RITCHIE S, TIBSHIRANI R: Controlled trial on mesangiocapillary glomerulonephritis (MCGN). *Abst 8th Int Cong Nephrol,* Athens, 1981 Abst CN-177
77. POLLAK VE, GLUECK HI, WEISS MA, LEBRON BERGES A, MILLER MA: Defibrination with ancrod in glomerulonephritis: Effects on clinical and histologic findings and on blood coagulation. *Am J Nephrol* 2:195–207, 1982
78. BORDER WA: Anticoagulants are of little value in the treatment of renal disease. *Am J Kidney Dis* 1984, pp 308–312
79. DONADIO J JR, ANDERSON CF, MITCHELL JC, HOLLEY KE, ILSTRUP D, FUSLER V: Membranoproliferative glomerulonephritis (MPGN): A prospective trial of platelet inhibitor therapy (*abstract*). *Kidney Int* 14:649, 1982
80. ZIMMERMAN SW, MOORTHY V, DREHER WH, FRIEDMAN A, VARANSI U: Prospective trial of warfarin and dipyridamole in patients with membranoproliferative glomerulonephritis. *Am J Med* 75:911–919, 1983
81. FUTRAKUL P, POSHYACHINDA M, MITRAKUL C: Focal sclerosing glomerulonephritis: A kinetic evaluation of hemostasis and the effect of anticoagulant therapy; a controlled study. *Clin Nephrol* 10:180–186, 1978
82. NEILD GH, IVORY K, HIRAMATSU M, WILLIAMS DG: Cyclosporin A inhibits acute serum sickness in rabbits. *Clin Exp Immunol* 52:586–594, 1983
83. ISENBERG A, SNAITH ML, MORROW WJW, AL-KHADER AA, COHEN SL, FISHER C, MOWBRAY J: Cyclosporin A for the treatment of systemic lupus erythematosus. *Int J Immunopharmacol* 3:163–169, 1981
84. LIANOS EA, ANDRES GA, DUNN MJ: Glomerular prostaglandin and thrombox-

ane synthesis in rat nephrotoxic serum nephritis. *J Clin Invest* 72:1439–1448

85. SAITO K, IDEURA T, TAKEUCHI J: Effects of a selective thromboxane A$_2$ synthetase inhibitor on immune complex glomerulonephritis. *Nephron* 36:38–45, 1984

86. CIABATTONI G, CINOTTI GA, PIERUCCI A, SIMONETTI BM, MANZI M, PUGLIESE F, BARSOTTI P, PECCI G, TAGGI F, PATRONO C: Effects of sulindac and ibuprofen in patients with chronic glomerular disease: Evidence for the dependence of renal function on prostacyclin. *N Engl J Med* 310:279–283, 1984

87. KUNKEL SL, ZANETTI M, SAPIN C: Suppression of nephrotoxic serum nephritis in rats by prostaglandin E. *Am J Pathol* 108:240–245, 1982

88. BERTANI T, REMUZZI G: Stagnations and regressions in the treatment of primary glomerulonephritis. *Lancet* 2:90–92, 1983

89. BRENNER BM, MEYER TW, HOSTETTER TH: Dietary protein intake and the progressive nature of kidney disease. *N Engl J Med* 307:652–659, 1982

90. KLAHR S, BUERKERT J, MURKERSON M: Role of dietary factors in the progression of chronic renal disease. *Kidney Int* 24:519–587, 1983

91. KLUTHE R, OECHSLIN D, QUIRIN H, JESDINSKY HJ: Six years' experience with a special low protein diet, in *Uremia: Pathogenesis, Diagnosis and Treatment,* edited by KLUTHE R, BERLYNE G, BURTON B, Stuttgart, Thieme Verlag, 1971, pp 250–257

92. WALSER M: Ketoacids in the treatment of uraemia. *Clin Nephrol* 3:180–186, 1975

93. BARSOTTI G, GUIDUCCI A, CIARDELLA F, GIOVANNETTI S: Effects on renal function of a low-nitrogen diet supplemented with essential amino acids and keto-analogues and of haemodialysis and free protein supply in patients with chronic renal failure. *Nephron* 27:113–117, 1981

94. MASCHIO G, OLDRIZZI L, TESSITORE N, D'ANGELO A, VALVO E, LUPO L, LOSCHIAVO C, FABRISO A, GAMMARO L, RUGIU C, PANZETTA G: Effects of dietary protein and phosphorus restriction on the progression of early renal failure. *Kidney Int* 22:371–376, 1982

95. ALVESTRAND A, AHLBERG M, FURST P, BERGSTROM J: Clinical results of long-term treatment with a low protein diet and a new amino acid preparation in patients with chronic uremia. *Clin Nephrol* 19:67–73, 1983

96. LEVY JA, MORROW WJW: Dietary regulation of the auto-immune process in murine lupus. *Immunol Today* 4:249–250, 1983

97. KINCAID-SMITH P: *The Kidney.* Oxford, Blackwell, 1975, p 193

98. RAMZY MH, CAMERON JS, TURNER DR, NEILD GH, OGG CS, HICKS J: The long-term outcome of idiopathic membranous nephropathy. *Clin Nephrol* 16:13–19, 1981

99. MOGENSEN CE: Long-term anti-hypertensive treatment inhibiting progression of diabetic nephropathy. *Br Med J* 285:685–688, 1982

100. KNOWLTON AL, STOERK H, SEEGAL BC, LOEB EN: Influence of adrenal cortical steroids upon the blood pressure and the rate of progression of experimental nephritis in rats. *Endocrinology* 38:315–324, 1946

101. TIKKANEN I, FYHRQUIST F, MIETTINEN A, TORNROTH T: Autologous immune complex nephritis and DOCA/NaCl load: A new model of hypertension. *Acta Pathol Microbiol Scand* [A] 88:241–250, 1980

102. IVERSEN BM: The effect of hypertension on experimental glomerulonephritis in rats. Thesis, Bergen University, 1981

103. BALDWIN DS: Chronic glomerulonephritis: Non-immunologic mechanisms of progressive glomerular damage. *Kidney Int* 21:109–120, 1982

104. OKUDA S, OHOYAMA K, FUJIMI S, OH Y, NOMOTO K, OMAE T: Influence of hypertension on the progression of experimental autologous immune complex nephritis. *J Lab Clin Med* 101:461–471, 1983

105. AZAR S, JOHNSON MA, HERTEL B, TOBIAN L: Single nephron pressures, flows and resistances in hypertensive kidneys with nephrosclerosis. *Kidney Int* 12:28–40, 1977
106. DWORKIN LD, HOSTETTER TH, RENNKE HG, BRENNER BM: Evidence for a hemodynamic basis for glomerular injury in hypertension. *Abst Am Soc Nephrol* Nov 1981, p 102

Use of Pulse Methylprednisolone in Primary and Multisystem Glomerular Diseases

W. Kline Bolton

Rapidly progressive glomerulonephritis (RPGN) is a clinical syndrome characterized by the presence of glomerulonephritis and a decrease in renal function of 50% or more within a 3-month period of time [1, 2]. This syndrome may result from primary glomerulopathies (for example, membranoproliferative glomerulonephritis [MPGN]), or from secondary renal involvement in multisystem diseases (for example, vasculitides) [3]. Although many, if not most, RPGN patients will have associated acute crescentic (AC) disease, this is not without exception; and patients with certain types of glomerulonephritis may have RPGN without crescents. We define patients as having AC-RPGN when the clinical course is present and 20% or more of glomeruli have associated crescents [3]. The idiopathic variety of AC-RPGN may be divided into subtypes consisting of patients with: (1) apparent glomerular immune complex deposition, (2) antiglomerular basement membrane (anti-GBM) antibodies along the basement membrane, or (3) minimal or absent immune deposits in the glomeruli, the no-immunoglobulin-deposit (NID) type of disease [4]. These may be considered to be primary glomerulopathies because no systemic effects of the underlying pathogenetic process are apparent, but actually are systemic diseases. Evidence for this is pulmonary involvement, which is frequently present not only with anti-GBM disease but with the other types as well, including recurrence of the disease in patients who receive transplants. The present chapter will address only the three categories of idiopathic AC-RPGN, polyarteritis nodosa (PAN) associated with AC-RPGN, and MPGN.

Numerous studies of RPGN describing the natural course and response to therapy have been of the melting pot variety and have nondiscriminantly included different histologic subtypes of nephropathies with the same clinical course. This lumping of diseases together makes an evaluation of their course and treatment difficult, if not impossible. Nonetheless, an assessment of the course of the disease, even with the old lumping classification, provides useful

This manuscript was presented as part of a Symposium on *The Treatment of Glomerulonephritis.*

Table 1. Prognosis of rapidly progressive glomerulonephritis with associated acute crescentic disease

Histologic diagnosis[a]	No. of patients	Improved	Death or dialysis
General	521	124 (24%)	397 (76%)
Proliferative (postinfectious) GN	47	23 (49%)	24 (51%)
NID and immune complex types	70	13 (19%)	57 (81%)
Anti-GBM	81	9 (11%)	72 (89%)
PAN-AC-RPGN	69	4 (6%)	65 (94%)

[a] Abbreviations are defined as follows: GN, glomerulonephritis; NID, no-immunoglobulin-deposit type of disease; GBM, glomerular basement membrane; PAN-AC-RPGN, polyarteritis nodosa associated with rapidly progressive glomerulonephritis and acute crescentic disease.

information about therapy in this group of devastating diseases. Table 1 summarizes the available information about the course of RPGN in more than 700 patients treated by conventional methods.[1] This includes all types of treatment or nontreatment, with the exception of plasma exchange and pulse methylprednisolone. Individual case reports are not included. The category indicated as "general" represents the lumping of all patients with the clinical syndrome and indicates that despite any therapy, death or dialysis intervenes in three-fourths of them. Even in proliferative (probably postinfectious) nephritis, half of the patients with renal failure and crescents do not recover. For NID and immune complex types of AC-RPGN, 81% fail to respond to treatment, as do 89% the patients with anti-GBM disease, including Goodpasture's syndrome and RPGN. For non-anti-GBM type RPGN with oliguria, 88% die or require dialysis. The prognosis is even worse in those cases of PAN associated with AC-RPGN, with essentially all of those patients requiring dialysis or dying. It is thus obvious that "conventional" therapy is unsuccessful.

In the following report, we shall present the results of pulse methylprednisolone therapy in patients with the histologic types of RPGN noted above and shall compare this to other modes of treatment.

Methods

Beginning in 1976, we began using i.v. pulse methylprednisolone therapy as a primary treatment of AC-RPGN [2, 3, 5, 6]. All patients meeting the histologic and clinical criteria for RPGN were offered the opportunity of receiving pulse or conventional therapy. The pulse was administered as previously described: 30 mg/kg given i.v. over a period of not longer than 20 min, with the dose not to exceed 3 g at a single time. This was given every

---

[1] Details of data for Tables, derivation of comparative information, and full description of therapeutic protocol are published in [2, 3, 5, 6].

Table 2. Response to pulse therapy compared to conventional treatment in granular and NID types of AC-RPGN[a]

Therapy	N	HD	Off HD	Improved
Conventional	9	6	1	4
Pulse	21	12	11[b]	18[b]

[a] HD refers to hemodialysis; N, to no. of patients. Other abbreviations are defined in footnote to Table 1.
[b] $P < 0.025$.

other day for three doses. We were always certain to ascertain that the patients did not have contraindications to pulse therapy, were volume-repleted, and did not receive diuretics before or after the pulse period. Pulse therapy was followed 48 hr later by alternating high doses of prednisone (orally administered) according to a tapering protocol to span a 5-year period with built-in steps for accelerated tapering after a good response. Patients had to survive 6 weeks or more after the start of pulse therapy to be considered as having responded to the therapy. Improvement was defined as a discontinuation of dialysis, a 30% improvement in glomerular filtration rate, or a decrease in serum creatinine by 30% or more.

Results

The study population was 47 patients with idiopathic AC-RPGN and 7 each with PAN-AC-RPGN and MPGN. Table 2 describes the response of our patients with granular and NID types of AC-RPGN to pulse therapy. The two types are combined because the response to therapy was identical. Of 30 patients, 9 were treated with modes of therapy other than pulse, and 6 of these required dialysis. One of these was able to discontinue it. A total of 4 patients were improved. Of 21 patients pulsed, 12 required hemodialysis; 11 of these 12 were able to discontinue dialysis. A total of 18 of the 21 patients were improved with pulse therapy. The difference between conventional and pulse therapy was significant statistically.

Because a high degree of crescent formation and the presence of oligoanuria are the classic indicators of a poor prognosis [1, 7], we analyzed the effects of pulse therapy relative to these two parameters. Table 3 presents the informa-

Table 3. Influence of percent crescents and oligoanuria on prognosis in pulsed patients: granular and NID types[a]

Prognosis	All	Percent crescents		Oligoanuria
		20 to 59%	60 to 100%	
Improved	18/21	7/8	11/13	10/11
	(86%)	(88%)	(85%)	(91%)
HD/Off HD	9/12	3/4	6/8	7/8
	(75%)	(75%)	(75%)	(88%)

[a] Abbreviations are defined in Table 1.

Table 4. Pulse methylprednisolone therapy of anti-GBM type AC-RPGN[a]

Therapy group	N	Age[b] (yr)	Oligoanuria	Cresc (%)[b]	Improved	HD	Off HD
Unpulsed	5	49 ± 8	4/5	94 ± 4	0	5	0
Pulsed	12	48 ± 3	7/12	68 ± 9	2	10	0

[a] HD refers to hemodialysis; N, to no. of patients. Other abbreviations are defined in footnote to Table 1.
[b] Values are the means $\pm$ SEM.

tion for patients pulsed relative to the percent of crescents and the presence of oligoanuria. Inasmuch as some centers use 60% or more crescents for evidence of significant disease, we divided our data into patients with 20 to 59% crescents and those with 60 to 100% crescents. As noted previously, 86% of all patients showed an improvement, and 75% of those on dialysis were able to discontinue dialysis. Among patients with 20 to 59% crescents, 88% were improved, with 75% of those on dialysis able to stop, whereas 85% of the patients with 60 to 100% crescents improved and 75% were off dialysis. Thus, the improvement rates were the same in patients with higher degrees of crescent formation as in those with lesser degrees. In the series of patients who were pulsed, 91% of all oligoanuric patients were improved, and 88% of oligoanuric patients on hemodialysis were improved.

The results of therapy of anti-GBM type AC-RPGN were completely different. Table 4 provides this information. Five patients have been treated with methods other than pulse therapy, including plasma exchange, and 12 patients received pulse methylprednisolone. All 5 patients treated with conventional measures required dialysis or died. Two patients treated with pulse therapy improved; neither of these two patients was oligoanuric, and neither was on dialysis. The other 10 patients did not respond to therapy. There was no statistical difference between these two groups. Table 5 presents the results of pulse therapy of patients with MPGN and PAN-AC-RPGN. Among 7 patients with MPGN who were pulsed, 6 improved. Of the 3 on hemodialysis, 2 were able to discontinue it. Two patients who improved later developed slowly progressive chronic disease and are now on dialysis. Among 7 patients with PAN-AC-RPGN, 4 received pulse therapy. Two of the pulsed patients also received cyclophosphamide. None of the 3 unpulsed patients improved, as opposed to improvement in all 4 patients who were pulsed. All 3 pulsed patients on hemodialysis were able to discontinue that support. One patient not treated with cyclophosphamide combined with pulse died of a ruptured mesenteric artery aneurysm after reactivation of his PAN.

Table 5. Pulse therapy of MPGN and PAN-AC-RPGN[a]

Disease group	N	Age (yr)	Pulse	HD	Off HD	Improved
MPGN	7	48.8 ± 4.7	7/7	3	2	6/7
PAN-AC-RPGN	7	62.6 ± 2.2	4/7	6	3[b]	4/4[b]

[a] HD refers to hemodialysis; N, to no. of patients. Other abbreviations are defined in footnote to Table 1.
[b] All pulsed.

Table 6. Follow-up data in patients with RPGN

Mean follow-up time	31.5 ± 5.1 months
Range	2 to 86 months
Patients responding initially, still off dialysis	85%
Long-term response rate	73%

Improvement in renal function in this series was noted after pulse therapy in patients with up to 90% of glomeruli in the biopsy sample demonstrating obsolescence or sclerosis. Of 15 patients with 20% or more glomerular sclerosis (mean, 44.3%), 10 (67%) improved. The side effects from pulse methylprednisolone therapy have been minimal in appropriately selected patients. There has been one death associated with pulse therapy; the death was related to a pre-existing undiagnosed process prior to methylprednisolone.

The follow-up information on RPGN patients treated with pulse methylprednisolone is given in Table 6. Most of the data applies to AC-RPGN patients. The mean follow-up time is 31.5 months, with a range from 2 to 86 months. Of those patients who responded initially to pulse methylprednisolone either with an improvement in creatinine clearance or with discontinuation of hemodialysis, 85% remain independent of dialysis, although several of them do have slowly decreasing renal function suggestive of chronic renal failure. The long-term response rate adjusted for patients who responded and then required dialysis is 73% of all patients with RPGN pulsed with methylprednisolone.

Discussion

Comparison to Other Treatment Modalities

Examination of the available series of various types of treatment of RPGN indicate that pulse methylprednisolone, plasma exchange with immunosup-

Table 7. Comparison of therapies for non-anti-GBM AC-RPGN[a]

Treatment	N	Death or dialysis	Improved
Quadruple therapy	41	12 (29%)	29 (71%)
Miscellaneous (conventional therapy)[b]	123	90 (73%)	33 (27%)
"Pure" idiopathic AC-RPGN (conventional therapy)	70	57 (81%)	13 (19%)
Pulse therapy	45	11 (24%)	34 (76%)
Plasma exchange and immunosuppression	43	13 (30%)	30 (70%)

Abbreviations are defined in footnote to Table 1 (N refers to patients).
[a] Excluding postinfectious patients.
[b] Includes mixed AC-RPGN.

Table 8. Comparison of therapies for anit-GBM AC-RPGN[a]

Treatment	N	Death or dialysis	Improved
Quadruple	3	3 (100%)	0
Miscellaneous	81	72 (89%)	9 (11%)
Pulse	12	10 (83%)	2 (17%)
Plasma exchange and immunosuppression	75	41 (55%)	34 (45%)[b]

[a] Abbreviations are defined in footnote to Table 1. *N* refers to patients.
[b] None improved with oligoanuria.

pression, and quadruple therapy appear to have the best overall effects in terms of improvement [3]. Data are derived from published series and our own experience. Table 7 compares the results of these types of therapy for non-anti-GBM AC-RPGN, excluding postinfectious nephritis. The "miscellaneous" category includes a variety of types of AC-RPGN, and the "idiopathic" category represents those series of patients in whom it was possible to establish that they had the NID and immune complex types of RPGN. Approximately 19 to 27% of patients with idiopathic AC-RPGN or RPGN of different categories improved with conventional therapy. This compares to a 71% improvement rate with quadruple therapy, 76% with pulse methylprednisolone, and 70% with plasma exchange and immunosuppression. Table 8 compares these same four types of therapy for anti-GBM AC-RPGN. Few patients have been treated with quadruple therapy, and none improved. Conventional therapy gave improvement to 11% of the patients; pulse methylprednisolone, to 17%. With plasma exchange and immunosuppression, 45% improved. It is important to note that the 2 patients treated with pulse and the 34 patients who improved with plasma exchange were not oligoanuric. None of the reported series of patients or our own patients with oligoanuria have improved with plasma exchange or with pulse therapy. Comparison of therapies in PAN-AC-RPGN is provided in Table 9. In a small series of patients, 17% responded to quadruple therapy, only 6% to miscellaneous therapy. All of our patients treated with pulse therapy improved, as did 88% of patients with plasma exchange and immunosuppression. Little information is available to assess different types of therapy on MPGN.

Table 9. Comparison of therapies for PAN-AC-RPGN[a]

Treatment	N	Death or dialysis	Improved
Quadruple	6	5 (83%)	1 (17%)
Miscellaneous	69	65 (94%)	4 (6%)
Pulse	5	0	5 (100%)
Plasma exchange and immunosuppression	8	1 (12%)	7 (88%)

[a] See Table 1 for abbreviations. *N* refers to patients.

Pathogenesis

Many processes, most of which have a rapidly progressive course, appear to result in a histologic picture that is termed *crescentic glomerulonephritis.* Regardless of the underlying pathogenetic process, there appear to be three basic patterns of immunoglobulin deposition: (1) antibody to the GBM, (2) deposition of apparent immune complexes within the glomerulus, and (3) minimal or no immunoglobulin deposits. In all of these situations, the crescentic nephritides have common histologic features consisting of a severe interstitial infiltrate with mononuclear cells, multinucleated giant cells, defects in Bowman's capsule, and gaps in the basement membrane [3]. These findings suggest that crescentic nephritis is a common final pathway for different pathologic insults. The similarity in the histologic picture and in the response to therapy for both rejection and certain types of glomerulonephritis suggests that similar mechanisms may be involved. Figure 1 provides an hypothesis for the development of rapidly progressive nephritis, whether it be crescentic or noncrescentic in origin [3]. Abundant supporting data are available for the concept of immunization and development of cellular and antibody-mediated immunity, as well as a role for macrophages, fibrin, and various humoral mediators [8, 9]. According to the present postulate, immune complexes, either the circulating soluble variety or the in situ type, may lead to disease with or without recruitment of cell-mediated immunity. Similarly, anti-GBM antibody may deposit in the kidney on the basement membranes, again with or without recruitment of cellular immunity. The degree and type of associated cellular immunity may well determine the ultimate histologic picture and course of the disease. In addition to cooperation between the various components of cell-mediated immunity in the development of nephritis, there may actually be some type of antibody-dependent cellular cytotoxicity as has been described in transplantation. Finally, cell-mediated immunity alone could produce glomerulonephritis [10]. It now seems quite apparent that there are overlaps in these syndromes. Patients with immune complex disease may progress to anti-GBM disease, and we have observed several patients with NID-AC-RPGN who later developed what appeared to be an immune-complex type of AC-RPGN.

Thus, an increasingly persuasive amount of evidence supports the concept of the role of cell-mediated immunity in the development of glomerulonephritis. Our supposition of the pivotal role of the cell in the pathogenesis of this process led to our use of therapy of demonstrated efficacy in a similar situation: transplant rejection. Pulse methylprednisolone therapy might be expected to have a beneficial effect on AC-RPGN mediated solely by steroid-sensitive cells and in humorally mediated AC-RPGN in which steroid-sensitive cells play a role. However, pulse therapy might not be expected to have a significant effect when the process is mediated by nonsteroid-sensitive cells or when the major portion of the damage is mediated by deposition of antibodies on structures in the kidney. While cell-mediated immunity appears to be of key importance in the development of experimental glomerulonephritides in association with deposition of immunoglobulin and, in certain models, in the absence of immunoglobulin deposition with proliferative nephritis [10],

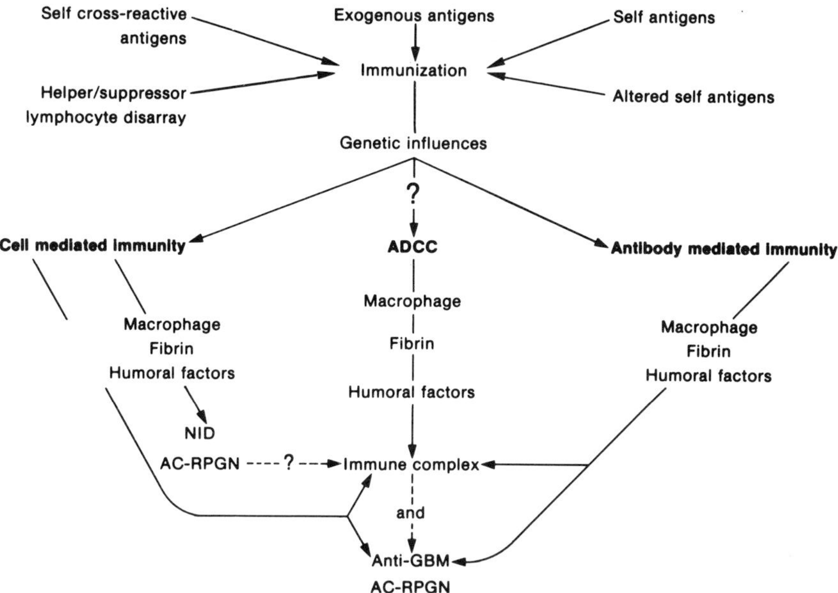

Fig. 1. Proposed mechanism for the development of rapidly progressive glomerulonephritis (RPGN). The development of antibodies to glomerular basement membrane (GBM), immune complexes, and cell-mediated immunity to renal antigens have been shown. Genetic influences have also been demonstrated in certain subtypes. Participation of macrophages, fibrin, and humoral mediators have been demonstrated in various forms of experimental and human glomerulonephritis. Conversion from immune complex to anti-GBM type disease has been well documented, and NID (no immunoglobulin deposits) also converts to immune complex RPGN. *ADCC* refers to antibody-dependent cellular cytotoxicity. The role and interaction of the three paths of the immune system illustrated are partly hypothetical, but based on information currently available both in human and experimental animal models of the immune system and renal disease. (Reproduced with permission of RG NARINS, editor of *Controversies in Nephrology and Hypertension* and *Current Therapy in Internal Medicine*)

these pathogenetic mechanisms remain to be verified in humans. Future studies will be needed to clarify the present hypothesis.

Risk–Benefit Relationship

In the final analysis, the efficacy of any therapy must be judged by the benefits accrued compared to the risks of treatment. In our hands, the risks seem justifiable relative to the outcome, especially in relation to the future risks of dialysis and transplantation. The monetary cost of therapy for methylprednisolone compared to plasma exchange is addressed in Table 10. The information is based upon a 70-kg patient and excludes laboratory, outpatient, and

Table 10. Cost of therapy[a]

1. *Methylprednisolone,* 7 vials @ $84.10	$ 589.00
Prednisone, 20 mg tablets per oral protocol	77.00
First year	$ 666.00
Prednisone, 20 mg tablets per protocol	
Second year	$ 60.00
2. *Plasma exchange,* 4 liters with colloid,	
per exchange	$ 1,100.00
2 months, 3 ×/wk, excluding hospital	
costs, cytotoxic medication	$26,400.00

[a] For a 70-kg patient, excluding laboratory, outpatient, and physician fees.

physician fees for pulse therapy. When the regimen of a 30-mg/kg pulse is used every other day with an alternate-day tapering schedule for oral prednisone, the cost of therapy for the first year is $666.00. In the second year, the cost of prednisone would be $60.00. For plasma exchange with 4 liters and colloid replacement, the cost at our institution is $1,100.00. If the 2-month period that we use for plasma exchange is followed in terms of ascertaining a response, the cost would be $26,400.00 for exchanges done three times a week; this cost excludes hospitalization and cytotoxic medications. Obviously, the number of exchanges that might be appropriate to result in a benefit would be greater than one exchange, and possibly less than the 2 months of exchanges illustrated here. Nonetheless, as is obvious, the cost of even one exchange is greater than 2 full years of pulse methylprednisolone and prednisone therapy, and the cost of multiple exchanges is considerably greater than the cost of methylprednisolone and prednisone. The money saved by successful treatment of patients who would otherwise require dialysis and transplantation is an additional consideration in analyzing benefits. We estimate that the net monetary savings for our series alone, by keeping patients off dialysis or getting them off dialysis with pulse therapy, are greater than $3 million. This figure does not in any way reflect the financial gain to society from the returns of individuals to their jobs, nor the social and emotional benefits to the patients and their families.

Conclusion

It is now apparent that aggressive therapy of these diseases will be successful in altering the natural course of progression. Several different types of therapy are comparable in response rate, but pulse methylprednisolone with alternate-day prednisone appears to be among the most effective, least expensive, and associated with few complications. We feel that pulse therapy is indicated for patients with idiopathic crescentic disease and the clinical course of RPGN as defined in the text; that it is effective, especially with cyclophosphamide for PAN-AC-RPGN; and that it appears efficacious in our small series of patients with MPGN. Additional studies will be needed to clarify additional benefits, if any, of quadruple therapy and plasma exchange relative to pulse methylprednisolone in these diseases.

Acknowledgments. This work was supported in part by USPHS grant #AM32530. I appreciate the participation of the members of the Charlottesville Collaborative Study: Drs. N. O. Atuk, W. Baker, F. J. Ballenger, C. Brooks, W. G. Couser, J. Cox, C. Culpeper, N. R. Falkinburg, R. D. Giles, J. C. Gretes, R. Lockridge, P. I. Lobo, T. L. Overby, I. Park, J. Richmond, J. Roman, B. C. Sturgill, and F. B. Westervelt, Jr.

References

1. GLASSOCK R. A clinical and immunopathologic dissection of rapidly progressive glomerulonephritis. *Nephron* 22:253–264, 1978
2. BOLTON WK, CHARLOTTESVILLE COLLABORATIVE STUDY: Pulse methylprednisolone therapy of rapidly progressive glomerulonephritis, in *Controversies in Nephrology,* edited by SCHREINER GE, Washington, DC, Nephrology Division, Georgetown University, 1981, vol 3, pp 213–221
3. BOLTON WK: The role of high dose steroids in nephritic syndromes: The case for aggressive use, in *Controversies in Nephrology and Hypertension,* edited by NARINS RG, New York, Churchill Livingstone (in press, 1984)
4. STILMANT MM, BOLTON WK, STURGILL BC, SCHMITT GW, COUSER WG: Crescentic glomerulonephritis without immune deposits: Clinicopathologic features. *Kidney Int* 15:184–195, 1979
5. BOLTON WK: Crescentic glomerulonephritis, in *Current Therapy in Nephrology and Hypertension,* edited by GLASSOCK RJ, Burlington, Ontario, BC Decker (in press, 1984)
6. BOLTON WK, COUSER WG: Intravenous pulse methylprednisolone therapy of acute crescentic rapidly progressive glomerulonephritis. *Am J Med* 66:495–502, 1979
7. COUSER WG: Idiopathic rapidly progressive glomerulonephritis. *Am J Nephrol* 2:57–69, 1982
8. McCLUSKEY RT, BHAN AK: Cell-mediated mechanisms in renal disease. *Kidney Int* 21(suppl. 11):S6–S12, 1982
9. FILLIT HM, ZABRISKIE JB: Cellular immunity in glomerulonephritis. *Am J Pathol* 109:227–243, 1982
10. BOLTON WK, TUCKER FL, STURGILL BC: A new avian model of experimental glomerulonephritis consistent with mediation by cellular immunity. *J Clin Invest* (in press, 1984)

Plasma Exchange for Glomerular Disease

Charles D. Pusey and C. Martin Lockwood

Intensive plasma exchange (PE) was introduced for the management of anti-glomerular basement membrane (anti-GBM) disease in 1974 [1]. After 10 years, the indications for [2] and hazards of [3] of this form of treatment for aggressive glomerulonephritis have been better defined. Additionally, the study of certain diseases treated by PE, such as autoantibody-mediated nephritis, has advanced our knowledge of pathogenetic mechanisms, and of the homeostatic processes that may normally control the evolution of autoantibody synthesis [2, 4]. A closer examination of the treatment regimens used has demonstrated the need to understand how the separate components work and interact. Our own experience indicates that in anti-GBM disease, cyclophosphamide (together with PE) is essential for the successful control of anti-GBM antibody synthesis [5]; other data attest to its beneficial effect (in combination with PE) in systemic lupus erythematosus (SLE) [6]. This drug also is an important component of treatment in nonantibody-mediated nephritis, when it occurs in the context of a systemic vasculitis such as Wegener's granulomatosis or microscopic polyarteritis [7]. Although many have advocated the use of high-dose steroids, both in patients with systemic vasculitis [7] and with idiopathic rapidly progressive nephritis [8–10], there is no controlled evidence of their value; indeed, there may be certain adverse effects, including an increased risk of infection [11]. One principal action, Fc receptor blockade, leads to impairment of the clearance of immune complexes [12], which may be undesirable in the clinical situations concerned.

Because of the need to know whether PE offers additional benefits for conventional immunotherapy in nonantibody-mediated rapidly progressive glomerulonephritis (RPGN), we have embarked on a randomized, prospective controlled trial. Patients entered in the trial are stratified according to levels of renal function, and then are randomized to receive conventional immunotherapy (high-dose steroids and cytotoxic drugs) in a regimen outlined below or the same together with a series of intensive PE. Interim analysis of the

---

This manuscript was presented as part of a Symposium on *The Treatment of Glomerulonephritis.*

trial will be discussed in this presentation. A similar prospective trial for PE in the management of anti-GBM antibody-mediated nephritis has not been carried out by us; largely because of the apparent benefit derived from PE when the outcome of our patients (see below) is compared with that of patients who were not treated [2] with PE.

The use of animal models has shown that homeostatic mechanisms may be available to control aberrant autoimmune responses. For example, in mercuric chloride-induced anti-GBM nephritis in the Brown Norway (BN) rat, we have found evidence that cellular (T-suppressor lymphocytes) [13] and humoral (autoanti-idiotypic antibodies) [14] factors may be important in controlling autoantibody synthesis. This work demonstrates the value of experimental models in renal disease, and also the need to search for similar regulatory mechanisms in humans that may be amenable to therapeutic manipulation.

In this review, we shall outline our experience with the use of PE in the management of the following groups of patients: (1) anti-GBM antibody-mediated nephritis, (2) microscopic renal vasculitis, (3) a controlled trial of patients with nonanti-GBM nephritis, and (4) lupus nephritis.

Anti-GBM Disease

Patients

There were 48 patients treated (25 male and 23 female), with ages ranging from 4 to 72 years. In 41 patients in whom immunofluorescence of renal biopsy specimens was available, IgG was deposited linearly along the GBM. Anti-GBM antibodies were detected by solid-phase radioimmunoassay [15] in the sera of all 48 patients.

Treatment

Four-liter PE was carried out daily by using antecubital veins or femoral vein catheters for vascular access. Plasma protein fraction (physiologic human albumin solution) was used as plasma substitute, except when exchanges were carried out within 48 hr of a renal biopsy or surgical procedure—when 2 U of fresh-frozen plasma were given to restore clotting factors. The PE was continued until control of anti-GBM antibody formation was achieved; our recent policy has been to perform at least 14 PE (see below). Cyclophosphamide (3 mg/kg/d), azathioprine (1 mg/kg/d), and prednisolone (60 mg/d) were used initially, except in patients over 55 years of age—in whom azathioprine was omitted and cyclophosphamide was given in a reduced dosage of 2 mg/kg/d. The cytotoxic drugs were continued at the same dosage for 8 weeks unless infection or leukopenia ($< 4 \times 10^9$/liter) necessitated their temporary withdrawal. Prednisolone therapy was reduced at weekly intervals by 15 mg for the first 2 weeks, 5 mg for the next 4 weeks, and

2.5 mg 1 week thereafter. In most patients with anti-GBM nephritis, cyclophosphamide and azathioprine were discontinued after 8 weeks, as discussed below.

Monitoring

Anti-GBM antibody levels were measured by a sensitive radioimmunoassay that was initially performed by Wilson at the Scripps Clinic in La Jolla, California. Since 1979, we have used a solid-phase radioimmunoassay that was developed in our laboratory [15].

Serial respiratory function tests were carried out to detect the presence of pulmonary hemorrhage [16]. A rise in the KCO > 30% of baseline value was taken as an indication of fresh lung bleeding. Standard laboratory measurements of plasma creatinine and creatinine clearance (C_{cr}) were performed, together with microscopic examination of the urine deposit.

Outcome

The results of the treatment regimen for renal function in these patients are shown in Table 1. The most important observation was that sustained recovery of renal function did not occur in any patient who was dialysis-dependent at the time of presentation. However, the treatment regimen appeared to substantially alter the prognosis of those patients who still had residual renal function (creatinine < 600 μmol/liter) at the time of referral. Long-term follow-up showed that recovery of renal function was maintained in the majority of patients for periods of up to 5 years [5]. Lung hemorrhage was controlled in 32 of 36 patients, and it provided a separate indication for use of PE. Sequential measurements of circulating anti-GBM antibody showed that effective control of autoantibody synthesis was achieved in patients treated with cytotoxic drugs, steroids, and intensive PE. Provided that serum antibody levels had fallen to near background values (less than twice the binding of normal serum), rebound did not occur even when immunosuppressive drugs were withdrawn [5]. Retrospective analysis showed that cyclophosphamide in combination with PE was essential for achieving this rapid control of antibody formation. In three oliguric patients treated by PE alone, there was little change in anti-GBM antibody levels, either in the short-term or during follow-up for 8 weeks.

Table 1. Outcome of treatment in 48 patients with anti-GBM disease

Presentation	N	Improved	No response
Creatinine (< 600 μmoles/liter)	18	16	2
Creatinine (> 600 μmoles/liter)	5	1	4
Dialysis-dependent	25	0	25

Microscopic Renal Vasculitis

Patients

Forty-nine patients were treated (35 male and 14 female), with ages ranging from 16 to 76 years. The diagnosis was Wegener's granulomatosis (WG) in 25 patients, microscopic polyarteritis (MP) in 18 patients, and idiopathic rapidly progressive glomerulonephritis (IRPGN) in 6 patients. Renal biopsy showed focal necrotizing glomerulonephritis in all cases, and granular deposits of IgG $\pm$ C3 were found in 24 of 40 specimens in which tissue was available for immunofluorescence. Circulating immune complexes were demonstrated in 23 of 29 by Clq or rheumatoid factor binding assays [17].

Treatment

Daily 4-liter PE for plasma protein fraction (PPF) were performed as described above. In the absence of a pathognomonic serum marker, discontinuation of treatment was determined by clinical assessment of the response; this group of patients received a mean of 10 exchanges. The steroid and cytotoxic drug dosage was initially the same as in the anti-GBM group. Steroid therapy was reduced in a similar manner; however, maintenance with cytotoxic drugs was usually required. Azathioprine was most commonly used for maintenance therapy, but some patients with Wegener's granulomatosis required long-term treatment with cyclophosphamide.

Monitoring

Although it was found that circulating immune complexes became rapidly undetectable during treatment, their levels did not always correlate with disease activity; and, they rarely proved to be a satisfactory method of judging treatment response [18].

More recently, we have found that serial measurement of C-reactive protein can be a valuable adjunct to determining disease activity in patients with systemic vasculitis. In the absence of intercurrent infection, the C-reactive protein value proved to be a better indicator of the degree of inflammation than (for example) measurements of erythrocyte sedimentation rate [19].

Renal disease was monitored as described above, with particular emphasis being placed on the finding of red blood cell casts in the urine deposit. As in anti-GBM disease, patients with pulmonary vasculitis and lung hemorrhage were monitored by serial tests of KCO.

Outcome

The outcome of treatment, when assessed at the end of the initial hospital admission, is shown in Table 2. The prognosis for recovery of renal function

Table 2. Outcome of treatment in 49 patients with microscopic renal vasculitis

Presentation	N	Improved	No response
Creatinine ($<$ 600 μmoles/liter)	16	14	2
Creatinine ($>$ 600 μmoles/liter)	10	8	2
Dialysis-dependent	23	17	6

in the dialysis-dependent group was clearly different from that of patients with antibody-mediated nephritis, although it was not possible to be sure that plasma exchange had contributed to this effect. Long-term follow-up of this group revealed that even in those patients who had originally required dialysis, improvement in renal function could be maintained for up to 5 years [20].

Controlled Trial of Plasma Exchange

Patients

Patients with the diagnoses described above were allocated to plasma exchange or control groups by randomized cards that were stratified for renal function. The criteria for entry to the trial excluded patients who had SLE, poststreptococcal nephritis, or Henoch-Schönlein purpura, because of the variable natural history and/or response to therapy. Patients whose RPGN developed on a background of primary glomerular disease also were excluded.

At the time of interim analysis, 32 patients had been entered into the trial: 17 in the PE group and 15 in the control group. Age and sex distribution in both groups was similar to that described above. Diagnosis in the PE group was: 9 WG, 5 MP, 3 IRPGN; and, in the control group: 8 WG, 6 MP, 1 IRPGN. Renal biopsy specimens confirmed focal necrotizing glomerulonephritis in 32 of 32 cases, with crescent formation in all but two of the least severely affected patients. Deposits of IgG and/or C_3 were found in renal biopsy specimens in 7 of 10 in the PE group and 6 of 9 in the controls.

Treatment

Treatment in the prospective trial was similar to that described for microscopic renal vasculitis, with all patients receiving full drug therapy for at least 8 weeks. In addition, the plasma exchange group received at least five 4-liter exchanges for plasma protein fraction (mean, 11). Therapy after 8 weeks was then determined by the clinical response; and, it was similar in both groups, usually including prednisolone and azathioprine for 6 months.

Table 3. Results of controlled trial: interim analysis

Presentation	Treatment	Patients	Improved[a]	RDT[b]	Died
Creatinine	PE	6	6	0	0
($<$ 500 μmoles/liter)	Drugs	6	5	0	1
Creatinine	PE	5	5	0	0
($>$ 500 μmoles/liter)	Drugs	4	4	0	0
Dialysis-dependent	PE	6	5	1	1[c]
	Drugs	5	1	2	2

[a] Defined as a sustained fall in plasma creatinine of $>$ 25% of the initial value, or recovery of independent renal function in those who were dialysis-dependent.
[b] RDT, regular dialysis therapy.
[c] One patient died despite recovery of renal function.

Monitoring

Patients were monitored as described above, with full assessment at 6 and 12 months.

Outcome

Interim analysis of patients in the trial, assessed by measurement of plasma creatinine or C_{cr} at 4 to 6 weeks, is shown in Table 3. There was no difference in outcome in those patients who were not dialysis-dependent at the start of treatment. However, there was a trend toward improvement in those dialysis-dependent patients who received PE, although this did not reach statistical significance ($P = 0.13$). A close comparison of these patients (Table 4) revealed no major differences in factors that may have been influential in determining outcome. Follow-up at 1 year showed that improvement was maintained in all patients who initially responded. The trial is continuing.

Table 4. Dialysis-dependent patients in controlled trial

	PE	Control
Patients	6	5
Sex (M/F)	3/3	3/2
Age	23 to 68 (50)	54 to 68 (59)
Diagnosis	3 WG, 2 MP, 1 IRPGN	2 WG, 2 MP, 1 IRPGN
Renal biopsy specimens		
% crescents	67 to 80 (74)	50 to 90 (63)
Ig deposits	2/5	2/2
Duration dialysis		
Days before first PE	1 to 13 (5)	1 to 5 (2.5)
Days after first PE	3 to 31 (12.5)	13

Parentheses denotes means.

Lupus Nephritis

Patients

We have treated 28 patients with lupus nephritis (25 female and 3 male), with ages ranging from 14 to 45 years. The diagnosis was confirmed by the finding of antibodies to double-stranded DNA in all cases. A study of this group of patients is necessarily complex, since many had already received long-term exposure to steroids and cytotoxic drugs. Their referral, unlike patients with other forms of severe nephritis, usually is late; assessment is complicated by such problems as hypertension, infection, drug toxicity, and renal vein thrombosis. We have used plasma exchange in lupus nephritis for three major reasons: (1) for progressive renal impairment that is unresponsive to drug therapy, (2) for treatment of nephritis when this occurs as part of life-threatening generalized vasculitis, and (3) to avoid complications of cumulative drug therapy; for example, in patients on steroids with avascular necrosis of the hip. In our studies, we have not used plasma exchange as initial therapy to study the possibility of steroid sparing, nor in mild lupus to study its effect on the evolution of the disease. Reversible complicating factors (as outlined above) were investigated and treated, where necessary, before commencement of PE.

Treatment

In 19 patients, plasma exchange was used as the sole additional therapy; these patients had received stable drug treatment for periods ranging from 1 week to 3 months before its introduction. All 19 patients had been maintained on prednisolone, and 13 had received cytotoxic drugs (9, azathioprine; 2, cyclophosphamide; and 2, both). The remaining nine patients received PE together with an increase in their steroid and/or cytotoxic therapy. A mean of seven 4-liter exchanges for PPF was performed. The duration of drug therapy was determined by the clinical response; steroid drugs were tapered as described above, and azathioprine generally was continued as maintenance therapy.

Monitoring

Anti-DNA antibodies were measured by a modification of the Farr technique [21]. Complement components C3 and C4 were measured by radial immunodiffusion and the CH_{50} via hemolytic plaque assay [22]. Renal function was assessed as described above. Specific tests of pulmonary function and regular neurologic assessment were performed when indicated.

Outcome

The outcome of treatment, as assessed at the end of the initial hospital admission, is shown in Table 5. The most striking feature was that 50% of the

Table 5. Outcome of treatment in 28 patients with lupus nephritis

Presentation	Drugs constant		Drugs increased	
	Patients	Improved	Patients	Improved
Creatinine (< 500 μmoles/liter)	6	3	2	1
Creatinine (> 500 μmoles/liter)	6	3	6	4
Dialysis-dependent	7	1	1	1

patients who were not dialysis-dependent improved following the introduction of plasma exchange alone, whereas recovery in dialysis-dependent patients was rare. In addition, we found that of 10 patients receiving both cyclophosphamide and PE, 7 improved—compared with 6 of 18 patients receiving prednisolone and/or azathioprine with PE. There was a significant overall fall in anti-DNA antibodies, which was sustained during a follow-up period of 1 month, and concomitant rise in C3 and C4 maintained for a similar period (Pusey, unpublished data). Of 12 patients in whom both of these indices improved, nine showed a parallel clinical response; whereas, of three patients in whom there was no serologic improvement, none responded. However, as other investigators have found [6], measurements of DNA binding and complement levels only were useful indicators of disease activity in certain patients.

Discussion

Treatment of glomerular disease by PE has provided the opportunity of determining whether removal of circulating nephrotoxic factors can be of significant therapeutic benefit. In anti-GBM antibody-mediated nephritis, sensitive radioimmunoassays have enabled the effects of treatment to be closely monitored; this allows analysis of antibody synthesis rates and the required duration of therapy. It has become clear that PE alone is unlikely to be of significant benefit, and also that the combination of an adequate course of PE and cytotoxic drug therapy is necessary to control autoantibody production [2]. Additionally, studies of this form of nephritis have defined factors other than anti-GBM antibody levels, which contribute to the severity of tissue injury. Examples of this are the contributions made by the patient's genetic background [23], role of intercurrent infection [24], and the influence of environmental agents (such as cigarette smoking) [25]. By contrast, in nonanti-GBM antibody-mediated nephritis, the difficulties inherent in monitoring treatment are clear; this form of nephritis will continue to present problems in management until the immunopathogenesis is better understood.

When considering the indications for PE, our results suggest that in anti-GBM nephritis, a combination of plasma exchange and cytotoxic drugs is of value in the management of nonoliguric patients; treatment also may be indicated for dialysis-dependent patients with lung hemorrhage or in whom early renal transplantation is desirable. In microscopic renal vasculitis, PE may be of particular value in those patients who are dialysis-dependent. It is too early to be sure whether their prognosis is improved by PE, although our uncontrolled data and the interim results of the trial strongly suggest a benefit. It is of interest that improvement can occur even after 1 month of dialysis, since duration of therapy has to be based on clinical experience. In lupus nephritis, we have found that some patients with severe disease unresponsive to drug therapy improved after PE was introduced. This retrospective study did not allow us to identify that subgroup of patients likely to benefit from PE. Despite the difficulty of assessing responses to treatment in other organ systems, extrarenal manifestations of systemic vasculitis may also respond to combination therapy. In particular, we have observed that cerebral, pulmonary, and digital vasculitis have improved more quickly than would be expected with conventional therapy; these findings clearly warrant further study.

Our clinical observations have underlined the importance of concomitant cytotoxic therapy in the control of antibody production in Goodpasture's syndrome; and, they are in agreement with studies in systemic lupus [6] and antibody-mediated allograft rejection [26]. Our experimental findings demonstrate that cyclophosphamide has a major role in the long-term regulation of autoantibody synthesis in anti-GBM nephritis in the BN rat [27]. There are several animal models of renal disease in which both the pathogenesis is well understood [28, 29] and autoregulatory mechanisms are under investigation [13, 14, 30, 31]. The application of PE and immunosuppressive drugs in these models should rapidly yield valuable information as to the effects of individual components of the treatment regimen; and, also the way in which they might interact with the immune system. For example, in the BN rat model, anti-idiotypic antibody synthesis follows the anti-GBM (idiotypic) response [14]; plasma exchange at an appropriate time, therefore, may selectively remove idiotype and allow earlier anti-idiotypic control. In situations where idiotype and anti-idiotype coexist in the circulation, specific immunoabsorption (using antigen) could perturb the balance of the immune network, leading to anti-idiotypic dominance. Our experimental studies of cyclophosphamide in the BN rat suggest that it may lead to functional deletion of those lymphocyte clones activated by mercuric chloride (Pusey et al, unpublished data); similar mechanisms may account for the synergy between PE and cyclophosphamide observed in our patients. This information should lead to the more rational design of treatment protocols in human glomerulonephritis.

Since the use of PE has become widespread, its risks have been better defined [3]; in particular, the hazards of allergic reactions, citrate toxicity, transfer of infection, and complications of vascular access. In our unit, 110 patients have been treated by 986 procedures between 1980 to 1982. The preferred routes of access have been antecubital venepuncture (66%) and femoral vein catheterization (26%); rarely have arteriovenous shunts (2%) or fistulae (4%) been employed [32]. As a result, there has been a marked reduction in the incidence of septicemia related to PE [33] and of inadequate treatment due to failure of access. Technical advances in the separation of blood components, including continuous flow centrifugation and membrane plasma filtration [34], have enabled selective removal of various defined cell populations and humoral factors (for example, cryoglobulins). It is likely that specific removal of pathogenetic macromolecules will shortly become possible, using a primary membrane separator in combination with a selective absorption device; this approach should overcome some of the problems described above.

Despite many reports of the value of PE in the treatment of glomerulonephritis (reviewed in [35, 36])—most of which are uncontrolled and retrospective—there remains a lack of controlled data to support its use. Nevertheless, our experience indicates that there are certain subgroups of patients in whom this form of treatment may radically alter the prognosis. In particular, PE probably is indicated for nonoliguric patients with anti-GBM nephritis, dialysis-dependent patients with microscopic renal vasculitis, and certain patients with severe drug-resistant lupus nephritis. Only carefully controlled clinical trials, together with basic research in experimental models, will provide more definite guidelines as to the future role of PE in the treatment of glomerular disease.

References

1. LOCKWOOD CM, BOULTON JONES JM, LOWENTHAL RM, SIMPSON IJ, PETERS DK, Wilson CB: Recovery from Goodpasture's syndrome after immunosuppressive treatment and plasmapheresis. *Br Med J* 2:252–254, 1975
2. PETERS DK, REES AJ, LOCKWOOD CM, PUSEY CD: Treatment and prognosis in antibasement membrane antibody mediated nephritis. *Transplant Proc* 14:513–521, 1982
3. EDITORIAL: Hazards of apheresis. *Lancet* 2:1025–1026, 1982
4. LOCKWOOD CM: Regulation of auto-antibody responses to glomerular basement membrane in man and experimental animals, in *Ciba Foundation Symposium 108,* edited by BERNFIELD M, London, Pitman in press
5. PUSEY CD, LOCKWOOD CM, PETERS DK: Plasma exchange and immunosuppressive drugs in the treatment of glomerulonephritis due to antibodies to the glomerular basement membrane. *Int J Artif Organs* 6:15–18, 1983
6. JONES JV: Plasmapheresis in SLE. *Clin Rheum Dis* 8:243–260, 1982
7. CUPPS TR, FAUCI AS: The vasculitic syndromes. *Adv Int Med* 27:315–339, 1982
8. BOLTON WK, COUSER WG: Intravenous pulse methyl prednisolone therapy of acute crescentic rapidly progressive glomerulonephritis. *Am J Med* 66:495–502, 1979
9. O'NEILL WM, ETHERIDGE WB, BLOOMER HA: High dose corticosteroids. Their use in treatment of idiopathic rapidly progressive glomerulonephritis. *Arch Intern Med* 139:514–518, 1979
10. OREDUGBA O, MAZUMDAR DC, MEYER JS, LUBOWITZ H: Pulse methyl prednisolone therapy in idiopathic rapidly progressive nephritis. *Ann Intern Med* 92:504–506, 1980
11. COHEN J, PINCHING AJ, REES AJ, PETERS DK: Infection and immunosuppression: a study of the infective complications of 75 patients with immunologically mediated diseases. *Q J Med* 51:1–15, 1982

12. HOYOUX C, FOIDART J, RIGO P, MAHIEU P, GEUBELLE F: Effects of methyl prednisolone on the Fc receptor function of human reticuloendothelial system in vivo. *Eur J Clin Inv* 14:60–67, 1984
13. BOWMAN C, MASON DW, PUSEY CD, LOCKWOOD CM: Autoregulation of auto-antibody synthesis in mercuric chloride nephritis in the Brown Norway rat. I. A role for T suppressor cells. *Eur J Immunol,* in press
14. CHALOPIN JM, LOCKWOOD CM: Auto-regulation of auto-antibody synthesis in mercuric chloride nephritis in the Brown Norway rat. II. Presence of antigen augmentable plaque-forming cells in the spleen is associated with humoral factors behaving as auto anti-idiotypic antibodies. *Eur J Immunol,* in press
15. LOCKWOOD CM, AMOS N, PETERS DK: Goodpasture's syndrome: radioimmunoassay for measurement of circulating anti-GBM antibodies (*abstract*). *Kidney Int* 16:93A, 1979
16. EWAN PW, JONES HA, RHODES CG, HUGHES JMB: Detection of pulmonary haemorrhage with carbon monoxide uptake. *N Engl J Med* 195:1391–1396, 1976
17. PUSSELL BA, LOCKWOOD CM, SCOTT DM, PINCHING AJ, PETERS DK: Value of immune complex assays in diagnosis and management. *Lancet* 2:359–363, 1978
18. LOCKWOOD CM, PUSEY CD, REES AJ, PETERS DK: Plasma exchange in the treatment of immune complex disease. *Clin Immunol Allergy* 1:433–455, 1981
19. HIND CRK, WINEARLS CG, LOCKWOOD CM, REES AJ, PEPYS MB: Objective assessment of disease activity in systemic vasculitis by serum C-reactive protein measurement: a prospective study of 38 patients. *Clin Nephrol,* in press
20. PUSEY CD, LOCKWOOD CM, PETERS DK: Plasma exchange and immunosuppressive drugs in the treatment of non-antibody mediated glomerulonephritis, in *Plasmapheresis,* edited by NOSE Y, MALCHESKY PS, SMITH JW, KRAKAUER RS, New York, Raven Press, 1983, pp 59–64
21. WOLD RT, YOUNG FE, TAU EM, FARR RS: Deoxyribonucleic acid antibody. A method to detect its primary interaction with deoxyribonucleic acid. *Science* 161:806, 1974
22. LACHMANN PJ, HOBART MJ: Complement technology, in *Handbook of Experimental Immunology,* edited by WEIR DM, Oxford, Blackwell Scientific Publishers, 1978, pp 5A1–5A23
23. REES AJ, PETERS DK, COMPSTON DAS, BATCHELOR JR: Strong association between HLA DRW2 and antibody mediated Goodpasture's syndrome. *Lancet* 1:966–968, 1978
24. REES AJ, LOCKWOOD CM, PETERS DK: Enhanced allergic tissue injury in Goodpasture's syndrome by intercurrent infection. *Br Med J* 2:723–726, 1977
25. DONAGHY M, REES AJ: Cigarette smoking and lung haemorrhage in glomerulonephritis caused by autoantibodies to glomerular basement membrane. *Lancet* 2:1390–1393, 1983
26. TAUBE DH, WILLIAMS DG, CAMERON JS, BEWICK M, OGG CS, RUDGE CJ, WELSH KI, KENNEDY LA, THICK MG: Renal transplantation after removal and prevention of resynthesis of HLA antibodies. *Lancet* 1:824–826, 1984
27. PUSEY CD, BOWMAN C, PETERS DK, LOCKWOOD CM: Effects of cyclophosphamide on autoantibody synthesis in the Brown Norway rat. *Clin Exp Immunol* 54:697–704, 1983
28. SUGISAKI T, KLASSEN J, MITGROM F, ANDRES GA, MCCLUSKEY RT: Immunopathologic study of an auto-immune tubular and interstitial renal disease in Brown Norway rats. *Lab Inv* 28:658–671, 1973
29. DRUET P, DRUET E, POTDEVIN F, SAPIN C: Immune type glomerulonephritis induced by $HgCl_2$ in the Brown Norway rat. *Ann Immunol (Inst Pasteur)* 129c:777–792, 1978

30. BROWN CA, CAREY K, COLVIN RB: Inhibition of autoimmune tubulointerstitial nephritis in guinea pigs by heterologous antisera containing anti-idiotype antibodies. *J Immunol* 123:2102–2107, 1979
31. NEILSON EG, PHILLIPS SM: Suppression of interstitial nephritis by auto-anti-idiotype immunity. *J Exp Med* 155:179–189.28, 1982
32. PUSEY CD: Vascular access for plasma exchange. *Apheresis Bull* i:87–91, 1983
33. SINGER D, COHEN J: Safety in plasma exchange. *Lancet* 2:1468, 1982
34. LYSAGHT MJ, SAMTLEBEN W, SCHMIDT B, GURLAND HJ: Contemporary technical issues in membrane plasmapheresis: controversies and reconciliation, in *Plasma Separation and Plasma Fraction,* edited by LYSAGHT MJ, GURLAND HJ, Basel, Karger, 1983, pp 315–328
35. RIFLE G, CHALOPIN JM, TANTER Y, DALAC S, CABANNE JF: Exchanges plasmatiques en nephrologie: etude critique. *Adv Neph* 12:243–313, 1983
36. HEAF JG, JORGENSEN F, NIELSEN LP: Treatment and prognosis of extracapillary glomerulonephritis. *Nephron* 35:217–224, 1983

Treatment of Glomerular Disease with Anticoagulant, Antiplatelet, and Nonsteroidal Anti-inflammatory Agents

James V. Donadio, Jr.

During the past 2 decades, important advances have been made in characterizing the pathogenesis, morphology, and clinical course of many varieties of human glomerular diseases. During the same time, however, no convincingly effective therapies were forthcoming to influence either the incidence or rate of renal failure from progressive forms of glomerulonephritis. Only corticosteroid drugs can alter the course of minimal-change glomerulopathy (so-called nil disease or lipoid nephrosis) in children [1] and adults [2] by inducing remission of the nephrotic syndrome in a predictable time course for therapy; usually 4 to 6 weeks. This discussion concerns the anticoagulant, antiplatelet, and nonsteroidal anti-inflammatory agents that have been used to treat various glomerular diseases.

Rationale for Use of Anticoagulant, Antiplatelet, and Nonsteroidal Anti-inflammatory Drugs

By historic perspective, treatment with anticoagulants, especially when combined with corticosteroids, immunosuppressive, and antiplatelet drugs—sometimes referred to as a "polypharmacy approach"—reached its peak of enthusiasm in the mid-1970s. The agents most often used were heparin via intravenous (i.v.) or subcutaneous injection, followed in frequency by the oral administration of sodium warfarin or phenindione. The purpose was to interfere with both the coagulation system and the formation of thrombin and fibrin. The approach to multiple drug use was based on evidence that fibrin or platelet microthrombi (or both) and immune complex formation in glomerular capillaries are the major pathogenetic mechanisms involved in the progression of most human glomerular diseases [3, 4]. Many forms of renal disease are

---

This manuscript was presented as part of a Symposium on *The Treatment of Glomerulonephritis.*

associated with deposition of fibrin in the glomeruli [5–9]. Concurrent intra-vascular coagulation can be systemic or focal; and yet, the role of intravascular coagulation in the pathogenesis of human renal disease is not fully established. Debate continues as to whether glomerular injury by intravascular coagulation is important. In experimental models of glomerular disease, evidence can be presented on both sides of the issue [10, 11]. Could it be that fibrin deposition within the glomeruli—even if secondary to immunologic mechanisms—is an important event leading to glomerular proliferation, necrosis, capillary wall thickening, and extracapillary crescents, as some experiments in animals suggest? Or is the secondary intravascular coagulation not directly involved in the progressive renal destruction? No definite answer to these questions is available. Also of concern is whether anticoagulant drugs have not only convincingly influenced models of immunologic glomerular disease, but also whether they have had an effect on human glomerulopathy [12, 13].

The rationale for the use of antiplatelet drugs in glomerulonephritis stems from demonstrating that platelets are activated in glomerular disease [14–16], that platelet factors can cause arterial smooth-muscle cell proliferation [17], and that increased platelet consumption occurs in various vascular [18–20] and renal [21, 22] diseases. In addition, platelet inhibitor drug treatment with dipyridamole and aspirin has been shown to improve shortened platelet survival, which has correlated with therapeutic benefit in patients with various cardiovascular diseases [18, 20, 23–25].

The inhibition of production of both platelet and renal prostaglandins may be the principal mechanism by which platelet inhibitor drugs reduce platelet aggregation and consumption. In clinical trials in which the daily dose of aspirin given to patients approaches or exceeds 1 g, the synthesis of both platelet thromboxane A_2 and vascular wall prostacyclin, in all likelihood, decreases [26–29]. However, 15 to 20 mg/kg/d of aspirin is the optimal dose that maximally potentiates dipyridamole to suppress the deposition and consumption of platelets in the flowing blood of animals and humans; and, the combination of these drugs is superior to aspirin alone [30–32].

Extensive investigations have demonstrated that naturally occurring prostaglandins of the E and F series significantly affect platelet function and are altered in renal disease. Thromboxane A_2 is a potent proaggregating agent in platelets and a potent vasoconstrictor, whereas prostacyclin (PGI_2) is a potent inhibitor of platelet aggregation and a potent vasodilator [26, 27]. Renal prostaglandin synthesis is increased both in various experimental models of glomerulonephritis and in human clinical conditions such as: (1) renal ischemia, in which vasoconstrictor peptides (angiotensin and vasopressin) stimulate prostaglandin synthesis, (2) extracellular fluid volume contraction after diuretic treatment or severe salt restriction, or (3) various glomerular diseases [33]. These are conditions in which prostaglandins fill a protective role in preserving renal hemodynamics.

Nonsteroidal anti-inflammatory drugs (NSAIDs) (such as aspirin, indomethacin, ibuprofen, naproxen, and meclofenamate) are potent inhibitors of the production of prostaglandins. Aspirin acetylates the enyzme fatty acid, cyclo-oxygenase, which converts arachidonic acid to labile endoperoxides that—when synthesized in kidney—are rapidly converted to prostaglandins

(PGE$_2$, PGF$_{2\alpha}$, PGI$_2$, and thromboxane A$_2$) [34, 35]. The effect of aspirin on platelets is irreversible, and its effect disappears only when a new enzyme is synthesized [36]. The other NSAIDs reversibly inhibit cyclo-oxygenase, with a gradually diminishing effect over 8 to 24 hr as they dissociate from the enzyme [37]. Thus, these drugs reduce urinary prostaglandin levels, and at the same time decrease glomerular filtration rate (GFR) and renal blood flow (RBF) under conditions in which the renal synthesis of prostaglandins is stimulated (as noted above).

Both in experimental models of nephritis and in human glomerular disease, treatment with NSAIDs—indomethacin has been the drug primarily used—reduces proteinuria [38]. The main hypothesis proposed for this effect is attributed to the inhibiting effects on the synthesis of prostaglandins and a concomitant decrease in GFR. Other possible mechanisms by which NSAIDs reduce proteinuria are by altering the capillary wall permeability itself, modifying the glomerular hemodynamics, and attenuating the inflammatory response secondary to immunologic glomerular injury [38]. These drugs not only impair GFR, they also cause renal toxicity, including the nephrotic syndrome and interstitial nephritis [39]; and, indomethacin can cause hyporeninemic hypoaldosteronism and elevated levels of serum potassium [40]. Thus, because of adverse effects, nephrologists have been reluctant to use these drugs in a therapeutic setting. Also, there have been no prospective studies to substantiate claims that there is no relationship between the effects of NSAIDs on proteinuria and renal function, and therefore on the long-term preservation of glomerular function [38].

Clinical Studies

Retrospective Treatment Studies

In a literature survey, covering 1975 to 1984, of retrospective or uncontrolled (or both) clinical studies involving five or more patients, there were nearly equal findings of favorable, equivocal, and unfavorable effects of various anticoagulants, NSAIDs, and combination regimens (Table 1) [41–66]. There were no studies on the use of antiplatelet drugs alone in the treatment of glomerular diseases. Furthermore, in those treatment studies, it is difficult to sort out the wide range of entities that were variously described and defined on both clinical and histopathologic bases (Table 2).

At the clinical level, justification for the use of anticoagulant, antiplatelet, and NSAID agents has been based on the severity of disease, which was generally defined by observing reduced renal function at the first examination or rapidly declining renal function in patients with glomerular disease. In some instances, aggressive disease was defined as the presence of crescents in a renal biopsy specimen; in other instances, it was the presence of persisting massive proteinuria, which has been shown to presage a poor prognosis in several forms of human glomerular disease [53, 67]. Multiple-entity therapy was most often used in patients who had renal failure due to more aggressive

Table 1. Treatment of glomerular disease with anticoagulant, NSAIDs, and various combinations in uncontrolled/retrospective studies (5 or more patients per study), 1975–1984 [36–60]

Drug	Results[a]		
	Favorable	Equivocal	Not favorable
Anticoagulant	2	—	3
Antiplatelet	—	—	—
NSAID[b]	2	3	2
Combinations[c]	6	3	6
Totals	10	6	11

[a] Favorable results attributed mostly to stable or improved renal function with anticoagulants and combinations of agents, and a reduction in proteinuria after NSAIDs. Complications of drug therapy were highlighted in four studies and were primarily bleeding due to anticoagulants.
[b] Nonsteroidal anti-inflammatory drugs (generally, indomethacin).
[c] Two to five drugs used: anticoagulant or antiplatelet (or both) agents plus immunosuppressive or corticosteroid (or both) drugs.

renal parenchymal lesions. Although platelet and fibrin deposits are found both in intra- and extracapillary locations in the renal glomeruli of patients with rapidly progressive glomerulonephritis (RPGN), treatment with continuous infusions or intermittent IV injections of heparin, alone or with other drugs, have not convincingly resolved crescentic lesions or improved renal function in a sustained manner in patients thus treated [44, 49, 50]. In two reports of children with RPGN and extensive crescent formation, renal function improved—especially in those children with apparent postinfectious nephritis—after anticoagulant and antiplatelet treatment [48, 57]. In the studies that reported favorable results with NSAIDs, reduction in proteinuria was the usual effect, while stable renal function or impaired renal morphology or both were reported with the combined drug programs. However, in all such studies, claims that renal function improved, renal failure was delayed, or proteinuria reduction was maintained without severely impairing renal function were not confirmed by prospective, controlled clinical trials. In four

Table 2. Categories of glomerular disease treated with anticoagulant, antiplatelet, NSAIDs reported in uncontrolled/retrospective studies

Acute anuric lupus nephropathy	Membranoproliferative GN
Chronic GN	Mesangioproliferative GN
"Collagenous" GN	Minimal-change glomerulopathy
Crescentic GN, some poststreptococcal, in children	Nephrotic syndrome—different glomerulopathies
Diffuse histologic forms of GN	Pre-eclampsia
Focal sclerosing GN, in children and adults	Rapidly progressive GN (RPGN)
"Histologically confirmed" GN	"Severe GN," in children
IgA nephropathy	"Various" GN
Lupus GN	

GN, glomerulonephritis.

of the retrospective treatment studies, complications of treatment were emphasized—in particular, bleeding due to anticoagulants [44, 49, 53, 54].

The use of ancrod, which is the purified fraction of the Malayan pit viper venom, has been shown to improve renal function and to decrease fibrin deposition and crescents in experimental glomerulonephritis [68, 69]. The agent acts by converting plasma fibrinogen to an unstable form of fibrin without an effect on other blood coagulation factors [70, 71]. In five patients with glomerulonephritis—four with systemic lupus erythematosus (SLE)— renal function remained stable or improved after treatment with ancrod [63]. However, prednisone treatment also was included in the treatment program, making it difficult to determine the additional effect of defibrination on the glomerular process.

On the venous side of the circulation, renal vein thrombosis is a well-known complication in patients with the nephrotic syndrome [72, 73]. Various coagulation abnormalities have been documented in nephrotic patients irrespective of the type of renal disease [72–76]. However, renal vein thrombosis most often is associated in idiopathic membranous glomerulopathy [72, 76, 77]. It is important to point out that coagulation abnormalities do not necessarily predispose nephrotic patients to renal vein thrombosis, and the incidence of thromboembolic phenomena appears to be low [76]. The use of anticoagulants has been reported to alter these complications [72]. Such treatment is advocated in individuals who clinically demonstrate thromboembolic events, especially pulmonary embolism. On the other hand, it remains uncertain whether the use of conventional anticoagulants or thrombolytic agents (such as prourokinase and streptokinase) influences the clinical course of the nephrotic patient, both in terms of preservation of renal function and reduction of proteinuria, even when renal vein thrombosis is present [76, 77]. No prospective studies are available. Perhaps the newer thrombolytic agents may be beneficial in patients with rapidly deteriorating renal function in whom complete main renal vein thrombosis could be a contributing and reversible influence [78, 79].

Prospective Clinical Trials

Only five prospective studies have been reported on the use of anticoagulant or antiplatelet drugs in glomerular disease—four on membranoproliferative glomerulonephritis (MPGN) and one on focal glomerulosclerosis. There are no prospective studies on the effects of NSAIDs on primary glomerular disease.

Futrakul et al [80] described 17 children with focal sclerosing glomerulonephritis and unusual clinical manifestations. These included what the authors termed a "hypercoagulable state" that was characterized by elevated fibrinogen and factor V levels and by platelet counts, but in which there were no clinical events such as bleeding or thrombosis. Also, one-third of the children had undisclosed types of peritonitis, and 82% had urinary tract infections. The study compared prednisolone and cyclophosphamide therapy with a quadruple-drug program of heparin, dipyridamole, prednisolone, and cyclophosphamide. Significant improvement in creatinine clearance (C_{cr}), ^{131}I-labeled para-aminohippurate to estimate RBF, and protein excretion were observed in the group with quadruple-drug treatment. However, methods of treatment assignment, the length of time (except for cyclophosphamide, 3 months), and complications of treatment were not mentioned. This lack of information both about the study design and the unusual clinical features overshadow the favorable results on renal parameters. It is difficult to recommend this form of treatment for either children or adults in view of the multiple dangers for severe drug toxicity.

As mentioned previously, four randomized therapeutic trials have been conducted in patients with MPGN. Two of the studies reported on triple-drug therapy with cyclophosphamide, dipyridamole, and sodium warfarin that, in an uncontrolled study, had been previously shown to benefit patients with MPGN. In 1972, Kincaid-Smith [81] reported on the use of this treatment regimen in 16 adults with type I or II MPGN and various degrees of renal failure, hypertension, and the nephrotic syndrome. Ten patients had clinical improvement, whereas six had renal function that either decreased or remained stable. Renal biopsy specimens were taken in all patients after treatment, and improvement was shown in glomerular morphologic features in four patients, with the improvement most striking in three of those who had had only mild renal functional impairment at the onset of treatment. The 30-month survival curves of the 16 treated patients were significantly better than those of the 13 patients who did not receive this form of treatment. The Australian Working Party in Glomerulonephritis reported their prospective, randomized therapeutic trial of the triple-drug regimen in 37 patients with both type I and type II MPGN [82]. In patients who completed 36 months of treatment, the authors concluded that no beneficial effects accrued; and, they were most disturbed about the high dropout rate of patients, most of whom were in the treatment group. Hemorrhagic cystitis, bone marrow depression, and other bleeding complications were the principal reasons for withdrawal from the study. In another independent controlled trial of cyclophosphamide, warfarin, and dipyridamole, the Metropolitan Toronto Glomerulonephritis Group reported on 63 adult patients with type I or type II lesions [83]. After a follow-up period of 18 months, they found no significant effects of treatment on proteinuria or renal function. Thus, the earlier uncontrolled observations by Kincaid-Smith were not confirmed by the prospective, randomized trials examining the use of this combination of agents.

Because evidence suggests that platelet activation and increased platelet consumption have a pathogenetic role in MPGN, two additional prospective trials examined the usefulness of platelet inhibitors. Zimmerman et al [84] combined treatment with sodium warfarin and dipyridamole in 18 adult patients (17 with type I, 1 with type II lesions) who completed either a control or treatment year—13 of whom completed both a control and treatment year. The study group received dipyridamole (400 mg/d) and warfarin, the dose of which was adjusted to maintain the prothrombin time at 1.5 to 2 times the control value. By determining the slopes of reciprocal serum creatinine values during control and treatment years, renal function was found to be better preserved in the treated group; but, only in the unpaired analysis of 18 patients comparing a control year first versus a treatment year first. In the paired analysis of renal function changes in the 13 patients who completed both a control and treatment year, differences in slopes of reciprocal creatinine favoring treatment were noted only for six patients, who demonstrated a change in renal function during 1 of the years of observation.

My colleagues and I [85] recently completed a study of 40 patients with type I MPGN who were treated for 1 year with dipyridamole (225 mg/d) and aspirin (975 mg/d) in a prospective, randomized, double-blind, and placebo-controlled study. Platelet survival, which was determined with ^{51}Cr-labeled autologous platelets, was shortened at the baseline in 12 of 17 patients. The shortened platelet survival was improved and renal function was stabilized in the treated group compared with the placebo group, which suggests a relationship between platelet consumption and aggregation on the glomerular disease. The GFR, which was determined by iothalamate clearance, was better maintained in the treated group—decreasing 1.3 ml/min/1.73 m^2/12 mo—than in the placebo group, which had an average decrease of 19.6 ml/12 mo. There was no effect of treatment on proteinuria. We followed-up our patients regularly for as long as 84 months, with the masked conditions of the controlled trial ending after 1 year of treatment. Fewer patients in the treated group progressed to terminal renal failure (3 of 21) after 62 months, compared with the placebo group (9 of 19) after 33 months. We concluded that dipyridamole and aspirin significantly slowed the deterioration of renal function and the development of terminal renal disease.

We believe there were several possible mechanisms by which the GFR was better maintained in the patients who were treated with dipyridamole and aspirin. First, a reduction in platelet-vascular wall interaction or platelet consumption might have stabilized the glomerulopathy, with this contention supported by the observed improvement in platelet survival in treated patients who maintained a satisfactory GFR. Also, the inhibition of both the platelet production and the renal production of prostaglandins could be another mechanism by which platelet-inhibitor drugs stabilized the GFR. The key to our study is whether the continued use of these agents will preserve renal function in a substantial number of patients with this generally progressive glomerulopathy. An analysis of the inter-relationships among renal prostanoids, platelets, glomerular function, and platelet inhibitors might provide a better understanding of the pathogenesis of this and other forms of progressive glomerulopathy and may lead to improved therapy.

References

1. INTERNATIONAL STUDY OF KIDNEY DISEASE IN CHILDREN: Nephrotic syndrome in children. Prediction of histopathology from clinical and laboratory characteristics at time of diagnosis. *Kidney Int* 13:159–165, 1978
2. COGGINS CH: Minimal change nephrosis in adults, in *Proceedings of 8th International Congress on Nephrology, Athens.* Basel, Karger, 1981, pp 336–344
3. VASSALLI P, MCCLUSKEY R: The pathogenetic role of fibrin deposition in immunologically induced glomerulonephritis. *Ann NY Acad Sci* 116:1052–1062, 1964
4. HAWIGEN J: Platelets, endothelium and immune reactions in renal disease, in

Hemostasis, Prostaglandins and Renal Disease, edited by REMUZZI G, MECCA G, DEGAETANO G, New York, Raven Press, 1980, pp 73–78

5. VASSALLI P, MCCLUSKEY RT: The coagulation process in glomerular disease. *Am J Med* 39:179–183, 1965

6. MCCLUSKEY RT, ET AL: An immunofluorescent study of pathogenetic mechanisms in glomerular diseases. *N Engl J Med* 274:695–701, 1966

7. STARZL TE, ET AL: Shwartzman reaction after human renal homotransplantation. *N Engl J Med* 278:642–648, 1968

8. DUFFY JL, ET AL: Intraglomerular fibrin, platelet aggregation, and subendothelial deposits and lipoid nephrosis. *J Clin Invest* 49:251–258, 1970

9. BOND RE, DONADIO JV JR, HOLLEY KE, BOWIE EJW: Fibrinolytic split products: a clinicopathologic correlative study in adults with lupus glomerulonephritis and various renal diseases. *Arch Intern Med* 132:182–187, 1973

10. VASSALLI O, MCCLUSKEY R: The pathogenetic role of the coagulation process in rabbit Masugi nephritis. *Am J Pathol* 45:653–678, 1964

11. THOMPSON NM, SIMPSON IJ, PETERS DK: A quantitative evaluation of anticoagulants in experimental nephrotoxic nephritis. *Clin Exp Immunol* 19:301–308, 1975

12. KINCAID-SMITH P: Anticoagulants are of value in the treatment of renal disease. *Am J Kidney Dis* 3:299–307, 1984

13. BORDER WA: Anticoagulants are of little value in the treatment of renal disease. *Am J Kidney Dis* 3:308–312, 1984

14. PARBTANI A, CAMERON JS: Platelet involvement in glomerulonephritis, in *Hemostasis, Prostaglandins and Renal Disease,* edited by REMUZZI G, MECCA G, DEGAETANO G, New York, Raven Press, 1980, pp 45–61

15. CLARK WF, FRIESEN M, LINTON AL, LINDSAY RM: The platelet as a mediator of tissue damage in immune complex glomerulonephritis. *Clin Nephrol* 6:287–289, 1976

16. GEORGE CRP, CLARK WF, CAMERON JS: The role of platelets in glomerulonephritis. *Adv Nephrol* 5:19–65, 1975

17. ROSS R, GLOMSET J, KARIYA B, HARKER L: A platelet-dependent serum factor that stimulates the proliferation of arterial smooth muscle cells *in vitro. Proc Natl Acad Sci USA* 71:1207–1210, 1974

18. HARKER LA, SLICHTER SJ: Platelet and fibrinogen consumption in man. *N Engl J Med* 287:999–1005, 1972

19. KAZMIER FJ, FUSTER V, CHESEBRO JH, O'FALLON WM, PALUMBO PJ: Platelet survival half-life (PS) in atherosclerosis and diabetes mellitus (*abstract*). *Circulation* 60(Suppl)2:270, 1979

20. FUSTER V, CHESEBRO JH, FRYE RL, ELVEBACK LR: Platelet survival and the development of coronary artery disease in the young adult: effects of cigarette smoking, strong family history and medical therapy. *Circulation* 63:546–551, 1981

21. CARRUTHERS JA, RALFS I, GIMLETTE TMD, FINN R: Platelet survival in acute proliferative glomerulonephritis. *Clin Sci Molec Med* 47:507–513, 1974

22. GEORGE CRP, SLICHTER SJ, QUADRACCI LT, STRIKER GE, HARKER LA: A kinetic evaluation of hemostasis in renal disease. *N Engl J Med* 291:1111–1115, 1974

23. STEELE P, RAINWATER J, VOGEL R: Platelet suppressant therapy in patients with prosthetic cardiac valves: relationship of clinical effectiveness to alteration of platelet survival time. *Circulation* 60:910–913, 1979

24. HARKER LA, ROSS R, SLICHTER SJ, SCOTT CR: Homocystine-induced arteriosclerosis: the role of endothelial cell injury and platelet response in its genesis. *J Clin Invest* 58:731–741, 1976

25. FUSTER V, CHESEBRO JH: Antithrombotic therapy: role of platelet-inhibitor drugs (second of three parts). *Mayo Clin Proc* 56:185–195, 1981

26. HAMBERG M, SVENSSON J, WAKABAYASHI T, SAMUELSSON B: Isolation and structure of two endoperoxides that cause platelet aggregation. *Proc Natl Acad Sci USA* 71:345–349, 1974

27. MONCADA S, VANE JR: Pharmacology and endogenous roles of prostaglandin endoperoxides, thromboxane A_2, and prostacyclin. *Pharmacol Rev* 30:293–331, 1978

28. MASOTTI G, GALANTI G, POGGESI L, ABBATE R, NERI SERNERI GG: Differential inhibition of prostacyclin production and platelet aggregation by aspirin. *Lancet* 2:1213–1216, 1979

29. WEKSLER BB, PETT SB, ALONSO D, RICHTER RC, STELZER P, SUBRAMANIAN V, TACK-GOLDMAN K, GAY WA JR: Differential inhibition by aspirin of vascular and platelet prostaglandin synthesis in atherosclerotic patients. *N Engl J Med* 308:800–805, 1983

30. MONCADA S, KORBUT R: Dipyridamole and other phosphodiesterase inhibitors act as antithrombotic agents by potentiating endogenous prostacyclin. *Lancet* 1:1286–1289, 1978

31. HANSON SR, HARKER LA: Evaluation of pharmacologic inhibitors of platelet function in baboons (*abstract*). *Thromb Haemost* 46:102, 1981

32. CHESEBRO JH, FUSTER V, NISHIMURA RA, STEELE PM, BADIMON L, ELVEBACK LR: Platelet survival in coronary patients: good response to dipyridamole plus aspirin, partial response to low-dose aspirin with or without dipyridamole; implications for trials (*abstract*). *Circulation* 68(Suppl III):105, 1983

33. DUNN MJ: Renal prostaglandins, in *Renal Endocrinology,* edited by DUNN MJ, Baltimore, Williams & Wilkins, 1983, pp 1–74

34. SMITH JB, WILLIS AL: Aspirin selectively inhibits prostaglandin production in human platelets. *Nature* 231:235–237, 1971

35. ROTH GJ, STANFORD N, MAJERUS PW: Acetylation of prostaglandin synthetase by aspirin. *Proc Natl Acad Sci USA* 72:6073–6076, 1975

36. ROTH GJ, MAJERUS PW: The mechanism of the effect of aspirin in human platelets. *J Clin Invest* 56:624–632, 1975

37. DUNN MJ, ZAMBRASKI EJ: Renal effects of drugs that inhibit prostaglandin synthesis. *Kidney Int* 18:609–622, 1980

38. MICHIELSEN P, VARENTERGHEM Y: Proteinuria and nonsteroidal anti-inflammatory drugs. *Adv Nephrol* 12:139–150, 1983

39. TORRES VE: Present and future of the nonsteroidal anti-inflammatory drugs in nephrology (*editorial*). *Mayo Clin Proc* 57:389–393, 1982

40. TAN SY, SHAPIRO R, FRANCO R, STOCKARD H, MULROW PJ: Indomethacin-induced prostaglandin inhibition with hyperkalemia. *Ann Intern Med* 90:783–785, 1979

41. CONTE JJ, MIGNON-CONTE MA, FOURNIE GJ: Lupus nephropathy. Treatment with the indomethacin-hydroxychloroquine combination and comparison with corticoids. *Nouv Presse Med* 4:91–95, 1975

42. PONTICELLI C, IMBASCIATI E, BRANCACCIO D, TARANTINO A, RIVOLTA E: Reversible acute anuric lupus nephritis. *Proc Eur Dial Transplant Assoc* 11:500–505, 1975

43. VANRENTERGHEM Y, ROELS L, VERBERCKMOES R, MICHIELSEN P: Treatment of chronic glomerulonephritis with a combination of indomethacin and cyclophosphamide. *Clin Nephrol* 4:218–222, 1975

44. SUC JM, DURAND D, CONTE J, MIGNON-CONTE M, ORFILA C, THAT HT, DUCHET JP: The use of heparin in the treatment of idiopathic rapidly progressive glomerulonephritis. *Clin Nephrol* 5:9–13, 1976

45. ARISZ L, DONKER AJ, BRENTJENS JR, VAN DER HEM GK: The effect of indo-

methacin on proteinuria and kidney function in the nephrotic syndrome. *Acta Med Scand* 199:121–125, 1976

46. MICHIELSEN P, ROELS L, VANRENTERGHEM Y, BOEL A, VAN DAMME B, VERMYLEN J: Significance of urinary excretion of fibrin degradation products during treatment of glomerulonephritis. *Clin Nephrol* 5:105–113, 1976

47. FAIRLEY KF, ADEY FD, ROSS IC, KINCAID-SMITH P: Heparin treatment in severe preeclampsia and glomerulonephritis in pregnancy. *Perspect Nephrol Hypertens* 5:103–112, 1976

48. ROBSON AM, COLE BR, KIENSTRA RA, KISSANE JM, ALKJAERSIG N, FLETCHER AP: Severe glomerulonephritis complicated by coagulopathy: treatment with anticoagulant and immunosuppressive drugs. *Pediatrics* 90:881–882, 1977

49. QUELLHORST E, REICHEL W, FERNANDEZ-REDO E, SCHELER F: Treatment of glomerulonephritis with heparin. *Med Klin* 72:981–987, 1977

50. WARDLE EN, ULDALL PR: Effect of heparin on renal function in patients with oliguria. *Br Med J* 4:135–138, 1972

51. THEBAULT JJ, LAGRUE G, BLATRIX CE, CHEYNIER L, CLUZAN R: Clinical pharmacology of flurbiprofen: a novel inhibitor of platelet aggregation. *Curr Med Res Opin* 5:130–134, 1977

52. GARIN EH, WILLIAMS RL, FENNELL RS, RICHARD GA: Indomethacin in the treatment of idiopathic minimal lesion nephrotic syndrome. *J Pediatr* 93:138–140, 1978

53. BEAUFILS H, ALPHONSE JC, GUEDON J, LEGRAIN M: Focal glomerulosclerosis: natural history and treatment. A report of 70 cases. *Nephron* 21:75–85, 1978

54. FUNISTUCK R, STEIN G, KROHS G, SPERSCHNEIDER H, STELZNER A, SUSSE I, WALDMANN G: Long-term treatment of glomerulonephritis with indomethacin with special regard to quantity and selectivity of proteinuria. *Urol Nephrol* 71:375–383, 1978

55. DONKER AJ, BRENTJENS JR, VAN DER HEM GK, ARISZ L: Treatment of the nephrotic syndrome with indomethacin. *Nephron* 22:374–381, 1978

56. SCHMITT E, KROGER E, LAKNER V, KLINKMANN H, RATNER M, TOMILINA N: Therapy of primary glomerulonephritis. Comparative study on the effect of cytostatics-prednisone and cytostatics-anticoagulant-aggregation inhibitor combination. *Gesamte Inn Med* 34:465–471, 1979

57. CUNNINGHAM RJ, GILFOIL M, CAVALLO T, BROUHARD BH, TRAVIS LB, BERGER M, PETRUSICK T: Rapidly progressive glomerulonephritis in children: a report of thirteen cases and a review of the literature. *Pediatr Res* 14:128–132, 1980

58. CHAPMAN SJ, CAMERON JS, CHANTLER C, TURNER D: Treatment of mesangiocapillary glomerulonephritis in children with combined immunosuppression and anticoagulation. *Arch Dis Child* 55:446–451, 1980

59. SCHMITT E, SINN W, LAKNER V, RATNER M, TOMILINA N: Glomerulonephritis therapy. Immunosuppression or coagulation inhibitor—a comparison. *Gesamte Inn Med* 35(Suppl):45–48, 1980

60. FUTRAKUL P: A new therapeutic approach of nephrotic syndrome associated with focal segmental glomerulosclerosis. *Int J Pediatr Nephrol* 1:18–21, 1980

61. ROY S, MURPHY WM, ARANT BS: Poststreptococcal crescenteric glomerulonephritis in children: comparison of quintuple therapy versus supportive care. *J Pediatr* 98:403–410, 1981

62. BELOVEZHDOV N, ROBEVA R: Controlled therapeutic trial in IgA glomerulonephritis. *Vutr Boles* 21:49–53, 1982

63. POLLAK VE, GLUECK HI, WEISS MA, LEBRON-BERGES A, MILLER MA: Defibri-

nation with ancrod in glomerulonephritis: effects on clinical and histologic findings and on blood coagulation. *Am J Nephrol* 2:195–207, 1982

64. BHUYAN UN, DASH SC, SRIVASTAVA RN, SHARMA RK, MALHOTRA KK: Immunopathology, extent and course of glomerulonephritis with crescent formation. *Clin Nephrol* 18:280–285, 1982

65. BELOVEZHDOV N, TSEKOVA D, DZHERASI R, GRUEN I, KIPEROVA B: Possibilities of combined treatment of diffuse collagenous glomerulonephritis. *Vutr Boles* 21:25–34, 1982

66. SINN W, SCHMICKER R, KLINKMANN H: Complications in the treatment of chronic glomerulonephritis. *Urol Nephrol* 76:497–502, 1983

67. VELOSA JA, HOLLEY KE, TORRES VE, OFFORD KP: Significance of proteinuria on the outcome of renal function in patients with focal segmental glomerulosclerosis. *Mayo Clin Proc* 58:568–577, 1983

68. NAISH P, EVANS DJ, PETERS DK: The effects of defibrination with ancrod in experimental allergic glomerular injury. *Clin Exp Immunol* 20:303–309, 1975

69. THOMSON NM, SIMPSON IJ, EVANS DJ, PETERS DK: Defibrination with ancrod in experimental chronic immune complex nephritis. *Clin Exp Immunol* 20:527–535, 1975

70. REID HA, CHAN KE, THEAN PC: Prolonged coagulation defect (defibrination syndrome) in Malayan viper bite. *Lancet* 1:621–626, 1963

71. ESNOUF MP, TUNNAH GW: The isolation and properties of the thrombin-like activity from Ancistrodon rhodostoma venom. *Br J Haemat* 13:581–590, 1967

72. LLACH F, PAPPER S, MASSRY SG: The clinical spectrum of renal vein thrombosis. *Am J Med* 69:819–827, 1980

73. HARRINGTON JT, KASSIRER JP: Renal vein thrombosis. *Ann Rev Med* 33:255–262, 1982

74. KANFER A, KLEINKNECHT D, BROYER M, JOSSO F: Coagulation studies in 45 cases of nephrotic syndrome without uremia. *Thromb Diath Haemorrh* 24:562–571, 1970

75. KENDALL AG, LOHMANN RC, DOSSETOR JB: Nephrotic syndrome: a hypercoagulable state. *Arch Intern Med* 127:1021–1027, 1971

76. WAGONER RD, STANSON AW, HOLLEY KE, WINTER CS: Renal vein thrombosis in idiopathic membranous glomerulopathy and nephrotic syndrome: incidence and signficance. *Kidney Int* 23:368–374, 1983

77. HARRINGTON JT: Thrombolytic therapy in renal vein thrombosis. *Arch Intern Med* 144:33–34, 1984

78. CROWLEY JP, MATARESE RA, QUEVEDO SF, GARELLA S: Fibrinolytic therapy for bilateral renal vein thrombosis. *Arch Intern Med* 144:159–160, 1984

79. BURROW CR, WALKER WG, BELL WR, GATEWOOD OB: Streptokinase salvage of renal function after renal vein thrombosis. *Ann Intern Med* 100:237–238, 1984

80. FUTRAKUL P, POSHYACHINDA M, MITRAKUL C: Focal sclerosing glomerulonephritis: a kinetic evaluation of hemostasis and the effect of anticoagulant therapy: a controlled study. *Clin Nephrol* 10:180–186, 1978

81. KINCAID-SMITH P: The treatment of chronic mesangiocapillary (membrano-proliferative) glomerulonephritis with impaired renal function. *Med J Aust* 2:587–592, 1972

82. TILLER DJ, CLARKSON AR, MATHEW T, ET AL: A prospective randomized trial in the use of cyclophosphamide, dipyridamole and warfarin in membranous and mesangiocapillary glomerulonephritis, in *Eighth International Congress of Nephrology: Advances in Basic and Clinical Nephrology*, edited by ZURUKZOGLU W, PAPADIMITRIOU M, SION M, Basel, Karger, 1981, pp 345–351

83. CATTRAN D, CHARRON R, CARDELLA C, ET AL: Controlled trial in mesangiocapillary glomerulonephritis (MCGN) (*abstract*), in *Eighth International Con-*

gress of Nephrology: Advances in Basic and Clinical Nephrology, edited by ZU-RUKZOGLU W, PAPADIMITRIOU M, SION M, Basel, Karger, 1981, p 287
84. ZIMMERMAN SW, MOORTHY AV, DREHER WH, FRIEDMANN A, VARANASI U: Prospective trial of warfarin and dipyridamole in patients with membranoproliferative glomerulonephritis. *Am J Med* 75:920–927, 1983
85. DONADIO JV, ANDERSON CF, MITCHELL JC, HOLLEY KE, ILSTRUP DM, FUSTER V, CHESEBRO JH: Membranoproliferative glomerulonephritis: a prospective clinical trial of platelet-inhibitor therapy. *N Engl J Med* (in press, 1984)

Nutrition in Renal Failure

Causes of Catabolism and Wasting in Acute or Chronic Renal Failure

Joel D. Kopple

Patients with acute or chronic renal failure are frequently hypercatabolic and may develop wasting and malnutrition. Usually, this is the result of superimposed illnesses. The occurrence of complicating illnesses is frequent in both acute renal failure and chronic uremia. In two recent surveys in the United States, the average number of days of hospitalization each year was 15.1 in patients treated with maintenance hemodialysis and 16.9 and 19.7 days, respectively, in patients undergoing continuous ambulatory peritoneal dialysis (CAPD) [1, 2].

Animal studies suggest that acute and chronic uremia, in themselves, may promote mild catabolism and protein wasting [3–5]. However, when patients with these disorders have associated underlying or superimposed illnesses, the degree of hypercatabolism can be profound [6, 7]; and, it may contribute to their high morbidity and—particularly for patients with acute renal failure—their high mortality. Even relatively mild illnesses may be surprisingly catabolic [6]. Intercurrent illnesses probably contribute to the high prevalence of wasting and malnutrition in nondialyzed patients with chronic renal failure and in patients undergoing maintenance dialysis. To this author's knowledge, every survey published in the past 6 years has indicated an increased incidence of wasting and malnutrition in these individuals [8–20].

There has been surprisingly little research concerning the adverse effects of wasting and malnutrition in renal failure. Acchiardo, Moore, and Latour studied the relationship between protein intake, as indicated by the net protein catabolic rate, and morbidity and mortality in 98 nondiabetic patients undergoing maintenance hemodialysis [21]. Patients were followed for 1 year, and they were assigned according to their calculated average net protein catabolic rate and mean serum urea nitrogen (SUN) level into four groups; these groups had a mean net protein catabolic rate of 0.63, 0.93, 1.02, and 1.2 g/kg/d, respectively. The group that had the lowest average net protein catabolic rate (0.63 g/kg/d), which indicates that they had the lowest protein intake, displayed the greatest frequency of hospitalization, the greatest number of

This manuscript was presented as part of a Symposium on *Nutritional Aspects of Renal Disease.*

days in the hospital, and the highest mortality rate. In the four groups, there was a rough inverse correlation between the protein intake and both the number of hospitalizations per patient per year and the mortality rate. Although this study suffers from the fact that protein intake was not varied randomly and independently, the data nonetheless are consistent with the thesis that poor nutrient intake and malnutrition adversely affect the prognosis in maintenance dialysis patients.

There are many factors that may promote wasting and malnutrition both in patients with acute renal failure and in chronically uremic patients, especially in a setting of intercurrent illnesses. This chapter will discuss these factors with an emphasis on those that lead to protein wasting. The possible causes of wasting in adult patients with acute or chronic renal failure and superimposed catabolic stress are listed in Table 1. The role of some of these

Table 1. Possible causes of wasting in patients with acute or chronic renal failure

Inadequate intake of nutrients
Factors that increase net degradation of protein and amino acids
   Catabolic illnesses
      Altered hormonal milieu
      Increased protease activity
      Microbial toxins (?)[a]
      Increased energy requirements
      Tissue hypoxia
      Acidosis (?)
   Altered hormonal activity of uremia (?)
      Insulin resistance
      Hyperglucagonemia
      Growth hormone—somatomedins
      Hyperparathyroidism
      Epinephrine
   Catabolic stimulus of hemodialysis
   Uremic toxins (?)
Nutrient removed by dialysis
   Protein (with peritoneal dialysis)—losses may be marked during peritonitis
   Amino acids
   Glucose (with hemodialysis with glucose-free dialysate)
   Water-soluble vitamins
Medicines that alter the digestion, absorption, excretion, or metabolism of nutrients
   Example: Anticonvulsants cause folate and vitamin D deficiency; isoniazid and hydralazine
   cause pyridoxine deficiency; and antibiotics in fasting patients may cause vitamin K deficiency
Losses of protein and other nutrients from blood drawing, intestinal malabsorption, enteric
   fistulas, and draining wounds
Impaired hormonal or metabolic activity of the kidney (?)
   1,25-dihydroxycholecalciferol deficiency
   Erythropoietin deficiency
   Impaired renal synthesis or degradation of amino acids, peptides (including hormones), and
   small proteins
Clinical or nutritional status prior to the onset of renal failure or intercurrent illness

[a] A question mark indicates that although these factors may contribute to wasting, at present, there is virtually no evidence supporting this possibility.

factors is well defined; for others, the evidence, although suggestive, is not definitive.

Inadequate Intake of Nutrients

Inadequate intake is a well-described and important cause of wasting in patients with renal failure [8]. An acute illness may impair the uremic patient's ability to eat, digest, absorb, or use nutrients. Some illnesses may simply depress mentation or induce anorexia; others may alter gastrointestinal function or metabolic processes. Diagnostic or therapeutic procedures may require patients to fast, sometimes for many hours or (in the case of surgical procedures) days.

The hemodialysis procedure and certain medicines offered to uremic patients may cause anorexia, nausea, or vomiting. The reduction in food intake by a sick patient may not be readily apparent. Such individuals frequently experience hunger. However, intake of even small quantities of food may cause satiety; and further food intake may promote nausea or vomiting. Patients are particularly likely to reject food when they are given the large quantities that often are necessary to maintain neutral protein and energy balance during superimposed illness. In our experience, when a dietary history is taken from sick patients, they not uncommonly overestimate their food intake, possibly because they fear displeasing their physician. The hospital dietician or food technologist can accurately estimate the daily food intake of hospitalized patients from interviews and examinations of the food left in their food trays when returned to the hospital kitchen. The physician may estimate the patient's oral intake by inspecting the patient's food tray at his or her bedside at the end of mealtime. In the hospitalized dialysis patient who is not hypercatabolic, the urea nitrogen appearance (UNA) [6] also may indicate the protein or amino acid intake.

Intercurrent Illnesses, Acute or Chronic Renal Failure

Infection, trauma, hypoxia, and burns that may occur in a setting of acute or chronic renal failure may increase net protein breakdown and urea generation. The catabolic rate may vary from mild to profound [6, 7]. In animal studies, uncomplicated acute renal failure also is a catabolic state (see below).

The altered hormonal milieu is one of the mechanisms responsible for the enhanced protein catabolism of acute stressful illness (Table 1). During acute catabolic stress, serum levels of epinephrine, glucagon, and cortisone often increase, and insulin resistance may occur [22–25]. These altered hormone levels or activities promote degradation of amino acids, gluconeogenesis, and urea formation. Epinephrine also increases basal energy expenditure [23]. Abnormal hormonal states have been largely investigated in acutely stressed patients without renal disease; and, there is a need to examine hormonal alterations during acute stress in acute and chronic renal failure.

Bacteremia and endotoxemia may have profound metabolic and physiologic effects on the host. These include hypotension, lactic acidosis, enhanced gluconeogenesis, and peripheral uptake of glucose [26, 27]. In extensively injured burn patients, gram-negative septicemia may suppress gluconeogenesis and glucose production [28].

Several studies suggest a causal role for proteases in the hypercatabolism of acutely ill patients with or without renal failure. Clowes et al reported that acutely traumatized or septic catabolic nonuremic patients may have increased serum levels of a peptide that promotes muscle protein degradation when assayed in vitro [29]. Horl et al found that ultrafiltrates of plasma from hypercatabolic patients with acute renal failure increase proteolytic activity in in vitro assays [30]. The increased protease activity may be related to reduced concentrations or to impaired function of proteinase inhibitors [31].

Baracos et al have identified a polypeptide from human leukocytes that appears to be identical to interleukin-1. This compound causes fever; in rat muscle, it enhances protein degradation [32]. The polypeptide may act by stimulating muscle synthesis of prostaglandin E_2 (PGE_2), which (in turn) promotes protein degradation in muscle by stimulating lysosomal proteolysis. Inhibition of PGE_2 synthesis with indomethacin or the use of an inhibitor of lysosomal thiol proteases blocks the stimulatory effects of this leukocytic pyrogen on muscle protein degradation. Going against the findings of a causal relationship between prostaglandins and muscle protein degradation are the observations of McKinley and Turinsky [33]. These investigators report that in rats, burn injuries stimulate PGE_2 release and muscle protein degradation. However, when PGE_2 synthesis is blocked, the enhanced rate of protein degradation does not fall.

Several researchers have examined muscle protein metabolism and proteolytic activity in acutely uremic rats. Flugel-Link et al [5], Clark and Mitch [34], and Pan et al [35] have reported increased protein degradation and reduced protein synthesis in hemicorpus, hindquarter, or isolated epitrochlearis muscle in these animals. Flugel-Link et al were unable to find increased activity of any of three muscle proteases examined: cathepsin B_1, cathepsin D, and alkaline protease [5]. It is possible that enhanced proteinase activity might be demonstrated with a different assay system. In their paper on these proceedings, Heidland and Horl report alterations in protease activity and protease inhibitors in acutely uremic rats [31]. Hepatic gluconeogenesis also is enhanced in acute renal failure [36].

It is well recognized that energy expenditure is increased in acute catabolic stress [23]. Mault et al observed that basal energy expenditure rose to an average of 37% above normal in patients with acute renal failure [37]. Those patients who died had significantly more negative energy balance than the surviving patients. However, it is possible that the higher mortality was not causally related to the more negative energy balance; both of these phenomena could be due to the greater severity of the underlying illnesses.

Feinstein et al found no relationship between energy intake (expressed as kcal/d or kcal/kg/d) and UNA in patients with acute renal failure who were receiving parenteral nutrition [7]. However, there was an inverse correlation between energy intake (expressed as a percentage of the patient's basal energy requirements calculated from the Harris Benedict equation) and UNA (F. Gotch, personal communication). This relationship suggests that net protein degradation may be reduced by providing more energy. A direct correlation also was observed between body weight and UNA, which may reflect an effect of protein mass on UNA [7]. Since the Harris Benedict equation for estimating energy expenditure is dependent on body weight, the inverse relationship between energy intake (as a fraction of estimated energy requirements) and UNA may merely reflect the direct relationship between body mass and UNA. In any event, since energy intake was not varied independently in this study, the relationship between energy intake and UNA in these sick, acutely uremic patients must be considered as not yet established.

It is relevant to the probable relationship between energy expenditure and net protein degradation that we observed a patient in whom hypoxia appeared to enhance net protein breakdown (Fig. 1). The patient was a 56-year-old man undergoing maintenance hemodialysis. He was ingesting a constant diet and undergoing nitrogen balance measurements in a clinical research center, when he suddenly developed acute pulmonary edema. His arterial P_{O_2} fell to 35 mm Hg, and the patient was given an emergency hemodialysis treatment during which 8 kg of water were removed. The patient improved dramatically during hemodialysis; several hours after the dialysis treatment he felt tired, but otherwise was normal. The cause of the acute pulmonary edema was never clearly established, but it was considered to be due to impaired cardiac output and overhydration obscured by the absence of peripheral edema or hypertension.

During the period of acute hypoxia, the patient's UNA rose markedly and nitrogen balance (adjusted for changes in body urea nitrogen [BUN]) became negative (Fig. 1). These developments were not due to changes in dietary intake. Within 12 to 24 hr after the episode of acute hypoxia, the UNA and nitrogen balance had returned to the prehypoxic levels.

Although the data do not definitely demonstrate that this patient's increased net protein degradation was due to hypoxia, there was no other apparent cause for the acute hypercatabolic response except, possibly, secondary changes in hormonal levels. As indicated above, a rise in blood catecholamine, glucagon, and cortisol concentrations could promote gluconeogenesis and hypercatabolism. This may be viewed as an adaptive and potentially beneficial response to hypoxia; anaerobic degradation of glucose to pyruvate and lactate generates much less adenosine triphosphate than the complete oxidation of glucose to carbon dioxide and water. When glucose is metabolized anaerobically, glycolysis and gluconeogenesis must increase markedly to generate the amount of energy that normally would be yielded by the complete oxidation of glucose.

Severe acidosis has profound effects on a variety of metabolic and physiologic processes, including oxygen delivery, enzyme activities, responsiveness to catecholamines, and bone reabsorption [38–40]. When rats fed a constant

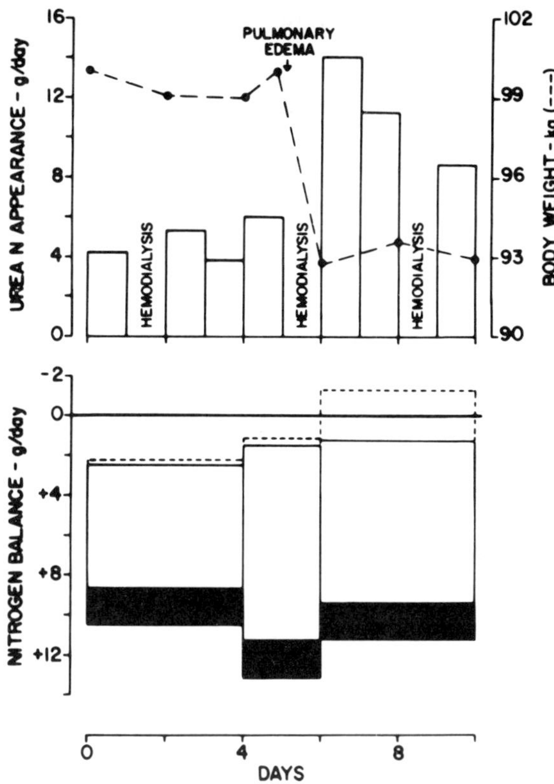

Fig. 1. Nitrogen balance, UNA, and body weight in a hemodialysis patient who developed acute pulmonary edema. In the *lower half* of the figure, the nitrogen balance data are shown, with intake plotted downward from the zero line and fecal and dialysate nitrogen output plotted upward from the intake line. Fecal and dialysate nitrogen are shown as *black* and *white areas,* respectively. Urinary nitrogen excretion was negligible. The *broken line* in the *lower half* of the figure indicates the nitrogen balance corrected for changes in body urea nitrogen, but not for unmeasured nitrogen losses. Urea nitrogen appearance is shown for days when the patient did not undergo hemodialysis.

diet are given an acid load, they increase their urinary ammonium excretion and develop a proportionate fall in urea excretion [41]. The many metabolic changes that occur with severe acidosis suggest that protein metabolism probably is also altered in this condition.

Metabolic studies of both uremic and nonuremic patients who sustain acute catabolic stress indicate that these individuals have undergone a complex and highly integrated response to their acute illness or injury. These are changes in plasma hormone levels and increased activities of proteinases. These and other mechanisms controlling the balance between synthetic and degradative processes—and between deposition and mobilization of proteins, amino acids, carbohydrates, and lipids from tissues—lead to a net outflow of these compounds and their metabolites, primarily from muscle and adipose tissue. These substances (along with the small endogenous pool of glycogen) are catabolized, yielding energy and providing substrates for formation of new proteins and peptides that are necessary for wound healing and host resistance. The liver plays a major role in the catabolism of these substrates and in the synthesis of new compounds. Thus, some of the amino acids released from catabolized protein may be used for synthesis of fibrinogen, collagen, acute phase proteins, complement, antibodies, hemoglobin, and albumin, and for formation of inflammatory cells, fibrocytes, and epithelial cells. The outpouring of minerals and vitamins from peripheral tissues during catabolic stress provides cofactors that are necessary for formation of new compounds and tissues.

Until the last 30 to 40 years, this response may have been critical for survival. The severely injured or diseased organism usually cannot procure, ingest, digest, absorb, and/or assimilate nutrients effectively. Hence, the mobilization of nutrients from endogenous pools is the only mechanism by which such acutely stressed mammals can generate fuel substrates for energy and precursors for the formation of new biologically valuable compounds, protoplasm, and tissues. Since most of the endogenous nutrients are generated from skeletal muscle or adipose tissue, the nutrient pools in more vital and smaller organs (for example, the heart or liver) may be somewhat spared.

The trade-off for these adaptive mechanisms is that the individual may develop profound wasting and debility; and, when renal failure is present, they may accrue more rapidly high plasma concentrations of minerals, hydrogen ions, and products of nitrogen metabolism. This adaptive response may also explain why administering enteral or parenteral nutrition to an acutely ill hypercatabolic patient often does not result in substantial improvement in nitrogen or protein balance; particularly, during the early days of the illness, when the individual is most catabolic. These patients are primed metabolically to degrade the infused amino acids, glucose, and lipids.

The challenge for the nutritional management of severely ill patients will be to devise methods for modifying intermediary metabolism, so that catabolic processes can be suppressed and anabolic pathways can be enhanced. Hopefully, this intervention will enable the patient to use exogenous nutrients more efficiently and to spare his or her endogenous nutrient reserves. It has yet to be shown that these interventions in intermediary metabolism— if they can be developed—will be beneficial to the patient. The ultimate test of the clinical value of such interventions is whether it decreases morbidity or mortality, or reduces the debility or duration of convalescence.

Endocrine Disorders in Stable Chronic Renal Failure

The multitude of endocrine disorders in clinically stable patients with chronic renal failure also may promote protein wasting. Insulin is the most potent, known anabolic hormone. Insulin stimulates protein synthesis, retards protein degradation, suppresses the release of amino acids from muscle, and has other anabolic actions. In renal failure, there is resistance to the actions of insulin on peripheral uptake of glucose and phosphorus [42], and glucose intolerance is common [43]. Most, but not all, resistance to the effects of insulin on glucose metabolism are removed by hemodialysis [43]. Glucagon, which antagonizes many of the actions of insulin and stimulates gluconeogenesis, is elevated in uremic sera [44]; both inactive moieties and the active fraction are elevated [45].

In renal failure, serum growth hormone concentrations usually are elevated [46]; serum levels of somatomedins, which are mediators of growth hormone actions, tend to be normal or increased [47]. However, bioassays indicate impaired biologic activity of the somatomedins in both children and adults with chronic renal failure [48, 49]; the biologic activity improves transiently after hemodialysis treatment [48, 49]. Since somatomedins have anabolic effects, it is possible that impaired somatomedin activity could lead to wasting in renal failure.

Parathyroid hormone (PTH) stimulates hepatic gluconeogenesis and urea synthesis [50]. Injection of PTH can increase urinary nitrogen excretion and cause negative nitrogen balance [51]. King and Stanbury described improved nitrogen balance in patients with primary hyperparathyroidism following parathyroidectomy [52]. Since hyperparathyroidism is common and often severe in uremia, it is possible that this disorder may contribute to wasting. Serum epinephrine levels are elevated in uremic serum [53]. Since epinephrine increases energy expenditure and gluconeogenesis, this disorder might also induce protein wasting. Currently, there are few experimental data regarding whether these endocrine disturbances promote protein wasting in chronic uremia; this would seem to be an important area for future investigation.

It has been speculated that uremic toxins, which accumulate in renal failure, may cause protein wasting. Delaporte et al has reported that dialysate from plasma of uremic patients impairs protein synthesis in a cell-free system derived from mouse Krebs II ascites cells [54]. Further studies clearly are needed to define this question.

Catabolic Stress of Hemodialysis

Several years ago, Borah et al and subsequently other investigators reported that net urea generation increases for several hours both near the end of hemodialysis and immediately afterwards [55, 56]. The cause of this phenomenon is not known. It could be an adaptive response to the amino acid and glucose losses into dialysate.

The study of Wathen et al is pertinent in this regard. They studied insulin and fuel substrate changes during a single hemodialysis treatment in 10 maintenance dialysis patients who were each studied twice—during dialysis with glucose-free dialysate and with glucose (200 mg/dl) in dialysate [57]. The patients fasted from 3 hr before hemodialysis until the end of the procedure. The investigators found that when the patients underwent hemodialysis with glucose-free dialysate, there was a fall in plasma glucose and insulin, a rise in blood β-hydroxybutyrate and acetoacetate, and a decrease in blood lactate and pyruvate. When hemodialysis was carried out in fasting patients by using dialysate containing glucose, these changes either were blunted or did not occur. There was a similar degree of rise in blood citrate and plasma-free fatty acids and a fall in plasma triglycerides in both groups. These observations suggest that the quantities of amino acids and glucose lost into dialysate, if not replaced during the dialysis procedure, lead both to a disruption in nutrient pools and to a plasma hormone profile that may cause the dialysis-induced gluconeogenesis and increased UNA described above. However, Farrell and Hone observed no reduction in net protein breakdown when patients underwent hemodialysis with 200 or 470 mg/dl of glucose in dialysate [56].

Hormonal alterations that occur during hemodialysis may also promote protein wasting. Alfred et al describe a tendency for serum concentrations of hormones that promote catabolism to rise, and for those that stimulate anabolism to fall, during hemodialysis treatment [58]. Another cause for dialysis-induced protein catabolism could be the release of proteinases from leukocytes that are sequestered in the lung during the initial min of hemodialysis treatment [59]. It has been suggested that the trapped leukocytes release proteinases that may stimulate protein catabolism [60, 61].

Nutrient Losses From Dialysis

During hemodialysis, there are average losses of 6 to 8 g of free amino acids and about 3 g of bound amino acids [62, 63]. With ingestion of food or intravenous (i.v.) nutrition, amino acid losses may increase modestly [63]. In the fasting patient, these losses are derived both from plasma and intracellular amino acid pools. Normoglycemic patients lose approximately 12 to 30 g of glucose during hemodialysis with glucose-free dialysate [56]. If patients do not eat during hemodialysis, which is a not uncommon event, serum glucose values usually fall to low normal or even below normal values. Normoglycemic patients exhibit virtually no loss or gain of glucose when they undergo hemodialysis with a dialysate containing dextrose, 100 mg/dl (90 mg/dl anhydrous dextrose).

The 10 to 15 ml of blood that is typically sequestered in the dialyzer at the end of hemodialysis treatment constitutes another source of nitrogen loss. In a patient with a serum total protein concentration of 7 g/dl and a hemoglobin level of 8 g/dl (hematocrit about 24%), a 15-ml blood loss constitutes a total protein loss of about 2 g.

In our experience, total protein losses with CAPD average 8.8 g/d [64]. Protein losses during acute intermittent peritoneal dialysis varied according to the duration of treatment and averaged 22.3 g/36 hr [64]. With intermittent peritoneal dialysis, much of the protein is removed during the first 2 or 3 hr of dialysis treatment from the washout of protein in ascitic fluid or that bound to the peritoneal membrane. Protein losses increase with the duration of the dialysate procedure. The frequency of dialysis exchanges has a much smaller effect on protein losses. The reason for this is that the protein concentrations in dialysate are far below serum concentrations; and, movement across the peritoneal wall appears to be the rate-limiting step in the dialysance of protein. Protein losses can increase markedly during peritonitis; we observed a protein loss into peritoneal dialysate of 106 g during a 24-hr period in a patient with severe untreated peritonitis [6]. With appropriate antibiotic therapy, protein losses fall rapidly, but they may not return to baseline values for many weeks [64]. Other factors that can affect protein losses include the tonicity of dialysate, the serum concentrations (for some proteins), the size of the patient, and interpersonal variations [64]. About 1.7 to 3.4 g of free amino acids are removed during 24 hr of CAPD therapy [65, 66].

Since dialysate solutions for CAPD contain dextrose, there is net accrual of dextrose during this treatment. A formula for estimating net glucose uptake in CAPD patients who receive four or five exchanges per day is as follows: Net glucose uptake $(g/d) = (0.89) \times$ the grams of glucose instilled each day -43, $r = 0.91$ [67].

The data used for these calculations are the anhydrous glucose concentrations, rather than the values for glucose monohydrate that are reported on the labels of parenteral or dialysate solutions. Peritoneal dialysate solutions that are listed as containing 1.5% and 4.25% glucose monohydrate contain 1.30 g/dl and 3.76 g/dl anhydrous glucose, respectively [67].

Small amounts of water-soluble vitamins are removed by hemodialysis and peritoneal dialysis [68]. The actual amounts removed have not been well defined, but they appear to be easily replaced with oral vitamin supplements. Since, in comparison to hemodialysis, peritoneal dialysis gives greater clearances for larger-sized molecules, there has been concern about the development of deficiencies in protein.

Medicines That Interfere with Nutrients

Many medicines interfere with the digestion, absorption, excretion, or metabolism of nutrients. This subject has been extensively reviewed by Roe [72]. Most drug nutrient interactions are believed to affect vitamins or minerals. Several medicines that affect vitamins are frequently used in patients with renal failure and could lead to vitamin deficiencies. Agents that may cause folate deficiency include diphenylhydantoin, barbiturates, oral contraceptives, methotrexate, and ethanol [68]. Isoniazid, hydralazine, oral contraceptives, and thyroxine (among other medicines) can lead to vitamin B_6 deficiency.

Losses of Protein and Other Nutrients From Blood Drawing, Draining Wounds, and Fistulas

These factors can lead to major losses of nutrients, particularly protein. Blood is a protein-rich fluid, especially because of its hemoglobin content. A person with a blood hemoglobin concentration and serum total protein concentration of 14 g/dl and 7 g/dl, respectively, would have a total protein concentration in blood of about 18 g/dl. It is not uncommon for acutely ill patients to have large quantities of blood drawn for diagnostic studies and to lose substantial quantities of blood from gastrointestinal bleeding or oozing at vascular puncture sites. The protein concentration in fistula drainage also may contribute to protein depletion. Albumin concentrations in ascitic fluid from patients undergoing intermittent peritoneal dialysis average 1.9 g/dl, and they correlate with serum albumin concentrations ($r = 0.67$) [64].

Impaired Endocrine and Metabolic Activity of the Kidney

The kidney is an endocrine organ that secretes 1,25-dihydroxycholecalciferol, erythropoietin, and renin. Prostaglandins synthesized by the kidney only appear to exert local effects. Kidney failure can perturb nutrient metabolism both by causing deficiencies of 1,25-dihydroxycholecalciferol and erythropoietin and by altering renin-aldosterone secretion. The kidney also synthesizes certain amino acids (particularly alanine, glutamate, and serine) and degrades other amino acids, peptides (including peptide hormones), and small proteins [8, 73]. It also is probable that in renal failure, the loss of renal metabolic activity exerts important actions on nutrient metabolism. However, the clinical effects resulting from these disorders have not yet been identified.

The Patients' Clinical Condition Prior to the Onset of Renal Failure or Intercurrent Illness

Clinical experience suggests that when either nondialyzed patients with chronic renal failure or patients undergoing maintenance dialysis become wasted or debilitated, their capacity for recovery and rehabilitation is abnormally limited. Salusky et al have examined this question in children undergoing CAPD, in whom nutritional status was repeatedly examined [74]. There was a high correlation between serum protein concentrations and anthropometric parameters (expressed as Z-stores) measured at the onset of CAPD therapy; and, between these respective measurements obtained in the same patients 1 year later. Those children who were rather well nourished at the onset of dialysis therapy tended to remain so 1 year later; the children who were wasted, malnourished, or short at the onset of CAPD exhibited roughly a similar degree of abnormality after 1 year of therapy. Recently, these same observations have been extended to 24 months of CAPD treatment (Salusky et al, unpublished observations). These data may indicate that the most effective way to avoid wasting and malnutrition in maintenance dialysis patients is to prevent them from developing these disorders before or at the time when maintenance dialysis is instituted.

Blumenkrantz et al evaluated nutritional status in a group of clinically stable patients at the time they commenced chronic dialysis therapy or during the first 3-month period after beginning such therapy [13]. These patients were part of a Veterans Administration cooperative study to evaluate the clinical response to home or self-care hemodialysis, as compared to home intermittent peritoneal dialysis. To be eligible for acceptance into the study, the patients had to be deemed capable of home hemodialysis or peritoneal dialysis. Hence, they were a healthy subpopulation of maintenance dialysis patients. Nonetheless, as a group, these patients demonstrated clear evidence of wasting or malnutrition [13]. Moreover, there was little or no deterioration or improvement in nutritional status in this group of patients during the next 1 to 3 years of dialysis treatment.

At present, there are little definitive data as to when wasting or malnutrition are most likely to occur in patients with chronic renal failure. However, some circumstantial evidence suggests that it is during or immediately before the time that patients begin maintenance dialysis. As indicated above, the data of Blumenkrantz et al suggest that patients are wasted or malnourished at the time that they begin maintenance dialysis or shortly afterwards [75]. Also, as previously stated, the data of Salusky et al indicate that their group of children are growth-retarded and wasted when they commence CAPD [74]; for many of these children, CAPD was their first form of dialysis therapy.

On the other hand, when Kopple et al evaluated the degree to which nondialyzed chronically uremic patients will adhere to dietary prescription, they observed normal nutritional status in these patients [76, 77]. The mean glomerular filtration rate (GFR) (mean of creatinine [C_{cr}] and urea clearances) was 7 ml/min at the start of the study; it fell during the 4-month period of evaluation to 5 ml/min. Nutritional status did not change during the course of treatment. The fact that these patients were able to participate in this study may indicate that they represented a somewhat healthier subpopulation of nondialyzed, chronically uremic patients. Nonetheless, the striking difference in nutritional status between the nondialyzed patients with a GFR of 5 ml/min and patients starting maintenance dialysis treatment suggests that some event or events during this brief period, between these two stages of advanced renal failure, produces wasting or malnutrition. Whether it is poor nutritional intake, intercurrent illnesses, uremic toxicity, or altered hormone function is not known. It is possible that earlier institution of maintenance dialysis, which might prevent anorexia and uremic toxicity, may diminish the likelihood of wasting and malnutrition in these patients. Carefully controlled prospective studies are clearly indicated to test whether wasting and malnutrition are most likely to occur between the time that the patient's GFR decreases below 5 to 6 ml/min and the first few days or weeks of dialysis treatment. If this hypothesis is confirmed, then studies will be needed to evaluate whether better nutritional intake, earlier dialysis, or other therapies will prevent the wasting.

Implications for Treatment of Patients with Acute or Chronic Renal Failure

The foregoing comments suggest that many steps can be taken to prevent or ameliorate the development of wasting and malnutrition in patients with acute or chronic renal failure. Clearly, it is necessary to ensure that the patient receives sufficient nutritional intake. As indicated above, in the hospitalized patient, inadequate oral nutrition is not always readily apparent; and, physicians may need to examine the patient's food trays or to institute calorie and protein counts. In clinically stable patients, the UNA will indicate the protein intake [78]. It is unfortunate that energy intake cannot be assessed by laboratory measurements, because low-energy intakes (if anything) appear to be a more common phenomenon than low-protein intakes in chronically uremic patients [8, 11, 13]. If the patient cannot be given sufficient nutrition through the enteral tract, partial or total parenteral nutrition may be necessary. The indications and techniques for parenteral nutrition in patients with acute and chronic renal failure have been recently reviewed [79, 80]. There is still controversy as to whether parenteral nutrition is of value during the first several days after the onset of acute renal failure or intercurrent illness. In this author's opinion, the data, although not conclusive, suggest that there are benefits to employing this treatment during this period [79–81]. On the other hand, for the patient who has been unable to receive oral or enteral nutrition for 2 to 3 weeks or longer, the benefits of parenteral nutrition are better established. In patients who undergo frequent dialysis treatments, the need for nutritional therapy is more crucial to replace nutrients that are removed by dialysis.

In the future, investigations of nutritional therapy for the stressed patient with acute or chronic renal failure probably will be focused on at least two areas. First, it is anticipated that there will be continued research to develop more optimal formulations for providing nutrition through the enteral tract, intravenously, and (possibly) through dialysate. In particular, the quantity and relative amounts of individual amino acids or amino acid substitutes, energy sources, vitamins (including vitamin D analogs), and trace elements should be investigated. Both the role of slow, continuous ultrafiltration to remove excess water and small quantities of solutes [82] and the use of nutritional hemodialysis [83] require further study. The second direction for future research involves intervention in intermediary metabolism to reduce catabolic processes and to promote anabolism. Further study is needed on the role of interleukin-1, lyzosomes, proteinases, and prostaglandins in both the degradation of protein and amino acids and the contribution of altered endocrine function, uremic toxins, and the dialysis procedure to protein wasting. The indications (if any) for anabolic steroids, insulin, or adrenergic blockers should be examined. Also, the use of protease inhibitors and other agents for reducing protein degradation, enhancing protein synthesis, or suppressing gluconeogenesis requires more investigation. Finally, the ultimate test of any new therapeutic technique will be whether it reduces morbidity, mortality, or the time for convalescence and rehabilitation in these patients.

References

1. BLAGG CR, WAHL PW, LAMERS JY: Treatment of chronic renal failure at the Northwest Kidney Center, Seattle, from 1960 to 1982. *ASAIO* 6:170–175, 1983

2. NISSENSON AR, GENTILE DE, SODERBLUM R, BRAX C: Long-term outcome of CAPD—regional experience. *Dialysis Transpl* 13:34–37, 1984

3. WANG M, VYHMEISTER I, KOPPLE JD, SWENDSEID ME: Effect of protein intake on weight gain and plasma amino acid levels in uremic rats. *Am J Physiol* 230:1455–1459, 1976

4. HOLLIDAY MA, CHANTLER C, MACDONNELL R, KEITGES J: Effect of uremic on nutritionally-induced variations in protein metabolism. *Kidney Int* 11:236–245, 1977

5. FLUGEL-LINK RM, SALUSKY IB, JONES MR, KOPPLE JD: Protein and amino acid metabolism in posterior hemicorpus of acutely uremic rats. *Am J Physiol* 244:E615–E623, 1983

6. GRODSTEIN GP, BLUMENKRANTZ MJ, KOPPLE JD: Nutritional and metabolic response to catabolic stress in chronic uremia. *Am J Clin Nutr* 33:1411–1416, 1980

7. FEINSTEIN E, BLUMENKRANTZ MJ, HEALY M, KOFFLER A, SILBERMAN H, MASSRY SG, KOPPLE JD: Clinical and metabolic responses to parenteral nutrition in acute renal failure. A controlled double-blind study. *Medicine* 60:124–137, 1981

8. KOPPLE JD: Abnormal amino acid and protein metabolism in uremia. *Kidney Int* 14:340–348, 1978

9. BIANCHI R, MARIANI G, TONI MG, CARMASSI F: The metabolism of human serum albumin in renal failure on conservative and dialysis therapy. *Am J Clin Nutr* 31:1615–1626, 1978

10. YOUNG GA, OLI HI, DAVIDSON AM, PARSONS FM: The effects of calorie and essential amino acid supplementation on plasma proteins in patients with chronic renal failure. *Am J Clin Nutr* 31:1802–1807, 1978

11. KLUTHE R, LUTTGEN FM, CAPETIANU T, HEINZE V, KATZ N, SUDHOFF A: Protein requirements in maintenance hemodialysis. *Am J Clin Nutr* 31:1812–1820, 1978

12. ATTMAN PO, EWALD J, ISAKSSON B: Body composition during long-term treatment of uremia with amino acid supplemented low-protein diet. *Am J Clin Nutr* 33:801–810, 1980

13. BLUMENKRANTZ MJ, KOPPLE JD, GUTMAN RA, CHAN YK, BARBOUR GL, ROBERTS C, SHEN FH, GANDHI VC, TUCKER CT, CURTIS FK, COBURN JW: Methods for assessing nutritional status of patients with renal failure. *Am J Clin Nutr* 33:1567–1585, 1980

14. GUARNIERI G, FACCINI L, LIPARTITI T, RANIERI F, SPANGARO F, GIUNTINI D, TOIGO G, DARDI F, VIDALI FB, RAIMONDI A: Simple methods for nutritional assessment in hemodialyzed patients. *Am J Clin Nutr* 33:1598–1607, 1980

15. BANSAL VK, POPLI S, PICKERING J, ING TS, VERTUNOLL, HANO JE: Protein-calorie malnutrition and cutaneous energy in hemodialysis maintained patients. *Am J Clin Nutr* 33:1608–1611, 1980

16. THUNBERG BJ, SWAMY AP, CESTERO RV: Cross-sectional and longitudinal nutritional measurements in maintenance hemodialysis patients. *Am J Clin Nutr* 34:2005–2012, 1981

17. YOUNG GA, SWANEPOEL CR, CROFT MR, HOBSON SM: Anthropometry and plasma valine, amino acids, and proteins in the nutritional assessment of hemodialysis patients. *Kidney Int* 21:492–499, 1982

18. HEIDE B, PIERRATOS A, JHANNA R, PETTIT J, OGILVJE R, HARRISON J, MCNEIL K, SICCION Z, OREOPOULOS DG: Nutritional status of patients undergoing CAPD. *PD Bull* 3:138–141, 1983

19. SALUSKY IB, FINE RN, NELSON P, BLUMENKRANTZ MJ, KOPPLE JD: Nutritional status of children undergoing continuous ambulatory peritoneal dialysis. *Am J Clin Nutr* 38:599–611, 1983

20. WOLFSON M, STRONG CJ, MINTURN D, GRAY DK, KOPPLE JD: Nutritional status and lymphocyte function in maintenance hemodialysis patients. *Am J Clin Nutr* 37:547–555, 1984

21. ACCHIARDO SR, MOORE LW, LATOUR PA: Malnutrition as the main factor in morbidity and mortality of hemodialysis patients. *Kidney Int* 24(Suppl 16):S-199–S-203, 1983

22. ROCHA DM, SANTEUSANIO F, FALOONA GR, UNGER RH: Abnormal pancreatic alpha-cell function in bacterial infections. *N Engl J Med* 288:700–703, 1973

23. WILMORE DW, LONG JM, MASON AD, SKREEN RW, PRUITT BA: Mediator of the hypermetabolic response to thermal injury. *Ann Surg* 180:653–668, 1974

24. DAHN M, BOUWMAN D, KIRKPATRICK J: The sepsis-glucose intolerance riddle: A hormonal explanation. *Surgery* 86:423–428, 1979

25. VITEK V, LANG DJ, COWLEY RA: The unexpected increase of serum insulin levels in patients soon after trauma. *Am Surg* 1979, pp 228–237

26. ADELEYE GA, AL-JIBOURI LM, FURMAN BL, PARRATT JR: Endotoxin-induced metabolic changes in the conscious, unrestrained rat: Hypoglycemia and elevated blood lactate concentrations without hyperinsulinemia. *Circ Shock* 8:543–550, 1981

27. KELLEHER DL, BAGBY GJ, FONG BC, SPITZER JJ: Glucose turnover five hours following endotoxin administration to normal and diabetic rats. *Circ Shock* 9:47–53, 1982

28. WILMORE DW: Impaired gluconeogenesis in extensively injured patients with gram-negative bacteremia. *Am J Clin Nutr* 30:1355–1356, 1977

29. CLOWES GH, GEORGE BC, VILLEE CA, SARAVIS CA: Muscle proteolysis induced by a circulating peptide in patients with sepsis or trauma. *N Engl J Med* 308:545–552, 1983

30. HORL WH, STEPINSKI J, SCHAFER RM, WANNER C, HEIDLAND A: Role of proteases in hypercatabolic patients with renal failure. *Kidney Int* 24(Suppl 16):S-37–S-42, 1983

31. HEIDLAND A, HORL WH: Contribution of proteases to hypercatabolism in acute renal failure, see Section on Acute Renal Failure, this volume

32. BARACOS V, RODEMANN P, DINARELLO CA, GOLDBERG AL: Stimulation of muscle protein degradation and prostaglandin E_2 release by leukocytic pyrogen (interleukin-1). *N Engl J Med* 308:553–558, 1983

33. MCKINLEY CJ, TURINSKY J: Dissociation of prostaglandin E_2 synthesis and protein degradation in postburn muscle (*abstract*). *Fed Proc* 43:703, 1984

34. CLARK AS, MITCH WE: Muscle protein turnover and glucose uptake in acutely uremic rats. *J Clin Invest* 72:836–845, 1983

35. PAN CS, INADOMI DW, LAIDLAW SA, JONES MR, KOPPLE JD: Oxandrolone enhances muscle protein synthesis in acutely uremic rats (*abstract 58*). *Kidney Int* 25:236, 1984

36. FROHLICH J, SCHOLMERICH J, HOPPE-SEYLER G, MAIER KP, TALKE H, SCHOLL-MEYER P, GEROK W: The effect of acute uremia on gluconeogenesis in isolated perfused rat livers. *Eur J Clin Invest* 4:453, 1974

37. MAULT JR, BARTLETT RH, DECHERT RE, CLARK SF, SWARTZ RD: Starvation: A major contribution to mortality in acute renal failure? *Trans Am Soc Artif Intern Organs* 29:390–395, 1983

38. RELMAN AS: Metabolic consequences of acid-base disorders. *Kidney Int* 1:347–359, 1972

39. MITCHELL JH, WILDENTHAL K, JOHNSON RL: The effect of acid-base disturbances on cardiovascular and pulmonary function. *Kidney Int* 1:375–389, 1972

40. WILLIAMSON JR, SAFER B, RICH T, SCHAFFER S, KOBAYASHI K: Effect of acidosis on myocardial contractility and metabolism. *Acta Med Scand* 587(Suppl):95–116, 1976

41. OLIVER J, BOURKE E: Adaptations in urea ammonium excretion in metabolic acidosis in the rat: a reinterpretation. *Clin Sci Mol Med* 48:515–520, 1975
42. WESTERVELT FB: Insulin effect in uremia. *J Lab Clin Med* 74:79–84, 1969
43. HAMPERS CL, SOELDNER JS, DOAK PB, MERRILL JP: Effect of chronic renal failure and hemodialysis on carbohydrate metabolism. *J Clin Invest* 45:1719, 1966
44. SHERWIN RS, BASTL C, FINKELSTEIN FO, FISHER M, BLACK H, HENDLER R, FELIG P: Influence of uremia and hemodialysis on the turnover and metabolic effects of glucagon. *J Clin Invest* 57:722–731, 1976
45. VALVERDE I, VILLANUEVA ML: Heterogeneity of plasma immunoreactive glucagon. *Metabolism* 25:1393–1395, 1976
46. FELDMAN HA, SINGER I: Endocrinology and metabolism in uremia and dialysis: A clinical review. *Medicine* 54:345–376, 1975
47. SCHIFFRIN A, GUYDA H, ROBITAILLE P: Increased plasma somatomedin reactivity in chronic renal failure as determined by acid gel filtration and radioreceptor assay. *J Clin Endocrinol Metab* 46:511–514, 1977
48. PHILLIPS LS, PENNISI AJ, BELOSKY DC: Somatomedin activity and inorganic sulfate in children undergoing dialysis. *J Clin Endocrinol Metab* 46:165–168, 1978
49. PHILLIPS LS, KOPPLE JD: Circulating somatomedin activity and sulfate levels in adults with normal and impaired kidney function. *Metabolism* 30:1091–1095, 1981
50. MOXLEY MA, BELL NH, WAGLE SR, ALLEN DO, ASHMORE J: Parathyroid hormone stimulation of glucose and urea production in isolated liver cells. *Am J Physiol* 227:1058–1061, 1974
51. CLARKSON B, KOWLESSAR OD, HORWITH M, SLEISENGER MH: Clinical and metabolic study of a patient with malabsorption and hypoparathyroidism. *Metabolism* 9:1093–1100, 1960
52. KING RG, STANBURY SW: Magnesium metabolism in primary hyper-parathyroidism. *Clin Sci* 39:281–303, 1970
53. CAMPESE VM, ROMOFF MS, LEVITAN D, LANE K, MASSRY SG: Mechanisms of autonomic nervous system dysfunction in uremia. *Kidney Int* 20:240–253, 1981
54. DELAPORTE C, GROS F, ANAGNOSTOPOULOS T: Inhibitory effects of plasma dialysate on protein synthesis in vitro influence of dialysis and transplantation. *Am J Clin Nutr* 33:1407–1410, 1980
55. BORAH M, SCHOENFELD PY, GOTCH FA, SARGENT JA, WOLFSON M, HUMPHREYS MH: Nitrogen balance in intermittent hemodialysis therapy. *Kidney Int* 14:491–500, 1978
56. FARRELL PC, HONE PW: Dialysis-induced catabolism. *Am J Clin Nutr* 33:1417–1422, 1980
57. WATHEN RL, KESHAVIAH P, HOMMEYER P, CADWELL K, COPMTY CM: The metabolic effects of hemodialysis with and without glucose in the dialysate. *Am J Clin Nutr* 31:1870–1875, 1978
58. ALFRED H, KIRKWOOD G, KUNITOMO T, WILLIAMS G, EMANUEL R, LOWRIE E: Acute hormone changes with conventional (CD) and high flux dialysis (HFD). *Trans Am Soc Artif Intern Organs* 8:37, 1979
59. CRADDOCK PR, FEHR J, DALMASSO AP, BRIGHAM KL, JACOB HS: Hemodialysis leukopenia: Pulmonary vascular leukostasis resulting from complement activation by dialyzer cellophane membranes. *J Clin Invest* 59:879–888, 1977
60. HORL W, JOCHUM M, HEIDLAND A, FRITZ H: Release of granulocyte proteinases during hemodialysis. *Am J Nephrol* 3:213–217, 1983
61. HEIDLAND A, HORL WH, HELLER N, HEINE H, NEUMANN S, HEIDBREDER H: Proteolytic enzymes and catabolism: Enhanced release of granulocyte protein-

ases in uremic intoxication and during hemodialysis. *Kidney Int* 24(Suppl 16):S-27–S-36, 1983

62. KOPPLE JD, SWENDSEID ME, SHINABERGER JH, UMEZAWA CU: The free and bound amino acids removed by hemodialysis. *Trans Am Soc Artif Intern Organs* 19:309–313, 1973

63. WOLFSON M, JONES MR, KOPPLE JD: Amino acid losses during hemodialysis with infusion of amino acids and glucose. *Kidney Int* 21:500–506, 1982

64. BLUMENKRANTZ MJ, GAHL GM, KOPPLE JD, KMDAR AV, JONES MR, KESSEL M, COBURN JW: Protein losses during peritoneal dialysis. *Kidney Int* 19:593–602, 1981

65. GIORDANO C, DESANTO NG, CAPODICASA G, DILEO VA, DISERAFINO A, CIRILLO D, ESPOSITO R, FIORE R, DAMIANO M, BUONADONNA L, COCCO F, DILORIO B: Amino acid losses during CAPD. *Clin Nephrol* 14:230–232, 1980

66. KOPPLE JD, BLUMENKRANTZ MJ, JONES MR, MORAN JK, COBURN JW: Plasma amino acid levels and amino acid losses during continuous ambulatory peritoneal dialysis. *Am J Clin Nutr* 36:395–402, 1982

67. GRODSTEIN GP, BLUMENKRANTZ MJ, KOPPLE JD, MORAN JK, COBURN JW: Glucose absorption during continuous ambulatory peritoneal dialysis. *Kidney Int* 19:564–567, 1981

68. KOPPLE JD, SWENDSEID ME: Vitamin nutrition in patients undergoing maintenance hemodialysis. *Kidney Int* 7(Suppl 2):S-79–S-84, 1975

69. DELMEZ JA, SLATOPOLSKY E, MARTIN KJ, GEARING BN, HARTER HR: Minerals, Vitamin D, and parathyroid hormone in continuous ambulatory peritoneal dialysis. *Kidney Int* 21:862–867, 1982

70. KURTZ SB, MCCARTHY JT, KUMAR R: Hypercalcemia in continuous ambulatory peritoneal dialysis (CAPD) patients: Observations on parameters of calcium metabolism, in *Advances in Peritoneal Dialysis,* edited by GAHL GM, KESSEL M, NOLPH KD, Amsterdam, Excerpta Medica, 1981, pp 467–472

71. GOKAL R, ELLIS HA, RAMOS JM, DEWAR J, SWEETING V, WARD MK, KERR DNS: Improvement in secondary hyperparathyroidism in patients on continuous ambulatory peritoneal dialysis, in *Advances in Peritoneal Dialysis,* edited by GAHL GM, KESSEL M, NOLPH KD, Amsterdam, Excerpta Medica, 1981, pp 461–466

72. ROE DA: Interactions between drugs and nutrients. Symposium on Applied Nutrition in Clinical Medicine. *Med Clin North Am* 63:985, 1979

73. KOPPLE JD, FUKUDA S: Effects of amino acid infusion and renal failure on the uptake and release of amino acids by the dog kidney. *Am J Clin Nutr* 33:1363–1372, 1980

74. SALUSKY IB, FINE RN, NELSON P, KOPPLE JD: Factors affecting growth and nutritional status in children undergoing CAPD (*abstract 54*). *Kidney Int* 25:260, 1984

75. COBURN JW, BLUMENKRANTZ MJ, KOPPLE JD: Controlled evaluation of maintenance peritoneal dialysis. NIH Grant No. 1-AM-5-2218 Technical Report, 1979

76. KOPPLE JD, ROBERTS CE, GRODSTEIN GP, SHAH GM, WINER RL, DAVIDSON WD, HENRY DA, FRANKLIN SS: Adherence to low protein diets by chronically uremic patients (*abstract*). *Kidney Int* 21:171, 1982

77. KOPPLE JD: Dietary maintenance of chronic uremic patients, final report. NIH Grant No. 1-AM-9-2220, 1983

78. KOPPLE JD: Nutritional therapy in kidney failure. *Nutr Rev* 39:193–206, 1981

79. KOPPLE JD, BLUMENKRANTZ MJ: Total parenteral nutrition and parenteral fluid therapy, in *Clinical Disorders of Fluid and Electrolyte Metabolism* (3rd ed), edited by MAXWELL MH, KLEEMAN CR, New York, McGraw-Hill, Inc, 1980, chap 10, pp 413–458

80. KOPPLE JD, CIANCIARUSO B: The role for nutrition in acute renal failure, in *Acute Renal Failure (ARF): Pathophysiology, Prevention, and Treatment,* edited by ANDREUCCI VE, Martinus Nijhoff, Chap 22 (in press, 1984)
81. ABEL RM, BECK CH JR, ABBOTT W JR, RYAN JA JR, BARNETT GO, FISCHER JE: Improved survival and acute renal failure after treatment with intravenous essential L-amino acids and glucose. *N Engl J Med* 288:695, 1973
82. KAPLAN AA, LONGNECKER RE, FOLKERT VW: Continuous arteriovenous hemofiltration. *Ann Intern Med* 100:358–367, 1984
83. FEINSTEIN EI, COLLINS JF, ROBERTS M, BLUMENKRANTZ MJ, KOPPLE JD, MASSRY SG: Nutritional hemodialysis. *Artif Organs* (in press, 1984)

Influence of Nutritional Therapy on Progression of Renal Insufficiency

William E. Mitch

It is a remarkable observation from both clinical and experimental studies that an injury to the kidney initiates a series of events that culminate in further loss of renal function. It is now indisputable that progressive deterioration in renal function occurs even when the initiating disease has resolved [1]. The implication that chronic renal failure (CRF) is a self-perpetuating disease is one of the most important therapeutic challenges facing the nephrologist today; if the autodestructive process were understood, a more rational and beneficial therapy could be designed for the large number of patients with CRF. Preliminary results of clinical studies published in recent years indicate that nutritional therapy, if initiated early, can break the vicious cycle that culminates in end-stage renal disease.

An accumulating mass of evidence in experimental animal models has shown that dietary manipulation of protein and phosphate intake can be very effective in interrupting the progressive downhill course of chronic renal insufficiency. As early as 1932, Bischoff summarized the data available at that time and concluded that there were toxic factors in the diet that affected the renal function of experimental animals [2]. Studies in rats have led to the formulation of three mechanisms that might account for the loss of renal function that characteristically accompanies CRF: (1) accumulated uremic toxins could cause progressive renal damage; (2) renal hemodynamic adaptations to loss of renal mass may cause progressive glomerular damage; (3) abnormal calcium and phosphorus metabolism and secondary hyperparathyroidism have been linked to progressive loss of renal function. It is now recognized that dietary intervention can be used to interrupt all these mechanisms.

This manuscript was presented as part of a Symposium on *Nutritional Aspects of Renal Disease.*

Experimental Renal Disease

Several investigators have demonstrated that excessive dietary protein is dele-terious to rats with experimental CRF induced either by subtotal nephrectomy or injection of antikidney antibodies. In 1927, Moise and Smith [3] reported that interstitial and glomerular lesions developed rapidly in uninephrecto-mized rats fed a high-protein diet. In 1932, Chanutin and Ferris [4] noted that varying the dietary protein of partially nephrectomized rats from 10 to 80% caused increasingly severe proteinuria, hypertension, renal insuffi-ciency, and histologic damage to the kidney; mortality also was higher [5]. By keeping the calorie intake constant, Kleinknecht et al were able to show that the nephrotoxic effects of protein were not related to concomitant changes in calorie intake [6]. Besides CRF produced by subtotal nephrectomy, it was reported in 1939 that feeding a 40% protein diet to rats with experimental allergic nephritis led to progressive renal failure and death, whereas a diet containing only 5% protein prevented progressive glomerular and tubular injury [7]. More recently, Friend et al [8] reported that there was significant protection from immune complex nephritis in the NZB × NZW mouse model of systemic lupus when dietary protein or calories were restricted. Not only was the diet associated with decreased immune complex deposition at the glomerular basement membrane, but there was also less mesangial damage. Taken together, these reports establish that high-protein diets accelerate histo-logic damage and the loss of renal function in rats with either surgically or immunologically induced CRF.

The hypothesis first proposed to explain these observations states that a nephrotoxic metabolite of protein accumulates in rats (or patients) with CRF because of impaired excretion. Accordingly, a high-protein diet must necessar-ily increase the circulating level of the toxin, leading to progressive loss of renal function [2]. This vicious cycle could be broken by feeding a low-protein diet.

The second hypothesis holds that dietary protein is responsible for the compensatory increase in the glomerular capillary hydrostatic pressure and for the "hyperfiltration" occurring in residual nephrons following renal dam-age. Micropuncture studies performed 1 week after a 90% reduction of renal mass in Munich-Wistar rats revealed a striking increase in glomerular plasma flow rate and hydraulic pressure caused by arteriolar vasodilatation, plus some increase in systemic arterial pressure [9]. The increases in glomerular plasma flow and pressure were virtually abolished by restricting dietary pro-tein content to 6%. In these studies, residual nephrons also displayed an adhesion of epithelial cells to Bowman's capsule, a detachment of epithelial cells from the underlying basement membrane, and a prominent increase in mesangial cells and matrix. A low-protein diet not only prevented the glomerular hemodynamic changes, but also the proteinuria, histologic abnor-malities, and alterations in physical properties of the glomerular capillaries [10]. These studies led Brenner, Myer, and Hostetter to propose that progres-sion of CRF is dependent on high pressures and plasma flow rates within the glomerular capillaries [11]. The lesion could be self-perpetuating if the consequent sclerotic process were to cause an adaptive increase in pressure and flow in less severely affected glomeruli, which would lead to further glomerular damage. The mechanisms whereby a low-protein diet attenuates the ongoing renal damage have not been identified, however.

The third hypothesis invokes the alterations in calcium and phosphate metabolism that occur in CRF as the cause of functional deterioration. Phosphate accumulation leading to secondary hyperparathyroidism and a high calcium × phosphorus product could cause an increasing calcium and phosphate deposition in the renal parenchyma and the accompanying inflammation and fibrosis. In support of this, patients with primary hyperparathyroidism often develop renal insufficiency [12], and rats with CRF following subtotal nephrectomy develop parathyroid gland hypertrophy and excessive calcium deposition in the kidney [13]. In such rats, parathyroidectomy has been shown to prevent renal calcification and reduce the severity of the accompanying interstitial nephritis. More recently, it was reported that dietary phosphate restriction following subtotal nephrectomy or immunologically induced CRF prevented progressive renal failure in rats [14, 15]. Other observations, however, suggest that calcium and phosphate deposition in the kidney does not play an important role in the progression of CRF [16]. For example, Laouari et al [17] found that feeding rats a phosphate-deficient diet produced marked anorexia and that the renal protective effect of this diet was more closely linked to a decrease in total food intake than to a lower phosphate intake. In fact, when dietary phosphate was restricted sufficiently to prevent phosphaturia and hyperparathyroidism without causing anorexia, there was little or no beneficial effect on the deterioration of renal function.

Some of the effects of restricting dietary protein could be mediated by the concomitant changes in the intake of dietary precursors of prostaglandins, thromboxanes, and leukotrienes. For example, a diet deficient in linoleic acid, a precursor of prostaglandins and leukotrienes, can retard progression of lupus nephritis in NZB × NZW mice [18]. On the other hand, a high linoleic acid intake protected rats from progressive proteinuria and glomerular sclerosis following their subtotal nephrectomy [19]. These reports are emphasized because of the striking results of Purkerson et al [20], who showed that an inhibitor of thromboxane synthesis prevented progression and hypertension in CRF rats, even though "hyperfiltration" persisted. Further work will be necessary to establish the importance of thomboxane in progressive renal insufficiency, but clearly, dietary manipulation could be used to modulate production of this or other prostaglandins.

In summary, available evidence indicates that protein intake may dramatically influence the rate of deterioration of residual renal function in many experimental models of renal disease. The evidence for a prominent effect of dietary phosphate in mediating progressive loss of renal function is less compelling. However, these studies have served to provide an additional stimulus for studying the effects of dietary manipulation in patients with CRF. To study large numbers of patients will require a simple design and a reliable method for assessing changes in renal function.

Measuring Progression of Renal Insufficiency

It is generally accepted that the most precise measure of renal function is the inulin clearance, but this is laborious and poorly suited for repeated studies in humans. Moreover, administering a water load to raise urine flow could be hazardous in patients with renal failure. Other methods of estimating GFR include the injection of compounds labeled with isotopes such as ^{51}Cr-EDTA, whose clearance is closely correlated with inulin clearance [21]. To avoid the errors associated with urine collections, investigators have used the rate of disappearance of ^{51}Cr-EDTA (or other radiolabeled compounds) from the serum after a single injection, but this method is not as precise as inulin clearance; it requires repeated blood samples, and the patient must remain recumbent throughout the 5-hr test [21]. GFR also has been estimated as the 24-hr, endogenous creatinine clearance or as the "calculated creatinine clearance" that is based on an average rate of creatinine excretion for persons of the same age, sex, and body habitus. Both methods yield less accurate results (compared with inulin clearance) than the mean of 24-hr creatinine and urea clearances in patients wih CRF [22]. The major limitation of creatinine clearance is the requirement for a 24-hr urine collection; the coefficient of variation of daily creatinine clearance in individual patients is as high as 10 to 15% [23, 24]. For these reasons and for convenience, most studies of dietary-induced changes in renal function in patients with CRF have relied on the serum creatinine concentration as an indirect measure of GFR.

A single value of serum creatinine is a relatively crude estimate of GFR. It does not take into account that patients with advanced renal failure have a reduced creatinine excretion owing to extrarenal creatinine clearance [25], nor does it take into account that in subjects with proteinuria, the excessive creatinine secretion may raise the creatinine clearance substantially above inulin clearance [26]. Although these factors limit the usefulness of a single value of serum creatinine as an estimate of GFR, serial values of serum creatinine in most patients can provide a reliable estimate of the rate of loss of renal function. By examining serum creatinine alone, it is difficult to quantify changes in renal function, but this difficulty is eliminated by calculating the rate of change of the reciprocal of serum creatinine concentration. This function decreases in a remarkably linear fashion with time in individual patients with progressive CRF [27]. We found that the decline was linear with time in over 90% of 31 CRF patients whose serum creatinine increased from an initial average value of 2.6 to a final value of 14.8 mg/dl and that the rate of change of the reciprocal serum creatinine varied widely among patients (from 0.0011 to 0.0152 dl/mg per month). The high variability in the rate of progression of CRF [27–29] emphasizes the importance of examining the course of each subject individually.

Rutherford et al [30] reported that the logarithm of serum creatinine can increase linearly with time in some patients with CRF and that this relationship occasionally fitted the observed data better than the reciprocal serum creatinine function. The slope of the logarithmic function often increased sharply late in the course of CRF, even though no associated clinical process could be identified coincident with the change. Thus, with this method, the future course of progression cannot be predicted accurately from observations made early in the disease. Recently, Gretz, Manz, and Strauch [31] examined whether the reciprocal or log serum creatinine method more accurately predicted the course of CRF. They found that the reciprocal method was substantially more accurate in the 110 patients studied. Because a linear decrease of reciprocal serum creatinine indicates that GFR is lost at a constant rate, whereas a linear rise in log serum creatinine means that a constant fraction of renal function is being lost per unit time, the two methods have different pathophysiologic implications.

The likely explanation for the linear decline in the reciprocal of serum creatinine with time is that creatinine clearance has decreased linearly with time. Barsotti et al [32] confirmed this by examining the course of renal insufficiency in 31 patients with moderately advanced CRF. This, in turn, suggests that GFR is lost at a constant rate, though apparently this has been established only for patients with diabetic nephropathy [33].

It is fortunate that the reciprocal relationship can be used to estimate the progression of CRF, because the day-to-day coefficient of variation in serum creatinine in patients with CRF is only 6.5% [34], which is no greater than the coefficient of variation of inulin clearance in a normal subject. This reproducibility contrasts sharply with the variability in 24-hr creatinine clearances [23, 24].

It is important to consider whether this method can be used in patients with CRF whose protein intake has changed. Creatinine production and, hence, steady-state excretion would change if creatine intake were varied by restricting meat in the diet. Creatinine excretion also might vary because of changes in the accumulation of meat-derived organic anions, which compete with creatinine for proximal tubular secretion. For example, ingestion of a large meal of boiled beef (225 g) caused a 52% increase in serum creatinine of normal subjects, which returned to control values after 24 hr [35]. The same quantity of meat eaten by patients with CRF would raise serum creatinine for a considerably longer period of time, depending on the degree of renal insufficiency. Conversely, reducing meat intake should lower creatinine production, but the reduction in serum creatinine would be expected to be less than 15%, the amount occurring on a creatine-free diet [36, 37]. Regardless, any decrease in serum creatinine would be only temporary if renal insufficiency continued to progress. After a new steady-state was established, the reciprocal of serum creatinine concentration would decrease again at a rate determined by the decrease in GFR. Similarly, if dietary protein restriction led to loss of lean body mass and, hence, a reduced creatinine production or if it led to a lower production of organic anions thereby increasing creatinine secretion, the change in the decline of the reciprocal of serum creatinine would be only transient if GFR continued to decrease.

The final issue is whether spontaneous changes in the slope of the reciprocal of serum creatinine occur in patients with CRF. Fortunately, this is unusual. About 20% of the 63 patients studied by Rutherford et al [30] had two slopes of their reciprocal serum creatinine plot; and of these patients, half (5 patients) had an apparent spontaneous slowing of progression. Hoffsten, Klahr, and Greenwalt [38] reported that only 1 of 32 untreated patients with glomerulonephritis and CRF had a spontaneous slowing of progression. Ledingham and Hart examined the course of renal insufficiency of 61 patients with CRF [39]. Six had apparent slowing of progression for unexplained reasons and another 9 had slowed progression associated with the release of urinary obstruction or successful treatment of hypertension, volume depletion, or glomerulonephritis. Finally, Oksa et al [29] noted that 19 of 73 patients had transient slowing of progression after initiating aggressive treatment of hypertension. Thus, spontaneous and persistent slowing of progression of CRF occurs rarely; that is, in only 12 (5%) of the 239 patients included in these reports. This indicates that changes in the reciprocal of serum creatinine can be used to evaluate the effects of treatment on progression of renal insufficiency.

Effect of Diet on Renal Function

In 1948, Addis reviewed the available experimental and clinical data and concluded that restricting dietary protein of patients with CRF might protect their kidneys from further damage [40]. He reasoned that the "renal work" required to excrete urea, sodium, potassium, acid, phosphate, and other catabolites might overtax the limited capacity of the diseased kidney. Although it is not known whether this explanation or those suggested by the animal experiments are correct, there is growing evidence that restriction of dietary protein may protect residual renal function of patients with CRF.

Long-term and acute changes in dietary protein have been shown to affect renal function in humans. Pullman et al reported that the GFR and effective renal plasma flow (RPF) of normal subjects decreased when dietary protein was restricted and increased when dietary protein was raised [41]. Bosch et al [42] restudied this question and found that the creatinine clearance of vegetarians was only 68 ml/min, 38% lower than that of control subjects (110 ml/min). Unfortunately, the protein content of the diets was not evaluated, so it is not clear that the differences in GFR were caused by differences in protein intake. However, after a single meal of 80 g of cooked meat, Bosch et al [42] noted a sharp increase in both inulin and creatinine clearances 2.5 hr later. In contrast, patients with CRF exhibited little or no change in clearance after the same meal. The authors concluded that the patients with CRF had lost their "renal functional reserve." This conclusion must be tempered because it was not established that GFR was maximally stimulated before the meat meal. In contrast to the effect of a meat meal on renal function of normal subjects, Levin and Cade [43] found that, in patients with moderate to severe CRF, a high-protein diet (1.5 to 2.0 g of protein/ kg per day) decreased both the GFR and the renal plasma flow (RPF) about 14%; a low-protein diet containing only 15 g of protein per day raised both GFR and RPF. Thus, in these patients, GFR could be increased by protein restriction, but not by feeding protein. It is unknown whether similar increases in GFR and RPF occur with other low-protein regimens that slow progression of chronic renal insufficiency.

Investigators from Italy, Germany, Sweden, and the United States have reported that dietary manipulation can slow the progression of CRF [1]. These studies used three dietary regimens: (1) For patients with mild CRF, the regimen was a low-protein (0.6 g/kg per day of predominantly high-quality protein), low-phosphate (less than 750 mg per day) diet supplemented with calcium and vitamins. (2) For patients with a more advanced CRF, the regimen was a further restriction of dietary protein and phosphate (protein, 20 to 25 g/d; phospate, less than 600 mg per day) plus a vitamin and calcium supplement and a mixture of essential amino acids. (3) The third regimen consisted of 20 to 25 g of protein per day plus vitamins and calcium, but the supplement used to meet the essential amino acid requirements was a mixture of amino acids and ketoacids.

In considering the impact of nutritional therapy on the progression of CRF, it is important to examine patients with mild CRF separately. Maschio et al [44] studied 75 such patients after dividing them into three groups. The 25 patients in group 1 had initial serum creatinine values of less than 3 mg/dl; the 20 patients in group 2 had serum creatinine values between 4 to 6 mg/dl. Both groups 1 and 2 ate a diet consisting of predominantly high-quality protein (0.5 g/kg per day), restricted phosphorus (less than 750 mg per day), and supplemental calcium (1.0 to 1.5 g per day). Group 3 (30 patients) represented a control population with initial serum creatinine values that ranged between 1.6 to 4.7 mg/dl. Their diet was unrestricted. The remarkable finding was that the average rate of loss of renal function of patients in the group eating an unrestricted diet was about 20 times higher than that of the patients in either of the two dietary restricted groups. No adverse effects of the dietary restriction were noted, and indices of nutrition were well maintained. These results are similar to those reported from the Mayo Clinic by Johnson et al [45], who treated 27 patients with CRF with a similar protein- and phosphate-restricted diet plus supplemental calcium. This regimen was successful in maintaining normal levels of serum phosphorus and ionized calcium and appeared to blunt the tendency for patients to develop secondary hyperparathyroidism. In addition, it induced a remarkable slowing of the progressive renal insufficiency. The average initial serum creatinine concentration (~5 mg/dl) did not change significantly over 27 months. This was totally unexpected considering the characteristic downhill course of patients with this degree of CRF [1]. Finally, Giordano reported that the survival to dialysis or transplantation of 12 patients with an average initial serum creatinine of 2.5 mg/dl who were being treated by dietary protein and phosphate restriction varied from 5 to 11 years [46]. This was markedly different from the 16-month average survival of the 13 patients who had a similar degree of impaired renal function but were reportedly unable to comply with dietary therapy. Thus, in these three studies of patients with mild CRF, dietary restriction induced a marked slowing of progression. These studies were retrospective and not fully randomized; therefore, the results, although impressive, will require confirmation before recommending it to all patients with mild CRF.

There also is convincing evidence that dietary therapy can benefit patients with more advanced CRF. Alvestrand et al have used a low-protein diet supplemented with a mixture of amino acids designed to correct the abnormal plasma amino acid profile of patients with CRF. In their initial report [47], two patients experienced a delay in progression lasting 6 to 8 months; two other patients had a halted progression lasting for 1.0 to 1.5 years. More recently, Alvestrand, Ahlberg, and Bergstrom studied 17 patients who had a well-established rate of decline of reciprocal serum creatinine, even though some were eating diets containing as little as 40 g of protein per day [48]. After beginning treatment with a 20-g protein diet supplemented with amino acids or ketoacids, there was a striking, 10-fold decrease in the rate of progression lasting an average of 355 days; only 3 patients did not have a substantial slowing of progression.

The effects of ketoacid-supplemented, low-protein, low-phosphate diets have been studied by several groups [1]. In a retrospective analysis of our early results using a diet containing 20 to 25 g of unselected protein per day and supplemented with calcium salts of keto and hydroxy analogues of essential amino acids, we identified a few patients with advanced renal failure who had a marked slowing of progression [49]. More recently, we analyzed the course of patients whose average initial serum creatinine was 10 mg/dl [50]. They received a diet containing 20 to 25 g of unselected protein per day supplemented with basic amino acid salts of ketoacids. For the group as a whole, deterioration of renal function was substantially slowed: 2 of the 3 patients with diabetic nephropathy had no deterioration of function for 8 and 18 months, respectively; 2 of 11 patients with glomerulonephritis had no further loss of renal function for 7 and 19 months; 5 of 11 patients with glomerulonephritis had a temporary slowing of progression lasting 6 or more months. However, 4 patients with glomerulonephritis and one patient with polycystic kidney disease experienced no slowing of progression with the ketoacid regimen; no patient experienced an accelerated deterioration of renal function. Therapy was clearly more effective if begun before the serum creatinine reached 8 mg/dl. In another report, Barsotti et al [32] examined the progression of renal insufficiency of 31 patients being treated with a low-protein (~0.5 g of high-quality protein/kg per day) and a low-phosphate diet. All these patients experienced a linear decline in creatinine clearance, in spite of the restricted diet. Twelve patients were then treated with a diet containing daily about 0.2 g of protein/kg, 300 mg of phosphorus, plus a supplement of calcium and ketoacids. Eleven of this group had marked slowing in the rate of loss of their renal function. Only one patient continued to lose renal function at the same rate. Gretz et al [51] studied the effects of a diet containing daily 30 g of unselected protein supplemented with calcium salts of ketoacids. The medium time for serum creatinine to increase from 6 to 10 mg/dl in the 45 patients treated with this regimen was 60 weeks. For the 45 other patients who served as a control group, the median time for the same increase to occur in serum creatinine (from 6 to 10 mg/dl) was only 25 weeks: a highly significant difference. Vetter et al [52] compared the effects of different low-protein regimens. The effects of a 0.6-g high-quality protein diet on the progression of renal insufficiency of 20 patients was compared with a 20-g protein diet supplemented with essential amino acids (20 patients) or ketoacids (20 patients). All three diets slowed progression when compared to the clinical course of a control group of patients eating an unrestricted diet. Apparently, the most benefit was obtained with the low-protein, ketoacid-supplemented regimen.

Summary

A restriction of dietary protein and phosphate can slow the rate of loss of residual renal function in mild chronic renal insufficiency; but for patients with more advanced CRF or for those who continue to lose renal function while being treated with the standard low-protein diet, the slowing of progression may require a restriction of the daily dietary protein to between 20 to 25 g plus a supplement of essential amino acids or ketoacids. Key questions that remain unanswered include: Which regimen is most frequently effective and acceptable to patients? Is there a specific beneficial effect of the ketoacid regimen? How can patients who will respond most favorably be identified? And, when should nutritional therapy be initiated?

References

1. MITCH WE: The influence of the diet on the progression of renal insufficiency. *Ann Rev Med* 35:249–264, 1984
2. BISCHOFF F: The influence of the diet on renal and blood vessel changes. *J Nutr* 5:431–450, 1932
3. MOISE TS, SMITH AH: Effect of high protein diet on the kidneys: Experimental study. *Arch Pathol* 4:530–542, 1927
4. CHANUTIN A, FERRIS EB: Experimental renal insufficiency produced by partial nephrectomy: I. Control diet. *Arch Intern Med* 49:767–787, 1932
5. CHANUTIN A, LUDEWIG S: Experimental renal insufficiency produced by partial nephrectomy: V. Diets containing whole dried meat. *Arch Intern Med* 58:60–80, 1936
6. KLEINKNECHT C, SALUSKY I, BROYER M, GUBLER MC: Effect of various protein diets on growth, renal function and survival of uremic rats. *Kidney Int* 15:534–541, 1979
7. FARR LE, SMADEL JE: The effect of dietary protein on the course of nephrotoxic nephritis in rats. *J Exp Med* 70:615–627, 1939
8. FRIEND PS, FERNANDES G, GOOD RA, MICHAEL AF, YUNIS EJ: Dietary restrictions early and late: Effects on the nephropathy of the NZB × NZW mouse. *Lab Invest* 38:629–632, 1978
9. HOSTETTER TH, OLSON JL, RENNKE HG, VENKATACHALAM MA, BRENNER BM: Hyperfiltration in remnant nephrons: A potentially adverse response to renal ablation. *Am J Physiol* 241:F85–F93, 1981
10. OLSON JL, HOSTETTER TH, RENNKE HG, BRENNER BM, VENKATACHALAM

MA: Altered glomerular permeability and progressive sclerosis following ablation of renal mass. *Kidney Int* 22:112–126, 1982

11. BRENNER BM, MEYER TW, HOSTETTER TH: Dietary protein intake and the progressive nature of kidney disease: The role of hemodynamically mediated glomerular injury in the pathogenesis of progressive glomerular sclerosis in aging, renal ablation, and intrinsic renal disease. *N Engl J Med* 307:652–659, 1982

12. ALBRIGHT F, BAIRD PC, COPE O, BLOOMBERG E: Studies on the physiology of the parathyroid glands: IV. Renal complications of hyperparathyroidism. *Am J Med Sci* 187:49–65, 1934

13. DONOHUE W, SPINGARN C, PAPPENHEIMER AM: The calcium content of the kidney as related to parathyroid function. *J Exp Med* 66:697–701, 1937

14. IBELS LS, ALFREY AC, HAUT L, HUFFER WE: Preservation of function in experimental renal disease by dietary restriction of phosphate. *N Engl J Med* 298:122–126, 1978

15. KARLINSKY ML, HAUT C, BUDDINGTON B, SCHRIER N, ALFREY AC: Preservation of renal function in experimental glomerulonephritis. *Kidney Int* 17:293–302, 1980

16. KLAHR S, BUERKERT J, PURKERSON ML: Role of dietary factors in the progression of chronic renal disease. *Kidney Int* 24:579–587, 1983

17. LAOUARI D, KLEINKNECHT C, COURNOT-WITMER G, HABIB R, MOUNIER F, BROYER M: Beneficial effect of low phosphorus diet in uremic rats: A reappraisal. *Clin Sci* 63:539–548, 1982

18. HURD ER, ZIFF M: Quantitative studies of immunoglobulin deposition in the kidney, glomerular cell proliferation and glomerulosclerosis in NZB/NZW F_1 hybrid mice. *Clin Exp Immunol* 26:261–268, 1976

19. BARCELLI UO, WEISS M, POLLAK VE: Effects of a dietary prostaglandin precursor on the progression of experimentally induced chronic renal failure. *J Lab Clin Med* 100:786–797, 1982

20. PURKERSON ML, VALDES A, YATES J, MORRISON A, KLAHR S: Inhibition of thromboxane synthesis prevents progressive renal disease in rats with 5/6 nephrectomy. *Kidney Int* 25:251, 1984

21. KAMPMANN JP, MOLHOLM-HANSEN J: Glomerular filtration rate and creatinine clearance. *Br J Clin Pharmacol* 12:7–14, 1981

22. LUBOWITZ H, SLATOPOLSKY E, SHANKAL S, RIESELBACH RE, BRICKER NS: Glomerular filtration rate: Determination in patients with renal disease. *JAMA* 199:252–256, 1967

23. MORGAN DB, DILLON S, PAYNE RB: The assessment of glomerular function: Creatinine clearance or plasma creatinine? *Postgrad Med J* 54:302–310, 1978

24. MORGAN DB, WILL EJ: Selection, presentation and interpretation of biochemical data in renal failure. *Kidney Int* 24:438–445, 1983

25. MITCH WE, COLLIER VU, WALSER M: Creatinine metabolism in chronic renal failure. *Clin Sci* 58:327–335, 1980

26. CARRIE BJ, GOLBETZ HV, MICHAELS AS, MYERS BD: Creatinine: An inadequate filtration marker in glomerular diseases. *Am J Med* 69:177–182, 1980

27. MITCH WE, WALSER M, BUFFINGTON GA, LEMANN J: A simple method of estimating progression of chronic renal failure. *Lancet* 2:1326–1328, 1976

28. JONES RH, HAYAKAWA H, MACKAY JD, PARSONS V, WATKINS PF: The progression of diabetic nephropathy. *Lancet* 1:1105–1106, 1979

29. OKSA H, PASTERNACK A, LUOMALA M, SIRVIO M: Progression of chronic renal failure. *Nephron* 35:31–34, 1983

30. RUTHERFORD WE, BLONDIN J, MILLER JP, GREENWALT AS, VAVRA JD: Chronic progressive renal disease: Rate of change of serum creatinine concentration. *Kidney Int* 11:62–70, 1977

31. GRETZ N, MANZ F, STRAUCH M: Predictability of the progression of chronic renal failure. *Kidney Int* 24:52–55, 1983
32. BARSOTTI G, GUIDUCCI A, CIARDELLA F, GIOVANNETTI S: Effects on renal function of a low-nitrogen diet supplemented with essential amino acids and keto-analogues and of hemodialysis and free protein supply in patients with chronic renal failure. *Nephron* 27:113–117, 1981
33. VIBERTI GC, BILIUS RW, MACKINTOSH D, KEEN H: Monitoring glomerular function in diabetic nephropathy. *Am J Med* 74:256–264, 1983
34. FRASER CG, WILLIAMS P: Short-term biological variation of plasma analytes in renal disease. *Clin Chem* 29:508–510, 1983
35. MAYERSOHN M, CONRAD KA, ACHARI R: The influence of a cooked meal on creatinine plasma concentration and creatinine clearance. *Br J Clin Pharm* 15:227–230, 1983
36. HEYMSFIELD SB, ARTEAGA C, MCMANUS C, SMITH J, MOFFITT S: Measurement of muscle mass in humans: Validity of the 24-hour urinary creatinine method. *Am J Clin Nutr* 37:494–498, 1983
37. WOLTHIUS FH: Balance studies on protein metabolism in normal and uremic men: Effect of diet, bed rest, and anabolic steroids. *Acta Med Scand* 171:1–150, 1961
38. HOFFSTEN P, KLAHR S, GREENWALT A: A comparison of reciprocal or logarithm serum creatinine vs time plots for predicting prognosis of glomerulonephritis. *Kidney Int* 14:653, 1978
39. LEDINGHAM JGG, HART G: The optimum time to start regular hemodialysis, in *Dialysis Review,* edited by DAVISON AM, Philadelphia, J.P. Lippincott, 1978, pp 22–31
40. ADDIS T: *Glomerular Nephritis: Diagnosis and Treatment.* New York, MacMillan, 1948, pp 265–309
41. PULLMAN TN, ALVING AS, DERN RJ, LANDOWNE M: The influence of dietary protein on specific renal functions in normal man. *J Lab Clin Med* 44:320–332, 1954
42. BOSCH JP, SACCAGGI A, LAUER A, RONCO C, BELLEDONNE M, GLABMAN S: Renal function reserve in humans: Effect of protein intake on glomerular filtration rate. *Am J Med* 75:943–950, 1983
43. LEVIN DM, CADE R: Metabolic effects of dietary protein in chronic renal failure. *Ann Intern Med* 63:642–653, 1965
44. MASCHIO G, OLDRIZZI L, TESSITORE N, D'ANGELO A, VALVO E, ET AL: Effects of dietary protein and phosphorus restriction on the progression of early renal failure. *Kidney Int* 22:371–376, 1982
45. JOHNSON WJ, GOLDSMITH RS, JOWSEY J, FROHNERT PP, ARNAUD CD: In *Second Workshop on Vitamin D, Wiesbaden,* edited by NORMAN AW, New York, Walter de Gruyter, 1975, pp 561–575
46. GIORDANO C: Early diet to slow the course of chronic renal failure, in *Proc 8th Int Congress Nephrol, Athens,* New York, Karger, 1981, pp 71–87
47. ALVESTRAND A, AHLBERG M, FURST P, BERGSTROM J: Clinical results of long-term treatment with a low protein diet and a new amino acid preparation in patients with chronic uremia. *Clin Nephrol* 19:67–73, 1983
48. ALVESTRAND A, AHLBERG M, BERGSTROM J: Retardation of the progression of renal insufficiency in patients treated with low protein diets. *Kidney Int* (in press, 1984)
49. WALSER M, MITCH WE, COLLIER VU: Essential amino acids and their nitrogen-free analogues in the treatment of chronic renal failure, in *Controversies in Nephrology,* edited by SCHREINER G, Washington, DC, Georgetown University, 1979, pp 404–413

50. MITCH WE, STEINMAN TI, WALSER M: The effect of protein restriction plus ketoacids on progression of chronic renal failure (*abstract*). *Clin Res* 31:437A, 1983
51. GRETZ N, MEISINGER E, GRETZ T, KORB E, STRAUCH M: Low protein diet supplemented by ketoacids in chronic renal failure: A prospective controlled study. *Kidney Int* (in press, 1984)
52. VETTER K, FROHLING PT, KASCHUBE I, GOTZ KH, SCHMICKLER R: Influence of ketoacid-treatment on residual renal function in chronic renal insufficiency. *Kidney Int* (in press, 1984)

Dialysis

Advantages and Disadvantages of Current Dialysis Techniques

Horst Klinkmann and Peter Ivanovich

For 4000 years, there has persisted in humans an intuitive belief that the majority of diseases results from impurities in the body. Therefore, correction of the body's humoral balance by purifying the blood through blood-letting was an accepted procedure in the concept of Talmudic medicine (100 to 200 BC); and, it has been used as a remedy for almost every illness in nearly every society and culture in the world. It is fascinating that with the exploitation of natural biologic laws, in combination with the latest development in technology in the twentieth century, this concept has been revived in a controlled and scientific way [1].

Dialysis treatment is entering its fifth decade of clinical application, and the number of living patients undergoing such treatment will soon reach 500,000 [2, 3]. The last two decades permitted not only the perfecting of conventional methods of hemodialysis, but also the introduction of new concepts into both experimental and clinical work. However, the main increase in the number of treatments, as well as in its quality, is simply the result of the development of conventional dialysis (Fig. 1). Except for continuous ambulatory peritoneal dialysis (CAPD) in certain regions and for special indications [3, 4], none of the recent innovations (hemofiltration, hemodiafiltration, and so on) have had a real impact on the number of patients treated or on the survival rate.

The treatment of end-stage renal disease (ESRD) accompanied by a variety of problems in different countries around the world is related to the available economic resources, as well as to differing ethical, religious, political, and—last but not least—personal points of view. I strongly oppose a judgment of treatment modalities based on an analysis of data from incomparable conditions in incomparable countries. This point of view is supported by two examples. First, the limited resources for hemodialysis in the United Kingdom are clearly the main reason for the recent significant increase in CAPD—not any medical preference. Second, in the German Democratic Republic, the

---

This manuscript was presented as a State-of-the-Art Lecture of the same title.

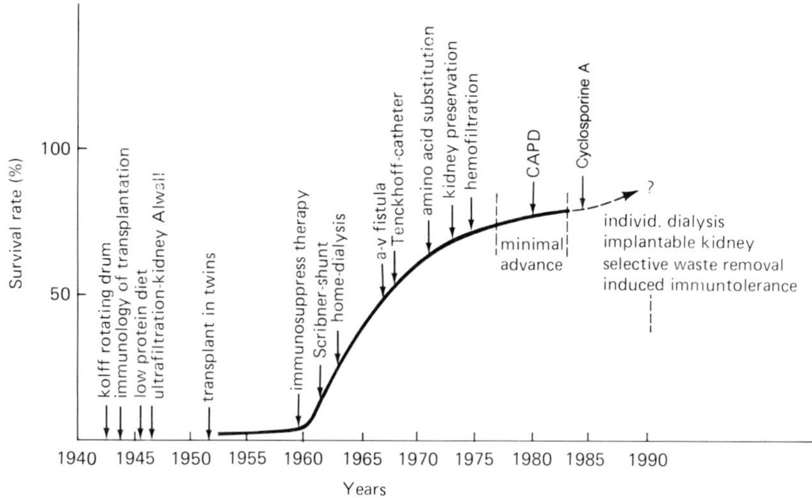

Fig. 1. Survival rate of dialysis patients in relation to the development of renal replacement therapy.

central organization of the health-care programs clearly favors center dialysis over home dialysis [2], despite the well-known advantages of a home dialysis system for certain patients. Therefore, this paper will not review the advantages and disadvantages of the currently available dialysis techniques exclusively on the basis of available statistics from different countries. We will try to express a more general view that is based on recent intensive discussions with leading experts in the field. We are fully aware that any report prepared by a single group of authors will always have a personal bias and provoke disagreement among specialists. Since controversies are the essence of further development, we hope that even such a biased review can contribute to progress.

At present, more than 85% of all patients treated worldwide are on a conventional hemodialysis program. In Europe, for example, less than 3% of the entire dialysis population are on hemofiltration; approximately 5% are on CAPD. Bicarbonate hemodialysis does not exceed 10%. All of the other treatment modalities—such as hemodiafiltration, high-sodium hemodialysis, combined hemodialysis and hemoperfusion, and different methods of peritoneal dialysis—collectively do not constitute more than 3% of the total dialysis population [3]. At present, there are more than 300 different hemodialyzers available on the world market, most of which are of hollow-fiber design; however, 10% of the world market still consists of coils and rebuildable plate hemodialyzers, primarily in countries with limited resources for renal replacement therapy.

This illustrates quite clearly that the greatest number of achievements, as measured by survival rate and quality of life, come from conventional hemodialysis. The statistics of the European Dialysis and Transplantation

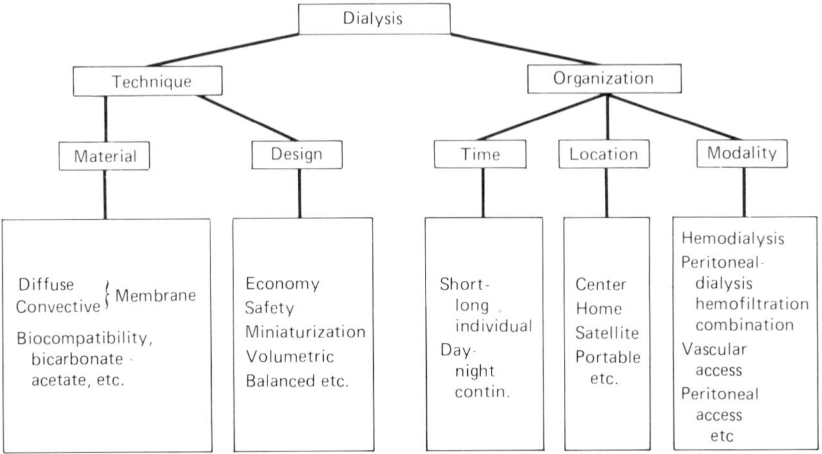

Fig. 2. Recent problem areas in dialysis therapy.

Association–European Renal Association provide an optimistic outlook for a life expectancy of 90% for a young hemodialysis patient without severe secondary complications for a 10-year period—demonstrating the efficacy of our presently available technique. Two fundamentals must be remembered: (1) we are treating a severe clinical condition—uremia—of which our knowledge is still extremely limited, and (2) the technical simulation of the natural kidney function is still imperfect. Figure 2 illustrates the different problem areas in our hemodialysis treatment facilities. A definitive answer is currently not available for any of these problems.

The quality concept for the advantages and disadvantages of different treatment modalities will be the assessment of adequacy of hemodialysis, as expressed in three major topics: survival rate, frequency of hospitalization, and work tolerance.

When to Start Hemodialysis

On a worldwide basis, this issue must be viewed in the perspective of a continuing disproportion between demand and available facilities. The major disadvantage in defining rational guidelines as to when to start dialysis is our ignorance with respect to the pathophysiology and pathobiochemistry of uremia. It would seem appropriate to correct uremic metabolic disturbances as early as possible via dialysis. Early hemodialysis as advocated by Bonomini et al [5] has been defined as the initiation of maintenance hemodialysis therapy in chronic uremia after minimal or no conservative low-protein dietary management, relying only on clinical signs and symptoms in patients with a residual renal function still relatively high (creatinine clearance [C_{cr}] 10 to 12 ml/min). By contrast, the majority of patients are referred for hemodialysis when their residual renal function is much lower (C_{cr} 5 ml/min), and often after a period of conservative management with a low-protein diet. With long-term results now available, this question again deserves our full attention based on ethical, clinical, and economic considerations [6]. We will review these problems, because they might become a future issue for the optimization of dialysis.

The two main criticisms of an earlier start of hemodialysis are: (1) a machine-dependent life, when the residual renal function is not life-threatening, and (2) a cost increase by 40 to 50% during the first year.

In addition, results from recent studies [7–9] seemed to indicate that properly conducted conservative management in the predialytic phase, which includes dietary measurement, can be helpful for the prevention of secondary uremic complications; therefore, it can be of benefit for the long-term results of dialysis treatment. The rational approach towards early dialysis takes into consideration that the available technology for treating our patients can counteract only the loss of the excretory function of the kidney, thus acting only as glomerulus. Since uremic symptoms are due to the suppression of both excretory and secretory renal functions, the present mode of treatment will never completely reverse uremic symptoms. A new philosophic motto, therefore, has been suggested [6]: dialysis is capable of a double miracle—keeping alive both the patient and the disease. The supporters of an earlier start of dialysis claim that most of the irreversible uremic problems can be prevented by starting treatment earlier. Despite initial high cost during the first and second year, they claim a 20% net saving in the ensuing years resulting from fewer hospitalization days and higher full-time working capacity [10].

Economic cost factors, feasibility of conservative dietary treatment, and bioethics—taking into consideration the quality of life and possible treatment-induced complications—have prevented wide acceptance of what is termed early dialysis.

The question of when to start dialysis still has to be considered from many different points of view, but the approach should no longer be disqualified as unrealistic.

Which Dialysis Technique Should Be Used?

The broad spectrum of treatment modalities currently available makes it difficult to reach a consensus among those concerned, regarding the advantages and disadvantages of current dialysis therapies. In recent extensive discussions with some of the leading pioneers of each treatment modality, basic agreement could be achieved for the following options [4].

Conventional Hemodialysis with Acetate

Advantages

This hemodialysis technique remains the standard treatment for more than 85% of the world dialysis population. It is a generally accepted, well-established treatment that is most widely available. The procedure is relatively simple and safe. Good clinical results in long-term treatment can be achieved, thus making life expectancy for a hemodialysis patient better than in many other chronic diseases [3, 11, 12]. Conventional hemodialysis with acetate may be performed in hospitals, satellite and free-standing outpatient hemodialysis centers, and in the home. It represents the most economical form of therapy in the United States. Costs are $116 and $148,[1] respectively, for free-standing and hospital units. Costs in the home are less when reimbursement of the assistant is not a factor.

Disadvantages

Like all other machine-dependent techniques, it limits the independence of the patient at least during the required treatment time—4 to 6 hr, three times weekly. Because of the use of buffers, there can be a delayed correction of the patient's metabolic acidosis and an "intolerance of acetate" [13]. The low clearance of so-called middle or larger molecules might become disadvantageous if our insight into uremia becomes more profound. The main disadvantage is related to cardiovascular instability, especially in combination with the use of large surface hemodialyzers and poorly controlled solute and fluid removal [14–17].

Conventional Hemodialysis with Bicarbonate

The current renaissance of bicarbonate hemodialysis is primarily related to the results obtained in the relatively small group of problem patients with cardiovascular instability and selected metabolic problems [14].

Advantages

From the metabolic point of view, bicarbonate hemodialysis is a more physiologic treatment alternative to acetate hemodialysis.

Disadvantages

The current drawbacks are still those that caused Mion et al [13] to switch from the original bicarbonate hemodialysis to acetate hemodialysis—the requirement for additional equipment for the preparation of bicarbonate; the problem of $CaCO_3$ precipitation in the equipment. The additional expense for equipment, preparation time, and special solution adds approximately $2 to $3 per treatment. The aforementioned problems and increased cost have limited the widespread use of bicarbonate hemodialysis.

---

[1] United States Health Care Finance Administration Statistical Analysis System, facility cost audit to develop August 1, 1983 reimbursement schedule.

Indications

Taking into account that bicarbonate hemodialysis may benefit the patient, but ruin the equipment, even the recent enthusiastic forecast for the use of bicarbonate would certainly not exceed 20% of all hemodialysis procedures performed at present. Clearly, it should be used in severe hemodialysis metabolic acidosis. Therefore, it is the method of choice in acute renal failure patients. Cardiovascular instability also is a clear indication for bicarbonate in the dialysate; this implies that its use is preferable in elderly patients. Finally, patients with insufficient metabolism of the liver require bicarbonate hemodialysis, as well as those who are hypoxic because of pulmonary dysfunction. In many cases, bicarbonate hemodialysis need only be applied during the acute phase of illness [17–20].

Sequential Ultrafiltration and Hemodialysis

With the availability of hemofilters or high-flux hemodialyzers, sequential ultrafiltration and hemodialysis remain of interest to those with access only to conventional hemodialyzers [19].

Advantages

It is a relatively simple procedure that increases the tolerance for fluid removal by using conventional equipment.

Disadvantages

Because of the necessary sequence in performing ultrafiltration and hemodialysis, the treatment time is prolonged. There is also a certain danger of an imbalance in electrolytes; for example, hyperkalemia, if the procedure is performed in the sequence of ultrafiltration first, and hemodialysis second.

Indications

Most of the indications overlap with those of hemofiltration or hemodiafiltration and will be addressed later.

Hemofiltration

Hemofiltration is an extracorporeal process by which uremic whole blood is cleansed by a combination of ultrafiltration and convective solute loss, and then rediluted with physiologic saline solution. Dilution may occur before or after the hemofiltration device. Despite many obvious benefits of the convective mass transfer process, especially for problem patients, the clinical use

of hemofiltration at present does not exceed 5% of the total dialysis population
[3, 21–23].

Advantages

The remarkable tolerance of the vascular system to fluid removal—and, therefore, the prevention of all of the intrahemodialytic complications caused by
cardiovascular instability—is the greatest advantage of this method [24, 25].
Materials used for hemofiltration membranes cause fewer problems of mem-
brane-related bioincompatibility than those used in hemodialyzers. The higher
clearance for middle-sized and larger molecules might prove to be of benefit
for long-term results [22, 23].

Disadvantages

The necessary special equipment, as well as the high cost of commercial
sterile replacement solution, together with the risk of their bacterial contamination have limited expansion of hemofiltration. However, the often-claimed
low efficiency in the removal of small molecules is questionable with the
introduction of new, highly efficient filters. The blood flow required from
the patient must always exceed 300 ml/min. The relative complexity of the
technique limits its application to academic institutions, hospitals, and dialysis
centers with specially qualified personnel. Its cost exceeds conventional hemodialysis by 50%.

Indications

Patients with vascular instability and serious intrahemodialytic episodes of
hyper- or hypotension, as well as patients with autonomic insufficiency and
persistent hypotension, are better treated with hemofiltration. Severe, constant
hyperhydration not only in renal patients, but also in edema or other origin,
also calls for hemofiltration or sequential ultrafiltration and hemodialysis.
   On-line high-efficiency hemofiltration seems to provide the possibility of
shortening treatment time by providing both adequate removal of toxic substances and cardiovascular stability. It could become a real challenge to all
other present treatment modalities of similar efficiency if it were not for its
expense.

Continuous Arteriovenous Hemofiltration (CAVH)

This rather recent development [26] has gained rapid acceptance worldwide
as an application for patients with acute problems [27].

Advantages

The ability to apply continuous treatment of fluid excess in metabolic disorders provides the physician with unique flexibility in controlling nutrition and fluid balance in patients requiring intensive care unit management. Such continuous treatment allows for precise fluid balance; and, ammonium carbonate substitution combined with the removal of intratubular nephrotoxins may provide a protective effect for the proximal tubules [28].

Disadvantages

Despite improvements in vascular access, there remains a considerable risk for infection in these patients. The continuous need for anticoagulation provides yet another risk. Despite the technical simplicity of the method, it requires well-qualified personnel or rather careful monitoring with adequate equipment.

Indications

The CAVH technique may be provided for patients with severly acute renal insufficiency as a physiologic continuous treatment of fluid and metabolic disturbances. It also enables the physician to use hyperalimentation without the limitations that otherwise are imposed by the volume of fluid necessary for total parenteral nutrition.

The CAVH technique should not be considered an alternative treatment to hemodialysis in patients with uncomplicated acute renal failure. In this case, the treatment of choice remains single-needle, venovenous, volume-controlled hemodialysis with bicarbonate dialysate.

Hemodiafiltration

Hemodiafiltration is an extracorporeal process by which uremic whole blood is cleansed by a combination of diffusive and convective transport of solute, with ultrafiltration and redilution of blood with physiologic saline solution. It uses a highly permeable membrane that is effective both as a hemodialyzer and hemofilter, thus combining hemofiltration and hemodialysis. Such simultaneous therapy is more efficient, and it usually allows for shorter treatment time when 8 to 10 liters of replacement solution are infused into the venous return limb of the extracorporeal circuit [29].

Advantages

This method combines the advantages of the diffusive and the convective transport mechanisms. It provides excellent efficiency for both small and large molecule removal, implying a shortening of treatment time.

Disadvantages

Special equipment and facilities are necessary. Since substitution fluid is required, the same serious risk exists as in hemofiltration. Its costs are less than those of hemofiltration; but, they are decidedly greater than those required for conventional hemodialysis with acetate dialysate.

Indications

Shortening of treatment time in hemodynamically unstable patients appears to be the only indication for hemodiafiltration with substitution fluid at present, in comparison with other available techniques.

High-flux Hemodialysis

The term high-flux hemodialysis is used for very efficient hemodialysis with high ultrafiltration that uses new, highly permeable membranes that combine convective and diffusive transport [4]. The term hemodiafiltration without substitution fluid has also been proposed for this method.

Advantages

The advantages listed under hemodiafiltration are true in this instance. By combining diffusion and convection, the natural kidney is more closely simulated in solute removal, and this can result in shorter treatment times. This is true because of the ability to use higher blood flow rates to achieve adequate solute removal. Despite high blood flows and higher clearances, vascular instability is less of a problem than conventional hemodialysis with acetate.

Disadvantages

The treatment only can be performed with the volumetric-balanced control equipment presently available only in hospital facilities and some free-standing units. The cost of this equipment is approximately twice that of conventional hemodialysis with acetate. However, the ability to reprocess the hemofilter reduces its cost. By shortening treatment time by 25%, it allows for better use of facilities, thus making the technique economically attractive and in the range of conventional hemodialysis. As with all other recently introduced treatment modalities, it lacks controlled long-term results. The risk of pyrogens entering the blood from dialysate is minimal, depending on the quality and the integrity of the membrane used.

Indications

For conventional hemodiafiltration with substitution fluid, there is no obvious indication at present in comparison with the other available techniques. However, high-flux hemodialysis combines the advantages of hemodialysis and hemofiltration; it could easily become the method of choice not only for all problem patients, but even as the prevailing procedure for appropriate treatment of ESRD. In concept, it comes closest to our goal of removing the most uremic toxins that are compatible with vascular stability in the shortest possible time, with the greatest physical and psychologic independence of the patient.

Controlled High-Sodium Hemodialysis

Despite repeated publication since 1978 of the beneficial effect of controlled high-sodium hemodialysis [30], the method has not gained general acceptance.

Advantages

There is better control of the basic humoral equilibrium via an adequate balance between the interhemodialytic load and intrahemodialytic removal of sodium (Na) and water (H_2O). The constant manipulation of Na^+ and H_2O transfer allows the equilibration of Na^+ and H_2O during treatment, which leads to both a reduction of intrahemodialytic symptoms and a possible correction of intrahemodialytic hypotension [31].

Disadvantages

In high-sodium hemodialysis, the single hemodialysis treatment is the reason for the next extreme fluid overload by excessive weight gain between hemodialyses. These extremes are to be avoided with respect to the long-term survival rate of hemodialysis patients.

Indications

Severe, repeated intrahemodialytic hypotensive episodes, as well as hypertension due to a sodium dysequilibrium, justify this treatment as a clinical trial. There seems to be general acceptance that the Na^+ in the dialysate solution could be varied during hemodialysis to allow quantification of sequential sodium therapy, correction of total exchangeable sodium, and establishment of stability criteria. A highly permeable membrane hemodialyzer in combination with a volumetric-controlled proportioning hemodialysis machine, where dialysate sodium can be varied during treatment, are the necessary prerequisites for this treatment modality, which might be a great advantage in the near future. This treatment requires special equipment, rendering it somewhat more expensive than conventional hemodialysis with acetate.

Peritoneal Dialysis

Peritoneal dialysis, being theoretically a more physiologic treatment than hemodialysis because of the avoidance of sudden changes in humoral balance, has gained a renaissance since the conception of CAPD by Popovich et al in 1976 [33] and its modifications by Oreopoulos et al in 1978 [34]. Despite serious medical complications and criticism, and a dropout rate of approximately 50% of patients entering CAPD at the end of the first year, its popularity is still growing [35, 36]. The reasons for its expansion include resource allocations (as in the United Kingdom), rationing decisions (as in diabetic patients [37]), and commercial promotion of an extent never seen in any other replacement therapy.

We prefer to view peritoneal dialysis not as an alternative to hemodialysis, but rather as an additional choice of methods among available renal replacement therapies. There might be enough evidence that certain treatment modalities may apply better to a certain group of patients. The key question is not which method of treatment is superior to the other, but when, how, and where to use one or another of the available modalities.

Continuous Ambulatory Peritoneal Dialysis (CAPD)

Advantages

At present, CAPD is the only true "wearable" renal replacement therapy. In addition to being a continous treatment, the patient's independence from equipment is greater than in any other treatment modality for ESRD, and the need for additional personnel is minimized. No vascular access is required. It allows for better control of extracellular fluid volume compared to intermittent hemodialysis, and no anticoagulation is required.

Disadvantages

The main complication in peritoneal dialysis [36] has always been bacterial peritonitis. Although there has been a significant reduction in the incidence of peritonitis with technologic advances (such as using plastic bags instead of glass bottles for the dialysate solution), improvement of peritoneal catheters, and the use of bacterial rejection filters, the average incidence of peritonitis is still fairly high; approximately two episodes per year. The lack of controlled long-term treatment data means a lack of information regarding a considerable number of acute problems. Also, many more hospitalizations are required with CAPD than with hemodialysis. Therefore, this home treatment—although less costly than hemodialysis with acetate—becomes less cost-effective when additional hospital expenses are included.

Indications

As with conventional hemodialysis, it is generally accepted that CAPD may be useful in diabetic and elderly individuals, especially those with cardiovascular problems [35, 37].

Continuous Cycling Peritoneal Dialysis (CCPD)

Advantages

In addition to the advantages listed under CAPD, CCPD does not require dialysate exchange during the daytime. Because sterile techniques are required only twice per day, CCPD has the potential to reduce the incidence of peritonitis.

Disadvantages

Special, rather expensive equipment is necessary; and, contrary to CAPD, the patient is "tied to a machine" even if only overnight. Bacterial peritonitis is the main complication of peritoneal dialysis [36], and it has resulted in more frequent hospitalizations than hemodialysis.

Indications

These are basically the same as in CAPD.

Intermittent Peritoneal Dialysis (IPD)

At present, IPD is mainly used for acute treatment. It requires longer treatment time, with lower efficiency than hemodialysis.

Additional Actual Problems in Peritoneal Dialysis Treatment

With the maintenance of many patients on long-term peritoneal dialysis, metabolic and nutritional effects (in addition to peritonitis) are emerging as critical limitations of this treatment.

The continuous absorption of glucose from the dialysate may lead to hypertriglyceridemia and to significant weight gain in patients. However, despite significant weight gain, protein malnutrition may occur as a consequence of the daily loss of albumin and amino acid in the dialysate. Recent investigations indicate that changes in dialysate composition, such as supplementation with amino acids, may be beneficial in reducing some of the critical effects [32]. For the correction of metabolic acidosis in peritoneal dialysis, organic base buffers (mostly acetate or lactate) are used in the procedure. To achieve a physiologic serum bicarbonate level, the buffer concentration in the dialysate should be approximately 40 to 50 mEq/liter.

Lactate and acetate are both fully metabolized to bicarbonate; however, lactate solutions obviously are better tolerated from the patient's standpoint. Regarding long-term results, alarming complications have been recently reported [38] via the occurrence of sclerosing peritonitis within a few weeks to several years after discontinuing peritoneal dialysis. This life-threatening complication is characterized by a progression to both complete intestinal obstruction and severe protein malnutrition. The etiology of sclerosing peritonitis remains obscure. The factors that can induce peritoneal inflammation are numerous. They comprise peritoneal infection, the content of dialysate solution or its contamination, as well as the mere presence of plasticizers, silicone rubber, and talc to initiate this specific inflammatory process. Most of the patients have been on acetate-containing hemodialysis fluid; therefore, our interest is focused on acetate per se or on characteristics of acetate-containing solutions. It would probably be an oversimplification to ascribe the pathogenesis of sclerosing peritonitis to a single etiologic factor. The multifactorial triggering of peritoneal fibrosclerosis may be one specific lesion of the peritoneum caused by the treatment. The main limitation for future expansion of CAPD—CCPD with long-term results comparable to hemodialysis—might be that the peritoneum as a living membrane is altered much more frequently and faster by repeated exposure to the physiochemic stresses of peritoneal lavage with many unphysiologic substances.

Whether chronic peritoneal dialysis treatment can ever achieve the same long-term results as the other hemodialysis techniques remains an open question in our opinion; and, it can only be answered about 5 years from now.

Dialysis Schedule—Short Versus Long Dialysis

The frequency and duration of hemodialysis has been a subject of interest as long as the treatment has been available. It generally is influenced by the availability of hemodialysis facilities and the hemodialysis techniques. A review of the history of changing hemodialysis schedules, according to the prevailing concepts, was given by Cambi et al [39].

The term "short or long dialysis" presently seems to be obsolete; the real challenge is between adequate and inadequate hemodialysis. Generally, the term "short hemodialysis" is applied to a 3 to 4 hr three times weekly schedule that can be adequate treatment with adequate equipment. The still remaining dilemma of choosing between highly efficient hemodialysis associated with cardiovascular instability or prolonged, safe hemodialysis might soon be resolved with highly efficient hemodialyzer-hemofilter using a volumetric-balanced control system. The hemodialysis schedule will remain time-dependent, but it should be adjusted to the patient's need; therefore, it calls for individualization of the treatment.

Individualization of Treatment

Although advanced hemodialysis technology generally provides a new lease on life in ESRD, only individualization of treatment would result in equal benefit for all [40, 43].

Individualization of treatment includes both the selection of a specific treatment for an individual patient as well as the adjustment of that specific treatment to the individual need; for example, by using kinetic modeling [41, 42].

We are still awaiting controlled and definitive studies as to which patients might benefit most from which treatment type. Omitting renal transplantation in this specific review, it is not easy to advise uremic patients about the choice for therapy. Our own point of view was expressed earlier. However, selection of uremic therapy worldwide is mostly determined by available resources, economic considerations, and physician-patient preference.

Individualization/Adequacy

The initial concern with therapy was mortality. Now, our focus is on morbidity and patient rehabilitation [43, 44]. To understand the complexity of interactions between treatment regimen and patient, it is essential to study the kinetics of interaction [42].

For any disease being managed by extracorporeal means, the most important causes of morbidity should be identified. High on the list of priorities in renal replacement therapy would be cardiovascular instability, electrolyte disorders, treatment fatigue, anemia, and bone disease [44–46].

Kinetic Modeling

Adjustment of independent treatment variables (hemodialyzer, dialysate composition, flow rates, treatment time, and nutrition) is the goal for optimization of treatment [47, 48]. Therefore, kinetic modeling seems to be a most logical procedure to improve the quality of treatment by providing elucidation and information on which to base clinical decisions. At present, our choice of the hemodialysis patient's treatment is quite arbitrary and is mainly based on the intuitive belief of the physician, who in the majority of renal units pays little attention to possible differences in individual patients. Most renal physicians would agree that the choice of hemodialysis regimens by intuition is far from satisfactory; yet, modeling is not widely accepted in renal units. Attempts to optimize hemodialysis therapy are as old as the treatment itself, whether they are called adequacy of hemodialysis or treatment individualization. Innovative studies from Seattle during the early 1970s hypothesized that uremic toxins might be "middle molecules"—metabolites with molecular weights between 300 to 2000 daltons. This induced indirect application of modeling concepts in different hemodialysis strategies [40]. These strategies involved studies of hemodialysis time, large surface hemodialyzers, and lowered hemodialysate flow rates. None of these approaches resulted in any significant elucidation of uremic toxicity or significant changes in long-term results. By using urea both as a market of protein catabolism and as an indicator of general metabolite production, Gotch et al [48] in the mid-1970s pioneered a further attempt at treatment individualization. It probably is not unfair to state that one of the main reasons for the slow acceptance of modeling is the limited understanding of the mathematics involved by many in the medical community. Some caution is justified, because a biologic system such as the human body is only incompletely represented by a physical model [45].

At present, a number of different approaches are used in the modeling of patient-hemodialyzer interaction. Urea and sodium are the most widely used markers to date. We will not outline the pros and cons of the different models, since most of them are still under clinical investigation [49]. The use of modeling for the individualization of treatment is now quite widespread and is increasing steadily [30, 50–52]. The advantages that can be concluded from a number of reported experiences are as follows:

1. It allows for adequacy of dialysis for the patient by prescribing the amount of therapy for each individual.
2. It decreases intradialytic morbidity.
3. It permits excellent nutritional counseling and monitoring.
4. It is extremely cost-effective and provides excellent quality control of the dialysis procedure in general.

Nutritional Aspects

For a long time, nutritional aspects of ESRD played a much more important role in the predialysis phase under conservative treatment than during the actual dialysis treatment phase. The importance of high caloric intake has never been denied in acute renal failure patients. The Diaphane Collaborative Study [11] from France, published in 1982, drew attention to the significant relationship between a poor nutritional state with insufficient protein intake and higher overall mortality. These data are based on a study of 1453 patients. The U.S. National Cooperative Dialysis Study also assessed study patients' nutritional status and stressed the importance of diet management, protein metabolism, and caloric intake [53]. A malignant combination, in the sense of morbidity and mortality in the dialysis population, is low protein intake and high blood urea nitrogen (BUN). We are glad that the dialysis community finally has accepted what has long been confirmed for the general population; that is, that low protein intake (1 g/kg/day) is one of the most dangerous limitations for life expectancy of our patients. One key problem that persists, even by using the most effective current hemodialyzer available, is the grossly inadequate removal of phosphate [54]. The only effective control of hyperphosphatemia in clinical routine remains the administration of aluminum-containing phosphate binders, which (in turn) can lead to long-term aluminum toxicity as manifested by the hemodialysis encephalopathy syndrome and by hemodialysis bone disease [55, 56].

Further optimization of nutritional management in renal replacement therapy will depend on greater phosphate removal during treatment, as neutral phosphate balance is required to avoid long-term complications in our patients.

Therapeutic Considerations

Dialysis used as renal replacement therapy is based on the assumption that sufficient elimination of various toxic or inhibiting substances is required for the adequate treatment of uremia [57, 58]. To date, there is still limited evidence to support this premise. Studies suggesting that the numerous side effects and complications of dialysis treatment are related (for example) to specific uremic toxins or to various other factors (such as bicarbonate, electrolyte disorders, biocompatibility, and depletion syndrome) have been largely inconclusive. To date, dialysis remains "unphysiologic" [59, 60]. The severe fluctuations in various ions and water may cause damage to the cells of the body that progresses with time of treatment. This continuous dysequilibration of the body cells induced by the machine, with a possible fatal effect on the self-regulation mechanism of our organism, was demonstrated by our group in 1970 [60].

Another explanation is offered by Bricker et al and his "trade-off hypothesis" [61]. This hypothesis assumes that high concentration of ions, phosphorus, and water may call for extreme levels of hormones designed to regulate these substances. These excessive hormones may have a detrimental effect for cells or cell membranes.

Our message is a warning against an oversimplification of certain clinical symptoms and their relationship to biochemistry and to biophysic or immunologic disturbances present in uremia before and during dialysis treatment. The following are typical examples.

Dialysis-induced Arterial Hypoxemia

The decreased arterial oxygen tension during hemodialysis treatment, together with the correction of metabolic acidosis, can cause impaired oxygen supply to tissues and organs. It may lead to hypotension, cardiac arrhythmia, acute myocardial infarction, and even sudden death in patients with cardiovascular lesions. There is no doubt that the pathophysiology is complex and multifactorial; and yet, investigations of bicarbonate dialysate, volumetric- or sodium-controlled ultrafiltration, or biocompatibility all claim to achieve the same results in decreasing these dangerous cardiovascular complications [62].

Bicarbonate Versus Acetate Hemodialysis

Studies comparing cardiovascular stability during acetate versus bicarbonate hemodialysis indicate that bicarbonate hemodialysis reduces the incidence of intradialytic cardiovascular episodes in the same manner as in isolated ultrafiltration or hemofiltration [15, 16, 20]. Considerable controversy exists regarding the pathophysiology of this phenomenon. The vasodilatory effect of acetate, its possible influence on myocardial contractibility as a positive inotropic effect, and autonomic dysfunction (as well as a vasoconstriction of the pulmonary vasculature) all have been considered to be responsible for cardiovascular episodes during hemodialysis [14, 17]. Also, the loss of carbon dioxide (CO_2) across the hemodialyzer membrane, causing hypocapnic hypoventilation by a decrease in the respiratory drive, has been blamed for the arterial hypoxemia in acetate dialysis [62].

Further controversy has been stirred by the findings that these hypotensive episodes during acetate hemodialysis could be avoided by keeping the serum osmolality rather high and stable during the treatment [30, 31, 51, 52]; for example, by use of high-sodium dialysate. To add to the confusion, hemofiltration (a convection-based therapy) has the well-known low incidence of intradialytic hypotension, despite the use of acetate as a buffer source and despite decreasing serum osmolality [24, 50]. In summary, if increased cardiac output can compensate in required magnitude for the change in peripheral resistance during acetate hemodialysis, it will not cause any clinical symptoms.

From a pragmatic point of view, taking into consideration the technically awkward and complex procedure of bicarbonate hemodialysis, acetate hemodialysis still accounts for the majority of the dialysis patient population. In our own experience, about 20% of present intermittent hemodialysis patients may be better treated with bicarbonate hemodialysis. This percentage increases with elderly and high-risk patients.

I am convinced that the availability of volumetric-controlled, high-flux hemodialysis or hemofiltration with on-line substitution, as well as Na$^+$-programmed hemodialysis, offers alternative solutions to the problem.

Another source for hemodialysis-induced arterial hypoxemia has been related to the biocompatibility of material used in the treatment and its interaction with blood and tissue.

Biocompatibility, Hypersensitive Reactions, First-use Syndrome

Early reports on a profound decrease in leukocyte count during hemodialysis were then considered to be a phenomenon of regular hemodialysis treatment without any clinical relevance [63]. The recent resurgence of interest in this material-related finding dates from the work of Craddock et al [64] on the relationships between leukopenia, complement system, pulmonary dysfunction, and arterial hypoxemia.

Since newer hemodialysis membranes have become available, it is possible to study differences between various membranes and different manufacturing processes. Despite the unavailability of a convincing study on the clinical implications of these findings, the biocompatibility of hemodialysis membranes has become an issue among the manufacturers of membranes for obvious commercial reasons.

According to the literature and our own results [65–68], cellulose membranes produce a more marked leukopenia and complement activation than their synthetic counterparts. The magnitude of changes is related to the manufacturing process, the surface area that comes in contact with the patient's blood, as well as the chemical derivative of the basic material. Without going into further detail, it should be stated that some of the long-term surviving patients have been exposed more than 3000 times to cellulosic membranes; and, consequently, to 3000 episodes of leukopenia and complement activation without any apparent clinical effect. This statement does not underestimate the problem of biocompatibility in extracorporeal treatment [69], but it calls for considerable caution in the interpretation of laboratory findings; especially since there are so many different synthetic substances involved in hemodialysis treatment.

Any of the substances listed in Figures 3 and 4, or a combination of them, could lead to the development of symptoms varying in severity from slight allergic reactions without clinical significance to life-threatening hypersensitivity syndrome with cardiovascular collapse.

The results of Tielemans et al [70] indicate that the use of different materials in hemodialysis can trigger different immune reactions that are not observed in conservatively treated patients. Interestingly, in 1981, the conclusion that immune reactions did not occur in patients undergoing peritoneal dialysis remained undisputed until recently, when peritoneal sclerosis was related to different materials used for peritoneal dialysis [38].

The complexity of the problem is demonstrated by additional evidence that residuals of ethylene oxide (the most widely used sterilization agent for hemodialyzers) in hemodialyzers or appropriate sets of tubing can be responsible for hemodialysis hypersensitivity reactions. Currently, ethylene oxide gas (ETO) has almost completely replaced formalin as a sterilizing agent. All of the earlier ascribed formalin-related sensations in patients at the onset of treatment seemed to be obsolete, since ETO sterilization is considered to be a safe process for hemodialysis disposables. However, with the ongoing discussion of biocompatibility in hemodialysis and the related allergic reactions, and even the hypersensitivity syndrome, a closer look at the literature since 1975 shows a different picture. Investigations have shown that the accused membrane may not even be the cause for these reactions, since it is deaerated and extracted considerably faster than (for example) the potted layer of the device, which is made of polyurethane [71].

As consequence, the careful preparation of the hemodialyzer before applying it to the patient must be stressed. It is well known in the hemodialysis

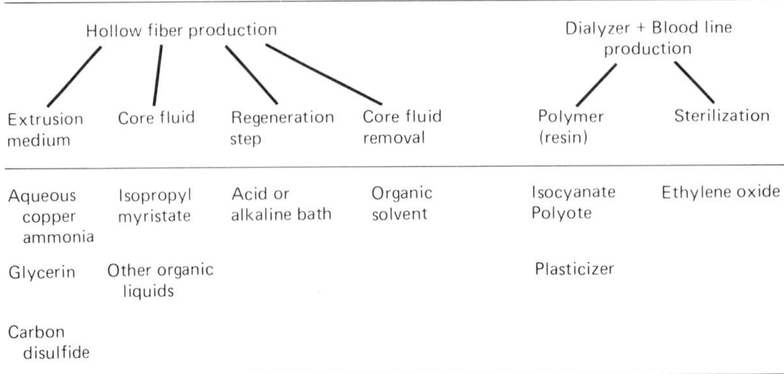

Fig. 3. (Toxic?) substances being used for production of cellulose hollow fiber dialyzers.

community that the use of a new brand of hemodialyzer can suddenly cause an anaphylactoid reaction. The reaction has also been reported with a fresh artificial kidney of the patient's usual brand of hemodialyzer [72, 73]. The term "first-use syndrome" has been introduced for these reactions [74]. Again, the clinical manifestations are numerous, and they range from light flushing of the skin to cardiopulmonary arrest—usually within the first 10 min of hemodialysis. The syndrome has been reported for all types of capillary and plate hemodialyzers made of cuprommonium cellulose, and to a lesser extent for cellulose acetate. The incidence rate has been estimated to be about 0.0035 to 0.06% of manufactured hemodialyzers, but it might be much higher because of the spontaneous recovery of most of the patients and the confusion with other hemodialysis-dependent complications [74, 75].

At present, the factors responsible for the first-use syndrome are unknown. Theoretically again, all of the substances listed in Figures 3 and 4 could be causative factors as well as complement activation, which may be well related to the syndrome.

It is our experience that the rinsing process of the hemodialyzer before

Dialysate	Heparin, Drugs, Infusion solutions (Substitute)	Reused dialyzer
Nitrate	Bacteria	Formaldehyde
Sulfate	and Pyrogens	Bacteria
Fluoride	Viruses	Pyrogens
Chloramines		Viruses
Heavy metals		
Bacteria and		
Pyrogens		

Fig. 4. (Toxic) substances being used for the hemodialysis procedure (hemofiltration).

its clinical use is important in preventing first-use reactions. In a new brand of hemodialyzer, we observed the first-use syndrome in 0.1% when rinsed with 1 liter of saline according to the manufacturer's instructions. The subsequent rinsing with 2 liters of saline eliminated first-use reactions with that brand of hemodialyzers.

Reused hemodialyzers obviously are more biocompatible than fresh cellulose-based artificial kidneys. The reused devices cause less leukopenia and complement activation, and no first-use reactions have been reported [76, 77]. The explanation favored mostly in the literature is that a protein layer covers the original membrane after the first use. While the protective coating may conceivably improve the biocompatibility, the beneficial effect may also be due to the extensive rinsing process in reused hemodialyzers.

There are many remaining open questions in the material-body interaction that cannot be covered in this chapter, but they might be as important as those reviewed: the still ongoing discussion about plasticizer migration from blood loss during hemodialysis, the role of trace elements, and the interleukin hypothesis—to mention a few of the possible sources of long-term complications.

There is an absence of clear evidence that any of the described complications is exclusively related to a single, specific origin (for example material, biocompatibility, dialysate composition, convective or diffusive process). We remain convinced that most of the hemodialysis-induced symptoms are of multifactorial origin. Quite a number of these so-called complications might be just the reaction of the human body to superimposed regulations by the machinery. We may even learn to accept them as a necessary pathophysiologic adjustment of the organism resulting from machine-patient interaction [60].

Summary

A review of the advantages and disadvantages of available methods of dialysis leads one to conclude that optimal treatment of chronic renal insufficiency is achieved by the greatest removal of toxins in the shortest possible time, which is compatible with vascular stability and physical and psychologic independence of the patient.

In our opinion, the following dialysis prescription comes closest: according to individual need, 3 to 5 hr of treatment three times weekly, with a biocompatible high-flux hemodialyzer operated on a volumetric-balanced control system, and preferably with bicarbonate dialysate of adjustable-dialysate Na^+ concentration. The development of dialysis is a prime example of the precept that personal relationships among scientific colleagues are strongly conducive to the growth and purpose of a professional discipline. This is especially important in extracorporeal technology, where progress much depends on cooperation between clinicians, engineers, and other natural scientists. Only 20 years ago, there were but 50 investigators worldwide who believed in hemodialysis as a major possibility to keep end-stage renal failure patients alive and well.

At present, we are treating more than 200,000 ESRD patients worldwide, and dialysis has proved to be more successful than even its most enthusiastic proponents had anticipated.

References

1. KOLFF WJ: *New Ways of Treating Uraemia.* London, J. & A. Churchill Ltd., 1947
2. SCHMITT E, KLINKMANN H: The epidemiological evaluation of active therapy of patients with renal failure, in *Economic and Medical Evaluation of Health Care Technologies, Part II: Dialysis,* edited by CULYER AJ, HORISBERGER B, Berlin, Heidelberg, New York, Tokyo, Springer-Verlag, 1983, pp 135–149
3. WING AJ, BROYER M, BRUNNER FP, BRYNGER H, BHALLAH S, DONCKER-WOKCKE RA, GRETZ N, JACOBS C, KRAMER P, SELWOOD NH: Combined report on regular dialysis and transplantation in Europe, XIII, 1982. *Proc Eur Dial Transplant Assoc (Europ Renal Assoc)* 20:5–75, 1983
4. KLINKMANN H, GURLAND H-J, WETZELS E, COLOMBI G: The role of controversies in the development of end-stage renal failure therapy, in *Controversies in the Treatment of Endstage Renal Failure,* edited by GURLAND J, WETZELS E, Basel, Karger, in press
5. BONOMINI V, VANGELISTA A, STEFONI S: Early dialysis in renal substitutive programs. *Kidney Int* 13:112–116, 1978
6. BONOMINI V, BALDRATI L, FELETTI C, STEFONI S, VANGELISTA A: Long-term early dialysis, in *Uremia—Pathobiology of Patients Treated for 10 Years or More,* edited by GIORDANO C, FRIEDMAN E, Milan, Wichtig, 1981, pp 133–137
7. KOPPLE JD, COBURN JW: Evaluation of chronic uremia: Importance of serum urea nitrogen, serum creatinine and their ratio. *JAMA* 227:41–44, 1974
8. ALVESTRAND A, AHLBERG M, BERGSTROM J: Retardation of the progression of renal insufficiency in patients treated with low-protein diets. *Kidney Int* 24(Suppl 16):S268–S272, 1983
9. MEYER TW, LAWRENCE WE, BRENNER BM: Dietary protein and the progression of renal disease. *Kidney Int* 24(Suppl 16):S243–S247, 1983
10. BONOMINI V, BALDRATI L, STEFONI S: Comparative cost/benefit analysis in early and late dialysis. *Nephron* 33:1–4, 1983
11. DEGOULET P, LEGRAIN M, REACH I, AIME F, DEVRIES C, ROJAS P, JACOBS C: Mortality risk factors in patients treated by chronic hemodialysis. Report of the Diaphane Collaborative Study. *Nephron* 31:103–110, 1982
12. LAURENT G, CALEMARD E, CHARRA B: Long dialysis: A review of fifteen years experience in one centre 1968–1983. *Proc Eur Dial Transplant Assoc (Europ Renal Assoc)* 20:122–135, 1983
13. MION CH, HEGSTROM RM, BOEN ST, SCRIBNER BH: Substitution of sodium acetate for bicarbonate in the bath fluid for hemodialysis. *Trans Am Soc Artif Intern Organs* 10:110–113, 1964
14. KESHAVIAH PR: The role of acetate in the etiology of symptomatic hypotension. *Artif Organs* 6:378–384, 1982
15. MEHTA BR, FISCHER D, AHMAD M, DUBOSE TD JR: Effects of acetate and bicarbonate hemodialysis on cardiac function in chronic dialysis patients. *Kidney Int* 24:782–787, 1983
16. WEHLE B, ASABA H, CASTENFORS J, GUNNARSON B, BERGSTROM J: Influence of dialysate composition on cardiovascular function in isovolemic hemodialysis. *Proc Eur Dial Transpl Assoc* 18:153–159, 1981
17. HAMPL H, PAEPRER H, UNGER V, FISHER V, RESA I, KEFSEL EM: Hemody-

namic changes during hemodialysis, sequential ultrafiltration and hemofiltration. *J Dialysis* 3:51–71, 1979

18. HAMPL H, MAHIOUT A, KESSEL M: Clinical effects in diabetic patients treated with acetate (HDA) and bicarbonate (HDB) dialysis. *Trans Am Soc Artific Intern Organs* (in press, 1984)

19. WEHLE B, ASABA H, CASTENFORS J, FURST P, GRAHN A, GUNNARSSON B, SHALDON S, BERGSTROM J: Hemodynamic changes during sequential ultrafiltration and dialysis. *Kidney Int* 15:411–418, 1979

20. SCHICK EC JR, IDELSON BA, LIANG C, REDLINE RC, BERNARD DB: Comparison of the hemodynamic response to hemodialysis with acetate or bicarbonate. *Trans Am Soc Artif Intern Organs* 29:25–28, 1983

21. QUELLHORST E, SCHUENEMANN B: Controlled study to compare hemodialysis and hemofiltration. Treatment in patients with chronic renal insufficiency. *NIH Report AK–1–8–2229–1* 1978

22. KOCH K, BALDAMUS C: Hemodialysis/hemofiltration: A comparison of medical, technical, and cost factors. *NIH Report AK–1–2227–F* 1981

23. HENDERSON LW, SAN FELEIPPO ML, STONEE RA: Comparison of hemodialysis and hemofiltration. *Proc 12th Annual Contractors' Conf Dept HEW, Publ. No NIH 81, 1979,* pp 112–115

24. SHALDON S, BEAU MC, DESCHOFT G, RAMPEREZ P, MION C: Vascular stability during hemofiltration. *Trans Am Soc Artif Intern Organs* 26:391–393, 1980

25. BALDAMUS CA, ERNST W, FASSBINDER W, KOCH KM, RAMPEREZ P, MION C: Differing hemodynamic stability due to differing sympathetic response. Comparison of ultrafiltration, hemodialysis and hemofiltration. *Proc Eur Dial Transpl Assoc* 17:205–218, 1980

26. KRAMER P, WIGGER W, RIEGER J, MATTHAEI D, SCHELER F: Arteriovenous haemofiltration, a new and simple method for treatment of over-hydrated patients resistant to diuretics. *Klin Wschr* 55:1121–1122, 1977

27. KAPLAN A, LONGNECKER RE, FOLKERT VW: Continuous arteriovenous hemofiltration—a report of six months' experience. *Ann Intern Med* 100:358–367, 1984

28. KRAMER P, KAUFHOLD G, GRONE HJ, WIGGER W, RIEGER J, MATTHAEI D, STOKKE T, BURCHARDI H, SCHELER F: Management of anuric intensive-care patients with arteriovenous hemofiltration. *Int J Art Org* 4:225–230, 1980

29. WIZEMANN V: Hemodiafiltration—an avenue to shorter dialysis? in *Contributions to Nephrology,* edited by WETZELS E, GUKLAND H, Basel Karger, in press

30. FUNCK-BRENTANO JL: Sodium-free water clearance in hemodialysis. *Artif Organs* 5:51–53, 1981

31. MAN NK, DI GIULIO S, ZINGRAFF J, SAUSSE A, FUNCK-BRENTANO JL: The role of sodium in the prevention of vascular instability during hemodialysis. *Proc Eur Dial Transpl Assoc* 18:255–265, 1981

32. OREN A, WU G, ANDERSON GH, MARLISS E, KHANNA R, PETITT J, MUPAS L, RODELLA H, BRANDES L, RONCARI DA, KAKIS G, HARRISON J, MCNEIL K, OREOPOULOS DG: Effective use of amino acid dialysate over four weeks in CAPD patients. *Trans Am Soc Artif Intern Organs* 29:604–609, 1983

33. POPOVICH RP, MONCRIEF JW, NOLPH KD, GHODS AJ, TWARDOWSKI ZJ, PYLE WK: Continuous ambulatory peritoneal dialysis. *Ann Intern Med* 88:449–456, 1978

34. OREOPOULOS DG, ROBSON M, IZATT A, CLAYTON S, DEVEBER GA: A simple and safe technique for continuous ambulatory peritoneal dialysis (CAPD). *Trans Am Soc Artif Intern Organs* 24:484–489, 1978

35. NOLPH KD, SORKIN M, RUBIN J, ARFANIA D, PROWANT B, FRUJO L, KENNEDY D: Continuous ambulatory peritoneal dialysis: Three years experience in one center. *Ann Intern Med* 92:609–613, 1980

36. OREOPOULOS DG, KHANNA R, WILLIAMS P, VAS SI: Continuous ambulatory peritoneal dialysis—1981 (*editorial*). *Nephron* 30:293–303, 1982
37. LEGRAIN M, ROTTEMBOURG J, BENTSCHIKAOU A, POIGNET JL, ISSAD B, BARTHELEMY A, STRIPPOLI P, GAHL GM, GROC FDE: Dialysis treatment of insulin dependent diabetic patients: ten years experience. *Clin Nephrol* 21:72–81, 1984
38. SLINGENEYER A, MION C, MONRAD C, CANAUD B, FALIER B, BERAUD JJ: Progressive sclerosing peritoneal dialysis. *Trans Am Soc Artif Intern Organs,* vol 29, in press, 1983
39. CAMBI V, GARINI G, SAVAZZI G, ARISI L, DAVID S, ZANELLI P, BONO F, GARDINI F: Short dialysis. *Proc Eur Dial Transplant Assoc (Europ Renal Assoc)* 20:111–121, 1983
40. BABB AL, STRAND JM, UVELLI DA, MILUTINOVIC J, SCRIBNER BH: Quantitative description of dialysis treatment: A dialysis index. *Kidney Int* 7(Suppl 2): S-23–S-29, 1975
41. FALKENHAGEN D: Kinetic modelling in artificial organs, in *Proc Int Symp Kinetic Modelling in Artificial Organs, Rostock-Warnemunde, 1982,* edited by KLINKMANN H, AHRENHOLZ P, BIESTER F-D, COURTNEY JM, FALKENHAGEN D, GAYLOR JD, Rostock, Int Soc Artif Organs, 1983, pp. 17–25
42. FARRELL PC: Kinetic modelling in extracorporeal treatment, in *Proc Int Symp Kinetic Modelling in Artificial Organs, Rostock-Warnemunde, 1982,* edited by KLINKMANN H, AHRENHOLZ P, BIESTER F-D, COURTNEY JM, FALKENHAGEN D, GAYLOR JD, Rostock, Int Soc Artif Organs, 1983, pp. 26–35
43. TESCHAN PE, GINN HE, BOURNE JR, WARD JW: Assessing adequacy of dialysis. *Artif Organs* 5(Suppl):65–67, 1981
44. LOWRIE EG, LAIRD NM, PARKER TF, SARGENT JA: Effect of hemodialysis prescription on patient morbidity. *N Engl J Med* 305:1176–1181, 1981
45. SARGENT JA, GOTCH FA: Principles and biophysics of dialysis, in *Replacement of Renal Function by Dialysis,* edited by DRUKKER W, PARSONS FM, MAHER IF, The Hague, Martinus Nijhoff Medical Division, 1978, pp 38–68
46. ROY T, STILLER S, AHRENHOLZ P, FALKENHAGEN D, MANN H, KLINKMANN H: Individual optimization of sodium and water removal during hemodialysis by means of a mathematical model, in *Proc Int Symp Kinetic Modelling in Artificial Organs, Rostock-Warnemunde, 1982,* edited by KLINKMANN H, AHRENHOLZ P, BIESTER F-D, COURTNEY JM, FALKENHAGEN D, GAYLOR JD, Rostock, Int Soc Artif Organs, 1983, pp 107–112
47. LOPOT F, VALEK A: A trial to define an optimal dialysis strategy, in *Proc Int Symp Kinetic Modelling in Artificial Organs, Rostock-Warnemunde, 1982,* edited by KLINKMANN H, AHRENHOLZ P, BIESTER F-D, COURTNEY JM, FALKENHAGEN D, GAYLOR JD, Rostock, Int Soc Artif Organs, 1983, pp 132–136
48. GOTCH F, SARGENT J, KEEN M, LAM J, PROWITT M: *The solute kinetics of intermittent dialysis therapy.* Annual Report, Artificial Kidney-Chronic Uremia Program, NIAMDD. National Institutes of Health, 1979
49. SHAPIRO JI, ARGY WP, RAKOWSKI TA, CHESTER A, SIEMSEN AS, SVHREINER GE: The unsuitability of BUN as a criterion for prescription dialysis. *Trans Am Soc Artif Intern Organs* 29:129–134, 1983
50. SHALDON S, BALDAMUS CA, BEAU MC, KOCH KM, MION CM, LYSAGHT MJ: Acute and chronic studies of the relationship between sodium flux in hemodialysis and hemofiltration. *Trans Am Soc Artif Intern Organs* 29:641–644, 1983
51. MURISASCO A, FRANCE G, LEBLOND G, STROUMZA P, DURAND D, REYNIER JP, CREVAT A, ELSEN R: Separation of Na^+ and H_2O transport during hemodialysis and quantification of high-low NA_{Di} levels during sequential sodium therapy. *Trans Am Soc Artif Intern Organs* 29:645–648, 1983

52. KLINKMANN H, HERRERA-VALDEZ R, HOLTZ M, SCHMIDT R: Experimentelle Untersuchungen zur Therapie hypotoner Kreislaufragulationsstorungen während der sequentiellen Ultrafiltration-Hämodialyse. *Z Ges Inn Med* 35:442–446, 1980

53. SCHOENFELD PY, HENRY RR, LAIRD NM, ROXE DM: Assessment of nutritional status of the National Cooperative Dialysis Study population. *Kidney Int* 23(Suppl 13):S80–S88, 1983

54. MASSRY SG, COBURN JW, PEACOCK M, KLEEMAN CR: Turnover of endogenous parathyroid hormone in uremic patients and those undergoing hemodialysis. *Trans Am Soc Artif Intern Organs* 18:416–422, 1972

55. SIDEMAN S, MANOR D: The dialysis dementia syndrome and aluminum intoxication. *Nephron* 31:1–10, 1982

56. BOURNERIAS F, MONNIER N, REVEILLAUD RJ: Risk of orally administered aluminum hydroxide and results of withdrawal. *Proc Eur Dial Transpl Assoc (Europ Renal Assoc)* 20:207–212, 1983

57. SCHREINER GE: The search for the uremic toxin(s). *Kidney Int* 7(Suppl 2):S270–S271, 1975

58. BERGSTROM J, GORDON A, FURST P, RYHAGE R: *A study of uremic toxicology.* Proceedings 7th Annual Contractors' Conference, Artificial Kidney-Chronic Uremia Program, NIAMDD, Bethesda, Maryland, 1974, pp 17–18

59. KJELLSTRAND CM, EVANS RL, PETERSEN RJ, SHIDEMAN JR, HARTITZSCH BV, BUSELMEIER TJL: The "unphysiology" of dialysis: A major cause of dialysis side effects? *Kidney Int* 7(Suppl 2):S30–S34, 1975

60. KLINKMANN H: The dysequilibrium syndrome in experimental hemodialysis. *Trans Am Soc Artif Int Organs* 16:523–533, 1970

61. BRICKER NS, BOURGOIGNIE J, WEBER H, SCHMIDT RW, SLATOPOLSKY E: Pathogenesis of the uremic state: A new perspective, in *Advances in Nephrology* (vol 2), edited by HAMBURGER J, CROSNIER J, MAXWELL MH, Chicago, Year Book Medical Publishers, 1972, chap 13, pp 263–276

62. KNUDSEN F, NIELSEN AH: Haemodialysis-induced arterial hypoxaemia. *Danish Med Bull* 31:154–157, 1984

63. KAPLOW LS, GOFFINET JA: Profound neutropenia during the early phase of hemodialysis. *JAMA* 203:1135–1137, 1968

64. CRADDOCK PR, FEHR J, DALMASSO AP, BRIGHAM KL, JACOB HS: Hemodialysis leukopenia: Pulmonary vascular leukostasis resulting from complement activation by dialyzer cellophane membranes. *J Clin Invest* 59:879–888, 1977

65. CHENOWETH DE, CHEUNG AK, HENDERSON LW: Anaphylatoxin formation during hemodialysis: Effects of different dialyzer membranes. *Kidney Int* 24:764–769, 1983

66. HOENICH NA, JOHNSTON SRF, WOFFINDIN C, KERR DNS: Haemodialysis leucopenia: The role of membrane type and re-use, in *Risk Profiles in Clinical Nephrology,* edited by BUCCIANTI G, Basel, Munchen, Paris, London, New York, Tokyo, Sydney, Karger, 1984, pp 120–128 (Contr Nephrol 37)

67. IVANOVICH P, CHENOWETH DE, SCHMIDT R, KLINKMANN H, BOXER LA, JACOB HS, HAMMERSCHMIDT DE: Symptoms and activation of granulocytes and complement with two dialysis membranes. *Kidney Int* 24:758–763, 1983

68. HAKIM RM, LOWRIE EG: Hemodialysis-associated neutropenia and hypoxemia: The effect of dialyzer membrane materials. *Nephron* 32:32–39, 1982

69. KLINKMANN H, WOLF H, SCHMITT E: Definition of biocompatibility, in *Risk Profiles in Clinical Nephrology,* edited by BUCCIANTI G, Basel, Munchen, Paris, London, New York, Tokyo, Sydney, Karger, 1984, pp 70–77

70. TIELEMANS C, BRENEZ D, DRATWA M: Eosinophilia in patients undergoing dialysis (*letter to the editor*). *Br Med J* 283:727–728, 1981

71. HENNE W, DIETRICH W, PELGER M, VON SENGBUSCH G: Residuals of ethylene oxide in hollow fiber dialyzers, in *Symposium on Hypersensitivity in Hemodialysis,* edited by WALTHEN RJ, KLEIN E, Louisville, Kentucky July 21–22, 1983

72. NICHOLLS AJ, PLATTS MM: Anaphylactoid reactions due to hemodialysis, hemofiltration, or membrane plasma separator. *Br Med J* 285:1607–1609, 1982

73. POPLI S, ING TS, DAUGIRDAS JT, KHEIRBEK AO, VIOL GW, VILBAR RM, GANDHI VC: Severe reactions to cuprophan capillary dialyzers. *Artif Organs* 6:312–315, 1982

74. ING TS, DAUGIRDAS JT, POPLE S, GANDHI VC: First-use syndrome with cuprammonium cellulose dialyzers. *Int J Artif Organs* 6:235–239, 1983

75. VILLARROEL F: Incidence of hypersensitivity in hemodialysis, in *Symposium on Hypersensitivity in Hemodialysis,* edited by WALTHEN RL, KLEIN E, Louisville, Kentucky July 21–22, 1983

76. HAKIM RM, LOWRIE EG: Effect of dialyzer reuse on leukopenia, hypoxemia and total hemolytic complement system. *Trans Am Soc Artif Intern Organs* 26:159–164, 1980

77. KANT KS, POLLAK VE, CATHEY M, GOETZ D, BERLIN R: Multiple use of dialyzers: Safety and efficacy. *Kidney Int* 19:728–738, 1981

Vascular Access for Hemodialysis

Chairpersons: Fred L. Shapiro and Robert Uldall
Discussants: Robert C. Anderson, Allan J. Collins, Howard Silberman,
Raymond Vanholder, and Alex Heaton

This Workshop started with a discussion of temporary access methods. It
began with the premise that subclavian cannulation with an indwelling catheter can be left in place for a few days or weeks, or even months, and that
it is now the preferred method for temporary vascular access in most parts
of the world. Two problems still give cause for concern: (1) patients are
still being injured during the use of this technique, and a number of deaths
have occurred; (2) single-lumen catheters, presently the most common type,
are best used with single-needle machines. Regrettably there is still widespread
ignorance about the principles underlying the use of single-needle machines.
Consequently subclavian dialysis may be less efficient than should be the
case.

Complications from Subclavian Cannulation

Vanholder discussed the isolated reports of serious or even fatal complications
from the use of subclavian cannulation for hemodialysis that have raised
questions about the safety of this technique. In view of the rising controversy
the following questions were considered: (1) What is the actual frequency
of fatal or potentially fatal complications? (2) What types of complications
occur most frequently? (3) What are the best ways to prevent complications
now and in the future?

An attempt was made to answer these questions from three series of data:
a personal experience with 386 patients at the University Hospital in Ghent,
a review of the literature including 10 published series (1,213 patients) and
an inquiry performed among Belgian nephrologists (2,000 patients). The
mortality in these three groups appeared to be 0 to 3 per thousand patients.
Of 12 fatal cases known to him, 8 were traumatic (hemothorax, hemoperi-

---

This is the summary of a Workshop by the same title.

cardium, pneumothorax) and occurred early after insertion of the catheter, whereas four were nontraumatic (septicemia, air embolism from a laceration in the catheter wall, bleeding) and these occurred later during the insertion episode. The incidence of early traumatic but nonfatal complications is estimated to be 1.0 to 1.4%. The incidence of late nontraumatic complications is higher, 1.9 to 7.25%, depending on the source.

Primary prevention of early traumatic complications depends on careful insertion by a skilled operator. In our unit a six-month experience of critical care medicine is required before a doctor is allowed to insert catheters in hemodialysis patients. A modified Seldinger technique is used and a chest X-ray to check the position of the radio-opaque catheter.

In patients who are at special risk by virtue of respiratory distress, pulmonary edema, or coagulation disorders, the femoral or internal jugular veins may be preferred. Some recent reports advocate the long-term use of surgically inserted Hickman or modified Tenckhoff catheters for patients with persistent access problems. Catheters with nonrigid tips are clearly desirable for the prevention of perforating injuries.

Late, nontraumatic complications, such as thrombosis and infection are rarely fatal but they may prolong hospitalization and every effort should be made to prevent them. Recent reports suggest that partial or total venous thromboses are more frequent than originally supposed. Clinical manifestations such as swelling of the limb and pulmonary edema are, however, surprisingly rare. Furthermore it may be that with the introduction of newer polymers in the manufacture of catheters that thrombotic complication will become less frequent. Infections, though relatively frequent, rarely give rise to fatalities and can easily be treated by catheter withdrawal and/or antibiotics. After withdrawal of a catheter, the tip should always be cultured. Special antiseptic and aseptic care should be given to immunosuppressed patients and patients on plasmapheresis.

In conclusion, subclavian catheter dialysis is not devoid of complications but deaths should be preventable and other complications should be reduced if the pitfalls are kept in mind by those making use of this technique.

The main guidelines to be used in the prevention of fatal or serious complications are as follows: (1) Catheters should be inserted only by carefully trained medical personnel. (2) All subclavian catheters in the future should have flexible or floppy tips, which are not capable of damaging vein walls even if they are misused. (3) Catheters should never be pushed back in without the use of a guide-wire if they are seen to be slipping out. (4) Catheters should be fabricated from high quality materials so that they do not split or break to allow hemorrhage or air embolus. They should also have high quality Luer-lock connections to prevent accidental disconnection of injection caps and infusion lines. Clamps on the catheters in the intervals between dialysis are an additional safeguard. (5) Hemodialysis with heparin should be avoided for at least 24 hours after accidental puncture of a subclavian artery. (6) Subclavian cannulation should not be attempted in acutely ill patients with pulmonary edema. Femoral cannulation is a safer alternative until the patient's condition has stabilized. (7) Meticulous aseptic and antiseptic techniques should be used by all medical and nursing staff to prevent infection.

Technology of Single-Needle Dialysis Using Subclavian Access

Heaton emphasized that cannulation of the subclavian vein provides rapid access to the circulation for temporary hemodialysis; the convenience and success of this route of access explain the rapid growth in its use. Dialysis can be accomplished either by a mechanical system using tidal blood flow or by the use of a double-lumen catheter with conventional continuous blood flow. Mechanical systems use either a single pump with clamps, or two occlusive peristaltic pumps, and the pumps may be triggered by time or pressure changes. Double pump systems can achieve better blood flow, less recirculation, and improved control of ultrafiltration as compared to single pump systems. A double pump system (Bellco BL760) has been used successfully for several years in Newcastle and it is now used routinely in over 75% of the home and hospital hemodialysis population.

The successful clinical application of any single-needle system depends on obtaining an efficient dialysis and maintaining patient safety. Adequate clearance of small molecules depends upon the mean blood flow through the dialyser. With single-needle dialysis blood flow is intermittent and the system must be able to accelerate blood rapidly through the extracorporeal circuit in order to achieve an acceptable mean of 200 ml/min. One should not be afraid to generate high pressures in order to achieve these flow rates. Good studies have shown that hemolysis is not a cause for concern. With an adequate blood flow the influence of recirculation only becomes clinically important above 10% with short dialysis schedules. Studies have shown no difference in the clearance of urea or creatinine between single and double-needle systems under conditions of equal flow; and blood flows of 200 ml/min can be achieved with the double pump system. The control of ultrafiltration during dialysis is achieved by controlling transmembrane pressure. In the occlusive double pump system the dialyser is isolated by the two pumps and blood flow can be adjusted independently of outlet pressure. Thus accurate ultrafiltration control is possible and this allows the use of high permeability membranes, hemofiltration, or sequential ultrafiltration, all without special equipment.

Some recirculation (arterial venous mixing) is inherent in all single-needle systems and depends upon a number of factors. Recirculation is increased when blood flow through the site of vascular access is poor and for subclavian lines this may occur when dialysing ill patients with poor cardiac output. In such patients, using the double pump system, recirculation is found. In the double pump system recirculation can be minimized by optimizing stroke volume (to 40 ml) and this is achieved when using noncompliant (hollow fiber) dialyzers by introducing an arterial expansion chamber. Catheter deadspace has only a minor effect in increasing recirculation.

The safety of double pump systems depends upon the control of blood flow by venous pump counting and by efficient air detection and monitoring of the venous return. Mechanical hemolysis is not a significant problem and splitting of the pump inserts has occurred rarely.

Safe effective dialysis in almost all patients can therefore be performed via a subclavian route using the single-needle system. In Newcastle they have also maintained a number of patients on long-term hemodialysis using a permanent in-dwelling superior vena caval catheter and they remain well dialysed without any change in treatment schedule.

It may be that double-lumen catheters may take over gradually from and obviate the need for single-needle systems, once these devices have been perfected and once it has been shown that the complication rate with double-lumen catheters is no higher than that with single-lumen catheters.

Shapiro next introduced the topic of permanent access methods. He stated that vascular access for regular hemodialysis remains a major concern of patients, nephrologists and vascular surgeons. After 24 years of experience, there is consensus that the simple arteriovenous fistula as described by Brescia and Cimino in 1966 is the most proven form of blood access and is the standard for comparison to other techniques of angio-access.

As the dialysis population increased in the proportion of patients who are aged or have other serious medical complicating diseases, the problems associated with establishing and maintaining usable simple arterio-venous (A-V) fistulas as blood access have also increased. Simple fistulas may not be able to be established initially because of problems with the native vessels and failure of the vein to enlarge even after prolonged intervals between creation and attempt to use. The simple fistula may become unusable for effective angio-access due to the development of poor blood flow secondary to stenosis within the vein with ultimate clotting or, rarely, infection of the vessel. Internal fistulas require the use of needles to access the blood and this may limit the frequency of use, as well as causing significant discomfort to the patient. This minimizes the potential for daily hemodialysis therapy.

Numerous innovative approaches have occurred over the years utilizing grafts of various materials and devices as substitute for angio-access. Angio-access has been created in many locations in the body including the arms, legs, subclavian area, across the chest, and the epigastric, iliac and cervical vessels. None of these other techniques have yielded better technical results than the simple A-V fistula, but some now approach the longevity of the simple A-V fistula. Other techniques offer other advantages not provided by the simple fistula, but do not have the longevity and may have more morbidity associated with their use.

The Workshop emphasized secondary access procedures that are applicable when a simple A-V fistula cannot be established, does not develop successfully, or fails. Problems encountered with secondary access procedures were stressed.

Conduit Grafts

When a simple A-V fistula cannot be established or fails, the most commonly employed technique is to utilize a vascular prosthesis. The most commonly utilized grafts are either bovine carotid arteries or some form of PTFE. Generally, the results obtained with either of these materials are quite comparable, as there appears to be no significant difference between the two relative to early and late patency, rate of infection, or the incidence of thrombosis. The University of Southern California compared 29 PTFE and 20 bovine grafts and found that 60.7% of the PTFE and 36.8% of the bovine grafts survived at the end of their study, 4 to 20 months post-implant. The Hennepin County Medical Center (HCMC) results utilizing bovine grafts were as follows: 185 patients had a one-year survival of 84%, a two-year survival of 73%, and a three-year survival of 69%. These latter results compare favorably to results reported for the A-V fistula.

The California group suggests that PTFE grafts may be more amenable to revision, are easier for the surgeon to handle and tailor to the specific requirements of the native vessels, and may be less prone to kink. The upper extremity is the preferred site of implantation as the procedure can generally be performed with local anesthesia and there are fewer complications with less morbidity. Although the California group prefers to use a straight forearm implant, the question remains as to whether or not looped grafts may have better survival. The HCMC group prefers the looped graft.

Several complications may occur with conduit grafts. Most complications are related to infection, venous stenosis with excessive bleeding, low flow, clotting and aneurysm formation, and, occasionally, excessive flow through the conduit leading to high output cardiac failure or distal ischemia.

Sepsis is one of the most serious problems that can develop with a conduit graft. It is usually manifested by redness along the graft, abscess formation, purulent drainage from a needle "stick" or a skin exit site, bleeding, and occasionally systemic symptoms. The earlier this problem is detected, the more likely it may be successfully treated. Initial treatment is appropriate antibiotics. Occasionally local surgical drainage or debridement is necessary. If this is not successful, the surgical removal or tying off of the graft is required.

An important aspect of removal of the conduit type of vascular access is to minimize the problem of sepsis at the arterial anastomosis. The HCMC group recommends removal of a segment from the arterial side of the graft, hopefully in an area without sepsis, while treating with large doses of antibiotics. This is done with the hope that some healing will occur between the divided graft in order to prevent contamination of the then isolated arterial section at the time of removal of the infected area. Fortunately, the venous side may usually be simply ligated. The segment removed to isolate the infected area is cultured in order to know if an arterial reconstruction or ligation may be needed. Occasionally if the infectious process is localized, the problem area may be totally excised, leaving the major portion of the conduit in place (tied off) to allow for later reconstruction, if possible.

The problems of bleeding "coming off" of dialysis, recirculation, clotting, low flow, and aneurysm formation are generally all related to venous obstruction. This obstruction is most frequently found just beyond the "venous" anastomosis. This high resistance and decrease in flow can be diagnosed by the presence of a pulse in the fistula where one would expect a bruit, or by a typical doppler signal of intermittent flow over the conduit or a high-pitched "jet" sound directly over the stenosis. An angio x-ray of the fistula can be of major assistance in repairing this problem. An x-ray post-declotting is of no use. Usually in the case of strictures the problem may be corrected by dilating the area, removal of the obstructing material, or a patch or jump graft.

In the case of aneurysms, if they are false aneurysms simple excision with repair of the defect is usually adequate. If the aneurysm is of the long fusiform variety, generally the stenosis is repaired downstream and nothing is done with the aneurysm itself. However, if that aneurysm is quite big, it may be excised and the flow to it is either ligated or a bypass graft is created. Better long-term results will be obtained if the bypass graft can return flow to the same vessel just above the stricture, as that vessel has already been modified to high flow and has a lesser likelihood of restenosing.

The problem of excessive flow manifested by heart failure and/or steal may usually be successfully managed by narrowing the "arterial" end of the conduit. The doppler may be useful to the surgeon in dealing with these types of problems. The lumen frequently must be reduced to a diameter one-fourth the size or less of the original diameter of the vessel in these situations.

Frequent surgical procedures usually lead to sepsis. Too early declotting may result in reclotting. The HCMC group prefers to wait 24 to 48 hours after a clotting episode to declot a graft. This allows time to correct some of the problems that may have led to the clotting. Also, the clot seems to hold together better and is easier to remove after a period of time.

Transcutaneous Vascular Access Devices

In 1980, two transcutaneous access devices for hemodialysis were introduced: the bioCarbon® vascular access system (American Bentley Company, CA) and the Hemasite™ vascular access device (Renal Systems, Inc., MN). These devices use PTFE grafts to create the arteriovenous fistula with a perpendicular metal transcutaneous part which is used to access the blood flow through the graft. The bioCarbon device uses a moveable plug to access the blood stream and the Hemasite a puncturable silicon septum.

Data for analysis were obtained from previous publications or provided by the individual companies. Data were available on 174 bioCarbon devices and 611 Hemasites.

Devices have been placed in the forearm, upper arm, thigh and subclavian position. There are few data comparing the placement sites, but the majority of the devices have been placed in the upper arm with each company indicating this to be the preferred location.

The overall survival at 24 months is 35% for the Hemasites and 24% for the bioCarbon devices. This difference may not be statistically significant. The HCMC cumulative survival experience with upper arm placement of 33 grafted Hemasites is 88% at one year and 68% at two years.

Equal percentages of the bioCarbon devices have been lost to infection and thrombosis. However, 23% of the Hemasite failures are related to infection compared to 12% of failures related to thrombosis. Outpatient declotting procedures have been performed through the transcutaneous part of the devices.

Survival results of these devices are less than published multicenter survival for bovine and PTFE grafts. With this information, the transcutaneous devices appear to have applications as a secondary access for some patients, but mostly as a tertiary access after failure of bovine and PTFE grafts. These devices also appear to be best suited to upper arm placement. Therefore, it would probably be most expedient to use forearm vessels first for simple fistulas, bovine, and PTFE grafts. After the forearm locations have been used, the upper arm placement of the transcutaneous devices would be an appropriate consideration.

Patient acceptance of these devices has been high related to the elimination of skin needle puncture. Some patients have received these devices over bovine and PTFE grafts due to excess anxiety related to skin needle puncture. In this setting, the patients' acceptance has been very high.

Further work is needed to define the most appropriate factors for patient selection for these devices. Infectious complications and their treatment need more careful study to develop recommendations for antibiotic selection and duration of treatment. The HCMC group, which had the best Hemasite survival and lowest failure rate from infections, treats their patients' infections with high-dose, specific antibiotics for a minimum of four weeks. Guidelines as to when to remove devices also need to be developed.

Overall, experience with transcutaneous devices suggests that they have an application as a blood access. With further work by investigators and manufacturers, these devices may offer broader applications in the area of hemodialysis blood access.

In summary, there are numerous factors that may influence blood access survival in a given patient. These include site selection, surgical technique, host factors, and needle puncture difficulties.

Factors to consider in access site selection include ease of use, depth of the vessels, and anatomy of the vessels. Previous vessel damage or scarring, multiple small run-off vessels, upper or lower extremity with normal rotation of the extremity and, thereby, the access, and propensity for external compression are some of the considerations that the prudent surgeon should make. Surgical technique aspects include experience of the surgeon, kinking or rotating the graft, too sharp a hairpin looped graft and avoiding incisions directly over the graft because they are more prone to early infection.

Several host factors may influence access survival. High venous pressure from venous stenosis and intimal reactions, increased venous pressure secondary to cardiac problems, and raising an intimal flap with the needle are possibilities. Conditions that decrease the blood throughout such as dehydration, hypertension, or impaired cardiac output states may predispose to clotting. Increased susceptibility to infection may emanate from immunologic incompetence or multiple access surgical procedures. Appropriate antibiotics in adequate doses and duration are important therapeutic considerations. The impact of the patient's personal hygiene is unclear on graft survival; however, with transcutaneous devices, hygiene is probably important. Hypercoagulable states may develop spontaneously and often occur in the postoperative period. Fragile skin with easy bruisability may be prone to infection and/or ulceration, which may lead to graft loss.

The trauma of needle punctures is more likely to impact on graft survival early in the use of the graft. Early use of the graft may predispose to later vessel scarring or hematoma formation and dissection along the tract of the graft, which may later develop into a false aneurysm.

Adequate preoperative planning, good surgical technique, and aggressive management of access complications, including the surgical placement of bypass grafts around diseased areas, may yield gratifying long-term results.

Anatomic and Physiologic Aspects of Peritoneal Dialysis

Karl D. Nolph

Peritoneal Anatomy and Membrane Resistances

Table 1 summarizes possible anatomic factors that contribute to membrane resistance during peritoneal dialysis. The importance of each of these resistance sites to the transport of solutes of differing molecular weight is unknown [1–3].

Endothelial and mesothelial resistances may relate to intercellular gap dimensions, particularly for solutes confined to the extracellular fluid space [4–15]. Intercellular gap width may differ in parietal and visceral peritoneum [12–15]. Lipid-soluble substances might move through lipid layers on cell surfaces [16]. If small solutes and water move transcellularly during peritoneal dialysis, then membrane resistance also could be effected by cell membrane permeability and cytoplasmic permeability. Numerous vesicles have been identified in endothelial and mesothelial cells in some species [14, 15]. The number and mobility of vesicles might have an impact on solute transport. Cell surface charges and intercellular-charged molecules could effect the transport of ionized or polarized solutes [3].

The permeability of, and charges within, capillary basement membranes may also contribute to the total resistance of the vascular wall.

The interstitium presumably is composed of aqueous tortuous channels separated by collagen and mucopolysaccharides. The resistance of interstitium may be influenced by the tortuosity, length, and width of the aqueous channels [17–20]. Polar molecules within the interstitial matrix may influence the movement of charged solutes.

Although the mesothelium is similar to the endothelium, in being a cell layer of resistance, surfaces of mesothelial cells have numerous microvilli projecting into the peritoneal dialysis solution [21–23]. The density and func-

This manuscript was presented as part of a Symposium on *Continuous Ambulatory Peritoneal Dialysis.*

Table 1. Possible anatomic factors contributing to membrane resistance

Capillary blood fluid films
Endothelium
    Intercellular gap dimensions, cell membrane permeability, cytoplasmic permeability; vesicle
        number and mobility, surface, and intracellular charges
Capillary basement membrane
    Permeability, charges
Interstitium
    Tortuosity, length, width of aqueous channels, charged molecules (collagen, mucopolysaccha-
        rides)
Mesothelium
    Same as endothelium plus microvilli density and function
Peritoneal cavity fluid films
    Channel width, mixing with peristalsis and body motion

tion of microvilli may influence the total effective surface area (if cell surface is important), thus altering dimensions and/or composition of fluid films adjacent to the mesothelial surface.

Fluid films within the peritoneal cavity most likely contribute to total resistance in a major way [24, 25]. Wide pools of fluid between adjacent folds of mesentery and poor mixing of that fluid must, in part, explain low clearances of small solutes during rapid-cycling peritoneal dialysis.

Figure 1 summarizes the anatomic resistances of the peritoneal dialysis system in diagrammatic fashion. Paths of solute movement across the peritoneal cellular layers are shown as occurring through multiple pathways (intercellular, transcellular, and vesicular). Additional work is necessary to determine the relative importance of these types of passive transport in all sites of the human peritoneum.

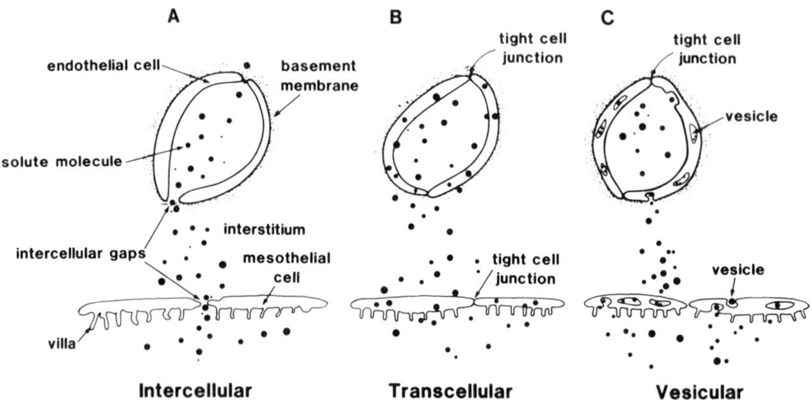

Fig. 1. Anatomic resistances and possible solute transport pathways during peritoneal dialysis are summarized. (Published with permission from [3])

Indexes of Solute Transport

Solute transport during peritoneal dialysis usually is quantitated as mass transfer, clearance, or as a mass transfer area coefficient [26–33].

Mass transfer is the net removal of solute per unit time. Since mass transfer, at any moment, is a function of the concentration gradient between peritoneal capillary blood and peritoneal dialysis fluid, mass transfer decreases exponentially as concentration equilibrium is approached. Thus, mass transfer per min represents an average value over the total time period measured. For a given peritoneal dialysis cycle, the net removal of the solute can be calculated as the difference between the amount removed in drainage (that is, drainage volume × drainage concentration) minus the amount instilled (that is, instillation volume × instillation fluid concentration). This net removal occurs from the time of initiation of instillation to the completion of drainage. Dividing the net removal by the total cycle time gives an average mass transfer per min.

Serum clearance represents the mass transfer rate divided by the solute concentration in serum during the cycle. During peritoneal dialysis, serum concentrations change slowly. If serum concentrations do change from the beginning to the end of the cycle, an average value can be used for the calculation. Clearance rates also decrease exponentially during a peritoneal dialysis cycle, and they approach 0 at concentration equilibrium. Clearance values usually are expressed as ml/min and represent average rates per cycle.

Calculations of the mass transfer area coefficient are much more complex and will not be reviewed here. The calculations reported in the literature differ, and all are based on some simplifying assumptions. This index of transport approximates the maximum clearance rate possible if an infinite concentration gradient (dialysis solution concentration, 0) could be maintained. Some calculations of the mass transfer area coefficient do not include solute transport secondary to convection; they focus only on the maximum clearance possible by diffusion [32]. The mass transfer area coefficient thus expressed is determined by membrane area and permeability.

Dedrick has recently stressed the importance of recognizing that solute movement during peritoneal dialysis occurs through complex tissue layers [34]. Classic thermodynamic analyses that are applicable to synthetic membrane systems in extracorporeal dialyzers may not accurately predict transport events in a complex biologic membrane.

Table 2 summarizes factors that influence each of these indices of solute transport. Mass transfer is affected by the blood or serum concentration of the solute, whereas clearance and the mass transfer area coefficient are independent of the serum concentration.

Evidence has been reviewed previously to support the contention that mass transfer rates and solute clearances are not subject to a major peritoneal capillary blood flow limitation [1, 35]. Clearances of hydrogen (H) and carbon dioxide (CO_2) gases usually are two to three times the maximum urea clearances with rapid cycling. If urea clearances were blood-flow limited, then gas clearances also should be blood-flow limited and approach clearances

Table 2. Factors influencing indices of solute transport

	Mass transfer (mg/min)	Clearance (ml/min)	Mass transfer area coefficient (ml/min)
Blood concentration	Yes	No	No
Blood flow	In shock?	In shock?	No
Dialysate flow	< 4 liters/hr	< 4 liters/hr	No
Ultrafiltration	Yes	Yes	No
Membrane area	Yes	Yes	Yes
Membrane permeability	Yes	Yes	Yes

of urea. Urea clearances seem to be very resistant to decreases in splanchnic blood flow [36]. In severe shock, splanchnic blood flow may decrease enough to have a significant impact on urea clearances [35, 36]. Calculations of mass transfer area coefficients usually have been based on the assumption that peritoneal capillary blood flow is not limiting solute transport. If this is not true, then calculations of the mass transfer area coefficient might be affected by variations in effective capillary flow.

Mass transfer rates and peritoneal clearances are limited by dialysis solution flow rates that are less than 4 liters/hr [1]. At flow rates in excess of 4 liters/hr, the ratio of urea clearance to dialysate flow rate usually is near 0.3, with a maximum urea clearance of less than 30 ml/min [37]. At these dialysis solution flow rates, urea clearances are more limited by the number of capillaries involved in both exchange and total membrane resistance. Mass transfer area coefficients are calculated from equilibration curves (dialysate-to-plasma concentration ratios as a function of cycle time), and they represent clearances extrapolated back to time 0 based on the early slope of the curve. Thus, the mass transfer area coefficient is independent of dialysis solution flow rate.

When ultrafiltration occurs, solute transport may be enhanced by the process of convection [38]. Solutes are swept along by the streaming effects of the bulk flow. Thus, mass transfer and clearance may include both convective as well as diffusive solute transport. As mentioned above, some calculations of mass transfer coefficient subtract convective components, thus focusing only on diffusion.

All three indexes of solute transport are affected by membrane area and membrane permeability. The total effective membrane area of the peritoneum may be only a fraction of the gross mesothelial surface area. This is especially true if the effective pores of the cellular layers are confined to intercellular gaps. Also, many portions of the mesentery are nearly avascular [39]. Thus, if most net solute removal originates in peritoneal capillaries, the endothelial surface area (particularly the effective endothelial pore area) may be very small [40]. On the other hand, some losses of albumin do occur during peritoneal dialysis, suggesting that there are at least some very large "pores" (compared to synthetic membranes) used for hemodialysis. Thus, the peritoneum behaves as if it is a membrane of relatively low total pore area that represents

Table 3. Clearances with various dialysis techniques

Technique	Treatment time (hr/ wk)	Dialysate inflow (liters/ hr)	(liters/ wk)	Curea (ml/ min)	(liters/ wk)	Cin (ml/ min)	(liters/ wk)
IPD	40	2	80	18	43	4	10
CAPD, CCPD	168	0.33	56	7	67	4	40
Hemodialysis	15	30	450	150	135	8	7

only a small fraction of the anatomic surface area, but it is a system of relatively high mean pore size.

Table 3 summarizes typical clearances of urea (60 daltons) and inulin (5200 daltons) during both peritoneal dialysis therapies and hemodialysis.

Treatment time for intermittent peritoneal dialysis (IPD) usually is at least 40 hr/wk [41]. Average clearance rates in ml/min during the treatments and in overall liters/wk are shown for IPD by using 2-liter/hr cycles. For continuous ambulatory peritoneal dialysis (CAPD) and continuous cycling peritoneal dialysis (CCPD), treatment time essentially is continuous, representing 168 hr/wk [42–44]. This figure is not corrected for brief interruptions during drainage and instillation of fresh fluid. Commonly, 8 liters/d are instilled, representing 56 liters/wk instilled.

Clearance rates per min for urea during therapy are markedly reduced because of the dialysate flow limitations imposed by the long-dwell exchanges. Minute clearances of inulin are minimally affected, because the clearances of larger solutes are affected primarily by membrane area and permeability. Weekly clearances for the continuous techniques exceed those of the intermittent technique, because the contributions of the total time of therapy per week outweigh the reductions of minute clearances with long-dwell cycles.

For comparison, typical values are shown for weekly treatments, with hemodialysis totaling 15 hr/wk. Dialysate flow rates per hr and per week are many times those of peritoneal dialysis. Urea clearances per min are much greater than maximum urea clearances with peritoneal dialysis; even with calculations of urea clearances per week and the much longer duration of therapy with peritoneal dialysis, weekly hemodialysis urea clearances are greater. By contrast, since the maximum inulin clearance rates per minute are similar for the dialysis techniques, the weekly time factor yields weekly inulin clearances with peritoneal dialysis (particularly the continuous techniques) that are in excess of those with hemodialysis. The relative importance of these weekly clearances of solutes in different molecular weight ranges is controversial, and a discussion of such is beyond the scope of this review.

In summary, the major limitation on urea clearances with hemodialysis probably relates to blood flow into the dialyzer. The system is not dialysis solution flow rate-limited. Membrane resistances, including fluid films, favor very high small solute clearances. On the other hand, the major limitation of urea clearance for IPD has to do with the low total pore area and multiple membrane resistances, including fluid films. For the continuous techniques, dialysate flow limitations predominate for smaller solutes. For the larger solutes, the minute clearances are limited by membrane area and permeability for all techniques.

These comparisons of peritoneal dialysis with hemodialysis are best understood in terms of the physiologic and anatomic limitations of the peritoneal dialysis system.

Peritoneal Ultrafiltration

Table 4 summarizes mean drainage volumes for 2-liter exchanges with dialysis solutions containing 1.5 or 4.25% dextrose in patients studied at our center. All of these dialysis solutions also contained sodium, chloride, calcium, and magnesium in concentrations approaching diffusible concentrations in serum. They did not contain potassium. The buffer anion-balancing difference between cations and chloride concentrations was lactate. The so-called 2-liter volumes indicated on containers are not precise, and they usually range from 25 to 50 ml in excess. For each type of solution, results with total cycle times of 4 and 8 hr are shown. Concentrations of dialysate glucose and dialysate protein are also indicated. Numbers of exchanges for each type of exchange are indicated.

For each dextrose concentration, drainage volume is less at 8 hr compared to 4 hr. This is due to the fact that osmotic equilibrium and peak peritoneal volume occur earlier than 4 hr with 1.5% dextrose solutions and near 4 hr for the 4.25% dextrose solution.

In most patients, serum glucose concentrations remain well below 200 with these types of cycles; therefore, osmotic equilibrium is reached before glucose equilibrium. Dialysate glucose concentrations at 8 hr are still well above typical serum glucose concentrations. Osmotic equilibrium can be reached before glucose equilibrium because of the low electrolyte content of ultrafiltrate; the so-called sieving effect [3, 45–49]. Electrolyte concentrations in dialysis solution decrease with ultrafiltration particularly early in the exchanges, as electrolyte-poor ultrafiltrate enters the peritoneal cavity.

With 1.5% dextrose solutions, dialysate glucose concentrations are 39%

Table 4. Drainage volumes, dialysate glucose, and dialysate protein in the absence of peritonitis (means)

Exchange type[a] (% dextrose, cycle time)	Drainage volume (ml)	Dialysate glucose (mg/dl)	Dialysate protein (mg/dl)	Number of exchanges
1.5 4 hr	2209	586	90	525
1.5 8 hr	2132	363	164	53
4.25 4 hr	2819	980	86	152
4.25 8 hr	2763	564	121	63

[a] All 2-liter instillations.

and 24% of instillation concentrations at 4 and 8 hr, respectively. (This is not a precise percentage, since actual glucose concentrations in instilled solutions are slightly less than indicated. The concentrations indicated on the label are in terms of weighed glucose monohydrate. For example, the true glucose concentration in a 4.25% dextrose solution is 3.86%.) Thus, there is a higher fractional absorption of glucose with prolonged time. With 4.25% dextrose solutions, drainage concentrations are 23% and 13% of the listed initial values. Again, greater fractional glucose absorption with prolonged time is noted. Also, for each respective cycle time, there is greater fractional absorption with the more hypertonic solution due to the steeper concentration gradient favoring more rapid uptake.

Dialysate protein concentrations increase with cycle time. During measurements in Table 4, patients were all on CAPD at the time of measurements; and, protein concentrations presumably represent entry of protein into the solution by infusion and convection across the peritoneal membrane, rather than a simple washout of protein in residual peritoneal fluid. It is important to note that dialysate protein concentrations with the 4.25% dextrose exchanges are lower than their respective counterparts with 1.5% dextrose. This is due to the fact that ultrafiltrate is very low in protein and tends to dilute the dialysate protein concentration. If one calculates net protein removal per exchange as being the product of drainage volume × dialysate protein concentration, the more hypertonic 4-hr cycle increases net protein removal approximately 20%, compared to the less hypertonic 4-hr exchange. For 8-hr cycles, there was no increase in the amount of protein removed with increased ultrafiltration. Thus, the augmentation of protein removal (representing mainly albumin) by convection with ultrafiltration must be quite low, suggesting significant "sieving effects."

Figure 2 summarizes intraperitoneal volumes as a function of cycle time for 2-liter exchanges containing 4.25% dextrose. The curves represent typical

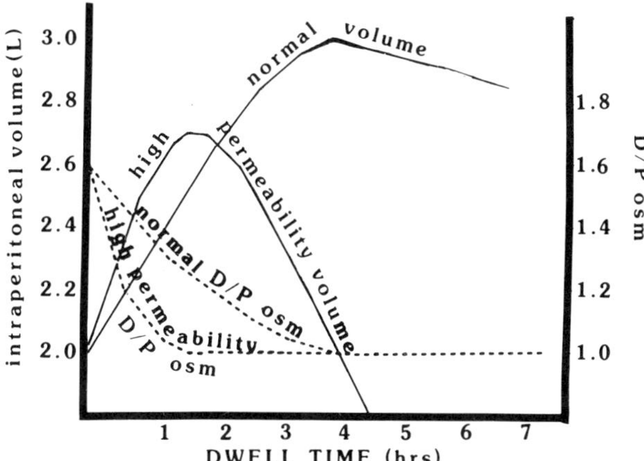

Fig. 2. Intraperitoneal volumes (*solid lines*) and dialysate/plasma osmolality (*D/P Osm*) (*broken line*) are related to dwell time. (Published with permission from [3])

values reported in the literature [50–52]. Dialysate-to-plasma osmolalities are also shown. Typical curves are shown for the usual adult who is undergoing peritoneal dialysis and for the patient with peritonitis. With peritoneal inflammation and/or injury, there is rapid glucose absorption, presumably secondary to increased membrane permeability (see below) [51, 52]. With more rapid osmotic equilibration, the peak of intraperitoneal volume occurs earlier. Changes in intraperitoneal volume are more rapid, while osmotic differences are present. Reabsorption of equilibrated fluid also seems to be more rapid with peritonitis. Not shown are the occasionally reported decreases in transient dialysate to plasma osmolality to values below 1 shortly before osmotic equilibrium is achieved. This may represent dilution by a very low electrolyte ultrafiltrate.

The distribution of glucose concentrations across the peritoneal membrane structures is not known. If mesothelium is an important barrier to glucose absorption, then transmesothelial osmotic pressure may mobilize interstitial fluid and may prevent distal capillary and venular reabsorption of physiologic proximal capillary ultrafiltrate resulting from hydrostatic pressure. On the other hand, if mesothelium is more permeable and high concentrations of glucose in peritoneal interstitium are achieved early in an exchange, then the osmotic pressure could be primarily across capillary walls, resulting in enhanced transcapillary ultrafiltration secondary to combined hydrostatic and osmotic pressure. It is not known whether hypertonic peritoneal dialysis solutions significantly enhance capillary ultrafiltration or mainly prevent reabsorption of the physiologic ultrafiltrate. There is increasing evidence that peritoneal injury confined to the mesothelium results in both rapid glucose absorption and reduced ultrafiltration (see below) [53].

There are numerous studies of the sieving effects of peritoneal ultrafiltration [47–49]. Clinically, rapid ultrafiltration can result in water removal from the extracellular fluid space without amounts of sodium that are proportional to extracellular fluid concentrations [47]. Severe hypernatremia can result. With slower rates of ultrafiltration, as in CAPD, this is less of a problem.

It is impossible to measure true sieving coefficients during peritoneal dialysis, since true sieving coefficients should be determined in the absence of diffusive transport. A common way of measuring a net sieving coefficient during peritoneal dialysis is to instill solutions containing solutes of interest in the same concentrations as their concentrations in serum water [38, 46]. The goal is to obliterate any concentration gradients for net diffusion at the beginning of the exchange, and also to depend on the convective effects of ultrafiltration to remove the solutes. The mass transfer of the solute can be calculated in the usual fashion. The mass transfer is then divided by the ultrafiltration volume to express the amount of mass transfer per unit volume of ultrafiltrate. Dividing this, in turn, by the serum water concentration expresses the ratio of the amount of solute per unit volume of ultrafiltrate to the amount of solute per unit volume of extracellular water. This is the so-called "net sieving coefficient." The true sieving coefficient probably is lower, since with sieving, the ultrafiltrate dilutes the solute concentrations within the peritoneal cavity and creates a concentration gradient for net diffusion. This results in a falsely high impression of the sieving coefficient.

For charged solutes, such as electrolytes, Gibbs-Donan effects must also be considered [54, 55]. Concentrations of the ions in extracellular fluid differ from those in serum water. For univalent cations, such as sodium and potassium, corrections to serum water concentrations (usually dividing by a value near 0.95) and predictions of Gibbs-Donan concentrations in interstitial fluid (usually multiplying by a value near 0.95) approximately cancel one another [54, 55]. Thus, net sodium-sieving coefficients can be estimated by dividing net removal per liter of ultrafiltrate via serum sodium concentration. For neutral solutes such as urea and inulin, mean net-sieving coefficients of 0.63 and 0.41, respectively, have been reported for 4.25% dextrose exchanges with a 30-min dwell time [46]. For sodium and potassium, mean values of 0.56 and 0.40, respectively, have been reported for similar-type exchanges [46].

A better understanding of these sieving effects during peritoneal ultrafiltration may improve our understanding of the physiology and the anatomy of peritoneal transport. Multiple explanations for the sieving effects have been proposed and are summarized in Figure 3.

Morphologic and functional evidence suggests that proximal capillaries are relatively low in permeability, compared to distal capillaries and venules [56–66]. Therefore, transcapillary ultrafiltration, whether primarily hydrostatic or hydrostatic and osmotic, may occur through a "tighter" section of the microcirculation. Water may move transcellularly or through very narrow intercellular gaps. Similarly, in the mesothelium, water may move transcellularly or through some narrow gap junctions. This may be quite different from the glomerulus, which is especially designed for both ultrafiltration with fenestrations through the endothelial cells and unique junctions between adjacent foot processes of epithelial cells.

It also has been suggested that countercurrent movement of glucose through the peritoneal membrane opposite to the direction of ultrafiltration may hinder convective solute transport as a result of molecular interference within the membrane pathways [67]. Comparisons of hydrostatic- and glucose-induced ultrafiltration in synthetic membrane systems has supported this hypothesis by demonstrating net sieving effects with osmotic-induced ultrafiltration that are not apparent with hydrostatic ultrafiltration [67].

The above mechanisms could effect charged and noncharged solutes. Charges within the peritoneal membrane might hinder the movement of charged solutes, such as ions. Endothelial and mesothelial cell surface charges (particularly within intercellular gaps), basement membrane charges on polarized molecules, and charged molecules within the interstitium all may interfere with electrolyte movements [68].

It is interesting that at least in some studies, the net sieving coefficient for urea does not approach unity [46]. If these observations can be confirmed, they suggest that water movement does occur in pathways where urea cannot readily follow. Also, it is interesting that the ratio of the inulin sieving coefficient to that of urea is relatively high [33, 46]. If urea and water could move transcellularly while inulin could not, the inulin sieving coefficient should be a very small fraction of that of urea. This is particularly true if a significant portion of endothelial and mesothelial cell surfaces would be

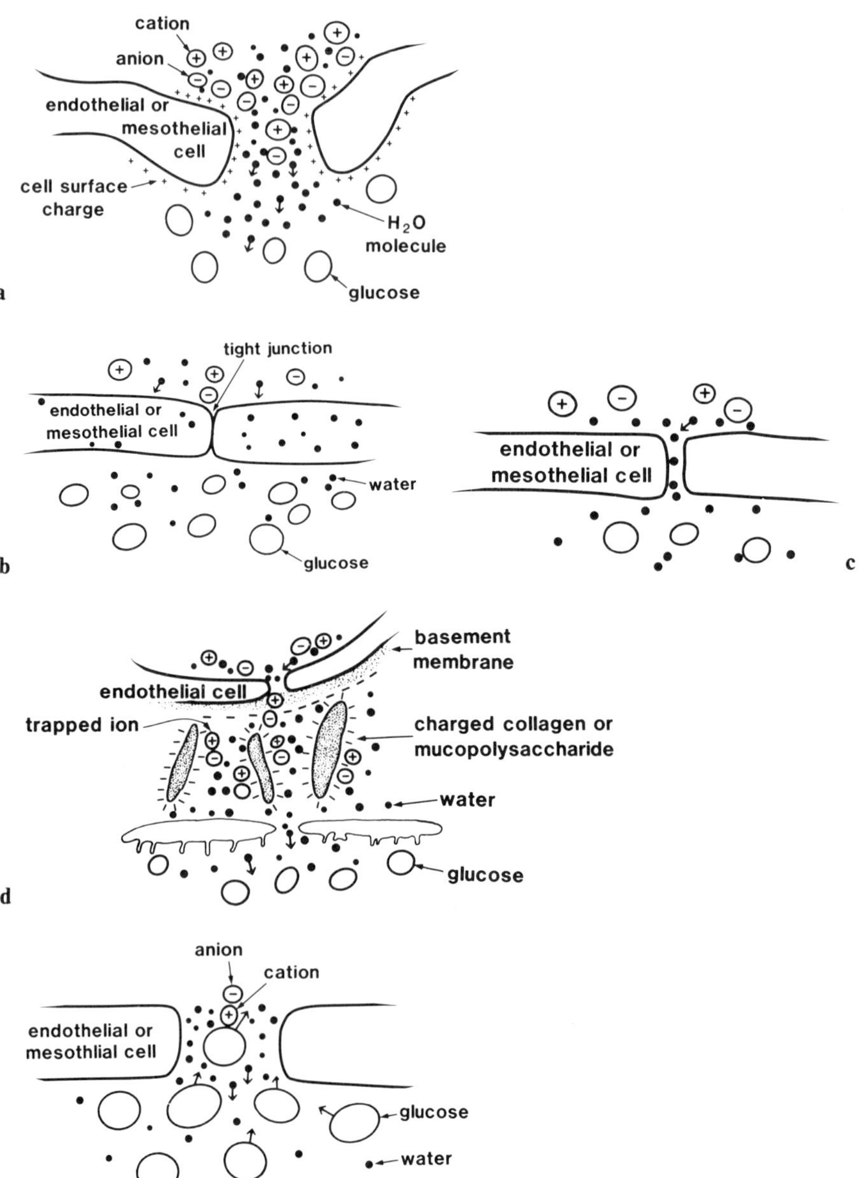

Fig. 3a-e. Five hypothetical mechanisms for solute sieving during peritoneal ultrafiltration are shown diagrammatically. **a** Surface charges in cell gaps. **b** Transcellular water movement. **c** Narrow cell junctions. **d** Interstitial and basement membrane charges. **e** Countercurrent glucose movement with molecular interference in gaps. (Reproduced with permission from [3])

available for urea and water movement, but not for inulin. The fact that the inulin sieving coefficient is two-thirds of that of urea seems to be more compatible with water movement through extracellular pathways of heterogeneous dimensions.

Thus, peritoneal ultrafiltration differs in many ways from ultrafiltration with extracorporeal systems. In general, during peritoneal dialysis, increased permeability results in reduced ultrafiltration. There is a sieving effect for small molecular weight-charged and neutral solutes that is not apparent with standard extracorporeal dialysis systems. We have previously reviewed the evidence that the source of the ultrafiltrate is extracellular and is predominantly from peritoneal capillaries [37]. Yet, we do not know whether physiologic capillary ultrafiltration is enhanced or mainly that reabsorption is prevented. Contributions of lymphatics are unknown.

Altered Transport of Solutes and/or Water

Exogenous Agents

Table 5 lists substances that have been reported to alter peritoneal transport of solutes and/or water. The vast literature on such studies has been reviewed elsewhere [69–73]. Only these general reviews will be cited in this section. The effects of most of the substances have been observed following their addition to peritoneal dialysis solution. Relatively high concentrations can

Table 5. Agents affecting peritoneal transport

Microcirculatory changes likely

Bradykinin	Glucagon	Phenytolamine
Cholecystokinin	Histamine	Puromycin
Diazoxide	Isoproterenol	Secretin
Dipyridamole	Nitroprusside	Serotonin
Dopamine	Norepinephrine	Tolazoline
Ethacrynic acid	Prostaglandins	Vasopressin
Furosemide		

Mesothelial, interstitial, or surface film changes likely

Amino proprionate	Insulin	THAM
Cetyl trimethyl NH_4CL	Protamine	Vasopressin
Dioctyl sodium sulfosuccinate	Puromycin	

Solute binding, ionic trapping, solubility

Albumin	Dialysate lipids	Specific chelates
Anthranilic acid	N-myristyl alanine	THAM
Alkaline dialysate		

Unknown site of action

Calcium	Phenazine-methosulfate	Streptokinase
Methylprednisolone		

be achieved within the peritoneal membrane, while concentrations within the systemic circulation remain relatively low. Some of the large gastrointestinal hormones have been reported to affect peritoneal transport when administered intravenously, and they have less or no effect when administered intraperitoneally. Substances of very large molecular weight may have difficulties in crossing the peritoneal mesothelium and interstitium and may fail to achieve adequate concentrations in the vascular walls when administered intraperitoneally.

A number of substances presumably exert at least some of their effects by altering the peritoneal microcirculation [37, 39]. Vasodilators tend to increase clearances of large molecular-weight solutes and to enhance protein losses. Since peritoneal dialysis solutions are, themselves, predominantly vasodilatory (and in rats appear to induce maximum arteriolar dilatation), effects of additional added vasodilators have been attributed primarily to their unique effects on venular permeability.

Peritoneal dialysis solutions cause a transient vasoconstriction in the parietal peritonium of rats (only several min in duration) followed by profound dilation of the parietal and visceral microcirculations [37, 39]. The substance responsible for the initial vasoconstriction has not been identified, but it does not appear to be a low pH or low PCO_2. The factors responsible for the vasodilation are the nonbicarbonate anions, lactate or acetate, and the hypertonicity of the solutions. Although arteriolar dilation is as great with solutions as with maximum doses of nitroprusside (a powerful vasodilator), nitroprusside induces more venodilation and directly alters venular permeability. Since small solute clearances during peritoneal dialysis presumably have minimal blood flow limitations, since solutions themselves probably cause maximum increases in blood flow, and since exogenous vasodilating drugs have marked effects on venules, it is not surprising that vasodilating substances primarily increase the clearances of large molecular weight substances.

Recent studies in our center with dipyridamole show increases in urea and inulin clearances that are proportional and most compatible with small increases in the total number of perfused capillaries and total effective capillary membrane area. Such findings, if confirmed, again suggest that urea and inulin use similar effective pore areas of the capillary walls that represent the same anatomic pathways—presumably extracellular.

Vasoconstrictors tend to reduce peritoneal clearances, particularly of large molecular-weight substances. Thus, rather than having major reductions in blood flow, effects may have more to do with reducing the number of capillaries perfused, decreasing effective membrane area, and decreasing permeability. The latter may be secondary to effects of the agents on vascular permeability directly, or as a result of selectively reducing perfusion of more permeable capillaries.

Some substances have been postulated to alter peritoneal transport by mechanisms that are not related to vasoactivity [69–73]. These might include mesothelial injury, alterations in the interstitial matrix, or changes in surface tension and surface fluid films. Evidence has been presented to suggest that vasopressin can induce effects that probably are related to vasoconstriction with relative preservation of large solute clearances in comparison to other vasoconstrictors. Simultaneous effects on permeability somewhere in the peritoneal membrane have been proposed.

Agents that bind solutes in peritoneal dialysis solution favor the conversion of a solute to an ionic form, or they alter solubility and may alter peritoneal transport. Such effects usually maintain a concentration gradient for net diffusion and enhance the average clearance achieved during a given exchange.

Some substances known to alter transport do so by unknown mechanisms.

Diseases

There are a number of clinical conditions in which peritoneal transport properties may be altered [74–78]. Reduced peritoneal clearances have been associated with advanced diseases that affect the microcirculation. These include collagen vascular diseases, diabetic vascular disease, and malignant hypertension. Unexplained low peritoneal clearances have been seen with heat- and exercise-induced rhabdomyolysis in acute renal failure. Possible microcirculatory alterations have not been proven.

Occasional patients on chronic peritoneal dialysis with IPD or CAPD have been reported to have decreases in peritoneal clearances over time [79–81]. This usually has been a small portion of the world CAPD population, focused mainly in France; in some patients (but not all), it seems to be associated with frequent and/or problematic peritonitis. On the other hand, there have been patients having many episodes of peritonitis over many years of chronic peritoneal dialysis therapy who have developed no apparent changes in transport characteristics [82].

It is helpful to analyze possible reasons for low ultrafiltration in CAPD. These reasons may include true membrane alterations or pseudomembrane alterations. Decreases in ultrafiltration or clearance may be incorrectly attributed to membrane failure. The development of edema in a patient on chronic peritoneal dialysis may reflect increased sodium and water intakes and/or a loss of residual renal function, rather than peritoneal membrane changes. Displacement of the catheter into the upper abdomen may result in poor drainage and build-up of a large reservoir of fluid in the peritoneal cavity. Glucose concentrations in instillate may be quickly diluted by the reservoir, resulting in low ultrafiltration. Poor drainage and poor mixing may result in low clearances. Patients in severe congestive heart failure or shock may drastically reduce effective peritoneal capillary area. In severe shock, reductions in blood flow may become important.

Table 6 categorizes reasons for low ultrafiltration into three groups, depending on dialysate glucose concentration. First, if ultrafiltration during a given cycle is below normal levels for the given concentration of dextrose in instillation fluid and (in addition) dialysate glucose concentration is low, consider a mechanical catheter malfunction with the build-up of a large residual volume diluting the instilled glucose concentration. Ultrafiltration will be low, because the osmotic gradient is low throughout the exchange and mechanical problems may interfere with adequate drainage of any ultrafiltrate that is formed and

Table 6. Reasons for low ultrafiltration in CAPD

With low dialysate glucose

Mechanical catheter malfunction (large residual volume dilutes osmotic gradient).
Increased peritoneal permeability or effective membrane area (as with peritonitis).

With normal dialysate glucose

Acute catheter malfunction (without a large residual volume at the time of instillation).

With increased dialysate glucose

Decreased peritoneal permeability or effective membrane area (as with very extensive reductions in transport subsequent to surgical removal or fibrosis of the membrane or reduced numbers of capillaries perfused, as in shock).
Severe hyperglycemia (enough to slow net glucose absorption and to simultaneously minimize the osmotic gradient).

sometimes even with adequate drainage of a volume equal to that instilled. Glucose concentrations will be low.

If there is no evidence of catheter malfunction or a large residual volume within the peritoneal cavity, then low-dialysate glucose concentrations and low ultrafiltration suggest either increased peritoneal permeability or an increase in effective peritoneal membrane area—or both. Peritonitis is associated with rapid glucose absorption that appears to be due to membrane alterations [53]. These include separation of mesothelial cells, loss of mesothelial microvilli, interstitial inflammation, and endogenous vasodilatation. Thus, with peritonitis, the mechanism for rapid glucose absorption could be microcirculatory, interstitial, and/or mesothelial. Verger has recently shown that superficial injuries to the peritoneum via brief heat drying of the mesothelial surface in rats result in rapid glucose absorption [53]. In this model, there were no obvious changes in the peritoneum deep to the mesothelium. In our own laboratories, we have also seen mesothelial injury that is secondary to polymer osmotic agents and secondary to microparticles of charcoal dispersed as a sorbent in peritoneal dialysis solution. Mesothelial changes were most obvious. Rapid glucose absorption was typical. All of these observations suggest that the mesothelial barrier may be an important controller of the glucose absorption rate; injury may result in loss of ultrafiltration. With this type of injury, there appears to be no reduction in peritoneal clearances. In fact, clearances and protein losses may be somewhat increased.

Reduced ultrafiltration with rapid glucose absorption in patients in the United States has mainly been seen with acute peritonitis. Usually, with acute peritonitis, the pattern disappears within 1 week of therapy. There are occasional patients, however, who develop this pattern chronically and who have had little or no peritonitis. Patients who have this chronic pattern have been most frequently seen in France [79–81]. Preliminary results of an international survey of ultrafiltration and glucose absorption, in 317 patients in 29 centers throughout Europe and North America, have revealed that the loss of ultrafiltration associated with rapid glucose absorption almost always is seen in patients using dialysis solutions manufactured by European-based companies [83]. More work is necessary to determine if there is membrane injury of a very subtle nature that is related to the choice of buffer anion, water purification methods, or plastic containers.

As in the second category of Table 6, if dialysate drainage volume is reduced and glucose concentration is normal, suspect acute catheter malfunction without a build-up of a large residual volume at the time of instillation.

Next, a loss of ultrafiltration with an increase in dialysate glucose concentration is very unusual. Severe decreases in peritoneal permeability and/or effective membrane area—subsequent to surgical removal or fibrosis of the membrane, or with severe reductions in the number of capillaries perfused (as in shock)—may result in both reduced peritoneal clearances and slow glucose absorption. However, the slow glucose absorption helps to protect the osmotic gradient and to somewhat buffer any changes in ultrafiltration. Nevertheless, if decreases in permeability or area are severe enough, ultrafiltration itself could be impaired, even with preservation of a good osmotic gradient.

Another rare cause of low ultrafiltration with an increased dialysate glucose could be severe hyperglycemia. The serum glucose concentration usually would need to be in excess of 500 mg/dl to have an impact on ultrafiltration with a 4.25% dextrose exchange [84]. In this case, glucose absorption would be slowed by the reduced concentration gradient, resulting in higher glucose concentrations in dialysate. However, the osmotic pressure gradient would be reduced because of the high osmolality of body fluids, resulting in a relatively low ultrafiltration.

There have been reports of sclerosing peritonitis in patients who are on IPD and CAPD [85–91]. It is not clear whether an early phase of this disease is associated with rapid glucose absorption and whether a later phase is associated with slow glucose absorption. Some anecdotal comments suggest this, but this needs further verification. It is not clear whether loss of ultrafiltration, as seen mainly in France, is an early form of sclerosing peritonitis. It is interesting that most cases of sclerosing peritonitis also have been reported in Europe among patients using brands of solution that also have been associated with loss of ultrafiltration. Some patients have had recurring or problematic peritonitis, but some cases have had no peritonitis. Beta-blocking drugs are known to cause the problem, but not all of these patients have been on beta-blocking drugs. Further work is necessary to clarify the etiology or etiologies of this sclerosing process, which results in a thickened fibrous peritoneum that eventually strangulates the bowel.

References

1. NOLPH KD, POPOVICH RP, GHODS AJ, TWARDOWSKI Z: Determinants of low clearances of small solutes during peritoneal dialysis. *Kidney Int* 13:117–123, 1978
2. NOLPH KD, MILLER FN, RUBIN J, POPOVICH R: New directions in peritoneal dialysis concepts and applications. *Kidney Int* 18:111–116, 1980
3. NOLPH KD: Solute and water transport during peritoneal dialysis, in *Perspectives in Peritoneal Dialysis,* edited by DIAZ-BUXO JA, Upper Montclair, New Jersey, Health Scan Inc, 1983, pp 4–8

4. SIMIONESCU N, SIMIONESCU M, PALADE GE: Structural basis of permeability in sequential segments of the microvasculature of the diaphragm. II. Pathways followed by microperoxidase across the endothelium. *Microvasc Res* 15:17–36, 1978

5. KARNOVSKY MJ: The ultrastructural basis of capillary permeability studies with peroxides as a tracer. *J Cell Biol* 35:213–235, 1967

6. JOHANSSON BR: Permeability of muscle capillaries to interstitially microinjected horseradish peroxidase. *Microvasc Res* 16:340–353, 1978

7. JOHANSSON BR: Permeability of muscle capillaries to interstitially microinjected ferritin. *Microvasc Res* 15:362–368, 1978

8. KARNOVSKY MJ: The ultrastructural basis of transcapillary exchanges, in *Biological Interfaces: Flows and Exchanges,* Boston,Little Brown & Co, 1968, pp 64–95

9. COTRAN RS: The fine structure of the microvasculature in relation to normal and altered permeability, in *Physical Bases of Circulatory Transport: Regulation and Exchanges,* edited by REVE EB, GUYTON AC, Philadelphia, WB Saunders & Co, 1967, pp 249–275

10. BARADI AF, RAYNS DJ: Mesothelial intercellular junctions and pathways. *Cell Tiss Res* 173:133–138, 1976

11. SIMIONESCU M, SIMIONESCU N: Organization of cell junctions in the peritoneal mesothelium. *J Cell Biol* 74:98–110, 1977

12. TSILIBRAY EC, WISSIG SL: Absorption from the peritoneal cavity; SEM study of the mesothelium covering the peritoneal surface of the muscular portion of the diaphragm. *Am J Anat* 199:127–133, 1977

13. DUMONT AE, ROBBINS E, MARTELLI A, ILIESCU H: Platelet blockade of particle absorption from the peritoneal surface of the diaphragm (41138). *Proc Soc Exp Biol Med* 167:137–142, 1981

14. GOITLOIB L, DIGENIS GE, RABINOVICH S, MEDLINE A, OREOPOULOS DG: Ultrastructure of normal rabbit mesentery. *Nephron* 34:248–255, 1983

15. FERIANI M, BIASIOLI S, CHIARAMONTE S, et al: Anatomical bases of peritoneal permeability: A reappraisal. Anatomy of peritoneum. *Int J Artif Organs* 5:345–348, 1982

16. WAYLAND H, SILBERBERG A: Blood to lymph transport. *Microvasc Res* 15:367–374, 1978

17. FOX JR, WAYLAND H: Interstitial diffusion of macromolecules in the rat mesentery. *Microvasc Res* 18:255–276, 1979

18. LAURENT TC: II. The ultrastructure and physical-chemical properties of interstitial connective tissue. *Pflügers Arch* 336(Suppl):S21–S42, 1972

19. WIEDERHIELM CA: The interstitial space, in *Biomechanics: Its Foundations and Objectives,* edited by FUNG YC, PERRONE N, ANLIKER M, Englewood Cliffs, New Jersey, Prentice Hall, pp 273–286

20. WATSON PD, GRODINS FS: An analysis of the effects of the interstitial matrix and plasma-lymph transport. *Microvasc Res* 16:19–41, 1978

21. ODOR DL: Observations of the rat mesothelium with the electron and phase microscopes. *Am J Anat* 95:433–465, 1954

22. BARADI AF, RAO SN: A scanning electron microscope study of mouse peritoneal mesothelium. *Tiss Cell* 8:159–162, 1976

23. ANDREWS PM, PORTER KR: The ultrastructure morphology and possible functional significance of mesothelial microvilli. *Anat Res* 177:409–426, 1973

24. RUBIN J, KIRCHNER K, BOWER J: Evaluation of stagnant fluid films during simulated peritoneal dialysis: In-vitro and in-vivo studies. *Clin Exper Dial Apher* 5:285–292, 1981

25. MCGARY TJ, NOLPH KD, RUBIN J: In vitro simulations of peritoneal dialysis:

A technique for demonstrating limitations on solute clearances due to stagnant fluid films and poor mixing. *J Lab Clin Med* 96(Suppl 1):148–157, 1980

26. POPOVICH RP, PYLE WK, MONCRIEF JW: Kinetics of peritoneal transport, in *Peritoneal Dialysis,* edited by NOLPH KD, The Hague, Martinus Nijhoff Publishers, 1981, pp 79–123

27. POPOVICH RP, PYLE WK, MONCRIEF JW, BOMAR JD: Peritoneal dialysis. Chronic replacement of kidney function. *AICHE Symp Series* 75:31–45, 1979

28. RANDERSON DH, FARRELL PC: Mass transfer properties of the human peritoneum. *ASAIO J* 3:140–146, 1980

29. POPOVICH RP, MONCRIEF JW: Kinetic modeling of peritoneal transport. *Contrib Nephrol* 17:59–72, 1977

30. NOLPH KD: Peritoneal clearances (*editorial*). *J Lab Clin Med* 94:519–525, 1979

31. BABB AL, JOHANSEN PJ, STRAND MJ, TENCKHOFF H, SCRIBNER BH: Bi-directional permeability of the human peritoneum to middle molecules. *Proc Eur Dial Transpl Assoc* 10:247–262, 1973

32. NOLPH KD, GHODS AJ, BROWN P, et al: Effects of nitroprusside on peritoneal mass transfer coefficients and microvascular physiology. *Trans Am Soc Artif Intern Organs* 23:210–218, 1977

33. HENDERSON LW, NOLPH KD: Altered permeability of the peritoneal membrane after using hypertonic peritoneal dialysis fluid. *J Clin Invest* 48:992–1001, 1969

34. DEDRICK RL, FLESSNER MF, COLLINS JM, et al: Is the peritoneum a membrane? *ASAIO* 5:1–8, 1982

35. AUNE S: Transperitoneal exchange 2. Peritoneal blood flow estimated by hydrogen gas clearance. *Scand J Gastroenterol* 5:99–104, 1970

36. ERBE RW, GREENE JA, JR, WELLER JM: Peritoneal dialysis during hemorrhagic shock. *J Appl Physiol* 22:131–135, 1967

37. NOLPH KD, SORKIN MI: The peritoneal dialysis system, in *Peritoneal Dialysis,* edited by NOLPH KD, The Hague, Martinus Nijhoff Publishers, 1981, pp 21–41

38. HENDERSON LW: Peritoneal ultrafiltration dialysis: Enhanced urea transfer using hypertonic peritoneal dialysis fluid. *J Clin Invest* 45:950–955, 1966

39. MILLER FN: The peritoneal microcirculation, in *Peritoneal Dialysis,* edited by NOLPH KD, The Hague, Martinus Nijhoff Publishers, 1981, pp 42–78

40. PAPPENHEIMER JR: Passage of molecules through capillary walls. *Physiol Rev* 33:387–423, 1953

41. AHMAD S, GALLAGHER N, SHEN F: Intermittent peritoneal dialysis: Status reassessed. *Trans Am Soc Artif Intern Organs* 25:86–89, 1979

42. POPOVICH RP, MONCRIEF JW, NOLPH KD, et al: Continuous ambulatory peritoneal dialysis. *Ann Intern Med* 88:449–456, 1978

43. NOLPH KD: Continuous ambulatory peritoneal dialysis (CAPD) (*editorial review*). *Am J Nephrol* 1:1–10, 1981

44. DIAZ-BUXO JA, WALKER PJ, CHANDLER JT, et al: Advances in peritoneal dialysis: continuous cyclic peritoneal dialysis. *Contemp Dial* 2(November):23–54, 1981

45. NOLPH KD, MILLER FN, PYLE WK, et al: An hypothesis to explain the ultrafiltration characteristics of peritoneal dialysis (*editorial review*). *Kidney Int* 20:543–548, 1981

46. RUBIN J, KLEIN E, BOWER JD: Investigation of the net sieving coefficient of the peritoneal membrane during peritoneal dialysis. *ASAIO* 5:9–15, 1982

47. NOLPH KD, HANO JE, TESCHAN PE: Peritoneal sodium transport during hypertonic peritoneal dialysis: Physiologic mechanisms and clinical implications. *Ann Intern Med* 70:931–941, 1969

48. NOLPH KD, SORKIN MI, MOORE H: Autoregulation of sodium and potassium

removal during continuous ambulatory peritoneal dialysis. *Trans Am Soc for Artif Int Organs* 26:334–338, 1980

49. BROWN ST, AHEARN DJ, NOLPH KD: Potassium removal with peritoneal dialysis. *Kidney Int* 4:67–69, 1973

50. RUBIN J, NOLPH KD, POPOVICH RP, MONCRIEF J, PROWANT B: Drainage volumes during CAPD. *ASAIO* 2:54–60, 1979

51. SMEBY LC, WIDEROE TE, SVARTAS TM, et al: Changes in water removal due to peritonitis during continuous peritoneal dialysis, in *Advances in Peritoneal Dialysis,* edited by GAHL GM, KESSEL M, NOLPH KD, Amsterdam, Excerpta Medica, 1981, pp 287–292

52. RUBIN J, MCFARLAND S, HELLEMS EW, et al: Peritoneal dialysis during peritonitis. *Kidney Int* 19:460–464, 1981

53. MALACH M: Peritoneal dialysis for intractable heart failure in acute myocardial infarction. *Am J Cardiol* 26:61–63, 1972

54. MANERY JF: Water and electrolyte metabolism. *Physiol Rev* 34:334–417, 1954

55. TARAIL R, HACKER ES, TAVMOR E: The ultrafiltrability of potassium and sodium in human serum. *J Clin Invest* 31:23–26, 1948

56. CASLEY-SMITH JR: Endothelial fenestrae in intestinal villi. Difference between the arterial and venous ends of the capillaries. *Microvasc Res* 3:49–68, 1971

57. WOLFF JR: Ultrastructure of the terminal vascular bed as related to function, in *Microcirculation,* edited by KALEY G, ALTURA BM, Baltimore, University Park Press, 1977, p 74

58. CLEMENT F, PALADE GE: Intestinal capillaries. I. Permeability to peroxidase and ferritin. *J Cell Biol* 41:33–58, 1969

59. NOLPH KD, MILLER FN, RUBIN J, POPOVICH R: New directions in peritoneal dialysis concepts and applications. *Kidney Int* 18:111–116, 1980

60. BRUNS RR, PALADE GE: Studies on blood capillaries. II. Transport of ferritin molecules across the wall of muscle capillaries. *J Cell Biol* 37:277–299, 1968

61. RENKIN E: Relation of capillary morphology to transport of fluid and large molecules: A review. *Acta Physiol Scand* 463(Suppl):81–91, 1979

62. CHAMBERS R, ZWEIFACH BW: Functional activity of the blood capillary bed, with special reference to visceral tissue. *Ann NY Acad Sci* 46:683–695, 1946

63. JACOBSON LF, NOER RJ: The vascular pattern of the intestinal villi in various laboratory animals and man. *Anta Res* 114:85–101, 1952

64. FOX J, GALEY F, WAYLAND H: Action of histamine on the mesenteric microvasculature. *Microvasc Res* 19:108–126, 1980

65. SMAJE L, ZWEIFACH BW, INTAGLIETTA M: Micropressures and capillary filtration coefficients in single vessels of the cremaster muscle in the rat. *Microvasc Res* 2:96–110, 1970

66. CASLEY-SMITH JR: Calculations relating to the passage of fluid and protein out of arterial-limb fenestrae through basement membrane and connective tissue channels, and into venous-limb fenestrae and lymphatics. *Microvasc Res* 12:13–34, 1976

67. TWARDOWSKI ZJ, NOLPH KD, POPOVICH RP, HOPKINS CA: Comparison of polymer glucose, and hydrostatic pressure induced ultrafiltration in a hollow fiber dialyzer; Effects on convective solute transport. *J Lab Clin Med* 92:619–633, 1978

68. AHEARN DJ, NOLPH KD: Controlled sodium removal with peritoneal dialysis. *Trans Am Soc Artif Intern Organs* 28:423–428, 1972

69. MAHER JF, HIRSZEL P: Augmenting peritoneal mass transport. *J Dialysis* 2:131–142, 1978

70. MAHER JF: Pharmacologic manipulation of peritoneal transport, in *Peritoneal Dialysis*, edited by NOLPH KD, The Hague, Martinus Nijhoff, 1981, pp 213–240
71. NOLPH KD: Peritoneal dialysis, in *Replacement of Renal Function by Dialysis* (1 ed), edited by DRUKKER, PARSONS, MAHER J, The Hague, Martinus Nijhoff, 1978, pp 277–321
72. NOLPH KD: Peritoneal dialysis, in *The Kidney* (3rd ed), edited by BRENNER B RECTOR FC, Philadelphia, WB Saunders & Co (in press, 1984)
73. NOLPH KD: Effects of intraperitoneal vasodilators on peritoneal clearances. *Dial Transpl* 7:812–817, 1978
74. NOLPH KD, MILLER L, HUSTED FC, HIRSZEL P: Peritoneal clearances in scleroderma and diabetes mellitus: Effects of intraperitoneal isoproterenol. *Int Urol Nephrol* 8:161–169, 1976
75. NOLPH KD, STOLTZ M, MAHER JF: Altered peritoneal permeability in patients with systemic vasculitis. *Ann Intern Med* 78:891–894, 1973
76. NOLPH KD, MILLER L, HUSTED FC, HIRSZEL P: Effects of intraperitoneal isoproterenol on reduced peritoneal clearances in patients with systemic vascular disease. *J Int Urol Nephrol* 8:161–169, 1976
77. BROWN ST, AHEARN DJ, NOLPH KD: Reduced peritoneal clearances in scleroderma increased by intraperitoneal isoproterenol. *Ann Intern Med* 78:891–894, 1973
78. NOLPH KD, WHITCOMB ME, SCHRIER RW: Mechanisms for inefficient peritoneal dialysis in acute renal failure associated with heat stress and exercise. *Ann Intern Med* 71:317–326, 1969
79. SLINGENEYER A, CANAUD B, MION C: Permanent loss of ultrafiltration capacity of the peritoneum in long-term peritoneal dialysis: An epidemiological study. *Nephron* 33:133–138, 1983
80. FALLER B, MARICHAL JF: Loss of ultrafiltration in CAPD: Clinical data, in *Advances in Peritoneal Dialysis* (Int Congr Ser No 567), edited by GAHL T, KESSEL G, NOLPH KD, Amsterdam, Excerpta Medica, 1981, pp 227–232
81. VERGER C, BRUNSCHVICG O, LE CHARPENTIER Y, LAVERGNE A, VANTELON J: Structural and ultrastructural peritoneal membrane changes and permeability alterations during CAPD. *Proc Eur Dial Transpl Assoc* 18:199–205, 1981
82. SORKIN MI, LUGER AM, PROWANT B, KENNEDY J, MOORE H, NOLPH KD: Histological and functional characteristics of the peritoneal membrane of a diabetic patient after 34 months on CAPD. *PD Bull* 2:24–27, 1982
83. AN INTERNATIONAL COOPERATIVE STUDY: Factors affecting ultrafiltration in continuous ambulatory peritoneal dialysis, First Report. *PD Bull,* in press
84. NOLPH KD: Continuous ambulatory peritoneal dialysis (CAPD) (*editorial review*). *Am J Nephrol* 1:1–10, 1981
85. GAHNDI VC, HUMAYUN JM, ING TS, et al: Sclerotic thickening of the peritoneal membranes in maintenance peritoneal dialysis patients. *Arch Intern Med* 140:1201–1203, 1980
86. GAHNDI VC, ING TS, DAUGIRDAS JT, HAGEN C, BLUMENKRANTZ MH, JABLOKOW FR: Failure to peritoneal dialysis due to peritoneal sclerosis (*letter to the editor*). Am J Artif Organs 6:97, 1983
87. SCHMIDT RW, BLUMENKRANTZ M: Peritoneal sclerosis: A "Sword of Damocles" for peritoneal dialysis? *Arch Intern Med* 141:1265–1267, 1981
88. ROTTENBOURG J, GAHL G, POIGNET JL, MERTANI E, STRIPPOLI P, LANGLOIS JP, LEGRAIN M: Severe abdominal complications in patients undergoing continuous ambulatory peritoneal dialysis. *Proc Eur Dial Transpl Assoc* 20:236–242, 1983

89. SLINGENEYER A, MION C, MOURAD G, CANAUD B, FALLER B, BERAUD J: Progressive sclerosing peritonitis: A late and severe complication of maintenance peritoneal dialysis. *Trans Am Soc Artif Intern Organs* 29:633–638, 1983
90. BRADLEY JA, MCWHINNIE DL, HAMILTON DN, STARNES F, MACPHERSON SG, SEYWRIGHT M, BRIGGS JD, JUNOR BJ: Sclerosing obstructive peritonitis after CAPD (*letter*). *Lancet* 2:113–114, 1983
91. BRADLEY JA, HAMILTON DN, MCWHINNIE DL, BRIGGS JD, JUNOR BJ: Sclerosing peritonitis after CAPD (*letter*). *Lancet* 2:572–573, 1983

Efficacy and Adequacy of Continuous Ambulatory Peritoneal Dialysis

George Wu, Donald Kim, and Dimitrios G. Oreopoulos

Continuous ambulatory peritoneal dialysis (CAPD) was introduced in 1976 [1], and it soon became one of the most popular modes of home dialysis. There is no single qualitative or quantitative index by which to evaluate the efficacy of CAPD. This paper will present evidence to suggest that CAPD provides adequate dialysis according to the following criteria:

1. It sustains life in patients with end-stage renal disease (ESRD).
2. It maintains patients in a satisfactory condition, while awaiting a kidney transplant, and it does not interfere with the results of transplantation; if the latter fails, it can keep the patients alive after transplant nephrectomy.
3. It provides an adequate and satisfactory quality of life, as indicated by adequate rehabilitation, sexual activity, and minimal "backup" hospitalization.
4. It can sustain children and can facilitate their growth.
5. It can provide adequate biochemical control.
6. It can arrest or even ameliorate uremic complications.
7. It is inexpensive.

In addition, the adequacy of CAPD will be demonstrated by comparing its results with those of the more firmly established dialysis modality—chronic hemodialysis.

Survival on CAPD

In Toronto Western Hospital, survival at the end of 1, 2, 3, 4, and 5 years is 90, 80, 70, 65, and 46%, respectively (Fig. 1). The attrition rate is about 10%/yr.

This manuscript was presented as part of a Symposium on *Continuous Ambulatory Peritoneal Dialysis.*

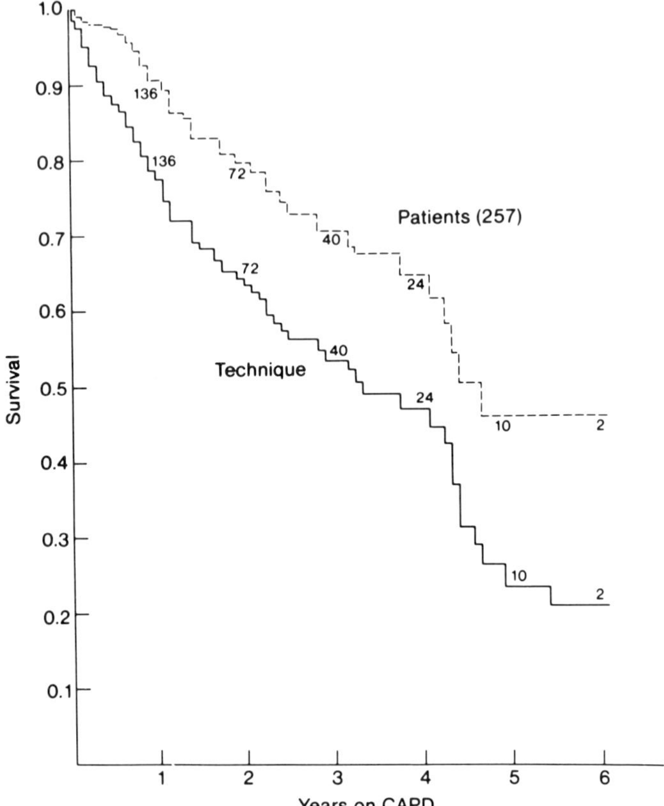

Fig. 1. Cumulative patient and technique survival in 257 CAPD patients at the Toronto Western Hospital.

Data concerning the various forms of dialysis used in Canada in 1981–1982 [2] show that the nondiabetic CAPD patients ($N = 596$), who were an average of 4 years older than those on hemodialysis, have a 90 and 80% chance of survival at the end of 12 and 24 months, respectively. During this same period, the nondiabetic patients on hemodialysis ($N = 1161$) had a survival rate of 85 and 75%, respectively. At the end of 2 years, the probability of dropout (failures and deaths together) was 48% for CAPD, and 41% for hemodialysis. Thus, by these criteria, the two modalities were comparable.

The European Dialysis and Transplant Association (EDTA) studied a large number of CAPD patients and compared them with patients on other replacement therapies [3]. They had 3607 patients registered on CAPD by the end of December 1982. Their data showed that the survival of CAPD patients from various age groups is comparable to that of patients on other modalities (Tables 1A and 1B). In all age groups, survival of diabetic patients on CAPD at 1 year was consistently better than that of the general diabetic

Table 1A. One-year survival among nondiabetic patients with end-stage renal disease being treated with replacement therapy in Europe

Age (yr)	Therapy (% of patients alive)			
	Hemodialysis[a]	CAPD	Cadaveric transplant	Any kidney replacement therapy[b]
15–34	—	97	93	93
35–44	—	96	90	91
45–54	90	92	84	90
55–64	—	84	77	85
65	—	75	77	76

[a] Value extracted from a figure.

[b] Irrespective of any subsequent changes in the mode of treatment.

Table 1B. One-year survival among diabetic patients with end-stage renal disease being treated with kidney replacement therapy in Europe

Age (yr)	Therapy (% of patients alive)			
	Hemodialysis[a]	CAPD	Cadaveric transplant	Any kidney replacement therapy[b]
15–34	—	92	72	77
35–44	—	77	77	73
45–54	72	80	63	71
55–64	—	71	—	70
65	—	—	—	58

[a] Number extracted from a figure.

[b] Irrespective of any subsequent changes in the mode of treatment.

population on renal replacement therapy, although they did not provide statistical analysis.

Of the factors that influence survival, the most important ones are age, diabetes, pre-existing cardiovascular disease, and depression at the onset of treatment. Survival at 4 years for patients younger than 40 years of age, those between 40 and 59, and those older than 60 were 95, 72, and 40%, respectively. This is not surprising, because younger patients generally are healthier and have fewer cardiovascular and metabolic complications.

Patients with ESRD due to diabetes mellitus are particularly difficult to treat. They have multiple system involvement and significant impairment of visual acuity. Their survival on intermittent peritoneal dialysis is poor [4]. Many diabetic patients with ESRD, even those who are blind, are now treated with CAPD [5]. At the Toronto Western Hospital, the overall survival of insulin-dependent diabetic patients on CAPD (type I) is 89, 65, 58, and

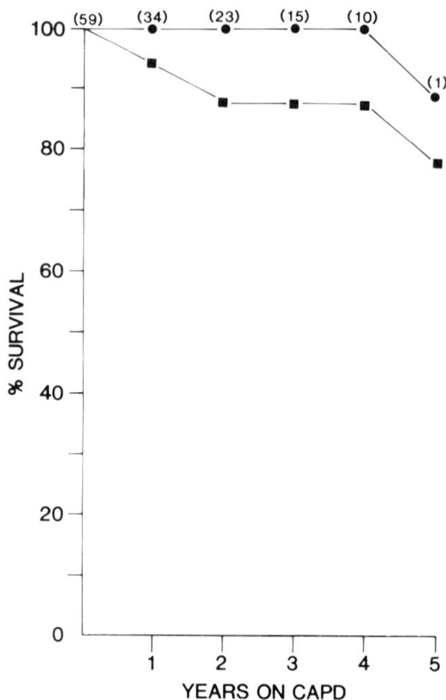

Fig. 2. Survival of low-risk patients on CAPD (See text for the definition of "low-risk"). Patient (●——●) and technique survival (■——■) among uncomplicated CAPD patients (20 to 60 yr without systemic disease, no known cardiovascular disease, and no history of angina or cardiomegaly) ($N = 59$). *Parentheses* indicate patients at risk.

58% at the end of 1, 2, 3, and 4 years (respectively), compared to 92, 81, 72, and 66% (respectively) for nondiabetic patients.

In a previous study [6], we demonstrated that patients with pre-existing cardiovascular disease have a lower survival than those who do not have cardiovascular disease at the start of CAPD.

Survival of Low-risk Patients

In a selected group of low-risk patients (those with ages between 20 to 60 years without coexisting systemic diseases such as diabetes mellitus, vasculitis, scleroderma, amyloidosis, and multiple myeloma, and without pre-existing cardiovascular complications such as angina pectoris, myocardial infarction, and hypertensive cardiomyopathy), we found a 100% survival at the end of 4 years on CAPD (Fig. 2).

CAPD and Kidney Transplantation

Among CAPD patients awaiting transplantation, the principal risk factors that are related to peritoneal dialysis and that may affect the outcome are peritonitis, perforation of peritoneal cavity during the procedure, and catheter skin exit infections. Patient and graft survival are comparable in patients who were maintained on hemodialysis or peritoneal dialysis before transplantation [7]. Problems with the catheter and exit site are uncommon, and they can be managed without complications [8]. If peritonitis develops in the postoperative period, it can be treated easily with antibiotics and early removal of the catheter. Immunosuppressive therapy does not increase the incidence and severity of peritonitis.

Patients in whom renal transplantation fails can be managed again by CAPD. Of 22 such patients who returned to our CAPD program, their survival was 84% at the end of the first year and 73% at the end of the second year. These figures are slightly lower than those for the general CAPD population, probably because these patients had multiple problems such as rejections, intensive treatment with cytotoxic drugs, and repeated episodes of severe infection. These patients did not have a higher incidence of peritonitis than the general CAPD population.

Quality of Life

It is difficult to quantify the quality of life. Sometimes, it can only be inferred from the patient's activity level, employment status, sexual activity, and relationship with other family members. The frequency of "backup" hospitalization provides a rough index of both morbidity and the quality of life.

A review of the level of rehabilitation among the patients in our program at the end of 1983 (Table 2) showed that 38% were working full-time—working men or women and homemakers with normal activity. The level of full rehabilitation in the work scale is low, because a large proportion of our patients were over the retirement age; and, it is not significantly different from that reported for a large population of ESRD patients on hemodialysis [9]. Among our patients, 63% claimed that their daily activity was normal. Among the 59 young patients without systemic complications (as defined previously), 64% were fully rehabilitated and 85% had normal daily activities.

Table 2. Rehabilitation of 86 patients on the CAPD program at Toronto Western Hospital on December 31, 1983

Occupational status	No. patients	(%)	Daily activity	No. patients	(%)
Full-time	12	14	Normal	54	63
Part-time	0		Restricted	26	
Sick leave	6		Requires care	5	
Homemaker (normal activity)	21	24	Confined to bed	0	
Homemaker (restricted)	10				
Unemployed	11				
Retired (normal activity)	11	13			
Retired (restricted)	14				

In a retrospective multicenter survey of the demography, physical activity, and employment status of CAPD and hemodialysis patients carried out via questionnaires, Fragola et al [10], found that 68% of the nondiabetic patients and 48% of the diabetic CAPD patients were capable of activities greater than self-care. Corresponding figures for hemodialysis patients were 59% and 23%, respectively. These differences were statistically significant. When the work scale of the CAPD patients was compared to that of hemodialysis, the trend was still better, but the difference was much less impressive. Thus, a better activity level did not translate into a better employment status; perhaps, because of factors related to the economy, workforce market, and a welfare system, which dissuades patients from gainful employment.

Churchill et al tried a new approach in quantifying the quality of life in dialysis and transplant patients, which they have called the "time trade-off" technique [11]. The patients were given a hypothetic choice: They could either continue in their present state of health with its physical, emotional, and social limitations for a lifetime (t) (determined from actuarial data), or they could choose a shorter time (x) in a state of full health, except for the normal aging process. The value (x/t) is an index of the health state or the perceived quality of life for the individual. They found that the mean values for hospital-based hemodialysis, CAPD, and transplantation patients were 0.57, 0.57, and 0.80, respectively.

Sexual Function

Sexual dysfunction is common in patients with chronic renal failure and those on dialysis [12]. The patient and the partner are under constant physical and psychological stress. They have to adjust every aspect of daily living to the restraints of dialysis. The patient's illness may force the spouse to change roles in earning income, assuming responsibility for housework, and raising the family. This change produces great stress and, frequently, the patient may not be able to accept the new role. In addition to these psychological factors, a concomitant abnormal metabolic and hormonal status may produce sexual dysfunction. Abnormal sexual hormonal homeostasis has been implicated in patients with renal failure [13–15]. Sexual dysfunction has been attributed to impaired pituitary function, with inadequate levels of follicle-stimulating hormone (FSH) and luteinizing hormone (LH), high levels of prolactin, and low levels of zinc [16–18]. In addition, CAPD patients may find the body image distorted by the presence of the catheter, the empty bag, and the dialysis solution in the abdomen; this may impair libido even further. Burton et al [19] showed that substantial numbers of dialysis patients, whether on hemodialysis or CAPD, reported marital strain, sexual dysfunction, and altered perceptions of sexual identity and attractiveness. However, patients undergoing hemodialysis complained significantly more often about all four of the above varieties of marital-sexual stress than did patients on CAPD.

Resumption of Menses

Most women do not menstruate while on maintenance hemodialysis. Galler et al [20] reported that 86% of women on CAPD and only 25% of those on hemodialysis have regular menses. Frequently, amenorrheic females on hemodialysis resume menstruation after being started on CAPD. Even though the ovulatory cycle is still rare, resumption of menstruation often has a beneficial psychological effect on women with renal disease.

Pregnancy is still a rare event among women on dialysis, and successful pregnancies with a live birth are even more unlikely. Kioko et al [21] described a successful pregnancy in a 26-year-old woman with advanced diabetic nephropathy who was treated with CAPD. The pregnancy was carried to 34 weeks, and an infant of 1.7 kg was delivered via Caesarian section. Two other women on CAPD became pregnant [22, 23], but both ended in spontaneous abortion at 13 and 32 weeks, respectively.

Backup Hospitalization

In the years up to and including 1982, our data showed both a gradual decrease in the need for hospitalization and a significant reduction in the need for hospitalization for peritonitis; but, this trend did not continue into 1983. On analyzing our data, it became obvious that the hospitalization pattern is highly skewed. Thus, during 1983, approximately one-third of the patients in the program did not require admission, whereas 10% of the patients accounted for one-half of all admission days. This small portion of CAPD patients were elderly and had multiple medical problems, which were difficult to manage and required long periods of convalescence. Of all CAPD patients, 68% required less than 2 weeks of hospitalization during 1983; and, they accounted for only 12% of all hospitalization days.

CAPD in Children with ESRD

Continuous ambulatory peritoneal dialysis has made an important contribution to the treatment of children with ESRD, especially very small ones [24].

Baum et al [25] compared two groups of children: one treated via CAPD and the other via hemodialysis. In the children on CAPD, protein and caloric intakes were higher and the growth rate was slightly faster, but the difference did not reach statistical significance. The CAPD treatment was more cost-effective than hemodialysis. In another report [26], Balfe reported that children treated by CAPD grew faster than those treated by hemodialysis, although the growth was still not as good as in children with successful renal transplants. It appears that children with ESRD would have a growth rate that would approach normal, if one controlled hyperparathyroidism and gave optimum nutrition. Kohaut et al [27], who described significant catch-up growth in children treated with CAPD, stressed both the importance of careful and intensive management of hyperparathyroidism and close attention to nutritional needs; the children in the latter study ingested about 2 g of protein/ kg of body wt. Thus, CAPD makes it possible to liberalize the diet and fluid intake in a group of patients who are particularly difficult to manage.

Biochemical Control

Generally, in most individuals, CAPD with 8 liters/d (four 2-liter exchanges) stabilizes the biochemical abnormalities (Table 3). The following observations about serum potassium and phosphorus may be of particular interest.

Potassium

Each day, CAPD removes approximately 25 to 35 mmoles of potassium, and some CAPD patients become hypokalemic despite a liberal potassium intake (60 to 80 mmoles/d). This may be due to increased potassium loss from the gastrointestinal tract [28], or intracellular accumulation of this ion associated with absorption of glucose from the dialysate or urinary loss (for example, in a patient receiving large doses of furosemide).

Phosphorus

Continuous ambulatory peritoneal dialysis alone does not remove enough phosphorus to keep the serum phosphorus at normal levels. Most patients

Table 3. The blood biochemical values of patients on four 2-liter exchanges per d after 1 year of CAPD treatment

	4-bag (days) (mean ± SD)
Blood urea nitrogen (mg%)	54.1 ± 16.6
Creatinine (mg%)	11.5 ± 1.50
Calcium (mg%)	9.3 ± 0.64
Phosphorus (mg%)	4.2 ± 0.75
Uric acid (mg%)	6.9 ± 1.03
Total protein (g%)	6.3 ± 0.93
Albumin (g%)	3.2 ± 0.44
Potassium (mEq/liter)	4.0 ± 0.59
Cholesterol (mg%)	237.2 ± 80.70
Triglycerides (mg%)	299.3 ± 134.20
Hemoglobin (g%)	9.3 ± 1.90
Platelets ($\times 100/mm^3$)	501.3 ± 106.41

also require a phosphorus-restricted diet and/or a phosphorus binder, but in a dose smaller than that required in hemodialysis. Aluminum binders are unpalatable, may aggravate constipation and even precipitate diverticulitis, and may contribute to the development of osteomalacia and dialysis dementia. The risk of these complications can be minimized by using a magnesium-free dialysate in combination with phosphorus binders containing a mixture of magnesium hydroxide and aluminum hydroxide. This mixture, which has a mild laxative effect, binds phosphorus with a lower dose of aluminum hydroxide and is more palatable.

Fluid Intake

One can be more liberal with fluid intake in CAPD than in hemodialysis, because ultrafiltration is continuous and thirst is decreased. Large volumes of ultrafiltrate can be removed by the use of hypertonic (4.25% dextrose) exchanges—600 to 800-ml per exchange. Recently, however, we advise our patients against the liberal use of water, because frequent hypertonic exchanges lead to increased glucose absorption with all of its consequences: lipid abnormalities, obesity, and possibly damage to the peritoneum. Patients who drink large volumes of fluid resort to frequent hypertonic exchanges, which (in turn) provokes more thirst [29]. This cycle can be broken by the deliberate reduction in intake of water and salt. This group of patients differs from those who have to use frequent hypertonic exchanges because of loss of ultrafiltration. Fortunately, such a loss, which usually leads to a discontinuation of CAPD, is rare in CAPD patients; it seems to develop mainly among those who use dialysis solutions buffered with acetate [30, 31].

CAPD and Uremic Complications

Control of Hypertension

Blood pressure is controlled easily in patients on CAPD, and it usually returns to normal during the first few weeks. We measured blood pressure in 197 patients, both before and after CAPD. Before starting CAPD, 77% of the patients had hypertension that was defined as a systolic pressure > 160 mm Hg and/or a diastolic pressure > 90 mm Hg; all patients were on antihypertensive medication and only 23% had a normal blood pressure. While on CAPD, 74% of those who were initially hypertensive became normotensive and required no further medication. Another 20% had normal blood pressure on antihypertensive medication, but the dosage was smaller than before. Of the patients who were initially hypertensive, 6% remained hypertensive. Because of the ease with which hypertension is occasionally brought under control, we have started CAPD on patients suffering from intractable hypertension, even though their renal failure had not advanced to the point where they required dialysis.

In view of the high incidence of cardiovascular deaths among dialysis patients (see below), it is of paramount importance to control even one of the major risk factors of coronary artery disease: hypertension, hypercholesterolemia, smoking, and diabetes mellitus. Leenen et al studied, with serial M-mode echocardiography [32], 17 CAPD patients—all of whom had a history of hypertension and echocardiographic evidence of increased left ventricular mass related to both concentric and eccentric hypertrophy. On CAPD, the blood pressure consistently returned to normal. In 14 of 17 patients, left ventricular mass decreased as a result of reduction in both left ventricular wall thickness and left ventricular dimension. Repeat echocardiography showed improvement in three of four patients who initially had impaired left ventricular function. These investigators concluded that CAPD improves left ventricular hypertrophy by normalizing pressure and volume overload of the left ventricle.

Control of Anemia

The average hematocrit is 30 to 35%, and the average hemoglobin is about 9 to 10 g/dl in CAPD patients. These patients require transfusions and anabolic steroids less frequently than patients on hemodialysis [33]. Frequently, it has been observed that hemoglobin and hematocrit increase in patients transferred from hemodialysis to CAPD [34].

In 34 patients on CAPD, DePaepe et al [35] found a significant increase in hemoglobin and hematocrit in the first 6 months of CAPD. The elevated hematocrit represents both a combination of true increase in red blood cell mass and a decrease in plasma volume. The serum parathyroid hormone (PTH) and ferritin remained unchanged. Zappacosta also found a significant increase in hematocrit in four of nine CAPD patients [36]; it appears that those patients who respond to CAPD are those who have high erythropoietein levels. Three of the four patients who did respond had polycystic kidney disease.

As yet, we have no explanation for the improvement of erythropoiesis in patients on CAPD. Lamperi et al confirmed the improved erythropoiesis by in vitro studies of the colony-formation capacity of the bone marrow cells, but found no correlation between the rise in hematocrit levels and the serum erythropoietein levels [37]. They suggested that the improved erythropoiesis results from the removal, by CAPD, of toxic factor(s) that suppress bone marrow. Hefti et al, who studied red blood cells survival in 11 CAPD patients, found that the reduction in red blood cell survival still persisted; the mean ^{51}Cr red blood cell half-life was 20 days [38].

Pericarditis

The incidence of pericarditis in patients with ESRD is reported to be 32 to 41% [39, 40]; however, with earlier initiation of therapy and more effective dialysis, uremic pericarditis can be prevented. The incidence of uremic pericarditis among patients on chronic hemodialysis has varied from 10 to 18% [41, 42]. Pericarditis was an infrequent complication among our CAPD patients. Since the beginning of our program, we have encountered only nine episodes of pericarditis among 257 patients. None of these developed tamponade; one developed pericarditis following a reactivation of systemic lupus erythematosus (SLE). The patients with pericarditis were treated with anti-inflammatory drugs and more frequent exchanges. None had other indications of inadequate dialysis.

Neuropathy

Neuropathy was identified as a complication of advanced renal failure in 1961 [43], but its cause still remains an enigma. Frequently, it has been attributed to an accumulation of uremic toxins of middle molecular size [44]. Initially, we hoped that CAPD patients might have a lower incidence and slower progression of uremic neuropathy than patients on hemodialysis or intermittent peritoneal dialysis, because it achieves a better clearance of middle-sized molecules.

We have studied the electrophysiologic parameters in 23 nondiabetic and 6 diabetic patients, who had been treated with CAPD for 3 years or more. Figure 3 shows the sequential motor and sensory nerve conduction velocities in these patients. Linear regression analysis of nerve conduction velocity as a function of time showed no significant change following dialysis. Motor nerve conduction velocities in diabetic patients also remained unchanged. These data suggest that peripheral neuropathy does not progress in patients on CAPD for prolonged periods. Contrary to our findings, Lindholm et al [45] showed that peripheral neuropathy may worsen during CAPD. However, the presence of a marked perdominance of males in their study may have influenced their results, because men are more prone to uremic neuropathy than women [46].

Cognitive Function

A large proportion of patients with advanced renal failure have a significant degree of cognitive dysfunction, which is attributed to neurotoxicity before treatment [47]. Kenny developed an "impairment index" to assess cognitive dysfunction in individual CAPD patients. This index, which ranges from 0.0 (no impairment) to 1.0 (severe impairment), is calculated on the basis of eight psychometric tests [47]. Kenny studied 46 patients over 1 year of CAPD treatment. In the beginning, only 37% of them had normal cognitive function (score 0.0 to 0.2), whereas 22.7% had markedly imparied function (score > 0.5). At the end of 1 year, 59% had normal cognitive function, and the proportion of those with markedly impaired scores dropped to 13%. The population of nonimpaired patients increased to 70% after treatment for 2 years or more.

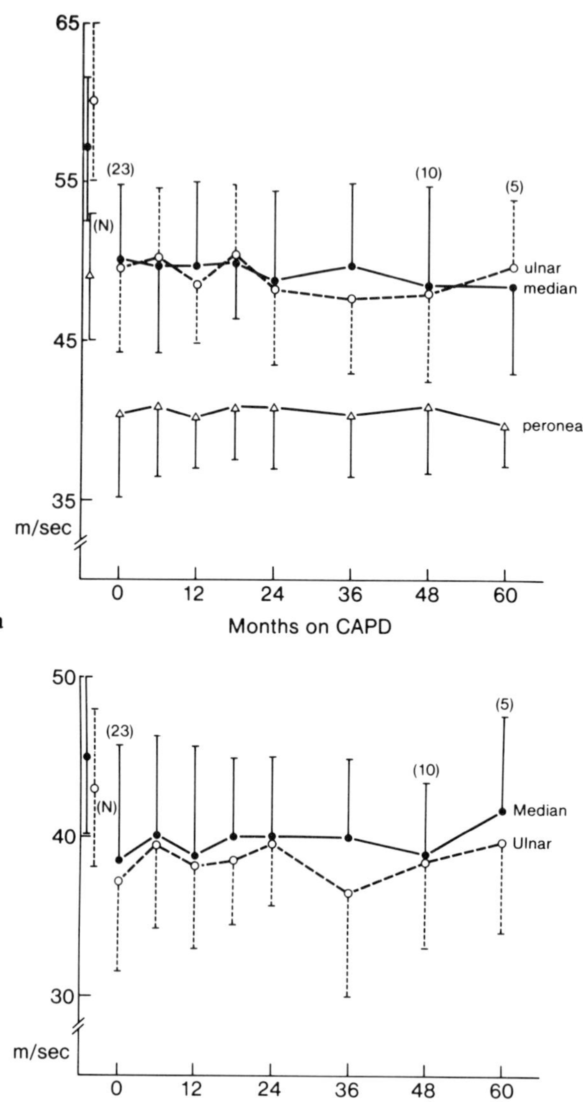

Fig. 3a. Sequential motor conduction velocities in nondiabetic patients on CAPD for more than 3 yr. **b.** Sequential sensory nerve conduction velocities in nondiabetic patients on CAPD for more than 3 yr.

Renal Osteodystrophy

Renal osteodystrophy is a major complication of long-term dialysis. With the better control of serum phosphorus, one would expect improvement in the course of renal osteodystrophy in CAPD patients. Thus far, the results have been conflicting. Tielmans et al [48] found that osteitis fibrosa progressed in 15 patients who were on CAPD for 7 to 28 months. Teitelbaum et al [49] studied six CAPD patients via repeat bone biopsy procedures and found that osteomalacia improved, whereas the osteitis fibrosa worsened. Gokal et al [50] studied 40 CAPD patients dialyzed with a dialysate calcium of 7 mg/dl; they found improvement of both osteomalacia and osteitis fibrosa during the first year. The PTH level declined in three-quarters of the patients. Digenis et al [51] reviewed the radiologic evidence of renal osteodystrophy in 27 patients who had been on CAPD for 3 years or more. According to the radiologic findings at the beginning of the treatment, they divided these 27 (10 males and 17 females) patients into two groups: Group A (10 patients) included those who had no subperiosteal resorption, and group B (17 patients) included those with increased subperiosteal resorption. In group A, the radiologic findings remained normal in eight and progressed in two patients. In group B, subperiosteal resorption remained unchanged or progressed in 14 patients, while it improved in the other three. Plasma PTH levels paralleled the radiologic changes. Of the 27 patients, 7 developed spontaneous fractures that healed with callus formation. Thus, secondary hyperparathyroidism persists in patients on long-term CAPD in our experience; this may be due to a low dialysate calcium and low oral calcium intake.

Abnormalities in Lipid Metabolism

Almost one-half of patients on CAPD develop hypertriglyceridemia, which has been attributed to the large load of glucose (150 to 200 g) absorbed daily from the dialysate.

In a prospective study of the effect of 3 to 6 months on CAPD treatment [52] on serum lipids, we found that patients with high triglycerides before starting CAPD continued to have high levels; in some patients, these levels rose even further. The very low-density lipoprotein (VLDL) cholesterol also increased, whereas high-density lipoprotein (HDL) cholesterol did not change. Serum triglyceride and cholesterol levels remained normal in patients who had normal lipid profiles at the start of CAPD. After 3 to 6 months of CAPD, the HDL cholesterol increased significantly in this group. Lindholm et al [53] also found that the serum lipids remained normal in a large proportion of their CAPD patients. It is difficult to determine whether these lipid abnormalities contribute to either the progression or development of atherosclerotic heart disease, because most of these patients already have this disease. In patients 40 to 59 years of age who had no evidence of angina or myocardial infarction before starting CAPD, 8% and 16% (respectively) developed these stigmata of atherosclerotic heart disease during the first and second year.

These incidences are similar to those observed in patients on chronic hemodialysis [6].

Hypotension and Peripheral Vascular Disease

Continuous ambulatory peritoneal dialysis controls blood pressure so effectively that these patients occasionally develop orthostatic hypotension. Brown et al [54] reported that a drop in both the systemic blood pressure and the already-impaired perfusion of the ischemic limbs could exacerbate symptoms of peripheral vascular disease. It may be necessary to remove patients from CAPD and to allow their blood pressure to increase, so as to alleviate the symptoms of peripheral vascular disease. Leenen et al [55] studied five symptomatic hypotensive CAPD patients before and after oral salt-loading, during which they did not allow a concomitant increase in body weight. The patients received between 85 to 170 mmoles/d of sodium in addition to the original daily intake. Salt-loading lasted 2 to 3 weeks. Supine blood pressure increased markedly after salt-loading, from 94/67 mm Hg to 121/78 mm Hg; and, the symptoms of orthostatic hypotension disappeared. Salt-loading appears to confer its benefits by increasing extracellular fluid volume and sympathetic tone, as assessed by both plasma norepinephrine levels and the pressor responsiveness to norepinephrine.

Causes of Death

Of 257 patients on our CAPD program, 42 had died; 16 died of cardiovascular causes and 10 died suddenly. We believe that most of those patients who died suddenly died of cardiac causes, because most of them had evidence of cardiac abnormalities and none had electrolyte disturbances on routine tests before death. Thus, cardiovascular deaths accounted for more than one-half of the deaths on CAPD. Seven patients died of peritonitis. They either had a *Staphylococcus aureus* infection or fecal peritonitis due to perforation of the viscus. The remaining nine deaths were due to causes such as pancreatitis, withdrawal from dialysis, and malignancies.

Comparison of the Costs of the Various Modes of Dialysis

The most expensive part of any dialysis therapy is the services of medical personnel and equipment. That is why CAPD achieves the most effective reduction in labor costs, because the patient carries out the entire procedure. This mode requires only minimal equipment. The Toronto ESRD Task Force has calculated that (per patient year) CAPD costs much less than center peritoneal dialysis and hemodialysis [56]. It is also cheaper than home hemodialysis [56, 57]. In Toronto (in 1983), CAPD costs $15,000 (Canadian) per patient year compared to $27,000 (Canadian) for center hemodialysis and $18,000 (Canadian) for home hemodialysis. Churchill et al (personal communication), who compared a 32-patient chronic hemodialysis program to a 12-patient CAPD program in 1982, showed that the annual cost for each CAPD patient was about $15,000 (Canadian) less than for patients on center hemodialysis. If the patients had required no hospitalizations, the cost per patient year would have been $40,502 (Canadian) for hemodialysis and $19,786 (Canadian) for CAPD.

Most centers refer patients of advanced age and patients with cardiovascular diseases to the CAPD program, because it achieves a stable hemodynamic and biochemical status. These patients tend to have multiple medical problems, and (hence) require frequent admissions that invariably add to the total cost of CAPD.

Even though CAPD is less expensive than hospital- or facility-based hemodialysis, it still remains relatively expensive; we should continue our efforts to lower the cost of dialysis solutions—the main expense. We can reduce the cost of CAPD by decreasing the frequency of exchanges from four to three per day, using either 2- or 3-liter bags. This modification would lower the total cost of dialysis solution; however, it also would reduce the cost of peritonitis treatment, because the frequency of peritonitis is much lower in patients using three exchanges per day [58]. At a time when economic resources are limited, reducing the cost of renal replacement therapy to a minimum will enable physicians to treat more patients with ESRD.

Conclusion

At this time, CAPD is known to provide adequate removal of metabolic wastes, ameliorates some of the common long-term complications, and restores disturbed physiology towards normal in ESRD. Thus, CAPD is an important treatment for patients with ESRD. While it is the treatment of choice for some patients, it may not be tolerated by others, who will then be maintained on hemodialysis. Centers that cannot provide both hemodialysis and CAPD with equally high standards function under a considerable handicap.

References

1. POPOVICH RP, MONCRIEF JW, DECHERD JP, BOMAR B, PYLE WK: The definition of a novel portable/wearable equilibrium peritoneal dialysis technique (*abstract*). *Trans Am Soc Artif Intern Organs* 5:64, 1976
2. KIDNEY FOUNDATION OF CANADA: *Canadian Renal Failure Register* (*1982 Report*). Ottawa, Ontario, K1V 6M8, pp 75–76
3. WING AJ, BROYER M, BRUNNER FP, BRYNGER H, CHALLAH S, DONCKEREWOLCKE RA, GRETZ N, JACOBS C, KRAMER P, SELWOOD NH: Combined report on regular dialysis and transplantation in Europe, XIII, 1982. *Proc EDTA* 20:5–76, 1983

4. KATIRTZOGLOU A, IZAATT S, OREOPOULOS DG, DOMBROS N, BLAIR GR, CHISHOLM L, MEEMA HE, OGILVIE R, VAS S, LEIBEL B, MCCREEDY W: Chronic peritoneal dialysis in diabetics with end-stage renal failure, in *Diabetic Renal-Retinal Syndrome,* edited by FRIEDMAN EA, L'ESPERANCE FA JR, New York, Grune & Stratton, 1980, pp 317–331

5. FLYNN CT: Why blind diabetics with renal failure should be offered treatment. *Br Med J* 287:1177–1178, 1983

6. WU GG, THE TORONTO COLLABORATIVE DIALYSIS GROUP: Cardiovascular deaths among CAPD patients. *Perit Dial Bull* 3(Suppl 3):23–26, 1983

7. CARDELLA CJ: Renal transplantation in patients on peritoneal dialysis. *Perit Dial Bull* 1:12–14, 1981

8. GOKAL R, RAMOS JM, VEITCH P, PROUD G, TAYLOR RMR, WARD MK, WILKINSON R, KERR DNS: Renal transplantation in patients on CAPD. *Dial Trans* 11:125–155, 1982

9. GUTMAN RA, STEAD WW, ROBINSON RR: Physical activity and employment status of patients on maintenance dialysis. *N Engl J Med* 304:309–313, 1981

10. FRAGOLA JA, GRUBE S, VON BLOCH L, BOURKE E: Multicenter study of physical activity and employment status on continuous ambulatory peritoneal dialysis (CAPD) patients in the United States. *Proc EDTA* 20:243–247, 1983

11. CHURCHILL DN, MORGAN J, TORRANCE GW: Quality of life in endstage renal disease. *Perit Dial Bull* 4:20–22, 1984

12. LEVY NB: Sexual adjustment to maintenance hemodialysis and renal transplantation: National survey by questionnaire, Preliminary report. *Trans Am Soc Artif Intern Organs* 19:138–143, 1973

13. LIM VS, FANG VS: Gonadal dysfunction in uremic men: A study of the hypothalamo-pituitary-testicular axis before and after renal transplantation. *Am J Med* 58:655–662, 1975

14. LIM VS, AULETTA F, KATHPALIA S: Gonadal dysfunction in chronic renal failure: An endocrinologic review. *Dial Transpl* 7:896, 1978

15. PROCCI WR, GOLDSTEIN DA, ADELSTEIN J, MASSRY SG: Sexual dysfunction in the male patient with uremia: A reappraisal. *Kidney Int* 19:317–323, 1981

16. LIM VS, KATHPALIA SC, FROHMAN LA: Hyperprolactinemia and impaired pituitary response to suppression and stimulation in chronic renal failure: Reversal after transplantation. *J Clin Endocrinol Metab* 48:101–107, 1979

17. LIM VS, HENRIQUEZ C, SIEVERTSEN G, FROHMAN LA: Ovarian function in chronic renal failure: Evidence suggesting hypothalamic anovulation. *Ann Intern Med* 93(Part I):21–27, 1980

18. MAHAJAN SK, ABBASI AA, PRASAD AS, RABBANI P, BRIGGS WA, MCDONALD FD: Effect of oral zinc therapy on gonadal function in hemodialysis patients. *Ann Intern Med* 97:357–366, 1982

19. BURTON HJ, KLATT HJ, CONLEY JA, LINDSAY RM, WAI L: Stresses associated with sexual adjustment of end-stage renal disease patients commencing home dialysis: A comparison between hemodialysis and CAPD. *Comtemp Dial* 2:25–30, 1981

20. GALLER M, SPINOWITZ B, CHARYTAN C, KABADI M, FREEMAN R: Reproductive function in dialysis patients: CAPD vs hemodialysis. *Perit Dial Bull* 3(Suppl 1):30–31, 1983

21. KIOKO EM, SHAW KM, CLARKE AD, WARREN DJ: Successful pregnancy in a diabetic patient treated with continuous ambulatory peritoneal dialysis. *Diabetes Care* 6:298–300, 1983

22. RUBIN J: Can a female patient on CAPD become pregnant? (*letter*). *Perit Dial Bull* 1:44, 1981

23. CATTRAN DC, BENZIE RJ: Pregnancy in a continuous ambulatory peritoneal dialysis patient. *Perit Dial Bull* 3:13–14, 1983
24. ALEXANDER SR: Pediatric CAPD update. *Perit Dial Bull* 3(Suppl 4):15–22, 1983
25. BAUM M, POWELL D, CALVIN S, MCDAID T, MCHENRY K, MAR H, POTTER D: Continuous ambulatory peritoneal dialysis in children. *N Engl J Med* 307:1537–1542, 1982
26. BALFE JW: Metabolic effects of CAPD in the child. *Perit Dial Bull* 3(Suppl 3):21–23, 1983
27. KOHAUT EC: Growth in children with end-stage renal disease treated with continuous ambulatory peritoneal dialysis for at least one year. *Perit Dial Bull* 2:159–160, 1983
28. BLUMENKRANTZ MJ, KOPPLE JD, MORAN JK, COBURN JW: Metabolic balance studies and dietary protein requirements in patients undergoing continuous ambulatory peritoneal dialysis. *Kidney Int* 21:849–861, 1982
29. COLE CH, PRICHARD S, WADDELL RW: Increased use of hypertonic dialysate by CAPD patients following repeated episodes of peritonitis. *Perit Dial Bull* 4:6–9, 1984
30. SLINGENEYER A, CANAUD B, MION C: Permanent loss of ultrafiltration capacity of the peritoneum in long-term peritoneal dialysis: An epidemiological study. *Nephron* 33:133–138, 1983
31. FIRST REPORT OF AN INTERNATIONAL COOPERATIVE STUDY: Factors affecting ultrafiltration in continuous ambulatory peritoneal dialysis. *Perit Dial Bull* 4:14–19, 1984
32. LEENEN FHH, SMITH DL, KHANNA R, OREOPOULOS DG: Changes in left ventricular anatomy and function on CAPD. *Perit Dial Bull* 3(Suppl 3):26–27, 1983
33. SPINOWITZ BS, SHERWOOD J, GALLER M, CHARYTAN C: Anemia and oxygen affinity in patients on continuous ambulatory peritoneal dialysis. *Perit Dial Bull* 3(Suppl 1):33–35, 1983
34. CANTALUPPI A, SCALAMOGNA A, CASTELNOVO C, GRAZIANI G, PONTICELLI C: Anemia in CAPD and Hemodialysis (*letter*). *Lancet* 2:1489, 1983
35. DEPAEPE MBJ, KAREL HG, SCHELSTRAETE L, RINGOIR SM, LAMEIRE NH: Influence of continuous ambulatory peritoneal dialysis on the anemia of endstage renal disease. *Kidney Int* 23:744–748, 1983
36. ZAPPACOSTA AR, CARO J, ERSLEV A: Normalization of hematocrit in patients with end-stage renal disease on continuous ambulatory peritoneal dialysis: The role of erythropoietin. *Am J Med* 72:53–57, 1982
37. LAMPERI S, CAROZZI S, ICARDI A: In vitro and in vivo studies of erythropoiesis during CAPD. *Perit Dial Bull* 3:94–96, 1983
38. HEFTI JE, BLUMBERG A, MARTI HR: Red cell survival and red cell enzymes in patients on continuous peritoneal dialysis (CAPD). *Clin Nephrol* 19:232–235, 1983
39. BAILEY GL, HAMPERS CL, HAGER EB, MERRILL JP: Uremic pericarditis. Clinical features in management. *Circulation* 38:582–591, 1968
40. SKOV PE, HANSEN HE, SPENCER ES: Uremic pericarditis. *Acta Med Scand* 186:421–428, 1969
41. MARINI PV, HULL AR: Uremic pericarditis: A review of incidence and management. *Kidney Int* 7(Suppl 2):163–168, 1975
42. MITCHELL AG: Pericarditis during chronic hemodialysis therapy. *Postgrad Med J* 50:741–745, 1974
43. HEGSTROM RM, MURRAY JS, PENDRUS JP, BURNELL JM, SCRIBNER BH: Hemodialysis in the treatment of chronic uremia. *Trans Am Soc Artif Intern Organs* 7:136–152, 1961

44. NOLPH KD: Short dialysis, middle molecules, and uremia. *Ann Intern Med* 86:93–97, 1977

45. LINDHOLM B, TEGNER R, TRANAEUS A, BERGSTROM J: Progress of peripheral uremic neuropathy during continuous ambulatory peritoneal dialysis (CAPD). *Trans Am Soc Artif Intern Organs* 28:263–268, 1982

46. NIELSEN VK: The peripheral nerve function in chronic renal failure. Longitudinal course during terminal renal failure and regular hemodialysis. *Acta Med Scand* 195:155–162, 1974

47. KENNY F: Neurotoxicity, cognitive function and the outcome of CAPD. *Perit Dial Bull* 3(Suppl 3):43–46, 1983

48. TIELMANS C, AUBRY C, DRATWA M: The effects of continuous ambulatory peritoneal dialysis (CAPD) on renal osteodystrophy, in *Advances in Peritoneal Dialysis*, edited by GAHL GM, KESSEL M, NOLPH KD, Amsterdam, Excerpta Medica, 1981, pp 455–460

49. TEITELBAUM S, FALLON MD, GEARING BK, DOUGAN CS, DELMEZ JA: The effects of CAPD on bone histomorphology. *Kidney Int* 21:180, 1982

50. GOKAL R, RAMOO JM, ELLIS HA, PARKINSON I, SWEETMAN V, DEWAR J, WARD MK, KERR DN: Histological renal osteodystrophy and 25 hydroxycholecalciferol and aluminum levels in patients on continuous ambulatory peritoneal dialysis. *Kidney Int* 23:15–21, 1983

51. DIGENIS G, KHANNA R, PIERRATOS A, MEEMA HE, RABINOVICH S, PETTIT J, OREOPOULOS DG: Renal osteodystrophy in patients maintained on CAPD for more than three years. *Perit Dial Bull* 3:81–85, 1983

52. KHANNA R, BRECKENRIDGE C, RONCARI D, DIGENIS G, OREOPOULOS DG: Lipid abnormalities in patients undergoing continuous ambulatory peritoneal dialysis. *Perit Dial Bull* 3(Suppl 1):13–15, 1983

53. LINDHOLM B, KARLANDER SG, NORBECK HE, FURST P, BERGSTROM J: Carbohydrate and lipid metabolism in CAPD patients, in *Peritoneal Dialysis*, edited by ATKINS RC, THOMSON NM, FARREL PC, Edinburgh, Churchill, 1981, pp 147–161

54. BROWN PM, JOHNSTON KW, FENTON SSA, CATTRAN DC: Symptomatic exacerbation of peripheral vascular disease with chronic ambulatory peritoneal dialysis. *Clin Nephrol* 16:258–261, 1981

55. LEENEN FHH, SHAH P, BOER WH, KHANNA R, OREOPOULOS DG: Hypotension on CAPD: An approach to treatment. *Perit Dial Bull* 3(Suppl 3):33–35, 1983

56. BULGIN RH: Comparative costs of various dialysis treatments. *Perit Dial Bull* 1:88–91, 1981

57. GOKAL R, McHUGH M, ROSEMARY F, WARD MK, KERR DN: Continuous ambulatory peritoneal dialysis: One year's experience in a UK dialysis unit. *Br Med J* 281:474–477, 1980

58. KIM D, KHANNA R, WU G, CLATON S, OREOPOULOS DG: Continuous ambulatory peritoneal dialysis with three-liter exchanges: A prospective study. *Perit Dial Bull,* vol 4 (in press, 1984)

Continuous Ambulatory Peritoneal Dialysis in Diabetic Patients

Marcel C. Legrain, Jacques B. Rottembourg, Belkacem Issad, Pierre-Yves Cossette, and Amar Boudjemaa

Continuous ambulatory peritoneal dialysis (CAPD), which is a recent alternative to hemodialysis in the treatment of end-stage renal disease (ESRD), is currently cited as a satisfactory dialysis method for treating insulin and noninsulin-dependent diabetic patients. Even if the reported series are still small with only a short follow-up, recently published data [1–5] clearly outline the advantages and drawbacks of what is an appealing dialysis procedure for treating this group—the only growing category of patients with ESRD in the industrialized countries.

Methods

Among 88 insulin-dependent diabetic (IDD) patients with ESRD treated between January 1978 and December 1983 by dialysis in the department of nephrology at the Hôpital de la Pitie in Paris, 51 patients were selected after August 1978 for treatment by CAPD. This technique was the first choice in 46 patients. The remaining five were transferred from hemodialysis because of ocular complications, (one patient), cardiovascular complications (three patients), and vascular access problems (one patient). Since October 1981, six patients who were unable to handle the CAPD procedure on their own were treated by continuous cycling peritoneal dialysis (CCPD). The data of the six patients on CCPD were included in the CAPD series. As of December 1983, the cumulative duration of treatment was 65.6 patient years, including 8.5 patient years on CCPD. The average duration of treatment per patient was 17.1 ± 11 months (mean ± SD) (range, 1 to 38 months). Fourteen patients were dialyzed for at least 3 years and four for more than 3 years.

This manuscript was presented as part of a symposium on *Continuous Ambulatory Peritoneal Dialysis.*

At the beginning of treatment, there were 27 males and 24 females whose mean age was 52.3 ± SD 13.5 years. The mean age at the time diabetes mellitus was discovered was 29.2 ± 15.2 years. The delay between the discovery of diabetes and the initiation of dialysis was 23.0 ± 17.6 years. The delay between the period when the serum creatinine concentration was 200 ± 50 μmoles/liter (mean ± SD) and the start of treatment by CAPD was 32.2 ± 12.8 months. There have been 35 patients treated with insulin since the discovery of diabetes mellitus; 16 have been treated temporarily with oral antidiabetic drugs. All patients were treated with insulin when dialysis was started.

At the initiation of dialysis therapy, all patients had severe extrarenal complications, including retinopathy in all patients (six of whom were totally blind), hypertension in 48 patients (94%), previous history of myocardial infarction in 26 patients (41%), severe peripheral vascular disease in 30 patients (59%), and clinical peripheral neuropathy in 38 patients (75%).

The CAPD training was performed in a separate unit with its own nursing staff especially devoted to this task. The mean training period lasted 22 days (range, 12 to 32 days). The CAPD was conducted through a double-cuff Tenckhoff catheter with a preferential use of the curled type [7]. The composition of the dialysate and the equipment used have been described previously [8]. Most patients performed four exchanges per day routinely, using three 2-liter bags with a 1.5% dextrose concentration during the daytime and one 2-liter bag with a 4.2 to 4.5% dextrose concentration overnight. The six patients on CCPD were treated with the aid of their relatives using a "cycler" that dispenses three to four 2-liter bags overnight, while 2 liters of 4.5% dextrose dialysis fluid was left in the peritoneal cavity during the daytime [9].

Water and salt intakes were adjusted according to the clinical status of hydration, the residual renal function, and the blood pressure values. Furosemide was administered to 41 patients in doses of 250 to 500 mg/d when dialysis therapy was begun.

Considering both the daily peritoneal absorption of about 100 to 130 g of dextrose and the daily loss of about 10 g of protein through the dialysate effluent, the patients were asked to eat a diet containing about 1.5 g protein per kg of body weight and 150 g/d of carbohydrates.

At home, patients were asked to measure their blood sugar concentration twice per day, once in the morning before breakfast (fasting) and once before supper, using a commercially available "finger-prick" kit (Glucometer®, Ames-Miles Labs, Elkhart, Indiana). Once a month, a series of six readings were made over 24 h, using the same technique. A determination of glycosylated hemoglobin was made every two months while the patient was attending the outpatient clinic.

In 36 of 40 patients treated by CAPD, regular insulin was injected directly into the connecting tubing after drainage of one bag and before installation of the next [6, 10]. The six patients on CCPD were treated twice daily by subcutaneous regular insulin, and once with a mixture of regular and long-acting insulin.

Results

Survival Rates, Cause of Drop-out, Technical Complications, and Hospitalization

The overall patient survival rate and the technical success rate according to age are given in Figure 1. At 2 years, the survival rate for all patients (mean age, 52.3 ± SD 13.5) was 63%. In patients under 50 years of age (mean age, 39 ± SD 8 years), the technique success rate at 2 years is 78%; it is only 50% in those over 50 years (mean age, 61.5 ± SD 8 years). The patient survival rate and technique success rate are almost identical among patients under 50 years of age. The dropout rate, including deaths and transfers, increased with age.

The causes of deaths and transfer are given in Table 1. The main cause of death remained a vascular one. Severe arteritis complicated by gangrene and sepsis and favored by malnutrition were lethal in six patients. Only one death occurring during CAPD was attributed to an acute abdominal complication; in this patient, it was related to the perforation of a sigmoid diverticulum.

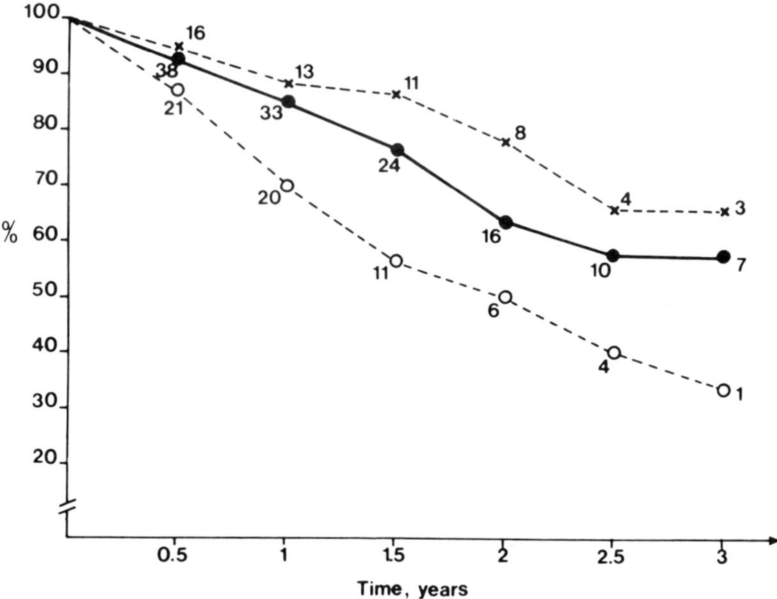

Fig. 1. Patient actuarial survival rate and technique success rate according to the ages of 46 IDD patients treated by continuous peritoneal dialysis from August 1978 to December 1983. (●——●, Patient survival rate, all cases. Technique success rate: x---x, 19 patients under 50 yr [mean age, 39.1 ± 8 yr]; ○--○, 27 patients over 50 yr [mean age, 61.5 ± 8 yr].)

Table 1. IDD patients treated by continuous peritoneal dialysis
(65.6 patient years), cause of transfer and death

Transfer to hemodialysis[a]		Deaths	
Unable to handle the technique	5	Myocardial infarct	3
Recurrent peritonitis	4	Cerebrovascular accident	1
Sclerosing peritonitis	2	Gangrene and sepsis	6
Malnutrition	1	Bowel perforation	1
Bowel perforation	1	Malnutrition	1
Loss of ultrafiltration	1	Liver insufficiency	1
Total	14		13

[a] Three patients died during the 2 mo following transfer.

From the Hôpital de la Pitie, Paris, France.

The causes of transfer differed according to the phase of treatment. Of
our 45 patients, 5 were transferred to hemodialysis during or immediately
after the training period because of the inability of the patient to handle
the technique on his or her own. Later on, transfer usually was attributed
to severe abdominal complications, including recurrent peritonitis, sclerosing
peritonitis, and loss of ultrafiltration; but, also to malnutrition. Three patients
died during hemodialysis within the 2 months following transfer from CAPD.
The causes of death were malnutrition and sepsis. Among the six patients
on CCPD, no death occurred, but one transfer was required because of recurrent peritonitis.

Peritonitis occurred once every 9.6 patient-months. Aseptic peritonitis was
observed in 18 episodes, including nine patients receiving antibiotics for other
reasons. There were 68 episodes that yielded a pathogen: 47 gram-positive,
26 gram-negative, and 5 fungi. Since October 1981, all cases of peritonitis
have been treated at home with intraperitoneal administration of antibiotics
without lavage [11]. Nevertheless, frequent consultations in our specialized
outpatient unit were required for clinical and bacteriologic controls during
the treatment of the peritonitis episodes [3]. Eight peritoneal catheters had
to be changed because of recurrent peritonitis in three patients, tunnel infection in one case, skin exit infection in two patients, and dislodgement in
two patients.

The duration of the in-hospital training period was $25 \pm$ SD 5 days. Patients
were subsequently hospitalized 23 ± 17 (mean $\pm$ SD) d/yr in the first year
of treatment and 18 ± 8 (mean $\pm$ SD) in the second year. The main causes
of hospitalization were, above all, severe abdominal complications and social-
familial factors, particularly in the elderly group. Most patients were already
retired when dialysis was initiated, but seven other patients were able to
maintain a professional occupation.

Main Clinical and Biologic Parameters

Results obtained are summarized in Table 2. A tendency to gain weight
was observed during the first years of dialysis, although to an extremely

Table 2. Evolution of major clinical and biologic parameters in IDD patients treated by CAPD

Months	0 to 1	6	12	24	30	36
Patients, N	46	37	31	14	8	4
Weight (kg)	63.6 ± 13.9	65.6 ± 12.4	66.9 ± 13.4	61.1 ± 9.5	62.4 ± 7.5	63.5 ± 6.
Blood pressure (mm Hg)						
Systolic	173 ± 42	150 ± 30	149 ± 30	146 ± 32	139 ± 32	137 ± 28
Diastolic	96 ± 27	85 ± 14	86 ± 17	83 ± 16	81 ± 16	89 ± 13
Diuresis (ml/day)	1060 ± 350	880 ± 320	680 ± 360	700 ± 350	650 ± 280	550 ± 300
Residual C_{cr} (ml/min)	4.3 ± 2.5	3.9 ± 2.8	3.8 ± 2.1	3.4 ± 2.7	3.2 ± 2.1	3.3 ± 1.
Peritoneal C_{cr} (ml/min)	—	4.6 ± 1.0	4.6 ± 1.3	4.4 ± 1.3	4.6 ± 1.5	4.7 ± 1.4
Protein losses (g/d)	—	10.7 ± 1.2	10.8 ± 1.5	9.8 ± 2.5	9.7 ± 2.6	9.9 ± 2.6
Serum hemoglobin (g%)	8.8 ± 2.2	11.1 ± 1.8	11.4 ± 1.8	10.3 ± 1.6	10.1 ± 1.9	10 ± 2
Serum albumin (g/liter)	33 ± 6	32 ± 5	32 ± 5	30 ± 5	30 ± 3	29 ± 4
Serum creatinine (μmoles/liter)	890 ± 230	741 ± 233	830 ± 243	861 ± 229	871 ± 134	887 ± 114
Serum uric acid (μmoles/liter)	650 ± 160	451 ± 110	455 ± 87	413 ± 74	405 ± 90	440 ± 70
Serum bicarbonate (mmoles/liter)	21 ± 4	25 ± 3	25 ± 3	25 ± 3	25 ± 2	25 ± 2
Serum calcium (mmoles/liter)	2.16 ± 0.50	2.31 ± 0.22	2.31 ± 0.18	2.21 ± 0.15	2.26 ± 0.12	2.27 ± 0.10
Serum phosphorus (mmoles/liter)	1.9 ± 0.8	1.6 ± 0.5	1.6 ± 0.5	1.6 ± 0.4	1.6 ± 0.4	1.5 ± 0.4
Serum alk Phosphatase (IU/liter)	108 ± 60	104 ± 60	113 ± 70	107 ± 53	129 ± 47	131 ± 60
Serum cholesterol (mmoles/liter)	5.8 ± 1.8	6.2 ± 1.3	6.3 ± 1.7	5.9 ± 1.9	6.1 ± 1.8	5.9 ± 1.4
Serum triglycerides (mmoles/liter)	2.6 ± 1.5	2.9 ± 1.7	3.0 ± 1.8	2.4 ± 1.9	2.0 ± 1.9	2.1 ± 0.8

varying degree on the individual level. After 6 months on CAPD, control of hypertension was obtained in most patients, although slightly more than 50% were still receiving antihypertensive drugs. In a few patients with major autonomic neurologic disorders, severe postural hypotension could be observed; and, it was increased when rapid ultrafiltration was induced by using high-dextrose concentration dialysate.

Residual Renal Function

Persisting residual renal function, although decreasing very slowly with time, was still detectable at least until the third year (see Table 2). A creatinine clearance (C_{cr}) between 3 to 4 ml/min was present in at least two-thirds of the patients. All patients with a persisting residual renal function were receiving furosemide orally.

Failing a randomized study, one cannot appreciate the exact value played by the oral administration of furosemide in such a situation.

Peritoneal Clearances

These include urea, phosphorus, and creatinine clearances, as well as protein losses in the peritoneal effluent (around 10 g/d); they remained stable during the period of observation. Loss of ultrafiltration requiring transfer to hemodialysis was observed in only one patient.

Evolution of Major Blood Parameters

From the initiation of dialysis treatment to the 36th month, these parameters are summarized in Table 2. After a sharp increase during the first month of treatment, hemoglobin levels stabilized around 10 g/liter. Despite permanent peritoneal protein losses, serum albumin levels remained around 30 g/liter after the first year. Serum creatinine and uric acid concentrations stabilized, respectively, around 900 and 400 μmoles/liter. Major serum electrolytes, including serum bicarbonate, remained in the normal range. Satisfactory calcium and phosphorus values were observed, although most patients were no longer taking aluminum phosphate binders. Nevertheless, a mild elevation of serum alkaline phosphatase around 115 U/liter (normal range, 30 $\pm$ 85 U/liter) was observed routinely. Cholesterol and triglycerides were elevated moderately throughout the observation period.

Blood Glucose Control and Nutrition

In 36 patients treated exclusively with CAPD by using the technique of injection of insulin into the connecting tube before instillation of the dialysis

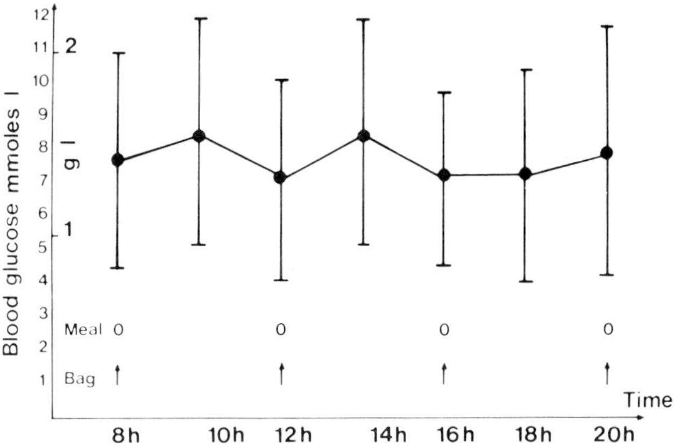

Fig. 2. Daily blood glucose concentrations in IDD patients on CAPD who are receiving insulin administered into the connecting tube four times per day before meals and instillation of dialysate; 132 serial daily studies in 21 patients.

fluid, on the average, 15 to 20 U of regular insulin were needed with the 1.5% dextrose concentration and 30 to 40 U with the 4.5% concentration. The mean total daily dose of administered insulin was 86 ± 32 U. The average total daily dose of insulin was commonly two to three times the pre-CAPD dose. The dose of regular insulin that was administered is either increased or decreased by 2 to 4 U to obtain a fasting blood glucose concentration around 7 mmoles/liter and also to avoid 2-hr postprandial sugar concentrations over 11 mmoles/liter. Such an objective is achieved routinely as shown in Figure 2. During peritonitis episodes, daily insulin doses were increased markedly. A clinical episode of acute ketosis never occurred during this study period. Hypoglycemia was seldom encountered, except when patients developed malnutrition and/or peritoneal infection. The mean serum glycosylated hemoglobin, Hb A1c, measured during the last year in 22 patients treated by CAPD for at least 1 year was 8.7 ± 1.3%.

Adequate nutrition was difficult to maintain in some diabetic patients with autonomic neuropathy that led to gastroenteropathy with nausea, vomiting, and diarrhea. Recurrent peritonitis leading to high protein losses was the main cause of severe and rapidly progressive hypoalbuminemia.

Visual Status

Sight was evaluated at start of treatment and after at least 6 months on CAPD (range, 6 to 38 months) in 31 patients. An improvement was observed in 14 patients, while aggravation was observed in 5 patients. Deterioration was due to vitreous hemorrhage and/or fibrosis and macula edema.

Peripheral Vascular Disease

During the period of observation, 11 of 46 patients required 23 amputations exclusively in the lower limbs, including 5 toes, 5 forefeet, 12 legs at different levels, and 1 thigh. Diffuse necrotic skin lesions were observed in four patients.

Neurologic Status

Clinical peripheral neuropathy, related to both diabetes and uremia, was present in 38 cases (75%) at the start of treatment. The peroneal nerve conduction velocity was 35.9 ± SD 5.8 meters/sec in 40 patients and was not measurable in 6 cases. In 14 patients at 12 years, the values were 36.3 ± SD 6.5 meters/sec in 12 cases and were not measurable in 2 patients.

Discussion

During the past 5 years, it has been well demonstrated that CAPD can offer excellent control of both uremia and blood glucose concentrations in insulin- and noninsulin-dependent diabetic patients with ESRD [1, 6, 12]. For these reasons, many institutions have selected CAPD since 1978 as a first-choice mode of home dialysis for diabetic patients with terminal uremia; the number of patients treated by CAPD is increasing regularly [13]. Nevertheless, an even wider application of the method has been limited by two major drawbacks. Some patients cannot handle the technique. Even if a special training program offers motivated blind patients an opportunity to take care of themselves successfully [12], partial or total blindness (a frequent complication associated with ESRD in diabetic patients) is a real barrier to the use of CAPD when the patient is in charge of his or her own treatment. The second limitation remains the high dropout rate in relation to the severe and sometimes lethal abdominal complications [14] induced by the technique.

However, the most recent results [2, 15] obtained with CAPD can compete very favorably with those obtained in a diabetic population of the same age that is treated not only by hemodialysis and intermittent peritoneal dialysis [15–18], but also by transplantation—with the only exception represented by the excellent graft survival rate when using a living related donor [19, 20].

The dropout rate including deaths and transfer (Table 1) is influenced largely by age, which is the major risk factor. In our series, the technical success rate at 2 years on CAPD was 78% for patients under 50 years of age, and only 50% for those over 50 years (see Fig. 1). The main cause of death was vascular in origin (Table 1), including severe arteritis complicated by gangrene and sepsis. Practically the only cause of transfer to other dialysis methods that was related to the CAPD procedure was either the inability to handle the technique or severe peritoneal complications, including bowel perforation, recurrent peritonitis, sclerosing peritonitis, or loss of ultrafiltration.

Excellent clinical status with good control of blood pressure, satisfactory values for major biologic parameters, and good nutritional conditions (see Table 2) were obtained routinely in many patients on CAPD during a four-exchange program that included only one 2-liter bag with 4.2 or 4.5% dextrose concentration. Adequate diet and good control of the glucose concentration avoided major lipid disorders. The persistence of a residual renal function with a C_{cr} between 3 to 4 ml/min in most of our patients, at least until the third year, was a major contributing factor to the feeling of well-being of the patients [10]; and it was a true advantage in comparison with what was observed among patients either on hemodialysis or intermittent peritoneal dialysis [3, 17]. In our series, the duration of hospitalization for both social and medical reasons was larger than in a nondiabetic population, but it was similar in both the hemodialyzed and the CAPD groups [3].

The best argument in favor of treating IDD patients with CAPD is the opportunity offered to the patient to administer insulin via the intraperitoneal route—a simple and efficient form of artificial pancreas [6, 12, 21] with excellent control of blood glucose concentrations (Fig. 2). The injection of insulin either into the dialysate bag or into the line [6, 21] is favored by most patients. In our experience, as in other series [1, 5, 6], the use of the intraperitoneal route to administer insulin does not significantly increase the rate of peritonitis. However, the average total daily dose of insulin is commonly two to three times the pre-CAPD dose, partly because of absorption of insulin to the material and losses in the dialysate effluent.

Abdominal complications remain the major drawback of the method and the first cause of the dropout rate (see Table 1). Although the peritonitis rate among diabetic patients is not superior to what is observed in a nondiabetic population [1, 3, 12], acute peritonitis is still a concern. Peritonitis may lead to severe complications in relation to a perforated bowel, to the organism involved such as fungi, or to frequent recurrences contributing to malnutrition through anorexia and high protein losses in the peritoneal effluent. Recently, unusual complications such as sclerosing peritonitis and decreased ultrafiltration [14, 22–24] have been reported in both diabetic and nondiabetic patients. Such complications seem to increase with time and can be observed with or without a past history of recurrent peritonitis. An acetate buffer has been suggested by epidemiologic studies [23, 25, 26] to be a contributing—although not exclusive—risk factor. The presence of a very low rate of such complications among patients using a dialysate from one brand with a lactate buffer is encouraging, and it allows already adequate prevention. However, the permanence of the quality of the peritoneal membrane in patients treated by CAPD for many years remains a challenging question.

In diabetic patients, mainly in the elderly, malnutrition can easily occur favored by protein losses in the dialysate effluent and gastroenteropathy that leads to nausea, vomiting, and diarrhea. Severe weight losses can be masked by a positive sodium balance and by overhydration. This situation requires the administration of nutriment in large amounts and the adjustment of insulin doses. Adequate control of water electrolyte balance often is difficult because of severe thirst. Hospitalization in an intensive care unit may be required. If transfer to other form of dialysis (mainly hemodialysis) is considered, the decision should not be made too late to avoid an irreversible situation leading to death in the months following transfer.

Vascular complications remain the main cause of death among diabetic patients treated by all forms of renal replacement therapy, including CAPD. Besides cardiac and cerebral vascular accidents, one must emphasize the severity of some peripheral vascular diseases leading to gangrene and (in some cases) to death via sepsis. The CAPD method has been considered to be a contributing factor to the acceleration of peripheral vascular disease [27]. In fact, a high rate of amputation (around 20 to 25%) among diabetic patients is observed with all dialysis methods [3] and after transplantation [19, 20]. Adequate prevention seems possible through an early foot care program. High caloric intake, sometimes through the venous route, is required to avoid septic complications if major surgery is required. Stabilization and (in some cases) radical improvement of the visual status of diabetic patients can be expected during CAPD. Peripheral nerve conduction velocity was stabilized in all of our patients treated for at least 2 years.

Exclusion of diabetic patients from treatment no longer is acceptable when the therapeutic facilities are available [28–30]. Thus, CAPD should be one of the choices.

An integrated CAPD-transplantation program could become the preferred supportive treatment for the juvenile diabetic patient. The CAPD method does not jeopardize the chance of successful transplantation, and it can be used in the postoperative period to control uremia if required, as illustrated by the experience of different groups [1, 31]. However, we have considered that CAPD should not exclude the use of other forms of dialysis. A free and informed choice between hemodialysis, either in the center or at home, and other forms of peritoneal dialysis should be offered to juvenile patients.

Although tedious precautions are required to avoid peritoneal infection, CAPD offers a unique opportunity to treat elderly diabetic patients at home. However, in this older age group, many patients will never handle the technique on their own due to social and medical reasons; and, we do not like to impose the burden of the daily exchange of bags on their families. For such patients, intermittent peritoneal dialysis (IPD) or CCPD should be available. They reduce the risk of peritonitis, compared to CAPD [9, 17], and diminish the technical burden of the dialysis procedure for the patient and/or the family—the machine or the cycler doing the dialysis during the night.

In conclusion, at least for some diabetic patients, CAPD offers the best mode of treatment; however, all modes should be made available to provide each patient with a free choice and to allow early transfer if required.

References

1. AMAIR P, KHANNA R, LEIBEL B, PIERRATOS A, VAS S, MEEMA E, BLAIR G, CHISHOLM L, VAS M, ZINGG W, DIBENIS G, OREOPOULOS D: Continuous ambu-

latory peritoneal dialysis in diabetics with end stage renal disease. *N Engl J Med* 306:625–630, 1982

2. KHANNA R, WU G, CHISHOLM L, OREOPOULOS D: Up date: Further experience with CAPD in diabetics with end stage renal disease. *Diabetic Nephrop* 2:8–12, 1983

3. LEGRAIN M, ROTTEMBOURG J, BENTCHIKOU A, POIGNET JL, ISSAD B, BARTHELEMY A, STRIPPOLI P: Dialysis treatment of insulin dependent diabetic patients. A ten year experience. *Clin Nephrol* 21:72–81, 1984

4. LAMEIRE N, DHAENE M, MATTHITS E, DE PAEPE M, VEREERSTRAETEN P, DRAWTA M, RINGOIR S: Experience with CAPD in diabetic patients, in *Prevention and Treatment of Diabetic Nephropathy,* edited by KEEN H, LEGRAIN M, Lancaster, MTP Ltd, 1983, pp 289–297

5. MADDEN MA, ZIMMERMAN S, SIMPSON DP: Continuous ambulatory peritoneal dialysis in diabetes mellitus. *Am J Nephrol* 2:133–139, 1982

6. ROTTEMBOURG J, EL SHAHAT Y, AGRAFIOTIS A, THUILLIER Y, DE GROC F, JACOBS C, LEGRAIN M: Continuous ambulatory peritoneal dialysis in insulin dependent diabetics: A 40 month experience. *Kidney Int* 23:40–45, 1983

7. ROTTEMBOURG J, JACQ D, VONLANTHEN M, ISSAD B, EL SHAHAT Y: Straight or curled Tenckhoff peritoneal catheter for continuous ambulatory peritoneal dialysis. *Perit Dial Bull* 1:123–124, 1981

8. RENAUX C, CERTAIN B, MOLLET M, ROTTEMBOURG J: La dialyse peritoneale continue ambulatoire: II Materiel, technique, formation. *Nouv Presse Med* 9:3154–3157, 1980

9. DIAZ-BUXO JA, WALKER PJ, FARMER CD, CHANGLER JT, HOLT KL, COX P: Continuous cyclic peritoneal dialysis. *Trans Am Soc Artif Intern Organs* 27:51–53, 1981

10. ROTTEMBOURG J, ISSAD B, POIGNET JL, STRIPPOLI P, BALDUCCI A, SLAMA G, GAHL G: Residual renal function and control of blood glucose levels in insulin-dependent diabetic patients treated by CAPD, in *Prevention and Treatment of Diabetic Nephropathy,* edited by KEEN H, LEGRAIN M, Lancaster, MTP Ltd, 1983, pp 339–352

11. DE GROC F, ROTTEMBOURG J, JACQ D, JARLIER V, N'GUYEN J, LEGRAIN M: Les péritonites au cours de la dialyse péritonéale continue ambulatoire. Traitement par lavage ou non. Etude prospective. *Nephrologie* 4:24–27, 1983

12. FLYNN C: The diabetic on CAPD, in *Diabetic Renal Retinal Syndrome* (vol 2), edited by FRIEDMAN E, L'ESPERANCE F, New York, Grune & Stratton, 1982, pp 320–330

13. JACOBS C, BRUNNER F, BRYNGER H, CHALLAH S, KRAMER P, SELWOOD N, WING A: The first five thousand diabetics treated by dialysis and transplantation in Europe. *Diabetic Nephrop* 2:11–16, 1983

14. ROTTEMBOURG J, GAHL GM, POIGNET J, MERTANI E, STRIPPOLI P, LANGLOIS P, TRANBALOC P, LEGRAIN M. Severe abdominal complications in patients undergoing continuous ambulatory peritoneal dialysis. *Proc Europ Dial Transpl Assoc* 20:236–242, 1983

15. KJELLSTRAND C, COMTY C, SHAPIRO F: A comparison of dialysis and transplantation in insulin dependent diabetic patients, in *Diabetic Renal Retinal Syndrome* (vol 2), edited by FRIEDMAN E, L'ESPERANCE F, New York, Grune & Stratton, 1982, pp 405–417

16. KJELLSTRAND C, WHITLEY K, COMTY C, SHAPIRO F: Dialysis in patients with diabetes mellitus. *Diabetic Nephrop* 2:5–17, 1983

17. MION C, SLINGENEYER A, CANAUD B, OULES R, BRANGER G, CHONG M, MOURAD G: Home intermittent peritoneal dialysis in the treatment of end-stage diabetic nephropathy. 1982 Update, in *Prevention and Treatment of Diabetic Ne-*

phropathy, edited by KEEN H, LEGRAIN M, Lancaster, MTP Ltd, 1983, pp 263–277

18. SHAPIRO FL: Haemodialysis in diabetic patients, in *Prevention and Treatment of Diabetic Nephropathy,* edited by KEEN H, LEGRAIN M, Lancaster, MTP, Ltd, 1983, pp 247–259

19. BRYNGER H, LARSSON O, ATTMAN PO, FRISK B, LUNDBERG M, MULEC M, SANDBERG L: Selection principles and outcome of renal transplantation in diabetics, in *Prevention and Treatment of Diabetic Nephropathy,* edited by KEEN H, LEGRAIN M, Lancaster, MTP Ltd, 1983, pp 213–217

20. SUTHERLAND D, FRYD DS, SIMMONS RL, FERGUSON RM, NAJARIAN JS: Current status of kidney transplantation in uremic diabetics at the University of Minnesota, in *Diabetic Renal Retinal Syndrome* (vol 2), edited by FRIEDMAN E, L'ESPERANCE F, New York, Grune & Stratton, 1982, pp 373–383

21. BALDUCCI A, SLAMA G, ROTTEMBOURG J, BAUMELOU A, DELAGE A: Intraperitoneal insulin in uraemic diabetics undergoing continuous ambulatory peritoneal dialysis. *Br Med J* 283:1021–1023, 1981

22. FALLER B, MARICHAL JF: Loss of ultrafiltration in CAPD: Clinical data, in *Advances in Peritoneal Dialysis,* edited by GAHL GM, KESSEL M, NOLPH K, Amsterdam, Excerpta Medica, 1981, pp 227–232

23. SLINGENEYER A, CANAUD B, MION C: Permanent loss of ultrafiltration capacity of the peritoneum in long term peritoneal dialysis: an epidemiological study. *Nephron* 3:133–138, 1983

24. SLINGENEYER A, MION C, MOURAD G, CANAUD B, FALLER B, BERAUD JJ: Progressive sclerosing peritonitis: a late and severe complication of maintenance peritoneal dialysis. *Trans Am Soc Art Intern Organs* 29:633–640, 1983

25. FALLER B, MARICHAL JF: Loss of ultrafiltration in continuous ambulatory peritoneal dialysis: a role for acetate. *Perit Dial Bull* 4:10–13, 1984

26. AN INTERNATIONAL COOPERATIVE STUDY: Factors affecting ultrafiltration in continuous ambulatory peritoneal dialysis. First report. *Perit Dial Bull* 4:14–19, 1984

27. BROWN PM, JONSTON KW, FENTON SSA, CATTRAN DC: Symptomatic exacerbation of peripheral vascular disease with chronic ambulatory peritoneal dialysis. *Clin Nephrol* 16:258–261, 1981

28. AVRAM MM: Diabetic renal failure. *Nephron* 31:285–290, 1982

29. FRIEDMAN E: Diabetic nephropathy. Strategies in prevention and management. *Kidney Int* 21:780–791, 1982

30. LEGRAIN M, ROTTEMBOURG J, GAHL G, BENTCHIKOU A, STRIPPOLI P: The treatment of renal failure in diabetic patients. The best buy, in *Prevention and Treatment of Diabetic Nephropathy,* edited by KEEN H, LEGRAIN M, Lancaster, MTP Ltd, 1983, pp 361–376

31. RYCKELYNCK JP, VERGER C, PIERRE D, SABATIER JC, FALLER B, BEAUD JM: Early post-transplantation infections in CAPD patients. *Perit Dial Bull* 4:40–41, 1984

Long-Term Metabolic Consequences of Continuous Ambulatory Peritoneal Dialysis

Bengt Lindholm, Anders Alvestrand, Hans Erik Norbeck, Anders Tranaeus, and Jonas Bergström

Continuous ambulatory peritoneal dialysis (CAPD) has been established as a viable alternative to intermittent peritoneal dialysis (IPD). While awaiting results concerning the long-term effects of CAPD, many centers have also accepted CAPD as a tentative alternative to intermittent hemodialysis. Since metabolic abnormalities and malnutrition are common among uremic patients, an essential part of the evaluation of CAPD is to clarify its metabolic long-term consequences.

Following the preliminary experiences with CAPD in the late 1970s, several favorable effects were reported. The patients appeared to thrive, they were well-controlled (with regard to urea, creatinine, electrolytes, acid-base equilibrium and fluid balance), and their body weight and hematocrit was increased [1–4]. These effects, which suggested an anabolic state, were attributed to the continuous dialytic process and to effective removal of uremic middle-sized molecules.

On the other hand, several potentially harmful metabolic factors were identified [5]. The removal of small nitrogenous waste products is inferior to that obtained with hemodialysis. Protein, amino acids, and other vital substances are lost into the dialysate. The continuous supply of glucose and lactate or acetate from the dialysate represents a sizeable and perhaps undesirable energy load that may induce or accentuate hyperglycemia, hyperinsulinemia, hypertriglyceridemia, and other metabolic abnormalities. Another concern was that some patients appeared to have an inadequate nutritional intake.

In this chapter, we will review the available literature, as well as report on some preliminary results concerning the effects of CAPD on carbohydrate, lipid, and protein metabolism in nondiabetic adult patients.

This manuscript was presented as part of a Symposium on *Continuous Ambulatory Peritoneal Dialysis*.

Results and Discussion

Effects of the Peritoneal Energy Supply on Carbohydrate Metabolism

The continuous absorption of glucose from the dialysate represents a unique situation that is not encountered in any other clinical condition. Most patients absorb between 100 to 200 g/24 hr of glucose (on the average, 70 to 75% of supplied amounts); the amount taken up depends on the quantity of glucose supplied per day in the dialysate and the rate of absorption [6–12]. In addition, 20 to 30 g of lactate is absorbed [12, 13]. The absorption of glucose increases during peritonitis [9, 14]. The absorption of glucose has been reported to increase over time in patients who have used dialysates containing acetate; in most patients, however, the absorption of glucose seems to be stable during long-term treatment [15, 16].

A major concern with CAPD is that the continuous supply of glucose may aggravate abnormalities in carbohydrate metabolism that are present in uremia. These abnormalities are characterized by glucose intolerance; often with normal fasting blood glucose, normal or elevated insulin levels, and raised circulating levels of glucagon and growth hormone [17]. The combination of glucose intolerance and normal or elevated insulin levels has been attributed to a decreased sensitivity of peripheral tissues to the action of insulin [18, 19].

During CAPD, a single dialysis cycle with hypertonic dialysate (anhydrous dextrose, 3.86 g/dl), blood glucose, and circulating insulin levels increases to peak values within 60 min, while the elevated glucagon levels decrease only slightly [6, 11, 13, 20–22]. These changes are similar to those observed after an oral glucose load in uremic patients, although an intraperitoneal supply of glucose has been reported to result in a more marked hyperglycemia and in a more long-lasting hyperinsulinemia than when the same amount of glucose is given orally [22].

A potential hazard with CAPD is that the intraperitoneal glucose load might exhaust the secretory capacity of the pancreatic beta cells. Indeed, a deterioration in insulin response has been reported in a few patients [23], and some patients may become insulin-dependent de novo during CAPD [24, 25]; this has occurred in 5 of our 110 CAPD patients (unpublished observation of the authors). However, in the majority of the patients, there is no further deterioration of glucose intolerance during long-term treatment; and, insulin and glucagon responses to an oral glucose load remain abnormal, but they are not altered during CAPD [12, 26, 27]. Thus, with the possible exception of individual subjects, CAPD patients do not become insulin-deficient.

By contrast, there is a constant tendency in CAPD patients towards hyperglycemia along with hyperinsulinemia, although exchanges with isotonic dialysates have only a marginal effect on blood glucose and insulin levels [13, 23]. This tendency is reflected by increased plasma C-peptide levels, as well as by an increased ratio between C-peptide and insulin in CAPD patients compared to hemodialysis patients; this indicates a continuously increased production of proinsulin [22]. Also, CAPD has been reported to be associated with raised levels of the gluconeogenic precursor lactate [13].

Since the sustained hyperinsulinemia may possibly increase atherogenesis [28], the elevated circulating insulin levels—rather than the apparently small de novo incidence of insulin-dependent diabetes mellitus—constitute a potential risk factor during long-term treatment with CAPD. Furthermore, the glucose load may lead to several other undesirable effects, such as lipid abnormalities and suppression of the spontaneous dietary intake of energy and protein (see below).

However, it should be pointed out that the peritoneal supply of energy is advantageous in patients with a compromised dietary intake as well as during acute illnesses such as peritonitis, in which case the energy demand is markedly increased [9, 29]. Dietary protein is better used when a nonprotein caloric source is provided simultaneously and when the continuous supply of glucose serves as an important source of nonprotein energy promoting nitrogen use [6, 30]. Moreover, insulin is an anabolic hormone; therefore, the stimulation of the pancreatic beta cell release of insulin may promote anabolism.

Protein Losses and Serum Proteins

The reported average losses of protein into the dialysate in CAPD vary between 5 to 15 g in different studies, with large interindividual differences [10, 15, 30–37]. Albumin accounts for 32 to 87% of protein loss [32, 34, 37]. Protein losses are mainly determined by the permeability of the peritoneum [34, 35]. During peritonitis, the losses usually increase considerably, and they may remain increased for several weeks [14, 34]. Dialysate protein losses are stable during long-term treatment [15, 33, 36, 38]; however, the combined urine and dialysate protein losses may actually fall over time [39].

During episodes of peritonitis, serum albumin levels sometimes may fall below 25 g/liter [40]; otherwise, few patients develop severe hypoproteinemia during long-term treatment with CAPD. On the contrary, most patients maintain stable serum levels of total protein, which are low to normal or slightly reduced [10, 15, 33, 36, 37]. Serum transferrin and C3 levels may increase to normal during the initial months of CAPD treatment [30, 36]. Kaysen et al have reported that plasma albumin mass, total albumin mass, and the distribution of albumin are normal in CAPD patients; and, that albumin homeostasis is maintained through decreased catabolism and increased synthesis of albumin [37].

Amino Acid Losses and Plasma Concentrations

While the protein losses during CAPD are unparalleled in hemodialysis, the losses of free amino acids into the dialysate during CAPD are of the same magnitude (per week) as with hemodialysis. The average dialysate loss of free amino acids during CAPD has been reported to be 1.2 to 3.4 g/24 hr [10, 23, 41–45]. Although peritoneal transport characteristics may differ between different amino acids [46], the main determinants of amino acid losses are plasma amino acid concentrations and the volume of dialysate outflow per 24 hr [41, 45, 46].

Although the losses of amino acids into the dialysate are too small to account for any major derangements, plasma amino acid concentrations are not restored to normal in CAPD patients. Kopple et al found that the sum of plasma essential and amino acid concentrations as well as the sum of nonessential and total amino acid concentrations was normal; however, valine, leucine, and serine were decreased and several amino acids were elevated [41]. In addition, others have reported: (1) decreased levels of lysine, threonine, tyrosine, and taurine, (2) a decreased sum of essential amino acids, (3) decreased ratios between valine and glycine and between tyrosine and phenylalanine, and (4) an increased ratio between glycine and serine [10, 23, 30, 42, 43, 45, 47, 48]. These abnormalities are commonly observed in untreated uremic patients; therefore, they probably reflect the metabolic and nutritional derangements of uremia, rather than depletion due to dialysate amino acid losses. In addition, the reduced plasma amino acid concentrations may, to some extent, reflect the sustained hyperinsulinemia during CAPD [45, 49] all the more, as insulin resistance of uremia patients does not involve the insulin effect on amino acids [50].

Plasma amino acid concentrations in uremic patients do not necessarily reflect the intracellular concentrations [51]. Therefore, we have investigated the intracellular concentrations of free amino acids in skeletal muscle tissue, which contains the largest pool of free amino acids. Our preliminary results in CAPD patients [48] show decreased plasma concentrations of most amino acids; however, aspartic acid, asparagine, glutamic acid, and citrulline were elevated. In muscle, the intracellular concentrations of tyrosine and taurine were markedly reduced, while the concentrations of lysine, asparagine, aspartic acid, glutamic acid, and citrulline were increased. Valine was low in plasma, but it was not significantly reduced in muscle. Since the intracellular muscle concentration of valine is markedly reduced in muscle in untreated uremic patients [52], our results suggest that this complication of uremia is relatively well controlled by CAPD. By contrast, the typically high citrulline concentrations observed in uremic plasma and muscle are not influenced by CAPD.

The low intracellular pools of taurine and tyrosine indicate depletion of these amino acids in CAPD patients [48]. Taurine has become increasingly acknowledged as a factor involved in the functional regulation of many organ systems [53]; tyrosine may be essential and limiting for protein synthesis in uremia [52]. Therefore, therapy with taurine and tyrosine may possibly be indicated in CAPD patients with muscle fatigue and protein depletion.

Protein and Energy Requirements

There are several signs indicating net anabolism in CAPD patients during the first year of treatment. The average increase in their body weight may exceed 5 kg without any clinical signs indicating fluid overload [10, 25, 33, 39]. Total body potassium also increases, and the increase is positively correlated to the weight gain [36, 39, 54]. Anthropometric measurements, including measurements of mid-arm muscle circumference and skinfold thickness, have shown stable values or slight improvements [15, 39]. Serum transferrin levels often rise and albumin homeostasis is well maintained through increased synthesis and decreased catabolism of albumin (see above). The hematocrit and hemoglobin levels usually increase during the initial months of treatment [33, 55–58].

Furthermore, several studies have shown that nitrogen equilibrium can be maintained or that positive nitrogen balance be achieved during the first year of CAPD treatment [30, 44, 59–63]. The daily protein intake of patients in these studies varied between 0.7 to 2.1 g/kg body wt. Nitrogen balance has been found to be positively correlated to both protein intake [30, 63] and the total energy intake [30]. Some patients with an intake of less than 1 g/kg body wt and 1 g/d of protein exhibited a clearly positive nitrogen balance [30, 44, 62, 63]. Nitrogen balance correlated with changes in body weight, indicating that the retention of nitrogen was associated with an increase in lean body mass with buildup of body protein [30, 60]. These results confirm early speculations [2, 3] that anabolism can be achieved with CAPD. However, the results also emphasize the important role of an adequate nutrition for improvement of metabolic status of CAPD patients.

The above-mentioned metabolic studies were of relatively short duration, and they comprised only stable patients during their first year on CAPD. Various factors, particularly an inadequate nutrition and frequent episodes of peritonitis, may negatively affect the long-term nitrogen balance. Peritonitis is associated with markedly negative nitrogen balance [30, 64]; and, in patients with a high incidence of peritonitis, total body potassium [54] as well as anthropometric measurements may show an impairment over time [15].

Nutritional problems may arise during CAPD because of an inadequate nutritional intake. Several studies have shown a decreased intake of both protein and total energy over time [21, 27, 36, 39, 65]. The average nutritional intake during the initial months on CAPD has been reported to exceed 1.2 g/kg body wt and 1 g/d of protein and total energy intake (including absorption of dialysate glucose) to exceed 150 kJ/kg body wt and 150 kJ/d [30, 36, 39, 65]. However, individual patients may have considerably lower initial intakes [12, 30, 62]. After about 1 year on CAPD, the average dietary protein intake has been reported to fall to about 1 g/kg and 1 g/d and average total energy intake to fall to about 125 kJ/kg and 125 kJ/d [27, 36, 39, 65]. Although some patients may exhibit a positive nitrogen balance with this relatively low nutritional intake (see above), it may be inadequate for the majority of the patients during long-term treatment.

The reduced nutritional intake during CAPD seems to be caused by a decrease in appetite. The dietary protein intake has been reported to decrease in patients after transfer from hemodialysis to CAPD; concomitantly, it increases in patients on transfer from CAPD to hemodialysis [66]. This suggests that the appetite is suppressed by factors related to CAPD; for example, due to absorption of dialysate glucose or abdominal distension by the dialysis fluid [12, 21, 67, 68]. Another explanation is that CAPD patients may become underdialyzed. Anorexia due to insufficient dialysis is a well-known complication in patients undergoing IPD [29]. A dietary protein intake over a certain level may become incompatible with the amount of dialysis during CAPD; if the total renal and peritoneal solute excretion falls (for example, due to a decrease in residual renal function), the patients may develop uremic symptoms, including anorexia [29]. Thus, it is possible that decreasing dietary intakes during CAPD may reflect anorexia due to both inadequate dialysis and a spontaneous dietary adaptation to a gradual decrease of the residual renal function over time.

Despite the protein loss into the dialysate and the relatively low and decreasing dietary intake of protein and energy, there are few reports of clinically overt malnutrition in CAPD patients. Only a few patients seem to develop severe hypoproteinemia [25, 38, 40] or other signs of protein-energy malnutrition [65]. However, indirect evidence of a gradual deterioration of the nutritional status of CAPD patients has emerged from prospective measurements of total body nitrogen by Oreopoulos et al [21, 36, 39]. The authors report that total body nitrogen decreases over time, during the initial 2 years of CAPD treatment, concomitantly with a stable nitrogen output and a decreasing protein intake. By contrast, body weight and total body potassium increased significantly in the same patients. The authors conclude that the increase of body weight and total body potassium may reflect an increase of intracellular water, while the combination of a stable nitrogen output and a declining protein intake result in a long-term negative nitrogen balance—which is reflected by decreasing total body nitrogen levels. The same group has reported that the use of amino acid-containing dialysates over 4 weeks in CAPD patients resulted in significantly increased total body nitrogen [47].

Lipid Abnormalities During CAPD

Uremic patients demonstrate several signs of a deranged lipid metabolism that are most obviously reflected in both the uremic dyslipoproteinemia [69, 70] and the altered fatty acid composition ofbody fat [71].

These abnormalities seem to occur early in the course of progressive chronic renal failure; and, except for transitory alterations during each hemodialysis session [72], they are only marginally affected by hemodialysis treatment [70, 73]. Although most of the etiology and much of the pathophysiology are unclear, evidence has been provided for both an increased hepatic production and an impaired removal of circulating triglyceride-rich VLDL-particles [73, 74].

The uremic dyslipoproteinemia share several similarities with both the type 3 and type 4 hyperlipoproteinemia [70, 75, 76]. The lipoprotein abnormalities include: (1) an increased concentration of lipids concurrently with a relative cholesterol enrichment of very low-density lipoproteins (VLDL), (2) an increased concentration and a relative enrichment of triglycerides in low-density lipoproteins (LDL), (3) a decreased concentration of cholesterol in high-density lipoproteins (HDL), and (4) an accumulation of an electrophoretic subclass of VLDL—late prebeta lipoproteins—which are thought to represent triglyceride-depleted remnants of VLDL and/or chylomicrons [69, 70, 73, 75]. These changes usually result in elevated serum triglycerides, whereas serum cholesterol often is normal. The different fatty esters in the body are composed of an increased proportion of saturated fatty acids, while the content of the essential fatty acid-linoleic acid is abnormally low [71].

Many of the described abnormalities, including the increased frequency of late prebeta lipoproteins and the low content of linoleic acid in fatty esters, are thought to promote arteriosclerosis [71, 75]. Among the etiologic factors of type 4 hyperlipidemia, an excessive supply of carbohydrates and derangements of glucose metabolism (including hyperinsulinemia and peripheral insulin resistance) may lead to an increased hepatic production of triglycerides [77–81]. Since these factors are present in CAPD patients, one may anticipate a further deterioration of their lipid status during CAPD.

A hyperlipidemic effect of CAPD has indeed been confirmed in several studies; however, the results differ considerably between different reports due to large interindividual variations, varying energy intakes, and fluctuations of serum lipids over time in the individual patient [8, 9, 25, 27, 40, 60, 82–89]. Nevertheless, the results may be summarized as follows. At the start of CAPD, many patients are hypertriglyceridemic, while most have normal serum cholesterol levels. During the first year of CAPD, both serum triglycerides and serum cholesterol usually increase, at least during the initial months of treatment. These changes are due to concurrently increased concentrations of these lipids in VLDL and LDL fractions. A significant rise of HDL cholesterol has been reported in some studies [86, 87], but the changes in HDL usually are less marked. Although some patients may develop very high triglyceride concentrations [83, 89], the changes of this variable often fail to reach statistical significance due to large interindividual differences in responses to CAPD. By contrast, cholesterol levels (in serum, VLDL, and LDL) usually increase significantly, although only about 20 to 30% of the patients are reported to develop hypercholesterolemia de novo [89].

The magnitude of the changes seems to be very dependent on individual reactions to the treatment, indicating important differences among the patients in lipoprotein metabolism [82]. Thus, the fractional removal rate of (exogenous) triglycerides from the blood (k_2) during intravenous (i.v.) fat tolerance tests, as well as the changes of k_2 during the treatment, vary considerably between the patients (unpublished observation of the authors). We have found that patients with stable or decreasing triglyceride levels after 1 year on CAPD often show an increase of k_2 values, while patients with continuously increasing triglycerides often "fail" to improve the fractional removal rate of exogenous triglycerides [83]. This suggests that a metabolic adaptation in some patients may prevent the development of increasing triglyceride levels [27]. However, the average fractional removal rate of triglycerides does not change significantly during the first year of CAPD [83, 85].

Another factor that may explain differences in circulating lipid levels between patients, and within individual patients over time, is the varying energy intake of the patients. Many centers recommend to their patients a restricted use of hypertonic dialysates, as well as a decreased dietary energy intake. These interventions seem to effectively reduce the development of hypertriglyceridemia; however, cholesterol levels still increase significantly [84, 85, 89]. By contrast, our patients are allowed a free use of hypertonic dialysates and a free diet. This may explain why we (and not others) have found a positive correlation between serum triglyceride levels and the amount of dialysate glucose supplied per day [83].

Several studies have shown that the changes in serum lipid concentrations during CAPD are transitory, except in a small group of patients with steadily increasing concentrations. Peak levels of serum cholesterol and triglycerides usually are reached within 3 to 12 months, with a subsequent fall during the following months to pretreatment levels [27, 88, 89]. This may indicate a metabolic adaptation to the treatment, but it also may be due to changes in energy intake over time [27]. Other factors, such as a decreasing use of beta-adrenergic blocking agents, among the patients over time also may play a role.

Although CAPD seems to induce potentially atherogenic alterations, especially during the initial months of treatment, the uremic dyslipoproteinemia remains essentially unchanged after 1 year compared to pretreatment status; again, with the exception of a small group of patients in whom serum triglyceride levels increase significantly [27, 40, 89]. In fact, lipid levels after 1 year of dialysis treatment are approximately the same in hemodialysis and CAPD patients [90]; CAPD patients may even show better (less reduced) HDL cholesterol levels than hemodialysis patients [91].

However, a certain concern is that the ratios between LDL and HDL cholesterol, as well as the ratios between VLDL plus LDL cholesterol and HDL cholesterol (which are considered to be atherogenic indices), increase significantly during the first year of treatment (unpublished observation of the authors).

Results from adipose tissue biopsy specimens show an increase of mean adipocyte diameters during the initial year on CAPD (unpublished observation of the authors). However, few patients become obese [25, 40]; instead, the body weights gradually return to levels recorded prior to the onset of renal failure [15].

The de novo incidence of cardiovascular diseases during CAPD has been reported to be similar to that reported on hemodialysis; and, serum lipid levels do not seem to discriminate between CAPD patients with and without these complications [92]. However, the mortality rates of CAPD patients are still high despite an excellent control of hypertension [93]. Furthermore, the long-term effects of increased serum lipids during CAPD are still uncertain, because the dropout rate from CAPD is high [89]. While awaiting the results of further studies, it seems prudent to evaluate the effects of various therapeutic approaches, such as a restricted use of hypertonic dialysates, attempts to replace glucose with other osmotic agents, lipid-lowering drugs including L-carnitine, dietary modification, and exercise [21, 85, 94–97].

Summary and Concluding Observations

Carbohydrate Metabolism

Despite the continuous peritoneal absorption of 100 to 200 g/d of glucose, few CAPD patients become insulin-dependent de novo; this may be due to an increased peripheral resistance to the action of insulin, especially in obese CAPD patients (unpublished observation of the authors). Thus, the glucose intolerance remains essentially unchanged in most patients, and the treatment does not seem to lead to an exhaustion of the pancreatic beta cells. Instead, there is a tendency towards constantly elevated serum insulin levels, especially in patients who frequently use the most hypertonic dialysis solutions. The peritoneal glucose load and the sustained hyperinsulinemia promote anabolism, but they may also lead to an increased atherogenesis.

Lipid Metabolism

The uremic dyslipoproteinemia persists during CAPD. It usually is worsened during the initial months of the treatment, and the changes—including increased concentrations of both serum triglycerides and cholesterol—are partly related to the peritoneal glucose load. However, the hyperlipidemic effect of CAPD seems to be transitory in most patients. This may indicate a metabolic adaptation to the glucose load and/or reflect changes in the nutritional intakes of the patients. However, some patients develop a severe hypertriglyceridemia, and some develop hypercholesterolemia de novo. Dietary interventions, as well as a decreased use of the most hypertonic dialysates, seem to effectively reduce the development of increasing serum triglycerides; however, these interventions may result in inadequate energy intakes (see below). The CAPD method induces certain potentially atherogenic alterations, but the patients do not appear to have an increased de novo incidence of cardiovascular diseases compared to hemodialysis patients.

Serum Proteins and Amino Acids

Despite heavy protein losses (about 5 to 15 g/24 hr) in the dialysate, most CAPD patients maintain only slightly reduced serum protein levels. The losses of free amino acids are about 15 to 30 g/wk and are approximately equivalent to losses reported in hemodialysis and IPD patients. The CAPD patients exhibit amino acid abnormalities that are similar to those observed in other uremic patients. Several patients had markedly reduced muscle intracellular concentrations of taurine and tyrosine, which may indicate depletion and a need for specific supplementation of these amino acids. By contrast, muscle intracellular valine concentrations were not significantly reduced.

Protein and Energy Requirements in CAPD

Several signs indicate a stable or improving nutritional status of CAPD patients during the initial year of treatment. Nitrogen balance studies have demonstrated nitrogen equilibrium or positive nitrogen balance; nitrogen balance was positively correlated with body weight increases, dietary protein intake, and total energy intake. During long-term treatment, few patients seem to develop clinically overt protein-energy malnutrition—except during bouts of severe peritonitis when patients may become markedly catabolic. However, a major concern is that nutritional intakes gradually decrease over time. In addition, one group has reported a gradual decrease of total body nitrogen during the initial 2 years of CAPD treatment; however, this finding is difficult to explain, because body weights as well as total body potassium increased in the same patients.

During long-term treatment with CAPD, many patients had dietary protein intakes below 1.2 g/kg body wt and 1.2 g/d and, perhaps more surprisingly, total energy intakes that fell below the recommended level of 150 kJ/kg body wt and 150 kJ/d. Although this cannot a priori be taken for granted as being harmful, it emphasizes the importance of prospective metabolic and nutritional studies in CAPD patients, and it gives reasons for attempts to improve nutritional intakes; for example, by supplementation of amino acids via the peritoneal dialysis solutions or by mouth.

Acknowledgment. This work has been supported by the National Institutes of Health, Grant No. RO1-AM-27519.

References

1. MONCRIEF JW, NOLPH KD, RUBIN J, POPOVICH RP: Additional experience with continuous ambulatory peritoneal dialysis (CAPD). *Trans Am Soc Artif Intern Organs* 14:476–483, 1978
2. NOLPH KD, POPOVICH RP, MONCRIEF JW: Theoretical and practical implications of continuous ambulatory peritoneal dialysis. *Nephron* 21:117–122, 1978
3. POPOVICH RP, MONCRIEF JW, NOLPH KD, GHODS AJ, TWARDOWSKI ZJ, PYLE WK: Continuous ambulatory peritoneal dialysis. *Ann Intern Med* 88:449–456, 1978
4. OREOPOULOS DG, ROBSON M, IZATT S, CLAYTON S, DE VEBER GA: A simple and safe technique for continuous ambulatory peritoneal dialysis (CAPD). *ASAIO* 24:484–489, 1978
5. BERGSTRÖM J: Potential metabolic problems associated with continuous ambulatory peritoneal dialysis, in *Continuous Ambulatory Peritoneal Dialysis,* edited by LEGRAIN M, Amsterdam, Excerpta Medica, 1980, pp 277–282
6. DE SANTO NG, CAPODICASA G, SENATORE R, CICCHETTI T, CIRILLO D, DAMIANO M, TORELLA R, GIUGLIANO D, IMPROTA L, GIORDANO C: Glucose utilization from dialysate in patients on continuous ambulatory peritoneal dialysis (CAPD). *Int J Artif Organs* 2:119–124, 1979
7. GRODSTEIN GP, BLUMENKRANTZ MJ, KOPPLE JD, MORAN JK, COBURN JW: Glucose absorption during continuous ambulatory peritoneal dialysis. *Kidney Int* 19:564–567, 1981

8. KEUSCH G, BAMMATTER F, MORDASINI R, BINSWANGER U: Serum lipoprotein concentrations during continuous ambulatory peritoneal dialysis (CAPD), in *Advances in Peritoneal Dialysis,* edited by GAHL GM, KESSEL M, NOLPH KD, Amsterdam, Excerpta Medica, 1981, pp 427–429

9. LINDHOLM B, KARLANDER SG, NORBECK HE, FÜRST P, BERGSTRÖM J: Carbohydrate and lipid metabolism in CAPD patients, in *Peritoneal Dialysis,* edited by ATKINS R, THOMSON N, FARRELL P, Edinburgh, Churchill Livingstone, 1981, pp 198–210

10. RANDERSON DH, CHAPMAN GV, FARRELL PC: Amino acid and dietary status in CAPD patients, in *Peritoneal Dialysis,* edited by ATKINS R, THOMSON N, FARRELL P, Edinburgh, Churchill Livingstone, 1981, pp 179–191

11. SPLENDIANI G, ACITELLI S, ALBANO V, GIANFORTE A, TANCREDI M: Metabolic aspects of CAPD, in *Advances in Peritoneal Dialysis,* edited by GAHL GM, KESSEL M, NOLPH KD, Amsterdam, Excerpta Medica, 1981, pp 449–451

12. VON BAEYER H, GAHL GM, RIEDINGER H, BOROWZAK R, AVERDUNK R, SCHURIG R, KESSEL M: Adaptation of CAPD patients to the continuous peritoneal energy uptake. *Kidney Int* 23:29–34, 1983

13. HEATON A, JOHNSTON DG, BURRIN JM, ORSKOV H, WARD MK, ALBERTI KGMM, KERR DNS: Carbohydrate and lipid metabolism during continuous ambulatory peritoneal dialysis (CAPD): the effect of a single dialysis cycle. *Clin Sci* 65:539–545, 1983

14. RUBIN J, RAY R, BARNES T, BOWER J: Peritoneal abnormalities during infectious episodes of continuous ambulatory peritoneal dialysis. *Nephron* 29:124–127, 1981

15. RUBIN J, KIRCHNER K, BARNES T, TEAL N, RAY R, BOWER JD: Evaluation of continuous ambulatory peritoneal dialysis. *Am J Kidney Dis* 3:199–204, 1983

16. NOLPH KD, RYAN L, MOORE RH, LEGRAIN M, MION C, OREOPOULOS DG: Factors affecting ultrafiltration in continuous ambulatory peritoneal dialysis. *Perit Dial Bull* 4:14–19, 1984

17. DEFRONZO RA, ANDRES R, EDGAR P, WALKER WG: Carbohydrate metabolism in uremia: A review. *Medicine* 52:469–481, 1973

18. WESTERVELT FB, SCHREINER GE: The carbohydrate intolerance of uremic patients. *Ann Intern Med* 57:266–276, 1962

19. DEFRONZO RA, ALVESTRAND A, SMITH D, HENDLER R, HENDLER E, WAHREN J: Insulin resistance in uremia. *J Clin Invest* 67:563–568, 1981

20. ARMSTRONG VW, FUCHS C, SCHELER F: Biochemical studies on patients undergoing continuous ambulatory peritoneal dialysis. *Klin Wochenschr* 58:1065–1069, 1980

21. OREOPOULOS DG, MARLISS E, ANDERSON GH, OREN A, DOMBROS N, WILLIAMS P, KHANNA R, RODELLA H, BRANDES L: Nutritional aspects of CAPD and the potential use of amino acid containing dialysis solutions. *Perit Dial Bull* 3:10–15, 1983

22. WIDERÖE TE, SMEBY LC, MYKING OL: Plasma concentrations and transperitoneal transport of native insulin and C-peptide in patients on continuous ambulatory peritoneal dialysis. *Kidney Int* 25:82–87, 1984

23. ARMSTRONG VW, BUSCHMANN U, EBERT R, FUCHS C, RIEGER J, SCHELER F: Biochemical investigations of CAPD: plasma levels of trace elements and amino acids and impaired glucose tolerance during the course of treatment. *Int J Artif Organs* 3:237–241, 1980

24. DE FREMONT JF, BATAILLE P, MORINIERE P, KACZMARECK P, FIEVET P, FOURNIER A: Metabolic tolerance of continuous ambulatory peritoneal dialysis (CAPD), in *Advances in Peritoneal Dialysis,* edited by GAHL GM, KESSEL M, NOLPH KD, Amsterdam, Excerpta Medica, 1981, pp 446–448

25. KURTZ SB, WONG VH, ANDERSON CF, VOGEL JP, MCCARTHY JT, MITCHELL

JC: Continuous ambulatory peritoneal dialysis. Three years' experience at the Mayo Clinic. *Mayo Clin Proc* 58:633–639, 1983

26. LINDHOLM B, BERGSTRÖM J, KARLANDER SG: Glucose metabolism in patients on continuous ambulatory peritoneal dialysis (CAPD). *Trans Am Soc Artif Intern Organs* 17:58–60, 1981

27. LINDHOLM B, KARLANDER SG, NORBECK HE, BERGSTRÖM J: Hormonal and metabolic adaptation to the glucose load of CAPD in nondiabetic patients, in *Prevention and Treatment of Diabetic Nephropathy,* edited by KEEN H, LEGRAIN M, Boston, MTP Ltd, 1983, pp 353–359

28. STOUT RW: The relationship of abnormal circulating insulin levels to atherosclerosis. *Atherosclerosis* 27:1–13, 1977

29. BLUMENKRANTZ MJ, SCHMIDT RW: Managing the nutritional concerns of the patient undergoing peritoneal dialysis, in *Peritoneal Dialysis,* edited by NOLPH KD, The Hague, Martinus Nijhoff Publishers, 1981, pp 275–308

30. LINDHOLM B, ALVESTRAND A, FÜRST P, TRANAEUS A, BERGSTRÖM J: Efficacy and clinical experience of CAPD—Stockholm, Sweden, in *Peritoneal Dialysis,* edited by ATKINS R, THOMSON N, FARRELL P, Edinburgh, Churchill Livingstone, 1981, pp 147–161

31. GAHL GM, SCHURIG R, BECKER H, SORGE F, PUSTELNIK A, BOROWZAK B, RIEDINGER R, VON BAEYER H, KESSEL M: Clinical and metabolic aspects of continuous ambulatory peritoneal dialysis (CAPD). *Int J Artif Organs* 3:245–249, 1980

32. KATIRTZOGLOU A, OREOPOULOS DG, HUSDAN H, LEUNG M, OGILVIE R, DOMBROS N: Reappraisal of protein losses in patients undergoing continuous ambulatory peritoneal dialysis. *Nephron* 26:230–233, 1980

33. NOLPH KD, SORKIN M, RUBIN J, ARFANIA D, PROWANT B, FRUTO L, KENNEDY D: Continuous ambulatory peritoneal dialysis: Three-year experience at one center. *Ann Intern Med* 92:609–613, 1980

34. BLUMENKRANTZ MJ, GAHL GM, KOPPLE JD, KAMDAR AV, JONES MR, KESSEL M, COBURN JW: Protein losses during peritoneal dialysis. *Kidney Int* 19:593–602, 1981

35. RUBIN J, NOLPH KD, ARFANIA D, PROWANT B, FRUTO L, BROWN P, MOORE H: Protein losses in continuous ambulatory peritoneal dialysis. *Nephron* 28:218–221, 1981

36. HEIDE B, PIERRATOS A, KHANNA R, PETTIT J, OGILVIE R, HARRISON J, MCNEIL K, SICCION Z, OREOPOULOS DG: Nutritional status of patients undergoing continuous ambulatory peritoneal dialysis (CAPD). *Perit Dial Bull* 3:138–141, 1983

37. KAYSEN GA, SCHOENFELD PY: Albumin homeostasis in patients undergoing continuous ambulatory peritoneal dialysis. *Kidney Int* 25:107–114, 1984

38. RANDERSON DH, FARRELL PC: Clinical assessment of CAPD. *Dial Transpl* 10:389–398, 1981

39. WILLIAMS P, KAY R, HARRISON J, MCNEIL K, PETTIT J, KELMAN B, MENDEZ M, KLEIN M, OGILVIE R, KHANNA R, CARMICHAEL D, OREOPOULOS D: Nutritional and anthropometric assessment of patients on CAPD over one year: Contrasting changes in total body nitrogen and potassium. *Perit Dial Bull* 1:82–87, 1981

40. THOMSON NM, ATKINS RC, HUMPHREY TJ, AGAR JM, SCOTT DF: Continuous ambulatory peritoneal dialysis (CAPD): An established treatment for endstage renal failure. *Aust NZ J Med* 13:489–496, 1983

41. KOPPLE JD, BLUMENKRANTZ MJ, JONES MR, MORAN JK, COBURN JW: Plasma amino acid levels and amino acid losses during continuous ambulatory peritoneal dialysis. *Am J Clin Nutr* 36:395–402, 1982

42. GIORDANO C, DE SANTO NG, CAPODICASA G, DI LEO VA, DI SERAFINO A, CIRILLO D, ESPOSITO R, FIORE R, DAMIANO M, BUONADONNA L, COCCO F, DI IORIO B: Amino acid losses during CAPD. *Clin Nephrol* 14:230–232, 1980

43. FÜRST P, BERGSTRÖM J, LINDHOLM B: Studies of amino-acid metabolism in continuous ambulatory peritoneal dialysis patients—preliminary results, in *Continuous Ambulatory Peritoneal Dialysis,* edited by LEGRAIN M, Amsterdam, Excerpta Medica, 1980, pp 292–297

44. VON BAEYER H, GAHL GM, RIEDINGER H, BOROWZAK B, KESSEL M: Nutritional behaviour of patients on continuous ambulatory peritoneal dialysis. *Proc EDTA* 18:193–198, 1981

45. DOMBROS N, OREN A, MARLISS EB, ANDERSON GH, STEIN AN, KHANNA R, PETTIT J, BRANDES L, RODELLA H, LEIBEL BS, OREOPOULOS D: Plasma amino acid profiles and amino acid losses in patients undergoing CAPD. *Perit Dial Bull* 2:27–32, 1982

46. DE SANTO NG, CAPODICASA G, DI LEO VA, DI SERAFINO A, CIRILLO D, ESPOSITO R, FIORE R, CUCCINIELLO E, DAMIANO M, BUONADONNA L, DI IORIO R, CAPASSO G, GIORDANO C: Kinetics of amino acids equilibration in the dialysate during CAPD. *Int J Artif Organs* 4:23–30, 1981

47. OREN A, WU G, ANDERSON GH, MARLISS E, KHANNA R, PETTIT J, MUPAS L, RODELLA H, BRANDES L, RONCARI DA, KAKIS G, HARRISON J, MCNEIL K, OREOPOULOS DG: Effective use of amino acid dialysate over four weeks in CAPD patients. *Perit Dial Bull* 3:66–73, 1983

48. LINDHOLM B, BERGSTRÖM J, ALVESTRAND A: Muscle free amino acids in patients treated with CAPD (*abstract*). *Third International Symposium on Peritoneal Dialysis,* Washington, DC, 1984

49. MARTIN-DU PAN R, MAURON C, GLAESER B, WURTMAN RJ: Effect of various oral glucose doses on plasma neutral amino acid levels. *Metabolism* 31:937–943, 1982

50. DEFRONZO RA, SMITH D, ALVESTRAND A: Insulin action in uremia. *Kidney Int* 24:S102–S114, 1983

51. BERGSTRÖM J, FÜRST P, NOREE LO, VINNARS E: Intracellular free amino acids in muscle tissue of patients with chronic uraemia: effect of peritoneal dialysis and infusion of essential amino acids. *Clin Sci Mol Med* 54:51–60, 1978

52. ALVESTRAND A, FÜRST P, BERGSTRÖM J: Plasma and muscle free amino acids in uremia: influence of nutrition with amino acids. *Clin Nephrol* 18:297–305, 1982

53. HAYES KC: Taurine in metabolism. *Ann Rev Nutr* 1:401–425, 1981

54. RUBIN J, FLYNN MA, NOLPH KD: Total body potassium—a guide to nutritional health in patients undergoing continuous ambulatory peritoneal dialysis. *Am J Clin Nutr* 34:94–98, 1981

55. KHANNA R, OREOPOULOS DG, DOMBROS N, VAS S, WILLIAMS P, MEEMA HE, HUSDAN H, OGILVIE R, ZELLERMAN G, RONCARI DAK, CLAYTON S, IZATT S: Continuous ambulatory peritoneal dialysis (CAPD) after three years: Still a promising treatment. *Perit Dial Bull* 1:24–34, 1981

56. SUMMERFIELD GP, GYDE OHB, FORBES AMW, GOLDSMITH HJ, BELLINGHAM AJ: Haemoglobin concentration and serum erythropoietin in renal dialysis and transplant patients. *Scand J Haematol* 30:389–400, 1983

57. DE PAEPE MBJ, SCHELSTRAETE KGH, RINGOIR SMG, LAMEIRE NH: Influence of continuous ambulatory peritoneal dialysis on the anemia of endstage renal disease. *Kidney Int* 23:744–748, 1983

58. ZAPPACOSTA AR, CARO J, ERSLEV A: Normalization of hematocrit in patients with end-stage renal disease on continuous ambulatory peritoneal dialysis. The role of erythropoietin. *Am J Med* 72:53–57, 1982

59. GIORDANO C, DE SANTO NG, PLUVIO M, DI LEO VA, CAPODICASA G, CIRILLO D, ESPOSITO R, DAMIANO M: Protein requirement of patients on CAPD: a study on nitrogen balance. *Int J Artif Organs* 3:11–14, 1980
60. LINDHOLM B, ALVESTRAND A, FÜRST P, KARLANDER SG, NORBECK HE, AHLBERG M, TRANAEUS A, BERGSTRÖM J: Metabolic effects of continuous ambulatory peritoneal dialysis. *Proc EDTA* 17:283–289, 1980
61. BRZOSTOWICZ M, SCHOENFELD P, KAYSEN G, MAPES D, NEWHOUSE Y, PIERCY L, HUMPHREYS M: Continuous ambulatory peritoneal dialysis (CAPD): Nitrogen balance is maintained or improved during initiation of therapy (*abstract*). *13th Annual Meeting, American Society of Nephrology* 1980, p 37A
62. GAHL GM, VON BAEYER H, AVERDUNK R, RIEDINGER H, BOROWZAK B, SCHURIG R, BECKER H, KESSEL M: Outpatient evaluation of dietary intake and nitrogen removal in continuous ambulatory peritoneal dialysis. *Ann Intern Med* 94:643–646, 1981
63. BLUMENKRANTZ MJ, KOPPLE JD, MORAN JK, COBURN JW: Metabolic balance studies and dietary protein requirements in patients undergoing continuous ambulatory peritoneal dialysis. *Kidney Int* 21:849–864, 1982
64. GRODSTEIN GP, BLUMENKRANTZ MJ, KOPPLE JD: Nutritional and metabolic response to catabolic stress in uremia. *Am J Clin Nutr* 33:1411–1416, 1980
65. RANDERSON DH, FARRELL PC: Metabolite generation and clearance variation in long-term CAPD, in *CAPD Update,* edited by MONCRIEF JW, POPOVICH RP, New York, Masson Publishing, Inc, 1981, pp 75–81
66. FARREL PC, RANDERSON DH: Comparison of CAPD with HD and IPD, in *Advances in Peritoneal Dialysis,* edited by GAHL GM, KESSEL M, NOLPH KD, Amsterdam, Excerpta Medica, 1981, pp 131–137
67. LINDHOLM B, AHLBERG M, ALVESTRAND A, FÜRST P, KARLANDER SG, BERGSTRÖM J: Nutritional aspects of continuous ambulatory peritoneal dialysis, in *Continuous Ambulatory Peritoneal Dialysis,* edited by LEGRAIN M, Amsterdam, Excerpta Medica, 1980, pp 199–206
68. GAHL GM, VON BAEYER H, RIEDINGER R, BOROWZAK B, SCHURIG R, BECKER H, KESSEL M: Caloric intake and nitrogen balance in patients undergoing CAPD, in *CAPD Update,* edited by MONCRIEF JW, POPOVICH RP, New York, Masson Publishing, Inc, 1981, pp 87–93
69. NORBECK HE, ORÖ L, CARLSON LA: Serum lipid and lipoprotein concentrations in chronic uremia. *Acta Med Scand* 200:487–492, 1976
70. NORBECK HE, CARLSON LA: The uremic dyslipoproteinemia: Its characteristics and relations to clinical factors. *Acta Med Scand* 209:489–503, 1981
71. NORBECK HE, WALLDIUS G: Fatty acid composition of serum and adipose tissue lipids in males with chronic renal failure. *Acta Med Scand* 211:75–85, 1982
72. NORBECK HE, OLSSON AG: Effect of intravenous heparin on serum lipoproteins with special reference to VLDL late pre-beta lipoprotein in uremic man, in *Chemistry and Biology of Heparin,* edited by LUNDBLAD RL, BROWN WV, MANN KG, ROBERTS HR, Amsterdam, Elsevier North Holland, Inc, 1981, pp 217–223
73. NORBECK HE: Serum lipoproteins in chronic renal failure (*thesis*). *Acta Med Scand* 649(Suppl):1–49, 1981
74. NORBECK HE, RÖSSNER S: Intravenous fat tolerance test with intralipid in chronic renal failure. *Acta Med Scand* 211:69–74, 1982
75. NORBECK HE, CARLSON LA: Increased frequency of late pre-beta lipoproteins (LP-beta) in isolated serum very low density lipoproteins in uraemia. *Eur J Clin Invest* 10:423–426, 1980
76. NORBECK HE: Lipoprotein metabolism in chronic renal failure, in *Lipoproteins and Coronary Atherosclerosis,* edited by NOSEDA G, FRAGIACOMO C, FUMAGALLI R, PAOLETTI R, Amsterdam, Elsevier Biomedical Press BV, 1982, pp 337–342

77. OLEFSKY JM, FARQUHAR JW, REAVEN GM: Reappraisal of the role of insulin in hypertriglyceridemia. *Am J Med* 57:551–560, 1974
78. SORGE F, CASTRO LA, NAGEL A, KESSEL M: Serum glucose, insulin, growth hormone, free fatty acids and lipids responses to high carbohydrate and to high fat isocaloric diets in patients with chronic, non-nephrotic renal failure. *Horm Metab Res* 7:118–127, 1975
79. SANFELIPPO ML, SWENSON RS, REAVEN GM: Response of plasma triglycerides to dietary change in patients on hemodialysis. *Kidney Int* 14:180–186, 1978
80. OKUBO M, TSUKAMOTO Y, YONEDA T, HOMMA Y, NAKAMURA H, MARUMO F: Deranged fat metabolism and the lowering effect of carbohydrate-poor diet on serum triglycerides in patients with chronic renal failure. *Nephron* 25:8–14, 1980
81. COULSTON AM, LIU GC, REAVEN GM: Plasma glucose, insulin and lipid responses to high-carbohydrate low-fat diets in normal humans. *Metabolism* 32:52–56, 1983
82. LINDHOLM B, BERGSTRÖM M, NORBECK HE: Lipoprotein (LP) metabolism in patients on continuous ambulatory peritoneal dialysis (CAPD), in *Advances in Peritoneal Dialysis,* edited by GAHL GM, KESSEL M, NOLPH KD, Amsterdam, Excerpta Medica, 1981, pp 434–436
83. LINDHOLM B, KARLANDER SG, NORBECK HE, BERGSTRÖM J: Glucose and lipid metabolism in peritoneal dialysis, in *Peritoneal Dialysis,* edited by LA GRECA G, BIASIOLI S, RONCO C, Milano, Wichtig Editore, 1982, pp 219–230
84. GOKAL R, RAMOS JM, MCGURK JG, WARD MK, KERR DNS: Hyperlipidaemia in patients on continuous ambulatory peritoneal dialysis, in *Advances in Peritoneal Dialysis,* edited by GAHL GM, KESSEL M, NOLPH KD, Amsterdam, Excerpta Medica, 1981, pp 430–433
85. TURGAN C, FEEHALLY J, BENNETT S, DAVIES TJ, WALLS J: Accelerated hypertriglyceridemia in patients on continuous ambulatory peritoneal dialysis—A preventable abnormality. *Int J Artif Organs* 4:158–160, 1981
86. RONCARI DAK, BRECKENRIDGE WC, KHANNA R, OREOPOULOS DG: Rise in high-density lipoprotein-cholesterol in some patients treated with CAPD. *Perit Dial Bull* 1:136–137, 1981
87. BRECKENRIDGE WC, RONCARI DAK, KHANNA R, OREOPOULOS DG: The influence of continuous ambulatory peritoneal dialysis on plasma lipoproteins. *Atherosclerosis* 45:249–258, 1982
88. KHANNA R, BRECKENRIDGE C, RONCARI D, DIGENIS G, OREOPOULOS DG: Lipid abnormalities in patients undergoing continuous ambulatory peritoneal dialysis. *Perit Dial Bull* 3(Suppl):S13–S15, 1983
89. RAMOS JM, HEATON A, MCGURK JG, WARD MK, KERR DNS: Sequential changes in serum lipids and their subfractions in patients receiving continuous ambulatory peritoneal dialysis. *Nephron* 35:20–23, 1983
90. NORBECK HE, LINDHOLM B: Long term effects of peritoneal versus hemodialysis on serum lipoproteins (*abstract*). *Eur J Clin Invest* 12:29, 1982
91. CHAN MK, BAILLOD RA, CHUAH P, SWENY P, RAFTERY MJ, VARGHESE Z, MOORHEAD JF: Three years' experience of continuous ambulatory peritoneal dialysis. *Lancet* I:1409–1412, 1981
92. KHANNA R, WU G, VAS S, OREOPOULOS DG: Mortality and morbidity on continuous ambulatory peritoneal dialysis. *ASAIO J* 6:197–204, 1983
93. WU G, ET AL: Cardiovascular deaths among CAPD patients. *Perit Dial Bull* 3(Suppl):S23–S26, 1983
94. CATTRAN DC: The significance of lipid abnormalities in patients receiving dialysis therapy. *Perit Dial Bull* 3(Suppl):S29–S32, 1983
95. BERTOLI M, BATTISTELLA PA, VERGANI L, NASO A, GASPAROTTO ML, RO-

MAGNOLI GF, ANGELINI C: Carnitine deficiency induced during hemodialysis and hyperlipidemia: effect of replacement therapy. *Am J Clin Nutr* 34:1496–1500, 1981

96. WU G: Osmotic agents for peritoneal dialysis solutions. *Perit Dial Bull* 2:151–154, 1982

97. VACHA GM, GIORCELLI G, SILIPRANDI N, CORSI M: Favorable effects of L-carnitine treatment on hypertriglyceridemia in hemodialysis patients: decisive role of low levels of high-density lipoprotein-cholesterol. *Am J Clin Nutr* 38:532–540, 1983

Transplantation

Renal Transplantation: Current Status

Peter J. Morris

Renal transplantation has become the treatment of choice for most patients with end-stage renal failure under the age of 60. This past decade has seen many exciting developments evolving through the laboratories to clinical practice, and the next decade promises to be no less exciting. One of the most important changes arising from better clinical care has been the striking improvement in patient survival seen after transplantation in most units. Many factors have led to improved graft survival, among which the transfusion effect, including donor-specific transfusions, must rank as the most important at this time. Matching for HLA-DR and the recognition that not all positive crossmatches between donor and recipient are an absolute contraindication to transplantation are two important developments in tissue typing. Cyclosporine represents the most exciting immunosuppressive agent since azathioprine, although nephrotoxicity is a major problem associated with its use. However, the low morbidity and acceptable graft survival associated with the fairly general adoption of protocols with low-dose steroids and azathioprine mean that this combination must now be considered the standard against which new therapy is compared. Heterologous antilymphocyte globulin (ALG) has been finally accepted as an effective therapy for the treatment of acute rejection, but the advent of monoclonal antibodies to T lymphocytes should allow a more precise attack on the cells involved in rejection. In addition, the gradual acceptance of brain death has led to the harvesting of better kidneys with a higher immediate graft function rate. Finally, the integration of dialysis facilities with transplantation remains an important concept in the provision of the most satisfactory care for the patient with end-stage renal failure. These, then, are some of the more important highlights of renal transplantation today which I shall enlarge on in the following pages.

This manuscript was presented as a State-of-the-Art Lecture of the same title.

Indications and Contraindications

The true incidence of end-stage renal failure which might be considered as treatable by dialysis has been estimated at anywhere from 50 to 100 patients per million population each year [1, 2]. The proportion of these new patients who might be treated by transplantation is difficult to assess accurately, for much of the growing incidence of patients presenting with end-stage renal failure is accounted for by elderly patients who are not considered suitable for transplantation. Thus, most units do not perform kidney transplantations on patients over the age of 60. However, to some extent this is dictated by the shortage of cadaver kidneys; and if this were to increase, then most units would extend their rather arbitrarily introduced age limits, especially when one remembers the relatively low morbidity associated with current immunosuppression.

The most common kidney disease in patients receiving a renal transplant is glomerulonephritis, followed by pyelonephritis and interstitial nephritis, cystic kidney disease, and multisystem disease, of which diabetes mellitus is the major example. Over recent years it has become apparent that no disease represents an absolute contraindication to transplantation [3]. Recurrence of the different histologic types of glomerulonephritis in the transplanted kidney varies widely, ranging from 5% for anti-GBM nephritis to over 80% for mesangiocapillary type II glomerulonephritis (or dense-deposit disease). However, even in the latter, where recurrence of the disease seems inevitable, the loss of grafts due to the recurrence is low [4]. Diabetes mellitus has been a relative contraindication to transplantation in many units, especially in Europe, but again attitudes have changed markedly in recent years, especially with the advent of continuous ambulatory dialysis, which is particularly suited to the diabetic patient awaiting a transplant. Even oxalosis can no longer be considered an absolute contraindication to transplantation for some successful transplants have been recorded [5], although recurrence is usually very rapid in most patients.

The Donor

There has been a major swing to cadaver transplantation over the past decade, but more recently, with the apparently excellent results being obtained with donor-specific transfusions between non-HLA identical family members, there has been renewed interest in the use of organs from living related donors in many centers. There has been concern for many years about the long-term outcome of a healthy donor who has provided 50% of his renal tissue. However, two long-term studies of over 600 living donors have failed to identify an increased incidence of hypertension or impaired renal function in these donors followed for as long as 19 years [6, 7]. Nevertheless, it is obvious that the bulk of the demand for kidneys must be met by cadaver donors. The gradual acceptance of the concept of brain stem death in most countries of the Western world [8] has led to an improved quality of kidneys with a higher immediate function rate than the previous ones. Often, the removal of the kidneys is now more complicated because other organs such as pancreas, liver, and heart may be removed from the same donor. Thus, a skilled surgical team responsible for this multiple organ harvesting is essential.

Pretreatment of the donor, or the kidney itself, in an attempt to reduce the immunogenicity of the transplanted organ is aimed at ridding the kidney of a passenger leukocyte population, which is thought to play a major role in the induction of the immune response to the graft. Although there is experimental data to support this approach, there is no convincing evidence that attempts to do this in clinical practice have been successful [9, 10].

Preservation

There has been a great shift away from machine preservation of kidneys to simple flushing with a cold preservation solution and storage in ice at 0° C. Most flushing solutions are either iso-osmolar or hyperosmolar electrolyte solutions. Recent experimental work has indicated that they owe their success to control of the cell volume and composition by modifying transmembrane movements of water and ions and their buffering capacity, for below 10° C the sodium pump is completely inhibited and the presence of permeant components in the flushing solution will diminish uptake of water by the hypothermic cell [11]. The two most popular flushing solutions are iso-molar or hyperosmolar Collins' and citrate solutions. Certainly satisfactory storage up to 48 hours can be obtained with flushing and ice storage, but for periods longer than this, preservation on a machine that perfuses the kidney with albumin at 4° C at low flow rates is necessary. The addition of other substances to albumin such as citrate, magnesium, and potassium seems to even further enhance machine preservation [11]. However, for most purposes the time available with ice storage is more than adequate for tissue typing, selection and preparation of a recipient, and transport of kidneys between centers.

HLA and Renal Transplantation

Matching

Matching for HLA within families can be very precise because the HLA region of the chromosome is generally inherited en bloc, and so assuming that two markers on that region of the chromosome can be determined, namely, the HLA-A and -B antigens, then the inheritance of the whole chromosome can be determined within the family [12]. Transplantation between HLA identical siblings is the ideal situation in which to perform transplantation (with the exception of monozygous identical twins), although immuno-suppression is still required. Indeed, rejection may occur owing to prior sensitization to minor histocompatibility antigens. However, as mentioned earlier, the use of donor-specific transfusions between non-HLA identical family members is producing results in this group of living related recipients similar to that of HLA identical sibling transplants. In both groups of living related transplants, graft survivals of 90% or even greater are now being achieved.

The role of matching in cadaver transplantation has had a more checkered course. Although considerable controversy has raged over many years about the role of matching for HLA-A and -B antigens, there is now a consensus of opinion that a kidney that is well matched for the A and B antigens (that is, 0 or 1 mismatch) has about a 10 to 15% better chance of survival at 1 year than a graft that is badly matched (3 or 4 mismatches) [13, 14]. Furthermore, some units have suggested that this influence of matching for these antigens is due predominantly to matching of the B series of antigens [15]. However, matching for the HLA-A and -B antigens has proved difficult because of the extreme polymorphism of the two series of antigens, and this has led to the development of national and regional organ sharing schemes based on matching.

The definition of the HLA-D and DR series of antigens in Oxford in 1978 [16] led to a new approach to matching. The DR system of antigens seemed to show a limited degree of polymorphism in comparison to the A and B series of antigens. This of course made matching much simpler, assuming one ignored the HLA-A and -B antigens. Indeed, the first report of matching for HLA-DR in cadaver transplantation suggested a strong influence on cadaveric graft survival [17], which has been confirmed since in our own unit and that of others [15, 18, 19]. Of interest is the observation made in Oxford that matching for HLA-DR produced the same graft survival in nontransfused recipients as transfusions did in HLA-DR mismatched recipients, but that the best survival of all was obtained in those patients who were both transfused and received HLA-DR compatible kidney [12] (Table 1). Similar results have been noted by Ayoub and Terasaki [20], but not by d'Apice et al [15]. Thus, the influence of matching for HLA-DR appears to be quite a strong one and theoretically simplifies the approach to matching. However, the definition of two other loci in the D/DR region (DC and SB) provides a question to be answered concerning their role in the induction of the immune response and, hence, their role in matching for cadaveric transplantation.

The observation by Hendriks et al [21] that recipients who were HLA-DRw6-positive had a much worse graft survival than HLA-DRw6-negative recipients has produced considerable interest. For they found that matching for HLA-DR was only significant in HLA-DRw6-positive individuals, and they suggested that HLA-DRw6 represented the product of an immune-response gene in man. Some support for their first observation was provided by Ting [12], but in general other groups have not been able to confirm this observation.

Table 1. The influence of matching for HLA-DR on the survival of first cadaveric grafts and the relation between matching for HLA-DR and pregraft transfusions on the survival of first cadaveric grafts

HLA-DR mismatches	N	Graft survival (%)		
		1 yr	3 yr	5 yr
0	92	79	74	69
1	127	62	55	45
2	64	60	54	50
Influence of pregraft transfusions[a]				
0 (+PGT)	46	87	79	79
0 (−PGT)	44	70	67	56
1,2 (+PGT)	108	74	63	54
1,2 (−PGT)	79	47	44	36

[a] "With pregraft transfusion" (PGT) is denoted by "+PGT"; "without," by "−PGT."

The Highly Sensitized Patient and the Positive Crossmatch

The highly sensitized patient (one with antibodies reacting with over 90% of the population) is a major problem in all renal units, for every waiting list has large numbers of such patients, most of whom have already rejected a previous transplant. For many years now, the accepted practice has been to regard a positive crossmatch between a potential recipient's serum and donor lymphocytes as an absolute contraindication to transplantation, because the outcome of a transplant in this situation was usually immediate graft failure known as hyperacute rejection [22, 23]. However, there have been significant developments in recent years showing that there are exceptions to the above dogma, which do allow a transplant to be performed safely. First, it was noted that a positive crossmatch that could be shown to be due to reactivity against only the donor B cells did allow a transplant to be performed safely in many instances [24, 25]. Second, it was shown that the apparent hypersensitization in many patients was due in part, or occasionally in whole, to autoantibodies against lymphocytes, either B lymphocytes alone or T and B lymphocytes, and that positive crossmatches due to such autoantibodies were also not a contraindication to transplantation [26]. The realization that a positive crossmatch could be due to antibodies that were not damaging to a subsequent graft has allowed some highly sensitized patients to be transplanted successfully. For example in Oxford 81 cadaveric transplants have been performed in the presence of a positive crossmatch, 47 of which were in highly sensitized patients, and 33 of those 47 were successful (Table 2).

A further development in this area of great importance is the recognition by Cardella and Falk [27] that a transplant may be successful in patients

Table 2. The function at 1 month of transplanted kidneys in highly sensitized patients (reactive with > 90% of the population) with a positive crossmatch against donor B or donor B and T lymphocytes[a]

Crossmatch					
T	B	Auto	No.	Functioning	Failed
−	+	+	11	8 (73%)	3
−	+	−	12	8 (67%)	4
−	+	nt	6	3 (50%)	3
+	+	+	16	14 (88%)	2
+	+	−	2	0 (0%)	2

[a] Positive crossmatch thought to result from autoreactive antibodies.

whose past sera gave a positive crossmatch with the donor but whose current sera gave a negative crossmatch, even though the antibody had been directed against HLA-A and -B antigens. Another approach that is being explored in the UK is the establishment of a panel of highly sensitized patients, with sera samples from such patients held in all units. All donors in the UK are tested against these sera samples, and if a negative crossmatch is found for any of these patients the kidney is transported to the center of that recipient.

Thus, there are now available for the highly sensitized patients several approaches that now give them some hope of a successful transplant. One can expect to see further advances in this area.

Immunosuppression

Azathioprine and Steroids

Azathioprine and steroids have been the backbone of immunosuppression in renal transplantation for 20 years, but with an appreciable morbidity owing mainly to the high doses of steroids used in all units. However, the demonstration by McGeown et al [28] that excellent results could be obtained with low doses of prednisolone and the confirmation of these observations in a randomized controlled trial in Oxford [29] have gradually led to the widespread use of low-dose steroid protocols in association with azathioprine throughout the world. This has led to a very significant reduction in the morbidity associated with the use of steroids, so that complications such as avascular necrosis of bone are now very uncommon [30]. Thus, any new immunosuppressive therapy must be compared against the graft survival and morbidity associated with an azathioprine and low-dose steroid protocol.

The treatment of acute rejection is high-dose steroids, either given as i.v. boluses of methylprednisolone (for example, 0.5 to 1.0 g 24-hourly over 3 to 5 days) or as an increased oral dosage of prednisolone (for example,

300 mg daily reduced over 10 days or so to the previous oral dose). Either approach is effective in two thirds of acute rejection episodes, but there may be more morbidity associated with the high oral dose regimen [31].

Cyclosporine

This exciting new immunosuppressive agent was first used clinically in renal transplantation in 1978 [32], following the demonstration of its potent immunosuppressive activity in many experimental models of vascularized organ allografts in different species (reviewed in Refs. 33 and 34). The drug is unique in its action in that its effect is directed primarily at T lymphocytes at an early stage of the induction of the immune response to an antigen. Much of this activity is related to the inhibition of the production of lymphokines, such as IL-2 and T helper factor by the T helper cell, thus preventing the IL-2 induced proliferation of cytotoxic T cell precursors and the proliferation of antibody-producing B cell precursors [35].

Considerable experience with the use of cyclosporine in renal transplantation has accumulated since the pioneer experience of Calne and colleagues in Cambridge [32]. Their early experience prompted a number of controlled trials of cyclosporine, namely single-center trials at Minneapolis, Oxford, Pittsburgh, and Sydney, as well as multicenter trials in Europe and Canada, together with uncontrolled studies of its efficacy in Denver, Pittsburgh, Stockholm, Houston, and Boston. Taken together, all these studies show an improvement in cadaveric graft survival at 1 year of up to 20%, and in no instance have the results proved worse in the cyclosporine-treated patients than in the conventionally treated patients (see Refs. 34, 35, and 36 for reviews of the clinical experience).

However, a number of side-effects of cyclosporine have become evident, as listed in Table 3. Most of these are dose related and will regress with lowering of the dose. The most serious side-effect associated with cyclosporine is nephrotoxicity, which provides problems in the management in the early months after transplantation and may also lead to permanent damage of the kidney. In the early weeks and months after transplantation, there can be considerable difficulty in distinguishing between rejection and nephrotoxic-

Table 3. Side-effects of cyclosporine therapy

Site	Side-effect	Site	Side-effect
Renal	Nephrotoxicity	Gastrointestinal	Anorexia
Hepatic	Hepatoxicity		Nausea
Neoplastic	Lymphomas		Weight loss
	Fibroadenomas of breast	Neurological	Tremor
Dermatological	Thickening of skin		Burning pain in limbs
	Rashes		Malaise, depression
	Hirsutism	Cardiovascular	Fluid retention
Dental	Gingival hypertrophy		Hypertension

ity, for the classical features of acute rejection seen in patients on azathioprine and steroids, such as fever, graft swelling and tenderness, together with a deterioration of renal function, are not seen in patients on cyclosporine, where there may only be a deterioration of renal function with little systemic evidence of rejection. The distinction between the two can be extremely difficult, and neither blood levels nor histologic findings provides reliable indications of the correct diagnosis. If the deterioration in renal function is due to nephrotoxicity it will respond to decreasing the dose or switching to azathioprine and prednisolone as is the practice in the Oxford trials of short-term use of cyclosporine.

The Oxford trials of cyclosporine are quite different from any other clinical trials, for patients who are randomly allocated to receive cyclosporine, receive cyclosporine only for 3 months, at which time they are converted to azathioprine and low-dose steroids, whereas the control group receives azathioprine and low-dose steroids. This trial of the drug was planned because of the concern about long-term renal damage and the possibility of an increased risk of lymphomas. The latter concern appears now unfounded, but the first certainly remains valid. In the first trial, only patients given diuresing kidneys and an HLA-DR imcompatible kidney were entered, but after some 35 patients had been randomized on this basis with no apparent ill effects of the strategy [37], a second trial was begun in which all patients were randomized to either cyclosporine alone, switching to azathioprine and low-dose steroids at 3 months, or conventional treatment with azathioprine and low-dose steroids. The strategy seems a successful one, at least in the short term as shown in Table 4. However, the long-term outcome will be awaited with considerable interest.

There is considerable controversy about the need to use steroids, albeit in low doses, with cyclosporine. In general, North American units have used steroids with cyclosporine, but European units have not. Some controlled trials of cyclosporine with and without steroids have been performed [36] or are in progress. To date, there is no evidence that graft survival is increased by the use of steroids with cyclosporine.

There is no question that cyclosporine represents a very significant addition to our immunosuppressive armamentarium, and should lead to substantial

Table 4. Short-term use of cyclosporine with conversion at 90 days to azathioprine and low-dose prednisolone in cadaveric renal transplantation

	N	Graft survival (%)			
		3 mo	6 mo	1 yr	2 yr
Oxford trial II					
Cyclosporine	50	79	79	74	74
Az. + Pred.	55	62	62	62	44
Oxford trials I and II					
Cyclosporine	73	77	76	72	68
Az. + Pred.	316	71	68	64	59

improvements in graft survival at least in the short term. The side-effects of the drug are not serious, apart from the nephrotoxicity, which does present a major problem immediately after transplantation and may result in permanent damage to the graft. The next few years will see efforts concentrated on defining the best method of using cyclosporine, but also one can expect other members of this drug family to be developed, some of which may be equally immunosuppressive but without the associated nephrotoxicity of the founder member of the family.

Antilymphocyte Globulin (ALG) and Monoclonal Antibodies

The role of heterologous ALG in renal transplantation has been a controversial one since its first use in the mid-60s [38]. It has been used either from the time of transplantation to prevent rejection or to treat an acute rejection episode. Variability between individual batches of antisera, lack of controlled trials, inadequate doses, and small numbers of patients evaluated have all contributed to the confusion. However, continuing improvements in production techniques and further careful trials have now established the clinical value of these heterologous antisera directed against human lymphocytes [39]. The prophylactic use of ALG from the time of transplantation in nine controlled trials has shown a significant improvement in graft survival at 1 year in five of the trials. However, in trials of its use for the treatment of rejection in comparison with steroids, there has been a reversal of rejection in 75 to 100% of patients given ALG compared to about 66% of those given steroids. Graft survival was also better in the patients given ALG for the treatment of acute rejection [39]. Thus, ALG does have a place in immunosuppressive therapy in renal transplantation, but this place is probably best reserved for the treatment of acute rejection episodes.

The advent of xenogeneic monoclonal antibodies to lymphocyte populations has provided a method of achieving the same ends as ALG but it enables the attack to be directed more precisely at the T lymphocytes that play such a prominent role in the rejection of a renal allograft [10]. Two such antibodies have been used clinically, OKT3 and an anti-T12, both of which are pan T monoclonal antibodies.

OKT3 has been shown to clear circulating T cells from the peripheral blood within minutes and reverse an acute rejection episode quite dramatically [39, 40]. A multicenter trial of its use confirmed its efficacy in reversing an acute rejection episode but pointed to other problems, namely, the development of antibody to mouse immunoglobulins in most patients and the early return of T lymphocytes with OKT4 and OKT8 markers in the absence of OKT3 determinants [39].

T12 is another pan T cell antibody directed against a different determinant and has been used clinically also with some success [41]. Acute rejection episodes, confirmed histologically, were completely reversed in 7 of 19 patients, and in all patients T12-positive cells were cleared immediately from the circulation.

A different type of monoclonal antibody, an antilymphoblast antibody, has been used in Japan in 19 patients undergoing acute rejection, with reversal of rejection in 17 of 19 episodes [42]. Thus, this approach to the treatment of rejection, which is at present in its infancy, might in time replace the use of heterologous ALG. But, in particular, it holds the promise of enabling clearance of the key cells involved in an acute rejection episode, as well as a more sophisticated manipulation of the immune response.

Other Methods

Many other methods of immunosuppression have been investigated over the last 20 years. These include thymectomy, splenectomy, irradiation of the graft, actinomycin, cyclophosphamide, thoracic duct fistula, and total lymphoid irradiation. Splenectomy before transplantation has been shown to improve graft survival in one controlled trial [43], but probably adds to the likelihood of severe infections after transplantation. Thoracic duct drainage is an effective method of immunosuppression if maintained for at least a month, but does provide very considerable logistic problems in its maintenance. Total lymphoid irradiation (TLI) before transplantation, a potent method of inducing immunosuppression in certain experimental models is being tested with some promise in Belgium [44], where diabetics receiving cadaver kidneys have been maintained after pretransplant TLI on no or minimal doses of steroids alone for up to a year.

Blood Transfusions

The beneficial effect of blood transfusions on graft survival is unquestioned, cadaveric graft survival being 10 to 20% better in transfused compared with nontransfused recipients. But very little is known about the mechanism of this effect [45]. Nor do we know the optimum number of transfusions, the component in the blood that produces the effect, the time that should elapse between the last transfusion and transplantation, or the appropriate age of the transfused blood. The fear that widespread sensitization of recipients would result from deliberate transfusion policies has not proved to be the case, for up to five transfusions lead to broad sensitization in very few patients and these mostly are multiparous women or previously transfused recipients.

Outstanding results have come from the use of donor-specific transfusions, generally three, in living-related transplantation where donor and recipient are not HLA-identical [46]. However, approximately one third of patients are sensitized against the donor following transfusion and so the transplant cannot be performed. For this reason two other approaches are being explored with promise: first, transfusion of stored donor blood [47] and, second, the administration of azathioprine to cover the time of transfusions before the transplant [48]. In both instances, the incidence of sensitization against the donor is very much lower, but the early results of transplantation are equally good. Of some interest is the suggestion that unrelated blood transfusions of the recipient are equally effective in avoiding donor-specific sensitization and in producing good graft survival [49].

Diagnosis of Rejection

Immediate function of a graft will occur in all living-related transplants and in about 60% of cadaver transplants. Barring the occurrence of an antibody-mediated hyperacute rejection or an accelerated rejection commencing within the first 72 hours, as seen in patients sensitized to their donor, the usual first-set type of rejection occurs between 7 and 14 days. The classical features of this rejection in a patient on azathioprine and prednisolone are a fever, swelling and tenderness of the graft, and a deterioration in renal function. Even in the presence of acute tubular necrosis, the clinical features usually make the diagnosis reasonably straightforward. If in doubt, a Trucut needle biopsy examination will confirm the diagnosis.

But in patients on cyclosporine the distinction between rejection, ATN, and nephrotoxicity presents a major problem. However, two approaches to the evaluation of the infiltrating cells within the graft itself may be of value. First, monoclonal antibodies are being used to identify the infiltrating leukocytes within a Trucut needle biopsy sample [50, 51], which may allow cellular patterns to be defined in different types of rejection in contrast to the pattern seen in patients on cyclosporine or in the presence of ATN without rejection. The frequency with which a Trucut biopsy can be performed is limited, and so a second approach is the technique of fine needle aspiration popularized by Häyry and von Willebrand [52, 55]. They have described a variety of morphologic patterns seen in rejection, as well as in ATN and cyclosporine toxicity. However, there is not general agreement about the validity of these patterns, but again the use of monoclonal antibodies may allow the easier identification of cells in the aspirate either by peroxidase labeling [53] or by the fluorescence-activated cell sorter [54]. The attraction of fine needle aspiration is that it can be performed daily if need be, and so it could prove a very valuable monitoring technique if it can be shown that it truly reflects the changes taking place in the kidney as shown by Trucut biopsies done at the same time.

Complications of Renal Transplantation

Technical complications are few after renal transplantation in experienced units, and the two major groups of complications are infections and cardiovascular complications [56, 57]. Although the infectious complications are no longer the major cause of death after renal transplantation, they remain a significant cause of morbidity and are the major cause of death in the first few months after transplantation when immunosuppression is at its maximum. The true incidence of infections after transplantation is unknown, but in one Oxford study 58% of patients after cadaveric transplantation suffered an infection within the first 6 months [29]. Many reasons can be advanced for the lower morbidity and mortality associated with infection in recent years, but probably the more conservative approach to immunosuppressive therapy is the major factor.

Cytomegalovirus (CMV) infection remains a major problem in the early months, and indeed many of the infectious deaths at this time can be related to a primary CMV infection. Prevention of CMV infection can be achieved by giving a seronegative recipient a kidney from a seronegative donor [57] (Table 5), but this is not always practical. Vaccination with live attenuated CMV has seroconverted 83% of negative recipients in the pretransplant period, on the assumption that reactivation of CMV is a less severe infection than primary CMV infection [58]. The availability of acyclovir for the treatment of severe herpes simplex infections and the development of a hepatitis B vaccine represent other significant developments in this area. However, the increased incidence of non-A non-B hepatitis poses a new threat to dialysis and transplant units. Overall, a more conservative approach to immunosuppression associated with a more aggressive approach to prevention, diagnosis, and treatment of infectious complications has led to a marked decrease in the mortality and morbidity of infection after renal transplantation.

Cardiovascular complications are now the major overall cause of death after transplantation, now that early deaths from infection are relatively few. As more elderly patients are transplanted, this trend is likely to increase. Although the seeds of cardiovascular complications have usually been sown well before transplantation, the hypertension and hyperlipidemia that occur after transplantation in many patients will enhance the progress of the vascular disease in these patients [56]. Ibbels et al [59] have shown that the cumulative incidence of nonfatal occlusive arterial disease in patients free of clinical evidence of such disease before transplantation was 0.42 at 6 years. This risk rate is comparable with that for smokers with hypertension, hyperlipidemia, and glucose intolerance in a nontransplant population. Thus, the treatment of hypertension, avoidance of smoking, and management of hyperlipidemia are essential in the transplant patient if the present unacceptably high cardiovascular mortality after transplantation is to be reduced.

Cancer after transplantation is being seen more frequently as more patients are surviving longer with a functioning graft. However, the two types of cancer that are seen with a much greater frequency are lymphomas and skin cancers, although all cancers are probably being seen with an increased

Table 5. CMV status of the donor and the recipient in 306 cadaveric donors and their recipients in Oxford and the number of primary or secondary CMV infections

	Donor/recipient status			
	CMV+/CMV−	CMV+/CMV+	CMV−/CMV+	CMV−/CMV−
No. of patients	60	84	98	64
No. infected	38 (63%)	52 (62%)	52 (53%)	0

incidence [60]. The Epstein-Barr virus (EBV) has been shown to cause a spectrum of B cell lymphoproliferative disease in the transplant patient ranging from an infectious mononucleosis-like, polyclonal B-cell proliferation (which responds to antiviral therapy with acyclovir) to a solid monoclonal B-cell lymphoma [61, 62]. Patients who have an infectious mononucleosis-like illness associated with polyclonal B cell proliferation (usually seen in the first 6 months after transplantation) may be successfully treated with acyclovir and reduction of immunosuppression, whereas patients with a monoclonal B-cell tumor are treated with conventional radiotherapy or chemotherapy, and immunosuppression is dicontinued, usually necessitating a transplant nephrectomy.

Results of Renal Transplantation

The growth and increasing success of renal transplantation can be considered one of the marvels of modern medicine, for the patient who receives a successful transplant can be fully rehabilitated in every sense of the word [63]. We are now achieving patient and graft survival rates that are highly acceptable, and indeed graft survival can be expected to continue to improve. However, it is now time to address more attention to the problems, both psychological and physical, that are associated with renal transplantation, for these are more common than we like to believe. This present decade will see more advances made in our understanding of the immune response and of rejection, which in turn will enable us to manipulate the response to a graft more intelligently than is possible at present. Again, more sophisticated agents, such as monoclonal antibodies, will be available for therapy, and other members of the cyclosporine family should appear. Provided the supply of kidneys can be increased, renal transplantation should be firmly established as the first line of treatment for patients of almost all ages with end-stage renal failure by the end of the current decade.

Acknowledgments. This work was supported in part by grants from the Medical Research Council of the United Kingdom and the National Kidney Research Fund.

References

1. LUKE RG: Renal replacement therapy. *N Engl J Med* 308:1593–1595, 1983
2. WING AH, SELWOOD NH: Achievements and problems in the treatment of end stage renal failure, in *Recent Advances in Renal Medicine,* edited by PETERS DK, Edinburgh, Churchill Livingstone, 1982, pp 103–119
3. BRIGGS JD: The recipient of a renal transplant, in *Kidney Transplantation: Principles and Practice* (2nd ed), edited by MORRIS PJ, New York, London, Orlando, Grune and Stratton, 1984, pp. 59–79
4. CAMERON JS: Glomerulonephritis in renal transplants. *Transplantation* 34:237–245, 1982

5. WHELCHEL JD, ALISON DV, LUKE RG, CURTIS J, DIETHELM AG: Successful renal transplantation in hyperoxaluria. *Transplantation* 35:161–164, 1983

6. VINCENTI F, AMAND W, FEDUSKA N, BIRNBAUM J, DUCA R, SALVATIERRA O, KAYSEN G: Long-term renal function in kidney donors: Sustained compensatory hyperfiltration with no adverse effects. *Transplantation* 36:626–629, 1983

7. WEILAND D, SUTHERLAND DER, CHAVERS B, SIMMONS RL, ASCHER N, NAJARIAN JS: *Transplant Proc,* in press

8. PALLIS C: Brainstem death: The evolution of a concept, in *Kidney Transplantation: Principles and Practice* (2nd ed), edited by MORRIS PJ, New York, London, Orlando. Grune and Stratton, 1984, pp 101–127

9. COSIMI AB: The donor and donor nephrectomy, in *Kidney Transplantation: Principles and Practice* (2nd ed), edited by MORRIS PJ, New York, London, Orlando, Grune and Stratton, 1984, pp 81–99

10. MORRIS PJ: The immunology of rejection, in *Kidney Transplantation: Principles and Practice* (2nd ed), edited by MORRIS PJ, New York, London, Orlando, Grune and Stratton, 1984, pp 15–32

11. MARSHALL VC: Renal preservation, in *Kidney Transplantation: Principles and Practice* (2nd ed), edited by MORRIS PJ, New York, London, Orlando, Grune and Stratton, 1984, pp 129–157

12. TING A: HLA and Renal Transplantation, in *Kidney Transplantation: Principles and Practice* (2nd ed), edited by MORRIS PJ, New York, London, Orlando, Grune and Stratton, 1984, pp 159–180

13. OPELZ G, TERASAKI P: Cadaver kidney transplants in N. America: Analysis 1978. *Dialysis Transplant* 8:167–170, 1979

14. PERSIJN GG, COHEN B, LANSBERGAN Q, D'AMARO J, SELWOOD N, WING A, VAN ROOD JJ: Effect of HLA-A and HLA-B matching on survival of grafts and recipients after renal transplantation. *N Engl J Med* 307:905–908, 1982

15. D'APICE AJF, SHEIL AGR, TAIT BD, BASHIR HV: Controlled trial of HLA-A,B versus HLA-DR matching in cadaveric renal transplantation. *Transplant Proc* 13:938–941, 1981

16. BODMER WF, BATCHELOR JR, BODMER JG, FESTENSTEIN H, MORRIS PJ (Eds): *Histocompatibility Testing 1977.* Copenhagen, Munksgaard, 1978

17. TING A, MORRIS PJ: Matching for B-cell antigens of the HLA-DR (D-related) series in cadaver renal transplantation. *Lancet* 1:575–577, 1978

18. MORRIS PJ, TING A: Studies of HLA-DR with relevance to renal transplantation. *Immunol Rev* 66:103–131, 1982

19. ALBRECHSTEN D, MOEN T, FLATMARK A, HALVORSEN S, JACOBSEN A, JERVELL J, SOLHEIM BG, THORSBY E: HLA-A,B,C,D, DR in clinical transplantation. *Transplant Proc* 13:924–929, 1981

20. AYOUB G, TERASAKI P: HLA-DR matching in multicenter, single-typing laboratory data. *Transplantation* 33:515–517, 1982

21. HENDRIKS GF, SCHREIDER GM, CLAAS FJ, D'AMARO J, PERSIJN GG, COHEN B, VAN ROOD JJ: HLA-DRw6 and renal allograft rejection. *Br Med J* 286:85–87, 1983

22. KISSMEYER-NIELSEN F, OLSEN S, PETERSON VP, FJELDBORG O: Hyperacute rejection of kidney allografts: Association with pre-existing humoral antibodies against donor cells. *Lancet* 1:662–665, 1966

23. WILLIAMS GM, HUME DM, HUDSON RP, MORRIS PJ, KANOK, MILGRIM F: Hyperacute renal homograft rejection in man. *N Engl J Med* 279:611–618, 1968

24. ETTENGER RB, TERASAKI PI, OPELZ G, MALEKZADEH M, PENNISI AJ, UITTENBOGAART C, FINE R: Successful renal allografts across a positive cross-match for donor B-lymphocyte alloantigens. *Lancet* 2:56–58, 1976

25. MORRIS PJ, TING A, DAAR AS, OLIVER D: B cell alloantibodies and renal allografts. *Lancet* 2:312–313, 1976
26. TING A, MORRIS PJ: Renal transplantation and a B-cell cross-match with autoantibodies and alloantibodies. *Lancet* 2:1095–1097, 1977
27. CARDELLA CJ, FALK JA: Graft outcome in patients with antibodies reactive with donor T and B cells. *Transplant Proc* 15:1142–1144, 1983
28. MCGEOWN MG, DOUGLAS JF, BROWN WA, DONALDSON RA, KENNEDY JA, LOUGHBRIDGE WG, MEHTA S, NELSON SD, DOHERTY CC, JOHNSTONE R, TODD G, HILL CM: Advantages of low dose steroid from the day after renal transplantation. *Transplantation* 29:287–289, 1980
29. MORRIS PJ, CHAN L, FRENCH ME, TING A: The case for low dose oral prednisolone in renal transplantation: A controlled trial. *Lancet* 1:525–527, 1982
30. D'APICE AJF: Non-specific immunosuppression: Azathioprine and steroids, in *Kidney Transplantation: Principles and Practice* (2nd ed), edited by MORRIS PJ, New York, London, Orlando, Grune and Stratton, 1984, pp 239–259
31. GRAY D, SHEPHERD H, DAAR A, OLIVER DO, MORRIS PJ: Oral versus intravenous high-dose steroid treatment of renal allograft rejection: The big shot or not? *Lancet* 1:117–118, 1978
32. CALNE RY, ROLLES K, WHITE DJ, THIRU S, EVANS DB, MCMASTER P, DUNN DC, CRADDOCK GN, HENDERSON RG, AZIZ S, LEWIS P: Cyclosporin A initially as the only immunosuppressant in 34 recipients of cadaveric organs: 32 kidneys, 2 pancreases and 2 livers. *Lancet* 2:1033–1036, 1979
33. MORRIS PJ: Cyclosporin A: An overview. *Transplantation* 32:349–354, 1981
34. MORRIS PJ: The impact of Cyclosporin A on Transplantation, in *Advances in Surgery*, edited by SHIRES T, Chicago, Year Book, 1984, pp 99–127
35. MORRIS PJ: Cyclosporine, in *Kidney Transplantation: Principles and Practice* (2nd ed), edited by MORRIS PJ, New York, London, Orlando, Grune and Stratton, 1984, pp 261–279
36. STILLER C, KEOWN P: Cyclosporine therapy in perspective, in *Progress in Transplantation: I*, edited by MORRIS PJ, TILNEY NL, Edinburgh, Churchill Livingstone, in press
37. MORRIS PJ, FRENCH ME, DUNNILL MS, HUNNISETT AG, TING A, THOMPSON JF, WOOD RFM: A controlled trial of cyclosporine in renal transplantation with conversion to azathioprine and prednisolone after 3 months. *Transplantation* 36:273–277, 1983
38. STARZL TE, MARCHIORO TL, PORTER KA, IWASKI Y, CERILLI GJ: The use of heterologous antilymphoid agents in canine renal and liver homotransplantation and in human renal homotransplantation. *Surg Gynecol Obstet* 124:301–318, 1967
39. JAFFERS GF, COSIMI AB: Antilymphocyte globulin and monoclonal antibodies, in *Kidney Transplantation: Principles and Practice* (2nd ed) edited by MORRIS PJ, New York, London, Orlando, Grune and Stratton, 1984, pp 281–299
40. COSIMI AB, BURTON RC, COLVIN RB, GOLDSTEIN G, DELMONICO FL, LA CUAGLIA MP, TOLKOFF-RUBIN N, RUBIN RH, HERRIN JT, RUSSELL PS: Treatment of acute renal allograft rejection with OKT3 monoclonal antibody. *Transplantation* 32:535–539, 1981
41. CARPENTER CB, MILFORD EL, STROM TB, KIRKMAN RL, TILNEY NL: Therapeutic use of monoclonal antibodies in transplantation, in *Progress in Transplantation: I*, edited by MORRIS PJ, TILNEY NL, Edinburgh, Churchill Livingstone, in press
42. TAKAHASKI H, OKAZAKI H, TERASAKI PI, IWAKI Y, KINUKAWA T, CHIN D, MIURA K, ISKIZAKA M, TAGUCHI Y, BILLING R: Reversal of transplant rejection by monoclonal antiblast antibody. *Lancet* 2:1155–1157, 1983

43. FRYD DS, SUTHERLAND DER, SIMMONS RL, FERGUSON RM, KJELLSTRAND CM, NAJARIAN JS: Results of a prospective randomized study on the effect of splenectomy versus no splenectomy in renal transplant patients. *Transplant Proc* 13:48–56, 1981

44. WAER M, VANRENTERGHEM Y, ANG KK, VAN DER SCHUEREN E, VANDEPUTTE M, MICHIELSEN P: Total lymphoid irradiation (TLI) as an immunosuppressive treatment for transplantation: A review of experimental and clinical data, in *Transplantation and Clinical Immunology,* edited by TOURAINE JL, et al, Amsterdam, Excerpta Medica, 1983, vol 15, pp 13–24

45. OPELZ G: Blood transfusions and renal transplantation, in *Kidney Transplantation: Principles and Practice* (2nd ed), edited by MORRIS PJ, New York, London, Orlando, Grune and Stratton, 1984, pp 323–334

46. SALVATIERRA O, VINCENTI F, AMEND W, GARAVOY M, IWAKI Y, TERASAKI PI, POTTER D, DUCA R, HOPPER S, SLEMMER T, FEDUSKA N: Four year experience with donor specific blood transfusions. *Transplant Proc* 15:924–931, 1983

47. LIGHT JA, METZ S, ODDENINO K: Donor-specific transfusion with minimal sensitisation. *Transplant Proc* 15:917–923, 1983

48. ANDERSON CB, SICARD GA, ETHEREDGE EE: Pretreatment of renal allograft recipients with azathioprine and donor-specific blood products. *Surgery* 92:315–321

49. FRISK B, BRYNGER H, SANDBERG L: Two random transfusions before primary renal transplantation: Four years' experience from a single center. *Transplant Proc* 14:386–388, 1982

50. PLATT JL, LEBIEN TW, MICHAEL AF: Interstitial mononuclear cell populations in renal graft rejection: Identification by monoclonal antibodies in tissue sections. *J Exp Med* 155:17–30, 1982

51. HANCOCK WW, THOMSON NM, ATKINS RC: Composition of interstitial cellular infiltrate identified by monoclonal antibodies in renal biopsies of rejecting human renal allografts. *Transplantation* 35:458–463, 1983

52. HÄYRY P, VON WILLEBRAND E, AHONEN J, EKLUND B, LAUTENSCHLARGER I: Monitoring of organ allograft rejection by transplant aspiration cytology. *Ann Clin Res* 13:264–287, 1981

53. WOOD RFM, BOLTON EM, THOMPSON JF, MORRIS PJ: Monoclonal antibodies and fine needle aspiration cytology in detecting renal allograft rejection. *Lancet* 2:278, 1982

54. WOOD RFM, THOMPSON JF, CARTER NP: Changes in lymphocyte subpopulations in blood and kidney after renal transplantation, in *Progress in Transplantation: I,* edited by MORRIS PJ, TILNEY NL, Edinburgh, Churchill Livingstone, in press

55. VON WILLEBRAND E, HÄYRY P: Composition and in vitro cytotoxicity of cellular infiltrates in rejecting human kidney allografts. *Cell Immunol* 41:358–372, 1978

56. RAINE AEG, LEDINGHAM JGG: Cardiovascular complications after renal transplantation, in *Kidney Transplantation: Principles and Practice* (2nd ed), edited by MORRIS PJ, New York, London, Orlando, Grune and Stratton, 1984, pp 469–489

57. WINNEARLS GG, LANE DJ, KURTZ J: Infectious complications after renal transplantation, in *Kidney Transplantation: Principles and Practice* (2nd ed), edited by MORRIS PJ, New York, London, Orlando, Grune and Stratton, 1984, pp 427–467

58. MARKER SC, SIMMONS RL, BALFOUR HH: Cytomegalovirus vaccine in renal allograft recipients. *Transplant Proc* 13:117–119, 1981

59. IBELS LS, STEWART JH, MAHONEY JF, WEALE FC, SHEIL AGR: Occlusive arterial disease in uraemic and haemodialysis patients and renal transplant recipients. *Q J Med* 46:197–214, 1977

60. SHEIL AGR: Cancer in dialysis and transplant patients, in *Kidney Transplantation: Principles and Practice* (2nd ed), edited by MORRIS PJ, New York, London, Orlando, Grune and Stratton, 1984, pp 491–507

61. HANTO DE, SIMMONS RL: Lymphoproliferative disease in immunosuppressed patients, in *Progress in Transplantation: I,* edited by MORRIS PJ, TILNEY NL, Edinburgh, Churchill Livingstone, in press

62. HANTO DE, GAJL-PECZALSKA KJ, FRIZZERA G, ARTHUR DC, BALFOUR HH, MCCLAIN K, SIMMONS RL, NAJARIAN JS: Epstein-Barr virus (EBV) induced polyclonal and monoclonal B-cell lymphoproliferative diseases occurring after renal transplantation: Clinical, pathologic, and virologic findings and implications for therapy. *Ann Surg* 198:356–369, 1983

63. MORRIS PJ: Results of renal transplantation, in *Kidney Transplantation: Principles and Practice* (2nd ed), edited by MORRIS PJ, New York, London, Orlando, Grune and Stratton, 1984, pp 547–563

Endocrine and Metabolic Dysfunctions Following Kidney Transplantation

Jacob Green and Ori S. Better

The transplanted kidney is exposed to a wide range of injuries. This may begin with the trauma, disease, and shock that caused the death of the donor. Further injury to the kidney is contracted during the extracorporeal handling and perfusion of the kidney with artificial solutions.

After transplantation, the kidney is also subjected to rejection and other deleterious conditions (summarized in Table 1). The resulting kidney damage may be generalized, with azotemia as its hallmark. Occasionally, however, despite this hostile environment, glomerular filtration rate is relatively spared, and the kidney damage is predominantly tubulointerstitial (see Table 2). These tubular syndromes may cause profound changes in acid-base balance and disturbances in electrolyte and mineral homeostasis. The resulting deranged metabolism of divalent ions may aggravate preexisting bone disease and lead to nephrocalcinosis or the formation of kidney stones. The recipient may also be subjected to several metabolic disturbances over and beyond tubular dysfunction. These are attributable to the presence of the original diseased kidneys of the host as well as to complications arising from the use of immuno-suppressive drugs and antibiotics.

The purpose of the present communication is to review the various tubular and metabolic defects that have been described following transplantation.

Renal Tubular Acidosis (RTA)

Renal tubular acidosis (RTA) after kidney transplantation was first reported in 1967 in a patient studied by Massry et al [1]. Subsequent studies reported similar findings of RTA in other post-transplant patients [2–10]. In those studies, most of the patients presented with mild spontaneous hyperchloremic

This manuscript was presented as part of a Symposium on *Endocrine and Metabolic Abnormalities in Renal Diseases.*

Table 1. Potential causes for tubular dysfunction following transplantation

Ischemic damage following acute tubular necrosis	Protein malnutrition
Acute and chronic rejection	Use of nephrotoxic agents
Unresolved hyperparathyroidism with or without hypercalcemia	Urinary tract infection
	Obstructive uropathy
	Ischemia due to renal artery stenosis

metabolic acidosis and an inappropriately high urinary pH. In some of the patients, however, the acid-base status was normal under basal conditions, and a defect in urinary acid excretion was unmasked only during oral ammonium chloride loading [4, 9]. Thus, they appeared to have an incomplete form of distal RTA. Proximal RTA with generalized proximal tubular dysfunction has also been described following transplantation [6–10].

In these early studies, the defect in urinary acidification was usually observed in the first few months after transplantation and in some cases appeared to be reversible [3, 5, 9]. It was suggested that the defective urinary acidification was related to acute rejection episodes or caused by ischemic tubular damage [2–5, 9]. Also implicated was bicarbonate wastage caused by secondary hyperparathyroidism [9]. In 1973 Wilson and Siddiqui [8] confirmed previous observations that defective urinary acidification commonly develops in the early post-transplant period. However, they also showed that in some cases distal RTA was either persistent or appeared de novo following a period of 1 to 3 years during which normal urinary acidification capacity had been documented. Furthermore, these investigators noticed that the occurrence of RTA in the late post-transplant period was often accompanied by the development of clinical features of chronic rejection.

Several studies in animals and in humans showed that an acquired distal acidification defect can result from a secretory or a nonsecretory defect in hydrogen ion transport [11–14]. Both defects can be distinguished by the acidification response to sodium sulfate or neutral phosphate administration. Using these maneuvers, Batlle et al [15] have recently described a secretory defect in acid secretion in five of six patients with persistent hyperchloremic

Table 2. Tubular dysfunction following kidney transplantation

Tubular acidosis (RTA): proximal RTA, distal RTA	Impaired ability to maximally concentrate and dilute the urine
Fanconi syndrome (defects in tubular reabsorption of bicarbonate, glucose, amino acids, phosphate, and uric acid)	Blunted intrinsic tubular ability to excrete potassium resulting in hyperkalemia ("nonazotemic hyperkalemia")
Urinary phosphate leak (PTH-dependent and PTH-independent types	Hypoaldosteronism resulting in hyperkalemia and acidosis ("type 4" RTA)
Diminished ammonium excretion relative to renal functional mass (subnormal $U_{NH_4}V/GFR$)	Nephrolithiasis and nephrocalcinosis
	Any combination of several disturbances described above

metabolic acidosis after kidney transplantation. The acidification defect was attributed to a functional expression of immunologically mediated allograft rejection because deposition of complement (C_3) along the tubular basement membrane was found. This impression was also strengthened by the similarity between the interstitial damage seen in histologic studies of rejected kidneys [16] and in autoimmune diseases complicated by RTA such as systemic lupus erythematosus [17] and Sjögren's syndrome [18]. In all these conditions, mononuclear cells infiltrate the renal interstitium, suggesting a cell-mediated immunologic reaction against tubulointerstitial tissues.

In recent years, the association of hyperchloremic metabolic acidosis with isolated aldosterone deficiency has been recognized [19–22]. In this syndrome, as contrasted with distal RTA, the ability to lower the urinary pH during acidosis is preserved ("type 4" RTA). The hyperkalemia of this syndrome contributes to the acidosis by augmenting proximal tubular bicarbonate loss, suppressing urinary ammonium secretion [23], and by exchanging plasma potassium for intracellular hydrogen ion. In fact, one of the patients in the series reported by Batlle et al [15] manifested the characteristic features of the syndrome. The patient's ammonium excretion was low during spontaneous systemic acidosis despite the fact that his urinary pH was below 5.5.

In summary, RTA (of divergent types) is the most prevalent tubular syndrome following kidney transplantation. It may encompass the entire spectrum of RTA: namely, proximal, distal (both secretory and nonsecretory), "type 3" (mixed proximal and distal), and "type 4" RTA. Acidification disorders may vary as a function of time after transplantation. As a general rule, the RTA that appears early following transplantation resolves spontaneously and is predominantly a sequel to acute renal failure ("acute tubular necrosis"). On the other hand, defects that exist in the late post-transplant period are due to chronic rejection. A contributory minor role in the pathogenesis of RTA may also be played by secondary hyperparathyroidism, reduced ammonium excretion (caused by protein malnutrition or hyperkalemia), urinary tract infection, and obstructive uropathy. Chronic RTA following transplantation may interfere with bone metabolism and rarely lead to nephrocalcinosis and nephrolithiasis. Therefore, if the condition is sustained, bicarbonate should be supplemented at least to protect the skeleton. Fortunately, in most patients RTA remits spontaneously and no special treatment seems to be indicated.

Non-Azotemic Hyperkalemia Following Kidney Transplantation

In the recovery stage after kidney transplantation, most patients have a tendency to become hypokalemic. Among contributing causes are the polyuria of the recovery phase from acute tubular necrosis in patients with cadaver kidney transplants, the administration of large doses of steroids, and, occasionally, the occurrence of renal tubular acidosis.

Table 3. Factors producing nonazotemic hyperkalemia by influencing the internal balance of potassium

Hypoinsulinism or end-organ refractoriness to the action of insulin	Acidosis
Hypoaldosteronism	Hyperglycemia in the presence of factors 1, 2, and 3
β-Adrenergic blockade	

In our experience, hyperkalemia is rare following a successful kidney transplantation. Yet, it remains a potential threat to patients without endogenous kidney function who undergo an emergency operation, such as cadaver kidney transplantation. Such a patient should receive potassium-binding resins rectally (Kayexalate) before the operation, particularly if time has elapsed since the previous dialysis. Transfusion of old, stored blood or administration of the muscle relaxant succinylcholine should be avoided because of their tendency to cause hyperkalemia [24].

The defense against hyperkalemia depends on the normal uptake of potassium by cells (internal balance), as well as on the elimination of excess potassium by the kidneys (external balance). The role of insulin and mineralocorticoids in the internal and external balance has recently been critically reviewed in depth [25]. A brief summary of the various influences on internal and external potassium balance is given in Tables 3 and 4.

Many reports of non-azotemic hyperkalemia have appeared since the original report of Hudson, Chobanian, and Relman [26], expanding the subject to include, namely, the hyperkalemia that may occur in patients with only modest kidney failure. This type of hyperkalemia has also been described in the particular setting of kidney transplantation.

The first report of a cluster of patients with kidney grafts and hyperkalemia came from Australia. The second communication describing this complication appeared recently in the U.S.A. [27]. In the experience of DeFronzo et al [27], hyperkalemia was observed in 23 of 75 patients in the first 3 months following transplantation. This hyperkalemia was unrelated to rejection, renal failure, oliguria, or acidosis. Urinary potassium excretion was sufficient to achieve potassium balance, but was inappropriately low relative to the hyperkalemia. In all patients, the hyperkalemia resolved spontaneously. An unusual feature was its refractoriness to furosemide. It responded, however, to thia-

Table 4. Factors producing non-azotemic hyperkalemia by interfering with the urinary excretion of potassium (external balance)

Hyporeninemic hypoaldosteronism
Impaired kaliuretic response to mineralocorticoids
Excessive distal tubular reabsorption of chloride leading to:
    Luminal potential difference unfavorable for distal K^+ secretion
    Systemic hypervolemia and suppression of the renin-angiotensin-aldosterone axis
Use of potassium-sparing diuretics (spironolactone, amiloride, triamterene)

zides, with an increase in urinary potassium excretion and a fall in serum potassium. When the renin-angiotensin-aldosterone axis was studied, it was found to be normal under basal conditions, and it responded adequately and appropriately to stimulation [27].

Because there was normal endocrine function and refractoriness to the kaliuretic action of acetazolamide and bicarbonate, the authors concluded that their hyperkalemic patients had an end-organ (distal tubular) defect of potassium excretion. The nature of this defect has not been elucidated [27]. It is, however, conceivable that medullary interstitial kidney damage, which is common after transplantation, accounts for the impairment of renal handling of potassium. A similar mechanism for hyperkalemia has been reported for patients suffering from systemic lupus erythematosus [28] and sickle cell disease [29].

In addition to end-organ refractoriness to the kaliuretic action of mineralocorticoids, some cases have been described in which the hyperkalemia following kidney transplantation resulted from hypoaldosteronism owing to suppression of the renin-angiotensin-aldosterone axis [15, 30]. Administration of mineralocorticoids in those instances corrected the hyperkalemia by augmenting urinary potassium excretion.

The instances of non-azotemic hyperkalemia just described were mainly due to an impaired elimination of potassium by the kidneys (positive external balance). Potassium loading from tissue catabolism caused by infection, hemolysis, massive blood transfusion, and acidosis is an additional factor aggravating the hyperkalemia.

An important impairment in the internal balance of potassium has recently been described in a diabetic patient [31]. In this patient, who was insulindependent and had an adequately functioning kidney graft, hyperglycemia was associated with hyperkalemia. Interestingly, plasma and urinary aldosterone levels were normal. It was considered that insulinopenia resulted in impaired cellular uptake of both glucose and potassium, leading to hyperglycemia and hyperkalemia. Solvent drag from the intracellular to the extracellular compartment under the influence of the hyperosmolality of hyperglycemia probably also contributed to the hyperkalemia.

In summary, transient hyperkalemia may be seen occasionally following kidney transplantation, even when the graft function is otherwise normal. Its etiology is obscure. The mechanism of this hyperkalemia may be (a) mineralocorticoid deficiency, (b) disturbed internal potassium balance reflecting diminished translocation of potassium from the extracellular to the intracellular compartment, or (c) end-organ (renal tubular) refractoriness to the action of aldosterone. The clinical implication of these phenomena is that following transplantation the use of potassium supplements or the use of potassium-sparing diuretics should be done under monitoring of serum potassium.

In the patients with post-transplant hyperkalemia, the response to diuretics may give a clue to its cause. Correction of the hyperkalemia with furosemide or exogenous mineralocorticoids suggests hypoaldosteronism with normal end-organ function. Refractoriness of the hyperkalemia to furosemide or mineralocorticoids, but its correction with thiazides, suggests a primary defect in the renal handling of potassium.

Disorders of Divalent Ion Metabolism Following Kidney Transplantation

Disturbances in divalent ion metabolism are common following renal transplantation. The occurrence of hypercalcemia after successful transplantation was first reported in 1964 [32] and has since been described by several authors [33, 34–39].

Hyperfunction of the parathyroid glands is the predominant factor implicated in post-transplant hypercalcemia. In fact, the hyperparathyroidism of chronic uremia often persists into the post-transplant period in spite of the resolution of the uremic state [37, 40]. The incidence of hypercalcemia following kidney transplantation has varied between 7% of patients according to some investigators [41] and more than one third of patients according to others [42]. Several factors may aggravate the hyperparathyroidism and accentuate hypercalcemia. Hypophosphatemia can potentiate hypercalcemia when phosphate depletion is produced by an overzealous antacid therapy with phosphate-binding gels or by increased urinary loss owing to high-dose glucocorticoid therapy [33]. Increased demand for phosphate by the skeleton because of the improved mineralization following successful transplantation may also contribute to hypophosphatemia and hypercalcemia. Hypercalcemia also could be caused by the transplanted kidney's capacity to hydroxylate 25-hydroxycholecalciferol to 1,25-dihydroxycholecalciferol, the most active metabolite of vitamin D. The latter restores the skeletal sensitivity to parathyroid hormone (PTH) and increases intestinal absorption of calcium. Normalization of the uremic environment may augment the tendency to hypercalcemia under these conditions.

Another possible cause of hypercalcemia after renal transplantation is the mobilization of metastatic calcifications after restoration of normal renal and parathyroid function [43].

The onset of hypercalcemia may be as early as one day and as late as one year post-transplant [42]. The occasional late onset of hypercalcemia might be explained by the time required for skeletal remineralization, after which there would be less demand for calcium by bone. Other factors responsible for the delayed appearance of hypercalcemia include the time required for the generation of phosphorus depletion [33], the slow establishment of normal renal function, and the dose of glucocorticoid used [34].

The post-transplant hypercalcemia may be transient or persistent. In the studies of David et al [42], persistent hypercalcemia of more than one year's duration was reported in 5 of the 22 hypercalcemic patients. Persistent hypercalcemia of more than 2 years' duration in renal transplant recipients is rare [34, 41]. Chatterjee et al [44] found persistent hypercalcemia for 2 to

4 years in 7 of 16 hypercalcemic patients, and in 2 other patients it persisted for 7 years. David et al [42] found a correlation between its time of onset and its severity and duration. Early-onset hypercalcemia (within the first 10 days after transplantation) was associated with a greater severity of hypercalcemia necessitating emergency parathyroidectomy. On the other hand, hypercalcemia that developed after the first month was significantly correlated with a persistent course (more than one year).

It is noteworthy that no correlation was found between the presence of renal osteodystrophy before transplantation and the occurrence of hypercalcemia following the transplantation [33]. However, a strong correlation was documented between kidney function in the early post-transplant period and the development of hypercalcemia. In none of the patients with creatinine clearance of less than 30 ml/min did hypercalcemia develop [42].

It is obvious that persistent hypercalcemia may be detrimental to the transplanted kidney. The main deleterious effects that hyperparathyroidism may have on the graft include metastatic calcium deposition, nephrolithiasis [45, 46], and renal tubular acidosis (both proximal and distal), which, by itself, may predispose the kidney to complications derived from hypercalciuria and recurrent infection. Severe hypercalcemia may also lead to oliguria or deteriorating GFR without any detectable organic lesion [37, 38].

Since the usual patient who reaches the stage of transplantation is already suffering from advanced bone disease, aggravated by complications of chronic dialysis, it is quite clear that persistent hyperparathyroidism coupled with hypophosphatemia, chronic acidosis (which is due to RTA), and steroid treatment may all act in concert to produce severe bone disease.

Several questions may arise concerning the handling and treatment of persistent hypercalcemia following transplantation. The main dilemma is predicting in which patient hyperparathyroidism will regress spontaneously, thus obviating the need for parathyroidectomy. The published opinions by Alfrey et al [33] and Johnson et al [36] have stated strongly that provision of adequate homeostasis with a well-functioning renal homograft should gradually correct the hypercalcemia. Based on their view that a state of phosphate depletion could contribute to the development of hypercalcemia, Alfrey et al [33] recommend a trial of repletion with phosphate-containing medications. This kind of phosphate supplementation probably is worth trying for a short period. However, if required chronically, it may stimulate the parathyroid by lowering the serum calcium level or it could, theoretically, aggravate soft tissue calcification. It is therefore recommended to try this treatment for a period of 3 months [34]. If hypercalcemia persists thereafter, or if metastatic calcifications develop, parathyroidectomy should be considered [34].

In establishing specific indications for parathyroidectomy, one must also consider total serum calcium values as well as any deterioration in kidney function. In fact, it has been shown that persistent elevation of serum calcium levels of less than 12 mg/dl does not damage the function of the renal graft [42]. On the other hand, serum calcium greater than 13.0 mg/dl may produce a decrease in creatinine clearance, which improves after subtotal parathyroidectomy [34, 42, 44]. Thus, it seems prudent to follow renal function carefully and frequently in renal transplant recipients who develop hypercalcemia, and once renal function deteriorates in the absence of evidence for rejection, parathyroidectomy should be performed.

Hypophosphatemia Following Kidney Transplantation

Hypophosphatemia occurs often following transplantation and is almost always associated with hypercalcemia in the early post-transplant period [3, 47, 48]. The introduction of normal kidney into an environment in which there is an excessive level of PTH in the circulation readily explains hypophosphatemia in this setting. However, hypophosphatemia is frequently observed also in the late post-transplant period [47, 48]. The factors that may play a role in this event include extrarenal mechanisms caused by an over-zealous use of phosphate binding antacids [33], reduced dietary intake, malabsorption, and vitamin D deficiency. These may act in concert with the phosphaturic action of steroids [49] and of autonomous hyperparathyroidism. However, renal phosphate leak may persist even after all of the above have been excluded. This suggests intrinsic tubular defect in phosphate reabsorption independent of PTH. These patients usually have reduced rates of renal phosphate reabsorption (TRP) [10, 50]. This has been attributed to increased sensitivity to PTH [48, 51], possible tubular action of immunosuppressive drugs [48], and an intrinsic tubular defect in phosphate reabsorption following immunologic injury [10]. The latter possibility is supported by the finding of structural damage to the early proximal tubule in microdissected tubules obtained from transplanted kidney in man [52]. The various possible causes for hypophosphatemia following transplantation are summarized in Table 5.

Whatever the cause of the hypophosphatemia following kidney transplantation, it has several deleterious effects on the recipient. These effects include increased osteolysis, unmasking of hypercalcemia associated with persistent secondary hyperparathyroidism, and a tendency to metabolic acidosis [53]. Chronic acidosis, by itself, may aggravate bone disease. It appears, therefore,

Table 5. Possible causes of hypophosphatemia following kidney transplantation

Extrarenal causes
    Use of phosphate-binding antacids
    Use of steroids
    Autonomous hyperparathyroidism
    "Hungry bone syndrome" following resolution of hyperparathyroidism
    Diminished circulating 1,25-dihydroxycholecalciferol leading to impaired intestinal or renal tubular transport of phosphate

Renal causes
    Intrinsic tubular defect in the reabsorption of phosphate
    Increased sensitivity to PTH

that early recognition and treatment of post-transplant hypophosphatemia
is essential for avoiding severe skeletal disease.

Hypertension Following Renal Transplantation

Sustained blood pressure elevation remains a serious problem in many patients
receiving an otherwise satisfactory renal allograft. It occurs in approximately
one third of all recipients. In patients who have not had bilateral nephrectomies before transplantation, the incidence of hypertension 6 months after
grafting approaches 80% [54, 55].

In the majority of patients, the cause of the hypertension is not clear.
Several mechanisms have been suggested: (1) hypersecretion of renin by the
host's kidneys [55–57] and activation of the renin-angiotensin-aldosterone
axis; (2) transplant rejection [54, 58, 59]; (3) transplant renal artery stenosis
[58, 60–64]; (4) corticosteroid therapy [65, 66]; (5) hypercalcemia [67]; (6)
inherent factors present in either donor or recipient.

Linas et al [56] gave clear evidence for the role of the host's kidneys in
post-transplant hypertension. They compared the effect of salt depletion and
saralasin between post-transplant patients with only one kidney to patients
with one or two original kidneys. They found that in patients with only
one kidney (the homograft), salt depletion and saralasin did not lower blood
pressure. In those with more than one kidney, salt depletion plus saralasin
lowered their blood pressure, suggesting that post-transplant hypertension is
more likely to be angiotensin-II-dependent in patients with more than one
kidney. Interestingly, one of the patients who showed a response to saralasin
had two transplanted kidneys but no host kidneys. It appears, therefore,
that the absolute number of kidneys available to release renin may determine
the renin dependency of post-transplant hypertension.

The donor kidney source may also influence post-transplant hypertension.
Thus, Whelton et al [68] found that in their transplanted hypertensive population the donor source was more frequently cadaveric and the patients were
more azotemic than nonhypertensive recipients. It is indeed likely that chronic
transplant rejection, which is more frequent among recipients of cadaveric
kidneys, plays a contributory role in the pathogenesis of post-transplant hypertension.

A peculiar role for renin secretion by the graft has been demonstrated
in the pathogenesis of excessive hypertension following transplantation. It
occurs with kidneys that are obtained from donors dying of the hepatorenal
syndrome and transplanted to anephric recipients. This type of hypertension
is probably due to the combination of high renin levels in the transplanted
kidney and the high plasma renin substrate in anephric recipients [69].

Stenosis of the renal artery has been reported to occur in from 1 to 10%
of patients undergoing kidney transplantation [58, 60–63]. Characteristic features of this group as compared with the remainder of the hypertensive population include the refractoriness of the high blood pressure to conventional

treatment, increased levels of plasma renin activity [63], and the presence of transplant bruit. It must be realized, however, that although transplant bruit is an important physical finding to the diagnosis of renal artery stenosis following transplantation, it is by no means an exclusive marker of transplant stenosis. In fact, transplant bruits have been associated with normotension, hypertension, transplant stenosis, good renal function, and poor renal function. Most commonly this physical finding is noted in patients with excellent renal function, and in this situation it is probably flow related. The disappearance of a bruit may indicate a reduction in renal blood flow and a worsening of renal function, whereas the appearance of a bruit that had not been present in the initial postoperative period and is associated with elevated blood pressure suggests the possibility of renovascular hypertension.

Finally, an important practical point that has recently gained recognition is that acute renal insufficiency may develop in patients receiving captopril for treatment of severe hypertension associated with post-transplant renal artery stenosis [70]. It was proposed that the azotemia in this context was functional and resulted from a disturbance in the autoregulation of glomerular filtration secondary to intrarenal blockade of the renin-angiotensin system in the presence of reduced renal artery perfusion pressure. Therefore, if renal function deteriorates shortly after captopril administration, arteriography should be considered.

Erythrocytosis after Renal Transplantation

Erythrocytosis has been reported as an uncommon and usually transient complication of transplantation [71–73]. There appear to be several mechanisms operative in the development of post-transplant erythrocytosis. In some patients, acute and chronic rejection presumably leads to intrarenal hypoxia and a resultant increase in erythropoietin secretion. In other patients, moderate to severe hypertension may lead to a contracted plasma volume with a resultant relative erythrocytosis. Also, some investigators have proposed that the patients' own kidneys may contribute to a transient increase in erythropoietin production and erythrocytosis.

Post-transplant erythrocytosis should raise the possibility of renal artery stenosis [62, 64]. It is possible but not proven that activation of the renin-angiotensin-aldosterone axis by reduced renal perfusion stimulates the production of erythropoietin [74].

Whenever the transplanted patient presents with erythrocytosis, hypertension, and azotemia, a clinical distinction is necessary between renal artery stenosis and graft rejection. However, absence of proteinuria and preserved ability to concentrate the urine despite azotemia (prerenal azotemia) are highly suggestive of renal artery stenosis rather than a diffuse parenchymal lesion secondary to rejection [64]. It is crucial to make a correct diagnosis of renal artery stenosis to avoid erroneous treatment with immunosuppressive drugs.

Complications of Antirejection Therapy

Transplant patients are subjected to numerous complications directly related to the prolonged use of immunosuppressive treatment. Some of these complications may lead to death.

Corticosteroids are responsible for the increased incidence of peptic ulcer and life-threatening gastrointestinal hemorrhage postoperatively. It has been recommended that patients who have evidence of peptic ulcer disease undergo prophylactic vagotomy and pyloroplasty or antrectomy before transplantation [75]. However, in general there has been a lack of correlation between the presence of preoperative peptic ulcers and postoperative bleeding [76]. The histamine H_2-receptor antagonist cimetidine has been used to control gastric hyperacidity and upper gastrointestinal ulceration in kidney transplantation patients [77]. Concern was raised, however, about the possibility of augmentation of delayed hypersensitivity in patients taking cimetidine [78]. In vitro data suggest that cimetidine is capable of increasing alloantigen-induced proliferation of lymphocytes from renal allograft recipients [79]. Furthermore, increased rejection episodes after kidney transplantation have been reported both in humans [80] and in experimental animals that received cimetidine postoperatively [81]. It is therefore recommended that the use of cimetidine in the transplant patient be abandoned and replaced by either conventional antacids or other H_2-receptor antagonists (e.g., ranitidine).

Hyperglycemia following kidney transplantation is a common complication of steroid use ("steroid diabetes"). Its frequency varies in different series [82–84], ranging up to half the number of renal transplant recipients [85]. Steroid diabetes is a dose-dependent complication, so that it is often first detected after increasing the dose of corticosteroids at rejection episodes [86], and it usually disappears when the steroid dose is reduced. In some patients, however, persistent diabetes requiring chronic insulin therapy may develop in spite of reduction of the steroid dosage to maintenance levels (10 to 15 mg/day of prednisone) [85].

Life-threatening hyperglycemia leading to hyperosmolar nonketotic states have been observed mainly after high-dose steroid therapy for the rejection of renal transplants [87, 88]. The treatment of this condition is based on rehydration with gradual lowering of blood osmolarity and small dosage of insulin.

The use of either azathioprine or cyclophosphamide in the conventional immunosuppressive regimens renders the transplant patient susceptible to various opportunistic infections. One type of disease is the cytomegalovirus (CMV) infection (which sometimes may be transmitted from the donor kidney). It is unique in that in addition to its potential for causing multisystem infection, it can produce a distinct glomerulopathy that clinically mimics rejection [89]. Only renal biopsy examination can differentiate between rejection and CMV glomerulopathy. Graft rejection is distinguished by vascular and tubulointerstitial changes as compared to the exclusive glomerular pathology caused by CMV.

Cyclosporine is a potent new immunosuppressive agent that selectively inhibits T-cell function, allowing survival of allografts without myelosuppression. This drug is a metabolic product of the fungi *Cylindrocarpon lucidium* and *Trichoderma polysporum.* After the original report of Borel et al [90, 91] on its biologic properties, further experience was added both in humans [92–94] and in experimental animals [95–97]. A recent study in cadaveric kidney transplant recipients has clearly shown that at 4 years post-transplantation, the rates of patient and graft survival with a cyclosporine regimen remain superior to those with conventional immunosuppression [98].

Higher serum creatinine concentrations have been observed in patients given cyclosporine than in those receiving conventional immunosuppressants [99–101]. Whether this elevation represents nephrotoxicity or subclinical rejection is unknown. However, some nephrotoxicity is reported to occur in almost 80% of the renal transplant patients using the drug [102], although the mechanism underlying this nephrotoxicity has not been clearly defined in experimental studies. It is difficult to differentiate nephrotoxicity from rejection, and a variety of techniques to help make this clinical distinction have been reported [103, 104]. None of these methods, however, provides a sensitive and specific tool for the diagnosis of cyclosporine-associated nephrotoxicity. For the present, a fall in the concentration of serum creatinine associated with a reduction in the dose of cyclosporine is the best retrospective evidence of nephrotoxicity. A unique, nephrotoxic complication related to cyclosporine is a sustained hyperkalemia out of proportion to the reduced glomerular filtration rate associated with hyperchloremic metabolic acidosis [105]. It has been suggested that both suppression of the renin-angiotensin-aldosterone axis and tubular damage produced defects in potassium and hydrogen ion secretion. Monitoring cyclosporine blood concentrations is believed to be essential for avoiding nephrotoxicity. Optimal trough serum concentrations are not yet known but an attempt should be made to keep them in the range of 100 to 500 ng/ml.

It appears that cyclosporine is a powerful immunosuppressant that provides a valuable alternative to conventional methods of antirejection therapy. However, 5- and 10-year survival results are still needed for determining the ultimate place of cyclosporine in the immunosuppressive armamentarium.

References

1. MASSRY SG, PREUSS HG, MAHER JF, SCHREINER GE: Renal tubular acidosis after cadaver kidney homotransplantation. *Am J Med* 42:284–292, 1967
2. MOOKERJEE B, GAULT MH, DOSSETOT JB: Hyperchloremic acidosis in early diagnosis of renal allograft rejection. *Ann Intern Med* 71:47–57, 1969
3. GYORY AZ, STEWART JH, GEORGE CRP, TILLER DJ, EDWARDS KDG: Renal tubular acidosis, acidosis due to hyperkalemia, hypercalcemia, disordered citrate metabolism and other tubular dysfunctions following human renal transplantation. *Q J Med* 38:231–254, 1969
4. BETTER OS, CHAIMOVITZ C, NAVEH Y, STEIN A, NAHIR AM, BARZILAI A, ERLIK D: Syndrome of incomplete renal tubular acidosis after cadaver kidney transplantation. *Ann Intern Med* 71:39–45, 1969

5. BETTER OS, CHAIMOVITZ C, ALROY GG, SISMAN I: Spontaneous remission of the defect in urinary acidification after cadaver kidney homotransplantation. *Lancet* 1:110–112, 1970
6. HENDERSON LW, NOLPH KD, PUSCHETT JB, GOLDBURG M: Proximal tubular malfunction as a mechanism for diuresis after renal homotransplantation. *N Engl J Med* 278:467–473, 1968
7. BRIGGS WA, KOMINAMI N, WILSON RE, MERRILL JP: Kidney transplantation and Fanconi syndrome. *N Engl J Med* 286:25–29, 1972
8. WILSON DR, SIDDIQUI AA: Renal tubular acidosis after kidney transplantation: Natural history and significance. *Ann Intern Med* 79:352–361, 1973
9. VERTUNO LL, PREUSS HG, ARGY WP, SCHREINER GE: Fanconi syndrome following homotransplantation. *Arch Intern Med* 133:302–305, 1974
10. VAZIRI ND, NELLANDS RE, BRUEGGMANN RM, BARTON CH, MARTIN DC: Renal tubular dysfunction in transplanted kidneys. *South Med J* 72:530–535, 1979
11. THIRAKOMEN K, KOZOLOV N, ARRUDA JAL, KURTZMAN NA: Renal hydrogen ion secretion following the release of unilateral ureteral obstruction. *Am J Physiol* 231:1233–1239, 1976
12. ARRUDA JAL, NASCIMENTO L, KUMAR SK, KURTZMAN NA: Factors influencing the formation of urinary carbon dioxide tension. *Kidney Int* 11:307–317, 1977
13. ARRUDA JAL, NASCIMENTO L, MEHTA PK, RADEMACKER DR, SEHY JT, WESTENFELDER C, KURTZMAN NA: The critical importance of urinary concentrating ability in the generation of urinary carbon dioxide tension. *J Clin Invest* 60:922–935, 1977
14. BATLLE DC, ARRUDA JAL, KURTZMAN NA: Hyperkalemia and distal renal tubular acidosis associated with obstructive uropathy. *N Engl J Med* 304:373–380, 1981
15. BATLLE DC, MOZES MF, MANALIGOD J, ARRUDA JAL, KURTZMAN NA: The pathogenesis of hyperchloremic metabolic acidosis associated with kidney transplantation. *Am J Med* 70:786–796, 1981
16. ANDERS GA, MCCLUSKEY RT: Tubular and interstitial renal disease due to immunologic mechanisms. *Kidney Int* 7:271–289, 1971
17. TU WH, SHEARN MA: Systemic lupus erythematosus and latent renal tubular dysfunction. *Ann Intern Med* 67:100–109, 1967
18. TALAL N, ZISMAN E, SCHUR PH: Renal tubular acidosis, glomerulonephritis and immunologic factors in Sjogren's syndrome. *Arthritis Rheum* 11:774–786, 1968
19. SCHAMBELAN M, STOCKIGT J, BIGLIER E: Isolated hypoaldosteronism in adults: A renin-deficiency syndrome. *N Engl J Med* 287:573–578, 1972
20. PEREZ G, SIEGEL L, SCHREINER GE: Selective hypoaldosteronism with hyperkalemia. *Ann Intern Med* 76:757–763, 1972
21. HULTER HN, ILNICKI LP, HARBOTTLE JA, SEBASTIAN A: Impaired renal H^+ secretion and NH_3 production in mineralocorticoid-deficient glucocorticoid-replete dogs. *Am J Physiol* 232:F136–F146, 1977
22. DITELLA P, SODHI B, MCCREARY J, ARRUDA JAL, KURTZMAN NA: The mechanism of the metabolic acidosis of selective mineralocorticoid deficiency. *Kidney Int* 14:466–477, 1978
23. SZYLMAN P, BETTER OS, CHAIMOVITZ C, ROSLER A: Role of hyperkalemia in the metabolic acidosis of isolated hypoaldosteronism. *N Engl J Med* 294:361–365, 1976
24. GRONERT GA, THEYE RA: Pathophysiology of hyperkalemia induced by succinylcholine. *Anaesthesiology* 43:89–99, 1975

25. Cox M, Sterns RH, Singer I: The defense against hyperkalemia: The roles of insulin and aldosterone. *N Engl J Med* 299:525–532, 1978
26. Hudson JB, Chobanian AV, Relman AS: Hypoaldosteronism: A clinical study of a patient with an isolated adrenal mineralocorticoid deficiency, resulting in hyperkalemia and Stokes-Adams attacks. *N Engl J Med* 257:529–536, 1957
27. DeFronzo RA, Goldberg M, Cooke CR, Barker C, Grossman RA, Agus Z: Investigations into the mechanism of hyperkalemia following renal transplantation. *Kidney Int* 11:357–365, 1977
28. DeFronzo RA, Cooke CR, Goldberg M: Impaired renal tubular potassium secretion in systemic lupus erythematosus. *Ann Intern Med* 86:268–271, 1977
29. DeFronzo RA, August P, Black H, McPhedran P, Cooke CR: Impaired renal tubular potassium secretion in sickle cell disease. *Abst Proc Am Soc Nephrol* 10:13A 1977
30. Roll D, Licht A, Rosler A, Durst A, Kleeman CR, Czaczkes J: Transient hypoaldosteronism after renal allotransplantation. *Isr J Med Sci* 15:29–34, 1979
31. Rosenbaum R, Hoffsten PE, Cryer P, Klahr S: Hyperkalemia after renal transplantation. *Arch Intern Med* 138:1270–1272, 1978
32. McPhaul JJ, Jr, McIntosh DA, Hammond WS, Park OK: Autonomous secondary (renal) parathyroid hyperplasia. *N Engl J Med* 271:1342–1345, 1964
33. Alfrey AC, Jenkins D, Groth CG, Schorr WS, Gecelter L, Ogden DA: Resolution of hyperparathyroidism, renal osteodystrophy and metastatic calcification after renal homotransplantation. *N Engl J Med* 279:1349–1356, 1968
34. Geis WP, Popovtzer MM, Corman JL, Holgrimson CG, Groth CG, Starzl TE: The diagnosis and treatment of hyperparathyroidism after renal homotransplantation. *Surg Gynecol Obstet* 137:997–1010, 1973
35. Hampers CL, Katz AI, Wilson RE, Merrill JP: Calcium metabolism and osteodystrophy after renal transplantation. *Arch Intern Med* 124:282–291, 1969
36. Johnson JW, Hattner RS, Hamper CL, Bernstein DS, Merrill JP, Sherwood LM: Secondary hyperparathyroidism in chronic renal failure: Effects of renal homotransplantation. *JAMA* 215:478–480, 1971
37. McIntosh DA, Peterson EW, McPhaul JJ: Autonomy of parathyroid function after renal homotransplantation. *Ann Intern Med* 65:900–907, 1966
38. Schwartz GH, David DS, Riggio RR, Saville PO, Whitsell JC, Stenzel KH, Rubin AL: Hypercalcemia after renal transplantation. *Am J Med* 49:42–51, 1970
39. Christensen MS, Nielsen HE, Torring S: Hypercalcemia and parathyroid function after renal transplantation. *Acta Med Scand* 201:35–39, 1977
40. Wilson RE, Bernstein DS, Murray JE, Moore FD: Effects of parathyroidectomy and kidney transplantation on renal osteodystrophy. *Am J Surg* 110:384–393, 1965
41. Cerilli J, Limbert JG, Ferris TF, Tzagournis M: Subtotal parathyroidectomy for tertiary hyperparathyroidism thirty-two months after renal transplantation. *Am J Surg* 125:636–638, 1973
42. David DS, Sakai S, Brennan BL, Riggio RA, Cheigh J, Stenzel KH, Rubin AL, Sherwood LM: Hypercalcemia after renal transplantation. *N Engl J Med* 289:398–401, 1973
43. Hornum I: Post-transplant hypercalcemia due to mobilization of metastatic calcifications. *Acta Med Scand* 189:199–205, 1971
44. Chatterjee SN, Friedler RM, Berne TV, Oldham SB, Singer FR, Massry SG: Persistent hypercalcemia after successful renal transplantation. *Nephron* 17:1–7, 1976
45. Rosenberg JC, Arnstein AR, Ing TS, Pierce JM Jr, Rosenberg B, Silva

Y, WALT AJ: Calculi complicating a renal transplant. *Am J Surg* 129:326–330, 1975

46. LEAPMAN SB, VIDNE BA, BUTT KMH, WATERHOUSE K, KOUNTZ SL: Nephrolithiasis and nephrocalcinosis after renal transplantation: A case report and review of the literature. *J Urol* 115:129–132, 1976

47. WARD HN, PABICO RC, MCKENNA BA, FREEMAN FB: The renal handling of phosphate by renal transplant patients: Correlation with serum parathyroid hormone, cyclic 3′,5′-adenosine monophosphate urinary excretion and allograft function. *Adv Exp Med Biol* 81:173–181, 1977

48. MOOREHEAD JF, AHMED KY, VARGHESE Z, WILLS MR, BAILLED RA, TATLER GLV: Hypophosphataemic osteomalacia after cadaveric renal transplantation. *Lancet* 1:694–697, 1974

49. INGBAR S, KON E, BURNETT C, RELMAN A, BURROWS B, SISSON J: The effects of cortisone on the renal tubular transport of uric acid, phosphorus and electrolytes in patients with normal renal and adrenal function. *J Lab Clin Med* 38:533–541, 1951

50. HERDMAN RC, VERNIER RL, MICHAEL AF, KELLY WP, GOOD RA: Renal function and phosphorus excretion after human renal homotransplantation. *Lancet* 1:121–123, 1966

51. ROSENBAUM RW, HRUSKA KA, KORKOR A, ANDERSON C, SLATOPOLSKY E: Decreased phosphate reabsorption after renal transplantation: Evidence for a mechanism independent of calcium and parathyroid hormone. *Kidney Int* 19:568–578, 1981

52. DARMADY EM, OFFER JM, STRANACK F: Study of renal vessels by microdissection in human transplantation. *Br Med J* 11:276–278, 1964

53. GOLD LW, MASSRY SG, ARIEFF AI, COBURN JW: Renal bicarbonate wasting during phosphate depletion: A possible cause of altered acid-base homeostasis in hyperparathyroidism. *J Clin Invest* 52:2556–2562, 1973

54. COLES GA, CROSBY DL, JONES GR, JONES J, MCVEIGH S: Hypertension following cadaveric renal transplantation. *Postgrad Med J* 48:399–404, 1972

55. COHEN SL: Hypertension in renal transplant recipients: role of bilateral nephrectomy. *Br Med J* 3:78–81, 1973

56. LINAS SL, MILLER PD, MCDONALD KM, STABLES DP, KATZ F, WEIL R, SCHRIER RW: Role of the renin-angiotensin system in post-transplantation hypertension in patients with multiple kidneys. *N Engl J Med* 298:1440–1444, 1978

57. MCHUGH MI, TANBOGA H, MARCEN R, LIANO F, ROBSON V, WILKINSON R: Hypertension following renal transplantation: The role of the host's kidneys. *Q J Med* 149:395–403, 1980

58. BENNETT WM, MCDONALD WJ, LAWSON RK, PORTER G: Posttransplant hypertension: studies of the cortical blood flow and the renal pressor system. *Kidney Int* 6:99–108, 1974

59. WEST TH, TURCOTTE JG, VANDER A: Plasma renin activity, sodium balance and hypertension in a group of renal transplant recipients. *J Lab Clin Med* 73:564–573, 1969

60. SMELLIE WAB, VINIK M, HUME DM: Angiographic investigation of hypertension complicating human renal transplantation. *Surg Gynecol Obstet* 129:963–968, 1969

61. LACOMBE M: Arterial stenosis complicating renal allotransplantation in man: A study of 38 cases. *Ann Surg* 181:283–288, 1975

62. BACON BR, ROTHMAN SA, RICANATI ES, RASHAD FA: Renal artery stenosis with erythrocytosis after renal transplantation. *Arch Intern Med* 140:1206–1211, 1980

63. MARGULES RM, BELZER FO, KOUNTZ SL: Surgical correction of renovascular hypertension following renal allotransplantation. *Arch Surg* 106:13–16, 1973
64. SCHRAMEK A, BETTER OS, ADLER O, TUMA S, HASHMONAI M, BARZILAI A, CHAIMOVITZ C: Hypertensive crisis, erythrocytosis, and uraemia due to renal-artery stenosis of kidney transplants. *Lancet* 1:70–71, 1975
65. SAMPSON D, KIRDANI RY, SANDBERG AA, MURPHY G: The aetiology of hypertension after renal transplantation in man. *Br J Surg* 60:819–824, 1973
66. POPOVTZER MM, PINNGGERA W, KATZ FH, CORMAN JL, ROBINETTE J, LANOIS B, HALGRIMSON CG, STARZL TE: Variations in arterial blood pressure after kidney transplantation: Relation to renal function, plasma renin activity and the dose of prednisone. *Circulation* 47:1297–1305, 1973
67. WEIDMAN P, MASSRY SG, COBURN JW: Blood pressure effects of acute hypercalcemia: Studies in patients with chronic renal failure. *Ann Intern Med* 76:741–745, 1972
68. WHELTON PK, RUSSELL RP, HARRINGTON DP, WILLIAMS GM, WALKER WG: Hypertension following renal transplantation: Causative factors and therapeutic implications. *JAMA* 241:1128–1131, 1979
69. MCDONALD FD, BRENNAN LA, TURCOTTE JG: Severe hypertension and elevated plasma renin activity following transplantation of "hepatorenal donor" kidneys into anephric recipients. *Am J Med* 54:39–43, 1973
70. CURTIS JJ, LUKE RG, WHELCHEL JD, DIETHELM AG, JONES P, DUSTAN HP: Inhibition of angiotensin-converting enzyme in renal transplant recipients with hypertension. *N Engl J Med* 308:377–381, 1983
71. NIES BA, COHN R, SCHRIER RW: Erythremia after renal transplantation. *N Engl J Med* 273:785–788, 1965
72. WU KK, GIBSON TP, FREEMAN RM, BONNEY WW, FRIED W, DEGOWIN RL: Erythrocytosis after renal transplantation: Its occurrence in two recipients of kidneys from the same cadaveric donor. *Arch Intern Med* 132:898–902, 1973
73. WESTERMAN MP, JENKINS JL, DEKKER A, KREUTNER A JR, FISHER B: Significance of erythrocytosis and increased erythropoietin secretion after renal transplantation. *Lancet* 2:755–757, 1967
74. ANAGNOSTOU A, BARANOWSKI R, PILLAY VKG, KURTZMAN N, VERCELLOTTI G, FRIED W: Effect of renin on extrarenal erythropoietin production. *J Lab Clin Med* 88:707–715, 1976
75. SPANOS PK, SIMMONS RL, RATTAZZI LC, KJELLSTRAND CM, BUSELMEIER TJ, NAJARIAN JS: Peptic ulcer disease in the transplant recipient. *Arch Surg* 109:193–197, 1974
76. CHISHOLM GD, MEE AD, WILLIAMS G: Peptic ulceration, gastric secretion and renal transplantation. *Br Med J* 1:1630–1635, 1977
77. JONES RH, RUDGE CJ, BEWICK M, PARSONS V, WESTON MJ: Cimetidine: Prophylaxis against upper gastrointestinal haemorrhage after transplantation. *Br Med J* 1:398–400, 1978
78. AVELLA J, BINDER HJ, MADSON JE, ASKENASE PW: Effect of histamine H_2-receptor antagonists on delayed hypersensitivity. *Lancet* 1:624–626, 1978
79. GIFFORD RRM, SCHMIDTKE JR, FERGUSON RM: Cimetidine modulation of lymphocytes from renal allograft recipients. *Transplant Proc* 13:663–667, 1981
80. PRIMACK WA: Cimetidine and renal allograft rejection. *Lancet* 1:824–825, 1978
81. ZAMMIT M, TOLEDO-PEREYRA LH: Cimetidine for kidney transplantation: Experimental observations. *Surgery* 86:611–619, 1979
82. SMYLLIE HC, CONOLLY CK: Incidence of serious complications of corticosteroid therapy in respiratory disease. *Thorax* 23:571–581, 1968
83. WOODS JE, ZINCKE H, PALUMBO PJ, JOHNSON WJ, ANDERSON CF, FROHMERT

PP, SERVICE FJ: Hyperosmolar nonketotic syndrome and steroid diabetes: Occurrence after renal transplantation. *JAMA* 231:1261–1263, 1975

84. DAVID SS, CHEIGH JS, BRAUN DW JR, FOTINO M, STENZEL KH, RUBIN AL: HLA-A 28 and steroid-induced diabetes in renal transplant patients. *JAMA* 243:532–533, 1980

85. ARNER P, GUNNARSSON R, BLOMDAHL S, GROTH CG: Some characteristics of steroid diabetes: A study in renal-transplant recipients receiving high-dose corticosteroid therapy. *Diabetes Care* 6:23–25, 1983

86. GUNNARSSON R, ARNER P, LUNDGREN G, MAGNUSSON G, OSTMAN J, GROTH CG: Steroid diabetes after renal transplantation—a preliminary report. *Scand J Urol Nephrol* 42:191–194, 1977

87. SPENNEY JG, EURE CA, KREISBERG RA: Hyperglycemic, hyperosmolar, nonketoacidotic diabetes: A complication of steroid and immunosuppressive therapy. *Diabetes* 18:107, 1969

88. DAOUK AA, MALEK GH, KAUFFMAN M, KISSEN WA: Hyperosmolar nonketotic coma in a kidney transplant recipient. *J Urol* 108:524–525, 1972

89. RICHARDSON WP, COLVIN RB, CHEESEMAN SH, TOLKOFF-RUBIN NE, HERRIN JT, COSIMI AB, COLLINS AB, HIRCH MS, McCLUSKEY RT, RUSSEL PS, RUBIN RH: Glomerulopathy associated with cytomegalovirus viremia in renal allografts. *N Engl J Med* 305:57–63, 1981

90. BOREL JF, FEURER C, GUBLER HU, STAHELIN H: Biological effects of cyclosporin A: A new anti-lymphocytic agent. *Agents Actions* 6:468–475, 1976

91. BOREL JF, FEURER C, MAGNEE C, STAHELIN H: Effects of the new anti-lymphocytic peptide cyclosporin A in animals. *Immunology* 32:1017–1025, 1977

92. CALNE RY, WHITE DJG, THIRU S, EVANS DB, McMASTER P, DUNN DC, CRADDOCK GN, PENTLOW BD, ROLLES K: Cyclosporin A in patients receiving renal allografts from cadaver donors. *Lancet* 2:1323–1327, 1978

93. CALNE RY, ROLLES K, WHITE DJG, THIRU S, EVANS DB, McMASTER P, DUNN DC, CRADDOCK GN, HENDERSON RG, AZIZ S, LEWIS P: Cyclosporin A initially as the only immunosuppressant in 34 recipients of cadaveric organs: 32 kidneys, 2 pancreases, and 2 livers. *Lancet* 2:1033–1036, 1979

94. CALNE RY, WHITE DJG, EVANS DB, THIRU S, HENDERSON RG, HAMILTON DV, ROLLES K, McMASTER P, DUFFY TG, McDOUGALL BRD, WILLIAMS R: Cyclosporin A in cadaveric organ transplantation. *Br Med J* 282:934–936, 1981

95. KOSTAKIS AJ, WHITE DJG, CALNE RY: Prolongation of rat heart allograft survival by cyclosporin A. *IRCS Med Sci* 5:280, 1977

96. CALNE RY, WHITE DJG: Cyclosporin A: A powerful immunosuppressant in dogs with renal allografts. *IRCS Med Sci* 5:595–596, 1977

97. CALNE RY, WHITE DJG, ROLLES K, SMITH DP, HERBERTSON BM: Prolonged survival of pig orthotopic heart grafts treated with cyclosporin A. *Lancet* 1:1183–1185, 1978

98. MERION RM, WHITE DJG, THIRU S, EVANS DB, CALNE RY: Cyclosporine: Five years' experience in cadaveric renal transplantation. *N Engl J Med* 310:148–154, 1984

99. FERGUSON RM, RYNASIEWICZ JJ, SUTHERLAND DER, SIMMONS RL, NAJARIAN JS: Cyclosporin A in renal transplantation: A prospective randomized trial. *Surgery* 92:175–182, 1982

100. HAKALA TR, STARZL TE, ROSENTHAL JT, SHAW B, IWATSUKI S: Cadaveric renal transplantation with cyclosporin-A and steroids. *Transplant Proc* 15:465–470, 1983

101. CANADIAN MULTICENTRE TRANSPLANT GROUP: A RANDOMIZED CLINICAL

TRIAL OF CYCLOSPORINE IN CADAVERIC RENAL TRANSPLANTATION. *N Engl J Med* 309:809–815, 1983

102. KAHAN BD: Meeting report: The First International Congress on cyclosporine, Houston, Texas, May 16–19, 1983. *Dialysis Transplant* 12:620–630, 1983
103. FRENCH ME, THOMPSON JF, HUNNISETT AGW, WOOD RFM, MORRIS PJ: Impaired function of renal allografts during treatment with cyclosporin-A: Nephrotoxicity or rejection? *Transplant Proc* 15:485–488, 1983
104. WAGNER E, PICHLMAYR R, WONIGEIT K, KLEMPNAUER J, BUNZENDAHL H, LAUCHART W: Differentiation between rejection and cyclosporin-A nephrotoxicity by monitoring interstitial pressure in human renal allografts. *Transplant Proc* 15:489–492, 1983
105. ADU D, TURNEY J, MICHAEL J, MCMASTER P: Hyperkalaemia in cyclosporin-treated renal allograft recipients. *Lancet* 2:370–372, 1983

Cyclosporine in Renal Transplantation

Rolf Loertscher, Mario Abbud-Filho, and Terry B. Strom

The Allograft Response

Activation of helper T cells by class II major histocompatibility complex antigens, such as HLA-DR, stimulates the release of a macrophage stimulant (perhaps the same molecule as colony-stimulating factor [1]) and the formation of receptors for insulin [2–4], transferrin [5], interleukin-1 (IL-1) [6], and interleukin-2 (IL-2) [7] (Fig. 1). Cytotoxic T lymphocytes stimulated by class I HLA antigens (such as HLA-A, -B, and -C) develop IL-2 receptors [7]. Subsequently, stimulated macrophages and other accessory cells release IL-1, which (in turn) stimulates the release of IL-2 [8]. Interleukin-2 interacts with specific IL-2 receptors expressed on activated helper and cytotoxic T cells [8]. This interaction stimulates both the initiation of DNA synthesis and eventual clonal proliferation of IL-2 receptor-bearing cells [8]. Moreover, the continued viability of activated T cell clones is IL-2-dependent. Interleukin-2, in turn, causes the release of gamma-interferon [9] (which activates macrophages [10]) as well as the release of B-cell growth factors that stimulate the proliferation of antigen-activated B cells [11, 12].

Another helper T cell product whose release might be stimulated by IL-2 is the cytotoxic differentiation factor (Fig. 1). Whereas IL-2 causes clonal growth of cytotoxic T cells, cytotoxic differentiation factor activates and (thereby) unleashes the cytotoxic potential of noncytotoxic T8-positive T cells. In brief, activation of helper T cells by alloantigen and IL-1 stimulates the release of a variety of lymphokines from helper T cells, which (in turn) activate macrophages, cytotoxic T cells, and antibody-releasing B cells (Fig. 1). These factors also support clonal expansion and viability of antigen-activated T and B cells. Unmodified rejection results from the cytodestructive effects caused by cytotoxic T cells, activated macrophages, and antibody

This manuscript was presented as part of a Symposium on *Immunomodulation for Transplantation: New Approaches.*

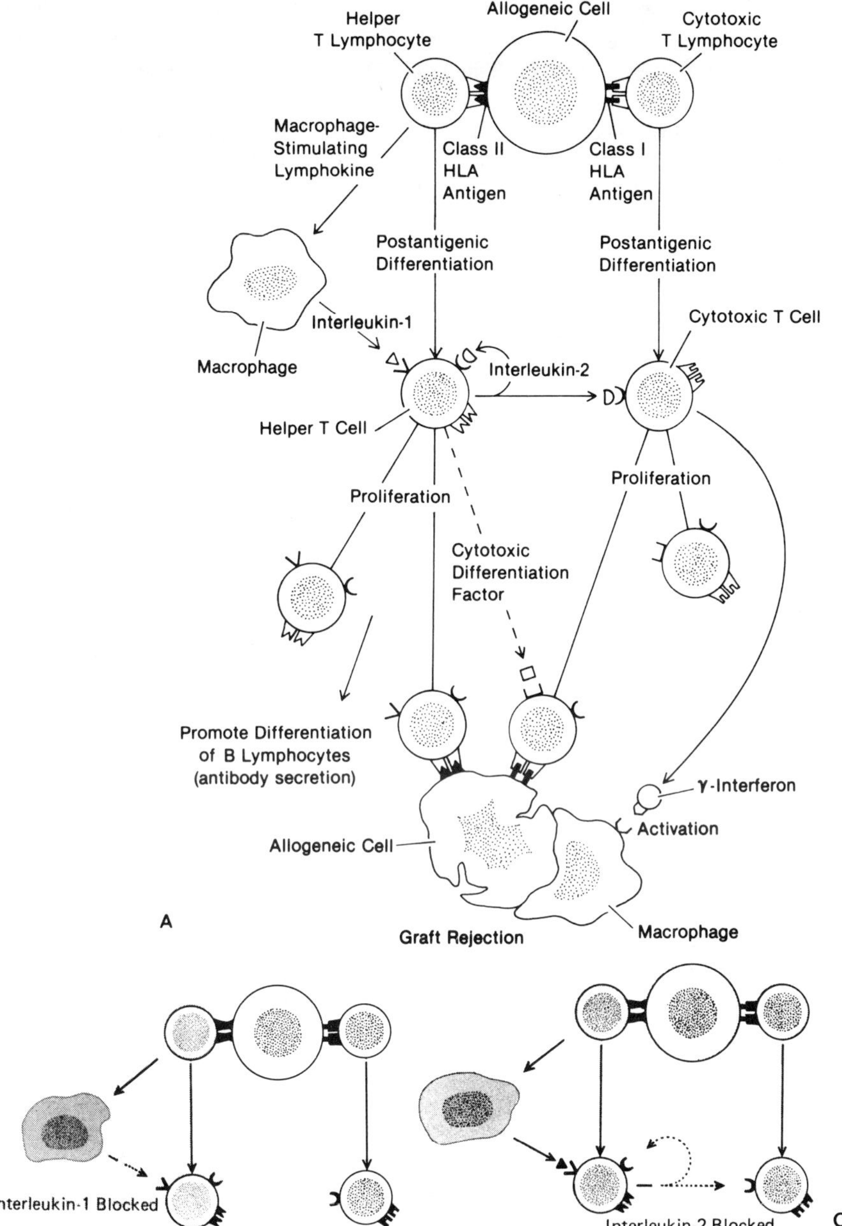

Fig. 1. a. The activation sequence that leads to the proliferation of alloreactive T cells includes antigen, interleukin-1 (IL-1) and interleukin-2 (IL-2). Macrophage activating factor has proven to be identical to gamma-interferon. Allograft rejection is a complex event that results from the cytodestructive effects of activated B lymphocytes, helper T cells, cytotoxic T cells, and activated macrophages. **b** Corticosteroids block the release of IL-1, thereby inhibiting the IL-1-dependent release of IL-2. **c** Cyclosporine prevents IL-2 release, and thus blocks antigen-driven T cell proliferation.

(Fig. 1). Although cytotoxic T cells are the dominant cell type that infiltrates the allograft during rejection episodes in experimental models—and in most clinical rejections—the transcendent importance of helper T cells in the events of rejection almost certainly derives from the "endocrine" role of helper T cells in providing the various soluble-growth and activation signals required during the allograft response (Fig. 1). The fact that helper T cells are pre-eminently important in rejection of vascularized organ transplants has been proven in our experiments, in which reconstitution of allograft immunity has been accomplished by injection of alloactivated helper T cells into T-cell-deficient experimental animals.

Mechanism of Action

Cyclosporine interferes with the activation sequence of lymphocytes, thus blocking the humoral and cellular effector mechanisms that participate in rejection. The drug inhibits both B and T lymphocyte activation, but the predominant effect appears to be its interference with the helper T cell function. While B lymphocytes participate in rejection, T lymphocytes are primarily responsible for rejection. The sites of influence of cyclosporine and corticosteroids on T cell activation are depicted in Figure 1. For most antibody responses, activation of antibody-producing B cells requires signals from helper T lymphocytes.

The fungal metabolite, cyclosporine, is a cyclic endecapeptide [13], that shares with corticosteroids the capacity to block the entry of activated T lymphocyte to the S phase of the cell cycle [14]. Unlike corticosteroids, cyclosporine does not inhibit the capacity of all, or even most, accessory cells to release IL-1 [15]. However, cyclosporine does block IL-2 release (Fig. 1) from activated helper T lymphocytes [15, 16]. The release of other lymphokines, such as gamma-interferon, by activated T cells also is inhibited by cyclosporine [17], whereas, the expression of IL-2 receptors [18] and the responsiveness of activated T lymphocytes to lymphokines are not blocked [19, 20]. Thus, under the influence of cyclosporine, helper T cell-dependent B cells are not fully activated due to a lack of necessary helper T cell stimulants.

Ample experimental evidence demonstrates that cyclosporine, in pharmacologic doses, does not grossly interfere with activation and proliferation of suppressor T lymphocytes [19–22]. Cyclosporine spares suppressor T lymphocytes. Indeed, in vitro studies have revealed the presence of a suppressor factor in the supernatants of cyclosporine-treated mixed lymphocyte cultures—an in vitro model of allograft rejection. This factor enhances the activity of suppressor cells. A study of heart-allografted rats demonstrated that cyclosporine inhibits in vivo release of IL-1 and IL-2, but it allows the release of a soluble mediator linked to the suppressor T cell induction [23]. Thus, while cyclosporine blocks the expansion of helper and cytotoxic T cells via interference with IL-2 release, liberation of suppressor cell-inducing factors is not affected. The preferential activation of suppressor cells under the umbrella of cyclosporine therapy may be the key to the induction of a state of tolerance in experimental animals.

Pharmacology

Cyclosporine is a metabolite of the fungal species, *Tolypocladium inflatum* (previously termed, *Trichoderma polysporum*) [13]. The drug is a neutral hydrophobic cyclic peptide consisting of 11 amino acids, including a previously unknown amino acid in position 9. The immunosuppressive activity depends on the presence of the carbon chains of amino acids in positions 1 and 11. For oral use, the drug is dissolved in olive oil. A gelenic formulation is used for intravenous (i.v.) administration.

Cyclosporine plasma or whole blood concentrations can be measured either by radioimmunoassay (which detects the parent drug and metabolites) or high-pressure liquid chromatography (HPLC) (which selectively measures the parent compound) [24–28]. The correlation between the two techniques is excellent, although values obtained by radioimmunoassay are approximately 1.3 times higher than those obtained by HPLC. The rate and degree of absorption after oral administration are extremely variable. Cyclosporine is metabolized by the liver and excreted via bile and feces.

Native cyclosporine, but none of 15 defined cyclosporine metabolites, is immunosuppressive. Approximately 10% of the metabolites are excreted in the urine; however, only 0.1% of the native drug is detected in the urine. These characteristics explain why an impaired renal function does not affect plasma or whole blood levels. However, liver dysfunction abnormalities do cause drug accumulation.

Controversy exists as to whether determinations of drug concentration aid in the management of renal transplant recipients. Between 40 to 60% of the drug concentration in whole blood is bound to red blood cells. Lymphocytes and granulocytes each bind approximately 5%; the remaining drug is associated with lipoproteins [25]. Drug binding to red blood cells is temperature-dependent. To obtain reproducible drug plasma levels, plasma must be separated from the red blood cells at 37° C. For convenience, the drug concentration of lysed whole blood often is determined, thus avoiding the temperature-dependent binding phenomenon.

Many kidney transplant groups have adopted a policy of keeping plasma cyclosporine levels between 100 to 400 ng/ml. These levels have been shown to be sufficient to prevent donor-specific immunoreactivity in in vitro assays that quantify recipient antidonor lymphocyte-proliferative and cytotoxic function [26]. Some groups recommend therapy aimed at producing even lower drug levels (that is, not exceeding plasma trough levels of 200 ng/ml), as they believe that plasma levels below 200 ng/ml are rarely associated with nephrotoxicity. Use of "low"-dose cyclosporine treatment does not seem to hamper the success rate of living-related or cadaver donor kidney grafts.

Cyclosporine catabolism is hastened by rifampicin and phenytoin. Both drugs lower plasma levels by inducing degradative hepatic enzymes. Cyclosporine, in turn, affects the metabolism of prednisolone by reducing the hepatic clearance via reducing the functional liver mass, or by competitive inhibition of the hepatic cytochrome, B 450. Concurrent therapy with aminoglycosides, trimethoprim/sulfa, ketoconazole, and amphotericin B elevates plasma drug levels and results in increased nephrotoxicity.

Clinical Trials

Following the first kidney transplant at Boston's Peter Bent Brigham Hospital in 1954, a series of important discoveries gradually improved the success rate of kidney transplantation. In the early 1960s, both the introduction of azathioprine for maintenance immunosuppression and the use of corticosteroids for the treatment of acute rejection were found to aid engraftment. In the 1970s, the salubrious effect of pretransplant blood transfusions on engraftment was recognized. Cyclosporine may be another milestone in clinical transplantation. Calne's group was the first to test cyclosporine therapy in recipients of mismatched cadaver kidney grafts [27]. The 1-year graft survival rate of these patients treated with cyclosporine alone reached 86%, which is a number clearly superior to historic controls. Similar results were obtained by Starzl et al [28] by using a combined cyclosporin and prednisone regimen. However, both groups observed a substantial number of patients with impaired graft function.

Subsequently, cyclosporine was tested in a number of randomized, controlled multicenter and single center studies in which cyclosporine therapy was compared to different established standard treatment protocols. Table 1 summarizes the results of these studies. One-year patient survival rates exceeded 90%, although the actuarial graft survival rates at 1 year differ considerably among the centers; however, 70 to 90% of grafts placed into cyclosporine-treated hosts can be expected to function after 1 year, whereas the standard treatment protocols yielded survival rates ranging from 50 to 85%. Cyclosporine immunosuppression was superior only in those studies in which the control group did not reach a 70% 1-year survival rate, that is, cyclosporine will be of greatest benefit in populations where the standard protocol has not yielded "optimal" survival rates. However, one must realize that these results obtained with cyclosporine were garnered during a learning period in which clinicians were unfamiliar with this drug. We can expect improved results as familiarity with the drug is achieved.

It is noteworthy that several centers using antilymphocyte globulin preparations in their standard protocol, either prophylactically or as antirejection treatment, did not observe a significant improvement in short-term graft and patient survival. By contrast, several categories of high-risk patients—such as recipients of haploidentical living-related donor kidneys with high-recipient antidonor in vitro assays [29], patients with prior immunologic loss of a renal allograft, as well as aged patients [30]—experience pronounced improvement in graft survival with cyclosporine therapy; that is, an increase of the

Table 1. Comparisons of cyclosporine with other immunosuppressive protocols

Trial	Number of patients	Immunosuppressive protocols	1-yr patient survival (%)	1-yr graft survival (%)	Graft function S-creatinine (μmoles/liter)	Rejection incidence/total episodes (%)	Infection incidence/total episodes (%)
Australian Multicenter[a] (*Transplant Proc* 15:2485, 1983)	30[b]/30[c] CAD	CsA vs A/P/ATG	93 vs 97	70 vs 80 *NS*	180 vs 119[g]	83 vs 93	31 vs 47[i] 7 vs 17[j]
Canadian Multicenter[a] (*N. Engl. J. Med,* 1983)	103/107 CAD	CsA/P vs A/P/(ATG)[d]	97 vs 89	80 vs 64 *P,* 0.003	195 vs 149 *P,* 0.03	159 vs 157[h]	81 vs 99 18 vs 27
European Multicenter[a] (*Lancet* 2:986, 1983)	117/115 CAD	CsA vs A/P	94 vs 92	72 vs 52 *P,* 0.001	184 vs 169 *P,* 0.001	86 vs 91	—
Birmingham[a] (*Transplant Proc* 15:2523, 1983)	35/33 CAD	CsA/P[e] vs A/P	94 vs 91	77 vs 85 *NS*	227 vs 121 *P,* 0.02	63 vs 64	48 vs 72 17 vs 15
Boston (*Ann Surg,* in press, 1984)	76/36 CAD	CsA/P vs A/P	95 vs 93	85 vs 60[k] 78 vs 53[l] *P,* 0.01	—	53 vs 72	30 vs 18 10 vs 7
Denver/Pittsburgh[a] (*Surg Gynecol Obstet* 157:309, 1983)	38/32 CAD	CsA/P vs A/P	99 vs 99	90 vs 50 *P,* 0.02	174 vs 142 *NS*	—	—
Minneapolis[a] (*Transplant Proc* 15:2463, 1983)	92/90 CAD + LRD	CsA/P vs A/P/ATG	92 vs 95	87 vs 80 *NS*	194 vs 133 *P,* 0.05	31 vs 58	47 vs 60 24 vs 63

[a] Randomized controlled studies.
[b] CsA group.
[c] Conventional control group.
[d] Part of control group with ATG.
[e] Short-term treatment (14 days).
[f] At 1 yr.
[g] Lowest level.
[h] Total episodes.
[i] Total infections.
[j] Viral infections.
[k] First transplants.
[l] All transplants.

Abbreviations: CAD, cadaveric transplantation; LRD, living related donor; A, azathioprine; P, prednisone; CsA, cyclosporine; S, serum; ATG, antithymocyte globulin; *NS,* not significant.

1-year graft survival from 40% to more than 70% in cyclosporine-treated patients.

In all series, the rate of engraftment is invariably better in cyclosporine-treated patients than with patients receiving azathioprine and prednisone alone. Nonetheless, graft dysfunction is common among cyclosporine-treated patients. It is still controversial as to whether most of these grafts undergo a smoldering rejection process or nephrotoxicity. In fact, graft biopsy specimens often show lymphocytic interstitial infiltrates. We believe that these infiltrates arise from rejection. On the other hand, trials in which patients are switched to conventional immunosuppression, after an initial induction period with cyclosporine treatment, show that improvements in graft function with this maneuver are frequently obtained. There can be no doubt that nephrotoxicity is common and reversible.

The combination of cyclosporine and corticosteroids appears to be particularly effective. It is likely that combined cyclosporine and steroid therapy is so effective because of the ability of both agents to abrogate IL-2 release through different sites of action. Whereas cyclosporine acts predominantly on helper cells, corticosteroids prevent IL-1 release from accessory cells (Fig. 1).

Overall, the incidence of infectious complications is comparable in standard- and cyclosporine-treated groups (Table 1). However, in our experience, Pneumocystis carinii pneumonia is more common in cyclosporine-treated kidney recipients. Consequently, our patients now receive low-dose trimethoprim/sulfa prophylaxis when the serum creatinine falls below 3 mg/dl.

Side Effects

Nephrotoxic effects of cyclosporine are readily observed in humans, but not in most animal models. Nephrotoxicity may become manifest in the early postoperative course as acute renal failure, or later in the course as an insidious decrease in glomerular filtration rate (GFR). At Cambridge in England, a number of patients were observed with initial diuresis who became oligoanuric after institution of cyclosporine [27]. These investigators suggested that cyclosporine should be delayed for 6 hours postoperatively to exclude these recipients from potentially nephrotoxic cyclosporine treatment in patients with primary oliguria. This policy was adopted in the European multicenter trial [31, 32]. After our ample clinical experience, we now believe that cyclosporine can be safely used in all kidney recipients as acute failure eventually resolves. In the Canadian trial [33], the following were noted as special risk factors for cyclosporine-treated patients with initial oliguria: (1) machine perfusion time of more than 24 hr, and (2) prolonged rewarming times of more than 45 min. These factors were associated with an increased incidence of primary nonfunction, as well as a higher number of acute rejection episodes. Consequently, these patients received more frequent prednisone pulses for antirejection treatment. More data are urgently needed to resolve this controversy, because we do not find these factors to preclude a satisfactory response to cyclosporine therapy. We wonder whether our routine use of corticosteroids spared oligoanuric patients from nephrotoxicity.

Each transplant group using cyclosporine has had to struggle to learn how drug-related chronic nephrotoxicity can be distinguished from acute rejection. Both conditions usually become manifest only as an impairment of graft function. Cyclosporine-treated recipients undergoing rejection episodes often lack the classic signs of fever, graft tenderness, and hypertension. The presence of other side effects may cause suspicion that a worsening graft function is due to cyclosporine toxicity. Hyperbilirubinemia invariably is a sign of high cyclosporine blood levels and often is an indicator of nephrotoxicity. However, the direct correlation of plasma or whole blood cyclosporine trough levels with the toxic effect is poor; there is no drug concentration that excludes the diagnosis of nephrotoxicity with certainty. On the other hand, acute rejection may occur despite high blood levels. Moreover, concurrent rejection and nephrotoxicity are common. A graft biopsy specimen can reveal only nonspecific evidence of the toxic effect of cyclosporine on tubular and interstitial cells. Vacuolization or focal necrosis of proximal tubular cells, interstitial edema or fibrosis and focal lymphocytic infiltrates all are common. We believe that these common cellular infiltrates are due to concomitant rejection. We rely heavily on renal biopsy specimens in addressing the possibility of rejection. Some groups report that much lower doses of cyclosporine than originally recommended, in conjunction with prednisone, yield a high graft survival rate with a low incidence of nephrotoxic episodes [34]. These investigators recommend keeping plasma trough drug levels below 200 ng/ ml. Some patients need doses as low as 2 mg/kg body wt to remain within this limit. Thiel et al found, in a group of 23 patients with cadaver kidneys treated according to these recommendations, that serum creatinine concentrations did not differ from those of a historic control group receiving azathioprine and prednisone [34].

The Oxford group and (more recently) our group at the Brigham and Women's Hospital and Beth Israel Hospital in Boston have approached the problem of nephrotoxicity differently. After 4 months of treatment with cyclosporine, patients are changed to azathioprine and prednisone. The results obtained with this protocol are very promising as well. A similar study in Oxford revealed a significant fall in serum creatinine by 45%, indicating the presence of a nephrotoxic component in almost 100% of their patients [35]. At Oxford, the change in immunosuppression was followed, in about one-third of their patients, by an acute rejection that led to graft loss only in patients with a previously compromised situation such as primary nonfunction. We have observed a more benign course following a switch to azathioprine in 60 patients given cyclosporine and steroids for 4 months. Rebound rejection was observed in 12% of the patients thus treated. Improved graft function 3 months following the switch was most ubiquitous. No grafts were lost, and only one patient lost graft function as a consequence of the switch. Our protocol differed from the Oxford regimen in that our patients were switched to azathioprine at 4 months rather than at 3 months post-transplantation; our patients received corticosteroids as well as cyclosporine. Future studies will concentrate on a comparison of a low-dose cyclosporine-prednisone regime versus a switch to conventional immunosuppression. Such a study will clarify the nature of long-term effects of cyclosporine on the kidney graft.

Hepatotoxicity

Cyclosporine affects the liver by an unknown mechanism. Serum bilirubin levels increase in relation to the sustained cyclosporine plasma trough concentrations [36]. It is our experience that trough levels about 500 ng/ml are accompanied by an elevated serum bilirubin—a phenomenon observed in about 20% of kidney graft recipients [37]. Serum transaminase levels occasionally rise in a dose-dependent fashion.

An intriguing finding is the persistent elevation of alkaline phosphatase in about one-third of the patients [36, 38] within the first 3 weeks of treatment; it remains elevated despite reductions in cyclosporine dosage. It is the bone-specific isoenzyme fraction that is elevated and not the liver-specific fraction [36, 38]. Furthermore, other indicators of chronic cholestasis remain normal in renal graft recipients. Nevertheless, cholestasis cannot be absolutely excluded, since heart transplant recipients exhibited dramatically increased bile acid (cholylglycine and sulfolithocholyglycine) concentrations in the serum [39]. Further studies including bone and liver biopsy procedures will have to assess the impact of cyclosporine on these two organs.

Lymphoma

It has been well documented that transplant recipients sustain an increased risk for the development of malignancies, especially those of lymphoreticular origin [40]. If cyclosporine is used alone or in combination with low doses of prednisone, the incidence of lymphoproliferative disease is 0.4% compared to 0.8% if other immunosuppressive agents are used in concert with cyclosporine. The manufacturer now recommends keeping plasma trough levels in a range of 50 to 200 ng/ml [41]. Starzl et al recently analyzed the outcome in 17 cyclosporine-treated organ recipients who developed a lymphoproliferative disorder 2 to 68 months post-transplantation [42]. In 16 of the 17 patients, the disease became manifest within 8 months. In 10 patients, the disease was localized to the gastrointestinal tract, and 11 of the 17 patients are alive and symptom-free after surgical treatment and reduction of cyclosporine doses. Most remarkably, four of seven kidney grafts were retained despite a 66% dose reduction, thus supporting the notion that good allograft survival may be achieved with much lower doses than originally recommended [42].

Epstein-Barr virus (EBV) infection may be important in the genesis of these lymphoproliferative disorders, because several tumors have been found to express EBV proteins. Excessive inhibition of T cell surveillance favors uncontrolled proliferation of EBV-infected B cells.

Miscellaneous

Hirsutism occurs in about 30 to 40% of the patients and sometimes poses a cosmetic problem, especially in women. However, it is a completely dose-dependent phenomenon and disappears after a change to azathioprine. Thus far, no hormonal abnormalities are implicated. Tremor is fairly frequent, as long as higher doses of cyclosporine are used. Paresthesias and burning sensations, mainly in the fingers, are other neurologic side effects that respond to lowered drug doses.

Discussion

Cyclosporine facilitates activation in allospecific suppressor T cells while blunting overall T cell proliferation. These actions may render an allograft recipient tolerant to the graft. Multiple clinical studies have confirmed increased graft survival rates in cyclosporine-treated patients, compared to patients given conventional immunosuppression with azathioprine and prednisone. We are still unable to recommend an optimal protocol. Reasonable regimens using low doses of cyclosporine combined with low doses of prednisone, or a change to azathioprine after an induction period of 3 to 6 months, emerge as alternative approaches. The long-term effect of cyclosporine on graft survival and function should be assessed in patients treated with one of these protocols. Most renal graft recipients are now treated over prolonged periods of time with excessive doses of this very promising drug.

References

1. MOORE RN, OPPENHEIM JJ, FARRAR JJ, CARTER CS JR, WAHEED A, SHADDUCK RK: Production of LAF (IL-1) by macrophages activated with colony stimulating factors. *J Immunol* 125:1302–1305, 1980
2. HELDERMAN JH, STROM TB: Specific insulin binding site on T and B lymphocytes as a marker of cell activation. *Nature* 174:62–63, 1978
3. HELDERMAN JH, STROM TB: Role of protein and RNA synthesis in the development of insulin binding sites on activated thymus-derived lymphocytes. *J Biol Chem* 254:7203–7207, 1979
4. HELDERMAN JH, STROM TB, GAROVOY MR: Rapid mixed lymphocyte culture testing by analysis of the insulin receptor on alloactivated T lymphocytes: implications for human tissue typing. *J Clin Invest* 67:509–513, 1981
5. TROWBRIDGE IS, OMARY MB: Human cell surface glycoprotein related to cell proliferation is the receptor for transferrin. *Proc Natl Acad Sci USA* 78:3039–3043, 1981
6. GILLIS S, MIZEL SB: T cell lymphoma model for the analysis of interleukin-1 mediated T cell activation. *Proc Natl Acad Sci USA* 78:1133–1137, 1981
7. ROBB RJ, MUNCK A, SMITH KA: T cell growth factor receptors quantitation, specificity, and biological relevance. *J Exp Med* 154:1455–1474, 1981

8. SMITH KA, LACHMAN LB, OPPENHEIM JJ, FAVATA MF: The functional relationship of the interleukins. *J Exp Med* 151:1551–1556, 1980

9. FARRAR WL, JOHNSON HM, FARRAR JJ: Regulation of the production of immune interferon and cytotoxic T lymphocytes by interleukin-2. *J Immunol* 126:1120–1125, 1981

10. PACE JL, RUSSELL SW, SCHREIBER RD, ALTMAN A, KATZ DH: Macrophage activation: priming activity from a T-cell hybridoma is attributable to gamma-interferon. *Proc Natl Acad Sci USA* 80:3782–3786, 1983

11. INABA K, GRANELLI-PIPERNO G, STEINMAN RM: Dendritic cells induce T lymphocytes to release B cell-stimulating factors by an interleukin-2-dependent mechanism. *J Exp Med* 158:2040–2057, 1983

12. HOWARD M, MATIS L, MALEK TR, SHEVACH E, KELL W, COHEN D, NAKANISHI K, PAUL WE: Interleukin-2 induces antigen-reactive T cell lines to secrete BCGF-1. *J Exp Med* 158:2024–2039, 1983

13. BOREL JF, FEUER C, GUBLER HU, STAHELIN H: The biological effects of cyclosporine A: A new antilymphocytic agent. *Agents Actions* 6:468–475, 1976

14. BOREL JF: Cyclosporin A—Present experimental status. *Transplant Proc* 13:344–348, 1981

15. BUNJES D, HARDT C, ROLLINGHOFF M, WAGNER H: Cyclosporin A mediates immunosuppression of primary cytotoxic T cell responses by impairing the release of interleukin-1 and interleukin-2. *Eur J Immunol* 11:657–661, 1981

16. HESS AD, TUTSCHKA PJ, SANTOS GW: Effect of cyclosporin A on human lymphocyte responses *in vitro*. III. CsA inhibits the production of T lymphocyte growth factors in secondary mixed lymphocyte responses but does not inhibit the response of primed lymphocytes to TCGF. *J Immunol* 128:355–358, 1982

17. KALMAN VK, KLIMPEL GR: Cyclosporin A inhibits the production of gamma interferon but does not inhibit production of virus-induced alpha/beta interferon. *Cell Immunol* 78:122–129, 1983

18. MIYAWAKI T, YACHIE A, OHZEKI S, NAGAOKI T, TANIGUCHI N: Cyclosporine A does not prevent expression of Tac antigen, a probable TCGF receptor molecule on mitogen-stimulated human T cells. *J Immunol* 130:2737–2742, 1983

19. WANG BS, HEACOCK EH, CHANG-XUE Z, TILNEY NL, STROM TB, MANNICK JA: Evidence for the presence of suppressor T lymphocytes in animals treated with cyclosporin A. *J Immunol* 128:1382–1385, 1982

20. WANG BS, ZHENG CX, HEACOCK EH, TILNEY NL, STROM TB, MANNICK JA: Inhibition of the production of a soluble helper mediator by cyclosporin A results in the failure to generate alloreactive cytolytic cells in mixed-lymphocyte culture. *Clin Immunol Immunopathol* 27:160–169, 1983

21. HUTCHINSON IF, SHADUR CA, DUARTE AJS, STROM TB, TILNEY NL: Cyclosporin A spares selectively lymphocytes with donor specific suppressor characteristics. *Transplantation* 32:210–216, 1981

22. KUPIEC-WEGLINSKI J, LEAR PA, BORDES-AZNAR J, TILNEY NL, STROM TB: Acute rejection in cyclosporin A treated graft recipients occurs following abrogation of suppressor cells. *Transplant Proc* 15:531–533, 1983

23. ABBUD-FILHO M, KUPIEC-WEGLINSKI JW, ARAUJO JL, HEIDECKE CD, TILNEY NL, STROM TB: Cyclosporine therapy of rat heart allograft recipients and release of interleukins (IL-1, IL-2, IL-3). A role for IL-3 in graft tolerance? *J Immunol,* in press

24. BEVERIDGE T, GRATWOHL A, MICHOT F, NEIDERBERGER W, NUESCH E, NUSSBAUMER K, SCHAUB P, SPECK B: Pharmacokinetics in man after a single dose and serum levels after multiple dosing in recipients of allogeneic bone marrow grafts. *Curr Therapeutic Res* 30:5–18, 1981

25. NIEDERBERGER W, LEMAIRE M, MAURER G, NUSSBAUMER K, WAGNER O:

Distribution and binding of cyclosporine in blood and tissues. *Transplant Proc* 15:2419–2421, 1983

26. KEOWN PA, STILLER CR, ULAN RA, SINCLAIR NR, WALL WJ, CARRUTHERS G, HOWSON W: Immunological and pharmacological monitoring in the clinical use of cyclosporine A. *Lancet* 1:686–689, 1981

27. CALNE RY, WHITE DJG, THIRU S, EVANS DB, MCMASTER P, DUNN DC, CRADDOCK GN, PENTLOW BD, ROLLES K: Cyclosporin A in patients receiving renal allografts from cadaver donors. *Lancet* 2:1323–1327, 1978

28. STARZL TE, WEIL R, IWATZUKI S, KLINTMALM G, SCHROTER GPJ, KOEP LJ, IWAKI Y, TERASAKI PI, PORTER KA: The use of cyclosporin A and steroid therapy in 66 cadaver kidney transplants. *Surg Gynecol Obstet* 151:17–26, 1980

29. KAHAN BD, VAN BUREN CT, FLECHNER SM, PAYNE WD, BOILEAU M, KERMAN RH: Cyclosporine immunosuppression mitigates immunologic risk factors in renal allotransplantation. *Transplant Proc* 15:2469–2478, 1983

30. RINGDEN O, OST L, KLINTMALM GBG, TILLEGARD A, FEHRMANN I, WILCZEK H, GROTH CG: Improved outcome in renal transplant recipients above 55 years of age treated with cyclosporine and low doses of steroids. *Transplant Proc* 15:2507–2512, 1983

31. EUROPEAN MULTICENTRE TRIAL GROUP: Cyclosporin A as sole immunosuppressive agent in recipients of renal allografts from cadaver donors. Preliminary results of a European Multicenter Trial. *Lancet* 2:57–60, 1982

32. EUROPEAN MULTICENTRE TRIAL GROUP: Cyclosporin in cadaveric renal transplantation: one year follow-up of a multicentre trial. *Lancet* 2:896–899, 1982

33. CANADIAN MULTICENTRE TRANSPLANT STUDY GROUP: A randomized clinical trial of cyclosporine in cadaveric renal transplantation. *N Engl J Med* 309:809–815, 1983

34. THIEL G, HARDER F, LOERTSCHER R, BRUNISHOLZ M, LANDMANN J, BRUNNER F, FOLLATH F, WENK M, MIHATSCH M: Cyclosporin A used alone or in combination with low dose steroids on cadaveric renal transplantation. *Klin Urschr* 61:991–1000, 1983

35. MORRIS PJ, FRENCH ME, DUNHILL MS, HUNNISETT AGW, TING A, THOMPSON JF, WOOD RFM: A controlled trial of cyclosporine in renal transplantation with conversion to azathioprine and prednisone after three months. *Transplantation* 36:273–277, 1983

36. LOERTSCHER R, THIEL G, HARDER F, BRUNNER FP: Persistent elevation of alkaline phosphatase in cyclosporin A treated renal transplant recipients. *Transplantation* 36:115–116, 1983

37. KLINTMALM GBG, IWATZUKI S, STARZL TE: Cyclosporin A hepatotoxicity in 66 renal allograft recipients. *Transplantation* 32:488–489, 1981

38. RODGER RSC, TURNEY JH, HAINES I, MICHAEL J, ADU D, MCMASTER P: Cyclosporine and liver function in renal allograft recipients. *Transplant Proc* 15:2754–2756, 1983

39. SCHADE RR, GUGLIELMI A, VAN THIEL DH, THOMPSON ME, WARTY V, GRIFFITH B, SANGHRI A, BAHNSON H, HARDESTY R: Cholestasis in heart transplant recipients treated with cyclosporine. *Transplant Proc* 15:2757–2760, 1983

40. PENN I: Lymphomas complicating organ transplantation. *Transplant Proc* 15:2790–2797, 1983

41. BEVERIDGE T, KRUPP P, MCKIBBIN C: Lymphomas and lymphoproliferative lesions developing under cyclosporine therapy (*letter*). *Lancet* 1:788, 1984

42. STARZL TE, NALESNIK MA, PORTER KA, HO M, IWATSUKI S, GRIFFITH BP, ROSENTHAL JT, HAKALA TR, SHAW BW, HARDESTY RL: Reversibility of lymphomas and lymphoproliferation lesions developing under cyclosporine therapy. *Lancet* 1:583–587, 1984

The Transfusion Effect in Renal Allograft Recipients

Sondra Perdue and Paul I. Terasaki

The enhancement of renal allograft survival by pretransplant blood transfusions was originally reported more than 1 decade ago. [1]. Subsequently, numerous studies have confirmed this observation. Although specific mechanisms have not been fully resolved, the strength of the transfusion effect has led many transplant centers to adopt a deliberate transfusion policy [2–4]. In this chapter, we offer an update on the transfusion effect in patients from a large registry and comment on several interactions regarding applicability of a deliberate transfusion policy to all transplant recipients.

Patients and Methods

A total of 8801 kidney transplant patients, reported to the UCLA Transplant Registry with pretransplant transfusion information, who were transplanted after January 1978 were included in this study.

Grant survival was evaluated by using actuarial estimates with clinical life table methods [5].

Results

Cumulative Effect of Individual Transfusions

The effects of multiple transfusions can be best seen by examining graft survival in patients subgrouped by numbers of pretransplant transfusions. The

This manuscript was presented as part of a Symposium on *Immunomodulation for Transplantation: New Approaches.*

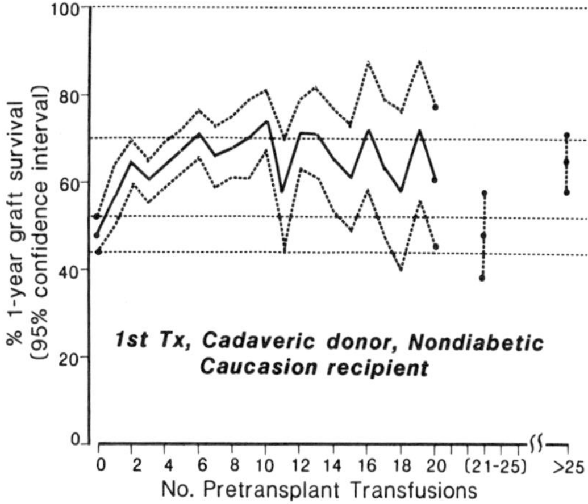

Fig. 1. One-year graft survival by number of pretransplant transfusions (1978–June 1984). The dotted curves (----) above and below the solid line (—) indicate the 95% confidence limits for the survival estimates. ($N = 4189$).

enhancement effect of multiple transfusions increased from a 1-year survival of about 48% with no transfusions to approximately 70% with six transfusions (Fig. 1). After about five or six transfusions, the effect levels off and does not continue to increase with up to 20 transfusions. In fact, increasing numbers of transfusions appear to yield *lower* graft survival after a peak of around 15 transfusions. This may be due to the deteriorated condition of recipients who require increased numbers of transfusions. The 95% confidence intervals indicated in the figure show that the transfusion effect is statistically significant at the 5% level, from 2 to about 14 transfusions; however, after that, it is not statistically different from nontransfused patients. This is partly a result of smaller numbers of patients in the 15 to 20 transfusion range, as indicated by the increased width of the confidence band.

Changing Impact of Transfusion Effect

Although multiple transfusions continue to have an overall enhancing effect on graft survival when compared with zero-transfused patients, there appears to be a transition within the last 2 years that has reduced the overall impact of transfusions (Fig. 2). In the period 1978 to 1981, zero-transfused patients showed a striking decline in graft survival during the first 6 months posttransplant, dropping to below 50% survival within that time period. By contrast, from 1982 to the present, the nontransfused group were more similar to the transfused group, although somewhat lower in overall survival. The major difference seems to be in the risk during the first 6 months. Comparison of the left and right figures (Fig. 2) shows that the graft survival in transfused patients has changed little, but the graft survival in zero-transfused patients has improved dramatically.

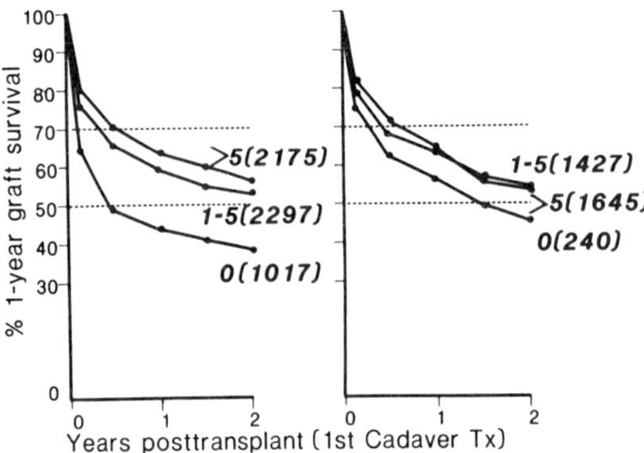

Fig. 2. Effect of pretransplant transfusions on first cadaveric grafts in two time intervals (*left panel:*1978–1981; *right panel:*1982–June 1984). Survival functions are shown for 0, 1–5, and > 5 transfusions. (The numbers in parentheses indicate the number of patients.)

Transfusions and Histocompatibility Effects

The efficacy of HLA-A,B matching can be evaluated within transfusion strata (Fig. 3). Although some effect of HLA matching is seen within the first year, the 3-year follow-up indicates more clearly the enhancing effect on graft survival of better-matched kidneys. Within each transfusion strata, zero or one mismatches do the best, with three or four mismatches doing the worst; and, two HLA-A,B mismatches are intermediate between those two extremes. The effect is most dramatic within the zero-transfused group, but the level of the effect is proportionately about the same within each transfusion group. In fact, the well-matched zero transfusion group has the same 3-year graft survival as the poorly matched one-to-five transfusion group.

The effect of HLA-DR matching within transfusion strata is less striking than for HLA-A,B matching (Fig. 4). Zero mismatches do better in each

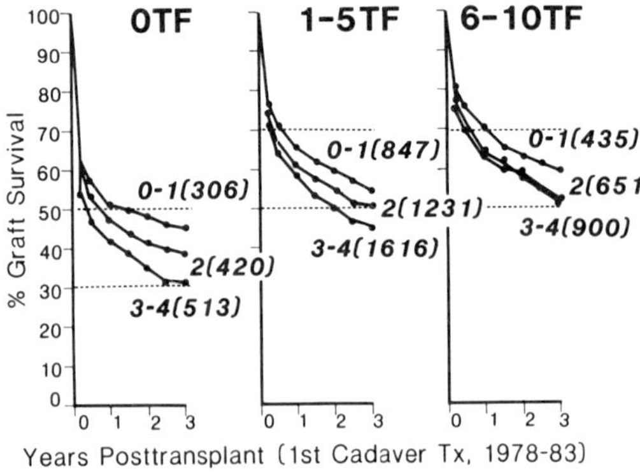

Fig. 3. Influence of HLA-A,B mismatches within transfusion strata. Survival functions are shown for 0 or 1, 2, and 3 or 4 mismatches for 3 years post-transplant.

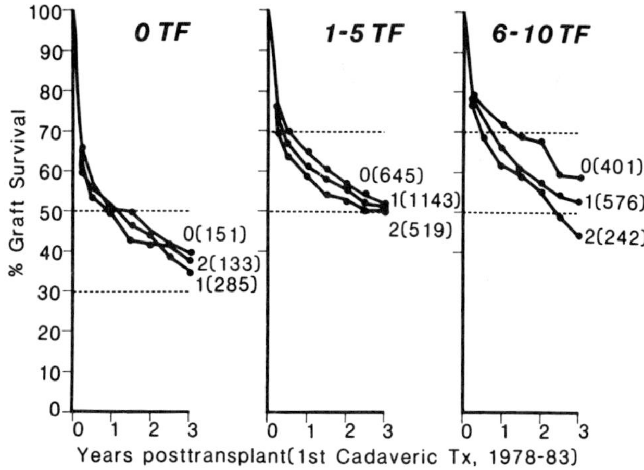

Fig. 4. Influence of HLA-DR mismatches within transfusion strata. Survival functions are shown for 0, 1, or 2 mismatches for 3 years post-transplant.

transfusion group, but the magnitude of the DR-matching effect is greatest for the multiply transfused patients.

Effect of Age at Transplant

In each transfusion strata, a decline of 1-year graft survival with increasing age at time of transplant can be seen (Fig. 5). Comparison across the transfusion strata shows that transfusions generally are effective in both genders and within all age strata. In general, males have a lower reponse with zero transfusions and a higher response with 6 to 10 transfusions than females; that is, the overall impact of transfusions is greater in males than in females. The one inconsistent point within this figure is the 0 transfusions for the

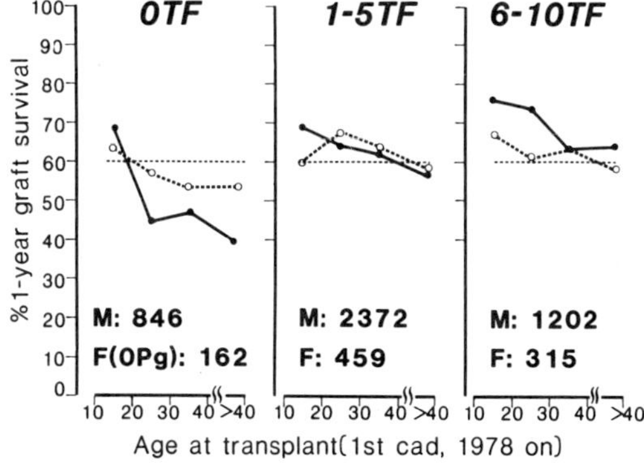

Fig. 5. One-year graft survival by recipient age group and gender within transfusion strata. The solid lines (●—●) represent males and the broken lines with open circles (○---○) represent female recipients.

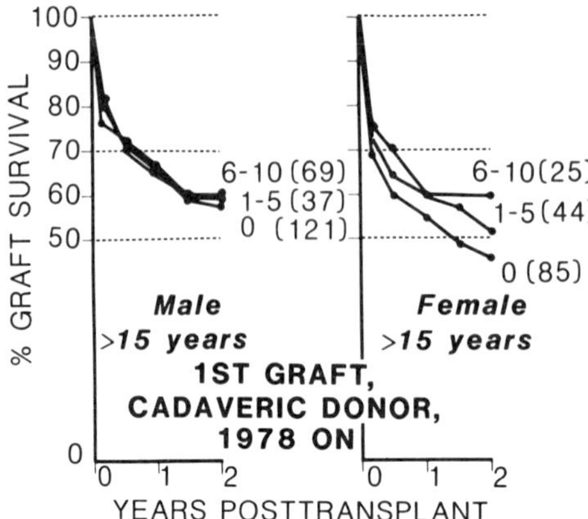

Fig. 6. Effects of 0, 1 to 5, or 6 to 10 pretransplant transfusions in pediatric recipients by gender.

10- to 20-year-old age group. This point is higher than expected in both males and females, and it was explored further.

Transfusion Effect in Pediatric Recipients

Detailed survival curves for 2 years post-transplant are shown separately for males and females who were all less than 15 years of age (Fig. 6). In marked contrast to other age groups, transfusions show no effect in males and little effect in females. Comparison with earlier figures shows that the difference is primarily in a lack of detrimental effect of 0 transfusions. Within this pediatric age group, we also can see clear differences between the genders in the risk of graft loss within the first post-transplant year. Males are at much lower risk for the first 2 to 6 months, with about 70% survival at 6 months, whereas females have a range of 60 to 70% graft survival in the same period.

Discussion

Evidence of beneficial effects of blood transfusions has widespread acceptance. Although the overall effect is still apparent in recent data, other factors are emerging that should cause reconsideration of some existing transfusion policies.

The effect of multiple transfusions seems to be bounded, with perhaps five transfusions as an optimal number for enhancing graft outcome. A similar bounded effect has been noted by other investigators [6], although Fehrmen did not see an increased survival effect until more than 20 transfusions [7].

The striking improvement in nontransfused cases during the past year must be due to recent factors that influence the overall graft survival. This trend change was not seen in an analysis covering quarterly results from

1975 to 1981 [8]. It is possible with a relatively short period of time, such as 1982 and 1983, that the upswing is not permanent, but rather is a temporary artifact. Alternatively, new factors in immunosuppression (for example, cyclosporine) may have started to show an effect in the overall data.

The effect of HLA histocompatibility matching is perhaps as important as the transfusion effect. The overall effect of matching in conjunction with transfusions has been shown by several investigators, although with some differences in specifics of the interaction between the two effects [9–11]. Although one study showed a stronger effect of matching in transfused than in nontransfused patients [9], the consensus is in agreement with our results, which show a somewhat weaker effect within the transfused patients [10, 11]. This effect has been found both in large registry studies in human allografts and in animal work with dogs and monkeys.

Although some studies have not shown an age effect in graft survival [10], this study clearly shows that a definite interaction of age and transfusion effect exists. The lack of a beneficial effect of transfusions in pediatric recipients suggests that deliberate transfusions of children (a policy now in effect at some centers) should be reconsidered [4].

Despite the indications that transfusions may not have an effect in pediatric cases and that zero-transfused patients tend to have a better transplant outcome, it would be premature to abandon the use of transfusions. As we have noted in a separate study (submitted for publication), the transfusion effect can be seen even in conjunction with cyclosporine treatment. Thus far, efforts to optimize the transfusion effect have not led to exceptionally high graft survival rates. Perhaps the use of donor-specific blood transfusions is an example of the possibility of enhancing the effect obtained with random transfusions. It is hoped that the critical antigens in a more purified form than blood transfusions will be used in the future.

References

1. OPELZ G, SENGAR DPS, MICKEY MR, TERASAKI PI: Effect of blood transfusions on subsequent kidney transplants. *Transplant Proc* 4:253–259, 1973
2. D'APICE AJF, TAIT BD: An elective transfusion policy: Sensitization rates, patient transplantability, and transplant outcome. *Transplantation* 33:191–195, 1982
3. GLASS NR, FELSHEIM G, MILLER DT, SOLLINGER HW, BELZER FO: Influence of pre-and perioperative blood transfusions on renal allograft survival. *Transplantation* 33:430–431, 1982
4. SQUIFFLET JP, PIRSON Y, VAN CANGH P, OTTE JB, VAN YPERSELE DE STRIHOU C, ALEXANDRE GPJ: Renal transplantation in children. *Transplantation* 32:278–281, 1981
5. MILLER RG JR: *Survival Analysis.* New York, John Wiley & Sons, 1981, pp 39–46
6. ZEICHNER WD, TOLEDO-PEREYRA LH: Lack of correlation between cadaver kidney transplant survival and the number of pretransplant transfusions. *Transplantation* 35:500–501, 1983
7. FEHRMAN I: Pretransplant blood transfusions and related kidney allograft survival. *Transplantation* 34:46–49, 1982

8. PERDUE ST, TERASAKI PI, CATS S, MICKEY MR: Kidney transplantation trends from UCLA registry data, 1975–1982. *Transplantation* 36:658–665, 1983

9. MOHANAKUMAR T, ELLIS TM, DAYAL H, DUVALL C, MENDEZ-PICON G, LEE HM: Potentiating effect of HLA matching and blood transfusions on renal allograft survival. *Transplantation* 32:244–247, 1981

10. SPEES EK, VAUGHN WK, WILLIAMS GM, FILO RS, McDONALD JC, MENDEZ-PICON G, NIBLACK G: Effects of blood transfusion on cadaver renal transplantation. *Transplantation* 30:455–463, 1980

11. BIJNEN AB, OBERTOP H, NIESSEN GJCM, JEEKEL J, WESTBROEK DL: Adverse effect of pretransplant blood transfusions on survival of matched kidney allografts in dogs. *Transplantation* 33:57–63, 1982

Antilymphocyte Globulin and Monoclonal Antibodies: Present Status as Therapy

A. Benedict Cosimi

The essential role of the immune system is to safeguard and maintain the integrity of the individual. The system's most striking feature is the exquisite specificity of each response. The ultimate objective of immunosuppressive therapy for allograft recipients, therefore, should be to block specifically the host's response to antigenic differences introduced by the graft, but spare reactivity to other antigens such as bacterial and viral pathogens. Until recently, the most widely used immunosuppressive protocols used a combination of cytotoxic agents and steroids as the basic regimen. Despite the nonspecific approach of these protocols, they have provided sufficiently effective suppression to make transplantation a routine treatment for many patients with end-stage renal disease. With such therapy, 1-year recipient survival of 90% and graft survival of 55 to 60% following cadaver donor transplantation can be expected [1]. Nevertheless, in view of the global suppression produced in these recipients, considerable morbidity must be anticipated, particularly in the form of infectious complications. Thus, the search for more effective and more specific agents continues.

Admittedly, the optimal approach to immunosuppressive therapy remains to be defined; yet considerable progress has been made away from the toxic, nonspecific suppression produced by cytotoxic agents and high-dose steroids, and toward more selective abolition of the rejection reaction. Figure 1 schematically depicts how various immunosuppressive modalities might be ranked in a "hierarchy of immunosuppression." The importance of increasing specificity is emphasized by the rather remarkable effects of the newest chemical immunosuppressive, cyclosporine. Interestingly, this agent appears to interfere rather selectively with the activation of T helper cells and the release of certain lymphokines [2]. This unexpected selective mechanism of action, identified long after the beneficial immunosuppressive qualities of cyclosporine have been observed, helps to clarify how such a compound could so effectively

This manuscript was presented as part of a Symposium on *Immunomodulation for Transplantation: New Approaches*.

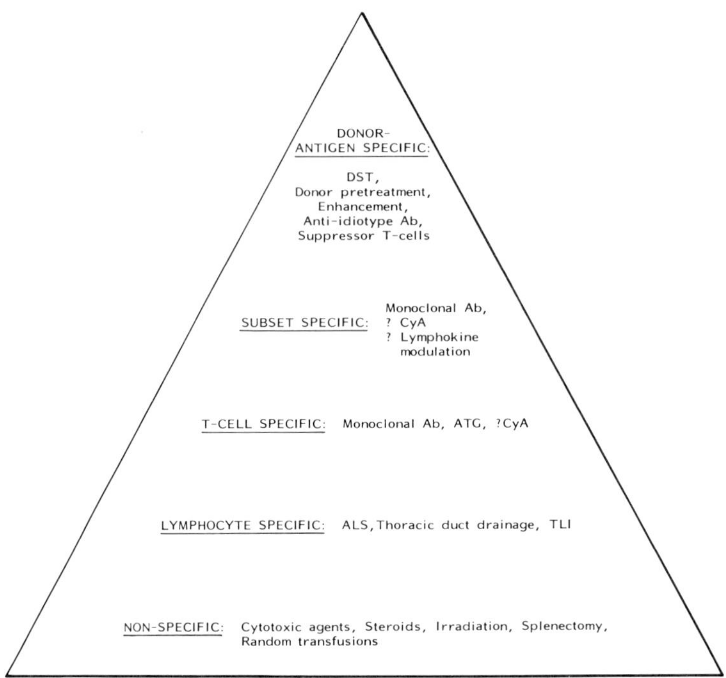

Fig. 1. Hierarchy of immunosuppression. A hierarchy of immunosuppressive modalities can be constructed demonstrating the increasing specificity of various approaches. The goal of clinical protocols is to apply measures nearer the apex so that improved suppression but reduced toxicity can be achieved. *DST* refers to donor-specific transfusions; *CyA,* to cyclosporine; *TLI,* to total lymphoid irradiation.

depress reactivity to allograft antigens without producing unacceptable infectious complications.

More specific immunosuppression can also be achieved by using antibodies against T lymphocytes. Although these agents impair most of the recipient's cellular responsiveness, humoral immunity, at least, is largely spared. To date, two generations of these agents have become available: polyclonal preparations, including such products as antilymphocyte globulin (ALG) or antithymocyte globulin (ATG), and monoclonal antibody preparations.

Polyclonal Antilymphocyte Preparations

Initial observations of destruction of leukocytes by xenotypic antisera were recorded by Metchnikoff near the turn of the century. However, it was only 2 decades ago that the capacity of antilymphocyte serum (ALS) to interrupt the immune sequence and prolong allograft survival was first reported [3].

Although extensive preclinical investigations since then have consistently demonstrated prolongation of allograft survival by these antibodies, their true clinical value was difficult to establish. Numerous controlled and uncontrolled clinical trials with ALS, ALG, or ATG have been reported. The agents have been administered to allograft recipients either prophylactically to avert rejection or, more recently, as treatment for ongoing rejection episodes. Several factors, including variability among individual batches of antisera, poorly controlled studies, limited numbers of appropriate patients, and inadequate dosages help to explain the inconsistent results observed in many of these trials. Continuing improvements in production techniques and more carefully designed trials, particularly trials using ATG or ALG for treatment of ongoing rejection, have now firmly established the clinical usefulness of these agents [4].

Despite the steroid-sparing effects and the increased specificity offered by these antilymphocyte preparations, they continue to fall short of the goal of optimal suppression. The use of conventional techniques to immunize animals provides a polyclonal product containing not only a heterogeneous group of antibodies to T-cell populations, but also some antibodies reactive with B cells or even with nonlymphoid cells. In addition, these products contain extraneous antibodies reflecting the animal's previous immunologic activity. The development of cell hybridization techniques that can provide monoclonal antibodies to single-cell membrane determinants [5] has now provided a methodology for producing reagents reactive with only T cells or, more importantly, with selected T-cell subsets. The recent utilization of this second generation of antilymphocyte antibodies for treatment of renal allograft rejection will be the subject of the latter part of this summary.

Production and Administration of Polyclonal Antilymphocyte Antibodies

Production of antibodies for clinical administration begins with the immunization of an animal through the use of human lymphoid cells. Many cell types have been evaluated. Currently, the most commonly used immunogens include either cultured lymphoblasts or human thymocytes. Cultured lymphoblasts offer the advantages of ready availability and freedom from contaminating erythrocytes or stromal elements, which might induce unwanted antibodies. A possible disadvantage arises from the fact that lymphoblasts are B cells rather than T cells. Human thymus tissue is an excellent source of T-cell antigens that are reasonably free of contaminating blood cells and stromal tissue. Thus, thymocytes are preferred by most manufacturers of antilymphoid preparations, but adequate amounts of tissue are not always available.

The selection of the heterologous species for immunization is based primarily upon practical considerations such as cost, animal size, and availability. Experience has indicated that either horses or rabbits can be stimulated to produce potent antilymphocyte antibodies, and thus these two species are currently the most commonly used.

The immunosuppressive potency of these antisera is confined almost exclusively to the IgG fraction that is usually isolated for use in humans, although the crude globulin fraction or even whole serum can be successfully administered. Preclinical assessment of immunosuppressive potency has been difficult. To date, no absolutely reliable in vitro test has been identified, but rosette inhibition assays do seem to provide a reasonably consistent means of selecting potent preparations. The capacity of the preparation to prolong allograft survival in nonhuman primates continues to be assessed in some products prior to clinical administration.

In general, it has been found that the route of ALG administration is of relatively little importance in determining the degree of suppression produced. Local inflammatory reactions, however, frequently result from s.c. or i.m. injections. As a result, many clinicians prefer i.v. administration, which has the added advantage of allowing an infusion of larger individual doses to be given and the agent to be presented through a less immunogenic route.

Prompt and usually profound lymphopenia usually follows the injection of antilymphocyte sera. Although absolute lymphopenia is apparently not necessary for immunosuppression, most effective preparations do provide at least some degree of cell depletion. In addition to the marked decrease in number of T cells, these preparations also produce a decrease in proliferative function. Upon cessation of treatment, the numbers of circulating T cells gradually increase, whereas the proliferative response remains impaired, possibly from the development of nonspecific suppressor T cells, which can be demonstrated in mouse [6] or monkey [7] models. These observations suggest that the initial interruption of cell-mediated graft destruction by ALG results from an elimination of T cells. More prolonged suppression may be provided by suppressor cell-mediated inhibition of proliferative responses. Undoubtedly, this sequence is an oversimplification and will remain so until the function of specific T-cell subpopulations is better clarified.

Use of Antilymphocyte Globulin in Renal Allograft Recipients

Initially, patient trials made use of various homemade preparations administered for a period of several days to weeks as part of the prophylactic suppressive protocol begun at the time of transplantation. More recently, larger and more consistent batches have become available from various pharmaceutical companies. The "prophylactic protocol" studies almost universally indicated fewer early rejection episodes and usually suggested improved 1-year allograft survival in the ALG-treated groups. However, the difference in survival from that achieved in conventionally treated patients often failed to reach statistical significance (Table 1). The multitude of variables involved in such clinical studies and the fairly high rate of survival already attained for kidney transplants using azathioprine and steroids alone help to explain why statistically significant improvement in survival was inconsistently demonstrated.

Table 1. Randomized trials comparing polyclonal antilymphocyte preparations to conventional prophylactic immunosuppression in cadaver donor renal allograft recipients

| Reference | No. of patients treated | 1-year function | | Significance ($P < 0.05$) |
		Control (%)	ATG (%)[a]	
21	100	63	80	+
22	179	55	62	*NS*
23	36	27	62	+
24	66	28	53	+
25	358	46	52	*NS*
26	104	57	70	*NS*
27	50	52	79	+
28	67	47	68	+
29	140	50	40	*NS*

[a] ATG refers to antithymocyte globulin.

Because earlier animal studies had suggested that ALG was most effective when administered at the time of, or even prior to, transplantation, evaluation of these agents for reversing an ongoing rejection was unfortunately delayed until recently. We reported in 1979 the first randomized clinical study comparing ATG to high-dose steroids for treatment of established rejection [8]. In that trial, involving recipients of living related donor (LRD) allografts, ATG proved to be as effective as high-dose steroids, and it had added benefits of more rapid reversal and fewer subsequent rejection episodes. We therefore continue to favor ATG as the primary mode of treatment for rejection in recipients of LRD allografts. With this approach, we have observed a graft survival rate essentially equal to that achieved in patients never suffering any rejection episodes [9]. As further studies have confirmed, acute rejection in cadaver donor (CD) allograft recipients is also responsive to ALG (Table 2), and because up to 20% of the patients receiving prophylactic azathioprine and steroids never experience rejection and, therefore, do not require ALG, many clinicians have now concluded ALG should be administered only in therapeutic regimens.

The reported incidence and severity of adverse clinical reactions following

Table 2. Randomized trials comparing steroids to antithymocyte globulin (ATG) plus steroids for treatment of acute renal allograft rejection

| Reference | No. of patients treated | Rejection reversal | | 1-year function | |
		Steroids (%)	ATG (%)	Steroids (%)	ATG (%)
30	52	62	91	49	74
31	64	75	100	61	82
32	52	75	84	47	73
33	40	65	75	65	70
34	23	83	100	75	91

ALG administration varies with the preparation being used. Fever, chills, and sometimes bronchospasm developing during the initial infusion have been observed in the majority of patients. Since subsequent infusions are usually tolerated without incident, it has been suggested that this initial reaction may result from endogenous pyrogens released during rapid lymphocytolysis. Prior to the initial administration of ALG, therefore, many clinicians recommend that a single i.v. bolus of prednisolone (250 to 500 mg) plus acetaminophen and diphenylhydramine be administered to ameliorate such reactions.

One of the main concerns during early ALG trials was the possibility that the host's immune response to the foreign protein might result in serum sickness or at least neutralization of the beneficial effects of the antiserum. Though anaphylactic reactions manifested by hypotension, respiratory distress, and chest or flank pain must be constantly anticipated, they have been exceedingly rare in ALG-treated patients. Pruritic skin eruptions have been noted in up to 20% of the patients. Although this might suggest the onset of serum sickness, the course of therapy has generally been continued without incident using antihistamines to control the skin rash. In fact, demonstration of antibody production to the foreign protein has been possible in a minority of patients receiving i.v. ALG, and numerous patients have been treated with ALG on multiple occasions without adverse effects. The lack of a troublesome immune response to the foreign IgG is in part due to careful deaggregation and to the use of the i.v. mode of administration, both of which present the foreign antigen in a less immunogenic fashion. In addition, ALG suppresses a variety of different lymphocyte populations so that the immune response to the foreign protein itself is also presumably depressed.

Thrombocytopenia of varying severity has been reported in approximately 50% of the patients treated. We have found this generally to be dose-related, occurring in patients who require more than 12 to 15 mg/kg/d to adequately depress T-cell levels. A modest reduction in ATG dosage or reduction in the azathioprine dosage usually resolves this problem without the need for discontinuing ATG. Although the thrombocytopenia is presumed to result from low levels of antiplatelet antibodies, reversible platelet aggregation within the pulmonary microcirculation has been demonstrated in dogs even in the absence of antiplatelet antibodies [10].

In earlier ATG trials, serious infectious complications, particularly with cytomegalovirus, were not infrequently encountered. We have found that reduction of the dosages of azathioprine and steroids during ATG therapy to approximately 50% of usually administered levels has resulted in a marked decrease in such infections [11]. The most frequently observed infection in ALG-treated patients is herpes labialis with approximately 60% of patients developing at least some evidence of this during or immediately after treatment. With the availability of acyclovir therapy, the herpes is relatively easily controlled.

Infection by other opportunistic agents obviously occurs in these patients as well. Again, however, when the dosages of concomitant immunosuppressive agents administered during ATG therapy are carefully limited, no increased incidence of such infections has been observed. Similarly, the incidence of neoplasia in ATG-treated patients is not increased over that observed in patients receiving only conventional suppression.

Monoclonal Antilymphocyte Preparations

The clinical usefulness and some of the limitations of ALG have been summarized above. Clearly, even the most meticulously prepared polyclonal product cannot be considered a standardized agent, so that some variability in immunosuppressive potency and in toxicity must be anticipated between batches. More importantly, because ALG necessarily produces a pan-T-cell depletion, these protocols cannot be further refined to achieve more specific immunosuppression.

The stage was set for another advance in this field by the clarification that lymphocytes, far from being identical to one another, can be divided into bursa-equivalent (B) cells and thymus-dependent (T) cells and further subdivided into functionally distinct subpopulations of T cells. In addition, distinctive cell surface antigens have been identified as being associated with the functional capacity of the T cells on which they reside. As a result, an antibody can be prepared against the suppressor/cytotoxic subset; for example, from one individual, anticipating it will react with that same subset in all individuals. Using hybridoma technology, it is now possible to produce such antibodies against these specific cell surface antigens.

With this approach, standardized products that react with only selected T-cell populations can be regularly produced without batch-to-batch variability. Because of the purity and specificity of the antibodies, milligram dosages can be expected to provide comparable T-cell depletion to that produced by much larger dosages of ALG. This both simplifies the clinical administration and limits the likelihood of toxic side effects in patients receiving monoclonal antibodies. The most important advantage offered by monoclonal antibodies is the opportunity to develop therapeutic protocols in which only selected subpopulations of the T-cell fraction are depleted.

Production and Administration of Monoclonal Antilymphocyte Antibodies

The steps involved in producing an immortal line of cells that will secrete a monomolecular species of antibody combine two previously recognized observations into a single effort. Lymphocytes from immunized animals, when cultured in vitro, can be readily isolated into separate clones, each producing a single antibody. Unfortunately, these clones have a very short lifespan. In contrast, myeloma cell clones can be grown permanently in culture, but produce antibodies with no predefined specificity. When the two types of cells are fused to form a hybridoma, both essential properties—secretion of antibodies with a predefined specificity and permanent growth—are retained.

Thus, splenic lymphocytes from mice previously immunized with human T cells are isolated, fused with mouse myeloma cells to obtain hybridomas, and then selected by random cloning to retain only those secreting the desired monoclonal antibodies. A number of these monoclonal antibody preparations, directed against human cell surface antigens, have now become available (Table 3).

The specificity of a monoclonal antibody is due to its purity. This does not preclude cross-reactivity with other cells owing to recognition by the antibody of a similar or identical epitope (reactive site) that might be present on different cell surface antigens. As a result, antilymphocyte antibodies must be thoroughly screened prior to their administration to exclude potentially toxic cross-reactivity with other normal human tissues [12]. On the other hand, cross-reactivity of antihuman monoclonal antibodies with lymphocytes of nonhuman primates fortunately allows preclinical studies that can evaluate toxicity, efficacy, and mechanisms of action.

We and others have begun to evaluate the immunosuppressive potency of some of these agents administered i.v. to allograft recipients. We initially studied the effects of OKT4 treatment of cynomolgus renal allograft recipients [13]. Immunologic monitoring of peripheral blood lymphocytes obtained from these animals revealed complete coating of the helper/inducer (OKT4-reactive) cells and an excess of OKT4 antibody in the serum of most animals. Nevertheless, the OKT4-reactive cells were not completely removed from the circulation, but were gradually depressed to approximately 20 to 30% of the pretreatment levels. Renal allograft survival was prolonged to as long as 47 days (control, 8 to 11 days) if the OKT4 treatment had been started prior to transplantation. This trial confirmed that effective immunosuppression can be achieved by depletion of only a single T-cell subpopulation.

We have also treated cynomolgus renal allograft recipients with OKT11A [14]. Following treatment with this antibody, the reactive antigenic site on the peripheral blood lymphocytes was modulated from the cell surface, and essentially no cell depletion occurred. Not unexpectedly, renal allograft survival in these animals was not prolonged, indicating that the type of reaction that occurs between the cell membrane antigenic site and the administered antibody is crucial in determining immunosuppressive efficacy.

Jonker, Goldstein, and Balner [15] have confirmed, in rhesus monkey skin allograft recipients, the significant immunosuppressive efficacy of OKT4

Table 3. Reactivity of monoclonal antibodies with peripheral blood leukocytes

Antibody	Reactive cell population	Reactive cells (%)
OKT3, Leu4, Anti-T12	Most circulating T cells	73 ± 8
OKT4, Leu3a	Helper/inducer T cells (HLA class II antigen-reactive)	46 ± 8
OKT8, Leu2a	Suppressor/cytotoxic T cells (HLA class I antigen-reactive)	25 ± 6
Leu7	Null cells, NK cells	15 ± 7
OKT11A, Leu5	E-rosetting cells	80 ± 8
CBL1	Activated "blast" cells, monocytes	<5

and the insignificant prolongation of graft survival by OKT11A. The monoclonal antibody OKT8A, specific for cytotoxic/suppressor T cells, was also
found to be without immunosuppressive efficacy in the rhesus model. In
contrast, we have found that treatment with Leu2a monoclonal antibody
(reactive with cytotoxic/suppressor T cells) prolongs the cynomolgus renal
allograft survival to as long as 5 weeks [16].

These studies emphasize that some monoclonal antibodies are more efficient
than others in activating mechanisms necessary for effective suppression of
the host's response to the allograft. A number of factors can be cited as
possible explanations for the variable efficacy observed, including antibody
isotype, antibody affinity with target antigen, target antigen density, efficiency
in activating complement, and mechanism of clearance of coated cells by
individual recipients. Continued screening of the numerous agents becoming
available, hopefully, will identify a group of clinically useful antibodies from
this second generation of antilymphocyte preparations.

Use of Monoclonal Antibodies in Renal Allograft Recipients

Therapeutic intervention by the IV administration of antilymphocyte monoclonal antibodies to renal allograft recipients has been undertaken to date
using three different preparations. We originally reported the use of OKT3,
an IgG2a monoclonal antibody, which reacts with an antigenic determinant
found on virtually all mature post-thymic T cells [17]. Because of our experience with ATG, we felt the most clear-cut evidence of efficacy would be
established if definite reversal of ongoing early rejection reactions could be
demonstrated. Prior trials with this particular antibody in nonhuman primates
were impossible, because it does not react with lymphocytes of any readily
available species.

To date, a total of 30 cadaveric renal allograft recipients have been evaluated. These patients were treated from the day of transplantation with standard doses of azathioprine and prednisone. At the onset of biopsy-confirmed
acute rejection, OKT3 antibody treatment was the sole addition to their
management. Azathioprine and prednisone dosages were further reduced,
based on the experience gained in the earlier ATG trials. In the first patients
treated, the daily dosage of OKT3 antibody was limited to the minimal amount
that completely cleared peripheral blood T cells. This usually required 1 to
2 mg/d. Subsequently, however, we have routinely used a daily dosage of
5 mg for a total of 10 to 14 days.

In each patient, circulating T-cell numbers plunged to undetectable levels
within minutes following the initial OKT3 injection. That the cells had actually been cleared from the circulation was supported by a corresponding
fall in total lymphocyte counts and an absence of cells bearing other independent T-cell markers. Approximately 5 to 7 days into the therapeutic course,
increasing numbers of cells, nonreactive with OKT3 but reactive with other
T-cell markers, became detectable in most patients treated. In vitro incubation

of these cells restored OKT3 reactivity, indicating that some degree of antigenic modulation had occurred. This, however, was apparently insufficient to interfere with the therapeutic effect, because in all instances the established rejection episode was reversed within 2 to 10 days without addition of any other immunosuppressive measures.

Despite this striking immunosuppressive efficacy, several limitations to OKT3 monoclonal antibody therapy have been identified. Virtually all patients have experienced chills and a febrile reaction beginning about 40 min after the first injection. Several patients were also noted to have dyspnea and mild bronchospasm. In our experience, all of these symptoms have resolved following treatment with antihistamines and antipyretics, and generally there was no recurrence after the initial infusion. Other investigators, however, have observed even more violent reactions with the initial infusion, and 2 patients were reported to develop severe bronchospasm and pulmonary edema leading to cardiopulmonary arrest [unpublished].

During the 4 to 38 month follow-up in our study, subsequent rejection episodes have occurred in two-thirds of the patients. Since some of these were irreversible with conventional therapy, long-term graft survival was retained in only 70% of the original group.

A third possible limitation has been the development in the recipients of both idiotypic and nonidiotypic antibodies to the OKT3 monoclonal reagent. Although no clinically evident reactions suggesting anaphylaxis have occurred in our experience, the formation of these antimouse antibodies would appear to contraindicate subsequent treatment of these patients with monoclonal antibodies. In an attempt to address these limitations, we have more recently altered the therapeutic protocol by adding increased steroid dosages on the first day of OKT3 therapy, limiting the period of OKT3 treatment to a maximum of 10 days, and administering i.v. cyclophosphamide infusions during the second week of OKT3 therapy. With these changes, we have noted both a marked reduction in the reactions to the initial infusion and a decrease in the host's immune response to the infused OKT3 [18].

A multiple-center prospectively randomized trial comparing OKT3 therapy with high-dose steroids, and ATG if necessary, for reversal of rejection has also been undertaken. Over 100 cadaveric renal allograft recipients were enrolled in this study. The preliminary results continue to show the remarkable efficacy of OKT3 in providing rapid depletion of peripheral blood T-cell levels and reversal of established rejection, with only two rejection episodes in the OKT3-treated group failing to respond [to be published]. In contrast, only about 70% of the rejection reactions responded to high-dose steroid therapy. Although subsequent rejection episodes have claimed some of the allografts in the OKT3 group, graft survival has continued to strongly favor this group because of the extremely high early reversal rate.

Evaluation of the effectiveness of another monoclonal antibody, anti-T12, has also been undertaken in renal allograft recipients [19]. This monoclonal reagent is an IgM antibody reactive with most mature post-thymic T cells, but directed against a different antigenic moiety than OKT3. In this trial, 19 patients undergoing acute rejection after either CD or living related (LRD) renal transplantation were studied. The allograft recipients were initially treated with azathioprine or cyclosporine and steroids. Rejection was treated with i.v. infused anti-T12 antibody. Seven of the recipients had clear-cut reversal of rejection activity within 10 days. Four additional patients had delayed responses after further immunosuppressive therapy had been added to their regimen. Eight patients failed to respond. In contrast to the patients treated with OKT3, no discernible febrile or systemic reactions to the initial infusion of anti-T12 were recorded. One patient did subsequently develop fever, lower back pain, and skin rash in association with the development of antimouse antibodies. No other significant side effects were identified. Of the seven patients who had prompt and complete resolution of the rejection episode by the anti-T12 therapy, only one required treatment for subsequent rejection activity during a follow-up period of 1 to 15 months.

A third clinical trial evaluating the usefulness of monoclonal antibody for reversing acute rejection has used a preparation with more limited T-cell reactivity [20]. In this trial, the monoclonal antibody, CBL1, which is directed against blast cells, was used to test the hypothesis that rejection might be reversed by specific clonal deletion of cells reacting against the graft. Eleven patients were recipients of donor-specific transfusions and LRD allografts. Eight patients received CD allografts. All recipients were initially treated with conventional immunosuppression. At the time of acute rejection, high-dose steroid therapy was administered to 15 of these patients. When rejection did not reverse after 3 to 5 days of steroid therapy, monoclonal antibody was added. Four patients received CBL1 antibody immediately because of the severity of the rejection episode.

Intravenous administration of this monoclonal antibody was found to be remarkably nontoxic. None of the patients developed fever, chills, or other significant side effects. There was no evidence of bone marrow toxicity, nor were peripheral blood lymphocyte counts decreased during treatment. Nevertheless, rejection was reversed in 17 of the 19 patients, and subsequent rejection episodes were infrequent during the limited follow-up period. As in the previous studies, formation of antimouse antibodies was observed in essentially all the patients studied.

Current Conclusions Regarding Antilymphocyte Therapy

The major complications of pharmacologic immunosuppression have been either infection or incomplete control of rejection. Through refinements in the use of conventional agents, primarily in the limitation of steroid dosages, a decrease in infectious complications and patient mortality has been achieved. The success rate, particularly following CD renal transplantation, however, has remained at a marginally acceptable and disturbingly stable level in patients treated with azathioprine and steroids alone. Further improvement in these results has more recently been reported for patients in whom ALG or ATG was added to the therapeutic regimen. The efficacy of these polyclonal preparations, especially for reversing acute rejection episodes, has now been firmly established. Despite the usefulness of such preparations, however, they are limited by lot-to-lot variability, contamination by extraneous antibodies, and the inability to refine their application beyond suppression of the entire T-cell response.

The availability of monoclonal antibodies now provides us with agents that may specifically suppress only T cells or even selected T-cell subsets. Initial clinical trials with the pan-T-cell reactive antibodies, OKT3 and anti-T12, have demonstrated truly impressive depletion of peripheral blood T cells and prompt reversal of established rejection episodes following administration of minute dosages. Although the long-term efficacy of these agents remains to be established, these observations have already confirmed the feasibility of using monoclonal antibodies to manipulate T-cell numbers precisely and to depress immune responses. An even more exciting aspect of this approach is the possibility of developing protocols directed against only selected T-cell subsets. The recently reported trial using CBL1 antibody is the first clinical venture into this area. Although the observations in these patients are preliminary, they are encouraging.

The tremendous potential of the powerful and sophisticated monoclonal technology has only begun to be applied to transplantation immunology. Undoubtedly, further refinements in the protocols currently being evaluated, as well as trials using other antibodies, will continue. The major question now being addressed is how these agents can or should be incorporated into cyclosporine protocols. With the arrival of both of these new immunosuppressive approaches at the same time, it is impossible to predict the precise role each will play in future therapeutic regimens. Because of their already demonstrated effects, however, one can anticipate both increased success rates and decreased toxicity for patients receiving renal allografts.

Acknowledgments. This work was supported by USPHS Grant HL/AM-18646 and by funds provided by the Ortho Pharmaceutical Corporation.

References

1. TERASAKI PI, PERDUE ST, SASAKI MA, MICKEY MR, WHITBY L: Improving success rates of kidney transplantation. *JAMA* 250:1065–1073, 1983
2. BRITTON S, PALACIOS R: Cyclosporin A: Usefulness, risks, and mechanism of action. *Immunol Rev* 65:5–22, 1982
3. WOODRUFF MFA, ANDERSON NF: Effect of lymphocyte depletion by thoracic duct fistula and administration of anti-lymphocyte serum on the survival of skin homografts in rats. *Nature (Lond)* 200:702, 1963
4. COSIMI AB: The clinical usefulness of antilymphocyte antibodies. *Transplant Proc* 15:583–589, 1983
5. MILSTEIN C: Monoclonal antibodies. *Scientific American* 243:66–74, 1980
6. MAKI T, SIMPSON M, MONACO AP: Development of suppressor T cells by antilymphocyte serum treatment in mice. *Transplantation* 34:376–381, 1982
7. THOMAS JM, CARVER FM, HAISCH CE, FAHRENBRUCK G, DEEPE RM, THOMAS FT: Suppressor cells in Rhesus monkeys treated with antithymocyte globulin. *Transplantation* 34:83–89, 1982

8. SHIELD CF, COSIMI AB, TOLKOFF-RUBIN N, RUBIN RH, HERRIN J, RUSSELL PS: Use of antithymocyte globulin for reversal of acute allograft rejection *Transplantation* 28:461–464, 1979

9. NELSON PW, COSIMI AB, DELMONICO FL, RUBIN RH, TOLKOFF-RUBIN NE, FANG L, RUSSELL PS: Antithymocyte globulin as the primary treatment for renal allograft rejection. *Transplantation* 36:587–588, 1983

10. HENRICSSON A, HUSBERG B, BERGENTZ SE: The mechanism behind the effect of ALG on platelets in vivo. *Clin Exp Immunol* 29:515–522, 1977

11. RUBIN RH, WOLFSON JS, COSIMI AB, TOLKOFF-RUBIN NE: Infection in the renal transplant recipient. *Am J Med* 70:405–411, 1981

12. GARSON JA, BEVERLEY PCL, COAKHAM HB, HARPER EI: Monoclonal antibodies against human T lymphocytes label Purkinje neurones of many species. *Nature* 298:375–377, 1982

13. COSIMI AB, BURTON RC, KUNG PC, COLVIN R, GOLDSTEIN G, LIFTER J, RHODES W, RUSSELL PS: Evaluation in primate renal allograft recipients of monoclonal antibody to human T-cell subclasses. *Transplant Proc* 13:499–503, 1981

14. GIORGI JV, BURTON RC, BARRETT LV, DELMONICO FL, GOLDSTEIN G, COSIMI AB: Immunosuppressive effect and immunogenicity of OKT11A monoclonal antibody in monkey allograft recipients. *Transplant Proc* 15:639–642, 1983

15. JONKER M, GOLDSTEIN G, BALNER H: Effects of in vitro administration of monoclonal antibodies specific for human T cell subpopulations on the immune system in a Rhesus monkey model. *Transplantation* 35:521–526, 1983

16. COSIMI AB: Anti-T-cell monoclonal antibodies in transplantation therapy. *Transplant Proc* 15:1889–1892, 1983

17. COSIMI AB, BURTON RC, COLVIN RB, GOLDSTEIN G, DELMONICO FL, LAQUAGLIA MP, TOLKOFF-RUBIN N, RUBIN RH, HERRIN JT, RUSSELL PS: Treatment of acute renal allograft rejection with OKT3 monoclonal antibody. *Transplantation* 535–539, 1981

18. THISTLETHWAITE R, COSIMI AB, DELMONICO FL, RUBIN RH, TOLKOFF-RUBIN N, FULLER TC, NELSON PW, FANG L, RUSSELL PS: Evolving use of OKT3 monoclonal antibody for treatment of renal allograft rejection. *Transplantation* (in press, 1984)

19. KIRKMAN RL, ARAUJO JL, BUSCH GJ, CARPENTER CB, MILFORD EL, REINHERZ EL, SCHLOSSMAN SF, STROM TB, TILNEY NL: Treatment of acute renal allograft rejection with monoclonal anti-T12 antibody. *Transplantation* 36:620–626, 1983

20. TAKAHASHI H, TERASAKI PI, KINUKAWA T, CHIA D, MIURA K, OKAZAKI H, IWAKI Y, TAGUCHI Y, HARDIWIDJAJA S, ISHIZAKI M, BILLING B: Reversal of transplant rejection by monoclonal antiblast antibody. *Lancet* 2:1155–1158, 1983

21. SHEIL AGR, KELLY GE, STOREY BG, MAY J, KALOWSKI S, MEARS D, ROGERS JH, JOHNSON JR, CHARLESWORTH J, STEWART JH: Controlled clinical trial of antilymphocyte globulin in patients with renal allografts from cadaver donors. *Lancet* 1:359–363, 1971

22. TAYLOR HE, ACKMAN CFD, HOROWITZ I: Canadian clinical trial of antilymphocyte globulin in human cadaver renal transplantation. *Can Med Assoc J* 115:1205–1208, 1976

23. LAUNOIS B, CAMPION JP, FAUCHET R, KERBAOL M, CARTIER F: Prospective randomized clinical trial in patients with cadaver-kidney transplants. *Transplant Proc* 9:1027–1030, 1977

24. BUTT KMH, ZIELINSKI CM, PARSA I, ELBERG AJ, WECHTER W, KOUNTZ

SL: Trends in immunosuppression for kidney transplantation. *Kidney Int* 13:S95–S98, 1978

25. WECHTER WJ, BRODIE JA, MORRELL RM, RAFI M, SCHULTZ JR: Antithymocyte globulin (ATGAM) in renal allograft recipients. *Transplantation* 28:294–312, 1979

26. COSIMI AB: The clinical value of antilymphocyte antibodies. *Transplant Proc* 13:462–468, 1981

27. KREIS H, MANSOURI R, DESCAMPS JM, DANDAVINO R, N'GUYEN AT, BACH JF, CROSNIER J: Antithymocyte globulin in cadaver kidney transplantation: A randomized trial based on T-cell monitoring. *Kidney Int* 19:438–444, 1981

28. NOVICK AC, BRAUN WE, STEINMULLER D, BUSZTA C, GREENSTREET R, KISER W: A controlled randomized double-blind study of antilymphoblast globulin in cadaver renal transplantation. *Transplantation* 35:175–179, 1983

29. BELL PRF, BLAMEY RW, BRIGGS JD, CASTRO JE, HAMILTON DNH, KNAPP MS, SALAMAN JR, SELLS RA, WILLIAMS G, GOWANS JL, PETO R, RICHARDS S, PHILLIPS AW, WEINBERG AL, FREESTONE DS: Medical research council trial of antilymphocyte globulin in renal transplantation. *Transplantation* 35:539–544, 1983

30. FILO RS, SMITH EJ, LEAPMAN SB: Therapy of acute cadaveric renal allograft rejection with adjunctive antithymocyte globulin. *Transplantation* 30:445–449, 1980

31. HOWARD RJ, CONDIE RM, SUTHERLAND DER, SIMMONS RL, NAJARIAN JS: The use of antilymphoblast globulin in the treatment of renal allograft rejection. *Transplant Proc* 13:473–474, 1981

32. NOWYGROD R, APPEL G, HARDY MA: Use of ATG for reversal of acute allograft rejection. *Transplant Proc* 13:469–472, 1981

33. HOITSMA AJ, REEKERS P, KREEFTENBERG JG, VAN LIER HJJ, CAPEL PJA, KOENE RAP: Treatment of acute rejection of cadaveric renal allografts with rabbit antithymocyte globulin. *Transplantation* 33:12–16, 1982

34. STREEM SB, NOVICK AC, BRAUN WE, STEINMULLER D, GREENSTREET R: Low-dose maintenance prednisone and antilymphoblast globulin for the treatment of acute rejection. *Transplantation* 35:420–424, 1983

Total Lymphoid Irradiation in Renal Transplantation: Reduction and Elimination of Maintenance Immunosuppressive Drugs

Samuel Strober, Richard T. Hoppe, Barry Levin, and Derek Sampson

Total lymphoid irradiation (TLI) has been used for more than 20 years to treat patients with Hodgkin's disease and non-Hodgkin's lymphomas [1]. The efficacy and side effects of this regimen have been studied extensively in several thousand patients with follow-up observation periods of up to 15 years [1]. Serious infectious complications requiring hospitalization are less than 1% [1]. There is no increased risk of hematologic malignancy or lymphoma when TLI (4400 rads) is used in the absence of adjuvant chemotherapy [2–5]. With adjuvant chemotherapy, there has been no synergism between TLI and chemotherapy with regard to the risk of leukemia or lymphoma [2–5].

TLI has been shown to be immunosuppressive in humans and laboratory animals [6–11]. It also increases the animals' susceptibility to tolerance induction for both allogeneic-transplanted tissues and heterologous proteins [6, 8, 9, 12–15]. This raises the possibility that TLI may be used in humans to induce specific transplantation tolerance with permanent acceptance of allogeneic organs without chronic immunosuppressive drug therapy. TLI has already been used in clinical organ transplantation as first reported by investigators at the University of Minnesota [10]. High doses of TLI (up to 4050 rads) were combined with conventional post-transplant immunosuppressive drugs (prednisone and azathioprine [Aza]) in a series of high-risk cadaver graft recipients given second or third transplants. Although graft survival was considerably increased as compared to conventional therapy, patient survival was not increased [10]. The maintenance immunosuppressive drug regimen was similar in patients given TLI and in patients given conventional therapy.

A subsequent study by investigators at the University of Leuven used lower doses of TLI (up to 2500 rads) followed by low doses of prednisone (approx. 0.2 mg/kg/d) as the sole maintenance immunosuppressive therapy

This manuscript was presented as part of a Symposium on *Immunomodulation for Transplantation: New Approaches.*

in a series of diabetic primary cadaver allograft recipients [11, 16]. Greater than 90% 1-year graft survival was observed with no mortality in this series. In a similar collaborative study involving Stanford University and the Pacific Medical Center, San Francisco (PMC), a series of unmatched cadaver kidney allograft recipients were given TLI (2000 rads), a brief course of antithymocyte globulin immediately post-transplant, and low doses of prednisone as the sole maintenance immunosuppressive drug regimen. The results of this study confirmed those reported by the investigators at the University of Leuven and support the conclusion that after TLI, cadaver renal allografts can be maintained by low doses of prednisone in the absence of dangerous second-line drugs, such as Aza or cyclosporine. In addition, the Stanford–PMC study suggests that maintenance immunosuppressive drugs can be eliminated in some renal allograft recipients given pretransplant TLI.

The subsequent sections review the immunosuppressive and tolerogenic effects of TLI in humans and laboratory animals, as well as the complications associated with this radiotherapy regimen. Details of the three clinical studies of TLI in renal transplantation are discussed and compared.

Radiotherapy Technique

The critical features of TLI that differ from single-dose whole body irradiation are: (1) the use of lead shielding to protect vital radiosensitive tissues, such as the central nervous system, lungs, kidneys, and bone marrow, and (2) the use of fractionated irradiation such that large cumulative doses are achieved by administering multiple small doses (150 to 250 rads each).

Figure 1 shows the radiation ports used to administer TLI to patients with Hodgkin's disease [1]. The supradiaphragmatic tissues (called the *mantle field*) includes the cervical, axillary, supraclavicular, and mediastinal lymph nodes, as well as the thymus. Subdiaphragmatic tissues include the spleen, para-aortic, iliac, and inguinal-femoral lymph nodes. Most Hodgkin's disease patients and some organ-transplant patients are splenectomized before radiotherapy, and only the splenic pedicle is irradiated. All tissues not in the ports are shielded with lead or are outside the perimeter of the x-ray beam. Irradiation is given to the mantle field in dosages of 150 to 250 rads per fraction until a total dose of 4400 rads is achieved over a period of 4 to 6 weeks [1]. A similar course of fractionated radiotherapy (4400 rads) is then administered to the abdominal fields to complete the regimen. The radiation source used most frequently is a megavoltage linear accelerator. In almost all cases, hospitalization is not required for the irradiation treatments, which are performed in the clinics during a period of 3 to 4 months.

Immune Changes in Patients with Hodgkin's Disease after TLI

In the course of investigating the cellular basis of the immunodeficiency of patients with Hodgkin's disease, Fuks et al examined the number and function

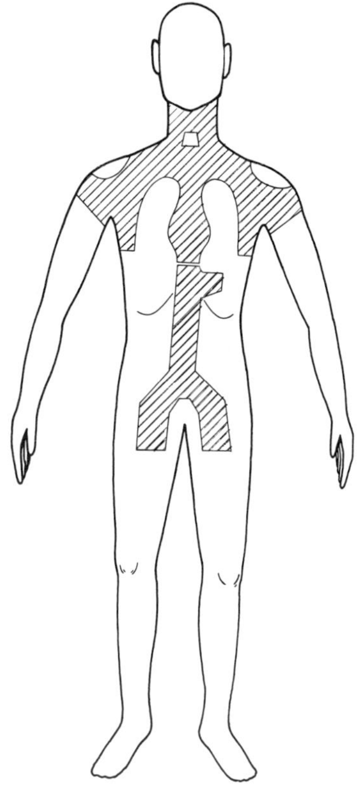

Fig. 1. Total lymphoid irradiation in the treatment of Hodgkin's disease. *Shaded areas* show ports for irradiation. Spleen is included in field if it has not been removed during staging laparotomy.

of lymphocytes in the peripheral blood before and after treatment with TLI [6]. Before radiotherapy, the total lymphocyte count and percentage of T and B cells in patients with Hodgkin's disease were not significantly different from those observed in normal controls. However, at the completion of TLI, the mean total peripheral blood lymphocyte count of 403/mm³ was 4 SDs below the mean of normal. Recovery of the lymphocyte count began shortly after completion of radiotherapy and reached pretreatment levels about 2 years later. After full recovery of the total count, the percentage of T cells as measured by an in vitro cytotoxicity assay with anti-T cell antiserum was approximately half the pretreatment value and remained at that level for at least 10 years. The T lymphocytopenia was associated with a B lymphocytosis and a reversal of the normal T:B ratio. Recently, it was shown that the reduction in T cell numbers observed after TLI was primarily due to a long-term reduction in the absolute number of helper T cells identified by the OKT4 monoclonal antibody [17]. Although both helper (OKT4$^+$) and suppressor/cytotoxic T cells (OKT8$^+$) were depleted immediately after radiotherapy, the OKT8$^+$ cells returned to normal levels within a few months. The helper cell repopulation was incomplete and resulted in a long-term decrease in the ratio of helper to suppressor/cytotoxic T cells [17].

The peripheral blood lymphocytes of untreated patients with Hodgkin's disease showed a decreased response to phytohemagglutinin (PHA) in vitro, measured by tritiated thymidine or tritiated leucine incorporation, as compared to normal controls [6]. This reversible defect might be secondary to the presence of inhibitory serum factor [18]. After radiotherapy, the PHA response of patients fell significantly below that of the pretreatment level [6]. The reduced PHA response after treatment was not reversible by incubation of cells in tissue culture medium and appeared to be an intrinsic functional deficit. The further reduction of the response persisted for at least 10 years after radiotherapy without the recurrence of disease.

The allogeneic mixed leukocyte response (MLR) of untreated patients with Hodgkin's disease was similar to that of normal persons as measured by incorporation of tritiated thymidine. However, after radiotherapy, the MLR was virtually eliminated and fell to background levels for about 20 months [6]. Thereafter, a slow recovery occurred such that normal responses were uniformly observed 5 or more years after treatment. The minority (27%) of untreated patients showed a delayed hypersensitivity skin reaction to dinitrochlorobenzene (DNCB). Of the responding group, almost all lost their skin reactivity immediately after the completion of TLI [6]. More than half of these treated patients had recovered a response to DNCB by 1 year after treatment. However, 29% of these patients remained anergic for at least 8 years after radiotherapy.

Complications Associated with TLI in Patients with Hodgkin's Disease

Despite the potent and long-lasting immunosuppression induced by TLI, it is an outpatient procedure that is tolerated extremely well. Less than 1% of Hodgkin's disease patients given TLI to a total dose of 4400 rads required hospitalization for irradiation complications [1]. Mild self-limited constitutional symptoms were frequent and included fatigue, anorexia, and nausea. Severe thrombocytopenia or leukopenia (less than 50% of baseline) persisting beyond 2 months after treatment was observed in less than 1% of the patients [1]. The incidence of severe bacterial infection requiring hospitalization was less than 1% and was not significantly increased above that associated with splenectomy performed at the time of staging of disease [1]. Approximately 20 to 30% of patients treated with TLI developed herpes zoster within 2 years after completion of therapy, but less than 1% of this group progressed to dissemination requiring hospitalization [1]. The risk of hematologic malignancy or lymphoma after TLI alone was not increased in over 1000 patients observed for up to 10 years in several different institutions [2–5]. The same studies indicate that chemotherapy is associated with an increased risk, but that a combination of TLI and chemotherapy results in an increase that is not statistically significantly higher than with chemotherapy alone [2–5].

Of Hodgkin's disease patients who received mantle-field irradiation, but no intended direct lung irradiation, 2.2% required treatment for symptomatic radiation pneumonitis [1]. Some of these patients received more direct lung irradiation because of the need to treat their enlarged mediastinal lymph nodes (not present in transplantation or autoimmune disease patients). There have been no documented cases of radiation-induced carditis or pericarditis in the treatment of several hundred patients when subcarinal lead shields are used [1]. Nearly two-thirds of the patients after TLI have evidence of chemical thyroid dysfunction, but less than one-third of these have true hypothyroidism as evidenced by a low T_4 level [1]. In many cases, thyroid damage may have been precipitated by a prior large iodide load (lymphangiography). The incidence of thyroid cancer is less than 1% even in patients followed for over 10 years after radiotherapy [1].

Possible local complications of subdiaphragmatic lymphoid irradiation include gastric ulcer, gastrointestinal bleeding, chronic radiation enteritis, and azospermia. Each has been seen in less than 1% of patients treated with TLI for Hodgkin's disease [1]. The expected incidence of amenorrhea after TLI is 100%, unless shields are used to protect the ovaries in menstruating females. With shielding of the ovaries, the expected incidence of amenorrhea is less than 1%.

Immune Changes in Patients with Rheumatoid Arthritis after TLI

Two studies of the use of TLI in patients with rheumatoid arthritis who have failed conventional treatment (nonsteroidal anti-inflammatory drugs, gold compounds, and penicillamine) have been reported [19–21]. In the Stanford University study, a total of 2000 rads was given using the two-field technique shown in Figure 1 [19, 21]; and in the Harvard University study, a total of 3000 rads was given using a three-field technique [20]. Improvement in joint disease activity after TLI was observed in both series of patients, as well as profound immunologic changes.

As in the studies of patients with Hodgkin's disease, there was a marked reduction in the absolute number of helper T cells in the peripheral blood after TLI, which persisted for at least 2 years [21]. The reduction in the number of suppressor/cytotoxic T cells was minimal during the same period of time, such that the ratio of helper to suppressor/cytotoxic T cells was decreased [19, 21]. These changes were due to poor repopulation of the helper T cell subset after radiotherapy and not due to selective depletion by TLI [22]. In vitro tests of T cell function were markedly reduced during the first 2 years (response to PHA, concanavalin A [Con A], allogeneic lymphocytes, tetanus toxoid, and herpes zoster antigen) [19, 21]. In addition, the in vitro secretion of immunoglobulins by peripheral blood lymphocytes stimulated with pokeweed mitogen was reduced by approximately 80% for at least 2 years after TLI [21]. Thus, the immune deficits observed after TLI in patients with Hodgkin's disease were also observed in patients with rheumatoid arthritis despite the reduction in the cumulative dose of radiation from 4400 rads to 2000 rads [19, 21].

Induction of Specific Transplantation Tolerance in Mice and Rats

In several experiments, BALB/c (H-2^d) mice were given TLI (3400 rads) and an i.v. injection of bone marrow cells from C57BL/Ka (H-2^b) donors 1 day later [23]. Skin grafts from the donors were also placed on the recipients at the same time. Approximately 90% of the TLI-treated recipients became stable chimeras as judged by the presence of donor-type lymphocytes in the peripheral blood more than 100 days after bone marrow transplantation. Chimerism was also found in the erythrocytes. Although allogeneic bone marrow engraftment was achieved, no clinical evidence of graft-versus-host (GvHD) was observed in the recipients. In contrast, nearly all mice prepared with single-dose lethal WBI developed GvHD and were dead by 60 days after bone marrow transplantation. Stable chimeras prepared with TLI permanently accepted skin grafts from the marrow donor strain, but rejected skin grafts from third-party (C3H, H-2^k) donors [23]. Thus, the chimeras were specifically tolerant to the alloantigens of the bone marrow donor.

In similar experiments, inbred rats were given TLI (3400 rads) and allogeneic bone marrow in combination with skin, heart, or pancreas grafts from the marrow donors [14, 24]. Donor and recipient strains were homozygous and differed at both major and minor histocompatibility genetic loci [14, 24]. Approximately 90% of the recipients became chimeras and permanently accepted the organ grafts [14, 24]. As in the studies with mice, the chimeras were specifically tolerant to the alloantigens of the marrow donor strain [14, 24]. Although TLI without marrow transplantation markedly prolonged the survival of skin, heart, or pancreas allografts, ultimately the large majority of these allografts were rejected. Thus, in the rodent model, TLI had to be used in combination with marrow transplantation to ensure tolerization.

Induction of Specific Unresponsiveness to Allogeneic Organ Transplants in Outbred Dogs and Baboons

The use of TLI alone (1800 rads total dose) or in combination with a brief course of other immunosuppressive agents was studied in adult mongrel dogs given heterotopic heart allografts from unmatched donors [8]. Maximum allograft survival with TLI alone was 28 days, and with six i.m. injections of rabbit antidog thymocyte globulin (ATG) alone, it was 33 days. However, marked synergy was observed with the combination of the two regimens such that four of eight allografts survived 200 days or more (Table 1). Three of eight dogs given TLI and ATG maintained their allografts with minimal or no cellular infiltrate during the entire observation period (360 to 495 days). All three animals rejected a third-party heart within 2 weeks. Thus, the latter recipients were specifically unresponsive to the initial allograft despite the withdrawal of all immunosuppressive reagents after day 10.

The addition of a 90-day course of Aza to the combination of TLI and

Table 1. Allograft survival in dogs treated with total lymphoid irradiation and antithymocyte globulin

Treatment	Heart allograft survival (days)
None	5, 5, 6, 6, 7
TLI alone[a]	6, 6, 8, 8, 9, 28
ATG alone	15, 16, 21, 28, 31, 33
TLI + ATG	45, 81, 89, 139, 200, >325,[c] >494,[c] >495[c]
TLI + ATG + Aza (90 days)[b]	113, 117, 120, 127, 140, 289, >538,[c] >538[c]
TLI + ATG + Aza (180 days)[b]	103, 132, 178, 181, 306, 313

[a] Abbreviations: TLI, total lymphoid irradiation; ATG, antithymocyte globulin; Aza, azathioprine.

[b] The parenthetical 90 and 180 days refer to azathioprine.

[c] Rejection of third-party heart allograft; the biopsy sample of the primary graft was normal at 9 months.

ATG had no further beneficial effect in increasing the fraction of recipients showing specific unresponsiveness (Table 1). Two of eight recipients given TLI, ATG, and Aza showed a pattern of specific unresponsiveness. Neither animal had abnormal findings upon biopsy examination of their allograft at 538 days, and they rejected third-party hearts transplanted at about 270 days. Addition of a 180-day course of Aza produced no long-term graft acceptance (Table 1). All dogs given a combination of ATG and Aza without TLI, or TLI and Aza without ATG, rejected their allografts by 40 to 178 days, respectively. Mortality in the groups given TLI, ATG, and Aza, or ATG and Aza without TLI, was 20 and 33%, respectively. Previous studies of TLI, ATG, and Aza in cynomolgus monkeys given orthotopic heart transplants showed a mortality rate of 60% [25]. In contrast, there were no deaths in dogs given TLI and ATG without Aza. Thus, the use of Aza increased the mortality rate of allograft recipients and decreased the fraction of recipients maintaining long-term grafts ($\geq$ 200 days) after the discontinuation of immunosuppressive agents. In conclusion, these results show that it is possible to achieve specific unresponsiveness in the absence of chronic immunosuppressive drugs or bone marrow transplantation in unmatched dogs given TLI and ATG.

Long-term acceptance of liver and kidney allografts in outbred baboons treated with TLI in the absence of marrow transplantation has been reported by Myburgh et al [9]. The most successful regimen involved the use of enlarged radiation fields, which included the whole abdomen as in previous rodent studies, but with a cumulative radiation dose of 800 rads given in 100-rad fractions. By this procedure, unmatched kidney allografts survived more than 200 days without post-transplant immunosuppressive drugs in 80% of the recipients [9]. Some animals in these studies were followed for as long as 4 years with intact kidney allografts [9]. Specific unresponsiveness in the latter graft recipients was demonstrated by the rapid rejection of a third-party graft transplanted 1 year after the initial graft [9].

The results of the outbred dog and baboon experiments show that it is possible to achieve specific unresponsiveness and long-term organ graft acceptance in the absence of marrow transplantation using TLI as a pretransplant preparative regimen. However, the radiation fields and fractionation procedures used to administer TLI to patients with Hodgkin's disease were insufficient to obtain marked prolongation of graft survival in these animal models. In the case of mongrel dogs, a six-injection course of ATG had to be given in combination with conventional TLI fields to induce specific unresponsiveness. In the case of baboons, the radiation fields had to be enlarged substantially (whole abdomen) as compared to conventional TLI fields to develop long-term graft acceptance.

Clinical Trials of TLI in Cadaver Renal Transplantation

The first study of the use of TLI in human renal transplantation was reported by investigators at the University of Minnesota [10]. Twenty-two high-risk patients were given TLI before transplantation, and azathioprine and prednisone as the maintenance regimen after transplantation. Twenty patients had previously rejected one to three kidney allografts and had developed cytotoxic antibodies. This increased the difficulties of finding a cross-match negative cadaver kidney. Eighteen patients received cadaveric grafts. Twenty-one patients were splenectomized before radiotherapy. Patients were treated with fractions of 100 to 125 rads each to supra- and subdiaphragmatic TLI fields (Fig. 1) simultaneously. The total dose of TLI varied from 1050 to 4050 rads, and the time interval between the completion of radiotherapy and transplantation varied between 1 and 330 days. Four patients had an interval of greater than 100 days owing to the difficulties in obtaining a cross-match negative graft. Full therapeutic doses of azathioprine (1.0 to 1.5 mg/kg/d adjusted to the white blood cell count) were given post-transplant in combination with prednisone, which was begun at 2 mg/kg/d, in 19 patients before tapering to lower maintenance doses.

At 24 months, 72% of the grafts were functioning in the TLI group as compared to 38% in a comparable group given conventional immunosuppression [10]. Five deaths were observed in 21 patients with technically successful transplants with a follow-up period of 5 to 36 months. A subsequent report of the 19 retransplant patients treated with TLI showed a 68% and 64% patient and graft survival, respectively (excluding technical failures), with a minimum of 22 months follow-up [26]. Of eight patient deaths in the latter study, four were associated with graft loss caused by rejection or to technical failure. Another four deaths were due to cytomegalovirus infection [1], lymphoma [2], and pneumococcal sepsis [1].

Immunologic studies showed a marked reduction in circulating T lymphocytes and in vitro tests of T lymphocyte function [10]. A review of the clinical outcome indicated that graft survival was optimum when the interval between radiotherapy and transplantation was within 2 weeks. Although five patients were given small numbers (approx. 0.5×10^8 nucleated cells/kg) of donor bone marrow cells treated in vitro with heterologous anti-T cell globulin, no chimerism or more favorable outcome was observed. These investigators concluded that TLI increased graft survival significantly as compared to conventional therapy, but was associated with similar patient survival [10] in this high-risk group.

In more recent studies, investigators at the University of Leuven treated eight diabetic recipients of cadaver kidney allografts with pretransplant TLI and low doses of prednisone as the sole maintenance immunosuppressive drug [11, 16]. All patients were splenectomized before radiotherapy, and supra- and subdiaphragmatic radiation fields were treated simultaneously. Fractions of 100 rads each were given until a total dose of 2000 to 2500 rads was achieved [11]. All patients received primary cadaver transplants within 11 days after TLI. After transplantation, prednisone (30 mg/d) was administered; the dosage was reduced to 15 mg/d by day 10 and to 10 mg/d after day 120. Rejection episodes were treated with increased doses of prednisone and a brief course of azathioprine. Interruption of TLI occurred in only one patient, who had blood element depression, and two patients required transient i.v. therapy for anorexia and vomiting. Eight out of eight patients maintained functioning grafts at 1 year, but six out of eight had at least one rejection episode during that time. Complications included a myocardial infarction in one patient, a cerebrovascular accident in another, a clinically apparent cytomegalovirus infection in one patient and *E. coli* septicemia with pyelonephritis in one. No deaths were observed.

Immunologic monitoring showed a marked reduction in the in vitro responses of peripheral blood T lymphocytes to mitogens and allogeneic lymphocytes during the entire follow-up period [11, 16]. However, natural killer cell activity was reduced only transiently and returned to the pretreatment range within 2 months after transplantation [16]. This pattern was opposite to that found in a group of nondiabetic transplant recipients treated with conventional prednisone and azathioprine. The latter patients showed substantially less reduction in the T cell responses, but a more marked and persistent reduction of natural killer cell activity [16].

The results of these studies suggest that excellent graft and patient survival can be obtained in high-risk diabetic cadaver transplant recipients after TLI. Since these studies were reported, an additional seven diabetic patients treated with TLI (3000 rads) received cadaver grafts (total 15) at the University of Leuven. Currently, 14 out of 15 patents are alive and maintain functioning grafts (M. Waer, personal communication). Differences between the results of the latter study and that of the University of Minnesota may be explained by several differences in the protocols, including: (1) use of primary versus secondary transplant recipients, (2) ability to perform transplantation within 2 weeks after TLI in all patients, (3) limitation of the maximum dose of radiation to 2500 to 3000 rads, and (4) elimination of maintenance azathioprine, and use of low-dose prednisone as the sole maintenance immunosuppressive therapy.

A recent collaborative study involving investigators at Stanford University and the Pacific Medical Center confirms the conclusion that cadaver renal allograft recipients given pretransplant TLI can be maintained on low-dose prednisone as the sole chronic immunosuppressive drug therapy. Twelve patients received 1800 to 2200 rads TLI in fractions of 100 rads each. Patients were not splenectomized as in the above two studies. Although supra- and subdiaphragmatic fields were irradiated simultaneously at the initiation of TLI, blood element depressions in the majority of patients necessitated interruption of therapy. On resumption, radiotherapy to the fields above the diaphragm was continued until a total of 2000 rads was achieved, and the subdiaphragmatic tissues were treated thereafter to the same dose. Subsequent weekly fractions of 100 rads were given until transplantation. All patients received unmatched cadaver grafts within 2 weeks after TLI. Ten patients with technically successful grafts received a total of six i.m. injections of rabbit antihuman thymocyte globulin during the first 10 days after grafting. Prednisone (10 mg/70 kg of body wt per day) was given from the day of transplantation. In the absence of rejection episodes during the first 8 months of maintenance, prednisone was reduced by approximately 25% per month and was eliminated at 1 year. Rejection episodes were treated with increased prednisone or prednisone and ATG. The use of ATG immediately post-transplant was based on the induction of specific unresponsiveness in approximately 40% of the dogs given TLI, ATG, and a heart allograft [8].

Of the 10 patients with technically successful grafts, four were diabetics and two had previously rejected a transplant within 6 months. Nine out of 10 patients are currently alive, and eight have functioning grafts during a follow-up period of 2 to 17 months post-transplantation. Four out of 10 patients have had rejection episodes (days 21, 62, and 365). None of the patients required hospitalization or IV therapy for side effects of the radiotherapy. Fatigue, nausea, and vomiting, mild neutropenia (<3000 cells/mm^3), and mild thrombocytopenia ($<150,000$ platelets/mm^3) occurred in almost all patients during and shortly after radiotherapy. Immunologic changes included a marked reduction of T lymphocytes, and a reduction in the proliferative response of peripheral blood lymphocytes to phyothemagglutinin, concanavalin A, pokeweed mitogen, and allogeneic lymphocytes. The responses to concanavalin A and allogeneic lymphocytes showed a gradual return toward pretreatment levels from 6 to 12 months after TLI. Infectious complications included two patients with transient herpes simplex infections of the oropharynx, and three patients with bacterial urinary tract infections. One patient developed a herpes viremia during treatment of a rejection episode and died of hepatic failure and diffuse intravascular coagulation. Clinically apparent cytomegalovirus infection or lymphoma was not observed. The first patient (diabetic) in the series has been followed for 17 months. He has received no immunosuppressive therapy after 12 months and maintains a serum creatinine concentration of approximately 1.4 mg/dl.

Conclusion

Although TLI has been used extensively during the past decade to treat cancer of the lymphoid tissues, the modification and use of this procedure in clinical organ transplantation has occurred only recently. It is clear from studies of laboratory animals that TLI can be used to induce specific unresponsiveness to allogeneic organ grafts. The results of clinical studies described above suggest that pretransplant TLI can be used most effectively to reduce the requirements for maintenance immunosuppressive drugs after transplantation. In particular, it appears that low doses of daily prednisone are sufficient to maintain allograft acceptance in the absence of potentially dangerous second-line drugs such as azathioprine or cyclosporine. In current practice, the latter drugs are usually added to low doses of prednisone and administered for an indefinite period of time. Thus, TLI may be helpful in eliminating cumulative side effects, such as nephrotoxicity, hepatotoxicity, neurotoxicity, and increased risk of lymphoma associated with the chronic administration of immunosuppressive drugs, such as cyclosporine [27–32]. Perhaps, the greatest promise afforded by TLI is the elimination of maintenance immunosuppressive drugs altogether. Although this can be achieved in a fraction of laboratory animals and humans, a major goal is to further modify TLI protocols to induce permanent and specific unresponsiveness uniformly in transplant recipients without maintenance drugs.

References

1. KAPLAN HS: *Hodgkin's Disease* (2nd ed). Cambridge, Harvard University Press, 1980, pp 366–441
2. BACCARINI M, BOSI A, PAPA G: Second malignancies in patients treated for Hodgkin's disease. *Cancer* 46:1735–1740, 1980
3. COLEMAN CN, BURKE JS, VARGHESE A, ROSENBERG SA, KAPLAN HS: Secondary leukemia and non-Hodgkin's lymphoma in patients treated for Hodgkin's disease, in *Malignant Lymphomas: Etiology, Immunology, Pathology, Treatment,* edited by ROSENBERG SA, KAPLAN HS, New York, Academic Press, 1982, pp 259–276
4. VALAGUSSA P, SANTORO A, KENDA R, FOSSATI-BELLANI F, FRANCHI F, BANFI A, RILKE F, BONADONNA G: Second malignancies in Hodgkin's disease: A complication of certain forms of treatment. *Br Med J* 280:216–227, 1980
5. PEDERSEN-BJERGAARD J, LARSEN SO: Incidence of acute nonlymphocytic leukemia preleukemia, and acute myeloproliferative syndrome up to 10 years after treatment of Hodgkin's disease. *N Engl J Med* 307:965–971, 1982
6. FUKS Z, STROBER S, BOBROVE AM, SASAZUKI T, MCMICHAEL A, KAPLAN HS: Long term effects of radiation of T and B lymphocytes in peripheral blood of patients with Hodgkin's disease. *J Clin Invest* 58:803–814, 1976
7. STROBER S, SLAVIN S, GOTTLIEB M, ZAN-BAR I, KING DP, HOPPE RT, FUKS Z, GRUMET FC, KAPLAN HS: Allograft tolerance after total lymphoid irradiation (TLI). *Immunol Rev* 46:87–112, 1979
8. STROBER S, MODRY EL, HOPPE RT, PENNOCK JL, BIEBER CP, HOLM BI, JAMIESON SW, STINSON EB, SCHRODER J, SOUMALAINEN H, KAPLAN HS: Induction of specific unresponsiveness to heart allografts in mongrel dogs treated with total lymphoid irradiation and anti-thymocyte globulin. *J Immunol* 132:1013–1018, 1984
9. MYBURGH JA, SMIT JA, STARK JH, BROWDE S: Total lymphoid irradiation in kidney and liver transplantation in baboon: Prolonged graft survival and alterations in T cell subsets with low cumulative dose regimens. *J Immunol* 132:1019–1025, 1984

10. NAJARIAN JS, FERGUSON RM, SUTHERLAND PER, SLAVIN S, KIM T, KERSEY J, SIMMONS RL: Fractionated total lymphoid irradiation as preparative immunosuppression in high risk renal transplantation. *Ann Surg* 196:442–452, 1982

11. VANRENTERGHEM Y, WAER M, VAN DER SCHUEREN E, ANG K, LENUT T, VANDEPUTTE M, GRUWEZ J, BOUILLON R, MICHIELSEN P: Renal transplantation in diabetes after total lymphoid irradiation (TLI). *Dialysis Transplant* 12:104–105, 1983

12. WAER M, ANG KK, VAN DER SCHUEREN E, VANDEPUTTE M: Allogeneic bone marrow transplantation in mice after total lymphoid irradiation: Influence of breeding conditions and strains of recipient mice. *J Immunol* 132:991–996, 1984

13. WAER M, ANG KK, VAN DER SCHUEREN E, VANDEPUTTE M: Influence of radiation field and fractionation schedule of total lymphoid irradiation (TLI) on the induction of suppressor cells and stable chimerism after bone marrow transplantation in mice. *J Immunol* 132:985–990, 1984

14. MULLEN Y, SHIBUKAWA RL: Use of total lymphoid irradiation in transplantation of rat fetal pancreases. *Diabetes* 31:69–74, 1982

15. ZAN-BAR I, SLAVIN S, STROBER S: Induction and mechanism of tolerance to bovine serum albumin in mice given total lymphoid irradiation (TLI). *J Immunol* 124:1400–1404, 1978

16. WAER M, VANRENTERGHEM Y, ANG KK, VAN DER SCHUEREN E, MICHIELSEN P, VANDEPUTTE M: Comparison of the immunosuppressive effect of fractionated total lymphoid irradiation (TLI) vs conventional immunosuppression (CI) in renal cadaveric allotransplantation. *J Immunol* 132:1041–1048, 1984

17. HAAS GS, HALPERIN E, DOSERETZ D, LINGGOOD R, RUSSELL PS, COLVIN R, BARRETT L, COSIMI AB: Differential recovery of circulating T cell subsets after nodal irradiation for Hodgkin's disease. *J Immunol* 132:1026–1030, 1984

18. FUKS Z, STROBER S, KAPLAN HS: Interaction between serum factors and T lymphocytes in Hodgkin's disease: Use as a diagnostic test. *N Engl J Med* 295:1273–1278, 1976

19. KOTZIN BL, STROBER S, ENGLEMAN EG, CALIN A, HOPPE RT, KANSAS GS, TERRELL CP, KAPLAN HS: Treatment of intractable rheumatoid arthritis with total lymphoid irradiation. *N Engl J Med* 305:969–979, 1981

20. TRENTHAM DE, BELLI JA, ANDERSON RJ, BUCKLEY JA, GOETZL EJ, DAVID JR, AUSTEN KF: Clinical and immunologic effects of fractionated total lymphoid irradiation in refractory rheumatoid arthritis. *N Engl J Med* 305:976–982, 1981

21. FIELD EH, STROBER S, HOPPE RT, CALIN A, ENGLEMAN EG, KOTZIN BL, TANAY AS, CALIN HJ, TERRELL CP, KAPLAN HS: Sustained improvement of intractable rheumatoid arthritis after total lymphoid irradiation. *Arthritis Rheum* 26:937–946, 1983

22. KOTZIN BL, KANSAS GS, ENGLEMAN EG, HOPPE RT, KAPLAN HS, STROBER S: Changes in T cell subsets in patients with rheumatoid arthritis treated with total lymphoid irradiation. *Clin Immunol Immunopathol* 27:250–260, 1983

23. SLAVIN S, STROBER S, FUKS Z, KAPLAN HS: Induction of specific tissue transplantation tolerance using fractionated total lymphoid irradiation in adult mice: Long-term survival of allogeneic bone marrow and skin grafts. *J Exp Med* 146:34–48, 1977

24. SLAVIN S, REITZ B, BIEBER CP, KAPLAN HS, STROBER S: Transplantation tolerance in adult rats using total lymphoid irradiation (TLI): Permanent survival of skin, heart, and marrow allografts. *J Exp Med* 147:700–707, 1978

25. PENNOCK JL, REITZ BA, BIEBER CP, AZIZ S, OYER PE, STROBER S, HOPPE R, KAPLAN HS, STINSON EB, SHUMWAY NE: Survival of primates following

orthotopic cardiac transplantation treated with total lymphoid irradiation and chemical immune suppression. *Transplant Proc* 32:467–473, 1981
26. SUTHERLAND DER, FERGUSON RM, AEDER MI, LEWIS WI, BENTLEY FR, ASCHER NL, SIMMONS RL, NAJARIAN JS: Total lymphoid irradiation and cyclosporine. *Transplant Proc* 15:2881–2888, 1983
27. KLINTMALM GBG, IWATSUKI S, STARZL TE: Nephrotoxicity of Cyclosporin A in liver and kidney transplant patient. *Lancet* 1:470–471, 1981
28. MARBET UA, GRAF U, MIHATSCH M, GRATWOHL A, MULLER W, THIEL G: Renale Nebenwirkungen der Therapie mit Cyclosporin A bei chronischer Polyarthritis and nach Knochenmarkstranplantation. *Schweiz Med Wochenschr* 110:2017–2020, 1980
29. CALNE RY, ROLLES K, WHITE DJG, THIRU S, EVANS DB, McMASTER P, DUNN DC, CRADDOCK GN, HENDERSON RG, AZIZ S, LEWIS P: Cyclosporin A initially as the only immunosuppressant in 34 recipients of cadaveric organs: 32 kidneys, 2 pancreas, and 2 livers. *Lancet* 2:1033–1036, 1979
30. KLINTMALM GBG, IWATSUKI S, STARZL TE: Cyclosporin A hepatotoxicity in 66 renal allograft recipients. *Transplantation* 32:488–489, 1981
31. EDITORIAL: Cyclosporin and neoplasia. *Lancet* 1:1083, 1983
32. EUROPEAN MULTICENTER TRIAL: Cyclosporin A as sole immunosuppressive agent in recipients of renal allografts from cadaver donors: Preliminary results of a European Multicenter Trial. *Lancet* 2:57–60, 1982

Adjuvant Methods of Immunomodulation for Transplantation

Tadeusz Orłowski

Immunosuppressive therapy with azathioprine and prednisone frequently prevents the irreversible rejection of kidney allografts. Nevertheless, a significant number of grafts are still rejected, even when adjuvant maneuvers such as kidney graft irradiation, thoracic duct drainage, splenectomy, or antithymocyte globulin infusions are used. Recently, a new immunosuppressive agent, cyclosporine, was shown to be more effective than azathioprine. Unfortunately, this drug has its own disturbing side effects, among which nephrotoxicity is especially undesirable. The use of a combination of low-dose cyclosporine with prednisone may decrease the incidence of this complication. Nevertheless, the high cost of the drug and the necessity of constant monitoring of its blood levels justify the search for less expensive and less troublesome methods.

Methods

The Warsaw Medical School Transplantation Center conducted controlled clinical trials of three adjunctive immunosuppressive agents: niridazole (N), promethazine (PM), and antiplatelet (AP) drugs.

There were 26 patients who completed the N trial; 102, the PM trial; and 62, the AP trial. In each study, half of the patients belonged to treated and half to a control group. There were no statistically significant differences between the groups with regard to age, sex, the primary renal disease, preformed antibody levels, dialysis age, pre- and perioperative blood transfusions, degree of HLA-A,B match, duration of graft ischemia, or frequency of postgrafting acute tubular necrosis. The basic regimen in N, PM, and their appropriate control groups consisted of prednisolone administered i.v. during the first 3 weeks postgrafting in the following doses: 1 g on day 1;

This manuscript was presented as part of a Symposium on *Immunomodulation for Transplantation: New Approaches.*

500 mg on day 2; 250 mg on day 3; 125 mg on days 4 through 21. Thereafter, oral prednisone was given in a single morning dose of 30 mg up to the end of the 3rd month, with slow tapering to 10 to 15 mg/d at the end of the first year. All recipients were given azathioprine (3 to 5 mg/kg) prior to transplantation and were then maintained on 1.0 to 2.5 mg/kg/d according to the WBC and platelet counts. When a diagnosis of acute rejection was established, prednisolone pulses of 1 g/d were given i.v. two to six times. The N group received 500 mg of N three times a day on alternate days for 2 weeks concomitantly with steroids and azathioprine. The PM group received 25 mg of PM twice a day in addition to standard immunosuppression. The same regimen was used in the AP control group. The AP group was treated with prednisone, azathioprine, promethazine, aspirin (75 mg/d), and dipyramidole (75 mg, 3×/d).

Results

Niridazole

Between December 1977 and May 1978, 26 patients received primary cadaveric kidney allografts: 13 were allocated randomly to N therapy and 13 to the control group. Six years after transplantation, no difference in patient survival was found, but only three recipients in the N group and five in the control group live with functioning grafts (Fig. 1). Nevertheless, graft survival was significantly higher statistically in the control group up to 4 years after transplantation. More rejection episodes were observed in the N group. Signs of mild hepatotoxicity were seen in patients given niridazole.

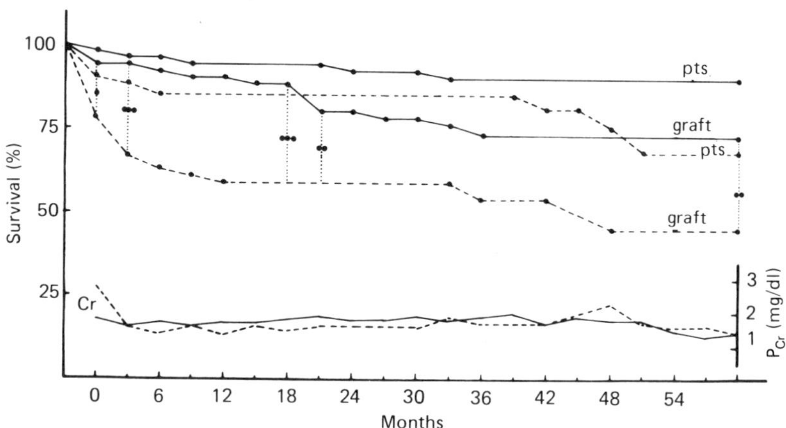

Fig. 1. Cumulative graft and recipient survival and serum creatinine concentrations in control (●---●) and promethazine groups (●——●). (●●●, $P < 0.001$; ●●, $P < 0.01$; ●, $P < 0.025$)

Since there was no beneficial effect of this drug on the clinical course of patients treated, this trial was discontinued.

Promethazine

At the time of trial analysis (March 1, 1984), no statistically significant difference between cumulative patient survival was found. However, 75% of the grafts in the PM group were functioning compared with 51% of the grafts in the control group. Actuarial graft survival was significantly higher in the PM group up to at least the 36th month (78 vs. 57%; $P < 0.025$). The function of surviving grafts as assessed by serum creatinine concentrations was comparable (Fig. 2).

About 20% of the recipients in both groups did not have rejection during the observation period. The number of irreversible rejections or deaths was significantly ($P < 0.05$) higher in the control (25/51) than in the PM (13/51) group. The fact that one of the control patients died in a car accident with a well-functioning graft did not alter these results.

The difference in graft survival was caused by a higher graft loss in the control group during the first 3 months after surgery (15/51 vs. 3/51, respectively). Thereafter, the frequency of graft failure was comparable in all recipients. No differences were observed in timing and frequency of reversible rejection episodes. The PM group of patients were given some more prednisone during the first 18 months of therapy (22.7 ± 5.7 vs. 19.9 ± 5.1; $P < 0.025$), and more boluses of prednisolone were required to control the rejection episodes occurring during the first 2 years after transplantation (7.9 ± 5.1 vs. 5.5 ± 3.8; $P < 0.05$). Nevertheless, this was not a decisive factor in explaining the better results obtained in the PM group because all but one

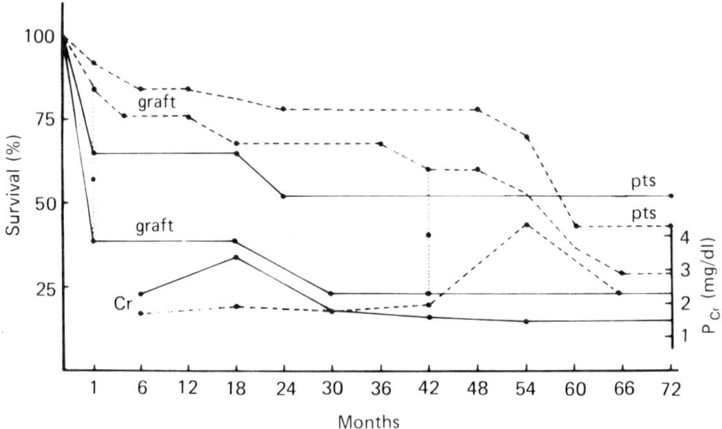

Fig. 2. Cumulative graft and recipient survival and serum creatinine concentrations in control (●---●) and niridazole groups (●——●). (●, $P < 0.05$)

of the control patients who rejected their graft received steroids in higher amounts than the average doses used in the PM group. In all but 3 of them, the number of prednisolone boluses given was higher than in controls. Although the irreversible graft rejections were almost twice as frequent in the control than in the PM group, the number of timing of the reversible rejection episodes were comparable in both groups of patients.

No serious side effects or complications related to the use of PM were encountered. The frequency of cardiovascular, gastrointestinal, bone, hepatic, and mental disorders, as well as bacterial, fungal, and viral infections, was comparable in both groups. The only significant difference was a higher rate of urinary tract infections; it was episodic during the first 3 months, and recurrent during the second year in the control group patients.

Antiplatelet Drugs

After 18 months of observation, cumulative patient and graft survivals were lower in the AP than in the control group (91 vs. 97% and 66 vs. 72%, respectively), but these differences did not reach statistical significance ($P > 0.2$ and $P > 0.5$). The frequency and timing of reversible rejections were comparable in both groups. At no time after the transplantation did the graft functions (evaluated on the basis of serum creatinine concentrations) differ significantly between the two groups (Fig. 3). The total doses of prednisone and the number of prednisolone boluses were comparable at least during the first year postgrafting.

The addition of AP drugs to standard PM therapy did not influence the frequency of postoperative complications of any kind. Early postoperative hemorrhage occurred in 5 AP and 6 AP control patients. In 2 and 5 patients,

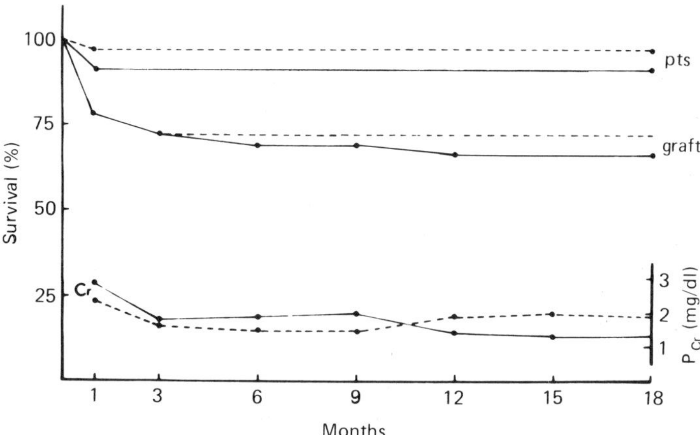

Fig. 3. Cumulative graft and recipient survival and serum creatinine concentrations in control (●---●) and antiplatelet drug groups (●——●).

respectively, it was caused by an early graft rupture and led to the loss of two transplanted kidneys in each group. Since no evidence of a beneficial effect of AP drugs on the post-transplant course was obtained, the regimen was discontinued.

Discussion

In rat [1], mouse [2, 3], guinea pig [4], and humans [5, 6], niridazole, a nitrothiazole derivative antischistosomal drug, was shown to be a potent long-acting immunosuppressive agent. It was especially effective when given concurrently with azathioprine and prednisolone [1, 6]. In patients treated with niridazole, a suppression of delayed hypersensitivity reactions and antigen-induced lymphocyte transformation was found [5]. This action is attributed not to the parent drug, but to its metabolites [3, 4, 6]. Given in combination with prednisolone and azathioprine, niridazole prevented cardiac allograft rejection in rat [1]. Sera and concentrated dialysates of urine from kidney allograft recipients inhibited in vitro mixed lymphocyte reaction [6] and significantly prolonged heterotopic heart allograft survival time in this species [6, 7]. Unfortunately, although the sera samples of most of our patients exhibited immunosuppressive action in mixed lymphocyte culture, no beneficial effect of niridazole on the post-transplant course was observed. Possibly, the dose applied was suboptimal, being much less than the most effective dosage of 50 mg/kg/d in rat [7]. But lack of precise information on the pharmacokinetics of niridazole and its metabolites in renal failure prevented us from using higher amounts of this drug.

Promethazine hydrochloride, an antihistaminic drug, has a weak immunosuppressive action on its own. Nevertheless, given i.p. it prevented early cardiac allograft rejection in the rat [8, 9]; and in combination with standard immunosuppressants it prolonged kidney allograft survival in rabbits and rats [10]. Up to now, only a few and rather negative results were obtained with promethazine treatment in human kidney allograft recipients [11].

The exact mode of immunosuppressive action of promethazine is not known. It probably prevents graft capillary endothelial damage, blocking platelet aggregation [8]. Its beneficial effects can also be partly associated with inhibition of antibody production and delayed hypersensitivity reactions. The present study confirms our previous suggestion that promethazine significantly improves the kidney graft survival rate in humans. This action does not appear to be related to less intensive corticoidtherapy in the control group, since all patients who rejected their graft received steroids in comparable, or even higher, amounts than the average doses given to the PM group. In an attempt to obtain still better results of graft survival by prevention of vascular damage of the transplanted kidney, antiplatelet drugs were added to the standard prednisone-azathioprine-promethazine regimen.

Aspirin and dipyridamole act on different phases of platelet function [12]. Aspirin blocks irreversibly thromboxane A_2 (TXA_2) synthesis, inhibits platelet aggregation and release, and prevents TXA_2 and serotonin-mediated vasoconstriction [13]. In higher doses, however, it also inhibits prostacyclin synthesis. It was shown that as little as 30 mg/d of this drug decreases TXA_2 activity for 2 weeks [12], and that a daily dose of 80 mg reduces TXA_2 synthesis [14] without inhibiting the endothelial production of prostacyclin [15]. This was the rationale for our use of low doses of aspirin, although according to most recent reports a higher dose of 325 mg/d may be preferred [16]. Dipyridamole diminishes platelet adherence to damaged endothelium and inhibits their aggregation induced by different stimuli. For this reason, it has been used (sometimes with beneficial results) in combination with aspirin to prevent intravascular clotting [17]. As it seems likely that the early application of antithrombotic drugs can be crucial for their beneficial effect on graft function [18], in our trial they were started before surgery. Unfortunately, no expected improvement in graft survival time was obtained. Possibly, it is due to the fact that the presumable inhibitory action of promethazine on platelet aggregation was so efficient that it could not be magnified by aspirin and dipyridamole.

Results obtained with triple-drug immunosuppression (prednisone, azathioprine, and promethazine) are comparable to that obtained with cyclosporine in several randomized studies [19–21]. This method may be the second best therapy in renal allograft transplantation.

References

1. SALAMAN JR, BIRD M, GODFREY AM, JONES B, MILLAR D, MILLER J: Prolonged allograft survival with niridazole, azathioprine, and prednisolone. *Transplantation* 23:29–32, 1977
2. MAHMOUD AAF, WARREN KS: Anti-inflammatory effects of tarter emetic and niridazole. *J Immunol* 112:222–228, 1974
3. MAHMOUD AAF, MANDEL MA, WARREN KS, WEBSTER LT JR: Niridazole, II. *J Immunol* 114:279–283
4. DANIELS JC, WARREN KS, DAVID JR: Studies on the mechanism of suppression on delayed hypersensitivity by the antischistosomal compound niridazole. *J Immunol* 115:1414–1421, 1975
5. WEBSTER LT JR, BUTTERWORTH AE, MAHMOUD AAF, MANGOLA EN, WARREN KS: Suppression of delayed hypersensitivity in schistosome-infected patients by niridazole. *N Engl J Med* 292:1144–1147, 1975
6. JONES BM, BIRD M, MASSEY P, MILLAR D, MILLER JJ, REEVES S, SALAMAN JR: Immunosuppressive properties of sera and urine dialysates from kidney-graft recipients treated with azathioprine, prednisolone, and niridazole. *Br Med J* 2:792–795, 1977
7. SALAMAN JR, BIRD M, GODFREY AM, JONES B, MILLAR D, MILLER J: Niridazole as an immunosuppressive agent. *Transplant Proc* 9:989–991, 1977
8. JAMIESON SW: Promethazine-hydrochloride (Phenergan) in the treatment of rat cardiac allografts. *Transplantation* 21:69–71, 1976
9. JAMIESON SW, BURTON NA, REITZ BA, STINSON EB: Survival of heart allografts in rats treated with azathioprine and sodium salicylate. *Lancet* 1:130–131, 1979
10. DUNN DC, WADE J: Prolonged kidney allograft survival with promethazine. *Transplant Proc* 9:871–873, 1979

11. CALNE RY: Pharmacological immunosuppression in clinical organ grafting. *Clin Exp Immunol* 35:1–9, 1979
12. PACKHAM MA, MUSTARD JF: Pharmacology of platelet-affecting drugs. *Circulation* 62 (Suppl U): 26–38, 1980
13. FIELDS WS: Aspirin for prevention of stroke. *Am J Med* 74:61–65, 1983
14. HARTER HR, BURCH JW, MAJERUS PW, STANFORD N, DELMEZ JA, ANDERSON CB, WEERTS CA: Prevention of thrombosis in patients on hemodialysis by low-dose aspirin. *N Engl J Med* 301:377–379
15. SALMAN EW: Aspirin to prevent arterial thrombosis. *N Engl J Med* 307:113–115, 1982
16. MARCUS AJ: Aspirin as an antithrombotic medication. *N Engl J Med* 309:1515–1517, 1983
17. CHESEBRO JH, FUSTER V, ELVEBACK LR, CLEMENTS IP, SMITH HC, HOLMES DR JR, BARDSLEY WT, PLUTH JR, WALLACE RB, PUGA FJ, ORSZULAK TA, PIEHLER JM, DANIELSON GK, SCHAFF HV, FRYE RL: Effect of dipyridamole and aspirin on late vein-graft patency after coronary bypass operations. *N Engl J Med* 310:209–214, 1984
18. GREEN RM, ROEDERSHEIMER R, DEWEESE JA: Effects of aspirin and dipyridamole on expanded polytetrafluoroethylene graft patency. *Surgery* 92:1016–1026, 1982
19. ORLOWSKI T, NIELUBOWICZ J, GORSKI A, GRADOWSKA L, JUSKOWA J, KLEPACKA J, MORZYCKA M, PODOBINSKA I, RANCEWICZ Z, ROWINSKA D, SZMIDT J, SMOGORZEWSKI M: A controlled prospective long term trial of promethazine as an adjustment immunosuppressant in 102 cadaver graft recipients. *Transplant Proc* 15:557–559, 1983
20. STILLER C: The Canadian trial of cyclosporine. *Transplant Proc* 15:2479–2489, 1983
21. SHEIL AJR, HALL BBT, STEPHEN MI, HARRIS JP, DUGGIN GG, HORVATH JS, JOHNSON JR, ROGERS JR, BONLAS J: Australian trial of CSA in cadaveric donor renal transplantation. *Transplant Proc* 15:2485–2489, 1983
22. SELLS RA: A prospective randomized substitute trial of cyclosporine as a prophylactic agent in human renal transplant rejection. *Transplant Proc* 15:2495–2500, 1983
23. LAND W, CASTRO LA, GUNTHER K, HAMMER C, HILLEBRAND C, ILLNER WD, SCHMELLER N, SCHNEIDER B, SIEBERT W, ZINK RA, ZOTTLEIN H: Cadaveric renal transplantation with cyclosporin. *Transplant Proc* 15:2517–2522, 1983
24. BUNZENDAHL H, WONIGERT K, KLAMPNAUER J, BROLSCH C, PILCHMAYR R: Cyclosporine and steroids: Effects on the clinical course after renal allotransplantation. *Transplant Proc* 15:2531–2534, 1983

Immunological Monitoring and Renal Transplantation

Chairpersons: Ronald D. Guttmann and Vittorio Bonomini
Discussants: Takahiro Oka, William E. Braun, Marvin R. Garovoy, Terry B. Strom, Fernando Valderrobano, Mark Waer, Louis Lanier, Wayne Hancock, and Mohammad Allajani

A new frontier in renal transplantation is the ability to provide relevant diagnostic measurements to assess a clinical state and monitor immunosuppressive therapy. There are a number of technical advances that have been made whereby it is possible to profile the immune response of patients before and after renal transplantation. This Workshop focused on the newest innovations in this, which are related to: (1) the use of flow cytometry to measure lymphocyte subsets in patients under various forms of immunosuppressive therapy including monoclonal antibody treatment, (2) the definition of multiple surface markers in activated cells, (3) the technical aspects and problems of subset measurement and their relationship to functional assays and clinical status, (4) the correlation between immunological findings in peripheral blood and infiltrate composition in renal tissue, (5) the measurement of delayed-type hypersensitivity responses and their clinical significance, (6) the relevance of prostaglandins as mediators during rejection, and (7) the utility of cyclosporine measurements to monitor therapy and recent monitoring data in total lymphoid irradiation (TLI). This emphasis is necessary since it is clear that oversimplification of complex broad phenomena analyzed by sophisticated tools has not provided critical insights to date.

Delayed-Type Hypersensitivity (DTH) and Renal Graft Survival

Valderrobano discussed the issue that in previous studies, the possible effect of cell-mediated immunity, measured by DTH, on the outcome of renal transplantation (Tx) has been investigated with dissimilar results. In order to elucidate this problem, DTH has been studied in 193 chronic dialysis

This is the Summary of a Workshop by the same title.

(CD) patients, using a new and easy multipuncture method to seven antigens: tetanus, diphtheria, streptococcus, tuberculin, Candida, trycophyton, and proteus (Multitest®). Anergy was defined by a score (sum of the induration to each antigen) lower than 5 mm. Patients were considered responsive when the score was higher than 10 mm, and intermediate between 5 and 10 mm. Anergy was found in 46% of CD patients (vs. 5.6% of healthy controls) and was related to time on dialysis, female sex, glomerulonephritis, younger age, and previous blood transfusions (BT). In CAPD patients, a correlation was found between anergy and the incidence of peritonitis (91% of anergic patients had some peritonitic episode, against 27% of responsive patients). As reported previously, a single unit of blood induces an important depression of the response. Transfusion-induced anergy persisted during a variable time, and nontransfused patients kept the same response up to 1 year. Since 1981, 47 previously tested patients were grafted from cadaver donors. The actuarial graft survival (AGS) at 1 year was 90% in anergic patients ($N=30$), versus 64% in responsive ones ($N=13$) ($P < 0.01$). There was no significant difference in the mortality rate, incidence of rejection, and of postoperative infections. Only one anergic patient lost the graft by rejection, but all the graft losses in the response group were as a consequence of acute irreversible rejection. Four patients died with a functioning graft. Three of them were anergic, and their serum creatinine concentration was < 1.3 mg/dl. The responsive patient who died with a functioning graft had a serum creatinine of 9.6 mg/dl and chronic rejection. As anergy is more frequent in transfused patients, we have tried to evaluate the relationship between pre-Tx BT and AGS. There was no significant difference between 1-year AGS in transfused and nontransfused patients. Moreover, there was no difference in AGS of patients that received more than 5 blood units and less than 10. On the other hand, in each group, anergic and responsive patients, 1-year AGS was similar independently of the number of transfusions received. We conclude that anergy measured by this method is a good predictive factor for the outcome of cadaver kidney transplantation irrespectively to pre-Tx BT. According to our results the controversy concerning the optimum number of pre-Tx BT would be solved using skin test as a marker, and the pre-Tx BT policy would be to transfuse only responsive patients in an attempt to induce a depression of cell-mediated immunity.

Monitoring the Humoral and Cellular Responses to Donor-Specific Transfusions

Braun and colleagues reported that antibodies to T and B lymphocytes, and in some cases to monocytes, have been monitored in 66 patients, 46 of whom have received their intended renal allograft. Several donor-specific protocols have been utilized: fresh whole blood × 3; stored whole blood × 3; fresh whole blood × 3 with azathioprine; leukocytes × 2 with RhoGam for Rh-incompatible recipients; and fresh whole blood × 1 with cyclosporine. The overall sensitization rate was 24.6% for T cell antibody; the highest frequency being in those with fresh whole blood without immunosuppression who had a 34.6% incidence. Sensitization that generally does not preclude transplantation (B cell and monocyte antibody) also had interesting clinical correlations; in 16 patients who developed B cell antibodies either prior to transplantation ($N = 15$) or immediately post-transplant ($N = 1$), the most important factor in their clinical correlation was not allo- or autoreactivity nor temperature reactivity, but rather the time of appearance. Those B cell antibodies that had only a transient appearance prior to transplantation were associated with a rejection episode in only 1 of 8 patients, whereas 5 of 7 B cell antibodies persistent at transplant and the solitary B cell antibody formed within 48 hr after transplantation were associated with rejections in the first 6 months. Two of 5 patients with monocyte antibodies (four with and one without associated B cell antibody) had rejection episodes in the first 6 months. Cellular responses to donor-specific transfusions were more complex. Phytohemagglutinin (PHA) stimulation indexes decreased from a mean of 115.2 ± 76.5 predonor-specific transfusion (DST) to 84.1 ± 72.7 post-DST ($P < 0.09$). However, 20 of the 34 PHA responses decreased in the course of the DST (152.7 ± 69.1 to 68.8 ± 40.4; $P < 0.0001$), while 14 increased (61.6 ± 51.1 to 117.3 ± 94.9; $P < 0.02$). Twelve of the 14 PHA responses that increased in the course of DST did so among patients receiving azathioprine with their fresh whole blood ($P < 0.05$), whereas the decrease in PHA response was significantly associated with the fresh whole blood without azathioprine ($P < 0.01$). One-way MLC S.I. and RR both decreased in the course of DST, but not significantly. Neither those with a decreased nor those with an increased S.I. or RR was associated with any particular DST protocol. Con-A-inducible suppressor cells could be demonstrated in 10 of 13 patients prior to transplantation, and suppression by a serum-mediated (? anti-idiotype antibody) mechanism could be demonstrated in 19 of 24 patients. Among the four cellular responses examined, the only one associated with a rejection-free period for the first 3 months was the presence of a serum-mediated possible anti-idiotype factor; rejection occurred in only 2 of 19 patients having this form of suppression as compared to the occurrence of rejection in 3 of 5 patients lacking it ($P < 0.04$). The serum-mediated suppression of the one-way MLC was typically not donor-specific. None of the different DST protocols was significantly associated with any clinical differences as measured by cumulative rejection episodes or serum creatinine. The most significant clinical correlations were related to the post-transplant immunosuppression protocols, with ALG and high oral prednisone giving the best results. A surprising finding was that immediate pre- or intraoperative *random* blood transfusions showed the strongest association with chronic rejection or failure and suggested that, even under immunosuppression, a new antigenic stimulation may have evoked a second signal (for example, IL-2) that could abrogate the DST effect.

Advances in Flow Cytometry

Lanier presented a review of flow cytometry and the utility of 2-color immunofluorescence. His studies demonstrate clearly how multiple antigen measurements can correlate with functional activity. The dissection of T cell subsets into cytotoxic, suppressor, helper, inducer, and various phenotypes responsible for natural killing is now possible using the Leu series (Becton-Dickinson) monoclonal antibodies. Multiple antigen studies exploit the fluorescent dyes fluorescein isothiocyanate, phycoerythrin (orange), and cyanines (red). The ability to measure multiple antigens represents a major advance.

Monoclonal Antibody Monitoring of Lymphocyte Subsets in Postrenal Transplant Patients

Guttman's group concluded their second study of long-term renal allograft recipients in order to characterize the chronic immunosuppressed state. Forty-two patients (aged 25 to 60 years) who were 5 or more years postrenal transplantation had their peripheral blood lymphocyte subsets measured using the monoclonal antibodies, Leu-1, Leu-2, Leu-3, and Leu-7 (Becton-Dickinson). There was a significant decrease in the number of T helper (Leu-3$^+$) cells and a decrease in the absolute level of T lymphocytes with no significant change in the number of T suppressor/cytotoxic (Leu-2$^+$) cells. On a relative basis, the "helper/suppressor ratio" was decreased in patients when compared to normals. This was due to the relative increase in Leu-2$^+$ cells. It was demonstrated that the Leu-7$^+$ subset, which marks the HNK1 population, was significantly elevated in relative proportion in peripheral blood when compared to controls. However, this was not seen on an absolute basis. The age dependence of the relative numbers of Leu-7$^+$ cells was seen in both the normal control population and the transplant cohort. There was no significant correlation between any of these lymphocyte subset measurements and delayed-type hypersensitivity skin tests in the transplant population. A finding of interest is that six of the patients who had been treated for malignant disease during their post-transplant course had significantly higher numbers of Leu-7$^+$ cells on an absolute and relative basis compared to the rest of the transplant group. The significance of this finding is not yet clear. Further studies subsetting the Leu-7$^+$ subset are necessary before an understanding of the long-term immune state is achieved and the finding of those patients successfully treated for malignancy having increased Leu-7$^+$ cells is clarified. Two-color fluorescence studies to split many of the subsets are now required before a system of classification and correlation with the clinical state is possible.

Presensitization and Enhancement: Detection by Flow Cytometry

Garovoy investigated whether accelerated rejection and early (3 to 6 month) graft loss continue to result from undetected presensitization and whether flow cytometry is able to measure antibodies currently missed by available lymphocyte cytotoxicity techniques. Flow cytometry was performed utilizing a modified Becton-Dickinson Fluorescent-Activated Cell Sorter (FACS II). Donor lymphocytes (0.5×10^6) from peripheral blood were incubated with 0.05 ml recipient serum at 22°C for 30 min, washed and incubated with FITC-conjugated goat antihuman immunoglobulin. Lymphocyte cytotoxicity cross-matches were performed using the modified Amos, long incubation, and antiglobulin techniques. The FACS histograms generated in normal human serum showed two peaks: a low intensity peak consisting of T lymphocytes and a higher intensity peak containing surface immunoglobulin (Ig) positive cells. Sera with known anti-HLA antibodies caused a measurable shift of the T cell peak proportionate to the amount of antibody binding. Flow cytometry detected these antibodies in serial dilution out to 1:1054 as compared to 1:16 by cytotoxicity. A preliminary retrospective analysis of 51 cadaveric recipients transplanted in 1979 and 1982 showed 7 of 51 to be FACS-positive (T cell peak shift; that is, anti-T cell antibody) despite negative cytotoxicity cross-matches. Six out of 7 had rejected their grafts by 3 months. In recipients of donor-specific transfusions (DST) we found that 20% of patients developed cytotoxic "B" cell antibodies (37°C or 4°C) whose sera by FACS analysis produced a shift of the T cell peak only (that is, anti-HLA-A,B,C antibodies) without shifting the B cell peak, suggesting that some of the deleterious effects attributed to "B cell" antibodies may have been due to undetected anti-HLA,A,B,C antibodies. To date, 20 DST recipients have been transplanted with positive B warm cytotoxicity cross-matches (titer less than or equal to 1:4) but without any HLA-A,B,C antibodies (no shift of the FACS T cell peak). All patients are doing well with follow-up ranging from 3 to 22 months. These results suggest that successful engraftment of DST recipients may be possible despite the presence of low-titered B warm cytotoxic antibodies (enhancing antibodies?) if the presence of anti-HLA-A,B,C locus antibodies can also be excluded reliably.

Immunohistological Analysis of Serial Biopsy Specimens Taken During Human Renal Allograft Rejection: Changing Profile of Infiltrating Cells and Monocyte Tissue Factor-Mediated Involvement of the Coagulation System

Hancock and colleagues presented a summary of recent research into the intragraft effector mechanisms associated with human renal allograft rejection, based on immunohistological analysis with antileukocyte monoclonal antibodies. Cellular infiltrates present within sequential renal biopsy specimens from 14 patients with allograft rejection were analyzed using a panel of monoclonal antibodies and a 4-layer immunoperoxidase technique. Thirty-six biopsy specimens, taken for assessment of episodes of renal failure post-transplantation, were studied. Comparison of specimens taken on days 2 to 3 post-transplantation with those taken either at days 10 to 12, or greater than 30 days, showed similar proportions of T cells, T cell subsets, B cells, and macrophages. By contrast, the proportion of NK cells was significantly increased at day 3 ($P < 0.01$), and the proportion of activated T cells bearing interleukin-2 receptors was significantly increased at days 10 to 12 ($P < 0.01$). Granulocytes were restricted to those biopsies that displayed areas of infarction, regardless of the timing at which this occurred. In addition, varying proportions of intragraft macrophages exhibited the membrane phenotype of activated macrophages, due to their expression of the procoagulant molecule termed human tissue factor-related antigen (HTF:RAg). Moreover, interstitial and perivascular collections of HTF:RAg$^+$ macrophages were closely associated with fibrin deposits and, in two cases, mononuclear cells harvested from rejected grafts were shown to contain significant procoagulant activity in vitro. These studies demonstrate a temporal variation in the types of cells contributing to human kidney rejection. Furthermore, the demonstration of macrophages with procoagulant antigen in close association with fibrin deposits suggests that macrophage infiltration and activation, possibly as a result of lymphokine stimulation, is an important mechanism in the initiation of intragraft fibrin deposition.

Specific In Vitro Reactivities of Lymphocytes Infiltrating Kidney Allografts

Oka and collaborators discussed the problem of the difficulty to demonstrate the in vitro-specific reactivities of peripheral blood lymphocytes (PBL) in kidney allograft recipients at the time of rejection, possibly because effector lymphocytes may be mobilized into the grafts. To elucidate in situ immunologic effector mechanisms of rejection in kidney transplantation, graft infiltrating lymphocytes (GIL) and PBL were expanded in culture in the presence of T-cell growth factor (TCGF), and their in vitro reactivities were examined in experimental animals and clinical case. Analysis of T lymphocyte subsets were also performed in clinical cases, using monoclonal antibodies. Kidney transplantations were performed using mongrel dogs and rats. At a certain time post-transplantation, small pieces of graft tissue were wedge-biopsied and then cultured in medium fed by 15% TCGF. At the time of biopsy, PBL of recipients were separated and cultured in the same way. On the 10th to 14th day after culture, the lymphocytes from the biopsied specimen, as well as PBL, which were expanded enough in number to be assayed, were harvested and tested for the reactivities in both mixed lymphocyte reaction (MLR) and cytotoxicity using the ^{51}Cr release method against the relevant donor and the third party. In a short-time MLR, GIL showed a proliferative response specifically against the donors, whereas PBL showed less reactivities. In the assay for cytotoxicity, GIL showed significantly higher reactivities against the donors than PBL in which the percent-specific release was below 7%. A 29-year-old male patient was transplanted with a kidney from his mother. On the 17th post-transplant day, he had an episode of severe acute rejection requiring hemodialysis, evidenced by massive interstitial cell infiltration in histology. A small piece of biopsy specimen and PBL was cultured in TCGF. After 1 week of culture, sufficiently expanded lymphocytes were harvested and submitted for analysis of T cell subsets with monoclonal OKT antibodies using flow cytometry and in vitro reactivities. The percentage of OKT4 cells and OKT8 cells in PBL was 43.4% and 42.7%, respectively, with a Th/Ts-c ratio of 1.02, which was similar to that in PBL prior to culture. In contrast, GIL had a decreased percentage of Th, 15.2%, and increased percentage of Ts-c, 93.0%, with a remarkably decreased Th/Ts-c ratio of 0.16. GIL showed a marked proliferative response in a short-term MLR and cytotoxic activity by the ^{51}Cr release method against the donor, and not at all against a panel of the third-party lymphocytes, except for one who shared one HLA antigen with the donor. These results indicate that kidney allografts are densely populated with effector cells at the time of rejection, and that it is necessary to use lymphocytes infiltrating grafts for the assay of specific in vitro reactivities in immunological monitoring of rejection.

Urinary Immunoreactive Thromboxane B2 (I-TXB2) in Allograft Rejection

Allajani presented the work of Foegh and collaborators (Washington) on the issue that are involved arachidonic acid (AA) metabolites in transplant rejection. Daily estimations were done of both urine i-TXB2 and serum beta-2-microglobulin (β2-MG) in a series of 80 consecutive patients for 20 to 40 days following kidney transplantation. Urine i-TXB2 was determined by radioimmunoassay; i-TXB2 is a mixture of TXB2 (the stable hydrolysis product of TXA2) and 2.3-dinor TXB2 (the major urinary metabolite of TXB2). In this retrospective study they found that an early rise in urine i-TXB2 occurs 2 to 5 days prior to the clinical diagnosis of rejection. Computer-based data analysis revealed a strong correlation between early increases in urine i-TXB2 and the late elevation of serum creatinine. Increases in serum β2-MG also correlate well with serum creatinine, but there is a larger incidence of false positive values. These data indicate that urinary i-TXB2 merits further evaluation in kidney transplant patients.

Cyclosporine Levels in Predicting Outcome of Conversion to Azathioprine Therapy

Strom discussed his group's study and concern with respect to prediction of therapy changes among 60 renal allograft recipients. Both the mean of all available serum cyclosporine concentrations and those obtained less than 1 month prior to conversion were analyzed with regard to predictive value of successful conversion to azathioprine. Poorer results were evident among those with low mean cyclosporine levels, but two of the eight patients had primary graft non-function while two others had ongoing rejection at the time of the switch. Of the 11 patients with recent serum cyclosporine concentrations < 100 ng/ml, four had primary nonfunction and two had ongoing rejection. The seven patients with recent serum cyclosporine concentrations > 500 ng/ml also fared more poorly than the overall group, but two had ongoing rejection and one had primary nonfunction prior to conversion. Thus, patients with cyclosporine concentrations outside of usual therapeutic range did less well after conversion than those with cyclosporine levels in desirable ranges (100 to 200 ng/ml). These results were unexpected as one might reason that those with optimal cyclosporine concentrations would have the least chance of cyclosporine nephrotoxicity and therefore less likelihood of improving renal function after conversion to azathioprine. The data, however, were more consistent with the hypothesis that many renal transplant recipients have some degree of cyclosporine-mediated nephrotoxicity, even at dose-giving concentrations of 100 to 200 ng/ml, the currently accepted optimal therapeutic range.

Comparison of Fractionated Total Lymphoid Irradiation (TLI) vs. Conventional Immunosuppression (CI) in Cadaveric Allotransplantation

Beginning in November 1981, Waer and colleagues studied eight patients with end-stage diabetic nephropathy who underwent renal cadaveric transplantation after TLI (*J Immunol* 132:1041, 1984). Transplantation was done between 2 to 11 days after the end of a fractionated TLI to a total dose of 20 to 30 Gy. During the same observation period, 60 nondiabetic patients with end-stage renal disease of different origin also received a cadaveric kidney graft, with a conventional regimen of immunosuppression that consists of antilymphocyte globulin, tapering high doses of prednisone, and azathioprine. In the TLI-treated group only a low maintenance dose of prednisone (15 mg) was given. Immunologic monitoring was performed after transplantation at regular intervals and was compared in both groups. Phytohemagglutinin (PHA)-, concanavalin A (con A)- and pokeweed mitogen (PWM)-induced blastogenesis, as well as the mixed lymphocyte reaction (MLR) and the cell-mediated lympholysis (CML) decreased progressively during the first few months after conventional immunosuppression up to 50% of the pretransplantation level and remained there for the first year after transplantation. These tests were much more impaired after TLI (less than 15% of pre-TLI value); and again no recovery occurred during the first year. Natural killer (NK) cell activity progressively decreased from a mean value of 53% lysis before transplantation to 15% lysis at the end of the first year after transplantation in the conventionally treated patients. In TLI-treated patients, however, the NK activity, which declined during irradiation from 46% specific lysis to 12% recovered rapidly after TLI to reach levels of 35 to 40% of specific lysis from the second month on after TLI. In both groups of patients, the ratio of helper-inducer (Th) to suppressor-cytotoxic (Ts-c) lymphocytes, as determined with monoclonal antibodies, progressively declined during the first 2 months after transplantation to a low value of about 1.2. In TLI-treated patients, however, this fall progressed further, so that very low levels (< 0.6) were noticed from the third month after TLI. The decline of the Th:Ts ratio after TLI is due to an absolute increase in the number of suppressor cells. This is in contrast to the conventionally treated patients, where the low ratio is due mainly to a decrease of the helper cell population. These changes in the balance between Th and Ts subpopulations are more frequently associated with positive functional suppressor cell assays in the TLI-treated patients. In the clinic, the more profound immunosuppression in TLI patients was more frequently associated with viral infections (cytomegalovirus and herpes zoster). The incidence of rejections, however, was somewhat less frequent in the TLI-treated group (mean: 1.5 rejections per patient vs. 1.8) and occurred significantly later (first rejection on day 141 vs. day 30). After TLI, the mean cumulative dose of steroids needed for kidney transplantation could be substantially reduced.

Index

Acetaminophen, 812–813
Acetate hemodialysis
    advantages of, 1531–1532
    vs. bicarbonate hemodialysis, 1544
    disadvantages of, 1532
Acid excretion
    control of, 251–268
    titratable, 1187–1188
Acidification, distal, PO_4 depletion and, 1191–1192
Acidification mechanism, 251–256
Acidosis
    metabolic, Na/H antiporter and, 72
    NH_3 production and, 274
    renal tubular, management of, 922
Acute crescentic-rapidly progressive glomulo-
        nephritis (AC-RPGN)
    definition of, 1464
    pathogenesis of, 1470–1471
Acute renal failure (ARF), 270, 273, 702–805
    ADH and, 1330
    calcitonin and, 1325–1326
    carbohydrate metabolism and, 1326–1327
    catabolism and wasting in, 1498–1510
    causes of, 702, 791–792
    cellular energy metabolism in, 801
    cellular mechanisms of protection in, 776–
        781
    divalent ion metabolism and, 1323–1324
    endocrine abnormalities in, 1322–1331
    endothelial fenestrae and, 723–724
    erythropoietin, 1331
    experimental
        backleak in, 737–739
        cellular events and, 741–742
        glomerular permeability in, 734–735
        hemodynamics in, 731–734, 739–740
        induction of, 711
        obstruction in, 735–737, 740–741
        pathophysiology of, 731–739
        protective maneuvers in, 739–742
        renin-angiotensin system and, 733
        vasopressin and, 732
    future directions in, 707–708
    gastrointestinal hormone and, 1330–1331
    glucagon and, 1327
    growth hormones and, 1327–1328
    historic perspective, 792
    HPG axis and, 1328–1330
    hypercatabolism in
        animal studies, 764
        assays, 764–765
        pathogenesis of, 763
        patients, 764
        proteases and, 763–772
    hypocalcemia and, 1324
    intercurrent illnesses and, 1500–1504
    metabolic abnormalities in, 1322–1331
    nephrotoxic, 797
    NSAID effect on, 823
    pathogenic mechanisms of, 703–707
    pathology of, 711–724
    phases of, 703
    pituitary adrenal axis and, 1330
    plasma $E\text{-}\alpha_1$ PI complex in, 766
    post-traumatic
        enhanced protease activity in, 767–768
        serum peptide fractions in, 765–766
    prevention of, 784–789
        adenine nucleotides in, 800–805
    principles of, 702–708
    PTH and, 1324–1325
    renal corpuscle in, 720–721
    serum $1,25(OH)_2D_3$ and, 1325
    study of, 702–703
    thyroid hormone metabolism and, 1328
    treatment of, 1509–1510
Acute tubular necrosis
    regeneration after, 751–753
    renal regeneration after, 748–758

Acute uric acid nephropathy (AUAN), 877–
    879
  diagnosis of, 878
  pathogenesis of, 878
  prophylaxis and, 879
  therapy for, 879
Adenine monophosphate deaminase deinhibi-
    tion, 1226–1228
Adenine nucleotide-MgCl$_2$ complex, and
    WKC$_{In}$, 802
Adenine nucleotides, 780
  energy metabolism and, 801
  in prevention of ARF, 800–805
  renal regeneration and, 750–751
Adenosine monophosphate, cyclic, see Cyclic-
    AMP
Adenosine triphosphate, see ATP
Adenosine-induced protein, 391–392
Adenylate cyclase, hormone-stimulated, 210–
    211
ADP-ribosylation reactions, in NaPO$_4$ co-
    transport, 60–62
Adrenal cortical cell, renin in, 332–333
Adrenal hormones, in distal nephron, 248–249
Adrenal medulla, renin in, 332
Adrenal steroids, Na-K-ATPase regulation by,
    367–370
  under basal conditions, 367–368
  under corticosteroid production conditions,
    369–370
Adrenergic inhibitors, for hypertension, 1165–
    1166
Adrenocorticotrophic hormone (ACTH), re-
    lease by AVP, 418–419
Adult respiratory distress syndrome (ARDS),
    BAL and, 764, 767
Adults, nephrotic syndrome in, 1034–1037
Aerobic energy production, 1219
  results of, 1220–1223
Afferent events, of cirrhosis, 449–454
Afferent renal nerve activity (ARNA), and me-
    chanoreceptor stimulation, 81–82
Afferent renal nerves
  hypertension and, 82
  neurophysiology of, 81
Age
  aminoglycoside nephrotoxicity and, 851–852
  and effect of transfusion in allograft, 1677–
    1678
  and renal scars, 960–961
Agonistic analog, of vasopressin, 417–423
Albumin, detection of, 1095
Albustix test, 1095
Aldosterone
  Na-K-ATPase activity, 381–382

effect on, 16, 364–370
  in CCT transport, 172
mechanism of action of, 380–385
  H transport and, 383–385
  K transport and, 382–383
  Na transport and, 380–382
  Na-K-ATPase and, 388–394
  Na pump and, 389–391
  pleiotropic response of, 388–389
Aldosterone receptor, localization of, along
    nephron, 372–378
Aldosterone-induced proteins, 388–389
Alkali, for Ca nephrolithiasis, 1020–1021
Alkalosis, NH$_3$ production and, 274
Allogenic disease, 543–544
Allogenic transplant, unresponsiveness in,
    1700–1702
Allograft, renal, see Renal allograft
Allopurinol, for Ca nephrolithiasis, 1018–1020
Allotransplantation, cadaveric, TLI vs.CI in,
    1722–1723
Alpha-ketoglutarate, low pH and, 275
1Alpha-(OH)vitamin D$_3$, in osteodystrophy,
    1364–1366
Alpha$_2$-adrenoceptors, sites of, 79–80
Alport syndrome, 577
Aluminum
  parenteral-nutrition-related bone disease
    and, 1386–1387
  removal with desferrioxamine, 1389
  sources of, in renal failure, 1387–1388
Aluminum absorption, in renal failure, 1417–
    1419
Aluminum accumulation, in osteodystrophy,
    1383–1391
Aluminum-loaded animals, observations in,
    1386
Aluminum-related osteomalacia
  bone biopsy features in, 1384–1385
  prevention of, 1391
  role of PTH in, 1385–1386
  treatment of, 1389–1391
Amiloride
  and aldosterone-induced ATPase synthesis,
    16–17
  Na/H antiporter interaction with, 75–76
  in Na-K-ATPase activity, 268
  and proximal acidification, 166–167
Amino acid
  loss during CAPD, 1613–1614
  renal regeneration and, 749–750
Amino acid metabolism, in uremia, 1344
Aminoaciduria, 930–931
  occurrence of, 931

Aminoglycoside antibiotics
  Na-K-ATPase and, 810
  toxicity of, 809–810
Aminoglycoside drug interaction, 854–855
  sex and, 855
Aminoglycoside, renal handling of, 846–849
Aminoglycoside nephrotoxicity, 776–778,
    809–810
  administration frequency and, 854
  age and, 851–852
  cellular mechanisms of, 858–860
  clinical aspects of, 855–857
  comparative, 853–854
  dehydration and volume contraction and,
    852
  dose and, 854
  drug related factors, 853–854
  K and Mg depletion and, 852
  molecular aspects of, 844–846
  morphologic patterns of, 849–850
  pathogenesis of, 857–860
  patient related factors, 851–852
  pharmacologic aspects of, 844–846
  prior renal insufficiency and, 852
  risk factors in, 851–854
Aminonucleoside nephrosis, proteoglycan syn-
    thesis in, 587–588
Ammonium excretion, 1187
Ammonium production
  pH changes and, 273–276
  metabolic alkalosis and, 274
  respiratory alkalosis and, 274
AMP, cyclic, see Cyclic AMP
Amphiuma kidney, cell volume regulation in,
    35–37
Amphotericin B, toxicity of, 810–811
Amyloidosis, in Hodgkin's disease, 906
Anaphylaxis, NSAID-induced, 827
Anemia, control of, CAPD and, 1590
Anerobic energy production, carbohydrate me-
    tabolism and, 1219
  results, 1223
Angioimmunoblastic lymphadenopathy, glo-
    merular lesions in, 908
Angiotensin II (AII), renal hemodynamics
    changes and, 159
Angiotensinogen analogs, 287–290
Anicteric renal failure, in leptospirosis, 1042
Animal models, pathogenic mechanisms of
    IgA nephropathy and, 645–650
Anionic components, in glomerular filtration,
    580–581
Anionic nonglomerular antigen, and subep-
    ithelial deposits, 512–514

Antagonist, specific, development of, 420–423
  importance of, 423
Antagonistic analog, of vasopressin, specificity
    of, 417–423
Anthracene-9-COO (A9C), inhibition of Cl
    conductance by, 235–236
Anti-GBM nephritis, and Goodpasture syn-
    drome, 494
Anti-glomerular basement membrane disease
    (anti-GBM)
  monitoring of, 1476
  outcome of, 1476
  treatment of, 1475–1476
Anti-gp333 IgG, induction of HN by, 565–567
Anti-idiotypic antibody, in circulating immune
    complexes, 535
Antibiotic-induced nephrotoxicity, 844–860
Antibody
  cationic, 554–555
  interaction with in situ antigen, 492–494
  and subepithelial deposits, 514
Anticoagulant therapy
  glomerulonephritis treatment and, 1454
  in glomerular disease, 1486–1487
  in MPGN, 1438–1439
Antidiuretic hormone (ADH)
  action on NaCl transport, 212–214
  and ARF, 1330
  effects on kidney, 246
  effects on rat kidney, 340–355
  effects on TALH, 349–352
  K secretion and, 263
Antidiuretic hormone analog, see dDAVP
Antidiuretic volume effect, vasopressin and,
    428–429
Antigen
  anionic nonglomerular, and subepithelial de-
    posits, 512–514
  cationic, 551–553
    nephritogenic potential of, 551–552
  cationic nonglomerular, and subepithelial
    deposits, 511–512
  exogenous-planted, 496–497
  glomerular
    and subendothelial deposits, 515
    and subepithelial deposits, 510–511
  Heymann, 510
  Heymann nephritis, 560–561
  in situ, interaction of antibody with, 492–
    494
  mesangial
    fixed, 517
    planted, 517–518
  planted nonrenal

Antigen (*cont.*)
  and subendothelial deposits, 515–516
  and subepithelial deposits, 511–515
Antigen elimination, glomerulonephritis treatment and, 1446–1447
Antigen-antibody systems, and immune complexes in glomeruli, 531–532
Antihypertensive drugs, 284–298
Antilymphoblast antibody, in transplantation, 1635–1636
Antilymphocyte globulin (ALG), 1635
  in allografts, 1684–1687
Antilymphocyte therapy, conclusions regarding, 1691–1692
Antiplatelet drugs, 1711–1712
Antiplatelet therapy, in glomerular disease, 1487
Antirejection therapy, complications of, 1654–1655
Apical membrane, hyperpolarization of, 12
Apical:basolateral cell membrane, resistance ratio of, 183–184
Aplastic bone disease, in hemodialysis patients, 1374–1381
Arachidonic acid (C_{20}:4), metabolism of, 277–280
Arachidonic acid metabolism, in nephrotoxic serum nephritis, 506, 601–607
  in tubuloglomerular feedback, 139–140
Arginine-vasopressin (AVP)
  ACTH release by, 418–419
  analogues of, 417–418
  antipyretic action of, 420
  and baroreceptor reflexes, 420
  behavioral effects of, 419–420
Arterial hypoxemia, dialysis-induced, 1543–1544
Ascites, overflow theory in, 451–452
Ask-Upmark kidney, 948
ATP
  exogenous, 780–781
  generation of, Na-K pump in, 233–234
ATP-MgCl$_2$
  SNC$_{In}$ and, 803
  and WKC$_{In}$, 802–803
ATP-MgCl$_2$ infusion, after cell injury, 717
ATPase, proton-translocating, in brushborder membrane vesicles, 164–165
ATPase activity, Na-K, *see* Sodium-potassium ATPase activity
Atrial natriuretic factor (ANF), 257–259
  furosemide and, comparative studies, 258–259
  mechanism of action of, 258

molecular weight distribution of, 258
  nature of, 257–258
Autocrine stimulation, 755
Autoimmune glomerulonephritis, 540
Autonomic nervous system, hypertension and, 1120–1121
Autoradiography, 373
5-Azacytidine nephrotoxicity, 876–877
Azathioprine, 1632
Azathioprine therapy, cyclosporine levels and, 1721–1722

Baboons, unresponsiveness to allogenic transplants in, 1700–1702
Bacteriuria, prevalence of, 969
Barium
  effect on basolateral membrane, 10
  inhibition of K conductance by, 234–235
Baroreceptor reflexes, AVP and, 420
Baroreflex function, modulation of, 429–430
Basolateral KCl cotransport, in TAL cell, 231–232
Basolateral cell membrane
  action of thyroid hormone on proximal tubule, 358–362
  effect on Ba, 10
  exit mechanism in, 58, 60
  K conductance of, 228–229
  Na-K pump in, generation of ATP and, 233–234
  properties of, Na-absorbing epithelium and, 7–17
  pump-leak properties of, 7–8
Basolateral potassium conductance, rate of Na entry and, 8–10
Basolateral sodium-potassium pump, function of, 7
Bence Jones proteinuria, 886–887
Bendroflumethiazide, in Ca nephrolithiasis, 1000
Berger's disease, *see* IgA nephropathy
Beta$_2$-adrenoceptors, sites of, 79–80
Bicarbonate conductance, in PCT, 167–168
Bicarbonate hemodialysis
  vs. acetate hemodialysis, 1544
  advantages of, 1532
  disadvantages of, 1532
  indications for, 1533
Bicarbonate reabsorption, by PCT, 161
Bicarbonate transport, 1203
Bile duct ligation
  in dog, 463–465
  in rats, 461–462
Biliary cirrhosis, primary, 467

Biliary obstruction, chronic, 461–465
Bioassay, in PTH measurements, 1278–1279
Biochemical analysis, of urine, 1425–1429
Biochemical control, CAPD and, 1588–1589
Biochemical mechanisms, regulation of Na/H antiporter by, 73–77
Biological fluids, states of saturation for, 991–993
Biosynthetic failure, uremia and, 1251
Blood drawing, protein loss from, 1507–1508
Blood glucose control, CAPD and diabetic patient, 1604–1605
Blood hyperviscosity, in leptospirosis, 1047
Blood parameters, CAPD and diabetic patient, 1604
Blood pressure, in diabetic nephropathy, 1097–1099
Blood pressure regulation, see also Hypertension
    Ca in, 1141–1143
    PTH in, 1145–1146
    therapy and, 1146–1147
Blood pressure response
    to Ca modification, 1142–1143
    to Ca-regulating hormones, 1145–1146
    to parathyroidectomy, 1145
Blood supply, medullary, see Medullary blood supply
Blood transfusion
    effect on allografts, 1674–1679
    in renal transplantation, 1636–1637
Blood volume, in nephrotic syndrome, 471–472
Bone biopsy features, in Al-related osteomalacia, 1384–1385
Bone disease
    in dialysis patients, 1374–1381
    parenteral-nutrition-related, 1386–1387
Bovine gamma globulin (BGG), mesangial IgA deposits, 646
Bovine serum albumin (BSA), native, 552–553
Bowel disease, 983–984
Bowman space, 506–507
Brain, renin in, intracellular actions of, 329–331
Bronchoalveolar lavage (BAL), in ARDS patient, 764, 767
Brushborder membrane vesicles
    biochemical modification in, 60
    cytochrome electron transport chain in, 165
    D-glucose transport in, 23–25
        overshoot phenomenon, 24
        physiologic rationale, 31
        results of, 25–31
        study methods used in, 25

$NaPO_4$ cotransport studies in, 57–62
OA/OH antiporter in, 164
phosphorylation with γ-^{32}P-ATP, 61
PO_4 transport across, effect of Na and pH on, 57–60
proton-translocating ATPase in, 164–165
thyroid hormone action on proximal tubule, 358–362
BSC-1 epithelial cell, 754–755
Budd-Chiari syndrome, 466
Bufo marinus, 388
Burkitt's lymphoma, glomerular lesions in, 908

Cadaver donor
    HLA matching in, 1630
    renal transplantation from, 1628–1629
    TLI trials of, 1702–1704
Cadaveric allotransplantation, TLI vs. CI in, 1722–1723
Calcitonin (CT)
    and ARF, 1325–1326
    effects on Henle's loop, 345–347, 349–352
    effects on plasma composition, 343–345
    effects on rat kidney, 340–355
    effects on TALH, 349–352
    glomerular and tubular effects, 345
Calcitriol, see also Vitamin D
    osteodystrophy and, 1400–1401
    uremia and, 1251
Calcium
    and disturbances in hypertension, 1142
    blood pressure response to, 1141–1143
        modification of, 1142–1143
    depolarizing agents and water transport, 412
    effects of quinidine on, 41–42
    effects on cytoskeleton, 41
    in ischemic injury, 794–795
    and parathyroid gland activity, 1267–1268
    and parathyroid hormone messenger RNA, 1268–1271
    in tubuloglomerular feedback, 135–138
    cytostolic, see Cytostolic calcium
    and vascular smooth muscle etiology, 1141–1142
Calcium absorption
    physiology of, in renal failure, 1412–1414
    after transplantation, 1415
    in uremia, 1414
Calcium antagonists, blood pressure regulation and, 1146–1147
Calcium binding protein (CaBP), in distal nephron, 249–250
Calcium-calmodulin complex, 44

Calcium channel blockers, 716–717, 779–780
  role of, 791–798
Calcium entry blockers, for hypertension, 1167
Calcium interaction, influence on feedback,
  138–139
Calcium ionophore (A23187), feedback response with, 136–137
Calcium metabolism, disturbances of, in nephrotic syndrome, 1349
Calcium oxalate crystallization
  glycosaminoglycan inhibitors of, 1027–1028
  growth inhibitors of, 1025–1026
  urinary inhibitors of, 1025–1029
Calcium oxalate nephrolithiasis
  alkali for, 1020–1021
    biochemical effects, 1020
    clinical effects, 1020
    side effects, 1020–1021
  allopurinol for, 1018–1020
    biochemical background, 1018–1019
    clinical effects, 1019
    side effects, 1019
  cellulose PO₄ for, 1014–1016
    biochemical effects, 1014–1015
    clinical effects, 1015–1016
    side effects, 1016
  choice of therapy in, 1003–1004
  DEAE cellulose for, 1021
  magnesium for, 1016–1018
    biochemical effects, 1016–1017
    clinical effects, 1017
    indications for, 1018
    side effects, 1017–1018
  orthophosphates for, 1011–1014
    biochemical effects, 1011–1012
    clinical effects, 1012
    side effects, 1013–1014
  pyridoxine for, 1021
  thiazide diuretics in, 999–1006
    efficacy of, 999–1001
    indications for, 1003
    mode of action of, 1001–1002
    side effects, 1005–1006
    treatment regimen, 1004–1005
  treatments for, 1021
Calcium oxalate urolithiasis
  physicochemical factors in, 990–996
  supersaturation in, 991–993
  treatment of, 996
Calcium-regulating hormone, blood pressure
  response to, 1145–1146
Calcium renal stones
  pathogenesis of, 980–987
  supersaturation and, 980–984

Calcium supplementation, osteodystrophy
  and, 1398–1399
Calcium transport, 1201–1202
Calculosis, intranephronic, 995–996
Calmodulin
  in cellular events, 44
  feedback responses and, 138
Cancer, after transplantation, 1638–1639
Cancer chemotherapy agents, nephrotoxicity
  caused by, 869–881
  direct, 869–877
  endogenous, 877–881
Capillary COPp, increase of, 443
Capillary plexus, 97
Captopril, for hypertension, 1166–1167
Carbohydrate metabolism
  anerobic energy and, 1219
  ARF and, 1326–1327
  disturbances of, in nephrotic syndrome, 1349
  effects of peritoneal energy supply on, 1612–
    1613
Carbonic anhydrase (CA-C), in distal nephron,
  249–250
Cardiac effects, vasopressin and, 429
Cardiovascular complications, after transplan-
  tation, 1638
Cardiovascular system, vasopressin and, 426–
  430
Catabolism
  in renal failure
    causes of, 1498–1510
    proteases of, 765–769
  and hemodialysis, 1505–1506
Catecholamine effect, in leptospirosis, 1047
Cationic antibody, 554–555
Cationic antigen, 551–553
  nephritogenic potential of, 551–552
Cationic immune complex, 555–556
Cationic molecules, and mesangium, 553–554
Cationic nonglomerular antigen, and subep-
  ithelial deposits, 511–512
Cationic protein, nephritogenicity of, 551
Cell
  control of renin action in, 336
  glucose requirement of, 4–5
  immortalized, 5
Cell-ATP, phosphorylation of, 1225–1226
Cell injury, along nephron, 718–719
Cell-mediated immunity (CMI), 497–499
Cell puncture technique, and microperfusion,
  180–184
Cell surface, Na-K-ATPase activity at, 392–
  394
Cell volume regulation, in epithelia, 34–38
Cellular electrophysiology, of K transport, 266

Cellular mechanisms
  regulation of Na/H antiporter by, 73
  of tubuloglomerular feedback, 130–140
Cellular mediator, of renal injury, 504–507
Cellular membrane-phospholipid synthesis,
    biochemical integrity of, 1220
  results, 1224–1225
Cellular response, to donor-specific transfu-
    sions, 1716–1717
Cellulose phosphate, for Ca nephrolithiasis,
    1014–1016
Cephalosporins, toxicity of, 811
Charge:substrate stoichiometry, static head
    method of, 30–31
Children
  allograft in, transfusion effect and, 1678
  CAPD in, with ESRD, 1587–1588
  nephrotic syndrome in, 1031–1034
  with reflux nephropathy, renal function in,
    961–962
Chloride conductance, inhibition of, by A9C,
    235–236
  by DPC, 235–236
Chlorpromazine, 717
Chlorthalidone, in Ca nephrolithiasis, 1000
Chondroitin sulfate proteoglycan (CSPG), 583
  mesangial cells and, 590
Chronic glomerulonephritis, immune complex
    disease and, 491–492
Chronic lymphocytic leukemia, glomerular le-
    sions in, 908–909
Chronic renal failure (CRF)
  catabolism and wasting in, 1498–1510
  endocrine disorders in, 1504–1505
  treatment of, 1509–1510
  intercurrent illness and, 1500–1504
Chronic renal insufficiency
  insulin metabolism in, 1345
  insulin resistance in, 1338–1339
    cellular mechanism of, 1340–1341
    site of, 1339–1340
  insulin secretion in, 1336–1338
  K metabolism in, 1345
Circulating immune complex see also Immune
    complex
  anti-idiotypic antibodies in, 535
  characteristics of, 527–537
  deposition of, 489
  mesangial deposits of, 518–519, 529–534
  removal of, by mononuclear phagocyte sys-
    tem, 528–529
  rheumatoid factors in, 534
  role of charge on, 532–533
  subendothelial deposits of, 529–534
  subepithelial deposits of, 535–537

trapping of, vs. in situ immune complex for-
    mation, 520
Circulation, medullary see Medullary circula-
    tion
Cirrhosis
  biliary, 467
  diminished effective volume in, 449–451
  edema in, pathogenesis of, 449–458
  Na homeostasis of
    afferent events, 449–454
    efferent events, 454–455
  overflow theory in, 451–454
Cis-platinum, 811–812
Cis-platinum nephrotoxicity, 870–872
  clinical manifestations of, 870–871
  histopathology of, 870
  pathogenesis of, 870
  prophylactic measures, 871–872
Citrate, crystal growth inhibitor, 987
Clinical disease, glomerular morphology and,
    674–675
Clonidine, ARF prevention and, 784–789
Cobra venom factor (CVF), complement deple-
    tion with, 504
Cognitive function, CAPD and, 1591
Computerized tomography, 1434–1435
  vesicoureteral reflux and, 943
Conduit grafts, 1556–1558
  complications of, 1557–1558
Continuous ambulatory peritoneal dialysis
    (CAPD)
  abnormal lipid metabolism and, 1593–1594
  advantages of, 1538
  amino acid losses during, 1613–1614
  anemia and, 1590
  cause of death, 1594
  in children, with ESRD, 1587–1588
  cognitive function and, 1591
  in diabetic patient, 1599–1608
    cause of death, 1601
    cause of transfer, 1602
    clinical and biological parameters, 1602–
      1606
    complications, 1602
    hospitalization, 1602
    methods, 1599–1600
    survival rates, 1601
  disadvantages of, 1538–1539
  efficacy and adequacy of, 1581–1595
  energy requirements and, 1614–1616
  fluid intake in, 1589
  hypertension control and, 1589–1590
  hypotension and, 1594
  indications of, 1539
  kidney transplantation and, 1584–1585

Continuous ambulatory peritoneal dialysis
    (*cont.*)
  lipid abnormalities during, 1616–1618
  metabolic consequences of, 1611–1620
  neuropathy and, 1591
  osteodystrophy and, 1593
  pericarditis and, 1590–1591
  peripheral vascular disease and, 1594
  protein losses during, 1613
  quality of life with, 1585–1587
  removal of K by, 1588
  removal of PO₄ by, 1588–1589
  serum proteins and, 1613–1614
  survival on, 1581–1584
    low-risk patients and, 1584
  uremic complications and, 1589–1594
Continuous arteriovenous hemofiltration
    (CAVH), 1534
  advantages and disadvantages of, 1535
  indications for, 1535
Continuous cycling peritoneal dialysis
    (CCPD), 1539
Continuous subcutaneous insulin infusion sys-
    tem (CSII), 1069
Contraluminal membrane, thyroid action on,
    360–361
Conventional immunosuppression (CI), vs.
    TLI, in cadaveric allotransplantation,
    1722–1723
Cortical collecting tubule (CCT)
  acidification in, 170–172
  aldosterone and, 172
  aldosterone binding sites in, 373–376
  antinatriuretic effect of aldosterone on, 380–
    381
  electrophysiologic studies of, 55
  K permeability of, 264–266
  K transport across, 382–383
  of rabbit, Na-Ca exchange process in, 53–
    55
Corticosteroid hormones
  binding along nephron, 364–367
  epithelial sensitivity to, 5–6
  glomerulonephritis treatment and, 1452–
    1453
Corticosterone
  binding along nephron, 364–367
  effect on Na-K-ATPase, 364–370
Corticotrophin releasing factor (CRF), 418
Cotransport mechanisms, 21–32
Cotransport systems, 229–233
Countercurrent multiplication, 398
Coupled transport, thermodynamics of, 21–23
Crane's gradient hypothesis, 21

Creatinine clearance, with glomerular pathol-
    ogy, 675, 677
Crescentic glomerulonephritis, 1470
  Hodgkin's disease and, 907
  non-Hodgkin lymphoma and, 907
Crush syndrome, 703
Crystal growth
  inhibitors of, 985–987, 993
    clinical significance of, 987
    metal citrate, 1028–1029
Crystal nucleation, urothelial membrane sur-
    faces on, 1026–1027
Cyclic AMP
  NaPO₄ transport in LLC-PK₁ cells, 63
  stimulation of NaCl reabsorption by, 237–
    238
  vasopressin and, 39
Cyclic AMP-dependent mechanism, 408
Cyclic AMP-independent mechanism, 408–
    409
Cyclic nucleotide, influence on feedback, 138–
    139
Cycloheximide, NaPO₄ cotransport and, 63–
    64
Cyclooxygenase, 278–280
  inhibition of, NSAID and, 820
Cyclosporin A, glomerulonephritis treatment
    and, 1454–1455
Cyclosporine, 1633–1635
  and azathioprine therapy, 1721–1722
  EBV infection and, 1670
  hepatotoxicity and, 1670
  lymphoma and, 1670
  Oxford trials of, 1634
  in transplantation allograft response, 1662–
    1664
    clinical trials, 1666–1668
    mechanism of action, 1664–1665
    pharmacology of, 1665–1666
    side-effects, 1668–1670
  side-effects of, 1633–1634
  steroids and, 1634
  toxicity of, 813–814
Cylindrocarpon lucidium, 1655
Cystography, vesicoureteral reflux and, 942
Cytochrome electron transport chain, in brush-
    border membrane vesicles, 165
Cytochrome P450, 280–282
Cytokinetics, of K-leak unit, 15–17
Cytomegalovirus, and ALG in allografts,
    1686
Cytomegalovirus infection
  after antirejection therapy, 1654
  after transplantation, 1638

Cytometry, flow, advances in, 1717–1718
  presensitization and enhancement, 1718–1719
Cytoskeleton, effect of Ca on, 41
Cytosolic calcium
  in feedback mechanism, 51–52
  in renal tubular transport, 51–55
  in vasopressin-sensitive epithelia, 39–47
Cytotoxic agents, glomerulonephritis treatment and, 1453

1,25-Dihydroxycholecalciferol
  in health, 1307–1309
  in kidney disease, 1309–1311
1,25-Diaydroxyvitamin D, osteodystrophy and, 1400–1401
D-glucose, and proximal tubular cell, 21–23
D-glucose flux, Na-dependent component of, 26
D-glucose transport
  in brushborder membrane vesicles, 23–25
    overshoot phenomenon, 24
    physiologic rationale, 31
    results of, 25–31
    study methods used in, 25
d-Penicillamine, 649
Dapsone, 649
dDAVP (ADH analog)
  effects on Henle's loop, 345–347, 349–352
  effects on plasma composition, 343–345
  effects on TALH, 349–352
  and glomerular and tubular effects, 345
Dehydration, aminoglycoside nephrotoxicity and, 852
Delayed type hypersensitivity (DTH), graft survival and, 1715–1716
  K secretion and, 383
Deoxycorticosterone acetate (DOCA)
  and K secretion, 383
  in K transport, 266
  Na-K-ATPase activity and, 267–268
Depolarizing agents, Ca and, 412
Desferrioxamine, aluminum removal with, 1389
Dexamethasone
  H_2O_2 production by mesangial cells, 612–614
  ^{125}I-STZ uptake by mesangial cells, 615
  and mesangial cell function in phagocytosis, 609–617
  PGE_2 production by mesangial cells, 612–614
Dextran, 647

Dextran-bound inhibitor (DBI), vs. unbound inhibitor, 251–252
Diabetes, experimental, proteoglycan synthesis in, 588–589
Diabetes mellitus
  altered glomerular metabolism in, 1074–1079
  diabetic nephropathy and, 1103–1104
  glucose regulation in, 1111
  insulin-dependent, kidney biopsy and, 1103–1107
  and kidney, 1053–1112
  PO_4, 1184–1185
  renal involvement in, stages of, 1055–1065
Diabetic glomerulopathy
  advanced, 1083
  intermediate, 1082–1083
  occult, 1081–1082
  patient population, 1083–1084
  study protocol in, 1084
  theoretic considerations, 1084–1085
Diabetic nephropathology, proteinuria in, 1081–1091
Diabetic nephropathy
  anionic charge in glomerular barrier and, 1065–1066
  antihypertensive treatment in, 1069–1070
  blood pressure in, 1097–1099
  clinical and renal studies in, 1053–1070
  and diabetes mellitus, 1103–1104
  early markers of, 1094–1100
    identification of, 1095
  incipient, 1054, 1060–1064
  intraglomerular pressure and, 1066
  kidney function tests in, 1054
  linear rate in morphogenesis and, 1065
  measurement of progression in, 1054–1055
  overt, 1064–1065
  pathogenesis and, 1065–1066
    general concepts, 1065
  pathogenesis as determinant of, 1109–1112
  proteinuria in, 1095–1097
  provocation tests in, 1055
  structural-functional relationships in, 1105
  systemic blood pressure and, 1066
Diabetic patient, CAPD in, 1599–1608
Diabetic renal lesions, glycemic control and, 1104–1105
Dialysate composition, osteodystrophy and, 1401
Dialysis, 1528–1620, *see also* Hemodialysis
  modes of, cost comparisons, 1594–1595
  nutrient losses from, 1506–1507
Dialysis schedule, 1540–1544

Dialysis techniques
  biocompatibility and, 1544–1547
  current, advantages and disadvantages of, 1528–1548
  first-use syndrome and, 1546–1547
  hypersensitive reactions to, 1544–1547
  types of, 1531–1540
Dialysis treatment
  individualization of, 1541
  individualization/adequacy in, 1541
  kinetic modeling and, 1541–1542
  nutritional aspects of, 1542–1543
  therapeutic considerations in, 1543
Dicyclohexylcarbodiimide (DCCD), 166
Diet
  blood pressure regulation and, 1147
  effect on renal function, 1521–1524
  eicosapentaenoic acid and, 1138–1139
  renal stones and, 984
Diethyl-amino-ethanol cellulose, for Ca nephrolithiasis, 1021
Diffuse mesangial proliferation (DMP), 637–638
Digital subtraction angiography, 1431
Diltiazem, for hypertension, 1167
Diphenylamine-2-COO (DPC), inhibition of Cl conductance by, 235–236
Distal convoluted tubule (DCT), aldosterone binding sites in, 373–377
Distal nephron, see Nephron, distal
Diuresis
  blood pressure regulation and, 1146
  pressure, 128
Divalent ion metabolism, and ARF, 1323–1324
DOCA-salt hypertension, protein restriction in, 1235–1236
Dogs, bile duct ligation in, 463–465
  unresponsiveness to allogenic transplants in, 1700–1702
Draining wounds, protein loss from, 1507–1508
Drug metabolites, toxic, acetaminophen and, 812–813
Drug nephrotoxicity
  alterations in GFR and, 807–808
  mechanisms of, 807–814, see also Nephrotoxicity
Drugs, tubular cell damage by, 808–809
DTPA Tc99m, vesicoureteral reflux and, 942

Eadie-Hofstee plots, 26
  curvilinear, 24

Edema, 435–479
  in cirrhosis, pathogenesis of, 449–458
  in heart failure, 443–444
  in hypoproteinemia, 443–444
  production of, equilibrium at capillary level in, 435–445
Edema-preventing mechanisms, 437–444
Efferent events, of cirrhosis, 454–455
Efferent renal nerve activity (ERNA), and mechanoreceptor stimulation, 81–82
Eicosanoid metabolism
  dietary fatty acids and, 1136–1137
  dietary fish oils and, 1136–1139
  after eicosapentaenoic acid enriched diets, 1138–1139
Eicosapentaenoic acid, diets enriched with, 1138–1139
Electrical charge, and glomerulus, 557–558
Electrolyte excretion, control of, 251–268
Electron microscopy, in TALH, 244–245
End-stage renal disease (ESRD), in children, CAPD and, 1587–1588
Endocrine abnormality, 1264–1355
  in ARF, 1322–1331
  in nephrotic syndrome, 1349–1355
Endocrine disorder, in CRF, 1504–1505
Endocrine dysfunction, after transplantation, 1644–1655
Endocrine failure, uremia and, 1251
Endocrine system, kidney and, 340–430
Endothelial fenestra(e), and ARF, 723–724
Endothia parasitica, 293
Energy metabolism, PO_4 depletion and, 1210–1213
Energy requirements, and CAPD, 1614–1616
Epithelium(ia), see also Renal epithelium cell
  calmodulin in, 44
  cell lines from, 3–4
  cell volume regulation in, 34–38
  changes in, 722–724
  in culture, 754–755
  growth, form and function in, 3–6
  growth control of, 751–755
  HSPG synthesis and, 590
  intact, 14
  leaky, 7
  Na-absorbing, 7–17
  Necturus, effect of galactose on, 8–9
  sensitivity to corticosteroids, 5–6
  of thin limbs of Henle's loop
    heterogeneity of, 197–199
    species differences, 198–199
  tight, 7
  transcellular solute transport in, 11
    physiologic importance of, 11–12

transport processes and, 3–77
  vasopressin-sensitive, 407–408
    role of cytosolic Ca in, 39–47
  volume regulatory responses in, 11
    physiologic importance of, 11–12
Epstein-Barr virus antigen, 908
Epstein-Barr virus infection
  cyclosporine and, 1670
  after transplantation, 1639
Erythrocytosis, after transplantation, 1653
Erythropoiesis, PTH in, 1253–1254
Erythropoietin, and ARF, 1331
Escherichia coli, P-fimbriated, 1442–1443
Essential hypertension, 1115
  manifestation of, 1123
  plasma renin activity in, 1122
  renin in, 286–287
Excretion
  acid and electrolyte, 251–268
  K, regulation of, 260–268
Excretion urography (IVU), vesicoureteral reflux and, 941
Excretory failure, acute toxicity of, 1248–1251
Excretory function, hormone mediated response of TALH and, 352–353
Exercise, and hypertension, 1163
Exogenous-planted antigen, 496–497
Experimental hypertension, Ca disturbances in, 1142
Extracellular fluid volume, regulation of, 435
Extracellular volume (ECV)
  changes in, 435
  constancy of, 435
Extrarenal buffering, effect of PO_4 depletion on, 1192

Fatty acids
  long-chain, 1220
  oxidation of, 1220
    biochemical integrity of, 1224–1225
  polyunsaturated
    effect of, 1137
    substitution of, 1137
    western diet supplementation with, 1137–1138
  short-chain, 1220
Feedback function, 146–148
Feedback loop, 144–146
  intact, 149–151
    altered feedback function and, 150–151
    altered feedforward function and, 150
    external forcing-autoregulation, 149–150
Feedback mechanism, cytosolic Ca in, 51–52

Fish oils, and eicosanoid metabolism, 1136–1139
Fistula, protein loss from, 1507–1508
Flow cytometry
  advances in, 1717–1718
  presensitization and enhancement, 1718–1719
Flow dependence, in TALH, 209–210
Flux, unidirectional, in juxtamedullary nephron, 188
  in superficial nephron, 188
Focal glomerulonephritis, Hodgkin's disease and, 906
Focal segmental glomerular sclerosis (FSGS), 636–637
  morphologic features of, 636
Franconi syndrome, with hypercalciuria, 929–930
Furosemide
  ANF and, comparative studies, 258–259
  and contrast-induced nephropathy, 840
  inhibition of $Na^+2Cl^-K^+$ cotransporter by, 236

Galactose, effect on Necturus epithelium, 8–9
Gamma-^{32}P-ATP, phosphorylation with, 61
Gastrointestinal hormone, and ARF, 1330–1331
Gentamicin, 777
  renal handling of, 846–847
  toxicity of, 809–810
Gentamicin nephrotoxicity, 855
  mitochondrial dysfunction and, 859
  resistance to, 859–860
Glomerular antigen, and subendothelial deposits, 515
Glomerular barrier
  function of, 1087–1088
  neutralization of, 557
Glomerular basement membrane (GBM)
  anionic site changes in, diseases and, 585–586
  antigens of, 486–488
  permeability properties of, proteoglycans and, 584–585
  plasma proteins in, 488
  proteoglycans association with, 582–584, 590
Glomerular capillary, characteristics of, 485–486
Glomerular capillary pressure, measurement of, 131
Glomerular capillary wall injury
  classification of, 1085–1087
  nature of, 1087–1089

Glomerular cell type, proteoglycan synthesis
     and, 590–591
Glomerular disease
  anionic site changes in GBM and, 585–586
  anticoagulant therapy in, 1486–1487
  antiplatelet therapy in, 1487
  biosynthesis of proteoglycans in, 587–589
  NSAID in, 1487–1488
  plasma exchange for, 1474–1483
  polypharmacy approach to
     prospective clinical trials, 1490–1492
     retrospective treatment studies, 1488–
       1490
  proteoglycan synthesis in, 587–589
  pulse methylprednisolone in, 1464–1472
  treatment of, 1445–1492
Glomerular filtration, 130–159
  anionic components in, 580–581
  effects of dDAVP, PTH, CT and glucagon
     on, 345
  intrarenal control of, 130–140
Glomerular filtration dynamics, 1088–1089
Glomerular filtration rate (GFR)
  drug nephrotoxicity and, 807–808
  and nephrotic syndrome, 475–476, 1351–
     1353
  NSAID effect on, 822
  effect of PO_4 depletion on, 1188–1189
  sickle cell anemia and, 916–917
Glomerular function, proteoglycans in, 580–
     597
Glomerular hyperfusion, and experimental re-
     nal disease, 1233–1236
Glomerular immune deposit formation, 510–
     519
Glomerular injury
  complement-mediated, 504
  and inhibition, 1450–1452
  O_2 preradicals in, 507
Glomerular lesions
  in leptospirosis, 1044–1045
  in leukemias, 908–910
  in lymphomas, 906–908
  treatment of, 974–975
Glomerular localization, of immune com-
     plexes, 489–491
Glomerular metabolism, in diabetes mellitus,
     1074–1079
Glomerular microcirculation, renal nerves in-
     fluence on, 154–159
Glomerular morphology, and disease, 674–675
Glomerular pathology
  creatinine clearance with, 675, 677
  proteinuria and, 677, 680

proteoglycans in, 580–597
sickle cell anemia and, 919–920
Glomerular permeability
  in experimental ARF, 734–735
  reduced, in ARF, 704–705
Glomerulonephritis, see also Specific types
  autoimmune, 540
  immune complex, 491–492
     pathogenesis of, 509
  immune complexes and, 491–492
  immunologically-mediated, 540–547
  intervention of hypertension in, 1456–1457
  monoclonal antibodies and, 505
  proliferative, 1034–1035
  syphilitic, 1035–1036
  treatment of, 1445–1457
  urinary erythrocyte counts in, 1426
  urinary fat and, 1426
  vascular disease in, 1456
  in Zimbabwe, 1030–1037
Glomerulopathy
  diabetic, see Diabetic glomerulopathy
  mercuric chloride, 542–543
Glomerulus(i)
  anti-idiotypic antibodies in, 535
  charge on circulating immune complex in,
     532–533
  electrical charge and, 557–558
  IgA immune complex in, 533–534
  immune complexes in, 508–520
     antigen-antibody systems and, 531–532
  juxtamedullary, 87
  lattice of immune complex in, 529–531
  localization of gp333 in, 564–565
  rat, antigenically distinct types of HSPG in,
     592–595
  rheumatoid factor activity in, 534
Glucagon
  and ARF, 1327
  effects on Henle's loop, 345–347, 349–352
  effects on plasma composition, 343–345
  effects on rat kidney, 340–355
  effects on TALH, 349–352
  glomerular and tubular effects, 345
  NaCl absorption and, 211
Glucagon metabolism, in uremia, 1344
Glucocortocoids, K secretion and, 263–264
Gluconeogenesis, 4–5
Glucose intolerance, in uremia, implications
     of, 1341–1344
Glucose metabolism, in uremia, 1335–1336,
     1344
Glucose regulation, in diabetes mellitus, 1111
Glucose transport, 1203

Glycemic control, and diabetic renal lesions, 1104–1105
Glycoproteins, crystal growth inhibitors, 985–986
Glycosaminoglycan (GAG) chain, 581–582
Glycosaminoglycans
    crystal growth inhibitors, 986
    as inhibitors of Ca oxalate crystallization, 1027–1028
Goldblatt hypertension, 82
Goldman equation, 181
Goodpasture syndrome, 494, 576
Gp300, vs. gp333, 567–568
Gp330
    characterization of, 563
    induction of Hn by, 562–563
    isolation of, 561–562
    in normal glomeruli, 564–565
Gp333
    localization in other organs, 568–570
    vs. maltase, 567–568
Granulocyte lysosomal function, in uremia, 766
Growth hormone, and ARF, 1327–1328

(^{3}H)-aldosterone, heterogeneity of, 377–378
Hagman factor-kallikrein system, 305–306
(^{3}H)-dexamethasone, binding sites of, 376–378
Health
    serum 1,25-(OH)$_2$-D in, 1307–1309
    vitamin D metabolism in, 1305–1306
Heart failure, localization of edema in, 443–444
Hematologic malignancy, 905–910
Hematopoietic system, 1406–1409
Hematuria
    asymptomatic microscopic, 687
    clinical management of, 921
    isolated episode of macroscopic, 687–688
    recurrent macroscopic, 688–689
Hemodiafiltration
    advantages of, 1535
    disadvantages of, 1536
    indications for, 1536
Hemodialysis, *see also* Dialysis
    catabolic stress of, 1505–1506
    high-flux, 1536–1537
    high-sodium, 1537–1538
    sequential filtration and, 1533
    vascular access in, 1553–1560
        trancutaneous device for, 1558–1560
    when to start, 1530–1531
Hemodialysis patients, osteodystrophy in, 1375–1381

Hemodialysis treatment, protease release during, 768–769
Hemodynamics, in experimental ARF, 731–734, 739–740
Hemofiltration, 1533–1534
    advantages and disadvantages of, 1534
    indications for, 1534
Hemolytic uremic syndrome, in leptospirosis, 1043
Hemorrhagic hypotension, saturation transfer NMR in, 273
Henle's loop
    changes in blood flow to, 123–124
    descending limbs of, function of, 201–203
    effects of dDAVP, PTH, CT and glucagon on, 345–347, 349–352
    regulation of NaCl transport by, 208–220
        complexities of, 209
    thick ascending limb of
        flow dependence in, 209–210
        NaCl reabsorption in, 224–238
    thin ascending limb of, 196–205
        functional heterogeneity, 201–204
        morphologic heterogeneity, 197–201
        physiological significance of heterogeneity of, 204–205
Heparin sulfate proteoglycan (HSPG), 583
    antigenically distinct types of, in rat glomeruli, 592–595
    epithelial cells and, 590
Hepatic disease, renal handling of Na in, 461–467
Hepatic venous outflow, obstruction to, 465–466
Hepatitis B virus, and membranous GN, 1032–1033
Hepatotoxicity, cyclosporine and, 1670
Herpes labialis, and ALG in renal allografts, 1686
Heterogeneity
    of ^{3}H-aldosterone, 377–378
    histotopographic, 200–201
    internephron, 197
    intranephron, 197
    nephron, physiological significance of, 204–205
    structural, of distal nephron, 243–250
    of thin limbs of Henle's loop
        functional, 201–204
        membrane particles, 199–200
        morphologic, 197–201
        physiological significance, 204–205
Heterogeneous nucleation, in crystal systems, 994
Heterogeneous nucleus(i), 985

Heymann antigen, 510
Heymann nephritis (HN), 540–541
  gp330 induction of, 562–563
    passive, 565–567
  pathogenic antigen of, 560–571
Heymann nephritis antigen, 560–561
Heymann nephritis model, 509
High flux hemodialysis
  advantages and disadvantages of, 1536
  indications for, 1537
High frequency stimulation, of renal nerves,
    156–157
High sodium hemodialysis
  advantages and disadvantages of, 1537
  indications for, 1537–1538
Histotopographic heterogeneity, 200–201
HLA antigen
  in renal allograft, 1676–1677
  matching for, 1629–1630
  renal transplantation and, 1629–1632
HLA system, IgA nephropathy and, 658–659
Hodgkin's disease
  glomerular lesions in, 906–907
  immune changes after TLI in, 1696–1698
  TLI therapy in, 1698–1699
Hormonal control systems, disruption of,
    1251–1257
Hormonal regulation, of NaCl absorption,
    210–212
Hormone, see Specific types
Hormone action, transport and, 361–362
Hormone mediated response, of TALH, excre-
    tory functions and, 352–353
Hormone-deprived rat, 343
Horse spleen ferritin, induced mesangial IgA
    deposits, 646
Hospitalization, backup, CAPD and, 1587
Human calcitonin (HCT), see Calcitonin (CT)
Human essential hypertension, renin in, 286–
    287
Human hypertension, Ca disturbances in, 1142
Human kidney tumor, ^{31}P-NMR of, 273
Human renal disease, see Renal disease
Human renal renin cDNA, 321
Human renal renin processing, 321–323
Human serum, characterization of antibodies
    and immunoreactive PTH components
    in, 1281–1282
Humans
  diabetic nephropathy in, clinical and renal
    studies of, 1053–1070
  immunologic aspects of IgA nephropathy in,
    652–660
  PTH measurements in, 1277–1287
Humoral mediator, of renal injury, 504–507

Humoral response, to donor-specific transfu-
    sions, 1716–1717
Hydrochlorothiazide, in Ca nephrolithiasis,
    1000–1001 1004
Hydrogen ion transport
  aldosterone action and, 383–385
  in CCT, 170–172
  in MCD, 172–174
  along nephron, 161–174
Hydrogen peroxide (H_2O_2), and mesangial
    cells, 611
  incubated with dexamethasone, 612–614
Hydrosmotic response, Vp-induced, 409–410
25 Hydroxyvitamin D3, osteodystrophy and,
    1399–1400
Hyperaldosteronism, role of, 456–458
Hypercalcemia
  acute, 1142–1143
  chronic, 1143
  after transplantation, 1649–1650
  thiazide treatment and, 1005
Hypercalciuria, 980
  Franconi syndrome with, 929–930
  idiopathic, 981
  thiazide diuretics in, 999–1001
Hypercatabolism, in ARF, pathogenesis of,
    763
  proteases and, 763–772
Hyperkalemia, non-azotemic, correction of,
    1648–1649
  factors producing, 1647
  after transplantation, 1646–1649
Hyperkelemia, NSAID-induced, 827
Hyperoxaluria, 983–984
  genetic, 984
Hyperparathyroidism, 981, 983
  glandular defect of PTH in, 1271–1274
  measurement of PTH in, 1299–1300
  thiazide treatment and, 1005–1006
  in uremia, pathogenic mechanisms of, 1358–
    1361
Hyperphosphatemia, PO$_4$ retention and, 1398
Hyperphosphatemic nephropathy, 880–881
Hypertension, 1115–1178, see also Blood pres-
    sure regulation
  autonomic nervous system and, 1120–1121
  control of, CAPD and, 1589–1590
  essential, see Essential hypertension
  Goldblatt, 82
  impaired Na excretion and, 1124–1125
  intervention of, in glomerulonephritis, 1456–
    1457
  kidney and, 1121–1125
  malignant, 1122
  management of, concepts of, 1125–1129

mechanisms of, current concepts, 1115–1129
mild, *see* Stratum I hypertension
portal, 466
reflux nephropathy and, 962–963
renal nerves in, 82
after transplantation, 1652–1653
resistance vessels in, 1116–1120
role of Na in, 1149–1151
role of PTH in, 1256–1257
role of renin-angiotensin system in, 1122–1123
smooth muscle hypertrophy and, 1116–1117
total peripheral resistance in, 1116
treatment of, 974
vesicoureteral reflux and, 943–944
Hyperuricosuria, thiazide treatment and, 1006
Hyperviscosity syndrome, 891
Hypocalcemia, and ARF, 1324
Hypophosphatemia, after transplantation, 1651–1652
Hypoproteinemia, localization of edema in, 443–444
Hypotension
CAPD and, 1594
hemorrhagic, saturation transfer NMR in, 273
Hypothalamic-pituitary-gonadal axis, 1328–1330
Hypovolemia, in leptospirosis, 1046–1047
Hypoxemia, arterial, dialysis-induced, 1543–1544

Icteric renal failure, in leptospirosis, 1042–1043
Idiopathic hypercalciuria, 981
Idiopathic IgA nephropathy, *see* IgA nephropathy
Idiopathic nephrotic syndrome (INS)
immunofluorescence findings in, 639
transplantation in, 639–640
IgA immune complex, in glomeruli, 533–534
IgA nephropathy
circulating immune complexes in, 654–655
clinical data in, 370–681
clinical prognostic markers of, 691–695
clinical signs of, 687–689
clinicopathologic correlations in, 665–682
electron microscopy in, 668–670
geographical distribution of, 686
glomerular morphology of, 667–668
histologic prognostic markers of, 691–695
history and outcome of, 689–691
HLA system and, 658–659
in humans, immunologic aspects of, 652–660
IgG immune complexes in, 655
immune cell abnormalities in, 656–658
as immune complex disease, 652–656
immunogenetic aspects of, 658–660
immunopathology of, 666–667
natural history of, 686–695
nature and origin of IgA in, 653–654
occurrence of, 686–687
pathogenic mechanisms of, 645–650
animal models and, 645–650
study of IgA complexes in, 653
tonsillectomy and, 696
treatment of, 695–696
upper respiratory tract infection and, 674
IgM mesangial nephropathy, 638–639
clinical presentation of, 638
Imaging techniques, new, 1430–1436
Immune cell abnormality, in IgA nephropathy, 656–658
Immune complex
cationic, 555–556
circulating, *see* Circulating immune complex
glomerular localization of, 489–491
in glomeruli
antigen-antibody systems and, 531–532
IgA, 533–534
mesangial zone and, 491
role of charge on, 532–533
and subendothelial deposits, 516–517
and subepithelial deposits, 514–515
Immune complex disease
antigen and antibody charge in, 550–558
chronic glomerulonephritis and, 491–492
IgA nephropathy as, 652–656
Immune complex formation
mechanisms of, 508–520
in situ, vs. circulating immune complex trapping, 520
proteoglycans and, 589
Immune response, glomerulonephritis treatment and, 1449–1450
Immunity, cell-mediated, 497–499
Immunization, in PTH measurements, 1280–1281
Immunocytochemistry, in distal nephron, 249–250
Immunohistological analysis, of biopsies during allograft, 1719–1720
Immunological monitoring, transplantation and, 1715–1723
Immunologically-mediated glomerulonephritis, 540–547

Immunosuppression, and transplantation, 1632–1636
Inactive renin, *see* Renin, inactive
Incipient diabetic nephropathy, 1054, 1060–1064
Increased interstitial fluid pressure (Pi), 440–442
Indirect cystography, vesicoureteral reflux and, 942
Indomethacin treatment, 825–826
Infants, pseudohypoaldosteronism in, 928–929
Infection, after transplantation, 1637–1638
Initial collecting tubule, K transport across, 263–264
Insulin, and ARF, 1326–1327
Insulin metabolism
  in chronic renal insufficiency, 1345
  and kidney, 1334–1335
Insulin pump treatment, perspective of, 1069
Insulin resistance, in chronic renal insufficiency, 1338–1339
  cellular mechanism, 1340–1341
  site of, 1339–1340
Insulin secretion, in renal insufficiency, 1336–1338
Insulin-dependent diabetes mellitus (IDDM), kidney biopsy and, 1103–1107
  future strategy, 1106–1107
Intact epithelium, 14
Interbundle capillary plexus, 93
Interbundle region, 97–98
Intercurrent illness, clinical condition prior to, 1508–1509
Intermittent peritoneal dialysis (IPD), 1539
Internephron heterogeneity, 197
Interstitial edema, in leptospirosis, 1045–1046
Interstitial fluid pressure (Pi), increased, 440–442
Interstitial nephritis, NSAID-induced, 826–827
Interstitial protein concentration
  estimates of, 439
  washdown of, 439–440
Interstitial-fluid-volume (IFV)
  constancy of, 435
  mechanisms opposing changes in, 437–438
  plasma volume vs., 444–445
Interventional radiology, 1433
Intestinal transport, of minerals, 1412–1421
Intra-arterial embolization, 1433
Intracellular pH, measurement of, 183
Intraglomerular pressure, diabetic nephropathy and, 1066
Intramembrane particle (IMP) aggregates, 410–411

Intranephron heterogeneity, 197
Intranephronic calculosis, 995–996
Intrarenal sodium retention, potential mechanisms of, 477
Intravascular coagulation, in leptospirosis, 1047
Intravascular hemolysis, in leptospirosis, 1047–1048
Intravenous digital subtraction angiography, 1431–1433
Ion metabolic disorder, after transplantation, 1649–1651
Ischemia, ^{31}P-NMR during, 270, 273
Ischemic injury
  role of Ca in, 794–795
  theory of mechanisms in, 795–796
Ischemic renal tubule injury, 778–779
Isobutyl methylxanthine (IBMX), and feedback response, 138–139
^{125}I-STZ uptake, with dexamethasone, 615

Jaundice, in leptospirosis, 1048
Juxtamedullary filtration rate, vasopressin and, 403–404
Juxtamedullary glomerulus(i), 87
Juxtamedullary nephron
  changes in blood flow to, 123–124
  K mass flow and, 191
  rubidium-86 fluxes in, 189–190
  tubuloglomerular feedback in, 125–126
  unidirectional fluxes in, 188

Kaposi's sarcoma, glomerular lesions in, 910
Kidney
  action of vasopressin on, 399–404
  diabetes mellitus and, 1053–1112
  effect of ADH on, 246
  endocrine system and, 340–430
  and hypertension, 1121–1125
    effect on, 1123–1124
  impaired endocrine activity of, 1508
  impaired metabolic activity of, 1508
  insulin metabolism and, 1334–1335
  ischemic insult to, cell volume regulation in, 37–38
  mammalian, anatomical features of, 397–398
  myeloma, 888–890
  PTH degradation by, 1297–1298
  rat
    effects of ADH, PTH, CT and glucagon on, 340–355
    renin in, intracellular actions of, 328–329
  thin-rim, 960

Kidney allograft, *see* Renal allograft
Kidney biopsy
  IDDM and, 1103–1107
  specimen studies of, 1106
Kidney disease, *see also* Renal disease
  evaluation and management of, 1425–1440
  in serum 1,25-(OH)$_2$-D in, 1309–1311
  in serum 24,25-(OH)$_2$-D, 1311–1312
  in tropics, 1030–1050
  urinary enzyme excretion in, 1427
  urine analysis in, 1425–1429
  urine solutes in, 1428–1429
  value of trials in, 1437–1440
  vitamin D in, 1305–1314
  vitamin D nutrition in, 1306–1307
Kidney function, *see also* Renal function
  effects of dDAVP, PTH, CT and glucagon
    on, 343–345
  excretory, TALH and, 352–353
  thyroid hormone and, 358–362
Kidney function tests, in diabetic patients,
    1054
Kidney glomerular filtration rate (KGFR),
    autoregulatory pattern for, 127
Kidney preservation, in transplantation, 1629
Kidney transplantation, *see* Renal transplanta-
    tion
Kinetic modeling, and dialysis treatment,
    1541–1542
Kinetics, of Na-dependent component of
    D-glucose flux, 26
Koefoed-Johnsen-Ussing double membrane
    model, 7
  for Na absorption, 7
Kupffer cell, 528–529

Lamina densa, immune complexes and, 535–
    537
Lattice of immune complex
  definition of, 529
  in glomerular deposition, 529–531
Leaky epithelium, 7
Lectin-gold cytochemistry, in distal nephron,
    249–250
Leptospira interrogans, 1041
Leptospires, in renal lesions, 1044
Leptospirosis
  immunologic mechanisms and, 1048–1049
  nephrotoxicity and, 1049–1050
  nonspecific effects of infection in, 1046–1048
  renal involvement in, 1041–1050
    clinical manifestations, 1041–1043
    pathogenesis, 1046–1050

  pathologic changes, 1043–1046
  treatment, 1043–1044
Leukemia, glomerular lesions in, 908–910
Light chain nephropathy, 898–902
  pathology of, 895–902
Lipid metabolism
  abnormalities in, CAPD and, 1593–1594,
    1616–1618
  role of PTH in, 1255–1256
Lipid synthesis, biochemical integrity of, 1220
Lipoid nephrosis, 640
Lipopolysaccharide (LPS), and anti-GBM an-
    tibody-induced injury, 505
Lipoxygenases, 280
Lithium, Na/H antiporter interaction with,
    73–75
Liver, PTH degradation by, 1298
LLC-PK$_1$ cells
  NaPO$_4$ cotransport regulation in, 62–64
Loop of Henle, *see* Henle's loop
Low frequency stimulation, of renal nerves,
    157
Luminal cell membrane, 227–228
  K conductance and, 227–228
Luminal membrane, thyroid action on, 358–
    360
Luminal potassium conductance, Ba inhibition
    of, 234–235
Lupus nephritis
  monitoring of, 1480
  outcome of, 1480–1481
  treatment of, 1480
Lymphocyte infiltration, of allograft, 1720–
    1721
Lymphoma
  cyclosporine and, 1670
  glomerular lesions in, 906–908
  after transplantation, 1638–1639

Macula densa signal, 143–144
Magnesium
  for Ca nephrolithiasis, 1016–1018
  interrelation of Ca and PTH with, 1144
Magnesium absorption, in renal failure, 1415–
    1417
Magnesium depletion, aminoglycoside nephro-
    toxicity and, 852
Magnesium transport, 1202–1203
Malaria, and nephrotic syndrome, 1033–1034
Malignancy, hematologic, 905–910
Malignant cell, growth of, 755
Malignant hypertension, plasma renin activity
    in, 1122
Maltase, vs. gp333, 567–568

Mammalian collecting duct, cell volume regulation in, 37
Mammalian kidney, anatomical features of,
397–398
Mannitol, and contrast-induced nephropathy,
840
Mantle field, 1696
Mass transfer area coefficient, in peritoneal
dialysis, 1563
Medulla
inner, 89, 98–99
solute escape from, 97
inner stripe of, 89, 93–95
species differences, 95
K recycling to, 217–219
effect on renal function, 218–219
outer stripe of, 89, 92–93
species differences, 93
O_2 supply to, 108–109
vascular organization of, 84–89
vascular-tubular relationships in, 89–92
Medullary blood flow
decrease in, 109–111
increase in, 109
intrarenal control of, 120–128
and urinary concentrating mechanism, 120–
128
sickle cell anemia and, 917
Medullary blood supply
measurement of, 100–101
regulation of, 99–101
modes of, 99–100
Medullary circulation
coupling of, 122–125
demands on, 107
organization of, 84–89, see also Medulla
pathophysiology of, 107–116
urine osmolarity and, 123–125
Medullary collecting tubule (MCT), aldosterone binding sites in, 373–377
H transport in, 172–174
Membrane particles, of thin limbs of Henle's
loop, heterogeneity of, 199–200
Membrane permeability, emerging concepts
on, 411–412
Membrane population, Na/H antiporter in,
71–72
Membrane resistance, in peritoneal dialysis,
1561–1562
Membranoproliferative glomerulonephritis
(MPGN)
anticoagulant therapy in, 1438–1439
Hodgkin's disease and, 907
non-Hodgkin lymphoma and, 907–908

prednisone therapy in, 1437–1438
treatment of, 1437–1440
Membranous glomerulonephritis (MGN)
in adults, 1036
Hodgkin's disease and, 906–907
role of hepatitis B virus and, 1032–1033
Menses, resumption of, CAPD and, 1587
Mercuric chloride glomerulopathy, 542–543
Mesangial antigen
fixed, 517
planted, 517–518
Mesangial cell
cationic molecules and, 553–554
circulating immune complex deposits in,
529–534
CSPG synthesis and, 590
culturing of, 610–611
function of, dexamethasone and, 609–617
H_2O_2 production by, 611
PGE_2 synthesis by, 611
role of, 724
Mesangial IgA deposition
active immunization, 646–647
extrapolations, 650
MCNS and, 680
mediation of injury, 648
natural history of, 648
passive models, 645–646
spontaneous models, 647–648
therapeutic considerations in, 648–650
Mesangial IgA nephropathy, see IgA nephropathy
Mesangial immune complex deposits, 517–519
circulating immune complexes and, 518–519
Mesangial proliferative glomerulonephritis,
637–638
Mesangial zone, immune complexes and, 491
Mesangium, see Measangial cell
Metabolic alkalosis, NH_3 production and, 274
Metabolic abnormalities, 1264–1355
in ARF, 1322–1331
in nephrotic syndrome, 1349–1355
Metabolic acidosis
effect on Na/H antiporter, 72
NH_3 production and, 274
Metabolic dysfunction, after transplantation,
1644–1655
Metabolic reaction, thyroid action and, 361
Metabolites, toxic drug, acetaminophen and,
812–813
Metal citrate inhibitor, of crystal growth,
1028–1029
Metastatic calcification, pathogenic mecha-
nisms of, 1362

Methotrexate nephrotoxicity, 872–875
  clinical manifestations of, 874–875
  histopathology of, 872–874
  pathogenesis of, 872–874
Methyl-CCNU nephrotoxicity, 875–876
3-0-Methylglucose, effect on Na activity, 14
Methylprednisolone, 1632–1633
Metolazone, in Ca nephrolithiasis, 1000
Mice
  mesangial IgA deposition in, 645–646
  transplantation tolerance in, 1700
Michaelis-Menten kinetics, 24
Microalbuminuria, 1081–1082
  Albustix-positive proteinuria and, 1095–
    1096
Microcirculation, glomerular, influence of re-
    nal nerves on, 154–159
Microperfusion, cell puncture technique and,
    180–184
Microscopic analysis, of urine, 1425–1429
Mineralocorticoids
  K secretion and, 263–264
  Na-K-ATPase activity and, 267–268
Minerals, intestinal transport of, in renal fail-
    ure, 1412–1421
Minimal change nephrotic syndrome, 635
Minor change nephrotic syndrome, and mesan-
    gial IgA deposits, 680
Mithramycin nephrotoxicity, 876
Mitochondrial cell injury, 796–797
Mitochondrial dysfunction, gentamicin
    nephrotoxicity and, 859
Mitochondrial energy transport, PO₄ depletion
    and, 1223
Mitomycin-C nephrotoxicity, 876
M-mTAL-1C cell line, 6
Monoclonal antibody
  glomerulonephritis and, 505
  as probes of renal structure, 575–579
  in allograft, 1689–1691
  in ransplantation, 1635–1636, 1687–1691
Monoclonal antibody monitoring, in post-
    transplant patient, 1718
Monoclonal antilymphocyte antibody
  preparation of, 1687
  production and administration of, 1687–
    1689
Mononuclear phagocyte system, circulating
    immune complex removal by, 528–
    529
Mouse, renin gene duplication in, 320
Mouse kidney renin, structure of, 323
Mouse SMG renin cDNA, 318–319
Mouse SMG renin processing, 319–320

Multiple myeloma
  electrolyte disturbances in, 885–886
  renal abnormalities in, 886–891
  renal involvement in, 885–892
  treatment of, 891–892
Mycoplasma pneumoniae, 656
Myelogenous leukemia, glomerular lesions in,
    909
Myeloma kidney, 888–890
  characteristics of, 895–897
  experimental models and, 897–898
  THP in, 897
Myocardial function, PTH in, 1254–1255
Myocardial injury, PO4 depletion and, 1217–
    1228
Myofibrillar energy usage, PO₄ depletion and,
    1223

Na:substrate stoichiometry, static head method
    of, 28–30
Natriuresis
  immersion-induced, 453–454
  renal nerve activity and, 80
Natriuretic factor, atrial, 257–259
Necturus epithelium, effect of galactose on,
    8–9
Necturus maculosus, 8
Neomycin, for mesangial IgA deposits, 649
Nephritis
  anti-GBM, and Goodpasture syndrome, 494
  Heymann, *see* Heymann nephritis
  interstitial, NSAID-induced, 826–827
  nephrotoxic serum, arachidonic acid metab-
    olism in, 506, 601–607
  Steblay's, 494
  streptococcal fractions triggering, 624
Nephritogenic streptococcus, 623–625
Nephritogenicity, of cationic proteins, 551
Nephrogenic diabetes insipidus, 928
Nephrolithiasis, Ca oxalate, thiazide diuretics
    in, 999–1006
Nephron
  binding of corticosteroid hormones along,
    364–367
  cell injury along, 718–719
  distal
    CA-C in, 249–250
    CaBP in, 249–250
    components of, 243
    cortical segment of, 247–248
    role of adrenal hormones in, 248–249
    structural heterogeneity of, 243–250
    TALH of, 243–247
    use of immunocytochemistry in, 249–250

Nephron (*cont.*)
  use of lectin-gold cytochemistry in, 249–
      250
  H ion transport along, 161–174
  localization of aldosterone receptors along,
      372–378
  structure and transport along, 161–250
Nephron acidification, distal, 1187–1188
Nephron heterogeneity, physiological signifi-
      cance of, 204–205
Nephropathy, *see also Specific types*
  combined light chain, 890
  contrast-induced
    clinical course of, 839
    diagnosis of, 839
    furosemide and, 840
    incidence of, 836
    laboratory findings of, 839
    mannitol and, 840
    pathogenesis of, 836–839
    prophylaxis and, 839
    risk factors for, 836
    therapy for, 839
  hyperphosphatemic, 880–881
  light chain, 898–902
    pathology of, 895–902
  xanthine, 880
Nephrosis, aminonucleoside, proteoglycan
      synthesis in, 587–588
Nephrotic syndrome
  in adults, 1034–1037
  blood volume in, 471–472
  in children, 1031–1034
  clinical management of, 921–922
  diagnostic tools and, 634–635
  endocrine and metabolic abnormalities in,
      1349–1355
  GFR in, 475–476
  malaria and, 1033–1034
  Na retention in, 477
    renal, 469–479
    tubular site of, 477–479
  platelet arachidonate metabolism in, 1407–
      1409
  renal response to volume expansion, 472–
      473
  renin-angiotensin-aldosterone and, 473–474
  in tropical Africa, 1030–1037
Nephrotoxic serum nephritis
  arachidonic acid metabolism in, 506, 601–
      607
  biochemical and physiologic alterations of,
      604–605
  heterologous response in, 603

Nephrotoxicity, 807–881
  acetaminophen and, 812–813
  aminoglycoside, *see* Aminoglycoside
      nephrotoxicity
  amphotericin B and, 810–811
  antibiotic-induced, 844–860
  5-azacytidine-induced, 876–877
  cancer chemotherapy induced
    direct, 869–877
    endogenous, 877–881
  cephalosporins and, 811
  cis-platinum induced, *see* Cis-platinum
      nephrotoxicity
  cyclosporine and, 813–814
  defining, 807–808
  drug
    alterations in GFR and, 807–808
    mechanisms of, 807–814
  gentamicin, 855
  leptospirosis and, 1049–1050
  methotrexate induced, *see* Methotrexate
      nephrotoxicity
  methyl-CCNU induced, 875–876
  mithramycin induced, 876
  mitomycin-C induced, 876
  nitrosoureas induced, 875–876
  of NSAID, 819–828
  streptozotocin induced, 875
Neuroblastoma cell, renin in, intracellular ac-
      tions of, 329–331
Neurologic status, CAPD and diabetic patient,
      1606
Neuropathy
  CAPD and, 1591
  membranous, induced, 494–496
Nifedipine
  for hypertension, 1167
  postischemic infusion of, 792–793
Niridazole, 1709–1710
Nitrosoureas nephrotoxicity, 875–876
Non-Hodgkin lymphoma, glomerular lesions
      in, 907–908
Non-steroidal anti-inflammatory drugs
      (NSAID), in glomerular disease, 1487–
      1488
Nonantibody-dependent complement activa-
      tion, 499
Nonrenal antigen
  and subendothelial deposits, 515–516
  and subepithelial deposits, 511–515
Nonsteroidal anti-inflammatory drugs
      (NSAID)
  anaphylaxis and, 827
  clinical syndromes and, 824–828
  cyclo-oxygenase inhibition and, 820

effect on ARF, 823
effect on GFR, 822
effect on RBF, 820–823
hyperkelemia and, 827
interstitial nephritis and, 826–827
Na retention and, 827
nephrotoxicity of, 819–828
renal insufficiency associated with, 825–826
water retention and, 827
Norepinephrine, vascular smooth muscle and,
    1117–1118
Nuclear magnetic resonance (NMR), 1431,
    1435–1436
  pulse and collect, 270
  quantitative, 270
  saturation transfer, 270
    in hemorrhagic hypotension, 273
  vesicoureteral reflux and, 943
Nutrients
  drug interference with, 1507
  inadequate intake of, 1500
  losses from dialysis, 1506–1507
Nutrition
  CAPD and diabetic patient, 1605
  and dialysis treatment, 1542–1543
  and experimental renal disease, 1517–1518
  influence on renal insufficiency, 1516–1524
  in renal failure, 1498–1524

3-O-methylglucose, effect on Na activity, 14
25(OH)D₃-1α-hydroxalase, activation of,
    1213–1214
Opsonized particles, preparation of, 611
Oral glucose tolerance test (OGTT), and
    nephrotic syndrome, 1353
Oral serum sickness, 646
Organic anion/hydroxyl antiporter, in brush-
    border membrane vesicles, 164
Orthograde microperfusion studies, 133–134
Orthophosphate, for Ca nephrolithiasis, 1011–
    1014
Orthostasis, vascular adjustments in, 442–443
Osmolality, effect on NaCl absorption, 215
Osmotic equilibration, of proximal fluid with
    interstitial osmolality, 192
Osteitis fibrosa, 1312
  dialysis and, 1362
  in hemodialysis patients, 1374–1381
Osteodystrophy, 1357–1401
  renal, see Renal osteodystrophy
Osteomalacia
  aluminum-related
    prevention of, 1391
    treatment of, 1389–1391

dialysis and, 1362–1364
  in hemodialysis patients, 1374–1381
  refractory dialysis, 1383–1384
  renal, 1361–1362
Ouabain, inhibition of Na-K-ATPase activity
    by, 237
Ovalbumin, induced mesangial IgA deposits,
    646
Overt diabetic nephropathy, 1064–1065
Oxygen, supply to medulla, 108–109
Oxygen preradicals, in glomerular injury, 507

Papillary necrosis, 922
Para-aminophenol, toxicity of, 813
Paracellular pathway
  cation selectivity of, 225–227
  conductances of, 226
  resistance of, 225
Paraproteinemia, electrolyte disturbances in,
    885–886
Parathyroid gland activity
  Ca and, 1267–1268
  regulation of, 1264–1275
    future investigations of, 1274–1275
Parathyroid hormone (PTH)
  alterations in CRF, 1292–1301
  in aluminum-related osteomalacia, 1385–
    1386
  bioassays of, 1278–1279
  in blood pressure regulation, 1145–1146
  Ca insensitivity, 1272–1274
  cardiovascular effect of, 1145
  concentration in uremia, 1252
  effects on Henle's loop, 345–347, 349–352
  effects on plasma composition 343–345
  effects on rat kidney, 340–355
  effects on TALH, 349–352
  hyperparathyroidism and
    glandular defect in, 1271–1274
    measurement of, 1299–1300
  glomerular and tubular effects, 345
  immunoreactive components of, 1281–1282
  measurement of, in hyperparathyroidism,
    1299–1300
  measurements in humans, 1277–1287
  N-RIA vs. C-RIA, 1285–1286
  peripheral metabolism of, 1297–1299
  postreceptor effects of, 1253
  radioimmunoassay of, 1279–1286
  regulation of, by vitamin D metabolites,
    1296–1297
  role in eyrthropoiesis, 1253–1254
  role in lipid metabolism, 1255–1256
  role in myocardial function, 1254–1255

Parathyroid hormone (*cont.*)
  secretion and synthesis of, regulation of, 1266–1271
  synthesis, structure and secretion of, 1293–1296
Parathyroid hormone messenger RNA, Ca and, 1268–1271
Parathyroidectomy
  blood pressure response to, 1145
  intravenous indications of, 1368–1369
Parathyroidism, role in hypertension, 1256–1257
Parenteral-nutrition-related bone disease, 1386–1387
Pars recta, 92–93
  transport properties of, 186–193
P-chloromercuribenzene sulfonate (PCMBS), in PCT, 179
Penicillamine, 649
Penicillin G, in leptospirosis, 1043
Pepstatin, and congeners, 287
Peptide hormones, 353–354
Percutaneous nephrostomy techniques, 1433
Percutaneous transluminal angioplasty, 1433
Pericarditis, CAPD and, 1590–1591
Peripheral disease, CAPD and diabetic patient, 1606
Peripheral vascular disease, CAPD and, 1594
Peritoneal clearances, CAPD and diabetic patient, 1604
Peritoneal dialysis, 1538–1539
  anatomic and physiologic aspects of, 1561–1575
  disease affecting, 1573–1575
  exogenous agents in, 1571–1573
  indexes of solute transport in, 1563–1566
  membrane resistances in, 1561–1562
  problems in, 1539–1540
Peritoneal energy supply, effects on carbohydrate metabolism, 1612–1613
Peritoneal ultrafiltration, 1566–1571
pH
  alpha-ketoglutarate and, 275
  changes in, renal NH_3 production and, 273–276
  effect on PO_4 transport, 57–60
  intracellular, 183
Phagocytosis
  mesangial cell function in, dexamethasone and, 609–617
  steroids and, 610
Phagocytosis assay, 612
Phenacetin, toxicity of, 813
Phenytoin, for mesangial IgA deposits, 649

Phloretin, inhibition of Na-K-ATPase activity by, 237
Phosphate absorption
  physiology of, in renal failure, 1412–1414
  after renal transplantation, 1415
  in uremia, 1414
Phosphate depletion, 1183–1228
  in diabetes mellitus, 1184–1185
  effect on glomerular filtration, 1188–1191
  effect on renal tubular transport, 1198–1205
  effect on urinary acidification, 1183–1193
  energy metabolism and, 1210–1213
  life threatening causes of, 1184
  mechanisms of myocardial injury in, 1217–1228
  and renal cell metabolism, 1209–1215
Phosphate retention
  and hyperphosphatemia, 1398
  in uremia, 1358
Phosphate transport, 1198–1200
  across brushborder membrane, effect of Na and pH on, 57–60
  in thyroidectomized rat, 358–359
Phospholipid precursors, 1220
Phosphorus
  interrelation of Ca and PTH with, 1143
  removal by CAPD, 1588–1589
Phosphorylation
  of cell-ATP, 1225–1226
  with γ-^{32}P-ATP, 61
  in Na/K cotransport, 60–62
Pituitary adrenal axis, and ARF, 1330
Pituitary gland, renin in, 331
Plasma, proteolytic enzyme systems in, 765
Plasma composition, effects of dDAVP, PTH, CT and glucagon on, 343–345
Plasma concentration, and CAPD, 1614
Plasma elastase α_1 protease inhibitor complex, in ARF, 766
Plasma exchange
  controlled trial of, 1478–1479
  outcome of, 1479
  for glomerular disease, 1474–1483
Plasma proteins, on GBM, 488
Plasma renin activity
  in essential hypertension, 1122
  in malignant hypertension, 1122
Plasma volume, vs. interstitial-fluid-volume, 444–445
Plasmodium malariae, 1033
Platelet abnormality, prostanoid-related, 1406–1409
Platelet arachidonate metabolism
  in nephrotic syndrome, 1407–1409
  in renal failure, 1406–1407

P³¹-NMR
  during ischemia, 270, 273
  of kidney tumor, 273
Podocyte, changes in, 722–724
Polyclonal antibody, in transplantation, 1682–
  1687
Polyclonal antilymphocyte antibody
  preparation of, 1682–1683
  production and administration of, 1683–
  1684
Portal hypertension, 466
Post-renal transplant patient, monoclonal antibody monitoring in, 1718
Poststreptococcal glomerulonephritis, 623–629
  epidemiology of, 626–627
  genetic considerations in, 627–628
  pathogenesis of, 625–626
  prognosis for, 628
Potassium
  homocellular, regulatory mechanisms for,
  14–17
  removal by CAPD, 1588
Potassium citrate therapy, therapeutic role of,
  1029
Potassium concentration, effect on NaCl absorption, 215–216
Potassium conductance
  Ba inhibition of, 234–235
  of luminal cell membrane, 227–228
  of basolateral cell membrane, 228–229
Potassium depletion, aminoglycoside nephrotoxicity and, 852
Potassium excretion, regulation of, 260–268
Potassium -42 flux, measurement of, 188
Potassium-leak unit, cytokinetics of, 15–17
Potassium mass flow
  and juxtamedullary nephron, 191
  and superficial nephron, 191
Potassium metabolism, in chronic renal insuffi-
  ciency, 1345
Potassium permeability, of CCT, 264–266
Potassium recycling, to medulla, 217–219
  effect on renal function, 218–219
Potassium secretion
  DOCA and, 383
  regulation of, Na-K-ATPase activity and,
  266–268
Potassium transport
  aldosterone action and, 382–383
  cellular electrophysiology of, 266
  DOCA in, 266
  across initial collecting tubule, 263–264
Pre-proparathyroid hormone, structure of,
  1265–1266
Prednisone therapy, in MPGN, 1437–1438

Pregnancy, reflux nephropathy and, 963–964
Pressure diuresis, 128
Primary biliary cirrhosis, 467
Primary glomerular disease, 623–696
Progressive IgA renal disease, 680–681
Proliferative glomerulonephritis, 1034–1035
Promethazine, 1710–1711
Pro-(Phe⁵Phe⁶)octapeptidyllysine, renin inhi-
  bition by 290–292
Propranolol, prevention of ARF, 784–789
Proprenin peptides, as renin inhibitors, 292–
  293
Prorenin, see Renin, inactive
Prostaglandin E₁ (PGE₁), for mesangial IgA
  deposits, 649
Prostaglandin E₂ (PGE₂)
  action of, on NaCl transport, 212–214
  mesangial cells and, 612–614
  mesangial cell synthesis of, 611
  NaCl absorption and, 210, 212
Prostaglandins
  glomerulonephritis treatment and, 1455
  and NSAID
    effects on Na excretion, 824
    effects on renin release, 823
    effects on water excretion, 824
  physiologic effects of, 819–824
  renal, biochemistry of, 277–282
  in tubuloglomerular feedback, 140
  vasodilatory role for, 821–822
Prostaglandin synthesis, stimuli of, 819–820
Prostanoid-related platelet abnormality, 1406–
  1409
Protease, in catabolic renal failure, 765–769
Protein
  adenosine-induced, late, 391–392
  aldosterone-induced, 388–389
  cationic, nephritogenicity of, 551
Protein loss, during CAPD, 1613
Protein matrix, renal stones and, 985
Protein restriction, in renal disease, 1240
Proteinuria
  Albustix-positive, microalbuminuria and,
  1095–1096
  anionic site changes in GBM and, 585–586
  anti-GBM antibodies and, 603
  Bence Jones, 886–887
  in diabetic nephropathology, pathophysiology of, 1081–1091
  in diabetic nephropathy, 1095–1097
  and glomerular pathology, 677, 680
  reflux nephropathy and, 964–968
Proteoglycans
  and GBM permeability properties, 584–585
  association with GBM, 590

Proteoglycans (*cont.*)
  biosynthesis of
    in aminonucleoside nephrosis, 587–588
    in glomerular disease, 587–589
  functions of, 584
  from GBM, 582–584
  in glomerular function and pathology, 580–597
  and immune complex formation, 589
  involvement in glomerular pathology, 585–586
  properties of, 581–582
Proteoglycan synthesis
  in aminonucleoside nephrosis, 587–588
  in experimental diabetes, 588–589
  glomerular cell type and, 590–591
  in glomerular disease, 587–589
Proteolytic enzyme systems
  in plasma, 765
  in uremic rat, 769–770
Proton-translocating ATPase, in brushborder membrane vesicles, 164–165
Proximal convoluted tubule (PCT), 161–169
  acidification of
    amiloride and, 166–167
    DCCD and, 166
  aldosterone binding sites in, 373–374
  bicarbonate conductance in, 167–168
  bicarbonate reabsorption by, 161
  distal segment, 169–170
  H ion transport mechanisms in, 162–165
  microperfusion and, 180–184
  Na/H antiporter in, 162–163
  Na transport in, 165–166
  PCMBS and, 179
  proximal segment, 161–169
  acidification in, 161–169
  transport in, 178–185
Proximal straight tubule (PST), cell volume regulation in, 34–35
Proximal tubular cell, D-glucose handling by, 21–23
Proximal tubular function, sickle cell anemia and, 919
Proximal tubule
  action of thyroid hormone on, 358–362
  regulation of Na/H antiporter of, 70–77
Proximal tubule bicarbonate reabsorption, 1185–1186
  effect of K depletion on, 1189–1191
Proximal tubule reflection coefficient, for NaCl, 179–180
Psammomys obesus, 247
Pseudohypoaldosteronism, in infants, 928–929

Pulse methylprednisolone, in glomerular disease, 1464–1472
Puromycin aminonucleoside (PAN), 474–475
Pyelonephritis, chronic atrophic, *see* Reflux nephropathy
Pyridoxine, for Ca nephrolithiasis, 1021
Pyrophosphate, crystal growth inhibitor, 986–987

Quinidine, effects on Ca ions, 41–42

Radioactive ligands, 1280
Radioimmunoassay, in PTH measurements, 1279–1286
  results, 1283–1285
Radiologic contrast media, damage induced by, 835–842
Rapidly progressive glomulonephritis (RPGN)
  characteristics of, 1464
  comparative treatments of, 1468–1469
    risk-benefit relationship, 1471–1472
  pulse methylprednisolone in, 1465–1466
    results of, 1466–1468
Rat
  bile duct ligation in, 461–462
  experimental uremia in, 769–772
  hormone-deprived, 343
  thyroidectomized
    K transport in, 358–359
    Na transport in, 359
  transplantation tolerance in, 959–961
  uremic
    proteolysis of skeletal muscle in, 770–772
    proteolytic activity in, 770
    proteolytic enzyme systems in, 769–770
Rat glomerulus(i), HSPG in, 592–595
Rat kidney, *see* Kidney, rat
R2 chemoreceptors, 81
Reflux nephropathy
  glomerular lesions in, 964–966
  hypertension and, 962–963
  natural history of, 959–970
  pregnancy and, 963–964
  proteinuria and, 964–968
  renal failure from, 968–970
  renal function and, 961–962
  scar formation in, 959–961
  therapeutic approaches in, 970–975
Refractory dialysis osteomalacia, 1383–1384
Relative supersaturation ratio (SS), 992
Renal acid excretion, sickle cell anemia and, 918–919

Renal afferent nerves, neurophysiology of, 81
Renal allograft
  biopsies taken during, immunohistological
      analysis of, 1719–1720
  HLA matching in, 1676–1677
  in vitro lymphocyte infiltration of, 1720–
      1721
  monoclonal antibodies in, 1689–1691
  rejection of, I-TXB2 in, 1721
  transfusion effect in, 1674–1679
    age and, 1677–1678
    changing impact of, 1675
    cumulative, 1674–1675
    histocompatability and, 1676–1677
    in pediatric recipients, 1678
  use of ALG in, 1684–1687
    clinical reactions and, 1686–1687
Renal autoregulation
  simulation study of, 127
  urine concentration mechanism and, 126–
      128
Renal basement membrane, components of,
    486–499
Renal blood flow (RBF)
  in experimental ARF, 731–732
  increased, 793–794
  NSAID effect on, 820–823
  sickle cell anemia and, 916–917
Renal cell injury
  amelioration of, 716–718
  ATP-MgCl$_2$ infusion and, 717
  Ca and, 716–717
  mechanisms of, 714–716
  stage 2, 712
  stage 3, 712–713
  stage 4, 713
  stage 5, 713–714
  stage 6, 714
  stage 7, 714
Renal cell metabolism, PO$_4$ depletion and,
    1209–1215
Renal circulation, 84–128
Renal compensatory growth, after uninephrec-
    tomy, 753–754
Renal concentrating mechanism, sickle cell
    anemia and, 917–918
Renal corpuscle, role in ARF, 720–721
Renal countercurrent system
  coupling of medullary circulation and, 122–
      125
  limitations of, 122
  mathematical model of, 121–122
Renal damage
  early indicators of, 1099–1100

radiologic contrast-induced, 835–842, see
    also Nephropathy
  vesicoureteral reflux and, 936–944
Renal denervation, renin-angiotensin-aldoster-
    one system and, 80–81
Renal disease, see also Kidney disease
  experimental glomerular hyperfusion and,
      1233–1236
  nutrition and, 1517–1518
  hematologic malignancies in, 905–910
  immunologic mechanisms in, 485–499
  mechanisms of progression of, 1233–1242
  progressive nature of, 1236–1238
    alternative explanations of, 1238–1240
    therapies interrupting, 1240–1241
  prostanoid-related platelet abnormalities in,
      1406–1409
Renal epithelial cell, see Epithelium(ia)
Renal failure
  acute, see Acute renal failure (ARF)
  aluminum absorption in, 1417–1419
  Ca absorption in, 1412–1414
  chronic, see also Chronic renal failure
    alterations in, 1292–1301
    pathogenesis and consequences of, 1233–
        1257
  clinical condition prior to, 1508–1509
  clinical management of, 922
  end-stage, 969–970
  evaluation and management of, 1425–1440
  indomethacin-induced, 825–826
  intestinal transport of minerals in, 1412–
      1421
  in leptospirosis, 1042–1043
  Mg absorption in, 1415–1417
    formula for, 1415
  nutrition in, 1498–1524
  platelet arachidonate metabolism in, 1406–
      1407
  PO$_4$ absorption in, 1412–1414
  from reflux nephropathy, 968–970
  sources of aluminum in, 1387–1388
  Zn absorption in, 1420–1421
Renal function, see also Kidney function
  effect of diet on, 1521–1524
  effect of K recycling on, 218–219
  reflux nephropathy and, 961–962
  residual, CAPD and, 1604
Renal glyconeogenesis, 1213
Renal graft survival, DTH and, 1715–1716
Renal hemodynamics, 857
  changes in, angiotensin II and, 159
Renal hyperfunction-hypertrophy, 1057–1060
Renal hypophosphatemic rickets, 926–927
Renal injury, 504–507

Renal insufficiency
   influence of nutrition on, 1516–1524
   measuring progression of, 1519–1521
   NSAID-induced, 825–826
   prior, aminoglycoside nephrotoxicity and,
      852
Renal ischemia
   medullary blood flow and, 110–111
   recovery phases of, 111
Renal mechanoreceptor stimulation
   ARNA and, 81–82
   ERNA and, 81–82
Renal medulla, see Medulla
Renal metabolism, contemporary issues in,
      269–276
Renal nerves, 79–83
   afferent, hypertension and, 82
   and changes in body Na, 80
   functions of, 79–83
   high frequency stimulation of, 156–157
   in hypertension, 82
   influence on glomerular microcirulation,
      154–159
   low frequency stimulation of, 157
   natriuresis and, 80
Renal NH$_3$ production, changes in pH, 273–
      276
Renal osteodystrophy
   1α-(OH)vitamin D$_3$ in, 1364–1366
   aluminum accumulation in, 1383–1391
   CAPD and, 1593
   Ca supplementation in, 1398–1399
   in CRF, treatment of, 1396–1401
   current issues, 1357–1369
   and dialysate composition, 1401
   and 1,25 dihydroxyvitamin D, 1400–1401
   general concepts, 1357–1369
   and 25 hydroxyvitamin D$_3$, 1399–1400
   pathophysiology of, 1357–1364
      before dialysis, 1357–1362
      during dialysis, 1362–1364
   treatment of, 1398–1401
   vitamin D metabolites in, 1312–1314
   vitamin D sterols in, 1367–1368
   and vitamin D$_2$, 1399
   and vitamin D$_3$, 1399
Renal osteomalacia, pathogenic mechanisms
      of, 1361–1362
Renal parenchymal hypertrophy, in scar for-
      mation, 961–962
Renal potassium excretion, abnormalities of,
      927–928
Renal prostaglandins, biochemistry of, 277–
      282

Renal regeneration
   after acute tubular necrosis, 748–758
   adenine nucleotides and, 750–751
   amino acids and, 749–750
   control of, an hypothesis, 755–758
   thyroxin and, 751
Renal renin cDNA, 321
Renal renin processing, 321–323
Renal salt retention, 474–475
Renal scars
   age and, 960–961
   caused by UTI, 1443–1444
   evolution of, 950–951
   parenchymal hypertrophy and, 961–962
   and vescoureteric reflux, 948–957
Renal segmental atrophy
   clinical background of, 949–950
   identification of, 949
   pathogenesis of, 948
   pathologic observations, 951–953
   pathology and pathogenesis of, 948–957
Renal sodium excretion, PGE and NSAID ef-
      fect on, 824
Renal stones, pathogenesis of, 980–987
Renal structure, monoclonal antibodies as
      probes of, 575–579
Renal transplantation
   blood transfusions in, 1636–1637
   Ca absorption after, 1415
   cadaver, trials of TLI in, 1702–1704
   CAPD and, 1581–1585
   complications of, 1637–1639
   current status, 1627–1639
   cyclosporine in, 1662–1671
   diagnosis of rejection in, 1637
   donor for, 1628–1629
   EBV infection after, 1639
   endocrine dysfunctions after, 1644–1655
   erythrocytosis after, 1653
   HLA and, 1629–1632
   hypertension after, 1652–1653
   hypophosphatemia after, 1651–1652
   immunological monitoring and, 1715–1723
   immunosuppression and, 1632–1636
   indications and contraindications, 1628
   ion metabolic disorders after, 1649–1651
   kidney preservation in, 1629
   metabolic dysfunctions after, 1644–1655
   monoclonal antibody therapy in, 1687–1691
   non-azotemic hyperkalemia after, 1646–
      1649
   PO$_4$ absorption after, 1415
   polyclonal antibody therapy in, 1682–1687
   results of, 1639

RTA after, 1644–1646
sensitized patient and positive crossmatch,
    1631–1632
TLI in, 1695–1705
Renal tubular acidosis (RTA)
    clinical management of, 922
    after renal transplantation, 1644–1646
Renal tubular cell damage, drugs and, 808–
    809
Renal tubular dysfunction, multiple myeloma
    and, 890–891
Renal tubular necrosis, acetaminophen and,
    812–813
Renal tubular transport
    effect of PO_4 depletion on, 1198–1205
    role of cytosolic Ca in, 51–55
Renal tubule injury, ischemic, 778–779
Renal vasculitis
    monitoring of, 1477
    outcome of, 1477–1478
    treatment of, 1477
Renal vasoconstriction, in ARF, 703–704
Renal water excretion, PGE and NSAID ef-
    fects on, 824
Renin
    in adrenal cortical cell, 332–333
    in adrenal medulla, 332
    in brain, intracellular actions of, 329–331
    in essential hypertension, 286–287
    inactive, 302–314
        activation of, 303–308
        cryoactivation of, 305
        factors influencing circulating levels of,
            308–312
        Hageman factor-kallikrein system and,
            305–306
        physiochemical characteristics of, 313–
            314
        trypsin and, 303–304
    intracellular actions of, 327–336
    in kidney, intracellular actions of, 328–329
    mouse kidney, structure of, 323
    in neuroblastoma cell, intracellular actions
        of, 329–331
    in pituitary gland, 331
    structure and processing of, 318–325
    in testis, 333
    three-dimensional structure of, 293–297
    in tissues, 331
    in vascular tissues, 333
Renin action, control of, in cell, 336
Renin gene, 318–325
    duplication of, in mouse, 320
    structural organization of, 324

Renin inhibition, 287–293
    animal studies in, 290
    human studies in, 290–292
    prorenin peptides and, 292–293
    research on, 284–298
    by RIP, 290–292
Renin messenger RNA, 318–323
Renin release, PGI_2 and NSAID effects on,
    823
Renin-angiotensin system, 333–334
    arterial smooth muscle and, 1117
    in experimental ARF, 733
    functional considerations in, 334–336
    interaction with sympathetic nervous sys-
        tem, 430
    physiologic role of, in hypertension, 1122–
        1123
Renin-angiotensin-aldosterone system
    nephrotic syndrome and, 473–474
    renal denervation and, 80–81
Renin-specific antibodies, 285–286
Renorenal reflexes, 81–82
Resistance vessels, in hypertension, 1116–1120
Respiratory alkalosis, NH_3 production and,
    274
Respiratory acidosis, NH_3 production and, 274
Retrograde microperfusion studies, 134–135
    with TMB-8, 137
Rheumatoid arthritis, immune changes after
    TLI in, 1699
Rheumatoid factor, in circulating immune
    complex, 534
Rhizopus chinensis, 293
Ribosylation reactions, in $NaPO_4$ cotransport,
    60–62
Rickets, renal hypophosphatemic, 926–927
RNA, renin messenger, 318–323
Rubidium-86 flux
    in juxtamedullary nephron, 189–190
    measurement of, 188

Salicylate, toxicity of, 813
Schistosoma hemotobium, 1036
Schistosoma mansoni, 1036
Schistosomiasis, 1036–1037
Sensing cells, 132
Sequential filtration, and hemodialysis, 1533
Serum 1,25-$(OH)_2$-D
    in health, 1307–1309
    in kidney disease, 1309–1311
Serum 1,25$(OH)_2$-D_3, ARF and, 1325
Serum 24,25-$(OH)_2$-D, in kidney disease,
    1311–1312
Serum clearance, in peritoneal dialysis, 1563

Serum phosphate, and ARF, 1323–1324
Serum proteins, and CAPD, 1613
Serum sickness, 527–528
  and ALG in renal allografts, 1686
Sex, gentamicin nephrotoxicity and, 855
Sexual function, CAPD and, 1586
Sickle cell anemia
  glomerular pathology and, 919–920
  renal circulation and, 916–917
  tubular function and, 917–919
Sickle cell nephropathy, 916–922
  reduced papillary flow and, 109–110
Single nephron glomerular filtration rate
    (SNGFR)
  determinants of, 155–156
  measurement of, 131
Single nephron inulin clearance (SNC$_{In}$), ATP-
    MgCl$_2$ and, 803
Single-needle dialysis, using subclavian access,
    1555–1556
Sjögren's syndrome, 655
Skin eruptions, and ALG in allografts, 1686
Sodium
  effect on PO$_4$ transport across vesicles, 57–
    60
  homocellular, regulatory mechanisms for,
    14–17
  interrelation of Ca and PTH with, 1144
  renal nerve activity and, 80
Sodium-absorbing epithelium, basolateral
    membrane properties of, 7–17
Sodium-calcium exchange process, in rabbit tu-
    bules, 53–55
Sodium chloride, proximal tubule reflection
    coefficient for, 179–180
Sodium chloride absorption
  effect of K concentration on, 215–216
  effect of osmolality on, 215
  glucagon and, 211
  hormonal regulation of, 210–212
  PGE$_2$ and, 210, 212
  regulation of, 216–217
  solute concentration effects on, 214–216
  by TALH, role of K in, 261–262
  vasopressin and, 210–211
Sodium chloride hormone, ADH and, 212–214
Sodium-chloride-potassium cotransport
  in TAL cell, 230–231
  furosemide and, 236
Sodium chloride reabsorption
  cyclic AMP stimulation of, 237–238
  effect of inhibitors of, 225–226
  increased, vasopressin and, 402
  in TAL cell, inhibitors of, 234–237
  in TALH, 218–219

Sodium chloride transport
  action of PGE$_2$ on, 212–214
  rate of, in TALH, 210
  regulation of, by Henle's loop, 208–220
  regulatory complexities of, 209
Sodium excretion, effect on hypertension,
    1124–1125
Sodium-glucose cotransport mechanisms, 21–
    32
Sodium homeostasis, of cirrhosis, afferent
    events, 449–454
  efferent events, 454–455
Sodium/hydrogen antiporter
  amiloride interaction with, 75–76
  asymmetrical distribution of, 70–72
  effect of metabolic acidosis on, 72
  external aspect of, 76
  lithium interaction with, 73–75
  in membrane populations, 71–72
  in PCT, 162–163
  regulation of, 72
    by cellular and biochemical mechanisms,
      73–77
    of proximal tubule, 70–77
Sodium phosphate cotransport
  cycloheximide and, 63–64
  kinetic parameters of, 58
  in LLC-PK$_1$ cells
    cyclic AMP and, 63
    regulation of, 62–64
  model for, 58
  properties of, 57–58
  phosphorylation and ribosylation reactions
    in, 60–62
  studies with vesicles, 57–62
Sodium-potassium-ATPase activity
  aldosterone action and, 388–394
  aldosterone and corticosterone effect on,
    364–370
  aldosterone induced, 16
  amiloride in, 16–17, 268
  aminoglycosides and, 810
  at cell surface, 392–394
  DOCA and, 267–268
  ouabain inhibition of, 237
  phloretin inhibition of, 237
  regulation by adrenal steroids,
    under basal conditions, 367–368
    under corticosteroid production condi-
      tions, 369–370
  regulation of K secretion and, 266–268
Sodium-potassium pump
  activity of, Na transport pool and, 13–14
  in basolateral membrane, generation of ATP
    and, 233–234

Sodium pump, aldosterone and, 389–391
Sodium retention
    evidence form 474–475
    in hepatic disease, 461–467
    in nephrotic syndrome, 469–479
    NSAID-induced, 827
    tubular site of, 477–479
Sodium:substrate stoichiometry, 28–30
Sodium transport, 1203–1205
    aldosterone action and, 380–382
    in PCT, 165–166
    in thyroidectomized rat, 359
Sodium transport pool, and pump activity, 13–
        14
Solute transport
    altered, 1571–1575
    indexes of, in peritoneal dialysis, 1563–1566
Steblay's nephritis, 494
Steroid diabetes, 1654
Steroid therapy
    cyclosporine and, 1634
    immunosuppression and, 1632–1633
Stimulus-hydrosmotic response, 409–410
Stoichiometry
    charge:substrate, 30–31
    Na:substrate, 28–30
Stone formation, theories of, 995–996
Stratum I hypertension
    analysis for and against treatment of, 1168–
        1178
    argument against treatment of, 1175–1177
    efficacy of treatment of, 1171–1175
    magnitude of problem of, 1169–1170
Streptococcal M protein, 624
Streptococcus, nephritogenic, 623–625
Streptozotocin nephrotoxicity, 875
Subclavian cannulation, complications from,
        1553–1554
Subclavian vein, single-needle dialysis using,
        1555–1556
Subendothelial cells, circulating immune com-
        plex deposites in, 529–534
Subendothelial immune deposits, 515–517
    fixed glomerular antigens and, 515
    immune complex and, 516–517
    planted nonrenal antigen, 515–516
Subepithelial immune deposits
    anionic nonglomerular antigens and, 512–
        514
    antibody localization and, 514
    cationic nonglomerular antigens and, 511–
        512
    circulating immune complex and, 535–537
    fixed glomerular antigens, 510–511

immune complex and, 514–515
    planted nonrenal antigens and, 511–515
Superficial nephron
    K mass flow and, 191
    unidirectional fluxes in, 188
Sympathetic nervous system, interaction with
        renin-angiotensin system, 430
Syphilitic glomerulonephritis, 1035–1036
Systemic blood pressure, diabetic nephropathy
        and, 1066
Systemic disease, kidney in, 885–922

TAL cell
    basolateral KCl cotransport in, 231–232
    carrier systems in, 232–233
    conductive properties of, 224–229
    cotransport systems in, 229–233
    diffusive fluxes in, 224–229
    Na+2Cl−K+ cotransport in, 230–231
    NaCl reabsorption in, inhibitors of, 234–
        237
    shunt pathway of, 225
TALH
    effects of ADH, PTH, CT and glucagon on,
        349–352
    electron microscopy in, 244–245
    flow dependence in, 209–210
    hormone mediated responses of, excretory
        functions and, 352–353
    transition to, 243
    vascular system of, 247
Tamm-Horsfall protein (THP), 3, 510, 889–
        890
    monoclonal antibodies to, 577
    myeloma kidney and, 897
Testis, renin in, 333
Thermodynamics, of coupled transport, 21–23
Thiazide, for idiopathic hypercalciuria, 981
Thiazide diuretics
    in Ca oxalate nephrolithiasis, 999–1006
    for hypertension, 1164–1165
    hypocalciuric action of, 1001–1002
Thick ascending limb of Henle, see TALH
Thrombocytopenia, and ALG in renal allo-
        grafts, 1686
Thromboxane B₂ (I-TXB₂), urinary immuno-
        reactive, in allograft rejection, 1721
Thyroid hormone
    action on metabolic reactions, 361
    effect on contraluminal membrane, 360–361
    effect on luminal membrane, 358–360
    in kidney function, 358–362
Thyroid hormone metabolism, 1328

Thyroidectomized rat
  K transport in, 358–359
  Na transport in, 359
Thyroxin, renal regeneration and, 751
Tight epithelium, 7
Tight junction, of thin limbs of Henle's loop,
    heterogeneity of, 197–199
Tissue
  characterization of 1431
  renin in, 331
TMB-8, retrograde microperfusion studies
    with, 137
Tolypocladium inflatum, 1665
Tonsillectomy, IgA nephropathy and, 696
Total lymphoid irradiation (TLI)
  in Hodgkin's disease, 1696–1698
    complications of, 1698–1699
  in renal transplantation, 1695–1705
  in rheumatoid arthritis, 1699
  technique of, 1696
  vs. CI, in cadaveric allotransplantation,
    1722–1723
Toxic drug metabolites, acetaminophen and,
    812–813
Transcapillary fluid flow, determinants of,
    436–437
Transcellular solute transport, in epithelia, 11
  physiologic importance of, 11–12
Transcutaneous vascular access device, for he-
    modialysis, 1558–1560
Transdermal clonidine, for hypertension, 1165
Transfusions, donor-specific, responses to,
    1716–1717
Transplantation, 1627–1723, see also Renal
    transplantation adjuvant methods of
    immunomodulation for, 1708–1713
Transplantation tolerance, in mice and rats,
    1700
Transport
  hormone action and, 361–362
  in PCT, 178–185
Transport processes, epithelia and, 3–77
Trichlormethiazide, in Ca nephrolithiasis,
    1004
Trichoderma polysporum, 1655, 1665
Trifluoperazine, 44
Tri-iodinated benzoic acid derivatives, 835–836
Tropics, kidney diseases in, 1030–1050
Trypsin, inactive renin activation with, 303–
    304
Tubular cell necrosis, aminoglycosides and,
    858–860
Tubular defects, isolated, 926–931
Tubular fluid compositional changes, feedback
    signals and, 133–135

Tubular leakage, in ARF, 706–707
Tubular lesions, in leptospirosis, 1045
Tubular necrosis, acute, regeneration after,
    748–758
Tubular obstruction, in ARF, 705–706
Tubular segment
  effects of dDAVP, PTH, CT and glucagon
    on, 345
  effect of peptide hormones on, 353–354
Tubulglomerular feedback, in subnormal flow
    range, 148–149
Tubulglomerular feedback loop, intact, 149–
    151
Tubuloglomerular feedback
  arachidonic acid metabolites in, 139–140
  Ca in, 135–138
  calmodulin and, 138
  cellular mechanisms of, 130–140
  characteristics of, 130–133
  fluid compositional changes and, 133–135
  function of, 146–148
  influence of Ca interaction on, 138–139
  influence of cyclic nucleotide on, 138–139
  in juxtamedullary nephrons, 125–126
  regulatory role of, 143–151
  response to IBMX, 138–139
  response with A23187, 136–137
Tubuloglomerular feedback loop, 144–146
Tubulointestinal nephritis (TIN), model of,
    505
Tupaia belangeri, 705, 732

Ultrasonography, 1434
Ultrasound, vesicoureteral reflux and, 943
Unidirectional flux
  in juxtamedullary nephron, 188
  in superficial nephron, 188
Uninephrectomy, growth after, 753–754
Upper respiratory tract infection, and IgA
    nephropathy, 674
Urea, medullary recycling of, vasopressin and,
    401–402
Urea permeability, increased, vasopressin and,
    400–401
Urease, effect on urine, 994–995
Uremia
  amino acid metabolism in, 1344
  antiproteolytic activity in, 766–767
  and biosynthetic failure, 1251
  calcitriol and, 1251
  Ca absorption in, 1414
  complications of, CAPD and, 1589–1594
  and endocrine failure, 1251

experimental, investigations in rats with, 769–772
glucagon metabolism in, 1344
glucose intolerance in, 1341–1344
glucose metabolism in, 1335–1336
granulocyte lysosomal function in, 766
hyperparathyroidism in, 1358–1361
pathogenesis of, 1247–1257
PO_4 absorption in, 1414
PTH involvement with, 1252–1257
Uremic rat
   proteolysis of skeletal muscle, 770–772
   proteolytic activity in, 770
   proteolytic enzyme systems in, 769–770
Ureteral obstruction, medullary blood flow in, 109
Uric acid, renal stones and, 985
Uridine triphosphate (UTP)
   specific activity of, 1076–1078
   synthesis of, 1074–1075
Urinary abnormality, in leptospirosis, 1041–1042
Urinary acidification
   mechanisms of, 1185–1188
   after transplantation, 1645–1646
Urinary albumin concentration, mortality and, 1062–1063
Urinary albumin excretion, rate of, 1060
Urinary concentrating mechanism, 120–128
   control of medullary blood flow and, 120–128
Urinary concentration, alterations in, 107–111
Urinary enzyme excretion, in kidney disease, 1427
Urinary erythrocyte counts, in glomerulonephritis, 1426
Urinary immunoreactive thromboxane B_2 (I-TXB_2), in allograft rejection, 1721
Urinary inhibitors, of Ca oxalate crystallization, 1025–1029
Urinary reflex, obstructive uropathy and, 932–975
Urinary tract infection, treatment of, 973–974
Urinary tract infections (UTI)
   kidney damage following, 1442–1443
   kidney scarring caused by, 1443–1444
   management of, 1441–1444
   symptoms of, 1441–1442
   treatment of, 1442
Urine
   concentration of, vasopressin and, 397–404
   microscopic and biochemical analysis of, 1425–1429
   states of saturation for, 991–993

Urine concentration mechanism, autoregulation and, 126–128
Urine osmolarity, medullary circulation and, 123–125
Urine solutes, in kidney disease, 1428–1429
Urine volume, and renal stones, 984
Urolithiasis
   Ca oxalate, physicochemical factors in, 990–996
   pathogenesis of, 1026
Uropathy, obstructive, pathophysiology of, 932–935
   urinary reflex and, 932–975
Urothelial membrane surfaces, and crystal nucleation, inhibitory properties of, 1026–1027

V1 antagonist, 421–422
V2 antagonist, 422–423
Vasa recta, 87, 92–93
   changes in blood flow into, 123
Vascular access, for hemodialysis, 1553–1560
Vascular bundles, 87, 95–97
Vascular disease, in glomerulonephritis, 1456
Vascular lesions, in leptospirosis, 1045
Vascular organization, of medulla, 84–89
Vascular smooth muscle
   etiology of, Ca and, 1141–1142
   hypertrophy of, 1116–1117
   ionic permeability disturbances in, 1118–1120
   norepinephrine and, 1117–1118
   renin-angiotensin system and, 1117
Vascular tissues, renin in, 333
Vascular-tubular relationship, in medulla, 89–92
Vasoconstriction, renal, in ARF, 703–704
Vasoconstrictor activity, 426–427
Vasopressin
   agonistic and antagonistic analogues of, 417–423
   antidiuretic volume effects and, 428–429
   baroreflex function and, 429–430
   cardiovascular effects of, 426–430
   cellular modes of action of, 407–413
   cyclic AMP and, 39
   and experimental ARF, 732
   increased juxtamedullary filtration rate and, 403–404
   increased NaCl reabsorption and, 402
   increased urea permeability and, 400–401
   increased water permeability and, 399–400
   medullary recycling of urea and, 401–402
   and messengers, 408–409

Vasopressin (*cont.*)
  NaCl absorption and, 210–211
  renal action of, 399–404
  and renin-angiotensin system, 430
  and sympathetic nervous system, 430
  and targets, 407–408
  urine concentration and, 397–404
Vasopressin receptor types, 417–418
Vasopressin-sensitive, epithelium, cytosolic Ca
    in, 39–47
Vasopressin vasoconstriction, 426–427
  physiologic importance of, 428
Verapamil, 716–717, 779–780
  for hypertension, 1167
  in vivo studies, 797
  postischemic infusion of, 792–793
  preischemic infusion of, 792
Vesicoureteral reflux
  advances in diagnosis, 941–943
  in antenatal period, 938–939
  basic pathophysiology of, 936–938
  from birth to 2 years, 939
  from 2 to 5 years, 939
  from 5 to 15 years, 939
  from 15 to 30 years, 940
  clinical age groups, 938–941
  clinical groups, 940–941
  complications of, early diagnosis of, 943–
    944
  hypertension and, 943–944
  over 30 years, 940
  renal damage and, 936–944
  renal scars and, 948–957
  surgical correction of, 970–971
    functional deterioration after, 971–972
    infection after, 971
    renal growth after, 972–973
    scar formation after, 971–972
Visual status, CAPD and diabetic patient, 1605
Vitamin D, *see also* Calcitriol
  and kidney disease, 1305–1314
Vitamin D metabolism
  altered, in uremia, 1358–1360
  in health, 1305–1306
  regulation of PTH by, 1296–1297
  in osteodystrophy, 1312–1314

Vitamin D nutrition
  in kidney disease, 1306–1307
Vitamin D sterols, in osteodystrophy, 1367–
    1368
Vitamin D_2, osteodystrophy and, 1399
Vitamin D_3, osteodystrophy and, 1399
Voiding cystourethrography (VCU), vesicour-
    eteral reflux and, 941–942
Volume contraction, aminoglycoside nephro-
    toxicity and, 852
Volume regulatory response, in epithelia, 11
  physiologic importance of, 11–12
von Willebrand factor, 578
V1-receptors, 418
V2-receptors, 418

Waldenstrom macroglobulinemia, glomerular
    lesions in, 910
Wasting, causes of, in renal failure, 1498–1510
Water immersion, effects of, 452–454
Water permeability, increased, vasopressin
    and, 399–400
Water retention, NSAID-induced, 827
Water transport, Ca and, 412
Weil's syndrome, 1042–1043
Whole kidney inulin clearance (WKCIn)
  adenine nucleotide-MgCl2 complex and, 802
  ATP-MgCl2 and, 802–803
Wounds, draining, protein loss from, 1507–
    1508
W-3 polyunsaturated fatty acid
  effect of, 1137
  substitution of w-6 fatty acid by, 1137
  western diet supplementation with, 1137–
    1138
W-6 polyunsaturated fatty acid, w-3 fatty acid
    substitution of, 1137

Xanthine nephropathy, 880

Zinc absorption, in renal failure, 1420–1421

Zinc absorption, in renal failure, 1420–1421